Dental Materials

Restorative Dental Materials

Edited by

Robert G. Craig, PhD
Marcus L. Ward Professor Emeritus
Department of Biologic and Materials Sciences
The University of Michigan School of Dentistry
Ann Arbor, Michigan

John M. Powers, PhD
Professor, Department of Restorative Dentistry and Biomaterials
Director, Houston Biomaterials Research Center
University of Texas Health Science Center at Houston
Dental Branch
Houston, Texas

Eleventh Edition

with 518 *illustrations*

Mosby
An Affiliate of Elsevier

Mosby
An Affiliate of Elsevier

Publishing Director: John Schrefer
Senior Acquisitions Editor: Penny Rudolph
Developmental Editor: Kimberly Frare
Editorial Assistant: Courtney Sprehe
Project Manager: Linda McKinley
Production Editor: Ellen Forest
Cover Design: Mark Oberkrom
Designer: Julia Ramirez

ELEVENTH EDITION

Printed in the United States of America

Mosby
11830 Westline Industrial Drive
St. Louis, Missouri 64146

Library of Congress Cataloging in Publication Data

Restorative dental materials / edited by Robert G. Craig, John M. Powers.—11th ed.
p. ; cm.
Includes bibliographical references and index.
ISBN 0-323-01442-9
1. Dental materials. I. Craig, Robert G. (Robert George), 1923- II. Powers, John M., 1946-
[DNLM: 1. Dental Materials. WU 190 R436 2002]
RK652.5 .P47 2002
617.6′95—dc21

04 05 06 GW/RRD 9 8 7 6 5 4

Contributors

George R. Baran, PhD
Professor
Department of Mechanical Engineering
Temple University
Philadelphia, Pennsylvania

Stephen C. Bayne, PhD
Professor of Dentistry
Section Head of Biomaterials
Department of Operative Dentistry
School of Dentistry
University of North Carolina
Chapel Hill, North Carolina

Robert G. Craig, PhD
Marcus L. Ward Professor Emeritus
Department of Biologic and Materials Sciences
School of Dentistry
University of Michigan
Ann Arbor, Michigan

Joseph B. Dennison, DDS, MS
Marcus L. Ward Professor of Dentistry
Department of Cariology, Restorative Sciences and Endodontics
School of Dentistry
University of Michigan
Ann Arbor, Michigan

Isabelle L. Denry, DDS, PhD
Associate Professor
Section of Restorative Dentistry, Prosthodontics and Endodontics
The Ohio State University
College of Dentistry
Columbus, Ohio

Glen H. Johnson, DDS, MS
Professor
Department of Restorative Dentistry
University of Washington
Seattle, Washington

David H. Kohn, PhD
Associate Professor
Department of Biologic and Materials Sciences and Biomedical Engineering
School of Dentistry
University of Michigan
Ann Arbor, Michigan

Andrew Koran, III, DDS, MS
Professor Emeritus of Dentistry
Division of Prosthodontics
Department of Biologic and Materials Sciences
School of Dentistry
University of Michigan
Ann Arbor, Michigan

John M. Powers, PhD
Professor
Department of Restorative Dentistry and Biomaterials
Health Science Center
Houston, Texas

John C. Wataha, DDS, PhD
Professor
Department of Oral Rehabilitation
Medical College of Georgia
School of Dentistry
Augusta, Georgia

Preface

The eleventh, and millennium, edition of *Restorative Dental Materials* continues to be a textbook designed for undergraduate dental students, and is also an excellent review of basic and applied information about restorative materials for dental practitioners and dental hygienists who are returning for graduate education. This text is also useful for general dental practitioners because it contains important information about recently developed dental materials.

Dr. John M. Powers is a coeditor of the eleventh edition. Dr. Powers earned a Ph.D. in the Dental Materials Department of the University of Michigan, was a faculty member of that department for a number of years, and is currently a professor in the Department of Restorative Dentistry and Biomaterials at The University of Texas Health Science Center at Houston Dental Branch. He is also a coeditor of *The Dental Advisor*.

We would like to welcome the following new contributors to the eleventh edition and thank them for their time and effort in improving the information presented: Dr. George R. Baran of Temple University, Dr. Stephen C. Bayne of the University of North Carolina, Dr. Joseph B. Dennison of the University of Michigan, Dr. Isabelle L. Denry of the Ohio State University, and Dr. Glen H. Johnson of the University of Washington. We also acknowledge and thank Dr. David H. Kohn and Dr. Andrew Koran III, both of the University of Michigan, for their continued valuable contributions, and Dr. John C. Wataha of the Medical College of Georgia for his increased contributions to the eleventh edition.

Two new chapters have been added to the eleventh edition: Chapter 8, *Preventive Materials*, and Chapter 10, *Bonding to Dental Substrates*. The increased importance of bonding to a variety of surfaces, not only tooth structure, in restorative dentistry has warranted a separate chapter for this topic. The basics of adhesion, the composition of bonding materials, and the application of materials to different surfaces are presented. Likewise, changes in chemotherapeutic agents, pit-and-fissure sealants, glass ionomers, and hybrid ionomers, plus improvements in athletic mouth protectors, justified placing these topics in a chapter entitled *Preventive Materials*.

All chapters have been updated; however, the ones that have undergone major revision are those discussing biocompatibility, dental alloys, casting of metals, composite restorative materials, impression materials, ceramics, metal-ceramics, and cements.

Special features, including problems and solutions, review paragraphs, and the addition of new and important literature references, continue to be presented. Outdated material has been deleted, and previous information has been condensed to provide space for new topics while maintaining the reasonable length of the textbook.

We especially thank Patricia J. Sellinger for her diligence and effort in preparing the final manuscript from such a variety of contributors.

Robert G. Craig
John M. Powers

Contents

10 Bonding to Dental Substrates, 259

Stephen C. Bayne

11 Amalgam, 287

Glen H. Johnson

12 Impression Materials, 329

Glen H. Johnson

18 | Ceramics, 551

Isabelle L. Denry

19 | Ceramic-Metal Systems, 575

Robert G. Craig

20 | Cements, 593

John M. Powers

Chapter 1

Scope and History of Restorative Materials

Humankind has always been plagued by the problem of restoring parts of the body lost as a result of accident or disease. Practitioners of dentistry have been confronted with this problem since the beginning of dental practice, and the means of replacing missing tooth structure by artificial materials continues to account for a large part of dental science.

The replacement of lost teeth is desired for two primary reasons: esthetics and restoration of function (partial or complete). The ability of the dentist to accomplish the desired results has been limited by certain basic factors. One is the availability of suitable materials for the construction of the restorative appliance; another is the development and control of a suitable technical procedure for using the materials that are available. This search for the correct materials, and for a method of manipulation or applied techniques, has continued from the beginning of dental art to the present. Throughout the ages, dentistry has depended to a great degree on advances of the contemporary arts and sciences for improvements in materials and procedures, and this relationship continues. The field of restorative materials is extensive with regard to not only the wide variety of materials and techniques of manipulation, but also the related sciences that are employed.

SCOPE OF MATERIALS COVERED IN RESTORATIVE DENTISTRY

Restorative dental materials include such items as noble and base metals, amalgam alloys, cements, composites, glass ionomers, ceramics, gypsum compounds, casting investments, dental waxes, impression-taking compounds, denture base resins, and other materials used in restorative dental operations. In describing these materials, comparisons are usually made on the basis of physical and chemical characteristics. The line dividing restorative dental materials from therapeutic agents often is not clear. For example, the distinction is not pronounced in such cases as medicated cements, cavity liners, or root canal–filling materials. Usually in such borderline instances the materials are included in both fields of study, with emphasis placed on the properties related to the application involved.

This subject should be approached from the point of view of determining what the material is chemically, why it functions as it does physically and mechanically, and how it is manipulated technically to develop the most satisfactory properties.

The application of dental materials is not limited to any one branch of dentistry. There is scarcely a dental procedure that does not make use of dental materials in one or more forms. The very existence of some phases of restorative dentistry depends largely on various materials and their favorable properties. Other branches of dentistry, such as minor oral surgery and periodontics, require less use of materials, but even in these fields the physical characteristics of the equipment and the chemical characteristics of materials used are important. However, because most materials are used in restorations, either directly or indirectly, the subject is described as one dealing with restorative dental materials.

Most restorative materials are measured by a set of physical, chemical, or mechanical tests that lend themselves to duplication, and as a result of these tests, efforts are being made to control the quality of and claims for the materials. This approach has led to a number of gradual improvements in the materials available to the profession. As improvements in properties have occurred, refinements in technique of application have become necessary.

BASIC SCIENCES APPLIED TO RESTORATIVE MATERIALS

The sciences of primary interest to the dentist are derived from the three basic scientific fields: biology, chemistry, and physics. No clear distinction can be made regarding the relative importance of these three sciences to dentistry, for two reasons: (1) the overlapping of these sciences tends to produce a continuous field of knowledge, and (2) investigations within each science are constantly encroaching on the others.

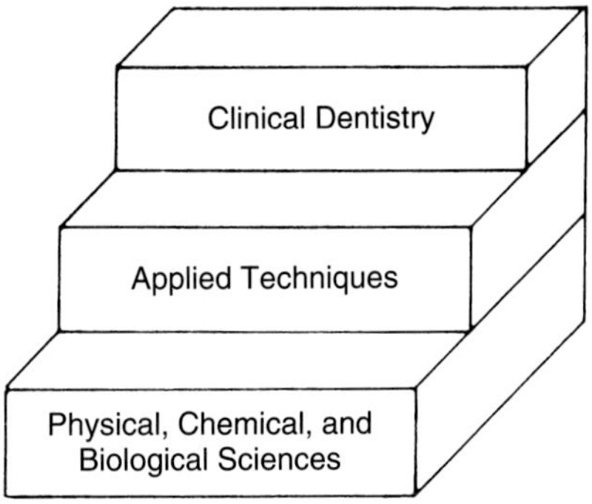

Fig. 1-1 Steps to understanding relations of materials science in dentistry.

Fig. 1-1 indicates the relationship of the three basic fields to applied techniques and clinical dentistry. The practice of clinical dentistry depends not only on a complete understanding of the various applied techniques but also on an appreciation of the fundamental biological, chemical, and physical principles that underlie the applied techniques. A failure to know the scientific principle on which a technique is established often leads to its incorrect application.

It is evident that chemistry, physics, and related engineering sciences serve as the foundation for the science of restorative materials. In no way are the physiological and biological aspects of dentistry subordinated by this physical science treatment of the materials, but rather the whole structure of restorative, corrective, and preventive dentistry is strengthened by its inclusion. Whereas the subject depends on one or more of these exact sciences, the chief problem in this field is to make the correct practical application and interpretation of information available from scientific studies. Most persons working with restorative materials believe that physical, chemical, and mechanical studies cannot be separated from physiological, pathological, or other biological studies of the tissue that support and tolerate the restorative structures. Certainly from the clinical standpoint it is desirable to keep the studies and interpretations as practical as possible. If practical clinical dentistry and the theoretical scientific aspects of restorative materials are allowed to develop without suitable correlation, neither is likely to progress as it should or be useful to the other.

APPLICATION OF VARIOUS SCIENCES

The fundamental principles of the physical sciences find application in the comparison of the physical characteristics with the structural applications of restorative materials. Often this situation is not fully appreciated because the application of the various scientific principles to dentistry has not been emphasized in undergraduate textbooks. In the chapters that follow, numerous practical examples of basic principles are presented, and throughout the discussions the fundamental characteristics are stressed, with a minimum of emphasis on test procedures and techniques of manipulation.

Not all the theoretical aspects and applications of physical, chemical, and engineering principles can be described in detail in the limited space available. Such treatment should not be necessary because predental training includes an understanding of many of the basic principles, even though the practical applications may have been neglected. Therefore emphasis is placed on applying significant fundamentals to dental operations.

A more complete understanding of these and other fundamental principles is important to the dentist as an aid in understanding such typical phenomena as the melting and freezing of casting alloys, the volatilization of liquids with the accompanying cooling action, or the crystal structure produced in solidified metals as compared with the essentially noncrystalline structure of hydrocolloid impression compounds and denture base materials. The branch of physical chemistry that considers the colloidal state of matter has been applied for years successfully to the sciences of medicine, physiology, botany, and engineering. Numerous illustrations of the application of colloid and surface chemistry to dentistry, oral conditions, and dental materials are also known.

To understand the complex nature of metals and alloys used for cast inlays or removable partial dentures, one should know something of the physical or chemical reactions that influence the combination of metals and alloys in liquid and solid states. Alloys that demand heat treatment to produce the optimum properties offer an example of the application of such physicochemical principles. With knowledge of physicochemical principles and the numerous principles of good metallurgical casting practices and fabrication of structures through soldering and assembly, it is possible to design and construct remarkably effective dental structures and appliances.

Knowledge of organic and polymer chemistry, the mechanics of restorative structures and mastication, and something of the biophysical principles involved in complete denture restoration is desirable for designing and constructing complete dentures. Stress analysis of the various types of restorations involves physical principles that are closely related to successful design as well as the biophysical analysis of the support structures.

The toxicity of and tissue reactions to dental materials are receiving more attention as a wider variety of materials are used and as federal agencies demonstrate more concern in this area. A further indication of the importance of the interaction of materials and tissues is the development of recommended standard practices and tests for the biological interaction of materials through the auspices of the American Dental Association (ADA).

After many centuries of dental practice, we continue to be confronted with the problem of replacing tooth tissue lost by either accident or disease. In an effort to constantly improve our restorative capabilities, the dental profession will continue to draw from contemporary arts and sciences to further develop an integrated science of dentistry.

HISTORY

An examination of the history of dentistry shows that the various materials available in any given period have always been important to contemporary restorative dental operations. Improvements came slowly and steadily over the centuries at about the same rate as related developments in other fields of science. It becomes evident therefore that many accepted techniques, materials, and practices have resulted from systematic evaluation and development, so that now the branch of restorative materials has become an accepted part of the science of dentistry.

During the past generation the quality of restorative dental materials has seen more improvement than during any other period of dental history. An understanding of the factors that contributed to this progress enables us to better appreciate the limitations, developments, and future possibilities of this phase of dentistry.

Although no complete history of restorative materials has been written, it is possible to follow the general development of the subject by the progress that was made in the art and science of restorative dentistry throughout the centuries. Until recently this subject was not a distinct science, but only an aspect of the art and science of dentistry. In the early development of dentistry the subject was sufficiently elementary that no separate study was devoted to materials. As dentistry developed and became more complex, so did the development of restorative materials. Therefore the accumulated mass of information regarding materials inevitably became so great as to be established as a separate science. As a science the subject is new, but as part of restorative practices, it is as old as dentistry itself.

EARLY HISTORY

Among the earliest recorded examples of dental prostheses are the gold structures of the Phoenicians, the Etruscans, and, a little later, the Greeks and Romans. Their restorations date back to a period several hundred years before the beginning of Christianity, and for practical purposes it makes little difference which of the civilizations produced the first prostheses. It is much more interesting to observe that many of the materials and practices now in common use were first used more than thousands of years ago.

Gold is one of the oldest materials used. It has been employed for prosthetic dental purposes for at least 2500 years. The ancient Babylonians, Assyrians, and Egyptians (4500 to 4000 BC) were familiar with gold, silver, copper, and lead. It remained for the Phoenicians (about 2700 BC) to spread the culture along the shores of the Mediterranean. They practically controlled the tin trade (which was important for the bronze industry) during the period 1000 to 300 BC, and were considered the most skillful metallurgists of the ancient world. Iron was known to them as early as 990 BC.

It seems reasonable to assume that the practice of using gold for dental appliances was common for centuries before the known examples. Evidence in favor of the antiquity of the art is found in the examination of the appliances. Many were prepared by soldering after reasonably careful assembly, and certainly this art was not developed for the convenience of only the few surviving examples.

It is not certain exactly how or by whom the appliances were constructed. Possibly they were made by skilled metalworkers and not by those who practiced the dental art. As pointed out by historians, the physicians and barber-surgeons probably performed the treatment and extractions, whereas goldsmiths and other artisans constructed the artificial restorations. The role played by the goldsmiths and other artisans is comparable to that of modern laboratory technicians. Persons qualified by practice and experience can often prepare a more artistic structure in less time than the one who visualized it, even though the functional design is the responsibility of the dentist.

The practice of using gold crowns and bridgework apparently flourished in Etruria and Rome as early as 700 to 500 BC. These people must have understood the arts of soldering and riveting to have prepared a restoration from pure gold rings soldered in correct relations, with the artificial tooth held in place by a pin that passed through both the artificial tooth and the gold ring. The extensive use of solder to prepare the appliance implies some knowledge of the simple alloying of gold and the preparation and use of fluxes and perhaps antifluxes.

The teeth used in the ancient appliances were either human or carved from the teeth of an animal. The early Phoenician restorations represent an interesting example of the use of wire to hold the teeth in a more or less fixed position. It appears therefore that the art of wire fabrication was known to this ancient civilization. Hippocrates, who was born in 460 BC, apparently used gold wire and linen thread for ligatures in the repair of bone fractures. He was likewise reported to be the inventor of a type of crude dental forceps and other dental instruments. In modern dentistry the oral surgeon is interested in the properties and behavior not only of ligature materials, but also of hypodermic needles, cobalt-chromium and titanium alloy screws and appliances, tantalum or titanium plates, and various instruments.

Filling carious teeth for preservation apparently was not practiced extensively by ancient civilizations. Celsus (first century AD) recommended the filling of large cavities with lint, lead, and other substances before attempting extraction to prevent the tooth from breaking under the pressure of the instrument. This may have been the beginning of filling materials for carious teeth.

Restorative dental materials were relatively simple in character and few in number at the end of this ancient period. However, a beginning had been made, and mankind was conscious of the desirability of replacing lost tooth tissue. Inasmuch as tools and supplies were simple, persons who practiced the dental art depended on nature to provide materials and on artisans to fashion restorations.

MEDIEVAL AND EARLY MODERN PERIOD

Dental historians describe little progress in the dental art from the beginning of the Christian era to about AD 1500. Historians doubt, however, that it was a period of retrogression or a "dark age" of inactivity. There was likely much activity, creative thought, and invention, but records either were not kept or were later destroyed through acts of superstition or religious fanaticism. The chief contribution to dentistry of this period appears to have been some shift in practice from prosthetic restorations to the restoration of carious teeth.

Some historians consider the sixteenth century to be the end of the Middle Ages. The invention of the printing press (1436), which aided in the dissemination of knowledge, and the emigration of Greek men of letters and science to Italy, were important events toward the close of this period. During the latter part of this period (between AD 1116 and 1289), universities with medical faculties were established at Bologna, Oxford, Paris, and Montpellier.

The development of books and writing on dental subjects was important to the progress of restorative dental materials. One of the first books to treat dentistry independently of medicine was written in German in 1548 by Walter Herman Ryff. This book, written in the language of the people, is significant because all previous works describing the teeth were in Latin.

The use of gold leaf to fill cavities was perhaps the most significant development of the period from the standpoint of restorative materials. The first authentic record of the use of gold fillings to preserve human teeth appears to have been about 1480 by an Italian, Johannes Arculanus, who was at the University of Bologna and later at Padua. A description of the removal of carious matter from the teeth before filling them with gold leaf was given by Giovanni de Vigo (1460-1520). The practice of using gold leaf for fillings probably was not original with either of these writers because there is some indication that the custom may have dated back to the Middle East, several centuries before. It is certain, however, that gold leaf has been used for the past 500 years.

Gold leaf was used for gilding and other commercial purposes in antiquity. The ancient Egyptians, Hebrews, and Greeks were familiar with the art, although the origin of gold leaf production was perhaps in the Far East. The early Greeks produced leaf of approximately 1/100,000-inch thickness, approaching the thickness of modern leaf or foil, which is approximately 1/300,000 inch. The methods for producing gold leaf have changed little through the ages.

Carious teeth were filled with ground mastic, alum, and honey or other substances during the period from about AD 1050 to 1122, according to the Arabian author Rhazes (al-Rãzi). Oil of cloves (eugenol) is mentioned by Riviére (1589) as being applicable to dental operations, but may have been used earlier (1562) by Ambroise Paré to alleviate toothache. Paré is also credited with having prepared artificial teeth from bone and ivory. Jacques Guillemeau, who was a pupil of Paré, prepared a substance by fusing together certain waxes, gums, ground mastic, powdered pearl, and white coral. This may have been the forerunner of esthetic fused porcelain.

Some Contemporary Arts of the Middle Ages

Contemporary arts were also being developed during this period. The writings of Pliny (AD 23-79), Theophilus (eleventh century), and Cellini (1558) describe how painters, goldsmiths, ceramists, metalworkers, and others applied their art. None of the authors claim credit for complete originality of all their practices, but rather indicate that the methods were routine.

In his *Natural History,* Pliny described bronze statuettes and other cast bronze or silver household articles such as candelabra and cups common to the period before AD 100. Pliny listed many dental practices that appear to be based on popular belief rather than on the practices of specialists.

In "An Essay Upon Various Arts," the priest and monk Theophilus shows certain improvements over the earlier writers and has omitted certain erroneous practices of the previous period. In Book One he deals primarily with painting and the allied arts. Of considerable interest is his description of the method for forming gold leaf from gold of high purity by hammering, which is similar to the recent practices of beating gold to form foil. Book Two deals predominantly with the ceramic art and gives a good description of early practices in glassworking.

In Book Three, Theophilus describes metalworking and devotes considerable space to the work of the goldsmiths. There is a description of the casting of handles for a silver cup in which the "lost wax" method is given in detail. The casting practice was so clearly described by Theophilus that it is possible to follow him in practice as well as in principle. After fashioning the handle in wax, a wax "sprue," which was described as being round like a slender candle and half a finger in length, was attached. It was somewhat thicker at the top. This wax, called the *funnel,* was made fast with a hot iron. Well-beaten clay was used to cover the wax carefully so that all details of the wax sculpture were filled. Afterward these molds were placed near warm coals, so when the molds became warm it was possible to pour out the wax. After the clay mold was well baked and still hot, the molten metal was poured in through the funnel. When the mold and casting became cold, the clay mold was removed, and a metal replica of the wax model remained.

If a suitable dental casting investment, or mold material, had been used with an appropriate inlay wax, a balanced casting alloy, and a modern casting machine, the description might well apply to the dental casting process of today.

A metal casting process very much like that of Theophilus is described by the Florentine artist Benvenuto Cellini in Chapter 41 of his *Memoires,* written in 1558. Cellini prepared a wax model and surrounded it with a plastic clay, which he allowed to dry and harden before attempting to melt the wax and pour the metal. He implied that he had frequently used wax patterns in previous castings. He claimed no originality for the casting method, though he indicated that the melting furnace he used was original.

Cellini, like Pliny and Theophilus, also soldered gold by using copper acetate, nitre, and borax, a method that was considered very effective. Thus it is seen that certain metals and materials were available to the artisans for use in their trades. The secrets of these practices were no doubt often guarded so they were not recognized outside the trade. Such dentistry was more an art than a science, so that full use possibly was not made of existing skills and techniques. Certainly the practice of casting restorations by the "lost wax" method was to wait several centuries before it was adopted by dentistry.

BEGINNING OF DENTAL SCIENCE—1600 TO 1840

During the period from 1600 to 1840, the foundations for the science of dentistry were established. So little progress had been made up to this time that dentistry was merely an art practiced largely by the barber-surgeons or artisans. Few records of results were kept, and little thought was given to the improvement of methods before the beginning of the seventeenth century. Nevertheless, a special type of medical-dental practitioner was recognized by the medical profession.

By the end of the sixteenth century a limited knowledge of dentistry had spread to most of the countries in Europe. France, England, and other nations had been established after the age of the feudal system. Carved bone and ivory teeth held to neighboring teeth with gold and silver wire were used in France, Germany, and Italy.

The contemporary sciences of chemistry and physics were being developed at the beginning of the seventeenth century. Galileo had stated his law of falling bodies and invented the telescope. The compound microscope and the printing press were in use. By the end of the century chemical elements had been defined by Robert Boyle, and Sir Isaac Newton had demonstrated the law of gravitation. Similar developments were taking place in the biological sciences of bacteriology, anatomy, and physiology.

Wax models used in prosthetic work are first mentioned by Matthaeus Gottfried Purmann about 1700. It is supposed that the wax was carved to the desired shape, after which it was reproduced in bone or ivory by a craftsman.

Much progress in dentistry was made during the eighteenth century. Pierre Fauchard described the materials and practices of his time in his book *Le chirurgien dentiste, ov Traité des dents,* published in 1728. He discussed many phases of dentistry, including operative and prosthetic procedures. He collected and catalogued much of the information that was good in dentistry at his time. There were dental texts before the time of Fauchard, but they were considerably more limited in extent and application.

Fauchard mentioned lead, tin, and gold as filling materials. He preferred tin because of the ease with which it could be adapted to cavity walls. Separate ivory or natural teeth with wood pivots were fastened in position with a cement compound of sealing wax, turpentine, and white copal, or were set into a low-melting-point alloy used to fill the canal. The use of the dental file had become common practice by the time of Fauchard, and emery wheels for grinding down teeth had been introduced by a Dutch physician, Kornelis van Soolingen, during the latter part of the seventeenth century. According to Vincenzo Guerini, it was Lorenz Heister (1683-1758) who first mentioned removable prosthetic appliances.

The early sixteenth century was the beginning of useful dental literature, whereas the seventeenth century was a period of rapid development of the art of dental practice with a coordination of the scientific knowledge that had evolved during the past centuries. The introduction of fused porcelain for teeth in 1789 is regarded as one of the most important events in the history of dentistry. It represents the beginning of scientific improvements in the restorative art of dental practice.

The first book to describe mechanical dentistry was that of Claude Mouton in 1746, *Essay d'odontotechnie, ou dissertation sur les dents artificielles.* He mentioned gold-shell crowns swaged from one piece of metal and the use of gold clasps instead of ligatures to retain artificial teeth. Clasps to retain partial dentures were in common use in 1796. Numerous other dental texts were written during the late eighteenth and early nineteenth centuries. Etienne Bourdet (1775) made the first reference to the use of a gold base to support artificial ivory teeth fixed with gold pins. Low-fusing metal alloy was introduced by Jean Darcet in 1770.

A baked-porcelain, complete denture made in a single block was first displayed by the French dentist Nicholas Dubois de Chemant in 1788. In 1797, he wrote a book in English, *A Dissertation on Artificial Teeth,* describing porcelain. The Italian dentist Guiseppangelo Fonzi, who lived in Paris, is credited with preparing the first baked-porcelain single tooth with attached platinum hooks about 1806 to 1808. He is also credited with preparing 26 shades of porcelain by using metallic oxides.

It is claimed that the first American book on dentistry was written by R.C. Skinner around 1801 *(A Treatise on the Human Teeth).* By this time dentistry was no longer entirely in the hands of barbers or artisans, but was practiced by professionally minded dentists or surgeons who warned the public against pretenders. Forty-four treatises on dentistry were published in the United States between 1800 and 1840. This is more than one per year, in addition to the numerous articles on dentistry that appeared in medical journals.

The combination of silver and mercury to form amalgam "silver paste" was announced by O. Taveau of Paris in 1826. This was the beginning of dental amalgam, which is recognized as one of the outstanding developments in the field of restorative materials.

Although French dentists may well be considered the leaders of this period, dentists in other countries of Europe were quick to adopt French practices or their equivalent, and in a few instances made additional contributions. In Germany there was little progress until the sixteenth century. Mention of the use of gold foil in German writings during this century is common. Philip Pfaff (1756) is credited with being the first to use plaster models prepared from sectional wax impressions of the mouth.

In Great Britain, dentistry did not develop much until the eighteenth century. The work of Fauchard was not generally known in Great Britain, and the first comprehensive textbook in English appeared in 1768, although in 1686 Charles Allen had written a book on teeth in which he described a method of transplantation. By the early part of the nineteenth century, dental practice had apparently improved somewhat in

Great Britain. Retentive cavities for gold fillings were prepared in Edinburgh in 1787.

James Snell (1832) wrote that he preferred forceps to the key for use in extractions. He chose gold for filling carious teeth, and he described two types of cement that might be used, although these cements offered little promise of success. Zinc oxychloride cement did not come into use until 20 years later.

Considerable progress was made toward the perfection of porcelain teeth in France, England, and the United States before 1840. These teeth had been introduced in the United States from France in 1817. By 1825, porcelain teeth were being produced and improved in America. The replacement of carved bone and ivory or natural teeth by the fused mineral product was another step forward for the profession and represents one of the first great improvements in dental materials. The Ash tube tooth introduced in 1838 was produced until recent times with only slight modification in form.

In the United States, Wooffendale is said to have introduced gold foil after he settled in New York in 1767 to practice dentistry. Tin and lead were also used as filling materials at this time. Carved ivory and bone dentures, ivory or natural teeth with metal pivots, silk and wire ligatures, and files for the removal of carious lesions were in common use. Paul Revere is credited with being a skilled ivory turner and goldsmith who applied his skill to the production of artificial teeth. Gold points were used to fill root canals in 1805 by Edward Hudson in Philadelphia. "Silver paste," the amalgam of silver with mercury, was introduced in the United States as a filling material by the Crawcour brothers in 1833.

Dental materials were beginning to be produced in America during the early part of the nineteenth century. Before that time they were imported from Europe. Gold coins were rolled into a noncohesive gold filling material in 1800, and by 1812 gold foil was being produced by the beating method by Marcus Bull in Hartford, Connecticut. He founded a company that later became the J.M. Ney Company, a leading dental gold alloy manufacturer. Thus the first American-made dental products were gold foil and dental porcelain.

By 1840 the practice of dentistry in America had reached a definite turning point. The first dental journal in the world, *The American Journal of Dental Science*, was established in 1839. The first national dental society, the American Society of Dental Surgeons, was established in 1840. The first dental school, the Baltimore College of Dental Surgery, was established the same year. H.H. Hayden and C.A. Harris were both active in these three institutions. This same year Charles Goodyear discovered the process of dry-heat vulcanization of rubber, in which he heated together caoutchouc, sulfur, and white lead, which later made possible the introduction of a most useful dental material—vulcanite.

With the establishment of a dental society, dental journal, and dental school, the foundation was laid for the development of a dental science in America. The coordination and practical application of the knowledge and practice of past centuries were begun, and uniform progress in all branches was seen. Dental materials in 1840 were still relatively simple, but such progress was being made in the industries that it could be expected that improvements would be forthcoming. Chemistry, physics, medicine, and the sciences were beginning to flourish in schools. These improvements helped promote dentistry and create a turning point for civilization generally. Numerous respected men were in the practice of dentistry in both America and Europe. Through the efforts of these men improvements were made in the profession, and the barber-surgeon was forced to discontinue his trade.

Progress still was not rapid in the early part of the nineteenth century, but dentistry was moving toward an improved and established science. It has been estimated that by 1830 the total number of dentists in the United States had increased to about 300, with an advancement in every department of dentistry as a science. The nineteenth century might be called a period of mechanical progress in contemporary fields and of the establishment of the dentist in society.

THE PERIOD OF MECHANICAL IMPROVEMENT—1840 TO 1900

Dentistry, like the allied arts and sciences, took full advantage of the mechanical developments of the last half of the nineteenth and the early twentieth centuries. The application of chemical, physical, and engineering principles, combined with advances in the biological sciences, was like a tonic to dentistry. The developments in related arts and sciences stimulated further growth in the field of restorative materials. During this period, applied mechanics was recognized as an essential supplement to the biological principles of dentistry. Apparently this was more quickly and completely recognized among American dentists than among those of other countries, thereby advancing American dentistry to the position it now holds. Few other nations had the early concept of coordination and balance between mechanical reconstruction and research and the biological fundamentals of dentistry.

Between 1839 and 1884, 44 dental journals were established in the United States, and between 1842 and 1884, 103 dental societies were organized. These assisted greatly in the dissemination of scientific dental information on practices and techniques throughout the profession. At the beginning of this period, dental materials were comparatively few in number, but this was the beginning of the application of physical principles to dental practices and processes, and the search had begun for better restorative materials.

By the end of the 60-year period from 1840 to 1900, many of the major present-day materials had been introduced to the profession, along with techniques for their manipulation and use. After 1840 America began to acquire leadership in creating and producing restorative dental materials, and a substantial industry developed in this field. From this industry dentistry derived many valuable contributions, relationships, and benefits in the form of research and scientific development.

Because of the great number of improvements and developments introduced by dentistry during this period, it is possible here to enumerate in chronological order only a few of the most important. In 1844, S.S. White became interested in the production of porcelain teeth and their improvements in color and form. White was later to become a leading manufacturer and distributor of dental materials, establishing the S.S. White Dental Manufacturing Company. The records indicate, therefore, that the Ney and White companies were among the oldest in the trade.

One of the early actions of the American Society of Dental Surgeons was to forbid its members to use silver amalgam for restoring lost tooth structure. Like many other acts of prohibition, this action apparently served to stimulate thought on the use and study of the nature of amalgam. Years later, after much study, an improved amalgam was developed that eventually became one of the most popular and useful of all restorative materials.

About the time the society started the "war" against the use of silver amalgam, a companion material in the form of copper amalgam was introduced (1844). Mouth impressions were being taken in plaster about this same time. Gutta-percha was discovered in India in 1842, and by 1847 it was being used as a root canal filling material when mixed with chloroform. This material, chloropercha, remained in use until recent times as a cavity liner and varnish in deep cavities. Gutta-percha was mixed with zinc oxide for filling purposes by Asa Hill in 1848. In 1883, gutta-percha was dissolved in eucalyptol and used as a root canal filler. This was perhaps the beginning of the present-day gutta-percha points for root canals. Platinum-gold alloys, consisting of three-fourths gold and one-fourth platinum, were introduced in 1847.

In 1851, Nelson Goodyear announced the development of a method for producing vulcanite, or hard rubber, based on Charles Goodyear's earlier discovery of a method of dry-heat vulcanization of rubber. The discovery of vulcanite and its subsequent use for "dental plates," patented on March 5, 1855, was another outstanding advance in dental materials. Although the material was not the most ideal as a denture base, and its use was covered by restricting patents for many years, vulcanite served well as the first substitute for carved ivory dentures. Not long afterward (1869) celluloid was introduced by

J. Smith Hyatt, who was searching for a suitable material for billiard balls, and soon it was used as a denture base material. Thus a substitute for vulcanite was sought soon after its introduction. It was not until about 80 years later (1937), however, that a satisfactory substitute for vulcanite was obtained in a material known as acrylic resin.

The second dental school in the United States was established in Cincinnati in 1845. By 1860 more than 200 dental books, in German, Spanish, Italian, French, and English, had appeared. The periodical literature had also increased, with journals in America, Germany, England, and France.

The restrictions on the use of amalgam had not been completely successful. A silver-tin-mercury alloy, or amalgam, was introduced in 1855 by Elisha Townsend, followed by another formula by J.F. Flagg in 1860. Gold foil was becoming increasingly popular at the same time, with the introduction of cohesive annealed foil by Robert Arthur of Baltimore in 1855. Zinc oxychloride cement was in common use by this time as a filling and cementing medium. Low–melting point alloy baseplates were developed by Alfred A. Blandy in 1856, and a flexible dental engine cable was introduced by Charles Merry of St. Louis in 1858, followed by the angle handpiece in 1862. The rubber dam to isolate teeth from saliva was put into use by Phineas Taylor Barnum of Monticello in 1864, and four years later the profession was to benefit by the expiration of the patents controlling the use of vulcanite. About 1870 zinc phosphate cements were first used, and they were introduced to the profession in 1879. Silicate cements were developed a few years later.

The practice of malleting for condensation of gold foil had been common since 1838, when it was introduced by E. Merrit of Pittsburgh. Since that practice started, numerous automatic mallets have been introduced, beginning with one developed by J.C. Dean in 1867. The introduction of automatic mechanical condensing devices has continued with varying degrees of success to the present time.

In 1850, the pivot crown was a crude structure with its wooden pin set into the tooth. The Richmond crown was introduced in 1878, followed by the Davis crown in 1885, with a modified form of the Davis crown in the same year by H.D. Justi, all making use of metal pins to replace the wood. These were only three of the many forms of porcelain pivot crowns common at that time. Much experimentation was being done with fused porcelain for inlays, jacket crowns, porcelain teeth set into vulcanite bases, and other modified porcelain structures. Some years later these ambitions were realized with the introduction of gas and gasoline furnaces for baking porcelain, porcelain jacket crowns, and high-fusing-point inlays by Charles Land (1889); an electric furnace for porcelain by Levitt Ellsworth Custer (1894); high-fusing-point porcelain inlays by W.E. Christensen (1895); the gingival shoulder for the porcelain jacket crown by E.B. Spalding (1903); and the summary of porcelain inlay construction in the technical publication of J.Q. Byram (1905).

Circular inlays that were ground and fitted to position were in common use from 1858 to 1890. Aguilhon de Saran of Paris is credited with melting 24k gold in an investment mold to form inlays about 1884. J.R. Knapp in America invented a blowpipe in 1887, but not until 1907 did W.H. Taggart of Chicago succeed in introducing a practical casting method for the gold inlay. This was a long-sought-for invention, and although there is some question in the records about the authenticity of Taggart's invention and the ethics of its marketing, there can be no question about the merit of the practice and the advantages it has given to restorative dentistry. Solbrig in Paris, independent of Taggart, cast gold inlays by a similar method during the same year, and B.F. Philbrook had described in 1897 a method of casting metallic fillings. This indicates that much study was given to the problem throughout the profession and that its solution was a natural result of investigation. Why it was not done at an earlier date is now interesting speculation, because it is known that Cellini and Theophilus used the same principles 1000 years before in their arts.

Continued progress was made in the work on

amalgam alloy throughout the last years of the nineteenth century. G.V. Black published the results of his studies in 1895, which marked the beginning of precision measurements on amalgam alloys. Black had previously published (1891) his theories on cavity design and preparation, which are only remotely related to dental materials but include certain principles of mechanics that involve properties of materials used for restorations.

These examples are only a few of the many techniques, practices, and principles that had their beginning in the late nineteenth century. This fact is often lost in the consideration of various materials and their use in the latter half of the twentieth century. The fundamental principles underlying such operations as shaping cavities for various restorations, impression-taking operations, wax patterns, models and indirect dies, the construction of complete and partial removable dentures, and many other types of structures were recognized before the beginning of the twentieth century. Current developments and additional consideration of the historical background of individual materials will be considered in other discussions in this book.

ADVANCES SINCE 1900

With the beginning of the twentieth century came many refinements and improvements in the quality of various materials and processes used in restorative dentistry. Physical and mechanical tests and the fundamentals of engineering practice were applied to structural designs and restorative materials. From studies of physical and mechanical behavior, certain shortcomings of structures and materials were observed. When these shortcomings were detected, the process of improvement began with studies of methods of chemical combination or physical improvement in fabrication. Thus for the first time a concentrated effort was made to develop and improve products with specific properties designed for a definite purpose.

Before 1900, relatively few persons specialized in the improvement of dental materials or were able to verify the claims made for available materials. Today, many individuals who have a background of training and experience in physics, engineering, chemistry, and dentistry are engaged in research and development in this field, and more than 65 universities offer graduate training in biomaterials. From 1900 to about 1925, frequent references to modifications, tests, and improvements of materials and structures appeared in the literature. Unfortunately, a lack of uniformity of testing conditions prevailed, and it can now be seen that this often caused failure to duplicate results and led to some misunderstanding of the science and studies as a whole. Since the early 1950s, much has been done to establish uniform standards, thanks to a cooperative effort among some of the dental schools; leaders in the profession; the American Dental Association Council on Dental Materials, Instruments, and Equipment (now the Council on Scientific Affairs); the National Bureau of Standards (now the National Institute for Standards and Technology); and the research departments of many reputable manufacturers.

Cooperative efforts among the workers in the field of restorative dentistry and materials appear to be stronger now than ever before. The researchers in this field, working in the profession, schools, and industries, are comparing results from tests and adopting a uniform method of testing. It is common practice now for schools to exchange data with research departments of manufacturers and for each to supply information to the profession. This is a most constructive sign. It means that dentists in practice have an opportunity to compare results of different investigators more easily than in the past, and they probably will receive fewer conflicting statements of properties from research investigators.

During the early part of the twentieth century, some of the persons engaged in improving the quality of restorative materials were associated with dental schools, and others were in practice or engaged in research with manufacturers. G.V. Black was still active in the profession and at Northwestern University Dental School. The various editions of his textbook *Operative Dentistry* contained references to various dental materials and in particular to the need for a balanced formula for an amalgam alloy. In addition, his rules on cavity design are still generally accepted, although there is a trend toward somewhat more conservative designs. In the related field of crown and bridge construction, F.A. Pesso was active in improving and modifying the technique and design of these restorations. At the University of Michigan School of Dentistry, M.L. Ward was active in improving methods to measure dimensional change, flow, and other properties of amalgam. The development of the optical lever micrometer for measuring dimensional change in amalgam was one of the first refinements in dimensional change–measuring equipment for this and related materials. Ward also studied cements, improved designs in instruments and cavities, and made numerous contributions to the literature. Many of these are described in several editions of the *American Textbook of Operative Dentistry*, which he edited.

The term *dental metallurgy* was commonly used during the early period of the twentieth century, and several books were written on the subject. The sixth edition of C.J. Essig and Augustus Koenig's book *Dental Metallurgy* was published in 1909. This book describes the metallurgy of various elements and procedures for melting and alloying. After a complete treatment of the methods of extracting metals from ore and refining various metals, there is a chapter on amalgam alloys with emphasis on their use in dentistry. The sixth edition of another popular book, *Practical Dental Metallurgy,* written in 1924 by J.D. Hodgen and G.S. Millberry, follows the same pattern of subject treatment. By that time, considerable information had been accumulated on the various metals, and particularly on amalgam and certain alloys used in dentistry, so the book is somewhat more complete than previous editions. Dental metallurgy at that time, however, was not highly specialized, but perhaps that is to be expected because the subject was only beginning to take form and a limited amount of information was available on various materials and dental alloys. Books in this field written in later years, such as those of O.E. Harder *(Modern Dental Metallurgy)*, K.W. Ray *(Metallurgy for Dental Students)*, J.S. Shell *(Hodgen-Shell Dental Materials)*, and E.W. Skinner *(The Science of Dental Materials)*, adopted an entirely different style and included a broader subject matter.

Among the contributors to the periodical literature during the early part of the century were A.W. Gray, Paul Poetske, R.V. Williams, and W.S. Crowell. Gray reported numerous studies on amalgam alloy and its behavior when subjected to various practices of manipulation. He first offered a theory for the dimensional change resulting from the hardening of the amalgam mass. Poetske reported studies on amalgam alloy and dental cement. Williams described methods of testing and improving dental gold alloys, and Crowell contributed reports of investigations on cements and various other materials, as well as test practices.

At about this same time, James McBain and co-workers in England were studying the behavior of amalgam alloy subjected to different mixing procedures. At a later date M.L.V. Gaylor, working in the same laboratory, made significant observations on the method by which mercury and silver combine. Studies in Germany during this period dealt with the investigation of the theoretical behavior of metals and various alloys when combined under varying conditions. The theoretical behavior of structural designs was also being studied and reported from Germany. Significant studies on the method of combining gold and copper were reported from Russian laboratories in the early part of the twentieth century and were subsequently verified by studies in the United States and Great Britain. The discovery of copper-gold compound formation was most significant in the development and improvement of dental casting alloys.

In 1919, the National Bureau of Standards in Washington was requested by the United States government to formulate specifications for the selection of dental amalgam to be used in the federal services. Wilmer Souder directed this research and presented a well-received report in 1920 that led to subsequent study of other materials. Shortly thereafter the Weinstein Research Laboratories established a research associateship at the National Bureau of Standards, and studies were started on other materials. The first associates included R.L. Coleman, W.L. Swanger, and W.A. Poppe, who were under the direction of Dr. Souder. Their studies included investigations of the physical and mechanical properties of casting gold alloys, wrought gold alloys, and accessory casting materials. As a result of this investigation, research paper No. 32, which contained much fundamental information, was published in December 1928.

Since April of 1928, the ADA has maintained a research fellowship at the National Bureau of Standards. Numerous reports presented on the progress of investigations made under this fellowship have stimulated the advancement of information on many dental restorative materials. This research body has formulated a number of specifications, based on qualified investigations into the characteristic properties of each type of material. These specifications have been of great value to the profession by ensuring greater uniformity and improved quality of restorative materials. The details of these specifications are described later in appropriate discussions.

Specifications have been developed in a number of countries, most notably in Australia and the United States. Specifications for materials and devices are important in the practice of dentistry throughout the world, as evidenced by the establishment of international standards. Currently, all American standards (specifications) are developed and approved by the ADA Standards Committee on Dental Products and are reviewed for adoption by the ADA Council on Scientific Affairs. All adopted standards are forwarded for approval by the American National Standards Institute and, if accepted, become American National Standards. These standards may be submitted for acceptance by the International Organization for Standardization and, if approved, become international standards. Of course, many countries contribute to the International Organization for Standardization, and specifications may be modified many times before they are finally accepted as international standards. The development of international standards will result in the improvement and reliability of materials and devices throughout the world and eliminates the need for each country to develop its own standards and specifications.

Because the development and acceptance of specifications often requires a number of years, the American Dental Association developed an Acceptance Program for dental materials in use but not covered by existing specifications. Manufacturers must submit test data that prove the materials function successfully for the specified application. Depending on the extensiveness of laboratory and clinical results, products may be given provisional or complete acceptance. In 1993, the American Dental Association published a report, *Clinical Products in Dentistry—A Desktop Reference*, which lists accepted, certified, and recognized dental materials, instruments, and equipment and accepted therapeutic products. It is designed to be a quick reference for dentists of the status of new products and to assist them in the selection of products.

The Medical Devices Amendments, signed into law in 1976, were designed to protect the public from hazardous and ineffective devices. Responsibility for commercially available medical devices was divided among 19 panels, one of which was a dental panel. Each panel is to classify devices, identify known hazards, recommend characteristics for which standards should be developed, advise on the formulation of protocols and review premarket approval applications, recommend exemption for certain devices, and respond to requests from the FDA relating to the safety and effectiveness of devices. The Dental Device Classification Panel classified life-sustaining and life-supporting devices, implants, and priority items for standards development. The list of dental devices included 11 in the diagnostic area, 1 in monitoring, 51 in prosthetics, 82 in the surgical field, 2 in therapeutics, and 166 in the category of other devices.

If one were to list the major new materials, techniques, or processes that have been developed or introduced since 1900, he or she would immediately realize that a continual search has been in progress for new and improved items and practices. The search has focused on ways to make restorative dentistry more acceptable and serviceable to the patient and convenient for the operator.

In the field of restorative materials and practices since 1900, several major items have been introduced, such as the casting process, the use of acrylic resins to replace vulcanized rubber in dentures, base-metal casting alloys for partial dentures, stainless steel for orthodontic and other appliances, and a variety of elastic impression materials. Each has made modern dental practice more acceptable to both the patient and the dentist. The development of carbide burs and diamond cutting instruments and the successful introduction of increased speeds for rotary instruments have aided materially in the operation of cutting tooth tissue. The development of resin composite, glass ionomer and compomer restorative materials, new and modified polymers for restorations and impressions, new phenolic and resin cements, pit and fissure sealants, improved base metal alloys and amalgams, low- or no-gold casting alloys such as palladium-based alloys, ceramics fused to metal systems, and improved ceramics for single restorations have contributed to the service and function of restorative materials.

The extensively used acid etching of tooth structure, base metals, and ceramics to provide adhesion of resin composites has had a dramatic effect on restorative and orthodontic dental treatment. The recent improvements in bonding agents for composites and metals to enamel and dentin has provided the opportunity for major changes in cavity design. The improvement in composites has resulted in their extended application to the restoration of posterior teeth. Clinical and biological evidence of the success of titanium and titanium alloys for dental implants has made it possible to replace a tooth lost as a result of extraction.

Biophysical applications such as experimental stress analysis studies have resulted in better guidelines for materials used in the design of restorations. Materials used for maxillofacial applications or as dental implants have received increased attention; the urgent need for improvement has stimulated research in both of these areas.

The interaction of materials with oral tissues has become increasingly important in the evaluation of these materials, as indicated by the interim acceptance by the Council on Dental Materials and Devices in November 1971 of recommended standard practices for the biological evaluation of dental materials. A series of handbooks has also been published reviewing the current knowledge about the biocompatibility of dental materials.

Many of the advances in biomaterials during the twentieth century occurred after 1950. These advances include high-speed cutting, carbide burs, metal-ceramic systems, rubber impression materials, chemical- and light-cured composites, pit and fissure sealants, acid etching of enamel and other surfaces, bonding agents, auto mixing of various materials, vacuum forming of athletic mouth protectors, titanium and its alloys for implants, glass ionomers, high copper amalgams, standardized endodontic instruments, strengthened ceramics, silicone maxillofacial materials, and compomers, to list only a few of the 100 or more major advances.

FUTURE DEVELOPMENTS IN BIOMATERIALS

Based on a 1996 report from the National Health and Nutrition Survey, it is expected that individuals less than 20 years of age will need fewer removable appliances but will require single or partial tooth replacement. For persons older than 20, maintenance and fabrication of appliances will be needed for those at the high end of this group and fixed bridges and single tooth restoration will be required for those at the low end of this age group. Thus single tooth replacement will become more important than fixed bridges or removable partial dentures.

With more emphasis on preventive treatment, future restorative needs will move in the direction of restoring teeth with intra-coronal and root caries. Thus it is expected that future research would be directed toward improvement in esthetic restorative materials for both anterior and posterior applications and for bonding systems to attach these materials to tooth structures. Also, the need for single tooth replacement will result in continued research on dental implants and surface treatments to produce satisfactory osseointegration.

In addition the interaction between the fields of biomaterials and biology will increase. Demands for ensuring the biocompatibility of restorative materials before they are marketed will be an incentive to develop in vitro short- and long-term tests. Studies on tissue regeneration will continue, as will studies controlling surface characteristics of materials. As the fields of cell and molecular biology continue to develop, applications of these technologies should have an impact on restorative dentistry and the development of biomaterials.

BIBLIOGRAPHY

American Dental Association: *Guide to dental materials and devices,* ed 8, Chicago, 1976, American Dental Association.

American Dental Association: *Dentist's desk reference: materials, instruments and equipment,* ed 2, Chicago, 1983, American Dental Association.

American Dental Association: *Clinical products in dentistry: a desktop reference,* Chicago, 1993, American Dental Association.

Coleman RL: Physical properties of dental materials, *J Res Nat Bur Stand* 1:868, 1928.

Council on Dental Materials and Devices, American Dental Association: Medical device legislation and the FDA Panel on Review of Dental Devices, *J Am Dent Assoc* 94:353, 1977.

Craig RG, Farah JW: Stress analysis and design of single restorations and fixed bridges, *Oral Sci Rev* 10:45, 1977.

Craig RG: Advances in biomaterials from 1957-1997, *J Oral Rehabil* 26:841, 1999.

Diefenbach VL: A national center for applied dental research, *J Am Dent Assoc* 73:587, 1966.

Docking AR: A critique of common materials used in dental practice, *Int Dent J* 12:382, 1962.

Essig CJ, Koenig A: *Dental metallurgy,* ed 6, Philadelphia, 1909, Lea & Febiger.

Gabel AB: The role of physics in dentistry, *J Appl Physics* 12:712, 1941.

Guerini V: *A history of dentistry,* Philadelphia, 1909, Lea & Febiger.

Harder OE: *Modern dental metallurgy,* Minneapolis, 1930, Burgess-Roseberry.

Hodgen JD, Millberry GS: *Practical dental metallurgy,* ed 6, St Louis, 1924, Mosby.

Kohn DH: Current and future research trends in dental biomaterials, *Biomat Forum* 19(1): 23, 1997.

Lufkin AW: *A history of dentistry,* ed 3, Philadelphia, 1948, Lea & Febiger.

McLean JW: Restorative materials for the 21st century, *Saudi Dent J* 9(3):116, 1997.

National Institute of Dental Research, National Institutes of Health: *International state-of-the-art conference on restorative dental materials,* Bethesda, Md, Sept 8-10, 1986.

Peyton FA: Significance of dental materials science to the practice of dentistry, *J Dent Educ* 30:268, 1966.

Ray KW: *Metallurgy for dental students,* Philadelphia, 1931, P Blakiston's Son.

Robinson JB: *The foundations of professional dentistry,* Baltimore, 1940, Waverly Press.

Shell JS: *Hodgen-Shell dental materials,* St Louis, 1938, Mosby.

Smyd ES: Bio-mechanics of prosthetic dentistry, *Ann Dent* 12:85, 1953.

Souder WH, Paffenbarger GC: Physical properties of dental materials, National Bureau of Standards Circular No. C433, Washington, DC, 1942, U.S. Government Printing Office.

Stanley HR: Biological testing and reaction of dental materials. In Craig RG, editor: *Dental materials review,* Ann Arbor, 1977, University of Michigan School of Dentistry, p 205.

Sturdevant CM, Barton RE, Sockwell CL, Strickland WD: *The art and science of operative dentistry,* ed 2, 1985, Mosby.

Taylor JA: History of dentistry, Philadelphia, 1922, Lea & Febiger.

Townsend RB: Porcelain teeth and the Chevalier Dubois de Chemant, *Dent Mag & Oral Topics* 58:249, 1941.

Tylman SD, Malone P: *Theory and practice of crown and fixed partial prosthodontics (bridge),* ed 7, St Louis, 1978, Mosby.

Von Recum AF, editor: *Handbook of biomaterials evaluation,* ed 2, Philadelphia, 1999, Taylor & Francis.

Weinberger BW: *Orthodontics, an historical view of its origin and evolution,* St Louis, 1926, Mosby.

Weinberger BW: The dental art in ancient Egypt, *J Am Dent Assoc* 34:170, 1947.

Weinberger BW: *An introduction to the histo of dentistry,* St Louis, 1948, Mosby.

Williams DF, editor: *Biocompatibility of dentc materials,* vols 1-4, Boca Raton, Fla, 1982, CRC Press.

Williams DF, editor: *Concise encyclopedia of medical and dental materials,* New York, 1990, Pergamon Press.

Chapter 2

Applied Surface Phenomena

Atoms or molecules at the surfaces of solids or liquids differ greatly from those in the bulk of the solid or liquid, and neighboring atoms may be arranged anisotropically. Also, some atoms or molecules may accumulate at the surface and thus cause unusual physical and chemical properties. The surfaces of solids may contain 10^{15} atoms or molecules per square centimeter plus or minus a factor of three, depending on the density. These solid surfaces have atoms of higher energy than bulk atoms because of the absence of some neighboring atoms and thus readily adsorb ambient atoms or molecules. It has been determined that to produce a clean solid surface, one with less than 1% of an adsorbed monolayer, a vacuum of 10^{-9} Torr or 1.33×10^{-7} Pa would be required to keep a surface clean for about an hour. At a vacuum of about 3×10^{-6} Torr, a newly cleaned surface would be coated with ambient atoms or molecules in only a few seconds. Therefore all dental materials and dental surfaces would be covered with a layer of ambient atoms or molecules and thus adhesives would be bonding to these adsorbed monolayers.

The surface layer usually is bonded to the substrate stronger than to adjacent adsorbed molecules. Thus the surface can be described as two layers: substrate layer and the adsorbed layer. The greatest interaction is between the substrate and the adsorbed layer, but interaction can involve several layers of adsorbed molecules. If the substrate is an insulator and an electrical charge exists at the interface between the solid and liquid, the charge may extend a number of layers into the solid and several layers into the liquid.

The energy involved in the adsorption of atoms or molecules onto the substrate may be of the level of a chemical reaction, or chemisorption, or may be of the level of van der Waal's reaction, or physiosorption. The former is irreversible whereas the latter is reversible.

Thus an important concept in surface chemistry is that critically important properties of a material may be more related to the chemistry of the surface layer and its composition than to the bulk properties. Such surface effects dominate the surface mechanical properties of adhesion and friction, the optical surface phenomena of the perception of color and texture, the tissue reaction to materials, the attachment of cells to materials, the wettability and capillarity of surfaces, the nucleation and growth of solids, and many other areas of crucial interest in biomaterials.

A few examples will convey the importance of surface chemistry to dentistry. Stainless steel used mainly in orthodontics is 72% to 74% iron, but has acceptable corrosion resistance in the mouth because the 18% chromium content forms an adherent oxide layer on the surface, which provides corrosion resistance. Titanium and its alloys, and noble alloys containing small amounts of indium and tin, have excellent biocompatibility properties as a result of oxides of titanium, indium, and tin on the surface.

Traditional methods and instrumentation allowed scientists and technicians to measure adsorption and desorption of atoms or molecules to surfaces, determine surface thermodynamic properties such as free energy and heats of adsorption and enthalpy, evaluate the contact angles of liquids on solid surfaces, and study adhesion, nucleation, friction, lubrication, and surface reactions.

Instrumentation and techniques developed over the past 20 years or so have permitted the study of surfaces on the atomic scale. The most common of these techniques involve scattering, absorption, or emission of photons, electrons, atoms, or ions. Of the many methods, here we will describe only three that have been applied to the study of dental biomaterials. Other techniques are adequately described in textbooks on surface chemistry and catalysis.

CHARACTERIZATION OF SOLID SURFACES

Several methods have been developed that facilitate routine surface analysis. Because tissues in contact with biomaterials have been found sensitive to contamination and surface composition, these approaches are used routinely in research. Three widely used methods for surface analysis are x-ray photoemission spectroscopy, electron spectroscopy for chemical analysis, and Auger electron spectroscopy.

X-ray photoemission spectroscopy (XPS) is often used because it is highly sensitive to small amounts of surface contamination since the x-ray beam does not penetrate deeply into the specimen. The specimen to be studied with XPS is bombarded with x-ray photons, which results in the emission of electrons from the surface atoms. The electrons are then analyzed according to energy level and a spectrum is obtained, as shown in Fig. 2-1, for a titanium dental implant. The spectrum shows the presence of titanium and oxygen peaks, which indicates titanium oxide. Small peaks for carbon, nitrogen, calcium, and phosphorus are probably the result of contamination, which may or may not be significant in tissue attachment to the implant.

Electron spectroscopy for chemical analysis (ESCA) also employs a beam of x-rays, which produce electron spectra characteristic of the atomic composition of the surface. The resolution of ESCA allows chemical analysis of areas as small as 200 μm by focusing the x-ray beam on a small spot. Fig. 2-2 shows an ESCA spectrum of a hydroxyapatite surface after plasma cleaning. The spectrum shows the presence of fluorine, silica, and sodium contamination, as well as the expected Ca, P, and O peaks. The C peak may be from carbonate.

Auger electron spectroscopy (AES) is another technique that can provide depth concentration profiles of elements. AES involves the bombardment of the specimen with electrons rather than x-ray beams and measurement of the secondary electrons emitted. At the same time, surface erosion is carried out by an ion bombardment process, called *sputtering*, to give the elemental analysis as a function of depth. Fig. 2-3 shows an AES spectrum from the surface of a titanium implant sample that shows the presence of Ti, O, and P as a function of sputter time and hence depth. The surface is dominated by TiO_2 with P

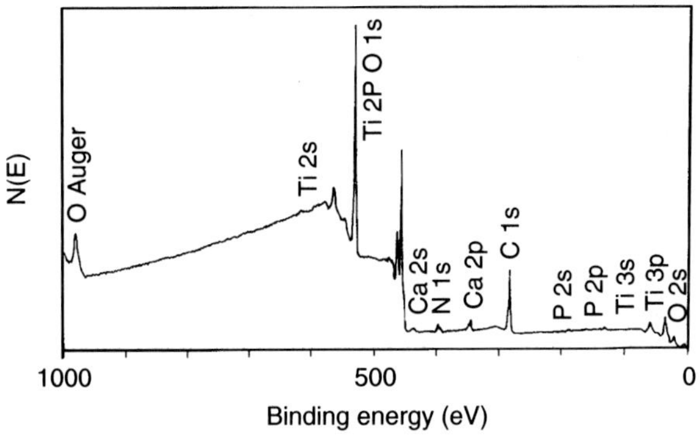

Fig. 2-1 XPS spectrum for Ti dental implant. The surface is dominated by TiO_2 peaks and smaller nitrogen, calcium, and phosphorous peaks resulting from surface contamination.
(From Kasemo B, Lausmaa J: *Int J Oral and Maxillofac Implants* 3:253, 1988.)

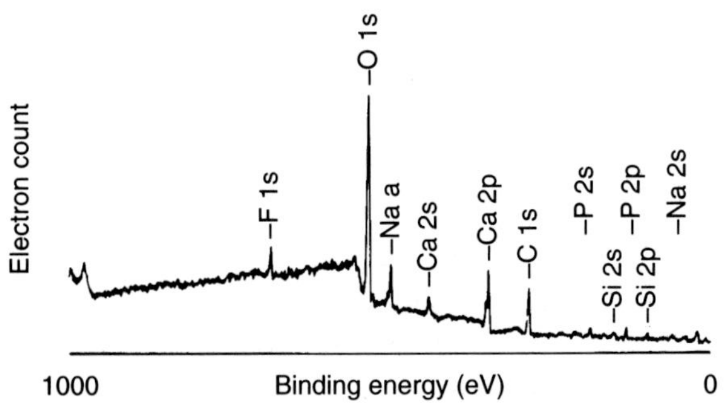

Fig. 2-2 ESCA spectrum from surface of hydroxyapatite after plasma cleaning.
(From Smith DC, Pilliar RM, Metson JB, McIntyre NS: *J Biomed Mater Res* 25:1080, 1991.)

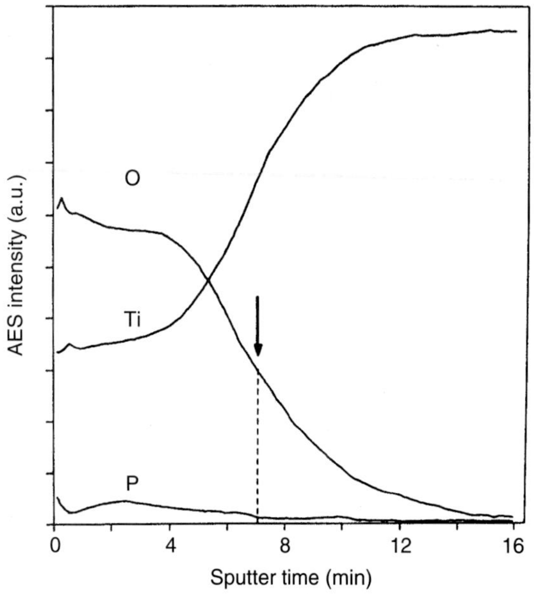

Fig. 2-3 AES depth profile for titanium implant surface as a function of depth removed by sputtering. (From Kasemo B, Lausmaa J: *Int Oral and Maxillofac Implants* 3:255, 1988.)

contamination from treatment with H_3PO_4. At deeper levels, sputtering uncovers the titanium under the oxide layer.

More recently, atomic force microscopy (AFM) has been used to study biomaterials interfaces and treated tooth surfaces. In the first study, diamond-knife microtomy was used to prepare specimens of adhesive tooth–biomaterials interfaces for examination by AFM, and the findings supported earlier XPS measurements demonstrating significant chemical bonding of glass ionomers to hydroxyapatite. In the second study, AFM was used to observe images of surfaces of polished, etched, dehydrated, and rehydrated dentin.

Nanoindentation of the surface of human enamel, filler particles of restorative materials, and the polymer-dentin bonding area of composites have been used to determine hardness and elasticity of these materials.

THE COLLOIDAL STATE

Colloids were first described by Thomas Graham (1861) as a result of his studies of diffusion in solutions. He observed that substances such as starch, albumin, and other gelatinous materials did not behave in the same manner as acids, bases, and salts. Because these substances were gluelike in nature, Graham described them as colloids, which was derived from the Greek word *kolla* for "glue" and *-oid-* meaning "like." As studies continued to increase the understanding of the subject of colloids and their nature, the name came to include more than the original term implied. The term *colloid* now is used to describe a *state* of matter rather than a *kind* of matter. The main characteristic of colloidal materials is their high degree of subdivision. These fine particles also have certain physical properties, such as electrical charges and surface energies, that control the characteristics of the colloids. It is not enough to confine the definition of colloids to particle size alone.

NATURE OF COLLOIDS

Substances are called colloids when they consist of two or more phases, with the units of at least one of the phases having a dimension slightly greater than simple molecular size. Although the range of size is somewhat arbitrary, it is usually recognized as being approximately 1 to 500 nm in maximum dimension.* Thus colloidal systems can be fine dispersions, gels, films, emulsions, or foams.

Except for a dispersion of a gas in a gas, which is a true solution, each of the three forms of matter—gas, liquid, and solid—may be dispersed as colloidal particles in the other and in itself as well. Each type has numerous examples of industrial and commercial importance, and many are known to have applications to dentistry, oral

*A micrometer (μm) is equal to 0.001 mm (10^{-3} mm), and a nanometer (nm) is equivalent to 0.000001 mm (10^{-6} mm); 100 nm is equal to 0.0001 mm, or 0.1 μm.

conditions, and restorative materials. The dispersed phase, which may be in the form of a gas, liquid, or solid, may also exist in a variety of conditions. Some examples of these dispersed phases are: (1) colloidal silica as a filler in resin composites, (2) colloidal silica in water to be mixed with high-strength dental stone to improve abrasion resistance, (3) droplets of oil in a water base used to prevent rusting of dental instruments during steam sterilization, (4) fillers used in rubber impression materials to control such properties as viscosity, and (5) agglomerates of detergent molecules in water that serve as wetting agents for wax patterns.

The colloidal state represents a highly dispersed system of fine particles of one phase in another, and a characteristic property of the dispersed phase is an enormous surface area. This is true whether a dispersed phase of oil droplets in an emulsion or a finely divided solid suspended in a liquid is considered. To visualize the increase in surface area and its relation to particle size, consider a solid in the form of a 1-cm cube having a total surface area of 6 cm^2. When this mass is cut into 1000 cubes, each being 1 mm on an edge, the surface area is increased to 60 cm^2. The same material reduced to cubes of 1 μm on an edge, which still is not within the range of colloidal particles, has a surface area of 60,000 cm^2. A further reduction in size to 0.1 μm, which is the upper limit for colloids, develops the enormous surface area of 600,000 cm^2 from the same mass that originally had an area of 6 cm^2. If it is assumed that the particles were of uniform size, the 1-cm cube produced 10^{15} particles. This increase in surface area gives rise to a corresponding increase in surface energy and surface reactions. A study of colloids is therefore a study of small particles and the related surface effects in the form of surface electrical charge or surface adsorption. Not only is the surface energy important, but the interface between the two phases also imparts important and characteristic properties to the system.

Suspended colloidal particles possess properties that permit the scattering of a beam of light. They also respond to superimposed electrostatic charges by being either attracted to or repelled by each other. Such a response is not characteristic of either true solutions or massive particles. It is often difficult to distinguish the colloidal range of substances from true solutions, or matter in the massive state, and therefore it is necessary to study not only the particle size but also the surface phenomena of the system.

TYPICAL COLLOID SYSTEMS

A few colloid systems are more important than others in relation to restorative materials. For example, the distinction between a sol and a gel is important because several of each find applications in dental operations. A sol resembles a solution, but it is made up of colloidal particles dispersed in a liquid. When a sol is chilled or caused to react by the addition of suitable chemicals, it may be transformed into a gel. In the gel form the system takes on a semisolid, or jellylike, quality.

The liquid phase of either a sol or a gel is usually water, but may be some organic liquid such as alcohol. Systems having water as one component are described as *hydrosols* or *hydrogels.* A more general term might be *hydrocolloid,* which is often used in dentistry to describe the agar or alginate gels used as elastic impression materials. A general term to describe a system having an organic liquid as one component would be *organosol* or *organogel.*

GELS

Two examples of materials that involve gel structures are the agar and alginate hydrocolloid impression materials.

Gels possess an entangled framework of solid colloidal particles in which liquid is trapped in the interstices and held by capillarity. Such a gel has some degree of rigidity, depending on the extent of the structural solids present.

Gels that are formed with water are hydrophilic (water loving) in character and tend to imbibe large quantities of water if allowed to stand immersed. The imbibition is accompanied by swelling and a change in physical dimensions. When allowed to stand in dry air, the gel loses water to the atmosphere, with an accompanying shrinkage. Such changes may be observed readily in agar or alginate gels.

A very common method for forming a gel is to add water to gelatin, agar, starch, or other substance that develops a dispersed colloid of the sol type. Such sols are often heated to aid the dispersion. Simple cooling of this sol results in the gel formation. Such a gel may contain as little as 2% to 10% solid colloids as interlaced and entangled filaments of molecular aggregates. The remainder of the gel is water held by capillarity. Gels produced in this manner are usually reversible in nature because they can be reconverted to a sol by heating and again to a gel by cooling. A common example of such a gel is agar. Within limits, gels of this type can be dehydrated by being allowed to stand in air and be rehydrated by being immersed in water.

Another common method of forming gels is by a reaction of two chemicals. The best-known example in dentistry is alginate gel, which results from the reaction of soluble potassium alginate with calcium ions to form an insoluble calcium alginate gel. This gel is thermally nonreversible, in contrast to the agar gel. Silicate-bonded dental investments set as a result of the formation of silica gel, which results from the reaction of sodium silicate and hydrochloric acid. This gel is an example of an inorganic nonreversible gel.

SYNERESIS

A characteristic of many gels is to contract on standing in closed containers and to exude or squeeze out some of the liquid phase. This process of accumulating an exudate on the surface is known as syneresis. The degree of attraction forces and the tenacity with which the filaments and fibers of the gel are held together have much to do with syneresis and the extent to which the exudate is formed. In dental impression-taking operations the formation of an exudate by syneresis is troublesome.

EMULSIONS

A uniform dispersion of minute droplets of one liquid within another constitutes an emulsion. The two liquids are highly insoluble and immiscible, but by mechanical means a colloidal dispersion of one liquid is produced in the other. Mechanical blenders, homogenizers, or grinders are used to prepare emulsions.

Most emulsions are either oil dispersed in water or water dispersed in oil. Usually an emulsion developed by the mechanical dispersion of pure liquids is unstable and soon breaks, with the droplets coalescing and separating into layers. The emulsion may be stabilized by the addition of a small quantity of a third substance known as an *emulsifier*. The emulsifier enters into the interface between the droplet and the dispersing liquid to give stability to the system. The action of the emulsifier is to lower the interfacial tension between the two liquids. Generally it is necessary to employ only a small quantity of emulsifier to produce a stable emulsion.

An emulsion of methyl methacrylate in water is obtained using a solid emulsifier; the small spheres of methyl methacrylate are polymerized to produce poly (methyl methacrylate) in the presence of an initiator, benzoyl peroxide. These polymer spheres are the powder used in acrylic denture materials and in the fabrication of orthodontic space maintainers.

DIFFUSION THROUGH MEMBRANES AND OSMOTIC PRESSURE

Osmotic pressure is the pressure developed by diffusion of a liquid or solvent through a membrane. The solvent passes from the dilute to the more concentrated solution through the membrane separating the two solutions. The presence of dissolved material in a solvent lowers the escaping tendency of the solvent molecules; the greater the concentration, the more the escaping tendency is lowered. Accordingly, the solvent will diffuse or pass through a membrane to a region of greater concentration, thus diluting the concentration of the solution.

The development of osmotic pressure has

been used to explain the hypersensitivity of dentin. It has been considered that the change in pressure (as the result of contact with saliva or concentrated solutions) of solutions present in natural tooth dentin in exposed carious teeth gives rise to diffusion throughout the structure to increase or decrease the pressure on the nerve system.

Just as diffusion through membranes is important, so also is the diffusion from a substance of a given concentration to that of another concentration important in many materials in dentistry. Studies have shown that salts and dyes will diffuse through human dentin. Stains and discoloring agents will diffuse through plastic restorative materials. Likewise, the diffusion of salts and acids through the organic-varnish type of cavity liners has been a problem.

ADSORPTION, ABSORPTION, AND SORPTION

It is common for liquids and solids to adsorb gases or other liquids on their surfaces; this process is always exothermic. In the adsorption process, a liquid or gas adheres firmly by the attachment of molecules to the surface of the solid or liquid, thus reducing their surface free energy. In a physical sense, if the two substances are alike, as, for example, two pieces of the same metal in the solid state pressed closely together, the mass is be said to *cohere*. When a dissimilar substance, such as a gas or liquid, is in intimate contact with the surface of the solid, it is said to *adhere* to the surface. The process of adsorption or adhesion to the surface of a substance is important in the wetting process, in which the substance is coated or wetted with a foreign substance such as a liquid. The degree to which saliva, for example, will wet or adhere to the surface of a resin denture depends on the tendency for surface adsorption. A substance that is readily wetted on the surface by water, as is glass or porcelain or the natural tooth surface, is considered to have adsorbed on its surface a layer of water molecules. When a wet, human enamel surface is desiccated, the first water to evaporate is bulk water, leaving physically and chemically adsorbed water. Considerable heat is required to remove physically adsorbed water, and even higher temperatures are needed to remove chemically adsorbed water. Thus any attempt to bond a restorative material to enamel must consider that adhesion will be to adsorbed water and not hydroxyapatite. High-energy surfaces such as metals will adsorb molecules more readily than low-energy surfaces such as waxes; oxides have intermediate surface energies.

The process of adsorption differs somewhat from the process of absorption. In the process of absorption, the substance absorbed diffuses into the solid material by a diffusion process and the process is not noted for concentration of molecules at the surface.

In instances in which both adsorption and absorption are known to exist and it is not clear which process predominates, the whole process is known as *sorption*. In measurement of the moisture content of dental resins, the process is described as one of sorption of moisture by the resin.

Numerous examples of these processes are found in the use of various restorative dental materials. The process of absorption of water by the hydrocolloid impression materials is particularly important to the stability of this type of compound. When the quantity of liquid absorbed into a substance is relatively large, there is likely to be an accompanying change in the dimensions of the absorbent.

SURFACE TENSION AND WETTING

Surface tension is measured in terms of force (dynes) per centimeter of the surface of liquid. In the case of water at 20° C, the value is 72.8 dynes/cm. At the same temperature, benzene has a value of 29 dynes/cm; alcohol, 22 dynes/cm; and ether, 17 dynes/cm. By contrast, mercury at 20° C has a surface tension of 465 dynes/cm. The values for each of these substances are influenced by factors such as temperature and purity. In general, there is a reduction in surface tension of all liquids as the temperature is increased. For

TABLE 2-1 Sodium Oleate in Water (Room Temperature, 22° C)

Solute Concentration	Concentration (%)	Surface Tension (dynes/cm)
Distilled water		72.8
1 part/500,000	0.0002	63.0
1 part/50,000	0.002	48.3
1 part/5000	0.02	35.3

example, the surface tension of water (in dynes per centimeter) is 76 at 0° C, 72 at 25° C, 68 at 50° C, and 59 at 100° C.

The surface tension of liquids is also reduced by the presence of impurities, some of which are exceedingly effective. Detergents, such as sodium lauryl sulfate, or the ingredients of soaps, including sodium stearate or sodium oleate, which have long hydrocarbon chains attached to hydrophilic groups (such as—COONa), are particularly effective in reducing the surface tension of water. An example of the effectiveness of sodium oleate in minute concentrations is shown in Table 2-1; notice that the surface tension is reduced approximately one half by the addition of only 0.02%, or 0.2 g/liter, of solute in water.

These surface-active agents affect the surface tension by concentrating at the liquid-air or other interfaces or surfaces. As these molecules occupy surface positions in the water-air surface, they displace surface water molecules, thus reducing the cohesive force between water molecules over the surface area, because the cohesion between water and surface active agent is less than that between water and water. This effect is demonstrated in Fig. 2-4, which represents two drops placed on wax, one of which is water and the other water with detergent. The presence of the surface-active agent molecules in the surface layer reduces the pull on the surface molecules toward the liquid mass. This reduces the surface tension to increase wetting. The soap molecules are oriented so that the hydrophilic end is in the water and the hydrophobic (hydrocarbon) end is oriented toward the wax or air.

The increased wettability of solids with liquids of reduced surface tension is important in numerous dental applications. The wetting power of a liquid is represented by its tendency to spread on the surface of the solid. In restorative dental operations it often is necessary to form wax patterns that are to be wetted by water or water suspensions of such materials as plaster or casting investment. Wax is not well wetted by water, for which reason a dilute solution of some wetting agent (such as 0.01% aerosol) is first painted on the wax in small quantities to aid in the spreading of water mixtures in subsequent operations.

Much can be learned about the spreading of liquids on solids, or the tendency for wetting surfaces, by measuring the angle of contact between the liquid and the solid surface. The angles of contact for different liquid droplets on a plane glass surface are illustrated in Fig. 2-5. The contact angle results from a balance of surface and interfacial energies. Notice that the surface energy of liquids is expressed as ergs per square centimeter, which is numerically equal to the surface tension in dynes per centimeter. Fig. 2-6 shows the balance of these energies for a solid and liquid where γ represents the surface energies and the subscripts *sa, sl,* and *lv* indicate solid-air, solid-liquid, and liquid-vapor interfaces. Notice that $\gamma_{sa} - \gamma_{sl}$ will be a maximum for a given liquid when the contact angle θ is 0 degree, because the cosine has a maximum value of 1 for that value of θ.

The greater the tendency to wet the surface, the lower the contact angle, until complete wetting occurs at an angle equal to zero.

Studies have been made to determine the contact angle of water and saliva on complete denture plastics because the angle relates to the retention of the denture (see Chapter 21). The contact angle and the tendency of a drop of water to spread on paraffin wax and dental methyl methacrylate plastic are shown for comparison in Fig. 2-7. The contact angle for water on wax is about 110 degrees, and for water on acrylic plastic around 75 degrees. The contact angle for saliva freshly applied to the acrylic plastic surface

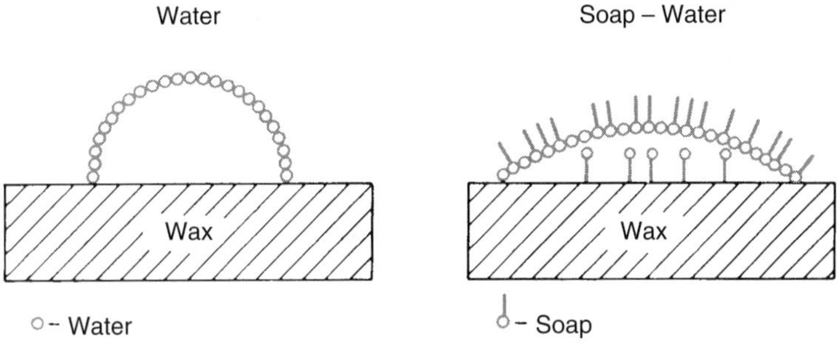

Fig. 2-4 Spreading of pure water and water containing soap molecules on wax.

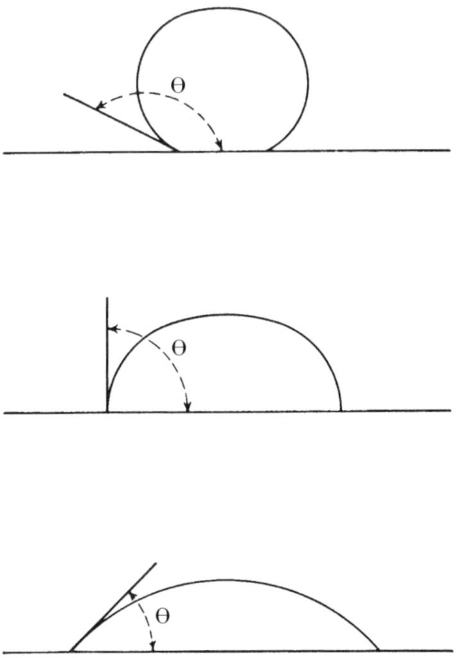

Fig. 2-5 Relation of contact angle to the spreading or wetting of a liquid on a solid.

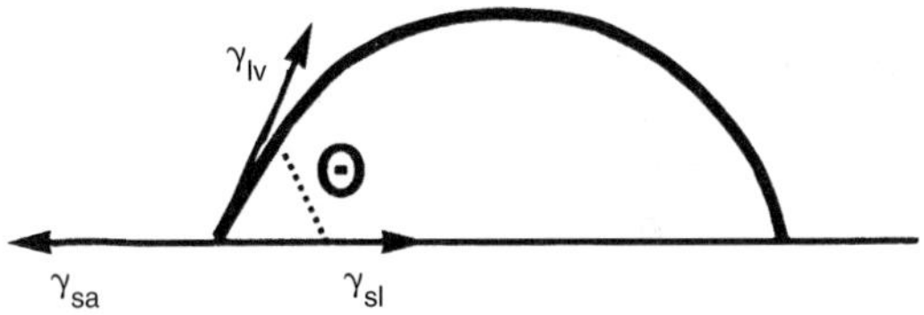

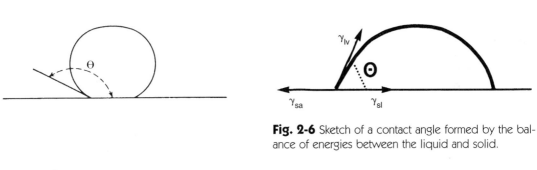

Fig. 2-6 Sketch of a contact angle formed by the balance of energies between the liquid and solid.

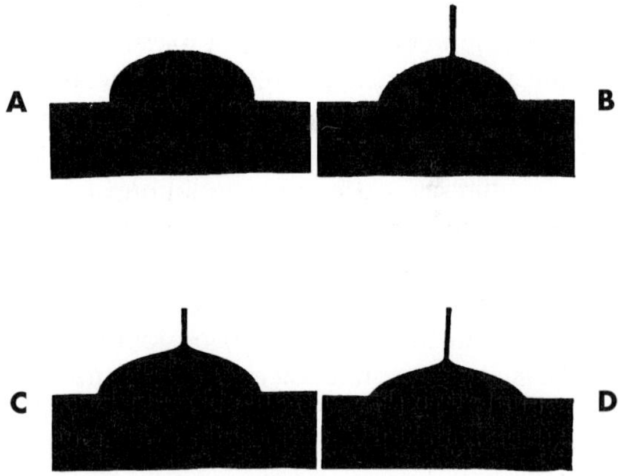

Fig. 2-7 Photographs to show the contact angle formed by a drop of water or saliva on wax and acrylic plastic. **A,** Water on wax. **B,** Water on plastic. **C,** Fresh saliva on plastic. **D,** Saliva after remaining in contact with plastic.

is 75 degrees, which is the same as that for water. When saliva was allowed to stand overnight in contact with the plastic material, the contact angle for saliva was reduced to approximately 68 degrees, which indicates that the surface wetting is somewhat improved after remaining in contact with the saliva. Table 2-2 gives contact angle values for water on selected materials.

The contact angles of water on various dental rubber impression materials are listed in Table 2-3, along with the castability of an impression of a very critical comb-like model. The ease of pouring a mix of dental stone and water to produce a model increases as the wettability (indicated by the contact angle) increases. The

TABLE 2-2 Contact Angles of Water on Solids at 27° C

Solid	Advancing Angle (degrees)
Acrylic polymer	74
Teflon	110
Glass	14
Amalgam	77
Acrylic filling material	38
Composite filling material	51

Adapted from O'Brien WJ: Capillary penetration of liquids between dissimilar solids, doctoral thesis, Ann Arbor, 1967, University of Michigan, p 40.

hydrophilic addition silicone differs from the hydrophobic type in that surfactants are added to the former, which reduce the surface tension of water in the mix of stone and increases the wetting of the impression material.

Other examples of wetting of surfaces by liquids include the spreading of molten flux on hot metal during melting or soldering operations. The spreading of molten solder on the surface of the parts to be assembled is an example of liquid metal wetting the surface of a solid metal. If the wetting is not adequate, the operation may be unsuccessful, and if the contact angle of the solder is too great, it will not penetrate into the fine detail of the structures to be joined. Antifluxes such as graphite are available, which can be painted on portions of metal surfaces where the solder is not wanted. Because the solder does not wet the graphite, it will not flow onto this treated surface.

The surface tension of metals is relatively high in comparison with that of other liquids, an indication that greater cohesive forces exist between the liquid metal atoms in the liquid-air surface than between molecules of liquid compounds such as alcohol or water. The surface tension of most metals, except mercury, cannot be measured at room temperature because of their high melting points. Typical values of a few metals are included in Table 2-4, which shows that there is a difference in the surface tension of various metals and that the values are much greater than for other liquids.

The surface tension of molten metals, like that of other liquids, is reduced with an increase in temperature. This is fortunate for the operation of casting molten metal, because some increase in the temperature will aid in producing sharp detail in the casting. This assumes, however, that the metal is not oxidized excessively or otherwise damaged by heating to the elevated temperature. The presence of a suitable flux will help prevent damage during heating.

Trituration of amalgam is important in amalgamation because of the degree of wetting of amalgam alloy by mercury. The contact angles of mercury on two common phases present in amalgam alloys, the silver-tin (γ) phase and the silver-copper eutectic phase, were found to be high and of the same order as those for commercial amalgam alloys. The high values are probably a result of the presence of silver and tin oxides on the surfaces of the alloys because the contact angle values for mercury on a set dental amalgam (Dispersalloy) are similar, as shown in Table 2-5. Trituration fractures the alloy particles, producing clean alloy surfaces that are readily wetted by mercury, and amalgamation can occur.

CAPILLARY RISE

The penetration of liquids into narrow crevices is known as *capillary action*.

The following equation relates the differential capillary pressure developed when a small tube of radius r is inserted in a liquid of surface tension γ (usually expressed in dynes/cm) and with a contact angle θ:

$$\Delta P = \frac{2\gamma \cos\theta}{r}$$

It follows that if the contact angle of the liquid on the solid is less than 90 degrees, as shown in Fig. 2-8, *A*, ΔP will be positive and the liquid will penetrate. If the contact angle is greater than 90 degrees (Fig. 2-8, *B*), ΔP will be negative and the liquid will be depressed.

TABLE 2-3 Wettability and Castability of Stone Models in Rubber Impression Materials

	Advancing Contact Angle of Water (degrees)	Castability of Water Mixes of High Strength Stone (%)
Condensation silicone	98	30
Addition silicone-hydrophobic	98	30
Polysulfide	82	44
Polyether	49	70
Addition silicone-hydrophilic	53	72

TABLE 2-4 Surface Tension of Metals

Metal	Temperature (° C)	Surface Tension (dynes/cm)
Lead	327	452
Mercury	20	465
Zinc	419	758
Copper	1131	1103
Gold	1120	1128

TABLE 2-5 Contact Angle of Mercury on Various Materials

Material	Contact Angle (degrees)
γ (73.2% Ag/26.8% Sn)	145
Eutectic (71.9% Ag/28.1% Cu)	138
Mynol	150
Dispersalloy	145
AgO	130
Ag_2O	135
SnO	107
SnO_2	130

From Baran G, O'Brien WJ: *J Am Dent Assoc* 94:898, 1977. Copyright by the American Dental Association. Reprinted by permission.

Most restorative materials used at present in dentistry do not adhere strongly to tooth structure. As a result, a crevice usually exists between the restoration and the tooth tissue into which mouth fluids penetrate because of capillary action. The importance of gap or width has long been recognized as a factor influencing the degree of marginal leakage. However, wetting is also an important factor in penetration. Fig. 2-9 describes the combined effects of gap width and contact angles on the capillary penetration of water between two plates. Two contact angles are involved, because one plate might be easily wetted, for example, glass, and the other might be a poorly wetted polymer.

PENETRATION COEFFICIENT

Another aspect of capillary phenomena involves the rate of penetration of a liquid into a crevice. An example is the penetration of a liquid prepolymer sealant into a fissure and the fine microscopic spaces created by etching of an enamel surface. The properties of the liquid affecting the rate of penetration may be related to the penetration coefficient *(PC)* where γ is the surface tension, η is the viscosity, and θ is the contact angle of the sealant on the enamel:

$$PC = \frac{\gamma \cos \theta}{2\eta}$$

The penetration coefficients for sealants have been shown to vary from 0.6 to 12 cm/sec. Narrow occlusal fissures can be filled almost completely if the penetration coefficient value is at least 1.30 cm/sec when the sealant is applied at a proximal edge of the fissure on the occlusal surface and allowed to flow to the other edge. If the sealant is painted over the occlusal surface, air trapped in the fissure prevents penetration beyond a certain depth. The same analysis applies to the penetration of liquid sealants into the

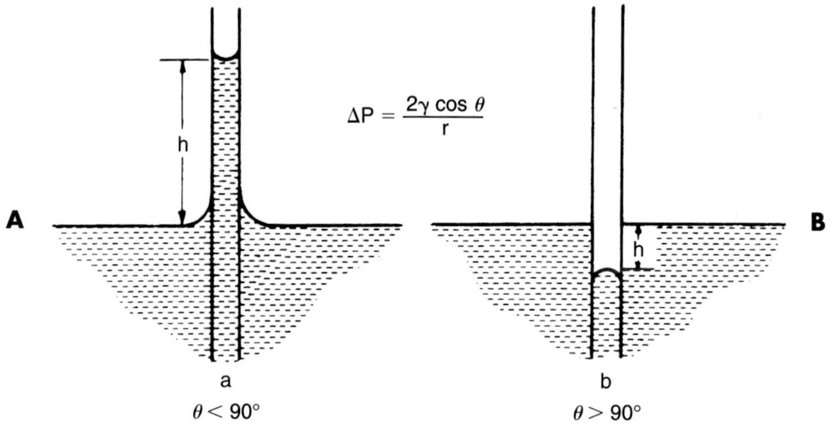

Fig. 2-8 Capillary penetration, **A,** and depression, **B.**
(From O'Brien WJ, Craig RG, Peyton FA: *J Prosthet Dent* 19:400, 1968.)

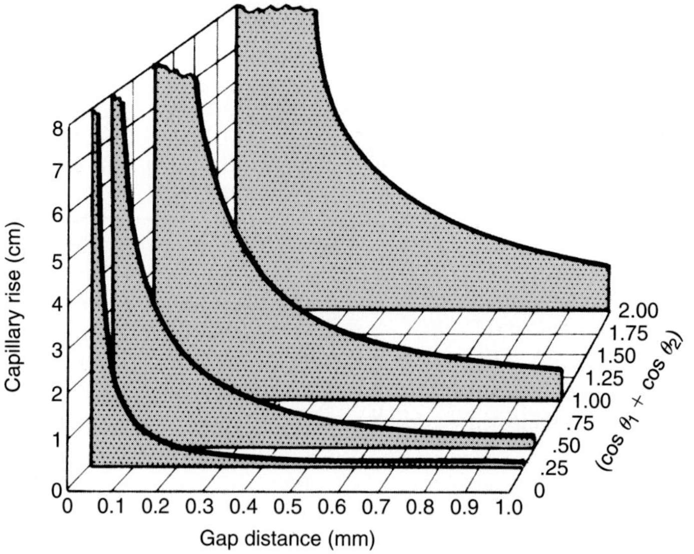

Fig. 2-9 Capillary rise curves for water between two plates of dissimilar materials.
(From O'Brien WJ, Craig RG, Peyton FA: *J Colloid Interface Sci* 26:507, 1968.)

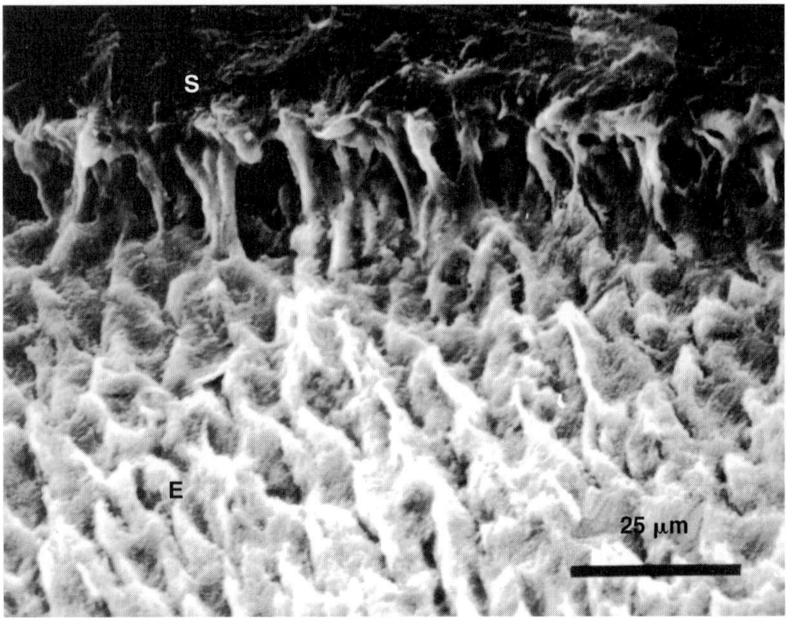

Fig. 2-10 Scanning electron micrograph of the interface of sealant *(S)* and enamel *(E)* showing sealant tags that had penetrated into the etched enamel surface.
(From O'Brien WJ, Fan PL, Apostolidis A: *Oper Dent* 3:53, 1978.)

etched surface of enamel to form tags, as shown in Fig. 2-10.

ISOLATED CAPILLARIES

Still another aspect of capillary phenomena is the adhesion of liquid bridges between solids. Liquid bridges are considered a contributing factor in denture retention (Fig. 2-11, *A*) when a thin film of saliva was present between the denture material and the mucosa. The source of capillary adhesion is the arrangement called an *isolated capillary*. As illustrated in Fig. 2-11, *C*, the differential pressure between a capillary and a connected reservoir is balanced by the hydrostatic pressure of capillary elevation. In capillaries isolated from a reservoir, as shown in Fig. 2-11, *A* and *B*, a negative differential pressure exerts an adhesive force. This force is partly responsible for denture retention, but it operates only if the film of saliva is isolated at the periphery of the denture. If the saliva film beneath the denture is connected to a reservoir of saliva beyond the borders of the denture, a negative differential pressure does not develop. Viscosity of the saliva film, however, offers some resistance to separation of the denture from the mucosa and thus contributes to retention.

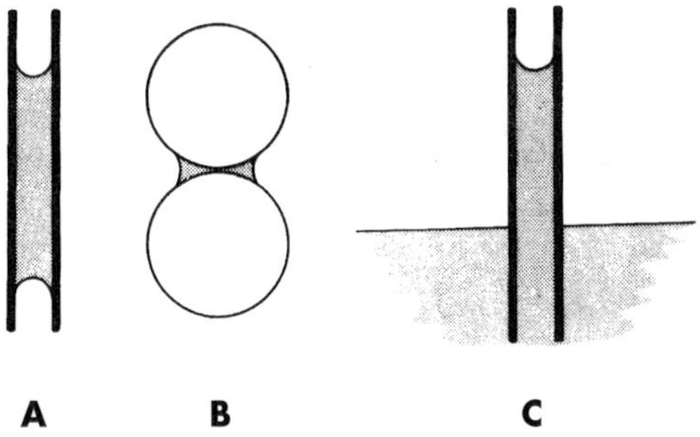

Fig. 2-11 Two classes of capillary systems. **A** and **B,** Isolated capillaries (isocaps). **C,** Connected capillary.
(From O'Brien, WJ: *J Dent Res* 52:545, 1973.)

Isolated capillaries form around teeth when small quantities of saliva are trapped in inter-

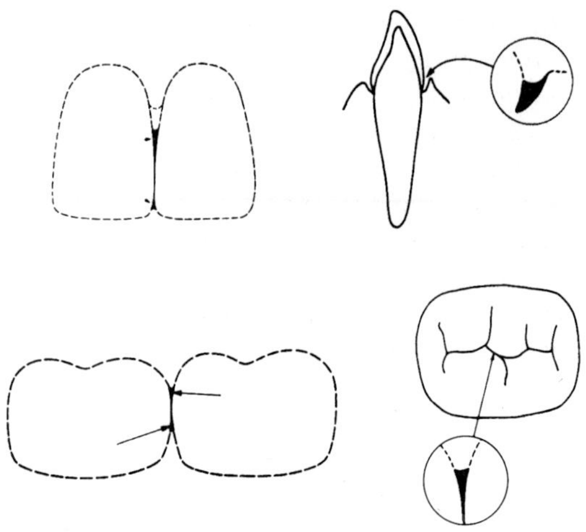

Fig. 2-12 Formation of isolated capillaries around teeth.
(From O'Brien WJ: *J Dent Res* 52:547, 1973.)

proximal spaces and occlusal fissures, as shown in Fig. 2-12. It is interesting that the growth rate of bacteria has been found to increase under these conditions of negative pressure.

FORCES INVOLVED IN DENTURE RETENTION

The accuracy of fit of a denture has been cited as an important factor in the retention of denture bases without any explanation as to why a better fit results in better retention. A technical discussion of all factors involved in the retention of dentures is not within the scope of this text, but a qualitative discussion is helpful in understanding the role of fit in denture retention. Factors include: (1) capillary forces involving the liquid film between the oral tissues and the denture base; (2) surface forces controlling the wetting of the plastic denture base by the saliva; (3) the seating force applied to the denture, which, for the most part, determines the thickness of the saliva film between the denture and the oral tissues; (4) the surface tension of the saliva; (5) the viscosity of the saliva; and (6) the atmospheric pressure.

The capillary force, *F*, responsible for retention of a denture can be expressed by the following equation:

$$F = \frac{\gamma A(\cos\theta_1 + \cos\theta_2)}{dg}$$

where γ is the surface tension of saliva, A is the surface area of the tissue surface of the denture, θ_1 and θ_2 are the contact angles of saliva against the plastic and the oral mucosa, d is the film thickness of the saliva between the denture and the tissue, and g is the gravitational constant.

Certain factors, such as wetting, are more important in the retention of a denture under static conditions, whereas other factors, such as capillarity and atmospheric pressure, are more effective when a force tends to dislodge the denture. The wetting of the plastic surface depends on the energy relationship between the solid and the liquid. If complete wetting occurs, the liquid will spread on the solid. If partial wetting occurs, the liquid will form droplets on the surface. The plastics used in dentistry are only partially wetted by saliva, but the wetting may improve after contact with oral fluids because of the adsorption of certain components of the saliva by the plastic surface.

The capillary force, which helps restrain any dislodging force on the denture, is increased by complete wetting of the denture surface, high surface tension of the saliva, and large tissue contact area of the denture. Patients with stringy (low surface tension) saliva experience difficulty with retention of dentures. The viscosity of saliva is low, and little difference in retention is observed regardless of whether the load is applied slowly or rapidly. The use of denture pastes, however, provides a film of increased thickness and viscosity; if they are used, greater retention is observed when the load is applied rapidly. It has been shown that the use of adhesives has no detrimental effect on the health of the supporting tissues.

The viscosity of saliva from dentate and edentulous patients differs, with edentulous patients demonstrating a lower viscosity. The lower viscosity may be caused by stimulation of salivary flow; the denture, acting as a foreign object, causes a larger flow of saliva with a lower mucin content. Another possibility is that the mandibular denture may obstruct the ducts of the submandibular glands, which produce a greater proportion of mucous glycoprotein. Saliva also appears to act as a non-newtonian fluid, exhibiting lower viscosities at higher shear rates or shear thinning.

The capillary force is diminished when the distance between the denture and the oral tissues is increased. It is reduced to a very small value if the periphery of the denture is immersed in saliva or other fluids. This explains some of the difficulty patients may encounter when drinking fluids and the variation in retention of the maxillary compared with the mandibular denture. At best, the role of atmospheric pressure is that of a temporary restraining force, because the pressure in the saliva film is only slightly less than atmospheric pressure. During the application of a dislodging force, however, a reduced pressure may occur under the denture, which may temporarily retard its movement.

The two factors just mentioned may explain in part the function of the peripheral seal. If all other factors are held constant for a particular patient, the fit of the denture controls the distance between it and the oral tissues, which in turn controls the force necessary to dislodge a denture. As a patient continues to wear a denture for a period of time, changes in the contour of the oral tissues and bone structure may eventually result in a poorer fit and decreased retention.

ADHESION

Adhesion is the bonding of dissimilar materials by the attraction of atoms or molecules. Because there is always some attraction between atoms, adhesive strength is a matter of magnitude. Stresses that weaken adhesive bonds are caused by differences in thermal expansion coefficients and dimensional changes during setting of the adhesive. Adhesion can also be reduced by hydrolytic degradation of the bond.

Two mechanisms of adhesion may be distinguished: chemical and mechanical. Chemical adhesion involves bonding at the atomic or molecular level. Mechanical adhesion is based on retention by the interlocking or the penetration of one phase into the surface of the other. In many cases chemical and mechanical adhesion occur together.

Adhesion with composites has been achieved by etching tooth enamel with acids such as phosphoric or acrylic acid. Adhesive bond strengths approaching the tensile strength of enamel have been found even after storage in water. Examination under high magnification shows the etched enamel to be greatly roughened. The adhesion of resins to etched enamel is a result of capillary penetration into surface irregularities. These polymer projections into enamel have been called *tags*. Enamel etching has been applied in the use of pit-and-fissure sealants to obtain adhesion and with composite filling materials to obtain adhesion to enamel margins.

Adhesion of hydrophobic composites to hydrophilic enamel and dentin, even with micromechanical etching, is improved by the use of an intermediate layer of a compound like hydroxyethyl methacrylate. One end of this molecule is hydrophilic while the other end is hydrophobic and has a polymerizable carbon double bond. Thus good wetting of tooth structure is obtained from the hydrophilic end, and good compatibility and reactivity with the resin in the composite at the hydrophobic end.

Glass ionomers with polymer acid groups can react with adsorbed water on the surface of teeth to produce a moderate and quite stable bond. However, the mechanical strengths of these materials are not as high as those of bonded composites.

SELECTED PROBLEMS

Problem 1

Why is mercury difficult to handle without contamination in the operatory?

Solution

The high surface tension of mercury and high contact angles on most surfaces cause mercury to cohere and roll off most surfaces. The vapor pressure of mercury at room temperature is high enough so that its concentration in air can be toxic. The solution is to handle free mercury over surfaces with lipped edges that can catch any spills or to use precapsulated amalgam systems.

Problem 2

Gold inlay castings made with the lost wax process were rough. What could have been the problem?

Solution

There could be several causes for the rough castings. A detergent or wetting agent may not have been used on the wax pattern prior to the investing procedure. Wax patterns are not readily wetted by the water-based gypsum investment unless a wetting agent is used; if one is not used, rough internal mold surfaces produce rough castings.

On the other hand, too much wetting agent placed on the wax will interfere with the setting of the investment and a rough surface will result. The wetting agent is painted on the wax pattern and the excess removed by painting with a dry brush. Very little wetting agent is needed (see Table 2-1).

Problem 3

The bond between a pit-and-fissure material that had just been removed from the refrigerator and etched enamel was found to be poor. Why?

Solution

The bonding of pit-and-fissure sealants to enamel depends on the capillary penetration of the sealant into the fine microscopic spaces produced by etching. The rate of capillary penetration is dependent upon the wetting and viscosity of the sealant. At lower temperatures, the viscosity of sealants is too high for rapid penetration. Therefore it is necessary to allow a refrigerated sealant to warm to room temperature before application.

Problem 4

An addition-silicone impression was poured in high-strength stone and it was difficult to reproduce the fine margins of cavity preparations. What might have been the problem?

Solution

In all probability, a hydrophobic addition-silicone impression material was used and wetting of the surface by the mix of high-strength stone was troublesome. Check the manufacturer's literature and it will probably not indicate that it is a hydrophilic type. Manufacturers will specify that it is hydrophilic, but not if it is hydrophobic.

Problem 5

A complete-denture patient is having difficulty with retention of a maxillary denture. What factors should you check to improve the retention?

Solution

Make sure there is adequate extension at the periphery so that on movement the seal is not broken.

The fit, especially at the periphery, is important because it will control the thickness of the saliva film between the denture and the tissue and the force needed to dislodge the denture. The thinner the film of saliva the greater the retention.

BIBLIOGRAPHY

Baier RE, Meyer AE: Surface analysis. In von Recum, AF: *Handbook of biomaterials evaluation,* New York, 1986, Macmillan.

Baran G, O'Brien WJ: Wetting of amalgam alloys by mercury, *J Am Dent Assoc* 94:897, 1977.

Craig RG, Berry GC, Peyton FA: Wetting of poly(methyl methacrylate) and polystyrene by water and saliva, *J Phys Chem* 64: 541, 1960.

Dental composites and adhesives in the 21st century; The Gunnar Ryge Memorial Symposium, *Quintessence Internat* 24(9):605, 1993.

Iler RK: *The chemistry of silica-solubility, polymerization, colloid and surface properties, and biochemistry,* New York, 1979, John Wiley & Sons.

Myers CL, Ryge G, Heyde JB et al: In vivo test of bond strength, *J Dent Res* 42:907, 1963.

Norman AL: Frictional resistance and dental prosthetics, *J Prosthet Dent* 14:45, 1964.

O'Brien WJ: Surface energy of liquids isolated in narrow capillaries, *J Surface Sci* 19:387, 1970.

O'Brien WJ: Capillary action around dental structures, *J Dent Res* 52:544, 1973.

O'Brien WJ: *Capillary effects in adhesion,* Proceedings of Conference on Dental Adhesive Materials, New York, 1973, New York University Press.

O'Brien WJ, Craig RG, Peyton FA: Capillary penetration around a hydrophobic filling material, *J Prosthet Dent* 19:400, 1968.

O'Brien WJ, Craig RG, Peyton FA: Capillary penetration between dissimilar materials, *J Colloid Interface Sci* 26:500, 1968.

O'Brien WJ, Fan PL, Apostolidis A: Penetrativity of sealants and glazes, *Oper Dent* 3:51, 1978.

Rosales JI, Marshall GW, Marshall SJ et al: Acid-etching and hydration influence on dentin roughness and wettability, *J Dent Res* 78: 1554, 1999.

Shaw DJ: *Electrophoresis,* New York, 1969, Academic Press.

Somorjai GA: *Introduction to surface chemistry and catalysis,* New York, 1994, John Wiley & Sons.

van Meerbeek B, Williams G, Celis JP et al: Assessment by mono-indentation of the hardness and elasticity of the resin-dentin bonding area, *J Dent Res* 72:1434, 1993.

van Pelt AWJ: *Adhesion of oral streptococci to solids,* Groningen, The Netherlands, 1985, Drukkerij Van Denderen B.V.

Willems G, Celis JP, Lambrechts P et al: Hardness and Young's modulus determined by nanoindentation technique of filler particles of dental restorative materials compared with human enamel, *J Biomed Mater Res* 27: 747, 1993.

Williams BF, von Fraunhofer JA, Winter GB: Tensile bond strength between fissure sealants and enamel, *J Dent Res* 53:23, 1974.

Yoshida Y, van Meerbeek B, Nakayama Y et al: Evidence of chemical bonding at biomaterial-hard tissue interfaces, *J Dent Res* 79:709, 2000.

Yoshida Y, van Meerbeek B, Snowwaert J et al: A novel approach to AFM characterization of adhesive tooth-biomaterials interfaces, *J Biomed Mater Res* 47:85, 1999.

Chapter 3

Optical, Thermal, and Electrical Properties

Restorative dental materials are developed by the producer and selected by the dentist on the basis of characteristic physical, chemical, mechanical, and biological properties of the material.

No single property can be used as a measure of quality of materials. Often several combined properties, determined from standardized laboratory and clinical tests, are employed to give a measure of quality. The information gained from an orderly laboratory investigation can assist greatly in the clinical evaluation of the particular product or technique by shortening the time required for clinical testing.

There are times when it is not possible to develop a test that is identical with clinical conditions because of the nature of the material or the equipment involved. In such instances a systematic study is conducted with as practical an approach as possible, and the results are then interpreted on a comparative basis.

Standardization of test practices is essential, however, to control quality and allow for duplication of results by other investigators. When possible, the test specimens should approach the size and shape of the structure employed in practice, with mixing and manipulating procedures comparable with routine clinical conditions.

Although it is important to know the comparative values of properties of different restorative materials, it is also essential to know the quality of the supporting tissue. Whereas many restorations fail clinically because of fracture or deformation, it is not uncommon for a well-constructed restoration to be useless because the supporting tissue fails. Consequently, in designing restorations and interpreting test results, remember that the success of a restoration depends not only on its physical qualities but also on the biophysical or physiological qualities of the supporting tissues.

The physical properties described in this chapter include color and optical properties, thermal properties, and electrical and electrochemical properties. The color and optical properties are color and its measurement, pigmentation, metamerism, fluorescence, opacity, index of refraction, and optical constants. The thermal properties are temperature, heat of fusion, thermal conductivity, specific heat, thermal diffusivity, and coefficient of thermal expansion. The electrical and electrochemical properties are electrical conductivity, dielectric constant, electromotive force, galvanism, corrosion, and zeta-potential. Other, less specific properties are tarnish and discoloration, water sorption, solubility and disintegration, setting time, and shelf life. These properties generally are not concerned with the application of force to a body as mechanical properties are.

OPTICAL PROPERTIES

COLOR

The perception of the color of an object is the result of a physiological response to a physical stimulus. The sensation is a subjective experience, whereas the beam of light, which is the physical stimulus that produces the sensation, is entirely objective. The perceived color response results from either a reflected or a transmitted beam of white light or a portion of that beam. According to one of Grassmann's laws, the eye can distinguish differences in only three parameters of color. These parameters are dominant wavelength, luminous reflectance, and excitation purity.

The dominant wavelength (λ) of a color is the wavelength of a monochromatic light that, when mixed in suitable proportions with an achromatic color (gray), will match the color perceived. Light having short wavelengths (400 nm) is violet in color, and light having long wavelengths (700 nm) is red. Between these two wavelengths are those corresponding to blue, green, yellow, and orange light. This attribute of color perception is also known as *hue*.

Of all the visible colors and shades, there are only three primary colors: red, green, and blue (or violet). Any other color may be produced by the proper combination of these colors. For example, yellow may be obtained by a correct mixture of green and red lights.

The luminous reflectance of a color permits an

object to be classified as equivalent to a member of a series of achromatic objects ranging from black to white for light-diffusing objects and from black to perfectly clear and colorless for transmitting objects. A black standard is assigned a luminous reflectance of 0, whereas a white standard is assigned 100. This attribute of color perception is described as *value* in one visual system of color measurement.

The excitation purity or saturation of a color describes the degree of its difference from the achromatic color perception most resembling it. Numbers representing excitation purity range from 0 to 1. This attribute of color perception is also known as *chroma*. Typical quantities for dominant wavelength, luminous reflectance, and excitation purity of materials and human tissues determined in reflected light are listed in Table 3-1.

MEASUREMENT OF COLOR

The color of dental restorative materials is most commonly measured in reflected light by instrumental or visual techniques.

Instrumental Technique Curves of spectral reflectance versus wavelength can be obtained over the visible range (405 to 700 nm) with a recording spectrophotometer and integrating sphere. Typical curves for a composite resin before and after 300 hours of accelerated aging in a weathering chamber are shown in Fig. 3-1. From the reflectance values and tabulated color-matching functions, the tristimulus values *(X, Y, Z)* can be computed relative to a particular light source. These tristimulus values are related to the amounts of the three primary colors required to give, by additive mixture, a match with the color being considered. Typically, the tristimulus values are computed relative to the Commission Internationale de l'Eclairage (C.I.E.) Source A (gas-filled incandescent lamp) or Source C (average daylight from overcast sky). The ratios of each tristimulus value of a color to their sum are called the *chromaticity coordinates (x, y, z)*. Dominant wavelength and excitation purity of a color can be determined by referring its chromaticity coordinates to a chromaticity diagram such as the one shown in Fig. 3-2. The luminous reflectance is equal to the value of the second *(Y)* of the three tristimulus values. Some typical quantities for color of dental materials are listed in Table 3-1.

A diagram of the C.I.E. *L*a*b** color space is shown in Fig. 3-3. The *L*a*b** color space is

TABLE 3-1 Typical Quantities for Color Determined in Reflected Daylight (C.I.E. Source C)

Material	Dominant Wavelength (nm)	Luminous Reflectance	Excitation Purity
Denture resins	601-623	22.5-28.6	0.30-0.38
Denture resin (Meharry shade)	−493*	22.2	0.15
Resin composites	576-580	51.6-78.9	0.16-0.31
Glass ionomer (class V restorative)	577-579	55.2-67.7	0.19-0.27
Human teeth	566-586	35.8-44.8	0.34-0.40
Human facial skin			
Black	588-594	9.8-33.4	0.25-0.44
White	584-599	19.1-44.9	0.20-0.44
Oriental	588-593	22.4-37.4	0.27-0.38
Veneering resin	577-580	56.0-64.4	0.26-0.31

*The negative sign indicates a complementary wavelength and a dominant wavelength in the purple hue.

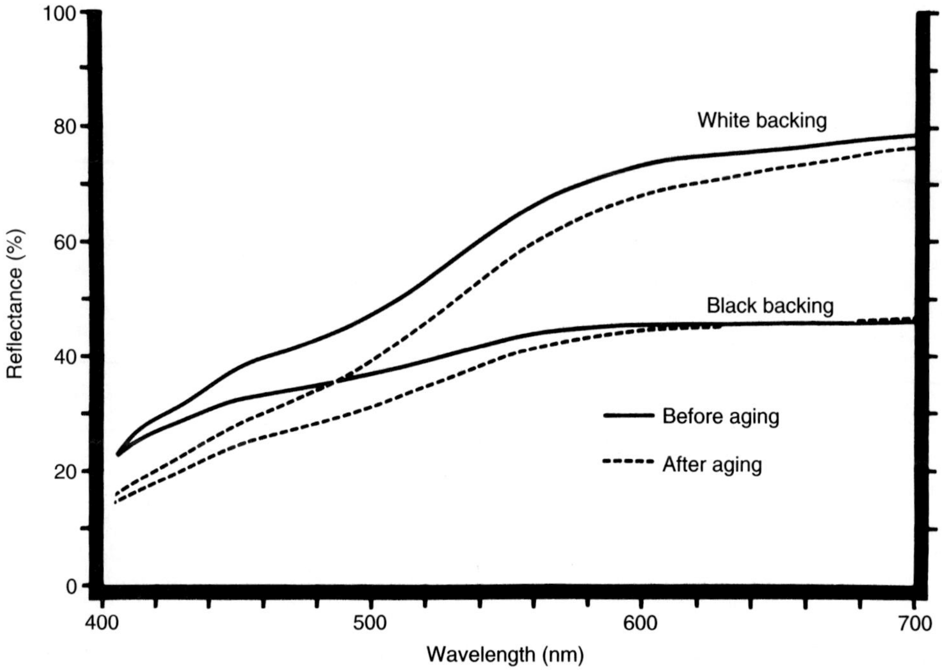

Fig. 3-1 Curves of spectral reflectance versus wavelength for a composite resin before and after exposure to conditions of accelerated aging. The specimen was exposed continuously for 300 hours to the radiation of a 2500-watt xenon lamp and intermittently sprayed with water. The aging chamber was held at 43° C and 90% relative humidity. Spectral reflectance curves for translucent specimens often are obtained with both black and white backings.

Fig. 3-2 Chromaticity diagram *(x, y)* according to the 1931 C.I.E. Standard Observer and coordinate system. Values of dominant wavelength determine the spectrum locus. The excitation purity is the ratio of two lengths *(AB/AC)* on the chromaticity diagram, where *A* refers to the standard light source and *B* refers to the color being considered. The point *C*, the intersection of line *AB* with the spectrum locus, is the dominant wavelength.

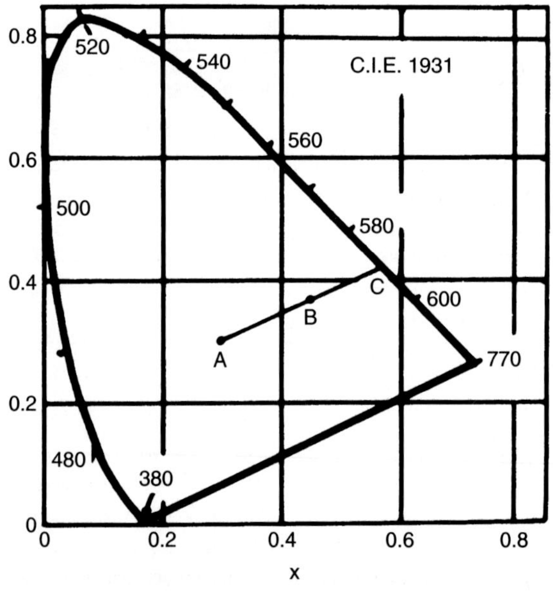

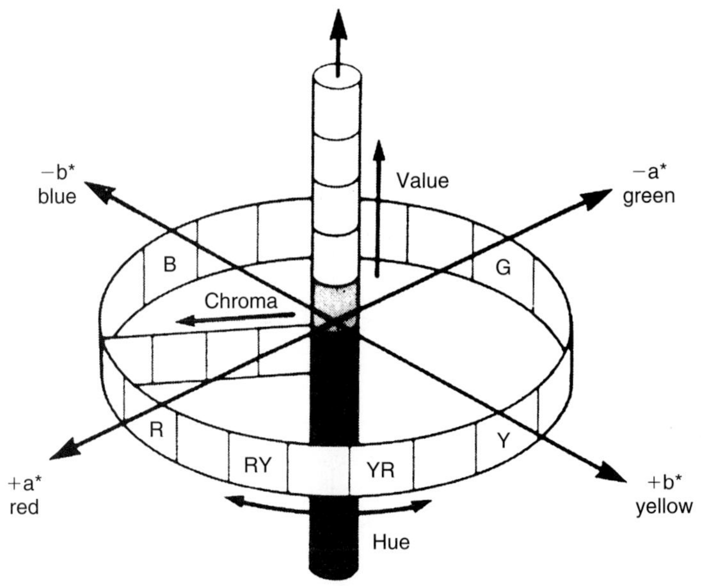

Fig. 3-3 C.I.E. $L^*a^*b^*$ color arrangement.
(From Seghi RR, Johnston WM, O'Brien WJ: *J Prosthet Dent* 56:35, 1986.)

characterized by uniform chromaticities. Value (black to white) is denoted as L^*, whereas chroma (a^*b^*) is denoted as red ($+a^*$), green ($-a^*$), yellow ($+b^*$), and blue ($-b^*$). Differences between two colors can be determined from a color difference formula. One such formula has the form:

$$\Delta E^*(L^*a^*b^*) = [(\Delta L^*)^2 + (\Delta a^*)^2 + (\Delta b^*)^2]^{1/2}$$

where L^*, a^*, and b^* depend on the tristimulus values of the specimen and of a perfectly white object. A value of ΔE^* of 1 can be observed visually by half of the observers under standardized conditions. A value of ΔE^* of 3.3 is considered perceptible clinically.

Visual Technique A popular system for the visual determination of color is the Munsell Color System, the parameters of which are represented in three dimensions, as shown in Fig. 3-4. The color considered is compared with a large set of color tabs. Value (lightness) is determined first by the selection of a tab that most nearly corresponds with the lightness or darkness of the color. Value ranges from white (10/) to black (0/). Chroma is determined next with tabs that are close to the measured value but are of increasing saturation of color. Chroma ranges from achromatic or gray (/0) to a highly saturated color (/18). The hue of the color is determined last by matching with color tabs of the value and chroma already determined. Hue is measured on a scale from 2.5 to 10 in increments of 2.5 for each of the 10 color families (red, R; yellow-red, YR; yellow, Y; green-yellow, GY; green, G; blue-green, BG; blue, B; purple-blue, PB; purple, P; red-purple, RP). For example, the color of the attached gingiva of a healthy patient has been measured as 5R 6/4 to indicate a hue of 5R, a value of 6, and a chroma of 4.

Two similar colors also can be compared in the Munsell Color System by a color difference formula such as one derived by Nickerson:

$$I = (C/5)(2\Delta H) + 6\Delta V + 3\Delta C$$

where C is the average chroma and ΔH, ΔV, and ΔC are differences in hue, value, and chroma of the two colors. For example, if the color of attached gingiva of a patient with periodontal disease was 2.5R 5/6, the color difference, I, between the diseased tissue and the aforementioned healthy tissue (5R 6/4) would be:

$$I = (5/5)(2)(2.5) + (6)(1) + (3)(2) = 17$$

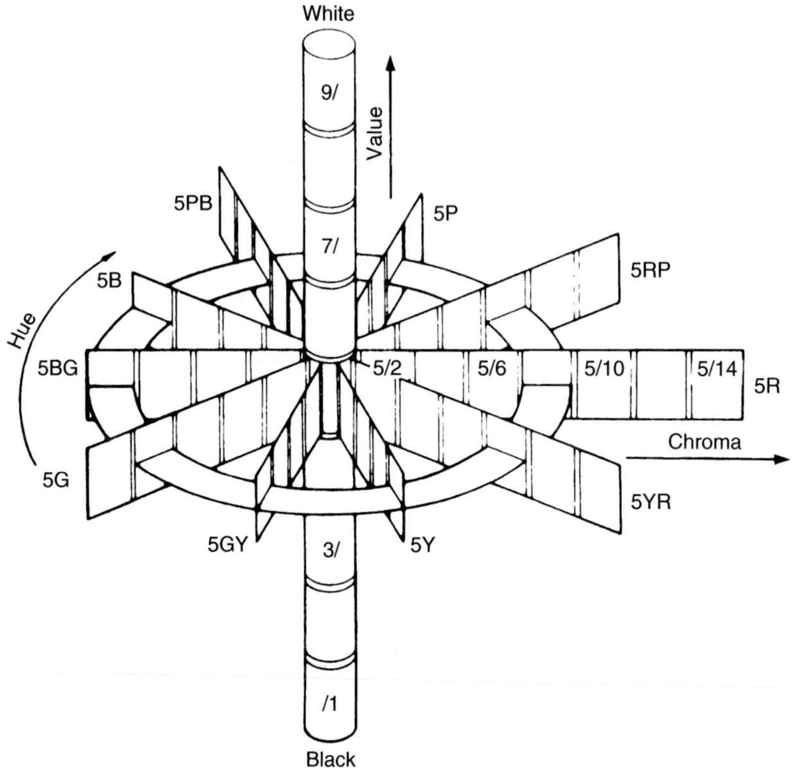

Fig. 3-4 Munsell scales of hue, value, and chroma in color space. (Adapted from Powers JM, Capp JA, Koran A: *J Dent Res* 56:112, 1977.)

A trained observer can detect a color difference, *I,* equal to 5.

Surface Finish and Thickness When white light shines on a solid, some of the light is directly reflected from the surface and remains white light. This light mixes with the light reflected from the body of the material and dilutes the color. As a result, an extremely rough surface appears lighter than a smooth surface of the same material. This problem is associated with unpolished or worn glass ionomer and composite restorations. For example, as the resin matrix of a composite material wears away, the restoration appears lighter and less chromatic (grayer).

The thickness of a restoration can affect its appearance. For example, as the thickness of a composite restoration placed against a white background increases, the lightness and the excitation purity decreases. The most dramatic change observed is the increase in opacity as the thickness increases.

PIGMENTATION

Esthetic effects are sometimes produced in a restoration by incorporating colored pigments in nonmetallic materials such as resin composites, denture acrylics, silicone maxillofacial materials, and dental ceramics. The color observed when pigments are mixed results from the selective absorption by the pigments and the reflection of certain colors. Mercuric sulfide, or vermilion, is a red pigment because it absorbs all colors except red. The mixing of pigments therefore involves the process of subtracting colors. For example, a green color may be obtained by mixing a pigment such as cadmium sulfide, which absorbs blue and violet, with ultramarine, which absorbs red, orange, and yellow. The only color reflected from such a mixture of pigments is green, which is the color observed.

Inorganic pigments rather than organic dyes are usually used because the pigments are more permanent and durable in their color qualities. When the colors are combined with the proper translucency, the restorative materials may be made to match closely the surrounding tooth structure or soft tissue. To match tooth tissue, various shades of yellow and gray are blended into the white base material, and occasionally some blue or green pigments are added. To match the pink soft tissues of the mouth, various blends of red and white are necessary, with occasional need for blue, brown, and black in small quantities. The color and translucency of human tissue shows a wide variation from patient to patient and from one tooth or area of the mouth to another.

METAMERISM

Metameric colors are color stimuli of identical tristimulus values under a particular light source but different spectral energy distributions. The spectral reflectance curves of two such colors would be complicated, with perhaps three or more crossing points. Under some lights such colors would appear to match, but under other lights they would not match.

The quality and intensity of light are factors that must be controlled in matching colors in dental restorations. Because light from incandescent lamps, fluorescent lamps, and the sun differs, the match in color between a pigmented dental material and tooth structure may also vary. Whenever possible, colors should be matched in light corresponding to that of use.

FLUORESCENCE

Fluorescence is the emission of luminous energy by a material when a beam of light is shone on it. The wavelength of the emitted light usually is longer than that of the exciting radiation. Typically, blue or ultraviolet light produces fluorescent light that is in the visible range. Light from most fluorescent substances is emitted in a single, broad, well-shaped curve, the width and peak depending on the fluorescing substance.

Sound human teeth emit fluorescent light when excited by ultraviolet radiation (365 nm), the fluorescence being polychromatic with the greatest intensity in the blue region (450 nm) of the spectrum. Some anterior restorative materials and dental porcelains are formulated with fluorescing agents (rare earths excluding uranium) to reproduce the natural appearance of tooth structure.

OPACITY, TRANSLUCENCY, AND TRANSPARENCY

The color of an object is modified not only by the intensity and shade of the pigment or coloring agent but also by the translucency or opacity of the object. Body tissues vary in the degree of opacity that they exhibit. Most possess a degree of translucency. This is especially true of tooth enamel and the supporting soft tissues surrounding the teeth.

Opacity is a property of materials that prevents the passage of light. When all of the colors of the spectrum from a white light source such as sunlight are reflected from an object with the same intensity as received, the object appears white. When all the spectrum colors are absorbed equally, the object appears black. An opaque material may absorb some of the light and reflect the remainder. If, for example, red, orange, yellow, blue, and violet are absorbed, the material appears green in reflected white light.

Translucency is a property of substances that permits the passage of light but disperses the light, so objects cannot be seen through the material. Some translucent materials used in dentistry are ceramics, resin composites, and denture plastics.

Transparent materials allow the passage of light in such a manner that little distortion takes place and objects may be clearly seen through them. Transparent substances such as glass may be colored if they absorb certain wavelengths and transmit others. For example, if a piece of glass absorbed all wavelengths except red, it would appear red by transmitted light. If a light beam containing no red wavelengths were shone on the glass, it would appear opaque, because the remaining wavelengths would be absorbed.

Measurement of Contrast Ratio The opacity of a dental material can be determined instrumentally or by visual comparison with opal glass standards. Opacity is represented by a contrast ratio, which is the ratio between the daylight apparent reflectance of a specimen (typically 1 mm thick) when backed by a black standard and the daylight apparent reflectance of the specimen when backed by a white standard having a daylight apparent reflectance of 70% (or sometimes 100%) relative to magnesium oxide. The contrast ratio ($C_{0.70}$) for a resin composite should lie between the values of 0.55 and 0.70. The spectral reflectance curves of a composite resin backed by black and white standards are shown in Fig. 3-1. The contrast ratio can also be calculated from optical constants, as discussed later.

INDEX OF REFRACTION

The index of refraction (ξ) for any substance is the ratio of the velocity of light in a vacuum (or air) to its velocity in the medium. When light enters a medium, it slows from its speed in air (300,000 km/sec) and may change direction. For example, when a beam of light traveling in air strikes a water surface at an oblique angle, the light rays are bent toward the normal. The *normal* is a line drawn perpendicular to the water surface at the point where the light contacts the water surface. If the light is traveling through water and contacts a water-air surface at an oblique angle, the beam of light is bent or refracted away from the normal. The index of refraction is a characteristic property of the substance (Table 3-2) and is used extensively for identification. One of the most important applications of refraction is the control of the refractive index of the dispersed and matrix phases in materials such as resin composites and dental ceramics, designed to have the translucent appearance of tooth tissue. A perfect match in the refractive indices results in a transparent solid, whereas large differences result in opaque materials.

TABLE 3-2 Index of Refraction of Various Materials

Material	Index of Refraction
Feldspathic porcelain	1.504
Quartz	1.544
Synthetic hydroxyapatite	1.649
Tooth structure, enamel	1.655
Water	1.333

OPTICAL CONSTANTS

Esthetic dental materials such as ceramics, resin composites, and human tooth structure are intensely light-scattering or turbid materials. In a turbid material the intensity of incident light is diminished considerably when light passes through the specimen. The optical properties of these materials are described by the Kubelka-Munk equations, which develop relations for monochromatic light between the reflection of an infinitely thick layer of a material and its absorption and scattering coefficients. These equations can be solved algebraically by hyperbolic functions derived by Kubelka.

Secondary optical constants (*a* and *b*) can be calculated as follows:

$$a = [R(B) - R(W) - R_B + R_W - R(B)R(W)R_B + R(B)R(W)R_W + R(B)R_BR_W - R(W)R_BR_W]/2[R(B)R_W - R(W)R_B]$$

and

$$b = (a^2 - 1)^{1/2}$$

where R_B is the reflectance of a dark backing (the black standard), R_W is reflectance of a light backing (the white standard), *R(B)* is the light reflectance of a specimen with the dark backing, and *R(W)* is the light reflectance of the specimen with the light backing.

These equations are used under the assumptions that (1) the material is turbid, dull, and of constant finite thickness; (2) edges are neglected; (3) optical inhomogeneities are much smaller than the thickness of the specimen and are distributed uniformly; and (4) illumination is homogeneous and diffused.

Scattering Coefficient The scattering coefficient is the fraction of incident light flux lost by reversal of direction in an elementary layer. The scattering coefficient, *S*, for a unit thickness of a material is defined as follows:

$$S = (1/bX)\ \mathrm{Ar\ ctgh}\ [1 - a(R + R_g) + RR_g/b(R - R_g)],\ \mathrm{mm}^{-1}$$

where *X* is the actual thickness of the specimen, *Ar ctgh* is an inverse hyperbolic cotangent, and *R* is the light reflectance of the specimen with the backing of reflectance, R_g.

The scattering coefficient varies with the wavelength of the incident light and the nature of the colorant layer, as shown in Fig. 3-5 for several shades of a resin composite. Composites with larger values of the scattering coefficient are more opaque.

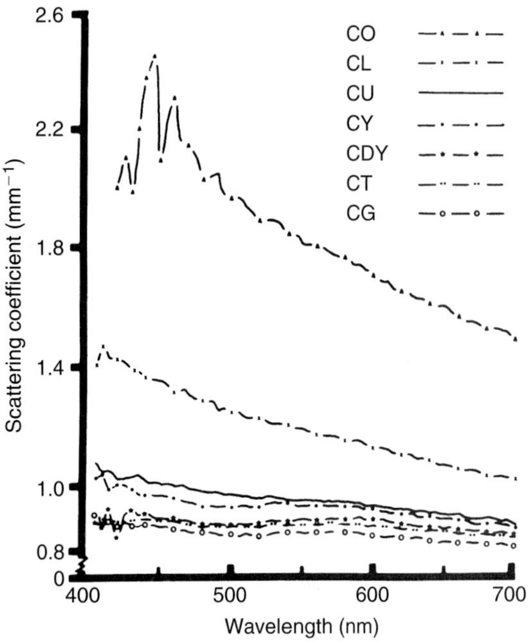

Fig. 3-5 Scattering coefficient versus wavelength for shades of a composite, *C*. Shades are *O*, opaque; *L*, light; *U*, universal; *Y*, yellow; *DY*, dark yellow; *T*, translucent; and *G*, gray.
(From Yeh CL, Miyagawa Y, Powers JM: *J Dent Res* 61:797, 1982.)

Absorption Coefficient The absorption coefficient is the fraction of incident light flux lost by absorption in an elementary layer. The absorption coefficient, *K*, for a unit thickness of a material is defined as follows:

$$K = S(a - 1),\ \mathrm{mm}^{-1}$$

The absorption coefficient also varies with the wavelength of the incident light and the nature of the colorant layer, as shown in Fig. 3-6 for several shades of a resin composite. Composites with larger values of the absorption coefficient are more opaque and more intensely colored.

Light Reflectivity The light reflectivity, *RI*, is the light reflectance of a material of infinite thickness, and is defined as follows:

$$RI = a - b$$

This property also varies with the wavelength of the incident light and the nature of the colorant layer.

The light reflectivity can be used to calculate a thickness, *XI*, at which the reflectance of a material with an ideal black background would attain 99.9% of its light reflectivity. The infinite optical thickness, *XI*, is defined for monochromatic light as follows:

$$XI = (1/bS)\ \mathrm{Ar\ ctgh}\ [(1 - 0.999aRI)/0.999bRI],\ \mathrm{mm}$$

The variation of *XI* with wavelength is shown in Fig. 3-7 for a composite resin. It is interesting that composites are more opaque to blue than to red light, yet blue light is used to cure light-activated composites.

Contrast Ratio Once *a*, *b*, and *S* are obtained, the light reflectance *(R)* for a specimen of

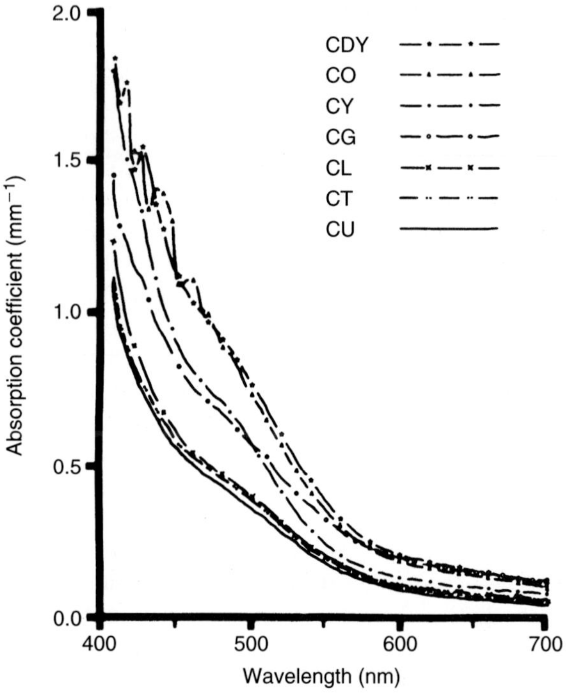

Fig. 3-6 Absorption coefficient versus wavelength for shades of a composite, *C*. Shades are *DY*, dark yellow; *O*, opaque; *Y*, yellow; *G*, gray; *L*, light; *T*, translucent; and *U*, universal.
(From Yeh CL, Miyagawa Y, Powers JM: *J Dent Res* 61:797, 1982.)

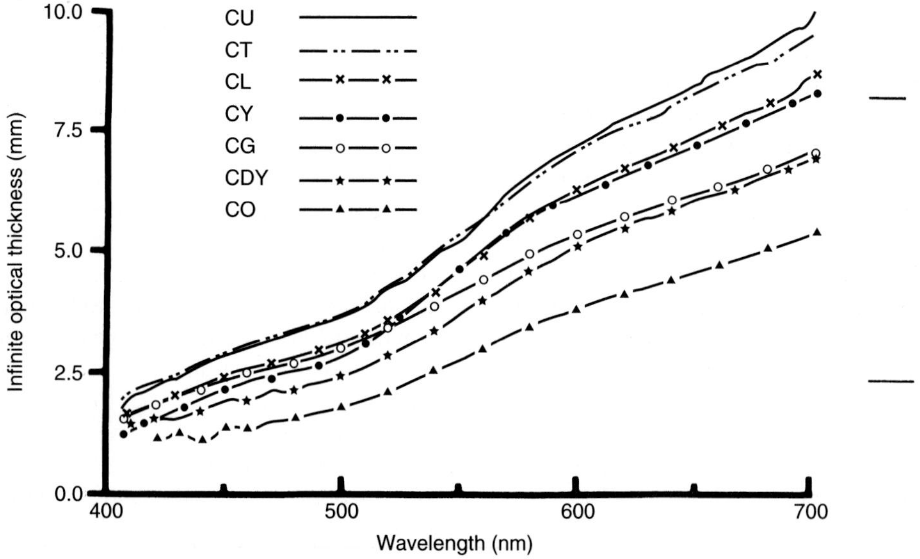

Fig. 3-7 Infinite optical thickness versus wavelength for shades of a composite, *C*. Shades are *U*, universal; *T*, translucent; *L*, light; *Y*, yellow; *G*, gray; *DY*, dark yellow; and *O*, opaque.
(From Yeh, CL, Miyagawa Y, Powers JM: *J Dent Res* 61:797, 1982.)

any thickness *(X)* in contact with a backing of any reflectance *(Rg)* can be calculated by:

$$R = [1 - R_g(a - b \text{ ctgh } bSX)] / (a + b \text{ ctgh } bSX - R_g)$$

An estimate of the opacity of a 1-mm-thick specimen can then be calculated from the contrast ratio *(C)* as:

$$C = R_0/R$$

where R_0 is the computed light reflectance of the specimen with a black backing. If R_g is 0.70, then $C_{0.70}$ can be calculated (see Measurement of contrast ratio).

THERMAL PROPERTIES

TEMPERATURE

The temperature of a substance can be measured with a thermometer or a thermocouple. An important application of temperature measurement in dentistry is the measurement of heat during the shaping of cavities in teeth. Numerous studies have been made of the effect of speed and force on the rise of temperature in teeth. The increase in temperature during the cutting of tooth structure with various types of steel burs, carbide burs, and rotary diamond instruments also has been investigated. In addition, the rise in temperature in the tooth at various distances from the cutting instrument has been determined. Examples of the effect of the speed of rotation and coolants on the increase in temperature in tooth structure are shown in Fig. 3-8. The temperature was measured by a thermocouple inserted into a small opening that extended into the dento-enamel junction. The tooth was then cut in the direction of the thermocouple and the maximum temperature recorded.

TRANSITION TEMPERATURES

The arrangement of atoms and molecules in materials is influenced by the temperature; as a result, thermal techniques are important in understanding dental materials. These techniques are differential thermal analysis, differential scanning calorimetry, thermogravimetric analysis, thermomechanical analysis, and dynamic mechanical analysis. Differential thermal analysis has been used to locate the temperature of transitions and to study the effect of variables, such as composition and heat treatment, on these transitions. Differential scanning calorimetry can determine the heats of transition and reaction. Thermogravimetric analysis measures the change in weight of materials as a function of temperature and environment and gives information related to the thermal decomposition of materials or their stability in various environments. Thermomechanical analysis measures the dimensional change with or without load as a function of temperature. Changes in the ease of deformation as the temperature increases indicate the presence of transitions. This method can also measure the coefficient of thermal expansion as a function of temperature. Dynamic mechanical analysis measures the changes in modulus of elasticity and loss tangent as a function of temperature. This technique can be used to measure the glass transition temperature of polymers.

Differential thermal analysis (DTA) has been used to study waxes used in the compounding of dental waxes. The DTA curve of a mixture of paraffin and carnauba wax is shown in Fig. 3-9. The thermogram was obtained when the difference in temperature between the wax and a standard was recorded under the same heating conditions in which thermocouples were used. The difference in temperature was recorded as a function of the temperature of the surroundings. A decrease in the value of ΔT indicated an endothermic process in the specimen. The endotherms at 31.5° and 35° C are solid-solid transitions occurring in the paraffin wax as the result of a change of crystal structure. The endotherm at 52° C represents the solid-liquid transition of paraffin wax, whereas the endotherms at 68.7° and 80.2° C result from the melting of carnauba wax. The heat of transition of the two solid-solid transitions is about 8 cal/g, and the

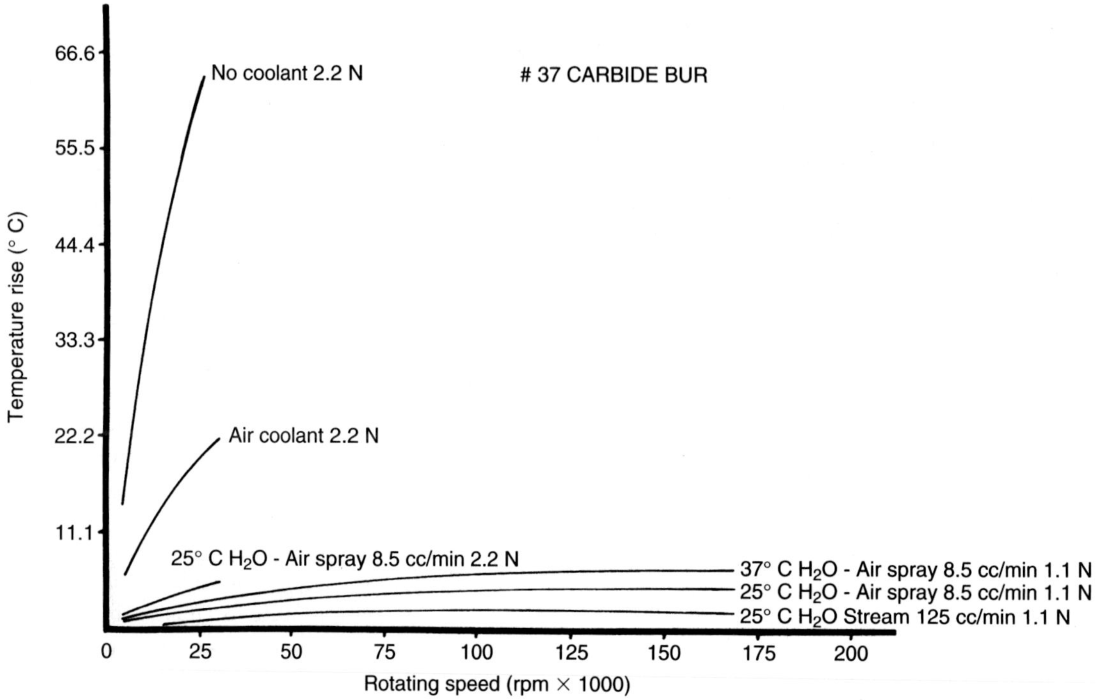

Fig. 3-8 Temperature rises developed by carbide burs during cutting of tooth tissue, operated at different speeds and with and without coolants.
(Adapted from Peyton FA: *J Am Dent Assoc* 56:664, 1958.)

melting transition of paraffin and carnauba wax is approximately 39 and 11 cal/g, respectively. These and other thermograms show that 25% carnauba wax added to paraffin wax has no effect on the melting point of paraffin wax but increases the melting range about 28° C.

Thermomechanical analysis (TMA) of the carnauba-paraffin wax mixture is also shown in Fig. 3-9. The percent penetration of the wax mixture by a cylindrical probe is shown for two stresses of 0.013 and 0.26 MPa. The penetration of the wax at the lower stress was controlled by the melting transition of the carnauba wax component, whereas the penetration at the higher stress was dominated by the solid-solid and solid-liquid transitions of the paraffin wax components. About 44% penetration, which is related to flow, occurred before the melting point of the paraffin wax was reached.

Other properties correlate with thermograms. The coefficient of thermal expansion of paraffin wax increases from about $300 \times 10^{-6}/°$ C to $1400 \times 10^{-6}/°$ C just before the solid-solid transition, and the flow increases greatly in this temperature range.

Dynamic mechanical analysis (DMA) of a dimethacrylate copolymer is shown in Fig. 3-10. A thin film of the copolymer was subjected to a sinusoidal tensile strain at a frequency of 11 Hz. As temperature was increased, values of modulus of elasticity (E') and loss tangent ($\tan \delta$) were obtained. The glass transition temperature (T_g) was determined from identification of the beginning of a rapid decrease in E' with temperature. The value of T_g identifies the temperature at which a glassy polymer goes to a softer, rubbery state upon heating. A lower value of T_g can result from a lower degree of conversion of

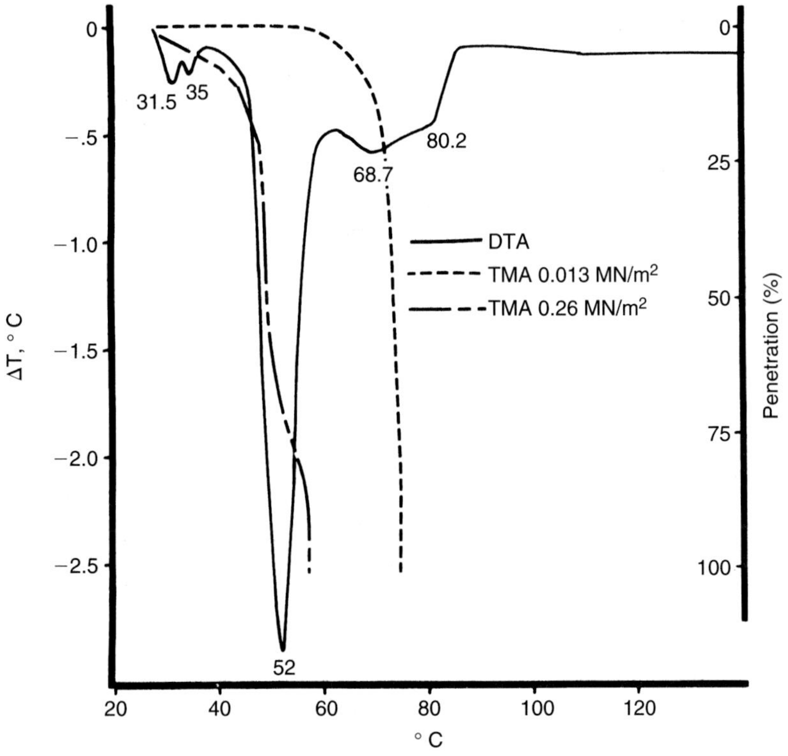

Fig. 3-9 Thermograms of a 75% paraffin–25% carnauba wax mixture.

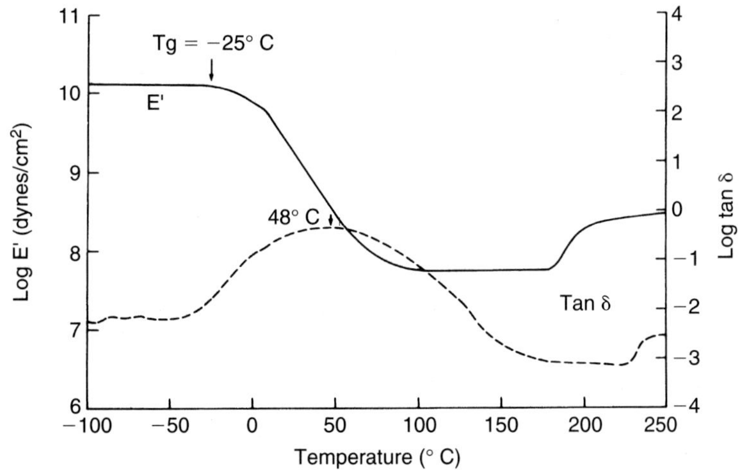

Fig. 3-10 Dynamic mechanical properties of a 75 wt% BIS-GMA/25 wt% TEGDM copolymer. (From Wilson TW, Turner DT: *J Dent Res* 66:1032, 1987.)

double bonds or from saturation by water. As discussed later, the value of the coefficient of thermal expansion of a polymer changes at T_g.

HEAT OF FUSION

The heat of fusion, *L,* is the heat in calories, or joules, *J,* required to convert 1 g of a material from solid to liquid state at the melting temperature. The equation for the calculation of heat of fusion is $L = Q/m$, where Q is the total heat absorbed and m is the mass of the substance melted. Therefore in practical applications it is apparent that the larger the mass of material being melted, the more heat required to change the total mass to liquid. The heat of fusion is closely related to the melting or freezing point of the substance, because, when the change in state occurs, it is always necessary to apply additional heat to the mass to cause liquefaction, and as long as the mass remains molten, the heat of fusion is retained by the liquid. When the mass is frozen, or solidified, the heat that was retained in the liquid state is liberated. The difference in energy content is necessary to maintain the kinetic molecular motion, which is characteristic of the liquid state.

The values for heat of fusion of some common substances (given in round numbers) are listed in Table 3-3. It may be seen that the values for heat of fusion of gold and the metals used for dental gold alloys (silver and copper) are below those of many other metals and compounds. This is true also for the specific heat of gold and its alloys.

TABLE 3-3 Heat of Fusion of Some Materials

Materials	Temperature (° C)	Heat of Fusion (cal/g [J/g])
METALS		
Mercury	−39	3 [12]
Gold	1063	16 [67]
Silver	960	26 [109]
Platinum	1773	27 [113]
Copper	1083	49 [205]
Cobalt	1495	58 [242]
Chromium	1890	75 [314]
Aluminum	660	94 [393]
COMPOUNDS		
Alcohol	−114	25 [104]
Paraffin	52	35 [146]
Beeswax	62	42 [176]
Glycerin	18	47 [196]
Ice	0	80 [334]

THERMAL CONDUCTIVITY

The thermal conductivity, *K,* of a substance is the quantity of heat in calories, or joules, per second passing through a body 1 cm thick with a cross section of 1 cm^2 when the temperature difference is 1° C. The units are cal/sec/cm^2/(° C/cm). The conductivity of a material changes slightly as the surrounding temperature is altered, but generally the difference resulting from temperature changes is much less than the difference that exists between different types of materials.

Common experience indicates that metals are better heat conductors than nonmetals. Several important applications of thermal conductivity exist in dental materials. For example, a large gold or amalgam filling or crown in proximity to the pulp may cause the patient considerable discomfort when hot or cold foods produce temperature changes; this effect is mitigated when adequate tooth tissue remains or nonmetallic substances are placed between the tooth and filling for insulation. Such filling materials as cements are relatively poor conductors and insulate the pulp area.

The difference in thermal conductivity of denture base materials likewise may cause differences in soft-tissue response. A metal base, a good conductor, causes a prompt tissue response, as shown in Fig. 3-11, whereas an acrylic denture base causes a more delayed response to thermal changes. Dental literature indicates that a good thermal conductor is preferred for denture bases to maintain good health in the supporting tissues by having the heat readily conducted to and from the tissue by the denture base. This concept has not been established on the basis of experimental data.

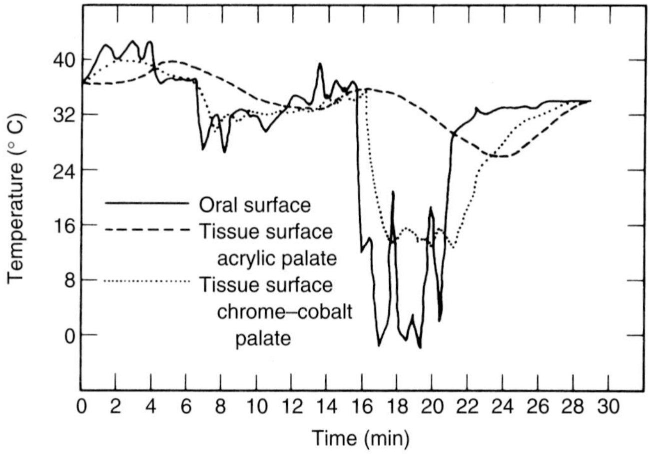

Fig. 3-11 Temperature on the oral surface and tissue surface of an acrylic palate and a cobalt-chromium palate while a subject was eating a meal.

(Adapted from Wehner PJ: Heat transfer properties of denture base materials, master's thesis, University of Michigan School of Dentistry, 1959.)

A better understanding of the conductivities of various restorative materials is desirable to develop an appropriate degree of insulation for the pulp tissue, comparable with that in the natural tooth, and to produce normal thermal stimulation in the supporting soft tissue under complete dentures. The conductivity of certain dental materials is listed in Table 3-4. Nonmetallic materials appear to be less effective as conductors than metals are, for which reason they serve as good insulators. Dental cements have a thermal conductivity similar to those of dentin and enamel. Note that the thickness of a cement base and its thermal conductivity are important in reducing the thermal transfer to the pulp, and remember that the temperature difference across an insulator depends on the extent of the heating or cooling period and the magnitude of the temperature difference.

SPECIFIC HEAT

The specific heat, *Cp*, of a substance is the quantity of heat needed to raise the temperature of one gram of the substance 1° C. Water is usually chosen as the standard substance and 1 g as the standard mass. The heat required to raise the temperature of 1 g of water from 15° to 16° C is 1 cal, which is used as the basis for the definition of the heat unit. Most substances are more readily heated, gram for gram, than water.

TABLE 3-4 Thermal Conductivity of Various Materials

Material	Thermal Conductivity	
	cal/sec/cm^2/(° C/cm)	J/sec/cm^2 (° C/cm)
METALS		
Silver	1.006	4.21
Copper	0.918	3.84
Gold	0.710	2.97
Platinum	0.167	0.698
Dental amalgam	0.055	0.23
Mercury	0.020	0.084
NONMETALS		
Gypsum	0.0031	0.013
Zinc phosphate cement	0.0028	0.012
Resin composite	0.0026	0.011
Porcelain	0.0025	0.010
Enamel	0.0022	0.0092
Dentin	0.0015	0.0063
Zinc oxide–eugenol cement	0.0011	0.0046
Acrylic resin	0.0005	0.0021
Beeswax	0.00009	0.0004

Obviously the total heat required to raise the temperature of a substance 1° C depends on the total mass and the specific heat. For example, 100 g of water requires more calories than 50 g of water to raise the temperature 1° C. Likewise,

TABLE 3-5 Specific Heat of Various Materials

Material	Specific Heat (cal/g/° C [J/g/° C])
SOLIDS	
Gold	0.031 [0.13]
Platinum	0.032 [0.13]
Silver	0.056 [0.23]
Copper	0.092 [0.38]
Enamel	0.18 [0.75]
Quartz	0.19 [0.79]
Aluminum	0.21 [0.88]
Porcelain	0.26 [1.09]
Dentin	0.28 [1.17]
Acrylic resin	0.35 [1.46]
LIQUIDS	
Water	1.000 [4.18]
Paraffin	0.69 [2.88]
Glycerin	0.58 [2.42]
Alcohol (ethyl)	0.547 [2.29]
Mercury	0.033 [0.14]

TABLE 3-6 Thermal Diffusivity of Various Materials

Material	Thermal Diffusivity (mm^2/sec)
Pure gold (calculated)	119.0
Amalgam	9.6
Resin composite	0.675
Porcelain	0.64
Enamel	0.469
Zinc oxide–eugenol cement	0.389
Zinc phosphate cement	0.290
Dental compound	0.226
Zinc polyacrylate cement	0.223
Glass ionomer cement	0.198
Dentin	0.183
Acrylic resin	0.123

because of the difference in specific heat of water and alcohol, 100 g of water requires more heat than 100 g of alcohol to raise the temperature the same amount. In general, the specific heat of liquids is higher than those of solids. Some metals have specific heat values of less than 10% that of water.

During the melting and casting process, the specific heat of the metal or alloy is important because of the total amount of heat that must be applied to the mass to raise the temperature to the melting point. Fortunately, the specific heat of gold and the metals used in gold alloys is low, so prolonged heating is unnecessary. The specific heat of both enamel and dentin has been found to be higher than that of metals used for fillings, as shown in Table 3-5.

THERMAL DIFFUSIVITY

The thermal diffusivity, Δ, is a measure of transient heat-flow and is defined as the thermal conductivity, *K*, divided by the product of the specific heat, *Cp*, times the density, ρ:

$$\Delta = K/Cp \times \rho$$

The units of thermal diffusivity are mm^2/sec.

The thermal diffusivity describes the rate at which a body with a nonuniform temperature approaches equilibrium. For a gold inlay or crown or a dental amalgam, the low specific heat combined with the high thermal conductivity creates a thermal shock more readily than normal tooth structure does. Values of thermal diffusivity of some materials are listed in Table 3-6. These values may vary somewhat with composition of the particular restorative material. For example, the thermal diffusivity of a zinc polyacrylate cement increases from 0.14 to 0.51 mm^2/sec as the powder/liquid ratio (by weight) increases from 0.5 to 5.0.

As mentioned in the discussion of thermal conductivity, thickness of the material is important. A parameter governing lining efficiency *(Z)* is related to thickness *(T)* and thermal diffusivity (Δ) as follows:

$$Z = \frac{T}{\sqrt{\Delta}}$$

COEFFICIENT OF THERMAL EXPANSION

The change in length ($l_{final} - l_{original}$) per unit length of a material for a 1° C change in temperature is called the linear coefficient of thermal expansion, α, and is calculated as follows:

$$\frac{(l_{final} - l_{original})}{l_{original} \times (°\,C_{final} - °\,C_{original})} = \alpha$$

The units are represented by the notation /° C, and because the values are usually small they are expressed in exponential form such as 22×10^{-6}/° C. A less common practice is to report the change in parts per million (ppm) and the previous number would be expressed as 22 ppm.

The linear coefficients of thermal expansion for some materials important in restorative dentistry are given in Table 3-7. Although the coefficient is a material constant, it does not remain constant over wide temperature ranges. For example, the linear coefficient of thermal expansion of a dental wax may have an average value of 300×10^{-6}/° C up to 40° C, whereas it may have an average value of 500×10^{-6}/° C from 40 to 50° C. The coefficient of thermal expansion of a polymer changes as the polymer goes from a glassy state to a softer, rubbery material. This change in the coefficient corresponds to the glass transition temperature (T_g).

Either the linear or volumetric coefficient of thermal expansion may be measured, and for most materials that function as isotropic solids, the volumetric thermal coefficient may be considered to be three times the linear thermal coefficient.

Both linear expansion and volume expansion are important in restorative materials and processes. It is obvious that with a reduction of temperature, or cooling, there is a contraction of the substance that is equal to the expansion that results from heating. Accordingly, tooth structure and restorative materials in the mouth will expand when warmed by hot foods and beverages but will contract when exposed to cold substances. Such expansions and contractions may break the marginal seal of an inlay or other filling in the tooth, particularly if the difference between the coefficient of expansion of the tooth and the restorative material is great. The high coefficient of expansion of pattern waxes is an important factor in the construction of properly fitting restorations. The change in volume as a result of cooling is responsible for the shrinkage spots or surface cracks that often develop in gold alloy castings during solidification. Compensation for the contraction that occurs during the cooling of gold alloys must be made if accurate gold castings are to result. Therefore in some materials and in certain operations, the coefficient of thermal expansion may be equally as important as the strength, hardness, or esthetic appearance of the material. The values in Table 3-7 show that with comparable temperature

TABLE 3-7 Linear Coefficient of Thermal Expansion of Various Materials

Material	Coefficient $\times 10^{-6}$/° C
Inlay waxes	350-450
Silicone impression material	210
Polysulfide impression material	140
Pit and fissure sealants	71-94
Acrylic resin	76.0
Mercury	60.6
Resin composites	14-50
Zinc oxide-eugenol cement	35
Amalgam	22-28
Silver	19.2
Copper	16.8
Gold	14.4
Porcelain	12.0
Tooth (crown portion)	11.4
Glass ionomer (type 2)	10.2-11.4

changes, materials such as acrylic resin and amalgam expand more than tooth tissue, whereas ceramic expands less. The coefficient of inlay pattern wax is exceptionally high when compared with that of other materials.

Of particular importance in casting investments is the property of thermal expansion of three crystalline polymorphic forms of silica. As a principal ingredient in dental investments that are to be heated before a metal casting is made, the amount of expansion at various temperatures is critical and important. This quality of silica compounds in relation to use in casting investments was described in 1932. Curves in Fig. 3-12 illustrate the relative percentage of thermal expansion of the four forms of silica at different temperatures below about 800° C. Of the crystalline forms, cristobalite shows the greatest expansion at the lowest temperature and quartz requires a higher temperature to develop an equal amount of expansion as cristobalite. Fused silica has long been recognized as having an exceedingly low thermal expansion.

ELECTRICAL PROPERTIES

ELECTRICAL CONDUCTIVITY AND RESISTIVITY

The ability of a material to conduct an electric current may be stated either as specific conductance or conductivity, or, conversely, as the specific resistance or resistivity. *Resistivity* is the more common term. The resistance of a homogeneous conductor of uniform cross section at a constant temperature varies directly with the length and inversely with the cross-sectional area of the specimen, according to the equation

$$R = \rho \frac{l}{A}$$

in which R is the resistance in ohms, ρ (rho) is the resistivity, l is the length, and A is the section area. The resistivity depends on the nature of the material. If a unit cube of 1-cm edge length is employed, the l and A are equal to unity, and in this case $R = \rho$. The resistivity is expressed as

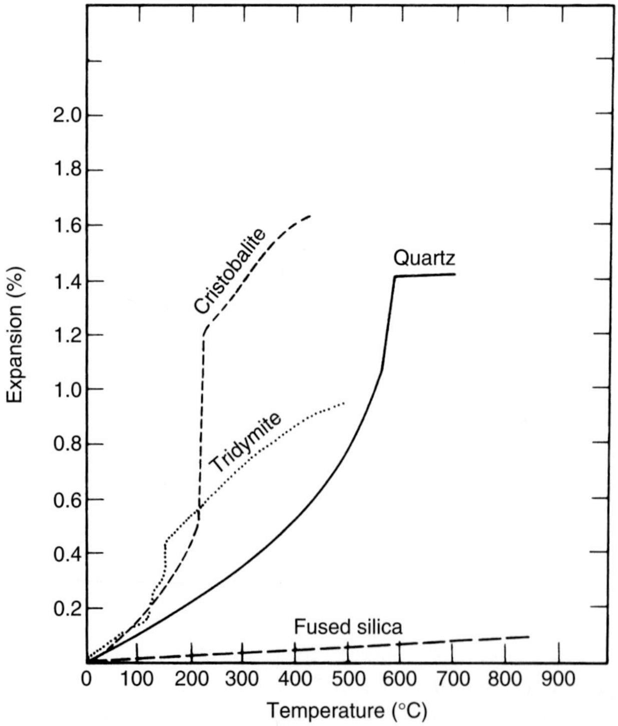

Fig. 3-12 Thermal expansion curves for four types of silica.
(Adapted from Volland RH, Paffenbarger GC: *J Am Dent Assoc* 19:185, 1932.)

ohm-centimeters where R is in ohms, l is in centimeters, and A is in square centimeters.

The change in electrical resistance has been used to study the alteration in internal structure of various alloys as a result of heat treatment. An early investigation of the gold-copper alloy system by electrical conductivity methods revealed a change in internal crystal structure with an accompanying change in conductivity. The correlation of these conductivity studies with related changes in other properties established the fundamental basis of structural changes associated with heat-treatment operations on dental gold alloys.

Values for the resistivity of human tooth structure are shown in Table 3-8. Resistivity is important in the investigation of the pain perception threshold resulting from applied electrical stimuli and of displacement of fluid in teeth caused by ionic movements. The electrical resistance of normal and carious teeth has been observed to differ, with less resistance offered by the carious tissue. Sound enamel is a relatively poor conductor of electricity, whereas dentin is somewhat better (see Table 3-8).

The conductivity of materials used to replace tooth tissue is of concern in restorative dentistry. The effectiveness of insulating cement bases and other nonmetallic restorative materials is not yet established. Several studies have measured the resistivity of dental cements (see Table 3-8). The zinc oxide-eugenol cements have the highest resistivity, followed by the zinc polyacrylate and zinc phosphate cements. The glass ionomer cements are the most conductive of the cements and have values most similar to dentin.

TABLE 3-8 Values of Resistivity of Human Tooth Structure and Several Dental Cements

Material	Resistivity (ohm • cm)
Human enamel	
Bjorn (1946)	$2.9\text{-}3.6 \times 10^6$
Mumford (1967)	$2.6\text{-}6.9 \times 10^6$
Human dentin	
Bjorn (1946)	$0.7\text{-}6.0 \times 10^4$
Mumford (1967)	$1.1\text{-}5.2 \times 10^4$
Dental cement	
Glass ionomer	$0.8\text{-}2.5 \times 10^4$
Zinc oxide-eugenol	$10^9 - 10^{10}$
Zinc polyacrylate	$0.4\text{-}4 \times 10^5$
Zinc phosphate	2×10^5

DIELECTRIC CONSTANT

A material that provides electrical insulation is known as a dielectric. The dielectric constant or relative permittivity, ε_r, compares the permittivity, ε, of the dielectric to the permittivity, ε_0, of empty space:

$$\varepsilon_r = \varepsilon / \varepsilon_0$$

where ε_0 of a vacuum is 8.854×10^{-12} farad/m. The dielectric constant varies with the temperature, bonding, crystal structure, and structural defects of the dielectric.

Values of the dielectric constant for human dentin and several dental cements are listed in Table 3-9. The dielectric constant of a dental cement generally decreases as the material hardens. This decrease reflects a change from a paste that is relatively ionic and polar to one that is less so. As shown by the high values of permittivity of the glass ionomer and zinc polyacrylate cements in Table 3-9, these cements have a high ionic content and are quite polar compared with zinc oxide-eugenol cements and human dentin.

Dielectric measurements have been used to

TABLE 3-9 Dielectric Constant for Human Dentin and Several Dental Cements

Material	Dielectric Constant
Human dentin	8.6
Dental cements (set)	
Glass ionomer	$2 \text{ to } 7 \times 10^5$
Zinc oxide-eugenol	10
Zinc polyacrylate	$4 \times 10^3 \text{ to } 2 \times 10^5$

study polymer-filler interactions in dental composites with and without silane coupling agents, and the effect of moisture on these interactions. The measurements showed that increasing the filler content restricted the mobility of the main polymer chains and that compatible silanes did not form a separate interphase at the polymer-filler interface. It was also shown that bulk water could exist at the interface if the filler was not silanated. Therefore correct silanation of fillers used in dental composites is essential for their successful application.

The problem of electrical insulation is made more complex by the presence of galvanic currents in the mouth, resulting from cells formed from metallic restorations. Recent studies indicate that a cement base does not effectively insulate the pulp from the electric current developed in a metallic restoration in the mouth. How much insulation is essential or how to effectively restore the tooth to its original status of equilibrium is currently not known.

ELECTROMOTIVE FORCE

Working with metals and alloys for dental restorations or with instruments that are susceptible to corrosion necessitates some understanding of the relative position of the metal in the electromotive force series. The electromotive series is a listing of electrode potentials of metals according to the order of their decreasing tendency to oxidize in solution. This serves as the basis of comparison of the tendency of metals to oxidize in air. Those metals with a large negative electrode potential are more resistant to tarnish than those with a high positive electrode potential. In general, the metals above copper in the series, such as aluminum, zinc, and nickel, tend to oxidize relatively easily, whereas those below copper, such

TABLE 3-10 Oxidation-Reduction Potentials for Corrosion Reactions in Water and Salt Water

Metal	Corrosion Reaction	In Water, Electrode Potential at 25° C (Volts versus Normal Hydrogen Electrode)	In Salt Water, Electrode Potential at 25° C (Volts versus 0.1 N Calomel Scale)
Aluminum	$Al \rightarrow Al^{3+} + 3e$	+1.662*	+0.83
Zinc	$Zn \rightarrow Zn^{2+} + 2e$	+0.763	+1.10
Chromium	$Cr \rightarrow Cr^{3+} + 3e$	+0.744	+0.4 to −0.18
Iron	$Fe \rightarrow Fe^{2+} + 2e$	+0.440	+0.58
Cobalt	$Co \rightarrow Co^{2+} + 2e$	+0.277	—
Nickel	$Ni \rightarrow Ni^{2+} + 2e$	+0.250	+0.07
Tin	$Sn \rightarrow Sn^{2+} + 2e$	+0.136	+0.49
Hydrogen	$H_2 \rightarrow 2H^+ + 2e$	0.000	—
Copper	$Cu \rightarrow Cu^{2+} + 2e$	−0.337	+0.20
	$4(OH^-) \rightarrow O_2 + 2H_2O + 4e$	−0.401	—
Mercury	$2Hg \rightarrow Hg_2^{2+} + 2e$	−0.788	—
Silver	$Ag \rightarrow Ag^+ + e$	−0.799	+0.08
Palladium	$Pd \rightarrow Pd^{2+} + 2e$	−0.987	—
Platinum	$Pt \rightarrow Pt^{2+} + 2e$	−1.200	—
	$2H_2O \rightarrow O_2 + 4H^+ + 4e$	−1.229	—
Gold	$Au \rightarrow Au^{3+} + 3e$	−1.498	—

Modified from Flinn RA, Trojan PK: *Engineering materials and their applications,* ed 3, Boston, 1986, Houghton Mifflin.
*A positive value indicates a strong tendency for the metal to go into solution. Higher positive values are more anodic, whereas higher negative values are more cathodic.

as silver, platinum, and gold, resist oxidation. A list of oxidation-reduction potentials for some common corrosion reactions in water and in salt water is given in Table 3-10. The values of electrode potential and the order of the series change when measured in a saline solution rather than water. The electrode potentials of some dental alloys measured in artificial saliva at 35° C are listed in Table 3-11.

Likewise, it is possible to determine from the electromotive force series that the reduction of the oxides of gold, platinum, and silver to pure metal can be accomplished more readily than with those metals that have a higher electromotive force value.

GALVANISM

The presence of metallic restorations in the mouth may cause a phenomenon called *galvanic action,* or galvanism. This results from a difference in potential between dissimilar fillings in opposing or adjacent teeth. These fillings, in conjunction with saliva or bone fluids such as electrolytes, make up an electric cell. When two opposing fillings contact each other, the cell is short-circuited, and if the flow of current occurs through the pulp, the patient experiences pain and the more anodic restoration may corrode. A single filling plus the saliva and bone fluid may also constitute a cell of liquid junction type. As shown in Fig. 3-13, ions capable of conducting electricity can easily migrate through dentin and around the margins of a restoration.

Studies have indicated that relatively large currents will flow through metallic fillings when they are brought into contact. The current rapidly falls off if the fillings are maintained in contact, probably as a result of polarization of the cell. The magnitude of the voltage, however, is not of primary importance, because indications support the fact that the sensitivity of the patient to the current has a greater influence on whether pain is felt. Although most patients feel pain at a value between 20 and 50 μamp, some may feel pain at 10 μamp, whereas others do not experience it

TABLE 3-11 Galvanic Series of Some Dental Alloys in Artificial Saliva at 35° C

Material	Electrode Potential at 35° C (Volts)*
Tin crown form	+0.048
Hydrogen/H^+	0.000
Amalgam	
Conventional spherical	−0.023
Dispersed high-copper	−0.108
Nickel-chromium alloy	−0.126 to −0.240
Cobalt-chromium alloy	−0.292
Gold alloy	
Au-Cu-Ag	−0.345
Au-Pt-Pd-Ag	−0.358 to −0.455

Modified from Arvidson K, Johansson EG: *Scand J Dent Res* 85:485, 1977.

*High positive sign indicates a strong tendency for the metal to go into solution.

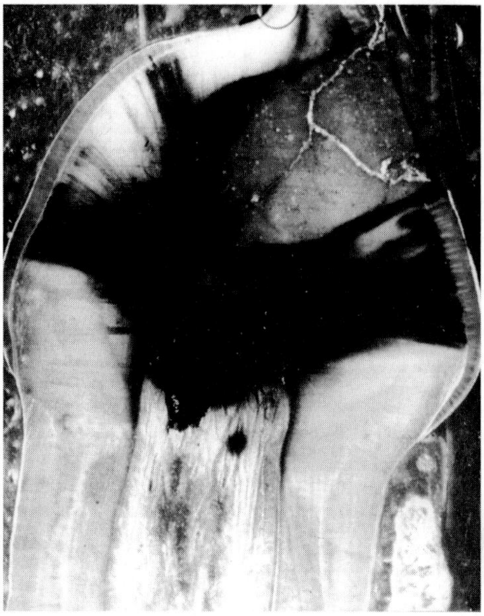

Fig. 3-13 Autoradiograph of a longitudinal section of a dog's permanent tooth in which the pulp has been capped with 45/20 Ca hydroxide. The dark areas in the tooth are evidence that migration of the Ca ions has occurred and that a circuit is possible.

(Courtesy Avery JK, University of Michigan School of Dentistry, 1958.)

until 110 μamp are developed. This is a possible explanation for the fact that some patients are bothered by galvanic action and others are not, despite similar conditions in the mouth.

The galvanic currents developed from the contact of two metallic restorations depend on their composition and surface area. An alloy of stainless steel develops a higher current density than either gold or cobalt-chromium alloys when in contact with an amalgam restoration. As the size of the cathode (such as a gold alloy) increases relative to that of the anode (such as an amalgam), the current density may increase. The larger cathode likewise can enhance the corrosion of the smaller anode. Current densities associated with non–γ_2-containing amalgams appear to be less than those associated with the γ_2-containing amalgams.

ELECTROCHEMICAL CORROSION

The corrosion and electrochemical behavior of restorative materials have received new interest with the study of multiphase systems such as gold alloys and amalgam. For example, the corrosion of γ, γ_1, and γ_2 phases in amalgam has been studied by electrochemical means. Anodic and cathodic polarization measurements indicated no strongly passive behavior of these phases in artificial saliva. The dental amalgam specimens became pitted at the boundaries between the phases or in γ_2 phase. Other studies, however, indicate that amalgam alloys exhibit decreasing electrochemical potentials, resulting in noble values when stored in neutral solutions. The addition of copper to amalgam alloys to form copper-tin compounds during hardening has improved the resistance of amalgam to chlo-

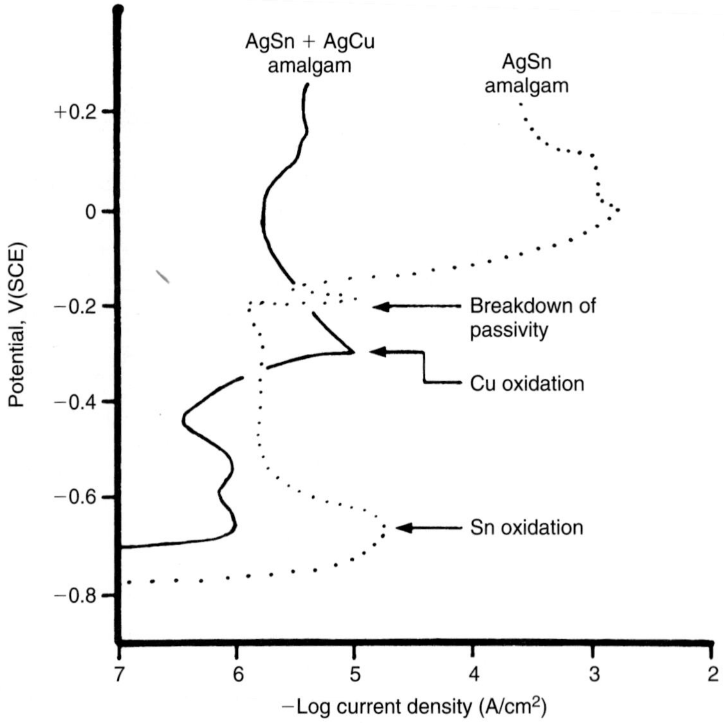

Fig. 3-14 Anodic polarization curves of two types of amalgam in synthetic saliva. (Adapted from Fairhurst CW, Marek M, Butts MB, Okabe T: *J Dent Res* 57:725, 1978.)

ride and galvanic corrosion. As shown in Fig. 3-14 the anodic activity of AgSn amalgam is quite different from AgSn + AgCu amalgams. The AgSn + AgCu amalgam remains passive under the testing conditions, whereas the AgSn amalgam does not.

Studies of corrosion of surgical stainless steel, stainless steel orthodontic brackets, and endodontic silver cones also have been reported. Corrosion of these alloys and others can result in decreased mechanical properties and the formation of corrosion products, which in some instances accumulate in the human organs. As shown previously in Table 3-10, corrosion can be affected by the environment, and certain metals such as cobalt and copper corrode more rapidly in a saline solution containing serum albumin and fibrinogen proteins.

ZETA-POTENTIAL

A charged particle suspended in an electrolytic solution attracts ions of opposite charge to those at its surface. The layer formed by these ions is called the *Stern layer.* To maintain the electrical balance of the suspending fluid, ions of opposite charge are attracted to the Stern layer. The potential at the surface of that part of the diffuse double layer of ions is called the *electrokinetic* or *zeta-potential.*

The zeta-potential, ζ, of a solid as a porous plug can be determined by measuring the streaming potential, *E,* which is the electric field caused when a liquid is made to flow along a stationary charged surface. The relation is as follows:

$$\zeta = (8.47 \times 10^8)(\eta/\varepsilon)(\Delta E/\Delta P)(R_{0.1\,N\,KCl} \cdot k_{0.1\,N\,KCl}/R_p)$$

where η is viscosity in poises, *E* is in millivolts, *Rp* is resistance in ohms of the porous plug, *k* is in $ohm^{-1}cm^{-1}$, and *P* is pressure in cm Hg. *Rk* is a cell constant for 0.1 N KCl. The term ϵ is the dielectric constant, which is 78.54 for water at 25° C.

Electrophoresis may be used to increase the stability of colloids, stimulate adsorption of ions, and characterize particle surfaces. Effects of pH, surface-active agents, and enzymes on zeta-potential are important. Zeta-potential may affect the near-surface mechanical properties (such as wear) of a material. The zeta-potentials of some materials are listed in Table 3-12.

TABLE 3-12 Zeta-Potential of Some Dental Materials

Material	Zeta-Potential (mV)
Hydroxyapatite	−9.0 to −10.9
Tooth structure*	
Calculus	−15.3
Cementum	
Exposed	−6.96
Unexposed	−9.34
Dentin	−6.23
Enamel	−9.04 to −10.3

Adapted from O'Brien WJ, editor: *Dental materials: properties and selection,* Chicago, 1989, Quintessence.
*Measured in Hanks' balanced salt solution at 30° C.

OTHER PROPERTIES

Certain properties often are highly important in the selection and manipulation of materials for use either in the mouth or for laboratory applications. Five such properties are tarnish and discoloration, water sorption, solubility and disintegration, setting time, and shelf life.

TARNISH AND DISCOLORATION

Discoloration of a restorative material from any cause is a very troublesome quality. The tarnish of metal restorations from oxide, sulfide, or any other materials causing a surface reaction is a critical quality of metal restorations in the mouth and of laboratory and clinical instruments. The process of steam sterilization of surgical instruments has long presented a serious problem of tarnish and corrosion. Many nonmetallic materials such as cements and composite restorations have displayed a tendency to discolor in service because colored substances penetrate the materials and continue chemical reactions in the composites.

Various in vitro tests have been proposed to study tarnish, particularly that of crown and bridge and partial denture alloys. Testing generally relies on controlled exposure of the alloy to a solution rich in sulfides, chlorides, and phosphates. Most recently the discoloration of alloys exposed to such solutions has been evaluated by spectrophotometric methods to determine a color-difference parameter discussed earlier in this chapter.

WATER SORPTION

Water sorption of a material represents the amount of water adsorbed on the surface and absorbed into the body of the material during fabrication or while the restoration is in service. Water sorption of denture acrylic, for example, is measured gravimetrically in $\mu g/mm^3$ after 7 days in water. The tendency of plastic denture base materials to have a high degree of water sorption is the reason this quality was included in American National Standards Institute/American Dental Association (ANSI/ADA) Specification No. 12 for this type of material. Usually a serious warpage and dimensional change in the material are associated with a high percentage of water sorption. The tendency of hydrocolloid impression materials to imbibe water if allowed to remain immersed and then to change dimensions has been a serious problem associated with their use.

SOLUBILITY AND DISINTEGRATION

Solubility and disintegration of crown and bridge cements can be measured gravimetrically by suspension of two disks, 20 mm in diameter and 1.0 mm in thickness, for 24 hours or longer in water at 37° C. The units are $\mu g/mm^2$. A conductimetric method for studying solubility and disintegration has the advantage of detecting the elution of volatile components and of using a smaller specimen. Care should be taken in predicting in vivo properties from tests in water because abrasion and attack from other chemicals often occur intraorally.

The lack of correlation between in vivo testing of the degradation of cements and the aforementioned test of solubility and disintegration in water has led to the development of other in vitro tests. One test involves placing cement between two, round, plane-parallel glass plates (16 mm in diameter) and exposing this specimen to various acidic media. Changes in the cement are recorded photographically. Observations suggest that degradation may follow a sequence of absorption, disintegration, and solution. Variables such as cement composition, thickness, molarity, and pH of the medium are important. More recently, an acid erosion test has been used for testing cements (see Chapter 20).

SETTING TIME

Setting time characteristics are associated with the reaction rates and affect the practical applications of many materials in restorative dentistry. Materials such as cements, impression materials, dental plaster, stone, and casting investments depend on a critical reaction time and hardening rate for their successful application. From the practical standpoint of manipulation and successful application, the time required for a material to set or harden from a plastic or fluid state may be its most important quality. The setting time does not indicate the completion of the reaction, which may continue for much longer times. The time varies for different materials, depending on the particular application, but duplication of results from one lot to another or from one trade brand of material to another is highly desirable. The influence of manipulative procedures on the setting time of various types of materials is important to the dentist and the assistant.

SHELF LIFE

Shelf life is a term applied to the general deterioration and change in quality of materials during shipment and storage. The temperature, humidity, and time of storage, as well as the bulk of material involved and the type of storage container, are significant factors that vary greatly from one material to another. A material that has exceptionally good properties when first produced may be quite impractical if it deteriorates badly after a few days or weeks. These qualities are discussed in chapters dealing with gypsum materials and impression materials. Some studies of these qualities of various materials have been made in recent years, and through accelerated aging tests, improvements in quality can sometimes be made. Radiographic film, anesthetics, and a few other products carry dates of expiration beyond which the product should not be expected to be serviceable. This practice assures the user that the material is not deteriorated because of age. Most materials that meet the requirements of the American Dental Association Specifications carry a date of production as a part of the serial number or as a separate notation.

SELECTED PROBLEMS

Problem 1

A hole was drilled in a gold crown to facilitate an endodontic procedure. Subsequently, the hole was filled with a dental amalgam. After several months the amalgam appeared discolored and corroded. What caused this problem, and how can it be avoided?

Solution

The dental amalgam is anodic to the gold alloy. Furthermore, the surface area of the gold restoration is much larger than that of the amalgam. Both of these factors will cause the amalgam to corrode by galvanic action. The hole should be filled with gold foil to minimize corrosion.

Problem 2

A ceramic veneer to be bonded on an anterior tooth matches the color of the shade guide but not the adjacent tooth. What most likely caused this problem, and how can it be avoided?

Solution a

If different light sources are used to match metameric shades, then the color could appear correct when observed under one light but not under the other. Be sure to match teeth and shade guides under appropriate lighting conditions.

Solution b

Ceramic is a translucent material, the color of which can be affected by the color of the cement retaining the restoration, particularly if the veneer lacks an opaque layer. Select a resin cement of an appropriate shade to bond the veneer.

Problem 3

A glaze applied to a ceramic restoration cracks on cooling. What caused the glaze to crack, and how can this problem be avoided?

Solution

Ceramics have a low thermal diffusivity and are subject to cracking as a result of thermal shock. Be sure to cool a ceramic restoration as recommended by the manufacturer to minimize larger thermal gradients.

Problem 4

A denture cleaned in hot water distorted and no longer fits the patient's mouth. Why?

Solution

If the temperature of the denture during cleaning exceeds the glass transition temperature of the resin, then distortion can occur readily. Be sure to use cool water to clean a denture.

BIBLIOGRAPHY

Color and Optical Properties

Asmussen E: Opacity of glass-ionomer cements, *Acta Odontol Scand* 41:155, 1983.

Baran GR, O'Brien WJ, Tien T-Y: Colored emission of rare earth ions in a potassium feldspar glass, *J Dent Res* 56:1323, 1977.

Colorimetry, official recommendations of the International Commission on Illumination (CIE), Publication CIE No 15 (E-1.3.1), 1971.

Crisp S, Abel G, Wilson AD: The quantitative measurement of the opacity of aesthetic dental filling materials, *J Dent Res* 58:1585, 1979.

Dennison JB, Powers JM, Koran A: Color of dental restorative resins, *J Dent Res* 57:557, 1978.

Hall JB, Hefferren JJ, Olsen NH: Study of fluorescent characteristics of extracted human teeth by use of a clinical fluorometer, *J Dent Res* 49:1431, 1970.

Johnston WM, O'Brien WJ, Tien T-Y: The determination of optical absorption and scattering in translucent porcelain, *Color Res Appl* 11:125, 1986.

Johnston WM, O'Brien WJ, Tien T-Y: Concentration additivity of Kubelka-Munk optical coefficients of porcelain mixtures, *Color Res Appl* 11:131, 1986.

Jorgenson MW, Goodkind RJ: Spectrophotometric study of five porcelain shades relative to the dimensions of color, porcelain thickness, and repeated firings, *J Prosthet Dent* 42:96, 1979.

Judd DB: Optical specification of light-scattering materials, *J Res Nat Bur Standards* 19:287, 1937.

Judd DB, Wyszecki G: *Color in business, science, and industry,* ed 3, New York, 1975, John Wiley & Sons.

Koran A, Powers JM, Raptis CN, Yu R: Reflection spectrophotometry of facial skin, *J Dent Res* 60:979, 1981.

Kubelka P: New contributions to the optics of intensely light-scattering materials, Part I, *Opt Soc Am J* 38:448, 1948.

Kubelka P, Munk F: Ein Beitrag zur Optik der Farbanstriche, *Z Tech Phys* 12:593, 1931.

Miyagawa Y, Powers JM: Prediction of color of an esthetic restorative material, *J Dent Res* 62:581, 1983.

Miyagawa Y, Powers JM, O'Brien WJ: Optical properties of direct restorative materials, *J Dent Res* 60:890, 1981.

Nickerson D: The specification of color tolerances, *Textile Res* 6:509, 1936.

Noie F, O'Keefe KL, Powers JM: Color stability of resin cements after accelerated aging, *Int J Prosthodont* 8:51, 1995.

O'Brien WJ, Johnston WM, Fanian F: Double-layer color effects in porcelain systems, *J Dent Res* 64:940, 1985.

O'Brien WJ, Johnston WM, Fanian F et al: The surface roughness and gloss of composites, *J Dent Res* 63:685, 1984.

O'Keefe KL, Powers JM, Noie F: Effect of dissolution on color of extrinsic porcelain colorants, *Int J Prosthodont* 6:558, 1993.

Panzeri H, Fernandes LT, Minelli CJ: Spectral fluorescence of direct anterior restorative materials, *Aust Dent J* 22:458, 1977.

Powers JM, Barakat MM, Ogura H: Color and optical properties of posterior composites under accelerated aging, *Dent Mater J* 4:62, 1985.

Powers JM, Capp JA, Koran A: Color of gingival tissues of blacks and whites, *J Dent Res* 56:112, 1977.

Powers JM, Dennison JB, Koran A: Color stability of restorative resins under accelerated aging, *J Dent Res* 57:964, 1978.

Powers JM, Dennison JB, Lepeak PJ: Parameters that affect the color of direct restorative resins, *J Dent Res* 57:876, 1978.

Powers JM, Koran A: Color of denture resins, *J Dent Res* 56:754, 1977.

Powers JM, Yeh CL, Miyagawa Y: Optical properties of composite of selected shades in white light, *J Oral Rehabil* 10:319, 1983.

Ruyter IE, Nilner K, Moller B: Color stability of dental composite resin material for crown and bridge veneers, *Dent Mater* 3:246, 1987.

Seghi RR, Johnston WM, O'Brien WJ: Spectrophotometric analysis of color differences between porcelain systems, *J Prosthet Dent* 56:35, 1986.

Specifying color by the Munsell system, D1535-68 (1974). In ASTM Standards, 1975, Part 20, Philadelphia, 1975, American Society for Testing and Materials.

Sproull RC: Color matching in dentistry. Part III. Color control, *J Prosthet Dent* 31:146, 1974.

Van Oort RP: *Skin color and facial prosthetic—a colorimetric study,* doctoral dissertation, The Netherlands, 1982, Groningen State University.

Wyszecki G, Stiles WS: *Color science,* New York, 1967, John Wiley & Sons.

Yeh CL, Miyagawa Y, Powers JM: Optical properties of composites of selected shades, *J Dent Res* 61:797, 1982.

Yeh CL, Powers JM, Miyagawa Y: Color of selected shades of composites by reflection spectrophotometry, *J Dent Res* 61:1176, 1982.

Thermal Properties

Antonucci JM, Toth EE: Extent of polymerization of dental resins by differential scanning calorimetry, *J Dent Res* 62:121, 1983.

Brady AP, Lee H, Orlowski JA: Thermal conductivity studies of composite dental restorative materials, *J Biomed Mater Res* 8:471, 1974.

Brauer GM, Termini DJ, Burns CL: Characterization of components of dental materials and components of tooth structure by differential thermal analysis, *J Dent Res* 49:100, 1970.

Brown WS, Christiansen DO, Lloyd BA: Numerical and experimental evaluation of energy inputs, temperature gradients, and thermal stress during restorative procedures, *J Am Dent Assoc* 96:451, 1978.

Brown WS, Dewey WA, Jacobs HR: Thermal properties of teeth, *J Dent Res* 49:752, 1970.

Civjan S, Barone JJ, Reinke PE et al: Thermal properties of nonmetallic restorative materials, *J Dent Res* 51:1030, 1972.

Craig RG, Eick JD, Peyton FA: Properties of natural waxes used in dentistry, *J Dent Res* 44:1308, 1965.

Craig RG, Peyton FA: Thermal conductivity of tooth structure, dental cements, and amalgam, *J Dent Res* 40:411, 1961.

Craig RG, Powers JM, Peyton FA: Differential thermal analysis of commercial and dental waxes, *J Dent Res* 46:1090, 1967.

Craig RG, Powers JM, Peyton FA: Thermogravimetric analysis of waxes, *J Dent Res* 50:450, 1971.

Dansgaard W, Jarby S: Measurement of nonstationary temperature in small bodies, *Odont Tskr* 66:474, 1958.

de Vree JH, Spierings TA, Plasschaert AJ: A simulation model for transient thermal analysis of restored teeth, *J Dent Res* 62:756, 1983.

Fairhurst CW, Anusavice KJ, Hashinger DT et al: Thermal expansion of dental alloys and porcelains, *J Biomed Mater Res* 14:435, 1980.

Henschel CJ: Pain control through heat control, *Dent Dig* 47:294, 444, 1941.

Lisanti VF, Zander HA: Thermal conductivity of dentin, *J Dent Res* 29:493, 1950.

Lloyd CH: The determination of the specific heats of dental materials by differential thermal analysis, *Biomaterials* 2:179, 1981.

Lloyd CH: A differential thermal analysis (DTA) for the heats of reaction and temperature rises produced during the setting of tooth coloured restorative materials, *J Oral Rehabil* 11:111, 1984.

McCabe JF, Wilson HJ: The use of differential scanning calorimetry for the evaluation of dental materials. I. Cements, cavity lining materials and anterior restorative materials, *J Oral Rehabil* 7:103, 1980.

McCabe JF, Wilson HJ: The use of differential scanning calorimetry for the evaluation of dental materials. II. Denture base materials, *J Oral Rehabil* 7:235, 1980.

McLean JW: Physical properties influencing the accuracy of silicone and thiokol impression materials, *Br Dent J* 110:85, 1961.

Murayama T: *Dynamic mechanical analysis of polymeric materials,* New York, 1978, Elsevier Science.

Pearson GJ, Wills DJ, Braden M et al: The relationship between the thermal properties of composite filling materials, *J Dent* 8:178, 1980.

Peyton FA: Temperature rise and cutting efficiency of rotating instruments, *NY J Dent* 18:439, 1952.

Peyton FA: Effectiveness of water coolants with rotary cutting instruments, *J Am Dent Assoc* 56:664, 1958.

Peyton FA, Morrant GA: High speed and other instruments for cavity preparation, *Int Dent J* 9:309, 1959.

Peyton FA, Simeral WG: The specific heat of tooth structure, *Alum Bull U Mich School Dent* 56:33, 1954.

Powers JM, Craig RG: Penetration of commercial and dental waxes, *J Dent Res* 53:402, 1974.

Powers JM, Hostetler RW, Dennison JB: Thermal expansion of composite resins and sealants, *J Dent Res* 58:584, 1979.

Rootare HM, Powers JM: Determination of phase transitions in gutta-percha by differential thermal analysis, *J Dent Res* 56:1453, 1977.

Soderholm KJ: Influence of silane treatment and filler fraction on thermal expansion of composite resins, *J Dent Res* 63:1321, 1984.

Souder WH, Paffenbarger GC: *Physical properties of dental materials,* National Bureau of Standards Circular No C433, Washington, DC, 1942, U.S. Government Printing Office.

Soyenkoff BC, Okun JH: Thermal conductivity measurements of dental tissues with the aid of thermistors, *J Am Dent Assoc* 57:23, 1958.

Tay WM, Braden M: Thermal diffusivity of glass-ionomer cements, *J Dent Res* 66:1040, 1987.

Walsh JP, Symmons HF: A comparison of the heat conduction and mechanical efficiency of diamond instruments, stones, and burs at 3,000 and 60,000 rpm, *NZ Dent J* 45:28, 1949.

Watts DC, Smith R: Thermal diffusivity in finite cylindrical specimens of dental cements, *J Dent Res* 60:1972, 1981.

Watts DC, Smith R: Thermal diffusion in some polyelectrolyte dental cements: the effect of powder/liquid ratio, *J Oral Rehabil* 11:285, 1984.

Wilson TW, Turner DT: Characterization of polydimethacrylates and their composites by dynamic mechanical analysis, *J Dent Res* 66:1032, 1987.

Electrical and Electrochemical Properties

Arvidson K, Johansson EG: Galvanic series of some dental alloys, *Scand J Dent Res* 85:485, 1977.

Bergman M, Ginstrup O, Nilner K: Potential and polarization measurements in vivo of oral galvanism, *Scand J Dent Res* 86:135, 1978.

Bjorn H: Electrical excitation of teeth, *Svensk Tandlak T* 39(Suppl):1946.

Braden M, Clarke RL: Dielectric properties of zinc oxide-eugenol type cements, *J Dent Res* 53:1263, 1974.

Braden M, Clarke RL: Dielectric properties of polycarboxylate cements, *J Dent Res* 54:7, 1975.

Cahoon JR, Holte RN: Corrosion fatigue of surgical stainless steel in synthetic physiological solution, *J Biomed Mater Res* 15:137, 1981.

Clark GCF, Williams DF: The effects of proteins on metallic corrosion, *J Biomed Mater Res* 16:125, 1982.

Fairhurst CW, Marek M, Butts MB et al: New information on high copper amalgam corrosion, *J Dent Res* 57:725, 1978.

Gjerdet NR, Brune D: Measurements of currents between dissimilar alloys in the oral cavity, *Scand J Dent Res* 85:500, 1977.

Holland RI: Galvanic currents between gold and amalgam, *Scand J Dent Res* 88:269, 1980.

Maijer R, Smith DC: Corrosion of orthodontic bracket bases, *Am J Orthodont* 81:43, 1982.

Marek M, Hochman R: *The corrosion behavior of dental amalgam phases as a function of tin content.* Microfilmed paper no 192, delivered at the Annual Meeting of the International Association for Dental Research, Dental Materials Group, Washington, DC, April 12-15, 1973.

Mohsen NM, Craig RG, Filisko FE: The effects of different additives on the dielectric relaxation and the dynamic mechanical properties of urethane dimethacrylate, *J Oral Rehabil* 27:250, 2000.

Mumford JM: Direct-current electrodes for pulp testing, *Dent Pract* 6:236, 1956.

Mumford JM: Direct-current paths through human teeth, master's thesis, Ann Arbor, Mich, 1957, University of Michigan School of Dentistry.

Mumford JM: Electrolytic action in the mouth and its relationship to pain, *J Dent Res* 36:632, 1957.

Mumford JM: Resistivity of human enamel and dentin, *Arch Oral Biol* 12:925, 1957.

Mumford JM: Path of direct current in electric pulp-testing, *Br Dent J* 106:23, 1959.

O'Brien WJ: Electrochemical corrosion of dental gold castings, *Dent Abstracts* 7:46, 1962.

Phillips LJ, Schnell RJ, Phillips RW: Measurement of the electric conductivity of dental cement. III. Effect of increased contact area and thickness: values for resin, calcium hydroxide, zinc oxide—eugenol, *J Dent Res* 34:597, 1955.

Phillips LJ, Schnell RJ, Phillips RW: Measurement of the electric conductivity of dental cement. IV. Extracted human teeth; in vivo tests; summary, *J Dent Res* 34:839, 1955.

Rootare HM, Powers JM: Comparison of zeta-potential of synthetic fluorapatite obtained by stepwise and continuous methods of streaming, *J Electrochem Soc* 126:1905, 1979.

Schreiver W, Diamond LE: Electromotive forces and electric currents caused by metallic dental fillings, *J Dent Res* 31:205, 1952.

Shaw DJ: *Electrophoresis,* New York, 1969, Academic Press.

Tay WM, Braden M: Dielectric properties of glass ionomer cements, *J Dent Res* 47:463, 1968.

Wilson AD, Kent BE: Dental silicate cements. V. Electrical conductivity, *J Dent Res* 47:463, 1968.

Zitter H, Plenk H, Jr: The electrochemical behavior of metallic implant materials as an indicator of their biocompatibility, *J Biomed Mater Res* 21:881, 1987.

Other Properties

German RM, Wright DC, Gallant RF: In vitro tarnish measurements on fixed prosthodontic alloys, *J Prosthet Dent* 47:399, 1982.

Koran A, Powers JM, Lepeak PJ et al: Stain resistance of maxillofacial materials, *J Dent Res* 58:1455, 1979.

Mesu FP: Degradation of luting cements measured in vitro, *J Dent Res* 61:655, 1982.

Raptis CM, Powers JM, Fan PL et al: Staining of composite resins by cigarette smoke, *J Oral Rehabil* 9:367, 1982.

Solovan DF, Powers JM: Effect of denture cleansers on partial denture alloys and resilient liners, *Mich Dent Assoc J* 60:135, 1978.

Walls AW, McCabe JF, Murray JJ: An erosion test for dental cements, *J Dent Res* 64:1100, 1985.

Wilson AD, Merson SA, Prosser HJ: A sensitive conductimetric method for measuring the material initially water-leached from dental cements. I. Zinc polycarboxylate cements, *J Dent* 8:263, 1980.

WEB SITES

Biomaterials Database:
www.lib.umich.edu/dentlib/dental_tables
(University of Michigan)

Chapter 4

Mechanical Properties

Most restorative materials must withstand forces during either fabrication or mastication. Mechanical properties are therefore important in understanding and predicting a material's behavior under load. Because no single mechanical property can give a true measure of quality, it is essential to understand the principles involved in a variety of mechanical properties to obtain the maximum service in a material. Quantities of force, stress, strain, strength, toughness, hardness, friction, and wear can help identify the properties of a material. In general, the stability of a solid under applied load is determined by the nature and strength of atomic binding forces. In this chapter, the concepts of elastic, viscoelastic, and surface mechanical properties are introduced, and the importance of these concepts in dentistry is emphasized.

FORCE

Force is generated through one body pushing or pulling on another. Forces may be applied through actual contact of the bodies or at a distance (e.g., gravity). The result of an applied force on a body is a change in position of rest or motion of the body. If the body to which the force is applied remains at rest, the force causes the body to deform or change its shape. A force is defined by three characteristics: point of application, magnitude, and direction of application. The direction of a force is characteristic of the type of force. The unit of force is the Newton, N.

OCCLUSAL FORCES

One of the most important applications of materials science in dentistry is in the study of forces applied to teeth and dental restorations. Numerous reports in the dental literature describe the measurement of biting forces on teeth. The maximum forces, measured by strain gauges, telemetric devices, or numerical simulations, range from 200 to 3500 N.

Biting forces on adult teeth decrease from the molar region to the incisors, with forces on the first and second molars varying from 400 to 800 N. The average force on the bicuspids, cuspids, and incisors is about 300, 200, and 150 N, respectively. A somewhat irregular but definite increase in force from 235 to 494 N occurs in growing children, with an average yearly increase the order of 22 N.

FORCES ON RESTORATIONS

Equally important to the study of forces on natural dentition is the measurement of forces and stresses on restorations such as inlays, fixed bridges, removable partial dentures, and complete dentures. One of the first investigations of occlusal forces showed that the average biting force on patients who had a fixed bridge replacing a first molar was 250 N on the restored side and 300 N on the opposite side, where they had natural dentition. For comparison, the average biting forces on permanent teeth were 665, 450, and 220 N on molars, bicuspids, and incisors, respectively.

Force measurements on patients with removable partial dentures are in the range of 65 to 235 N. For patients with complete dentures, the average force on the molars and bicuspids was about 100 N, whereas the forces on the incisors averaged 40 N. The wide range in results is possibly caused by age and gender variations in the patient populations. In general, the biting force applied by women is 90 N less than that applied by men.

These studies and others indicate that the chewing force on the first molars of patients with fixed bridges is about 40% of the force exerted by patients with natural dentition. A further decrease in force is obtained in patients with complete or removable partial dentures. Patients who wear such appliances exert only about 15% of the force applied by persons with normal dentition.

Recent measurements made with strain gauges are more precise, but, in general, the conclusions are similar. The distribution of force between the first bicuspid, second bicuspid, and the first molar of a complete denture is about 15%, 30%, and 55% of normal, respectively. The average force on the first bicuspid, second bicuspid, and first molar while the patient chewed peanuts, coconut, or raisins was 6.6, 12.0, and 22.6 N, respectively. These values are low because they are forces required to chew the food rather than average maximum forces. A patient wearing a complete denture therefore may facilitate the chewing of tough foods by increasing the force or the number of chewing thrusts or by shifting the food to the small bicuspids, where the stress is greater. Because the range of force application is small, shifting the food forward would be a better solution.

SUMMARY OF OCCLUSAL FORCES

The studies cited above were for small patient populations or patients of different ages. Based on the range of data reported, research on forces of mastication should be conducted on a large number of controlled patient groups for more accurate quantification. However, we may surmise that the forces of occlusion and the response of underlying tissue change with anatomic location, age, malocclusion, and placement of a restorative appliance. Therefore a material or design sufficient to withstand the forces of occlusion on the incisor of a child may not be sufficient for the first molar of an adult with a malocclusion or bridge.

STRESS

When a force acts on a body tending to produce deformation, a resistance is developed to this external force application. The internal reaction is equal in intensity and opposite in direction to the applied external force, and is called *stress*. Both the applied force and internal resistance (stress) are distributed over a given area of the body, so the stress in a structure is designated as the force per unit of area. In this respect, stress resembles pressure, because both stress and pressure are represented by the following equation:

$$\text{Stress} = \frac{\text{Force}}{\text{Area}}$$

Because the internal resistance to force applications is impractical to measure, the more convenient procedure is to measure the external force (F) applied to the cross-sectional area (A), which can be described as the stress, typically denoted as S or σ. The unit of stress therefore is the unit of force (N) divided by a unit of area or length squared, and is commonly expressed as Pascal (1 Pa = 1 N/m^2 = 1 MN/mm^2). It is common to report stress in units of megaPascals (MPa), where 1 MPa = 10^6 Pa.

Because the stress in a structure varies directly with the force and inversely with area, it is necessary to recognize that the area over which the force acts is an important consideration. This is particularly true in dental restorations in which the areas over which the forces are applied often are extremely small. For example, the clasps on removable partial dentures, orthodontic wire structures, or small occlusal restorations may have cross-sectional areas of only 0.16 to 0.016 cm^2.

As a numerical example, a 20-gauge orthodontic wire has a diameter of 0.8 mm and a cross-sectional area of 0.5 mm^2. If a 220 N force is applied to a wire of this diameter, the stress developed is equivalent to 220 N/0.5 mm^2, or 440 N/mm^2 (MPa).

Stress is always stated as though the force were equivalent to that applied to a 1-m^2 section, but a dental restoration obviously does not have a square meter of exposed occlusal surface area. A small occlusal pit restoration may have no more than 4 mm^2 of surface area, if it were assumed that the restoration were 2 mm on a side. If a biting force of 440 N should be concentrated on this area, the stress developed would be 100 MPa. Therefore stresses equivalent to several hundreds of MPa occur in many types of restorations.

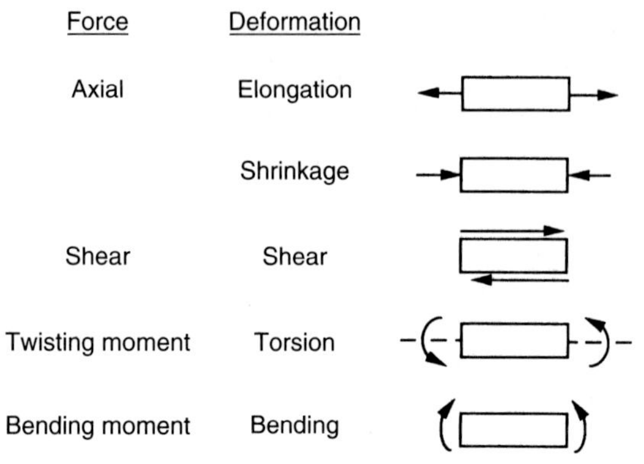

Fig. 4-1 Schematic of the different types of stresses and their corresponding deformations.

TYPES OF STRESS

A force can be directed to a body from any angle or direction, and often several forces are combined to develop complex stresses in a structure. In general, individually applied forces may be axial (tensile or compressive), shear, bending, or torsional. These directional forces are illustrated in a simplified manner in Fig. 4-1. All stresses, however, can be resolved into combinations of two basic types—axial and shear.

Tension results in a body when it is subjected to two sets of forces directed away from each other in the same straight line. *Compression* results when the body is subjected to two sets of forces directed toward each other in the same straight line, and *shear* is the result of two sets of forces directed parallel to each other. *Torsion* results from the twisting of a body, and *bending* results from an applied bending moment. When tension is applied, the molecules making up the body must resist being pulled apart. When compression is applied, they resist being forced more closely together. As a result of a shear stress application, one portion of the body must resist sliding past another. These resistances of a material to deformation represent the basic qualities of elasticity of solid bodies.

An example of the complexity and varying direction and magnitude of stresses in the oral cavity is shown in Fig. 4-2, in which a photoelastic model of a three-unit bridge has been loaded in compression by the opposing occlusion. The arrows in Fig. 4-2, *A*, indicate locations of contact that are under compressive stress. Fig. 4-2, *B*, shows the type of stress at the periphery of the model and illustrates that the occlusal surface of the bridge is subjected alternately to areas of compression and tension, whereas the gingival portion of the pontic is under tensile stress. The soldered joints, however, are under both tensile and shear stress.

STRAIN

In the discussion of force, it was pointed out that a body undergoes deformation when a force is applied to it. It is important to recognize that each type of stress is capable of producing a corresponding deformation in a body (see Fig. 4-1). The deformation resulting from a tensile or pulling force is an elongation of a body in the direction of applied force, whereas a compressive or pushing force causes compression or shortening of the body in the direction of loading. Strain, ϵ, is described as the change in length ($\Delta L = L - L_o$) per unit length (L_o) of the body when it is subjected to a stress. Strain has no unit of measurement, but is represented as a pure number obtained from the following equation:

$$\text{Strain } (\epsilon) = \frac{\text{Deformation}}{\text{Original length}} = \frac{L - L_o}{L_o} = \frac{\Delta L}{L_o}$$

Thus if a specimen with an original length of 2 mm is pulled to a new length of 2.02 mm, it has deformed 0.02 mm and the strain is 0.02/2 = 0.01, or 1%. Strain is therefore reported as an absolute value or as a percentage. The amount of strain will differ with each type of material subjected to stress and with the magnitude of the stress applied. Note that regardless of the composition or nature of the material, and regardless of the magnitude and type of stress applied to the material, deformation and strain result with each stress application. The importance of strain in dentistry is as follows: a restorative material, such as a clasp or an orthodontic wire, which can withstand a large amount of strain before failure,

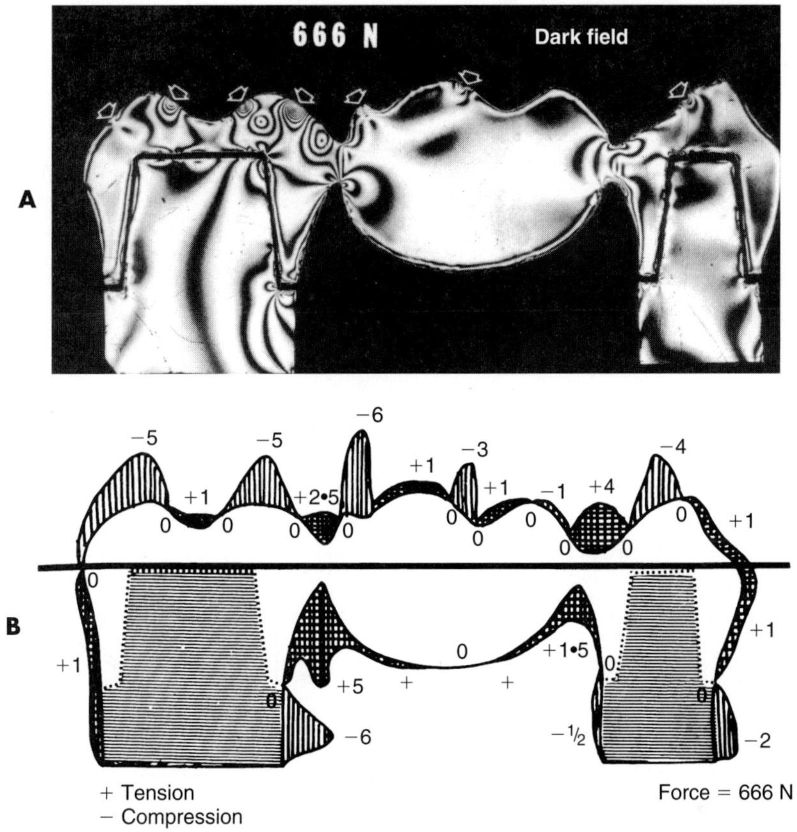

Fig. 4-2 Stress distribution in a model of a dental bridge showing **A,** the isochromatic fringes or lines of constant stress when loaded in compression, and **B,** the fringe order or a measure of the magnitude of the stress at the periphery.

(From El-Ebrashi MK, Craig RG, Peyton FA: *J Prosthet Dent* 23:177, 1970.)

can be bent and adjusted with less chance of fracturing.

STRESS-STRAIN CURVES

Consider a bar of material subjected to an applied force, *F*. We can measure the magnitude of the force and the resulting deformation (δ). If we next take another bar of the same material, but different dimensions, the force-deformation characteristics change (Fig. 4-3, *A*). However, if we normalize the applied force by the cross-sectional area *A* (stress) of the bar, and normalize the deformation by the original length (strain) of the bar, the resultant stress-strain curve now becomes independent of the geometry of the bar (Fig. 4-3, *B*). It is therefore preferential to report the stress-strain relations of a material rather than the force-deformation characteristics. The stress-strain relationship of a dental material is studied by measuring the load and deformation and then calculating the corresponding stress and strain.

The testing of many materials necessitates loads of 2220 N or more and the measurement of deformations of 0.02 mm or less. A further requirement may be that the load should be applied at a uniform rate or that the deformation should occur at a uniform rate. A typical machine that permits testing of tension, compression, or

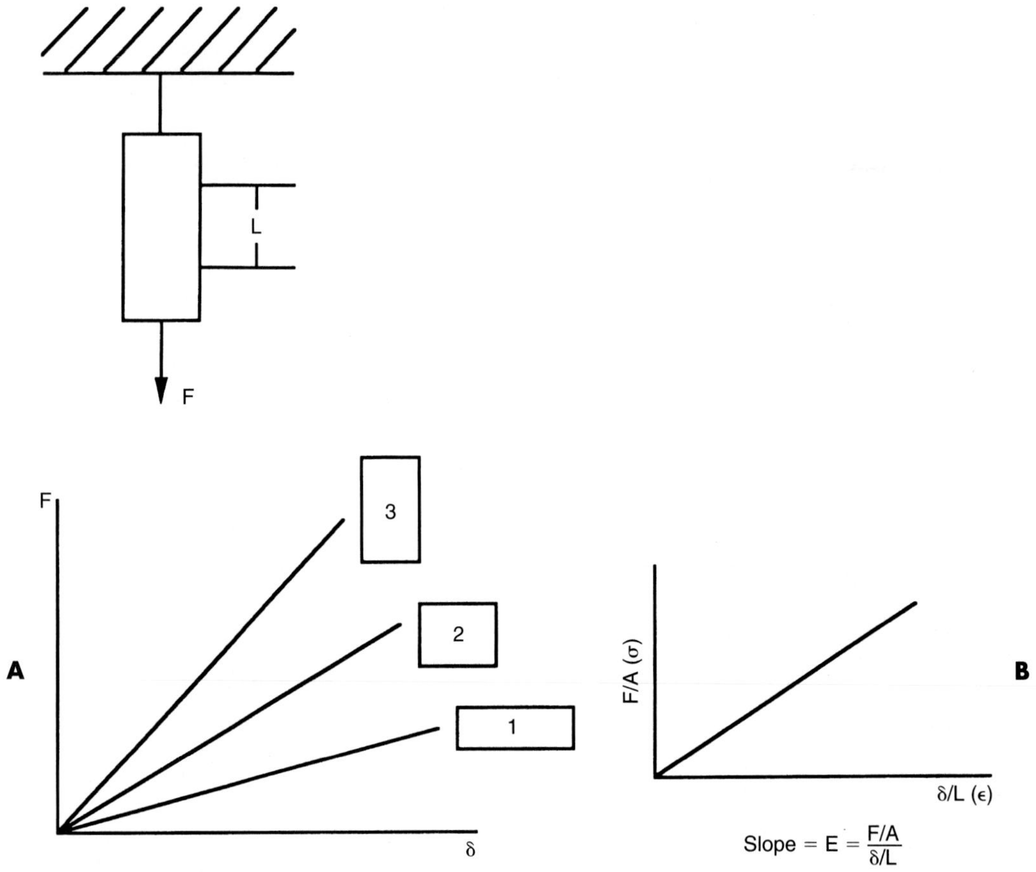

Fig. 4-3 A, Force-deformation characteristics for the same material but having different dimensions. **B,** Stress-strain characteristics of the same group of bars. The stress-strain curve is independent of the geometry of the bar.

shear is shown in Fig. 4-4. In the figure, a rod is clamped between two jaws and the tensile properties are measured by pulling the specimen. The load is measured electronically with a force transducer and the deformation is measured with an extensometer clamped over a given length of the specimen. One obtains a plot of load versus deformation, which can be converted to a plot of stress versus strain (Fig. 4-5) by the simple calculations described previously.

In the calculation of stress, it is assumed that the cross-sectional area of the specimen remains constant during the test. The resulting stress-strain curve is called an *engineering stress-strain curve,* and stresses are calculated based on the original cross-sectional area. For many materials, significant changes in the area of the specimen may occur as it is being deformed. A stress-strain curve based on stresses calculated from a non-constant cross-sectional area is called a *true stress-strain curve.* A true stress-strain curve may be quite different from an engineering stress-strain curve at high loads because significant changes in the area of the specimen may occur. For example, if a specimen is being tested in tension and the area decreases, the engineering stress will be lower than the true stress. The engineering stress-strain curve is used throughout the remaining chapters.

A stress-strain curve for a hypothetical mate-

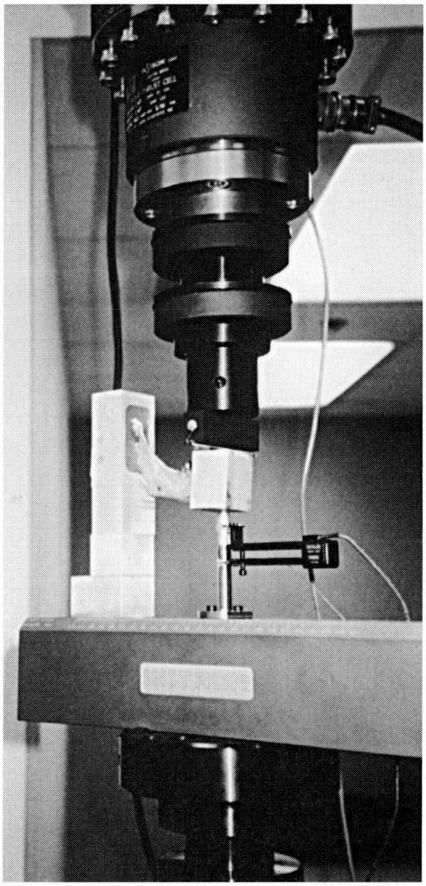

Fig. 4-4 Servo-hydraulic mechanical testing machine capable of applying axial, shear, bending, and/or torsional loads to a material.

rial that was subjected to increasing tensile stress until fracture is shown in Fig. 4-5. The stress is plotted vertically, and the strain is plotted horizontally. As the stress is increased, the strain is increased. In fact, in the initial portion of the curve, from 0 to *A,* the strain is linearly proportional to the stress, and as the stress is doubled, the amount of strain is also doubled. When a stress that is higher than the value registered at *A* is achieved, the strain changes are no longer linearly proportional to the stress changes. Hence the value of the stress at *A* is known as the *proportional limit.*

PROPORTIONAL AND ELASTIC LIMITS

The *proportional limit* is defined as the greatest stress that a material will sustain without a deviation from the linear proportionality of stress to strain. Below the proportional limit, no permanent deformation occurs in a structure. When the stress is removed, the structure will return to its original dimensions. Within this range of stress application, the material is elastic in nature, and if the material is stressed to some value below the proportional limit, an elastic or reversible strain will occur. The region of the stress-strain curve before the proportional limit is called the *elastic region.* The application of a stress greater than the proportional limit results in a permanent or irreversible strain in the specimen; the region of the stress-strain curve beyond the proportional limit is called the *plastic region.*

The *elastic limit* is defined as the maximum stress that a material will withstand without permanent deformation. Therefore for all practical purposes the proportional limit and elastic limit represent the same stress within the structure, and the terms are often used interchangeably in referring to the stress involved. Keep in mind, however, that they differ in fundamental concept, in that one deals with the proportionality of strain to stress in the structure, whereas the other describes the elastic behavior of the material. The proportional limit of the material in Fig. 4-5 is approximately 330 MPa. The proportional and elastic limits are quite different for different materials. Values for proportional or elastic limits in either tension or compression can be determined, but the values obtained in tension and compression will differ for the same material.

The concepts of elastic and plastic behavior can be illustrated with a simple schematic model of the deformation of atoms in a solid under stress (Fig. 4-6). The atoms are shown in Fig. 4-6, *A,* with no stress applied, and in Fig. 4-6, *B,* with an applied stress that is below the value of the proportional limit. When the stress shown in *B* is removed, the atoms return to their positions shown in *A*. When a stress is applied that is greater than the proportional limit, the atoms can move to a position as shown in

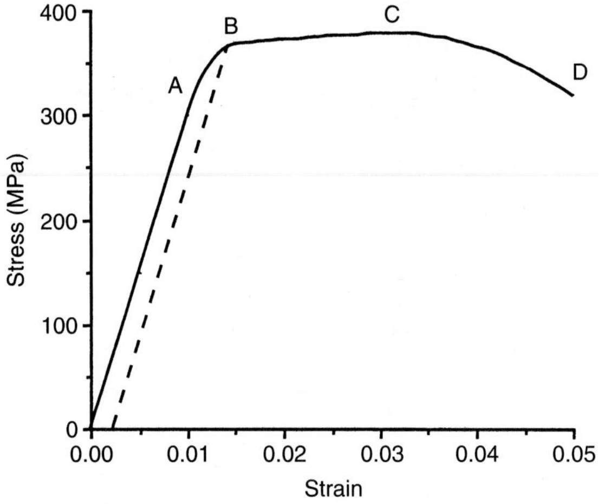

Fig. 4-5 Stress-strain curve for a material subjected to a tensile stress.

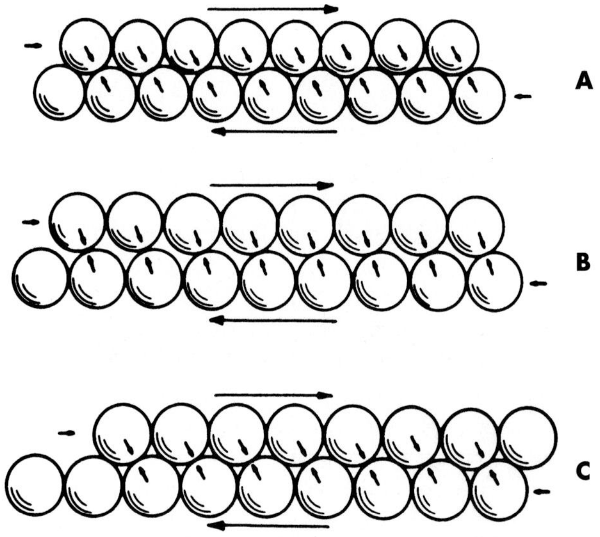

Fig. 4-6 Sketch of an atomic model showing atoms in **A,** original position, **B,** after elastic deformation, and **C,** after plastic deformation.
(Adapted from Cottrell AH: *Sci Am* 217[3]:90, 1967.)

Fig. 4-6, *C,* and, on removal of the stress, the atoms remain in this new position. The application of a stress less than the proportional or elastic limit results in a reversible strain, whereas a stress greater than the proportional or elastic limit results in an irreversible or permanent strain in the specimen.

The model described in Fig. 4-6 is considerably oversimplified; a more realistic but more complicated model of plastic deformation is shown in Fig. 4-7. In this schematic the atoms can move to new stable positions, resulting in plastic deformation by the movement of dislocations or imperfections (as indicated by the black circles in Fig. 4-7) in the structure of the solid. These imperfections allow the consecutive movement of atoms without the need for an entire row or plane of atoms to move.

YIELD STRENGTH

Stress-strain curves determined in the laboratory are rarely as ideal as the curve shown in Fig. 4-5. Therefore it is not always feasible to explicitly measure the proportional and elastic limits. The *yield strength* or *yield stress (YS)* of a

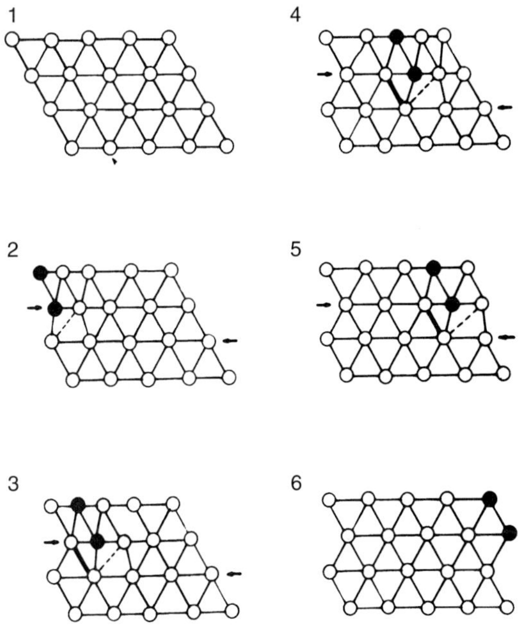

Fig. 4-7 Sketch of an atomic model showing plastic deformation taking place by the movement of dislocations.
(Adapted from Cottrell AH: *Sci Am* 217[3]:90, 1967.)

material is a property that can be determined readily and is often used to describe the stress at which the material begins to function in a plastic manner. At this stress, a limited permanent strain has occurred in the material. The yield strength is defined as the stress at which a material exhibits a specified limiting deviation from proportionality of stress to strain. The amount of permanent strain is arbitrarily selected for the material being examined and may be indicated as 0.1%, 0.2%, or 0.5% (0.001, 0.002, 0.005) permanent strain. The amount of permanent strain may be referred to as the *percent offset*. Many specifications use 0.2% as a convention.

The yield stress is determined by selecting the desired offset and drawing a line parallel to the linear region of the stress-strain curve. The point at which the parallel line intersects the stress-strain curve is the yield stress. On the stress-strain curve shown in Fig. 4-5, for example, the yield strength is represented by the value B. This represents a stress of about 360 MPa at a 0.25% offset. This yield stress is slightly higher than that for the proportional limit and also indicates a specified amount of deformation. Again, note that when a structure is permanently deformed, even to a small degree (such as the amount of deformation at the yield strength), it does not return completely to its original dimensions when the stress is removed. For this reason, the proportional limit, elastic limit, and yield strength of a material are among its most important properties.

Any dental structure that is permanently deformed through the forces of mastication is usually a functional failure to some degree. For example, a bridge that is permanently deformed through the application of excessive biting forces would be shifted out of the proper occlusal relation for which it was originally designed. The prosthesis becomes permanently deformed because a stress equal to or greater than the yield strength was developed. Recall also that malocclusion changes the stresses placed on a restoration; a deformed prosthesis may therefore be subjected to greater stresses than originally intended. Usually a fracture does not occur under such conditions, but rather only a permanent deformation results, which represents a destructive example of deformation. A constructive example of permanent deformation and stresses in excess of the elastic limit is observed when an appliance or dental structure is adapted or adjusted for purposes of design. For example, in the process of shaping an orthodontic appliance or adjusting a clasp on a removable partial denture, it may be necessary to introduce a stress into the structure in excess of the yield strength if the material is to be permanently bent or adapted. Values of yield strength for some partial denture alloys are listed in Table 4-1.

ULTIMATE STRENGTH

In Fig. 4-5, the test specimen is subjected to its greatest stress at point *C*. The *ultimate tensile strength or stress* is defined as the maximum stress that a material can withstand before failure in tension, whereas the *ultimate compressive strength or stress* is the maximum stress a material can withstand in compression. If the direction

TABLE 4-1 Values of Yield Strength for Some Partial Denture Alloys

Material	Yield Strength, 0.2% Offset MPa
Nickel-chromium alloy	690
Cobalt-chromium alloy	572
Gold (type IV) alloy	621*

*0.1% offset.

of loading has previously been specified, then the term *ultimate strength* (stress) is often used. The ultimate stress is determined by dividing the maximum load in tension (or compression) by the original cross-sectional area of the test specimen. The ultimate tensile strength of the material in Fig. 4-5 is about 380 MPa.

The ultimate strength of an alloy is used in dentistry to give an indication of the size or cross section required for a given restoration. Note that an alloy that has been stressed to near the ultimate strength will be permanently deformed, so a restoration receiving that amount of stress during function would be useless. Therefore, although data on materials used in dentistry usually specify values for ultimate strength, the use of ultimate strength as a criterion for evaluating the relative merits of various materials should not be overemphasized. The yield strength is of greater importance than ultimate strength because it is a gauge of when a material will start to deform.

FRACTURE STRENGTH

In Fig. 4-5 the test specimen fractured at point D. The stress at which a material fractures is called the *fracture strength* or *fracture stress*. Note that a material does not necessarily fracture at the point at which the maximum stress occurs. After a maximum stress is applied to some materials, they begin to elongate excessively, and the stress calculated from the force and the original cross-sectional area may drop before final fracture occurs. Accordingly, the stress at the end of the curve is less than at some intermediate point on the curve. Therefore in the most general case the ultimate and fracture strengths are different. However, for the specific cases of many dental alloys subjected to tension, the ultimate and fracture strengths are the same, as is seen later.

ELONGATION

The deformation that results from the application of a tensile force is *elongation*. Elongation is extremely important because it gives an indication of the workability of an alloy. As may be observed from Fig. 4-5, the elongation of a material during a tensile test can be divided conveniently into two parts: (1) the increase in length of the specimen below the proportional limit (from 0 to A), which is not permanent and is proportional to the stress applied; and (2) the elongation beyond the proportional limit and up to the fracture strength (from A to D), which is permanent. The permanent deformation may be measured with an extensometer while the material is being tested and calculated from the stress-strain curve. A common method to express total elongation is in percentage, such as 20% elongation for a 5-cm test specimen. The percent elongation would be calculated as follows:

$$\%\ \text{Elongation} = \frac{\text{Increase in length}}{\text{Original length}} \times 100\%$$

We see that elongation and axial strain are similar.

The total percent elongation includes both the elastic elongation and the plastic elongation. The plastic elongation is usually the greater of the two, except in materials that are quite brittle or those with very low elastic moduli. A material that exhibits a 20% total elongation at the time of fracture has increased in length by one fifth of its original length. Such a material, as in many dental gold alloys, has a high value for plastic or permanent elongation and, in general, is a ductile type of alloy, whereas a material with only 1% elongation would possess little permanent elongation and be considered brittle.

TABLE 4-2 Values of Percent Elongation of Some Crown and Bridge and Partial Denture Alloys

Alloy	% Elongation
Crown and bridge	
Gold (type III)	34.0
40% Au-Ag-Cu	2.0
Nickel-chromium	1.1
Partial denture	
Gold (type IV)	6.5
Nickel-chromium	2.4
Cobalt-chromium	1.5
Iron-chromium	9.0
Cobalt-nickel-chromium	8-10

Values of percent elongation of some crown and bridge and partial denture alloys are compared in Table 4-2. An alloy that has a high value for total elongation can be bent permanently without danger of fracture. Clasps can be adjusted, orthodontic appliances can be prepared, and crowns or inlays can be burnished if they are prepared from alloys with high values for elongation. When selecting alloys for specific clinical purposes, therefore, it is necessary to recognize that because they may be subjected to permanent deformation and adaptation during the construction or assembly of the restoration, it is necessary to have an acceptable amount of elongation. In other restorations in which permanent deformation is not anticipated, it is possible to employ materials with a lower value for elongation. A relationship exists between elongation and yield strength for many materials, including dental gold alloys, where, generally, the higher the yield strength, the less the elongation.

ELASTIC MODULUS

The measure of elasticity of a material is described by the term *elastic modulus,* also referred to as *modulus of elasticity* or *Young's modulus,* and denoted by the variable *E.* The elastic modulus represents the stiffness of a material within the elastic range. The elastic modulus can be determined from a stress-strain curve (see Fig. 4-5) by calculating the ratio of stress to strain or the slope of the linear region of the curve. The modulus is calculated from the equation

$$\text{Elastic modulus} = \frac{\text{Stress}}{\text{Strain}} \text{ or } E = \frac{\sigma}{\epsilon}$$

Because strain is dimensionless, the modulus has the same units as stress, and is usually reported in MPa or GPa (1 GPa = 1000 MPa).

The elastic qualities of a material represent a fundamental property of the material. The interatomic or intermolecular forces of the material are responsible for the property of elasticity (see Fig. 4-6). The stronger the basic attraction forces, the greater the values of the elastic modulus and the more rigid or stiff the material. Because this property is related to the attraction forces within the material, it is usually the same when the material is subjected to either tension or compression. The property is generally independent of any heat treatment or mechanical treatment that a metal or alloy has received, but is quite dependent on the composition of the material.

The elastic modulus is determined by the slope of the elastic portion of the stress-strain curve, which is calculated by choosing any two stress and strain coordinates in the elastic or linear range. As an example, for the curve in Fig. 4-5 the slope can be calculated by choosing the following two coordinates:

$$\sigma_1 = 150 \text{ MPa}, \epsilon_1 = 0.005; \text{ and } \sigma_2 = 300 \text{ MPa}, \epsilon_2 = 0.010$$

The slope is therefore

$$(\sigma_2 - \sigma_1)/(\epsilon_2 - \epsilon_1) = (300 - 150)/(0.010 - 0.005) = 30{,}000 \text{ MPa} = 30 \text{ GPa}$$

Stress-strain curves for two hypothetical materials, *A* and *B,* of different composition are shown in Fig. 4-8. Inspection of the curves shows that for a given stress, *A* is elastically deformed less than *B,* with the result that the elastic modulus for *A* is

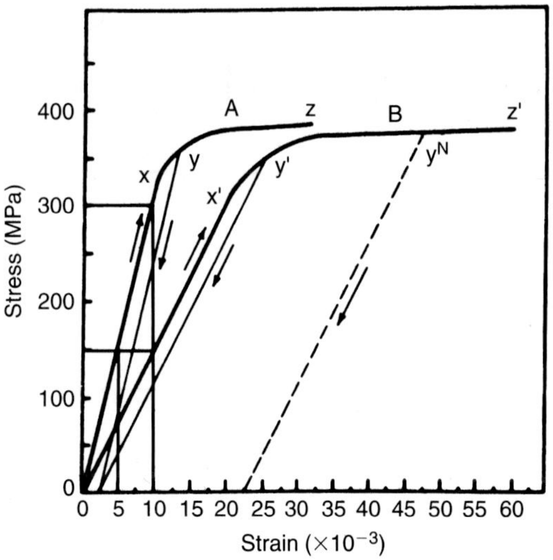

Fig. 4-8 Stress-strain curves of two hypothetical materials subjected to tensile stress.

greater than for *B*. This difference can be demonstrated, numerically, by calculating the elastic moduli for the two materials subjected to the same stress of 300 MPa. At a stress of 300 MPa, material *A* is strained to 0.010 (1%) and the elastic modulus is

$$E = \frac{300 \text{ MPa}}{0.010} = 30{,}000 \text{ MPa} = 30 \text{ GPa}$$

On the other hand, material *B* is strained to 0.02 (2%), or twice as much as material *A* for the same stress application. The equation for the elastic modulus for *B* is

$$E = \frac{300 \text{ MPa}}{0.020} = 15{,}000 \text{ MPa} = 15 \text{ GPa}$$

The fact that material *A* has a steeper slope in the elastic range than material *B* means that a greater stress application is required to deform material *A* to a given amount than for material *B*. From the curves shown in Fig. 4-8, it can be seen that a stress of 300 MPa is required to deform *A* to the same amount elastically that *B* is deformed by a stress of 150 MPa. Therefore *A* is said to be stiffer or more rigid than *B*. Conversely, *B* is more flexible than *A*. Materials such as rubber and plastics have low values for the elastic modulus, whereas many metals and alloys have much higher values, as shown in Table 4-3.

TABLE 4-3 Values of Elastic Modulus of Some Restorative Dental Materials

Material	Elastic Modulus GPa*
Cobalt-chromium partial denture alloy	218.0
Gold (type IV) alloy	99.3
Enamel	84.1
Feldspathic porcelain	69.0
Zinc phosphate cement (base)	22.4
Amalgam	27.6
Dentin	18.3
Resin composite	16.6
Zinc phosphate cement (luting)	13.7
Acrylic denture resin	2.65
Silicone rubber (maxillofacial)	0.002

*1 gigapascal (GPa) = 103 MPa.

POISSON'S RATIO

During axial loading in tension or compression there is a simultaneous axial and lateral strain. Under tensile loading, as a material elongates in the direction of load, there is a reduction in cross section. Under compressive loading, there is an increase in the cross section. Within the elastic range, the ratio of the lateral to the axial strain is called *Poisson's ratio* (ν). In tensile loading, the Poisson's ratio indicates that the reduction in cross section is proportional to the elongation during the elastic deformation. The reduction in cross section continues until the material is fractured.

Poisson's ratios of some dental materials are listed in Table 4-4. Brittle substances such as hard gold alloys and dental amalgam show

TABLE 4-4 Values of Poisson's Ratio of Some Restorative Dental Materials

Material	Poisson's Ratio
Amalgam	0.35
Zinc phosphate cement	0.35
Enamel	0.30
Resin composite	0.24

little permanent reduction in cross section during a tensile test. More ductile materials such as soft gold alloys, which are high in gold content, show a high degree of reduction in cross-sectional area.

DUCTILITY AND MALLEABILITY

Two significant properties of metals and alloys are ductility and malleability. These properties cannot always be determined with certainty from a stress-strain curve. *Ductility* is the ability of a material to be plastically deformed; it is indicated by the plastic strain.

A high degree of compression or elongation indicates good malleability and ductility, although certain metals show some exception to this rule. The reduction in area in a specimen, together with the elongation at the breaking point, is, however, a good indication of the relative ductility of a metal or alloy.

The ductility of a material represents its ability to be drawn into wire under a force of tension. The material is subjected to a permanent deformation while being subjected to these tensile forces. The malleability of a substance represents its ability to be hammered or rolled into thin sheets without fracturing.

Ductility is a property that has been related to the workability of a material in the mouth. It has also been related to burnishability of the margins of a casting. Although ductility is important, the amount of force necessary to cause permanent deformation during the burnishing operation also must be considered. A burnishing index has been used to rank the ease of burnishing alloys and is equal to the ductility (elongation) divided by the yield strength.

TABLE 4-5 Relative Ductility and Malleability of Metals in Decreasing Order

Ductility	Malleability
Gold	Gold
Silver	Silver
Platinum	Aluminum
Iron	Copper
Nickel	Tin
Copper	Platinum
Aluminum	Lead
Zinc	Zinc
Tin	Iron
Lead	Nickel

Note: Some authorities consider tungsten to be the most ductile metal.

The relative malleability and ductility of 10 metals used in dentistry and industry are given in Table 4-5. It is interesting that gold and silver, used extensively in dentistry, are the most malleable and ductile of the metals, but other metals do not follow the same order for both malleability and ductility. In general, metals tend to be ductile, whereas ceramics tend to be brittle.

RESILIENCE

Resilience is the resistance of a material to permanent deformation. It indicates the amount of energy necessary to deform the material to the proportional limit. Resilience is therefore measured by the area under the elastic portion of the stress-strain curve, as illustrated in Fig. 4-9, *A*. Resilience can be measured by idealizing the area of interest as a triangle and calculating the area of the triangle, (1/2)bh. The resilience of the material in Fig. 4-5, for example, would be $1/2 \times 0.011 \times 330 = 1.82$ m MN/m^3. The units are m MN/m^3 (meter × megaNewtons per cubic meter), which represents energy per unit volume of material.

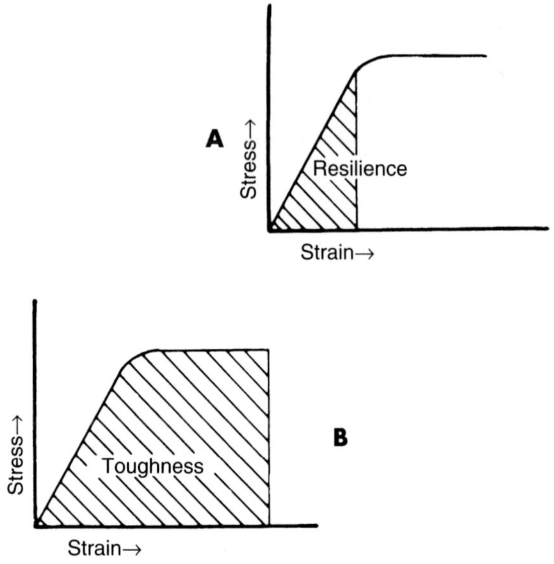

Fig. 4-9 Stress-strain curves showing **A,** the area indicating the resilience, and **B,** the area representing the toughness of a material.

Resilience has particular importance in the evaluation of orthodontic wires because the amount of work expected from a particular spring in moving a tooth is of interest. There is also interest in the amount of stress and strain at the proportional limit because these factors determine the magnitude of the force that can be applied to the tooth and how far the tooth will need to move before the spring is no longer effective. For example, Fig. 4-10 illustrates the load-deflection curve for a nickel-titanium (Ni-Ti) orthodontic wire. Note that the loading (activation) portion of the curve is different from the unloading (deactivation) portion. This difference is called *hysteresis.*

TOUGHNESS

Toughness, which is the resistance of a material to fracture, is an indication of the amount of energy necessary to cause fracture. The area under the elastic and plastic portions of a stress-strain curve, as shown in Fig. 4-9, *B,* represents the toughness of a material. Toughness is not as easy to calculate as resilience, and the integration is usually done numerically. The units of toughness are the same as the units of resilience—m MN/m^3 or mMPa/m. Toughness therefore represents the energy required to stress the material to the point of fracture. Note that a material can be tough by having a combination of high yield and ultimate strength and moderately high strain at rupture, or by having moderately high yield and ultimate strengths and a large strain at rupture.

FRACTURE TOUGHNESS

Recently the concepts of fracture mechanics have been applied to a number of problems in dental materials. Fracture mechanics characterizes the behavior of materials with cracks or flaws. Flaws or cracks may arise naturally in a material or nucleate after a time in service. In either case, any defect generally weakens a material, and, as a result, sudden fractures can arise at stresses below the yield stress. Sudden, catastrophic fractures typically occur in brittle materials that don't have the ability to plastically deform and redistribute stresses. The field of fracture mechanics provides an analysis of and design basis against these types of failures.

Two simple examples illustrate the significance of defects on the fracture of materials. If one takes a piece of paper and tries to tear it, greater effort is needed than if a tiny cut is made in the paper. Analogously, it takes a considerable force to break a glass bar; however,

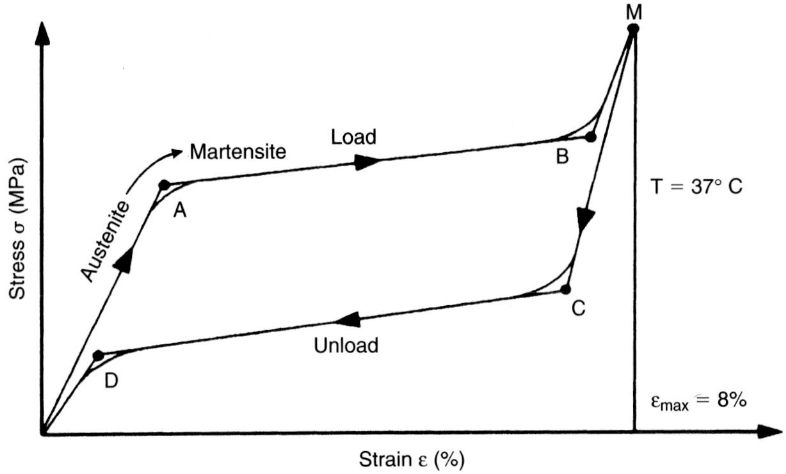

Fig. 4-10 Load-deflection curve for Ni-Ti orthodontic wire. Note that the loading (activation) portion of the curve is different from the unloading (deactivation) portion, indicating hysteresis in the material.

if a small notch is placed on the surface of the glass bar, less force is needed to cause fracture. If the same experiment is performed on a ductile material, we find that a small surface notch has no effect on the force required to break the bar, and the ductile bar can be bent without fracturing (Fig. 4-11). For a brittle material such as glass, no local plastic deformation is associated with fracture, whereas for a ductile material, plastic deformation, such as the ability to bend, occurs without fracture. The ability to be plastically deformed without fracture, or the amount of energy required for fracture, is the *fracture toughness.*

In general, the larger a flaw, the lower the stress needed to cause fracture. This is because the stresses, which would normally be supported by material, are now concentrated at the edge of the flaw. The ability of a flaw to cause fracture depends on the fracture toughness of the material. Fracture toughness is a material property and is proportional to the energy consumed in plastic deformation.

A material is characterized by the energy release rate, *G,* and the stress intensity factor, *K.* The energy release rate is a function of the energy involved in crack propagation, whereas the stress intensity factor describes the stresses at the tip of a crack. The stress intensity factor changes with crack length and stress according to

$$K = Y\sigma a^{1/2}$$

where Y is a function which is dependent on crack size and geometry. A material fractures when the stress intensity reaches a critical value, K_c. This value of the stress intensity at fracture is called the fracture toughness. Fracture toughness gives a relative value of a material's ability to resist crack propagation. The units of K_c are units of stress (force/length^2) × units of length$^{1/2}$, or force × length$^{-3/2}$, and are typically reported as MN m$^{-3/2}$ or MPa m$^{1/2}$.

As will be discussed later in this chapter, nano-indentation techniques have recently been introduced as a means of measuring mechanical properties of micron-sized phases in a material. For brittle materials, one of the properties that may be measured is fracture toughness. By selectively indenting specific regions of a microstructure, the relative effects of different microstructural constituents may be identified. The spatial variation in properties may also be

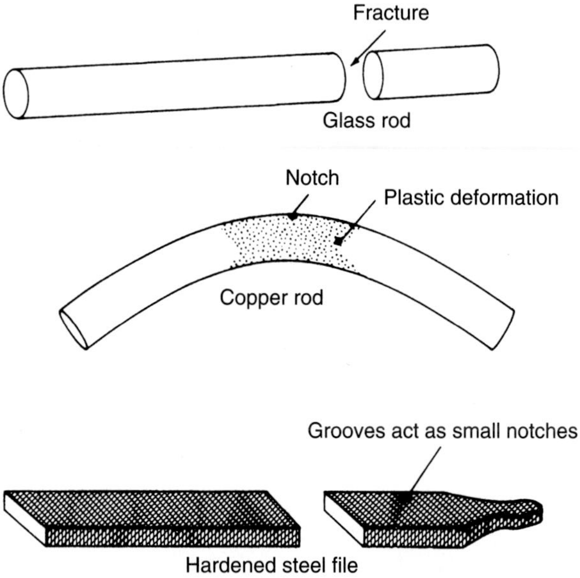

Fig. 4-11 Schematic of different types of deformation in brittle (glass, steel file) and ductile (copper) materials of the same diameter and having a notch of the same dimensions.
(From Flinn RA, Trojan PK: *Engineering materials and their applications,* Boston, 1981, Houghton Mifflin, p 535.)

determined. For example, amalgams show significant differences in fracture toughness as a function of distance from the margin.

Fracture toughness (K_{IC}) has been measured for a number of important restorative materials, including amalgams, acrylic denture base materials, composites, ceramics, and orthodontic brackets, cements, and human enamel and dentin. Typical values for composites, ceramics, enamel, and dentin are indicated in Table 4-6.

The presence of fillers in polymers substantially increases fracture toughness. The mechanisms of toughening are presumed to be matrix-filler interactions but are not yet established. Similarly, the addition of up to 50 wt% zirconia to ceramic increases fracture toughness. As with other mechanical properties, aging or storage in a simulated oral environment or at elevated temperatures can decrease fracture toughness, but there is no uniform agreement in the literature. Attempts to correlate fracture toughness with wear resistance have been mixed, and therefore it is not an unequivocal predictor of the wear of restorative materials. Also, numerical analysis techniques have been applied to composites and the tooth-denture base joint to determine energy release rates in the presence of cracks.

TABLE 4-6 Fracture Toughness of Selected Dental Materials

Material	K_{IC} (MN $m^{-3/2}$)
Amalgam	1.3
Ceramic	1.5–2.1
Resin composite	0.8–2.2
Porcelain	2.6
Enamel	0.6–1.8
Dentin	3.1

K_{IC}, Fracture toughness.

PROPERTIES AND STRESS-STRAIN CURVES

The shape of a stress-strain curve and the magnitudes of the stress and strain allow classification of materials with respect to their general properties. The idealized stress-strain curves in Fig. 4-12 represent materials with various combinations of physical properties. For example, materials *1* to *4* have high stiffness, materials *1, 2, 5,* and *6* have high strength, and materials *1, 3, 5,* and *7* have high ductility. If the only requirement for an application is stiffness, materials *1* to *4* would all be satisfactory. However, if the requirements were both stiffness and

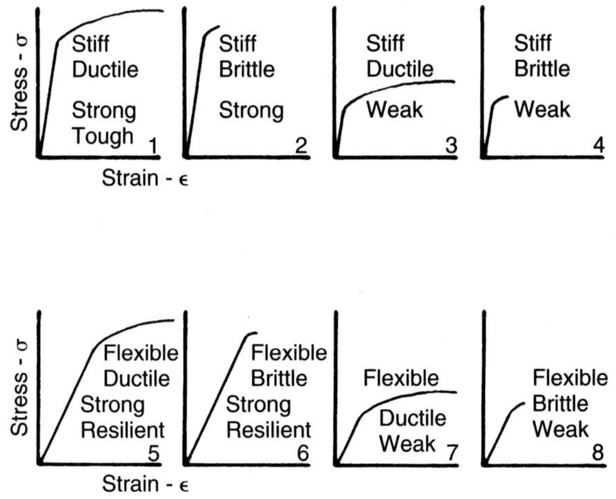

Fig. 4-12 Stress-strain curves for materials with various combinations of properties.

strength, only materials *1* and *2* would now be acceptable. If the requirements were to also include ductility, the choice would be limited to material *1*. It is clear that the properties of stiffness, strength, and ductility are independent, and materials may exhibit various combinations of these three properties.

OTHER MECHANICAL PROPERTIES

TENSILE PROPERTIES OF BRITTLE MATERIALS

A variety of brittle restorative materials, including dental amalgam, cements, ceramics, plaster and stone, and some impression materials, is important to dental practice. In many instances the material is much weaker in tension than in compression, which may contribute to failure of the material in service. Such material should therefore be used only in areas subjected to compressive stresses.

Previously, test methods were described for the development of stress-strain curves resulting from tensile measurements on ductile materials such as metals, alloys, and some types of plastics. Similar test methods have been applied to brittle materials. However, brittle materials must be tested with caution, and any stress concentrations at the grips or anywhere else in the specimen can lead to premature fracture. As a result, there has been large variability in tensile data on brittle materials. Although special grips have been used to permit axial tensile loading with a minimum of localized stress concentrations, obtaining uniform results is still difficult, and such testing is relatively slow and time consuming.

An alternative method of testing brittle materials, in which the ultimate tensile strength of a brittle material is determined through compressive testing, has become popular because of its relative simplicity and reproducibility of results. The method is described in the literature as the *diametral compression test for tension,* the *Brazilian test,* or the *indirect tensile test.* In this test method, a disk of the brittle material is compressed diametrically in a testing machine until fracture occurs, as shown in Fig. 4-13. The compressive stress applied to the specimen introduces a tensile stress in the material in the plane of the force application of the test machine. The tensile stress is directly proportional to the load applied in compression through the following formula:

$$\text{(Tensile stress) } \sigma_x = \frac{2P}{\pi \times D \times T} \quad \frac{\text{(Load)}}{\text{(Diameter} \times \text{Thickness)}}$$

Note that if the specimen deforms significantly before failure or fractures into more than two equal pieces, the data may not be valid. Some materials yield different diametral tensile

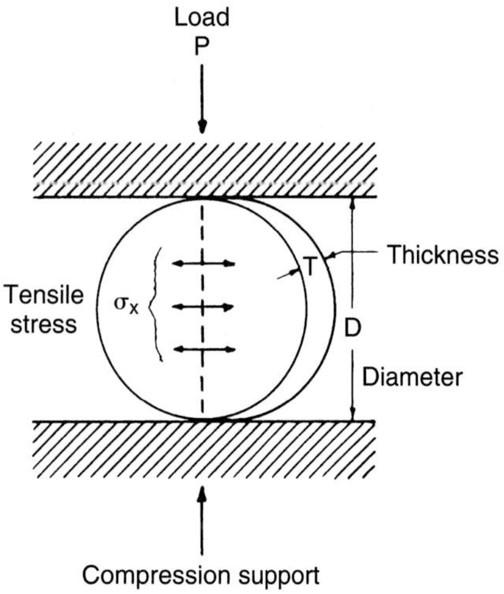

Fig. 4-13 Drawing to illustrate how compression force develops tensile stress in brittle materials.

TABLE 4-7 Values of Tensile Strength for Some Restorative Dental Materials

Material	Diametral Tensile Strength (MPa)	Ultimate Tensile Strength (MPa)
Gold alloy	—	448
Amalgam	65.7	—
Dentin	—	98.7
Resin composite	45.5	—
Feldspathic porcelain	—	24.8
Enamel	—	10.3
Zinc phosphate cement	8.1	—
High-strength stone	7.66	—
Calcium hydroxide liner	0.96	—

strengths when tested at different rates of loading and are described as being strain-rate sensitive. Strain-rate dependence is discussed later in the chapter. The diametral tensile test is not valid for these materials, and thus the strain-rate sensitivity of a material should be determined before this test is used to evaluate the tensile strength. Values of diametral and ultimate tensile strengths for some dental materials are listed in Table 4-7.

COMPRESSIVE PROPERTIES

Compressive strength is important in many restorative dental materials and accessory items used in dental techniques and operations. This property is particularly important in the process of mastication because many of the forces of mastication are compressive. Compressive strength is most useful for comparing materials that are brittle and generally weak in tension and that are therefore not employed in regions of the oral cavity where tensile forces predominate. It is somewhat less useful to determine the compressive properties of ductile materials such as gold alloys. Compressive strength is therefore a useful property for the comparison of dental amalgam, resin composites, and cements and for determining the qualities of other materials such as plaster, investments, and some impression materials. Typical values of compressive strength of some restorative dental materials are given in Table 4-8.

Certain characteristics observed in materials subjected to tension are also observed when a material is in compression. For example, a stress-strain curve can be recorded for a material in compression similar to that obtained in tension. Such a curve represents a material that has both elastic and plastic characteristics when subjected to compressive stress, although the plastic region is generally small. The modulus of elasticity of a material in compression can be determined from the ratio of stress to strain in the elastic region. Such a modulus value is usually similar for a material whether tested in compression or tension. A proportional limit or yield strength in compression can also be observed. The ultimate compressive strength is calculated from the original cross-sectional area of the specimen and the maximum applied force, in a similar manner to the ultimate tensile strength.

When a structure is subjected to compression, note that the failure of the body may occur as a result of complex stress formations in the

TABLE 4-8 Compressive Strength of Some Restorative Dental Materials

Material	Compressive Strength (MPa)
Enamel	384
Amalgam	388
Dentin	297
Resin composite	277
Feldspathic porcelain	149
Zinc phosphate cement	117
High-strength stone	81
Calcium hydroxide liner	8

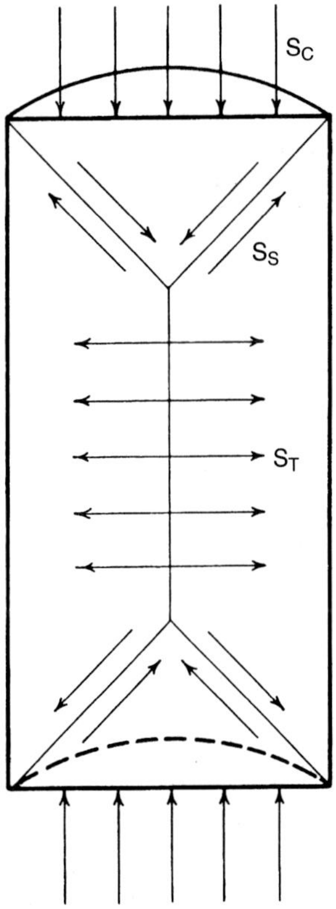

Fig. 4-14 Drawing of complex stress pattern developed in cylinder subjected to compressive stress.

body. This is illustrated by a cross-sectional view of a right cylinder subjected to compression, as shown in Fig. 4-14. It is apparent from Fig. 4-14 that the forces of compression applied to each end of the specimen are resolved into forces of shear along a cone-shaped area at each end and, as a result of the action of the two cones on the cylinder, into tensile forces in the central portion of the mass. Because of this resolution of forces in the body, it has become necessary to adopt standard sizes and dimensions to obtain reproducible test results. Fig. 4-14 shows that if a test specimen is too short, the force distributions become more complicated as a result of the cone formations overlapping in the ends of the cylinder. If the specimen is too long, buckling may occur. Therefore the cylinder should have a length twice that of the diameter for the most satisfactory results.

SHEAR STRENGTH

The shear strength is the maximum stress that a material can withstand before failure in a shear mode of loading. It is particularly important in the study of interfaces between two materials, such as porcelain fused to metal or an implant-tissue interface. One method of testing the shear strength of dental materials is the punch or push-out method, in which an axial load is applied to push one material through another. The shear strength (τ) is calculated by

$$\text{Shear strength}(\tau) = F/\pi dh$$

where F is the compressive force applied to the specimen, d is the diameter of the punch, and h is the thickness of the specimen. Note that the stress distribution caused by this method is not "pure" shear and that results often differ because of differences in specimen dimensions, surface geometry, composition and preparation, and mechanical testing procedure. However, it is a simple test to perform and has been used extensively. Alternatively, shear properties may be determined by subjecting a specimen to torsional

TABLE 4-9 Values of Shear Strength Tested by the Punch Method for Some Restorative Dental Materials

Material	Shear Strength (MPa)
Amalgam	188
Dentin	138
Acrylic denture resin	122
Porcelain	111
Enamel	90
Zinc phosphate cement	13

loading. Shear strengths of some dental materials are listed in Table 4-9.

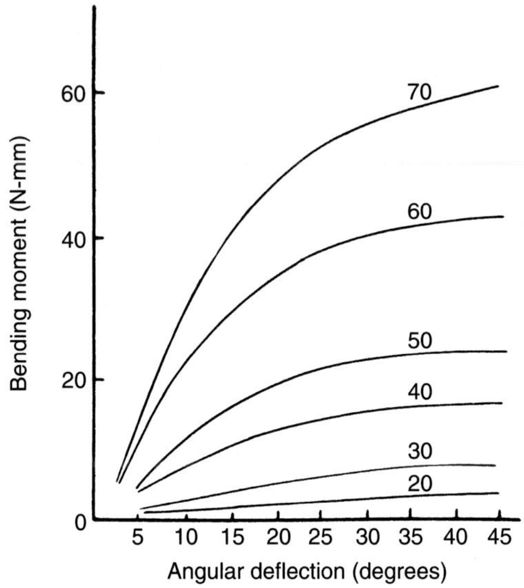

Fig. 4-15 Bending moment–angular deflection curves for endodontic reamers sizes 20 through 70.

BOND STRENGTH

A variety of tests have been developed to measure the bond strength between two materials, such as porcelains or laboratory composites to metal; cements to metal; or polymers, ceramics, resin composites, and adhesives to human enamel and dentin. Most of the tests are designed to place the bond in tension, although a few, especially for ceramics to metals, place the bond in shear. To simulate oral conditions, many of the test specimens are subjected to cycles of varying temperature, ranging from 5° to 50° C, before measuring bond strength. These bond-strength values may not simulate the clinical situation because of differences between the geometry of the test specimens and the clinical application. Bond strength values typically overestimate the bond strength obtained in clinical usage and should therefore be viewed with caution.

BENDING

The bending properties of many materials are as or more important than their tensile or compressive properties. The bending properties of stainless steel wires, endodontic files and reamers, and hypodermic needles are especially important. For example, ANSI/ADA Specification No. 28 for endodontic files and reamers requires bending tests.

Bending properties are usually measured by clamping a specimen at one end and applying a force at a fixed distance from the face of the clamp. Specimens are subjected to conditions that resemble pure bending, and cantilever beam theory has been used to analyze the data. As the force is increased and the specimen is bent, corresponding values for the angle of bending and the bending moment (force × distance) are recorded. Graphic plots of the bending moment versus the angle of bending are similar in appearance to stress-strain curves. As an example, a series of plots for various sizes of endodontic reamers is shown in Fig. 4-15. An instrument will be permanently bent if the bending angle exceeds the value at the end of the linear portion of the curve. The larger instruments are stiffer, as shown by the initial steeper slope. The initial linear portion of the curve is shorter for the larger instruments and thus the deviation from linearity occurred at lower angular bends.

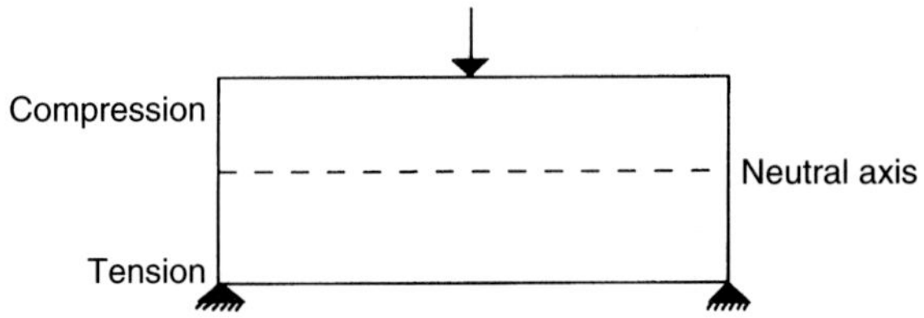

Fig. 4-16 Schematic of a three-point bending (transverse strength, flexural strength, modulus of rupture) test.

The maximum bending stress σ in a wire is

$$\sigma = My/I$$

where M is the bending moment, y is the distance from the neutral axis (plane of the specimen which is stress free) to the outer surface of specimen, and I is the moment of inertia, which indicates the distribution of forces relative to the specimen geometry.

The maximum angle of bending, θ_{max}, of a wire fixed at one end may be determined by the following formula:

$$\theta_{max} = Ml/EI$$

where l is the distance from the point of force application to the fixed end, and E is the modulus. For round wires with $l/d \sim 15$ and $l = 25$ mm, the elastic modulus in bending (also called *modulus of stiffness*) approximates the elastic modulus in tension. The equation is

$$E = (32\,l/\pi d^4)M/\theta$$

where l is the span length of the wire, d is the diameter of the wire, and M/θ is the slope of a plot of bending moment versus angular deflection in radians. The use of cantilever beam theory to calculate E results in values about two thirds those determined in tension.

TABLE 4-10 Values of Transverse Strength for Some Restorative Dental Materials

Material	Transverse Strength (MPa)
Gold foil	292
Resin composite	139
Lathe-cut amalgam	124
Feldspathic porcelain	65
High-strength stone	17

TRANSVERSE STRENGTH

The transverse strength of a material is obtained when one loads a simple beam, supported at each end, with a load applied in the middle (Fig. 4-16). Such a test is called a *three-point bending (3PB) test* and transverse strength is often described in technical, dental, and engineering literature as the *modulus of rupture* (MOR) or *flexural strength*. The transverse strengths for several dental materials are shown in Table 4-10. The transverse strength test is especially useful in comparing denture base materials in which a stress of this type is applied to the denture during mastication. This test determines not only the strength of the material indicated, but also the amount of distortion expected. The transverse strength test is a part of ANSI/ADA Specification No. 12 (ISO 1567) for denture base resins. The transverse strength and accompanying deformation are important also in long bridge spans in which the biting stress may be severe.

The stresses and deflections in three-point bending can be determined as specific cases of the more general formulae presented in the last section. A beam having a rectangular cross section of width, *b,* and height, *d,* has a moment of inertia of

$$I = bd^3/12$$

For a load, *P,* applied in the center, the bending moment is

$$M = \frac{1}{4Pl}$$

Substituting these relations for *I* and *M* into the general equation $\theta = My/I$, the equation for the maximum stress developed in a rectangular beam loaded in the center of the span becomes

$$\text{Stress} = \frac{3 \times \text{Load} \times \text{Length}}{2 \times \text{Width} \times \text{Thickness}^2}$$

or

$$\sigma = \frac{3Pl}{2bd^2}$$

The resulting deformation or displacement in such a beam or bridge can be calculated from

$$\text{Deformation} = \frac{\text{Load} \times \text{Length}^3}{4 \times \text{Elastic modulus} \times \text{Width} \times \text{Thickness}^3}$$

or

$$\delta = \frac{Pl^3}{4Ebd^3}$$

The significance of the length, thickness, and width of the restoration in relation to the strength and deformation is evident from these formulae. Both the length and the thickness of the span are critical, because the deformation varies as the cube of these two dimensions.

As a numerical example, consider a simple beam, such as the one shown in Fig. 4-16, with a rectangular cross section of 6.4 mm in thickness and 25.4 mm in height and a concentrated load of 666 N applied in the center. The total length of the beam is 102 mm, and the distance between supports is 89 mm. Because this is a static situation (i.e., the beam does not move), the reactant forces at the supports in this symmetrical loading are 333 N each. The solution for this beam may be calculated as follows:

$$M = \frac{1}{4}Pl = \frac{1}{4} \times 666\ \text{N} \times 89\ \text{mm} = 14{,}800\ \text{mmN}$$

The moment of inertia is determined by

$$I = (6.4)(25.4)^3/12 = 8740\ \text{mm}^4$$

Thus at the lower surface of the beam, y = 12.7 mm and

$$\sigma = \frac{14{,}800\ \text{mmN} \times 12.7\ \text{mm}}{8740\ \text{mm}^4}$$

or 21.5 MPa. The lower surface of the beam is under a tensile stress of 21.5 MPa, and the upper surface is under a compressive stress of 21.5 MPa. The maximum deflection is

$$\frac{-PL^3}{48EI} = -0.36\ \text{mm}$$

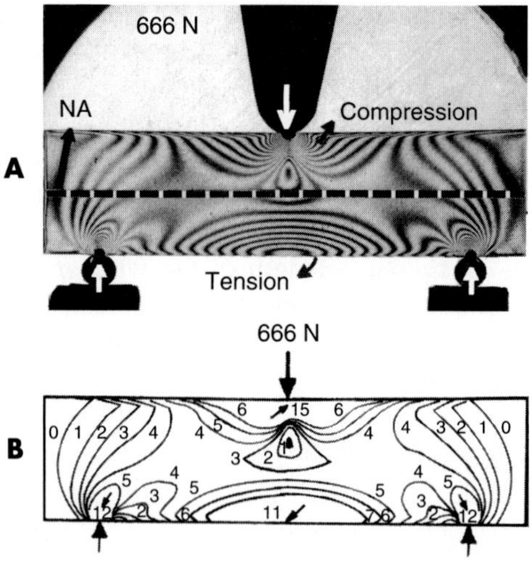

Fig. 4-17 Analysis of transverse bending. **A,** Photoelastic model with isochromatic fringes. **B,** Drawing to illustrate isochromatic fringe order.

The transverse strength of a beam can also be determined by the photoelastic method of analysis. A model of the simple beam used in this example is shown in Fig. 4-17, *A*. The isochromatic fringes, or lines of constant principle stress, are shown in Fig. 4-17, *A*, with the neutral axis, *NA*. The fringe order of the isochromatics is shown in Fig. 4-17, *B*, and the isotropic point can be seen in the center. Below the loading point and above the support points, the beam is in compression, whereas in the center of the lower portion of the beam it is in tension. Along any isochromatic fringe the difference in the principal stresses is constant, and the difference in the state of stress between fringes is 0.41 MPa/fringe.

PERMANENT BENDING

During fabrication, many dental restorations are subjected to permanent bending. The adjustment of removable partial denture clasps and the shaping of orthodontic appliances are two examples of such bending operations. Bends are also often introduced into hypodermic needles or root canal files in service. Comparisons of wires and needles of different compositions and diameters subjected to repeated 90-degree bends are often made. The number of bends a specimen will withstand is influenced by its composition and dimensions, as well as its treatment in fabrication. Such tests are important because this information is not readily related to standard mechanical test data such as tensile properties or hardness. Severe tensile and compressive stresses can be introduced into a material subjected to permanent bending. It is partly for this reason that tensile and compressive test data on a material are so important.

TORSION

Another mode of loading important to dentistry is torsion or twisting. For example, when an endodontic file is clamped at the tip and the handle is rotated, the instrument is subjected to torsion. Because most endodontic files and reamers are rotated in the root canal during endodontic treatment, their properties in torsion are of particular interest. ANSI/ADA Specification No. 28 for endodontic files and reamers describes a test to measure resistance to fracture by twisting with a torque meter. Torsion results in a shear stress and a rotation of the specimen. In these types of applications, we are interested in the relation between torsional moment (M_t = shear force × distance) and angular rotation π. A series of graphs in which the torsional moment was measured as a function of angular rotation is shown in Fig. 4-18. In this example, the instruments were twisted clockwise, which results in an untwisting of the instrument. As was the case with bending, the curves appear similar to stress-strain curves, with an initial linear portion followed by a nonlinear portion. The instruments should be used clinically so that they are not subjected to permanent angular rotation; thus the degrees of rotation should be limited to values within the linear portion of the torsional moment-angular rotation curves. The larger instruments are stiffer in torsion than the smaller ones, but their linear portion is less. The irregular shape of the curves at high angular rotation results from the untwisting of the instruments.

The resultant shear stress in a wire of radius *r* may be calculated from

$$\tau = M_t \times r/I_z$$

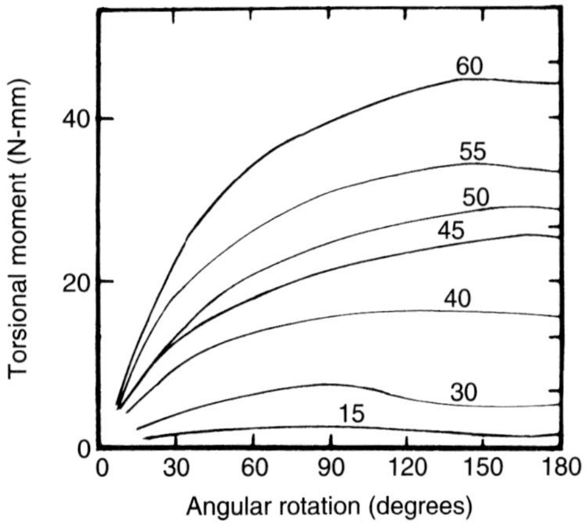

Fig. 4-18 Torsional moment-angular rotation curves for endodontic files sizes 15 through 60.

TABLE 4-11 Viscosity of Some Dental Materials Soon after Mixing

Material	Temperature (° C)	Viscosity (cp)
Cements		
Zinc phosphate	18	43,200
	25	94,700
Zinc polyacrylate	18	101,000
	25	109,800
Endodontic sealers	37	7000-678,000
Fluid denture resins	23	67-575
Impression materials		
Agar	45	281,000
Alginate	37	252,000
Impression plaster	37	23,800
Polysulfide, light	37	57,200
Polysulfide, heavy	36	1,360,000
Silicone, syringe	37	95,000
Silicone, regular	36	420,000
Zinc oxide-eugenol	37	99,600

listed in Table 4-11. As a basis for comparison, the viscosity of water at 20° C is 1 cp.

Rearranging the equation for viscosity, we see that fluid behavior can be described in terms of stress and strain, just like elastic solids.

$$\tau = \eta[d\epsilon/dt]$$

In the case of an elastic solid, stress (σ) is proportional to strain (ϵ), with the constant of proportionality being the modulus of elasticity *(E)*. The above equation indicates an analogous situation for a viscous fluid, where the (shear) stress is proportional to the strain rate and the constant of proportionality is the viscosity. The stress is therefore time dependent because it is a function of the strain rate, or rate of loading. To better comprehend the concept of strain rate dependence, consider two limiting cases—rapid and slow deformation. A material pulled extremely fast ($dt \rightarrow 0$) results in an infinitely high stress, whereas a material pulled infinitesimally slow results in a stress of zero.

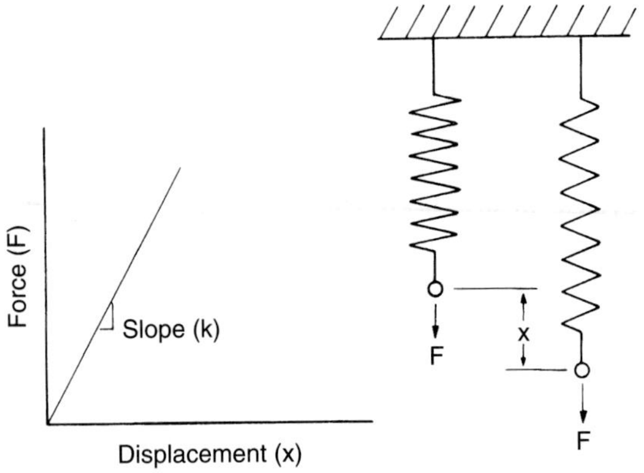

Fig. 4-20 Force versus displacement of a spring, which can be used to model the elastic response of a solid.
(From Park JB: *Biomaterials science and engineering,* New York, 1984, Plenum Press, p 26.)

The behavior of elastic solids and viscous fluids can be understood from simple mechanical models. An elastic solid can be viewed as a spring (Fig. 4-20). When the spring is stretched by a force, *F,* it displaces a distance, *x*. The applied force and resultant displacement are proportional, and the constant of proportionality is the spring constant, *k*. Therefore

$$F = k \times x$$

Note that this relation is equivalent to

$$\sigma = E \times \epsilon$$

Also note that the model of an elastic element does not involve time. The spring acts instanta-

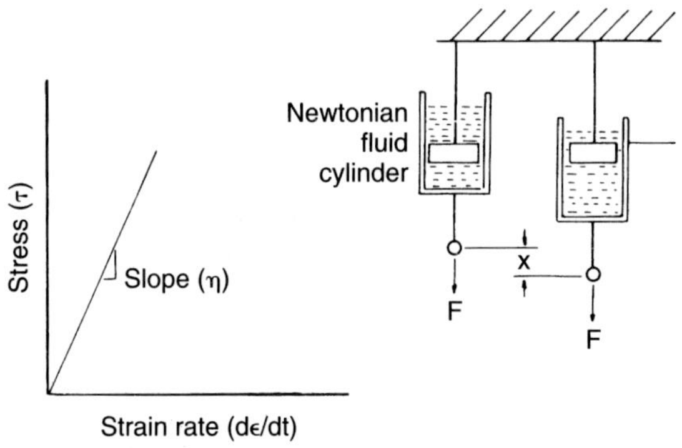

Fig. 4-21 Stress versus strain rate for a dashpot, which can be used to model the response of a viscous fluid.

(From Park JB: *Biomaterials science and engineering*, New York, 1984, Plenum Press, p 26.)

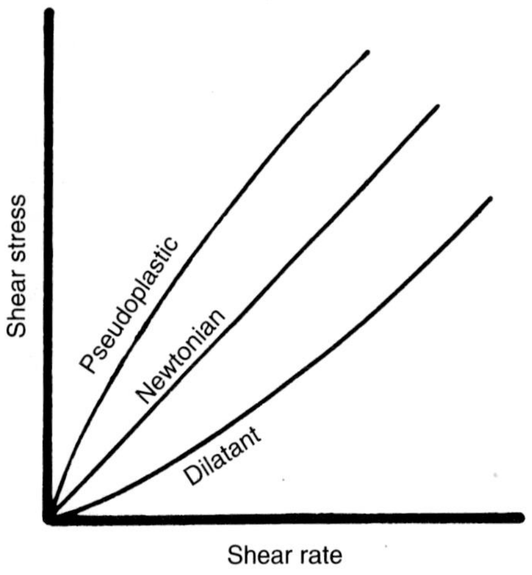

Fig. 4-22 Shear diagrams of Newtonian, pseudoplastic, and dilatant liquids. The viscosity is shown by the slope of the curve at a given shear rate.

neously when stretched. In other words, an elastic solid is independent of loading rate.

A viscous fluid can be viewed as a dashpot, or a shock absorber with a damping fluid (Fig. 4-21). When the fluid-filled cylinder is pulled, the rate of straining *(dε/dt)* is proportional to the stress *(τ)* and the constant of proportionality is the viscosity of the fluid *(η)*.

Although the viscosity of a fluid is proportional to the shear rate, the proportionality differs for different fluids. Fluids may be classified as Newtonian, pseudoplastic, or dilatant depending on how their viscosity varies with shear rate, as shown in Fig. 4-22. The viscosity of a Newtonian liquid is constant and independent of shear rate. Certain dental cements and impression materials are Newtonian. The viscosity of a pseudoplastic liquid decreases with increasing shear rate. Several endodontic cements are pseudoplastic, as are monophase rubber impression materials. When subjected to low shear rates during spatulation or while an impression is made in a tray, these impression materials have a high viscosity and possess "body" in the tray. These materials, however, can also be used in a syringe, because at the higher shear rates encountered as they pass through the syringe tip, the viscosity decreases by as much as tenfold. The viscosity of a dilatant liquid increases with increasing shear rate. Examples of dilatant liquids in dentistry include the fluid denture-base resins.

Two additional factors that influence the viscosity of a material are time and temperature. The viscosity of a non-setting liquid is typically independent of time and decreases with increasing temperature. Most dental materials, however, begin to set after the components have been mixed, and their viscosity increases with time, as evidenced by most dental cements and impression materials. A notable exception is a zinc oxide–eugenol material that requires moisture to set. On the mixing pad, these materials maintain a constant viscosity that is described clinically as a long working time. Once placed in the mouth, however, the zinc oxide–eugenol materials show rapid increases in viscosity because exposure to heat and humidity accelerates the setting reaction.

In general, for a material that sets, viscosity increases with increasing temperature. However, the effect of heat on the viscosity of a material that sets depends on the nature of the setting reaction. For example, the initial viscosities of a zinc phosphate cement (material *A*) and a zinc polycarboxylate cement (material *B*) are compared at three temperatures in Fig. 4-23. The setting reaction of *A* is highly exothermic, and mixing at reduced temperatures results in a lower viscosity than when mixed at higher temperatures. The setting reaction of *B* is less affected by temperature. Clinically, additional working time is achieved for these cements by the use of cool- or frozen-slab mixing techniques.

VISCOELASTIC MATERIALS

For viscoelastic materials, altering the strain rate alters the stress-strain properties. The tear strength of alginate impression material, for example, is increased about four times when the rate of loading is increased from 2.5 to 25 cm/min. Another example of strain-rate dependence is the elastic modulus of dental amalgam, which is 21 GPa at slow rates of loading and 62 GPa at high rates of loading. A viscoelastic material therefore may have widely different mechanical properties depending on the rate of load application, and for these materials it is particularly important to specify the loading rate with the test results.

Materials that have properties dependent on the strain rate are better characterized by relating stress or strain as a function of time. Two properties of importance to viscoelastic materials are stress relaxation and creep. *Stress relaxation* is the reduction in stress in a material subjected to constant strain, whereas *creep* is the increase in strain in a material under constant stress.

As an example of stress relaxation, consider how the load-time curves at constant deformation are important in the evaluation of orthodontic elastic bands. The decrease in load (or force) with time for a latex and a plastic band of the same size at a constant extension of 95 mm is shown in Fig. 4-24. The initial force was much greater with the plastic band, but the decrease in force with time was much less for the latex band. Therefore plastic bands are useful for applying high forces, although the force decreases rapidly with time, whereas latex bands apply lower

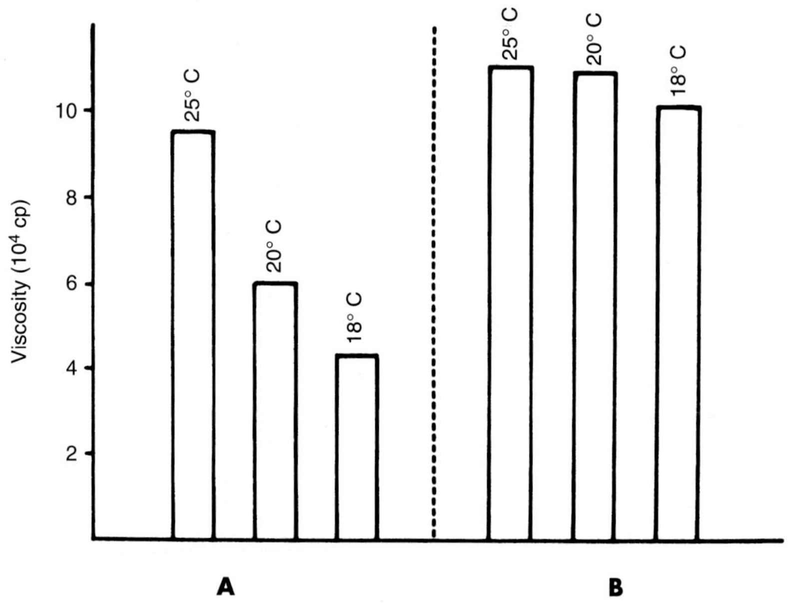

Fig. 4-23 Changes in initial viscosity with temperature of **A,** a zinc phosphate cement, and **B,** a zinc polycarboxylate cement.
(Adapted from Vermilyea S, Powers JM, Craig RG: *J Dent Res* 56:762, 1977.)

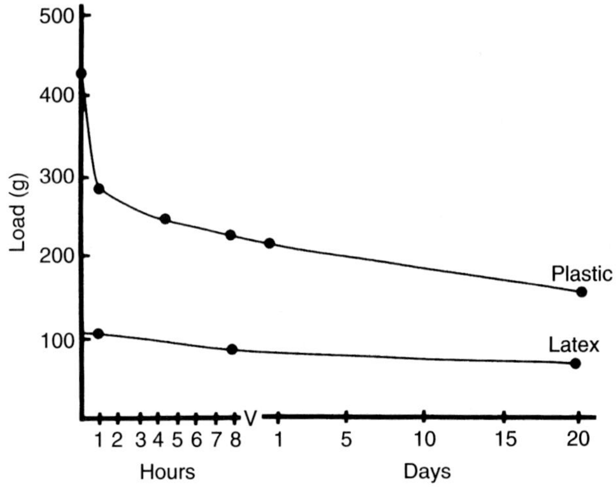

Fig. 4-24 Decrease in load of latex rubber and plastic bands as a function of time at a constant extension of 95 mm.
(From Craig RG, editor: *Dental materials: a problem-oriented approach,* St Louis, 1978, Mosby-Year Book.)

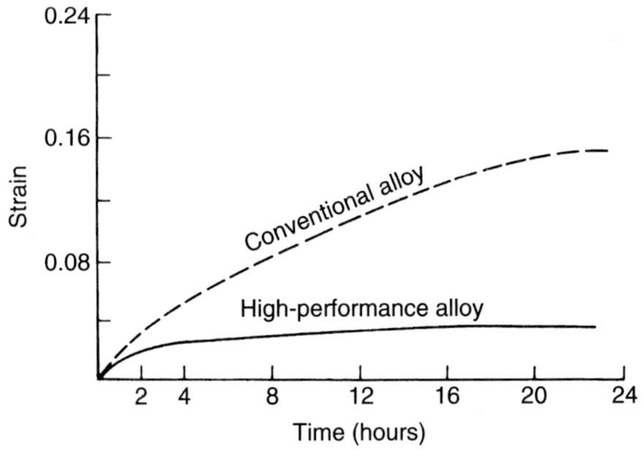

Fig. 4-25 Creep curves for conventional (low copper) and high-performance (high copper) amalgams.
(From O'Brien WJ: *Dental materials: properties and selection,* Chicago, 1989, Quintessence, p 25.)

forces, but the force decreases slowly with time in the mouth; latex bands are therefore useful for applying more sustained loads.

The importance of creep can be seen by interpreting the data in Fig. 4-25, which shows creep curves for low- and high-copper amalgam. For a given load at a given time, the low-copper amalgam has a greater strain. The implications and clinical importance of this are that the greater creep in the low-copper amalgam makes it more susceptible to strain accumulation and fracture, and also marginal breakdown, which can lead to secondary decay. Note that low-copper amalgam is no longer commonly used in dentistry.

MECHANICAL MODELS OF VISCOELASTICITY

Because a viscoelastic material may be viewed as a material exhibiting characteristics of both a solid and a fluid, we may also understand the behavior of a viscoelastic material in terms of combinations of the simple mechanical models of a spring and dashpot, introduced previously. Strain as a function of time for the various combinations is shown in Fig. 4-26. When a constant load is applied (at time t_0) to a spring (an ideal elastic element), an instantaneous strain occurs and the strain remains constant with time; when the load is removed (at time t_1), the strain instantaneously decreases to zero. When a constant

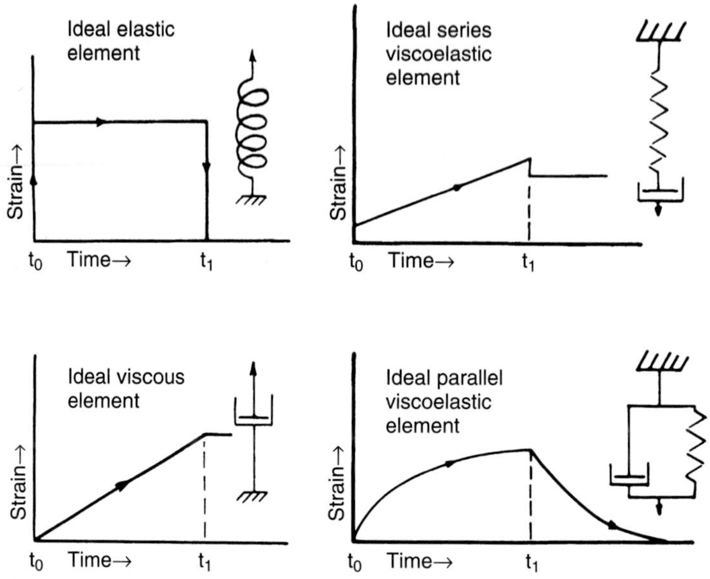

Fig. 4-26 Strain-time relationship of combinations of springs and viscous elements. A constant load is applied at time t_0 and removed at time t_1.

load is applied to an ideal viscous element, the strain increases linearly with time, and when the load is removed, no further increase or decrease in strain is observed. The elastic element reacts instantaneously (changes strain) to a change in load, and the viscous element reacts after a finite time.

The relative time-course of spring and dashpot reactions is observed when the two ideal elements are combined. When a spring and viscous element are in series (a Maxwell model) and a fixed load is applied, a rapid increase in strain occurs and is followed by a linear increase in strain with time. The resultant strain, often referred to as the *viscoelastic strain,* represents a combination of elastic and viscous responses. The rapid increase in strain represents the elastic portion of the strain (i.e., response of the elastic spring), whereas the linear increase represents the viscous portion of the strain (i.e., response of the viscous component). When the load is removed an instantaneous recovery of the elastic strain occurs, but the viscous strain remains.

A constant load applied to a spring and viscous element in parallel (a Kelvin or Voigt model) causes a nonlinear increase in strain with time as a result of the viscous element and reaches a constant value as a result of the spring. On removal of the load, the spring acts to decrease the strain to zero. However, the strain does not instantaneously diminish to zero because of the action of the dashpot. Note that real materials exhibit more complex behavior than these simple models predict, and modeling the strain-time properties requires a combination of the elements described. Impression materials such as agar, alginate, polysulfide, and silicone have been modeled by a Maxwell model in series with a Kelvin model.

An example of the importance of viscoelasticity lies with impression materials. Because these materials are viscoelastic, they do not immediately lose their strain when a load is removed. Therefore on removal from the mouth, these materials remain stressed, and thus time is required for the material to recover before a die can be poured.

The viscoelasticity of the oral tissues also has important clinical implications. The palatal mucosa has little resistance to loading compared

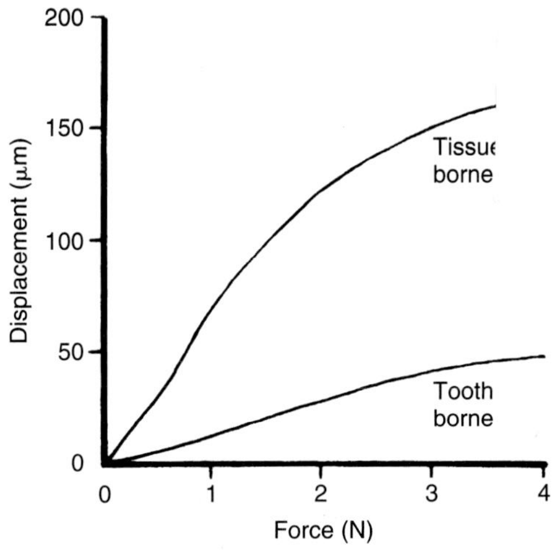

Fig. 4-27 Displacement versus force for denture baseplates supported by six teeth and by mucosa alone. Loading rate was 4 N/sec.

(Adapted from Wills DJ, Manderson RD: *J Dent* 5:310, 1977.)

with the periodontal ligament. Thus denture baseplates supported by palatal mucosa show substantially more displacement as a function of load than those supported by teeth (Fig. 4-27). The creep of the palatal mucosa under load is sustained and recovery is prolonged and variable because the mechanism of deformation and recovery is controlled by physiological and physical factors. Making an impression of the mucosal tissues in their resting state therefore requires that the tissues be allowed to recover free of the denture for several hours. Teeth, on the other hand, will recover from load within minutes. Recording the mucosal tissues under load will result in recoil of these tissues, initially displacing the denture base and artificial teeth to a position superior to the natural teeth. However, the tissues will return to their displaced state on loading of the denture.

CREEP COMPLIANCE

A creep curve yields insight into the relative elastic, viscous, and anelastic response of a viscoelastic material; such curves can be interpreted in terms of the molecular structure of the associated materials, which have structures that function as elastic, viscous, and anelastic elements. On removal of a load, a creep recovery curve can be obtained (Fig. 4-28). In such a curve, after the load is removed there is an instantaneous drop in strain and a slower strain decay to some steady-state strain value, which may be nonzero. The instantaneous drop in strain represents the recovery of elastic strain. The slower recovery represents the anelastic strain, and the remaining, permanent strain represents the viscous strain. A family of creep curves can be determined by using different loads. A more useful way of presenting these data is by calculating the creep compliance. *Creep compliance* (J_t) is defined as strain divided by stress at a given time. Once a creep curve is obtained, a corresponding creep compliance curve can be calculated. The creep compliance curve shown in Fig. 4-29 is characterized by the equation

$$J_t = J_0 + J_R + (t/\eta)$$

where J_0 is the instantaneous elastic compliance, J_R is the retarded elastic (anelastic) compliance, and t/η represents the viscous response at time t for a viscosity η. The strain associated with J_0 and J_R is completely recoverable after the load is removed; however, the strain associated with J_R is not recovered immediately but requires some finite time. The strain associated with t/η is not recovered and represents a permanent deformation. If a single creep compliance curve is calculated from a family of creep curves determined at different loads, the material is said to be linearly viscoelastic. Then the viscoelastic qualities can be described concisely by a single curve.

The creep compliance curve therefore permits an estimate of the relative amount of elastic, anelastic, and viscous behavior of a material. J_0 indicates the flexibility and initial recovery after deformation, J_R the amount of delayed recovery that can be expected, and t/η the magnitude of permanent deformation to be expected. Creep compliance curves for elastomeric impression materials are shown in Chapter 12, Fig. 12-25.

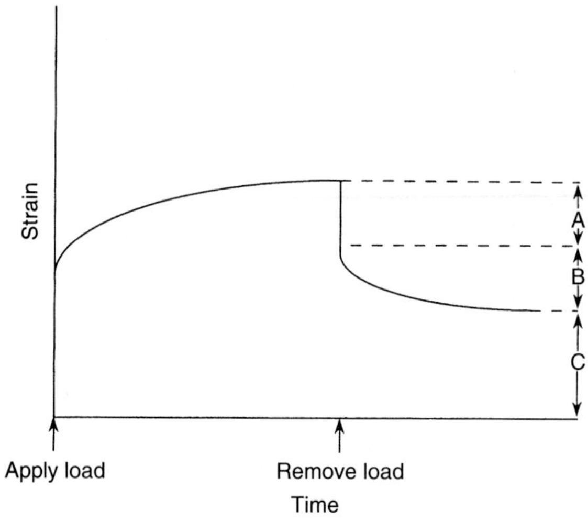

Fig. 4-28 Creep recovery curve, showing *A*, elastic, *B*, anelastic, and *C*, viscous strain.

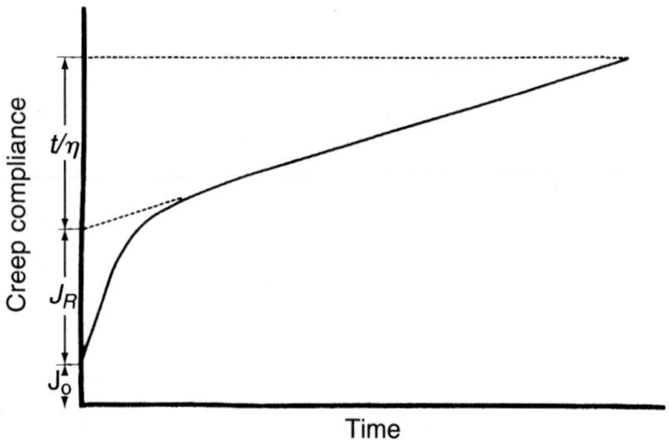

Fig. 4-29 Creep compliance versus time for a viscoelastic material.

(Adapted from Duran RL, Powers JM, Craig RG: *J Dent Res* 58:1801, 1979.)

DYNAMIC MECHANICAL PROPERTIES

Although static properties can often be related to the function of a material under dynamic conditions, there are limitations to using static properties to estimate the properties of materials subjected to dynamic loading. *Static testing* refers to continuous application of force at slow rates of loading, whereas *dynamic testing* involves cyclic loading or loading at high rates (commonly referred to as *impact*). Dynamic methods, including a forced oscillation technique used to determine dynamic modulus and a torsion pendulum used for impact testing, have been used to study viscoelastic materials such as dental polymers. Ultrasonic techniques have been used to determine elastic constants of viscoelastic materials such as dental amalgam and dentin. Impact testing has been applied primarily to brittle dental materials.

DYNAMIC MODULUS

The *dynamic modulus* (E_D) is defined as the ratio of stress to strain for small cyclical deformations at a given frequency and at a particular point on the stress-strain curve. When measured in a forced oscillation instrument, the dynamic modulus is computed by

$$E_D = mqp^2$$

where m is the mass of the vibrating yoke, q is the height divided by twice the area of the cylindrical specimen, and p is the angular frequency of the vibrations.

In conjunction with the dynamic modulus, values of internal friction and dynamic resilience can be determined. For example, cyclical stretching or compression of an elastomer results in irreversibly lost energy that manifests itself as heat. The internal friction of an elastomer is compara-

TABLE 4-12 Values of Dynamic Modulus and Dynamic Resilience as a Function of Temperature for Some Dental Elastomers

Material	Temperature (° C)	Dynamic Modulus (MPa)	Dynamic Resilience (%)
Maxillofacial materials			
Polyurethane	−15	5.98	15.0
	37	3.06	19.9
Polyvinylchloride	−15	12.2	6.0
	37	2.51	19.6
Silicone	−15	2.84	16.0
	37	2.36	23.2
Polyvinylacetate-polyethylene mouth protectors			
New	37	9.39	23.4
Worn	37	7.23	20.2

ble with the viscosity of a liquid. The value of internal friction is necessary to calculate the *dynamic resilience,* which is the ratio of energy lost to energy expended.

The dynamic modulus and dynamic resilience of some dental elastomers are listed in Table 4-12. These properties are affected by temperature (−15° to 37° C) for some maxillofacial elastomers, such as plasticized polyvinylchloride and polyurethane, but not so much for silicones. As shown in Table 4-12, the dynamic modulus decreases and the dynamic resilience increases as the temperature increases. As a tangible example, the dynamic resilience of a polymer used for an athletic mouth protector is a measure of the ability of the material to absorb energy from a blow and thereby protect the oral structure. Once the mouth protector has been worn, however, deterioration in properties is observed.

IMPACT STRENGTH

A material may have reasonably high static strength values, such as compressive, tensile, and shear strengths, and even reasonable elongation, but may fail when loaded under impact. Materials such as fused glasses, cements, amalgam, and some plastics have low resistance to breakage when a load is applied by an impact. Such a sudden blow might correspond to the energy of impact resulting from an accident to a person wearing a restoration or from dropping the restoration on a floor.

The impact resistance of materials is determined from the total energy absorbed before fracture when struck by a sudden blow. Often a bar of material is supported as a beam and struck either at one end or in the middle with a weighted pendulum. A test specimen in an impact instrument is shown in Fig. 4-30. The energy absorbed by the blow can be determined by measuring the reduction in swing of the pendulum compared with the swing with no specimen present. The values are usually reported in joules, J (1 J = 1 N m), for a specimen of a specific shape. Some substances offer relatively little resistance to the shock, whereas others of different composition may not fracture under the same impact. For example, the Charpy impact strength of unnotched specimens of denture resins ranges from 0.26 J for a conventional denture acrylic to 0.58 J for a rubber-modified acrylic resin.

TEAR STRENGTH AND TEAR ENERGY

Tear strength is a measure of the resistance of a material to tearing forces. Tear strength is an

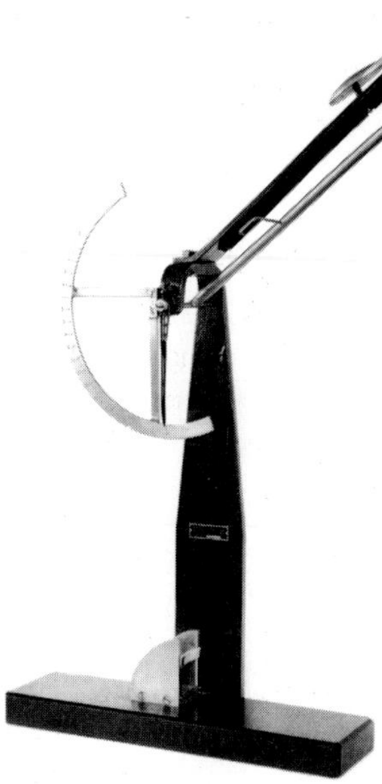

Fig. 4-30 Impact-testing instrument.

TABLE 4-13 Tear Strength of Some Dental Materials

Material	Tear Strength* kN/m
Agar duplicating material	0.22
Denture liners	2.6-45
Impression materials	
Agar	0.99
Alginate	0.47
Polysulfide	4.0
Polyvinylacetate-polyethylene mouth protectors	114

*Crosshead speed, 25 cm/min.

important property of dental polymers used in thin sections, such as flexible impression materials in interproximal areas, maxillofacial materials, and soft liners for dentures. Specimens are usually crescent shaped and notched. The tear strength of the notched specimen is calculated when the maximum load is divided by the thickness of the specimen, and the unit of tear strength is N/m.

Because of the viscoelastic nature of the materials tested, tear strength depends on the rate of loading. More rapid loading rates result in higher values of tear strength. Clinically, the rapid (or snap) removal of an alginate impression is recommended to maximize the tear strength and also to minimize permanent deformation. Typical values of tear strength are listed in Table 4-13 for some dental materials. The table indicates that the elastomeric impression materials have superior values of tear strength compared with agar and alginate hydrocolloids.

The tear energy *(T)* is a measure of the energy per unit area of newly torn surface and is determined from the load *(F)* required to propagate a tear in a trouser-shaped specimen by

$$T = (F/t)(\lambda + 1)$$

where t is the specimen thickness and λ is an extension ratio. Typical values of tear energy determined for some dental impression materials and maxillofacial materials are listed in Table 4-14.

MECHANICAL PROPERTIES OF COMPOSITES

Many materials used in dentistry are not homogeneous solids but consist of two or more essentially insoluble phases. There may be one continuous phase and one or more dispersed phases, or there may be two or more continuous phases, with each of these phases containing one or more dispersed phases. These materials are called *composites*. A composite can be generally defined as a combination of two or more different materials still present as separate entities in the final material. Although composites take advantage of selected properties of each material, the physical and mechanical properties of the composites are different from those of the

TABLE 4-14 Tear Energy of Some Dental Materials

Material	Tear Energy* (J/m^2 [$Mergs/cm^2$])
Impression materials	
Alginate	66 [0.066]
Polyether	640 [0.64]
Polysulfide	1100-3000 [1.1-3.0]
Silicone	390-1150 [0.39-1.15]
Maxillofacial materials	
Polyurethane	1800 [1.8]
Polyvinylchloride	11,000 [11]
Silicone rubber	660 [0.66]

*Crosshead speed, 2 cm/min.

separate phases. The trend in the development of materials for various applications is toward composites rather than completely new classes of materials. There can be metal, ceramic, and polymer-based composites. Important examples of dental composites include posterior resin composite used as direct esthetic restorative materials. Such composites are made from an organic polymer matrix (usually a diacrylate) filled with an inorganic phase, such as borosilicate or strontium glass, lithium or barium, aluminum silicate, or colloidal silica.

Factors that affect the properties of composites include: (1) the state of matter of the second (dispersed) phase; (2) the geometry of the second phase; (3) the orientation of the second phase; (4) the composition of the dispersed and continuous phases; (5) the ratio of the phases; and (6) bonding of the phases. Examples of properties that can be changed (improved if the composites are judiciously developed) are: (1) modulus, (2) strength, (3) fracture toughness, (4) wear resistance, (5) thermal expansion, and (6) chemical and corrosion resistance.

A simple example of how adding a second phase affects properties is now illustrated. Consider a series of continuous parallel glass fibers oriented in the same direction in a plastic matrix. If a tensile load is applied to the specimen in the direction of the fibers, the elastic modulus of the composite E_c is

$$E_c = E_f V_f + E_m V_m \quad \text{or} \quad E_f V_f + E_m (1 - V_f)$$

where E_c and E_m and V_f and V_m represent the elastic modulus and volume fraction of the fiber and matrix. If, on the other hand, the tensile load is applied in the direction transverse to the fibers, the composite elastic modulus would be

$$E_c = \frac{E_f E_m}{E_m E_f + E_f V_m}$$

If the volume fraction of fibers is zero (i.e., the material is strictly a polymer), the modulus is that of the polymer, and if the volume fraction is 100%, the material is a glass and has the modulus of glass. Thus the moduli of the polymer and glass serve as lower and upper bounds on the composite modulus. Furthermore, from the above two equations, we see that in addition to the ratio of the two phases, the orientation of the second phase also plays an important role in the composite properties.

The basis for the function of a dispersed phase in a matrix is shown in Fig. 4-31. A single fiber is shown surrounded by a matrix, and the tensile stress in the fiber is plotted versus the distance along the fiber. The load is applied to the matrix and is transferred to the fiber by shear at the interface. The elastic and plastic deformation in the matrix can be transferred to the fiber if the modulus of the matrix is less than that of the fiber. Also, the bond between the matrix and the fiber must be maintained or the stress will drop to the frictional force. As the load is increased, the tensile stress in the fiber may reach the ultimate shear stress and the fiber will fail.

Continually increasing the volume fraction of the fibers should continue to increase the strength of the composite. However, as the concentration of fibers increases, more and more contact of the fibers with each other occurs, and

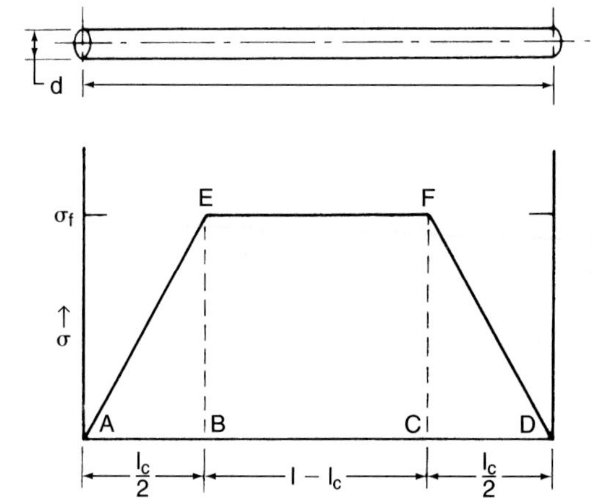

Fig. 4-31 Stress on a glass fiber in a plastic matrix. (Adapted from Titelman AS, McEvily AJ, Jr: *Fracture of structural materials,* New York, 1967, John Wiley & Sons, pp 635-661.)

premature rupture results. Therefore for many composites, the maximum strength occurs at a volume fraction of 80% for the dispersed phase.

As a further illustration of the factors that affect the properties of a composite, consider the filled resins used in dentistry. For many of these dental composites a random arrangement of the dispersed phase is used, even though a random orientation results in about a sixfold lower strength compared to an oriented dispersed phase. However, the resultant lower strength due to random second phase orientation can be counteracted in several ways. The use of a fine (e.g., <1 μm) dispersed phase increases strength. Also, the selection of the shape of the dispersed particles is important, with rods and plates being more effective than spheres in improving the strength. The principal factors needed are (1) a high-strength dispersed phase; (2) a more ductile matrix phase; (3) fine dispersed particles at the optimum volume fraction; and (4) adhesion between the dispersed and matrix phases. The last requirement is usually accomplished by treating the dispersed phase with an organosilane. The silanes, often called *coupling agents,* react with the glass or water adsorbed on the glass and form a bond with the resin.

SURFACE MECHANICAL PROPERTIES

In our discussion so far, we have introduced and discussed mechanical properties that are mainly dependent on the bulk characteristics of a material. In this section, mechanical properties that are more a function of the surface condition of a material are presented. In particular, the concepts of hardness, friction, and wear are summarized.

HARDNESS

The property of hardness is one of major importance in the comparison of restorative materials. *Hardness* may be broadly defined as the resistance to permanent surface indentation or penetration.

Formulating a more rigorous definition of hardness is difficult because any test method will, at a microscopic level, involve complex surface morphologies and stresses in the test material, thereby involving a variety of qualities in any single hardness test. Despite this condition, the most common concept of hard and soft substances is their relative resistance to indentation. Hardness is therefore a measure of the resistance to plastic deformation and is measured as a force per unit area of indentation (Fig. 4-32).

Based on this definition of hardness, it is clear why this property is so important to dentistry. Hardness is indicative of the ease of finishing of a structure and its resistance to in-service scratching. Finishing or polishing a structure is important for esthetic purposes and, as discussed previously, scratches can compromise fatigue strength and lead to premature failure.

Some of the most common methods of testing the hardness of restorative materials are the Brinell, Knoop, Vickers, Rockwell, Barcol, and Shore A hardness tests. Each of these tests differs slightly from the others, and each presents certain advantages and disadvantages. They have a common quality, however, in that each depends on the penetration of some small, symmetrically shaped indenter into the surface of the material being tested. The various hardness tests differ in the indenter material, geometry, and load. The indenter may be made of steel, tungsten carbide or diamond, and be shaped as a

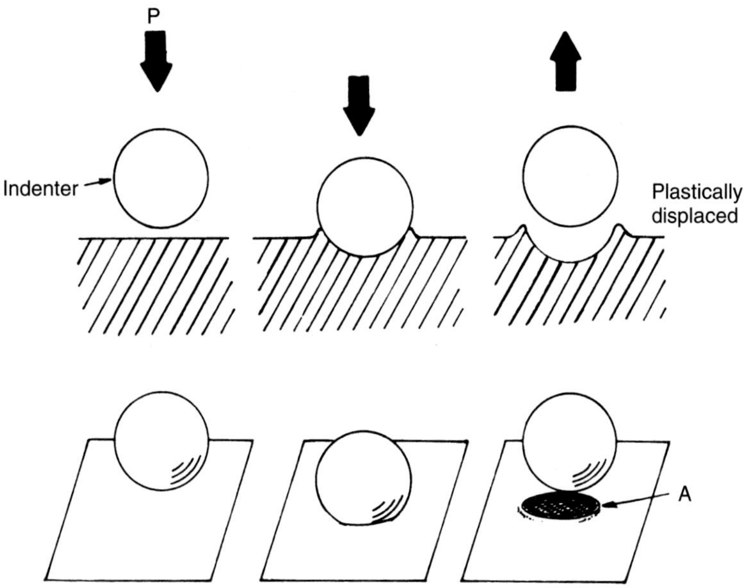

Fig. 4-32 Schematic representation of a hardness test. *A*, Area of plastic deformation; *P*, normal load.
(From Park JB: *Biomaterials science and engineering,* New York, 1984, Plenum Press, p 18).

sphere, cone, pyramid, or needle. Loads typically range from 1 to 3000 kg. The choice of a hardness test depends on the material of interest, the expected hardness range, and the desired degree of localization.

The general procedure for testing hardness, independent of the specific test, is as follows. A standardized force or weight is applied to the penetrating point. Applying such a force to the indenter produces a symmetrically shaped indentation, which can be measured under a microscope for depth, area, or width of the indentation produced. The indentation dimensions are then related to tabulated hardness values. With a fixed load applied to a standardized indenter, the dimensions of the indentation vary inversely with the resistance to penetration of the material tested. Thus lighter loads are needed for softer materials.

Brinell Hardness Test The Brinell hardness test is among the oldest methods used to test metals and alloys used in dentistry. The method depends on the resistance to the penetration of a small steel or tungsten carbide ball, typically 1.6 mm in diameter, when subjected to a weight of 123 N. In testing the Brinell hardness of a material, the penetrator remains in contact with the specimen tested for a fixed time of 30 seconds, after which it is removed and the indentation diameter is carefully measured. A diagram showing the principle of Brinell hardness testing, together with a microscopic view of the indentations into a gold alloy, is shown in Fig. 4-33. The resulting hardness value, known as the *Brinell hardness number* (BHN), is computed as a ratio of the load applied to the area of the indentation produced. The formula for computing the BHN is as follows:

$$\mathrm{BHN} = \frac{L}{\frac{\pi D}{2}\left(D - \sqrt{D^2 - d^2}\right)}$$

In this formula *L* is the load in kilograms, *D* is the diameter of the ball in millimeters, and *d* is the diameter of the indentation in millimeters, thus the units for BHN are kg/mm^2. The smaller

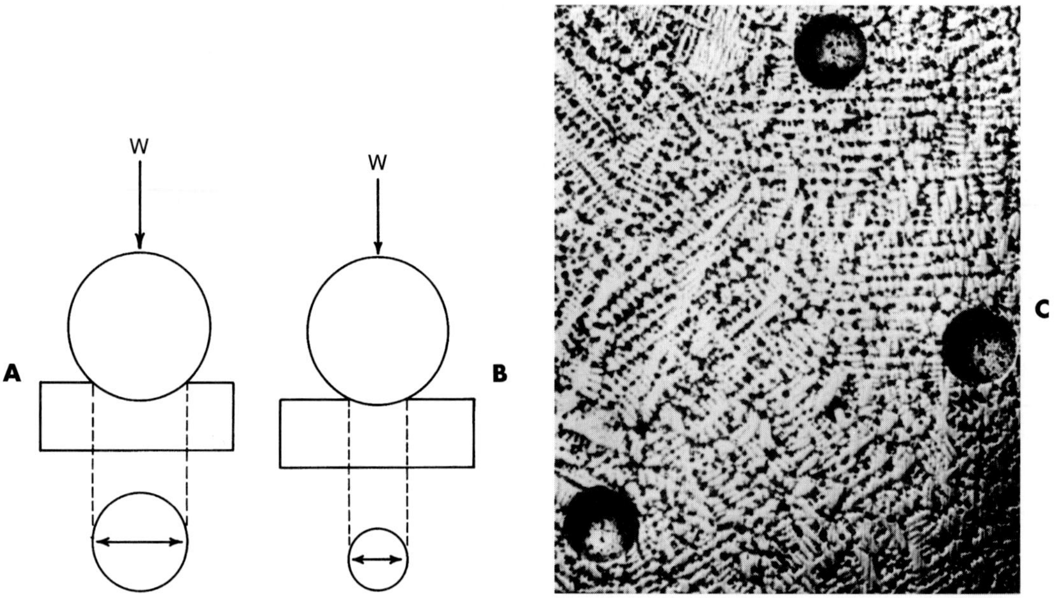

Fig. 4-33 Brinell hardness test. **A,** Indentation in soft material. **B,** Indentation in harder material. **C,** Microscopic view of indentations.

TABLE 4-15 Brinell Hardness Number (BHN) of Some Dental Casting Alloys and Condensed Gold

Material	BHN (kg/mm^2)
Condensed gold	
Foil	69
Powdered	46
Gold alloys*	
Type I	45
Type II	95
Type III	120
Type IV	220
40% Au-Ag-Cu	252
99% noble alloy†	165

*Alloys that are hardenable by heat treatment are in the hard condition.
†For metal-ceramic restorations.

the area of indentation, the harder the material and the larger the BHN value. Tables of Brinell hardness values have been developed from this formula for indentations of different diameters. Because the Brinell hardness test yields a relatively large indentation area, this test is good for determining average hardness values and poor for determining very localized values. The Brinell hardnesses of some dental casting alloys and condensed gold are listed in Table 4-15.

Knoop Hardness Test The Knoop hardness test was developed to fulfill the needs of a microindentation test method. A load is applied to a carefully prepared diamond indenting tool with a pyramid shape, and the lengths of the diagonals of the resulting indentation in the material are measured. The shape of the indenter and the resulting indentation are illustrated in Fig. 4-34, *A*. The Knoop hardness number (KHN) is the ratio of the load applied to the area of

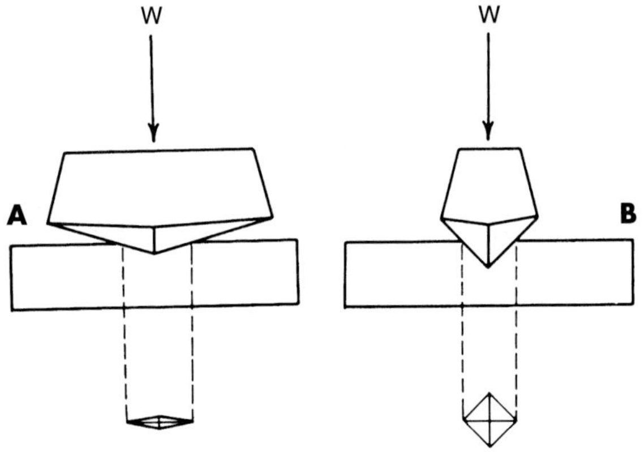

Fig. 4-34 A, Principle of the Knoop hardness measurement; **B,** the diamond pyramid (Vickers) indentation test.

the indentation calculated from the following formula:

$$KHN = \frac{L}{l^2 C_p}$$

In this equation L is the load applied, l is the length of the long diagonal of the indentation, and C_p is a constant relating l to the projected area of the indentation. The units for KHN are also kg/mm^2. Similar to the Brinell method, higher values for KHN represent harder materials.

The Knoop method is designed so varying loads may be applied to the indenting instrument. The resulting indentation area, therefore, varies according to the load applied and the nature of the material tested. The advantage of this method is that materials with a great range of hardness can be tested simply by varying the test load. Because very light load applications produce extremely delicate microindentations, this method of testing can be employed to examine materials that vary in hardness over an area of interest. For example, the Knoop method has been used extensively in testing the hardness of both enamel and dentin in extracted teeth and in determining the hardness of metals and alloys that have isolated hard and soft phases throughout the material. The chief disadvantages of the method are the need for a highly polished and flat test specimen and the time required to complete the test operation, which is considerably greater than that required for some other, less precisely controlled methods. The KHNs of some dental materials are listed in Table 4-16.

TABLE 4-16 Knoop Hardness Number (KHN) of Dental Materials

Material	KHN (kg/mm^2)
Silicon carbide abrasive	2480
Feldspathic porcelain	460
Cobalt-chromium partial denture alloy	391
Enamel	343
Gold foil	69
Dentin	68
Cementum	40
Zinc phosphate cement	38
Denture acrylic	21

Vickers Hardness Test The Vickers hardness test, or 136-degree diamond pyramid, is also suitable for testing the surface hardness of materials. It has been used to a limited degree to test the hardness of restorative dental materials. The method is similar in principle to the Knoop and Brinell tests, except that a 136-degree diamond pyramid-shaped indenter is forced into the material with a definite load application. The indenter produces a square indentation, the diagonals of which are measured as shown in Fig. 4-34, *B*. Equipment for Knoop hardness testing has been adapted to use the 136-degree indenter. Loads are varied from 1 to 120 kg, depending on the hardness of the tested material. The Vickers test is especially useful in measuring the hardness of small areas and for very hard materials.

Rockwell Hardness Test The Rockwell hardness test was developed as a rapid method for hardness determinations. A ball or metal cone indenter is normally used, and the depth of the indentation is measured with a sensitive dial micrometer. The indenter balls or cones are of several different diameters, as well as different load applications (60 to 150 kg), with each combination described as a special Rockwell scale, Rockwell A-G, denoted R_A, R_B, etc.

The superficial Rockwell method has been used to test plastics used in dentistry. This method uses a relatively light (30 kg) load and a large-diameter (12.7 mm) ball in comparison with the standard Rockwell methods. The test is made by first applying a preload (minor load) of 3 kg. A major load of 30 kg then is applied to the specimen for 10 minutes before a reading is taken. Because dental plastics are viscoelastic, recovery of the indentation occurs once the major load has been removed. The percent recovery can be determined on the same specimen by the following equation:

$$\text{Percent recovery} = \frac{A - B}{A} \times 100\%$$

where *A* is the depth of the indentation caused by application of the major load for 10 minutes, and *B* is the depth of the indentation after the major load has been removed for 10 minutes. Values of indentation depth and percent recovery for some dental plastics are listed in Table 4-17. The advantages of the Rockwell hardness test are that hardness is read directly and it is good for testing viscoelastic materials. The disadvantages are that a preload is needed, greater time is required, and the indentation may disappear immediately on removal of the load.

TABLE 4-17 Indentation Depth and Percent Recovery of Some Dental Plastics

Material	Indentation Depth (μm)	% Recovery
Acrylic denture teeth	93	88
Pit and fissure sealants	85-158	74-86
Resin composite	56-72	70-83

Barcol Hardness Test Barcol hardness is one method used to study the depth of cure of resin composites. The Barcol indenter is a spring-loaded needle with a diameter of 1 mm that is pressed against the surface to be tested. If no penetration of the needle into the surface occurs, the scale reads 100. The reading on the scale decreases as the indenter penetrates the surface. Depth of cure of a resin composite is tested by preparing specimens varying in thickness from 0.5 to 6.0 mm or more in increments of 0.5 mm. Then the top surface of a specimen is activated by a light-curing unit. The Barcol hardness of the top surface is compared with that of the bottom surface. The depth of cure is defined as the maximum thickness at which the Barcol reading of the bottom surface does not change by more than 10% of the reading of the top surface. Research has shown that a 10% decrease in Barcol hardness of a resin composite results in a 20% decrease in the flexural strength.

Shore A Hardness Test The hardness measurements described previously cannot be used to determine the hardness of rubbers, because the indentation disappears after the removal of the load. An instrument called a *Shore A Durometer* is used in the rubber industry to

TABLE 4-18 Values of Shore A Hardness for Some Dental Materials

Material	Shore A Hardness
Resilient denture liners	48-85
Polyvinylacetate-polyethylene mouth protector	67
Silicone maxillofacial elastomer	25

determine the relative hardness of elastomers. The instrument consists of a blunt-pointed indenter 0.8 mm in diameter that tapers to a cylinder 1.6 mm. The indenter is attached by a lever to a scale that is graduated from 0 to 100 units. If the indenter completely penetrates the specimen, a reading of 0 is obtained, and if no penetration occurs, a reading of 100 units results. Because rubber is viscoelastic, an accurate reading is difficult to obtain because the indenter continues to penetrate the rubber as a function of time. The usual method is to press down firmly and quickly on the indenter and record the maximum reading as the Shore A hardness. The test has been used to evaluate soft denture liners, mouth protectors, and maxillofacial elastomers, values of which are listed in Table 4-18.

NANO-INDENTATION

Traditional indentation tests use loads as high as several kilograms and result in indentations as large as 100 μm. Although valuable for screening materials and determining relative values among different materials, these tests are subject to limitations. Many materials have microstructural constituents or, in the case of microfilled composites, filler phases substantially smaller than the dimensions of the indenter. To accurately measure the properties of these microphases, it is necessary to be able to create indentations of a smaller size scale and to spatially control the location of the indentations. In this regard, special indentation techniques have recently been introduced. These techniques, commonly referred to as nano-indentation, are able to apply loads in the range of 0.1 to 5000 mg, resulting in indentations approximately 1 μm in size. In addition, indentation depth is continuously monitored, obviating the need to image the indentation to compute mechanical properties. Although most commonly used to measure hardness of micron-sized phases, the technique is also useful for measuring modulus. For brittle materials, yield strength and fracture toughness may be determined.

The nano-hardness, dynamic hardness, and elastic moduli values of human enamel and dentin are listed in Table 4-19, along with the nano-hardness and elastic modulus for the region of the dentin-enamel junction. The nano-hardness of dentin of 71 kg/mm^2 agrees well with the Knoop value of 68 kg/mm^2 reported in Table 4-16; however, the nano-hardness of 457 kg/mm^2 for enamel is considerably higher than the Knoop value of 343 kg/mm^2. This difference may result from the much smaller indentation used in the nano-indentation test in relation to the size of the enamel rods. The dynamic hardness values are lower than those for the corresponding nano-hardness because they are calculated from the maximum displacement, whereas the nano-hardness values are calculated from the permanent deformation. The elastic moduli of 87.7 and 24.0 GPa for enamel and dentin by nano-indentation are in reasonable agreement with the values from compressive test specimens of 84.1 and 18.3 GPa, respectively. Of special interest is the elastic modulus of 53.2 GPa for the region of the dentin-enamel junction, which is intermediate to the values for enamel and dentin. The nano-indentation test is especially useful in studying this small region, which was not possible with compressive or tensile tests.

FRICTION

Friction is the resistance to motion of one material body over another. If an attempt is made to move one body over the surface of another, a restraining force to resist motion is produced

TABLE 4-19 Properties of Tooth Tissues from Nano-indentation Tests

	Nano-hardness		Dynamic Hardness		Elastic Modulus
Tissue	**GPa**	**kg/mm²**	**GPa**	**kg/mm²**	**GPa**
Enamel	4.48 (0.44)	457 (45)	2.90 (0.23)	295 (23)	87.7 (5.9)
DEJ	2.37	242			53.2
Dentin	0.70 (0.12)	71 (12)	0.55 (0.09)	56 (9)	24.0 (3.9)

Adapted from Urabe I, Nakajima M, Sano H et al: *Am J Dent* 13:129, 2000.
Numbers in parentheses represent standard deviations.
DEJ, Dento-enamel junction.

(Fig. 4-35). This restraining force is the (static) frictional force and results from the molecules of the two objects bonding where their surfaces are in close contact. The frictional force, F_s, is proportional to the normal force ($F_\perp$) between the surfaces and the (static) coefficient of friction (μ_s).

$$F_s = \mu_s \times F_\perp$$

The coefficient of friction varies between 0 and 1 and is a function of the two materials in contact, their composition, surface finish, and lubrication. Similar materials have a greater coefficient of friction, and if a lubricating medium exists at the interface, the coefficient of friction is reduced.

The conditions for motion are for the applied force to be greater than F_s. Once motion occurs, molecular bonds are made and broken, and microscopic pieces break off from the surfaces. With motion, a sliding or kinetic friction is produced, and the force of kinetic friction opposes the motion.

$$F_k = \mu_k \times F_\perp$$

Frictional behavior therefore arises from surfaces that, because of microroughness, have a small real contact area (see Fig. 4-35). These small surface areas result in high contact stresses, which lead to local yielding. The resistance to shear failure of the junctions results in the frictional force. When static friction is overcome and relative motion takes place, it is accompanied by the modification of the interface through kinetic friction and wear.

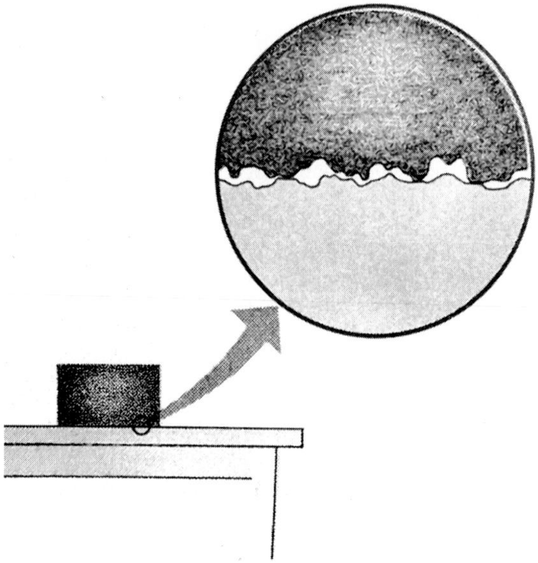

Fig. 4-35 Microscopic area of contact between two objects. The frictional force, which resists motion, is proportional to the normal force and the coefficient of friction.
(Adapted from Tipler PA: *Physics,* 1976, Worth, p 156.)

An example of the importance of friction in dentistry lies in the concept of roughening the surface of a dental implant to reduce motion between the implant and adjacent tissue. It is perceived that a rough surface and resultant less motion will provide for better osseointegration. Friction is also important in sliding mechanics used in the orthodontic movement of teeth.

WEAR

Wear is a loss of material resulting from removal and relocation of materials through the contact of two or more materials. When two solid materials are in contact, they touch only at the tips of their highest asperities (see Fig. 4-35). Wear is usually undesirable, but under controlled conditions during finishing and polishing procedures, wear is highly beneficial.

Several factors make wear of biomaterials unique. Most importantly, wear can produce biologically active particles, which can excite an inflammatory response. The wear process can also produce shape changes that can affect function. For example, wear in the oral cavity is characterized by the loss of the original anatomical form of the material. Wear of tooth structure and restorative materials may result from mechanical, physiological, or pathological conditions. Normal mastication may cause attrition of tooth structure or materials, particularly in populations that consume unprocessed foods. Bruxism is an example of a pathological form of wear in which opposing surfaces slide against each other. If improperly performed, tooth brushing with a dentifrice may cause an abrasive form of wear.

Wear is a function of a number of material and environmental factors, including the nature of wearing surfaces (i.e., inhomogeneity, crystal orientation, phases, and inclusions present); the microscopic contact; interaction between sliding surfaces (i.e., elevated stress, temperature, and flow at contact points, leading to localized yielding, melting, and hardening); lubrication; and different material combinations. In general, wear is a function of opposing materials and the interface between them. The presence of a lubricating film, such as saliva, separates surfaces during relative motion and reduces frictional forces and wear.

In general, there are four types of wear: (1) adhesive wear; (2) corrosive wear; (3) surface fatigue wear; and (4) abrasive wear. Adhesive wear is characterized by the formation and disruption of microjunctions. The volume of wear debris, *V*, is determined by

$$V = \frac{kF_{\perp}x}{3p}$$

where x is the total sliding distance, k is the wear coefficient, $F_{\perp}$ is the perpendicular force, and p is the surface hardness (of the softer material).

Abrasive wear involves a soft surface in contact with a harder surface. In this type of wear, particles are pulled off of one surface and adhere to the other during sliding. There can be two types of abrasive wear: two- and three-body abrasion (wear). This type of wear can be minimized if surfaces are smooth and hard and if particles are kept off the surfaces. Corrosive wear is secondary to physical removal of a protective layer and is therefore related to the chemical activity of the wear surfaces. The sliding action of the surfaces removes any surface barriers and causes accelerated corrosion. In surface fatigue wear, stresses are produced by asperities or free particles, leading to the formation of surface or subsurface cracks. Particles break off under cyclic loading and sliding.

In general, metals are susceptible to adhesive, corrosive and three-body wear, whereas polymers are susceptible to abrasive and fatigue wear.

Wear has been studied by (1) service or clinical testing, (2) simulated service measurements, (3) model systems using various wear machines, (4) measurements of related mechanical properties such as hardness, and (5) examination of the amount and type of surface failure from a single or low number of sliding strokes.

Two-body abrasion tests have been used to rank the wear resistance of restorative materials. As shown in Table 4-20, the resistance of composite resins to abrasion depends on the nature of the filler particles (glass or quartz) and on silanation of the filler. Three-body abrasion tests are often used to compare the abrasion resistance of tooth structure with that of dentifrices and

TABLE 4-20 Two-Body Abrasion of Restorative Dental Materials

Material	Two-Body Abrasion (10^{-4} mm^3/mm of Travel)
Amalgam	
Spherical	7.0
AgSn + AgCu	5.6
Composite resin	
Glass-filled	7.7
Glass-filled–no silane	13.8
Quartz-filled	3.8
Quartz-filled–no silane	5.6
Microfilled	12.0
Diacrylate resin	17.0
Pit and fissure sealant	21.5
Unfilled acrylic resin	13.3

prophylaxis materials. Enamel is about 5 to 20 times more resistant to abrasion than dentin. Cementum is the least resistant to abrasion. Measurements of enamel loss during a 30-second prophylaxis have shown that fluoride is removed from the enamel surface and have allowed estimation of the removal of enamel to be 0.6 to 4 μm, depending on the abrasive.

Unfortunately, a 1:1 ratio between wear observed clinically and that measured in the laboratory seldom exists. Thus most tests strive to rank materials in an order that is seen clinically. Traditional wear tests measure the volume of material lost but do not reveal mechanisms of wear, whereas a single-pass sliding technique may characterize modes of surface failure. In general, wear data do not correlate well with other mechanical property data, making it more difficult to infer wear properties from other, simpler, laboratory tests.

In the study and evaluation of wear, note that multiple processes occur simultaneously, and materials, mechanics, and environment have combined effects on wear. Most important is the fate of the wear particles. Are these particles dissolved or distributed? If they are distributed, is their migration local or systemic, and what biological consequences can arise?

STRESS ANALYSIS AND DESIGN OF DENTAL STRUCTURES

The mechanical properties of dental restoration materials must be able to withstand the stresses and strains caused by the repetitive forces of mastication. The design of dental restorations is particularly important if the best advantage of a material is to be taken. The necessary designs are those that do not result in stresses or strains that exceed the strength properties of a material under clinical conditions.

Stresses in dental structures have been studied by such techniques as brittle coatings analysis, strain gauges, holography, two- and three-dimensional photoelasticity, finite element analysis, and other numerical methods. Stress analysis studies of inlays, crowns, bases supporting restorations, fixed bridges, complete dentures, partial dentures, endodontic posts, and implants have been reported, as well as studies of teeth, bone, and oral soft tissues. The stress analysis literature is too extensive and beyond the scope of this text to review. Only brief summaries of two-dimensional photoelasticity and finite element analysis, and the advantages and disadvantages of both, are provided.

TWO-DIMENSIONAL PHOTOELASTICITY

The procedure for two-dimensional models is to prepare a transparent plastic or other isotropic model of the restoration or appliance. The material becomes anisotropic (its properties exhibit a directional dependence) when stressed, so the behavior of light is affected by the direction it takes. As a result of the applied stress, the plastic model exhibits double refraction because of its anisotropic structure. The light from a source passes through a polarizer, which transmits light waves parallel to the polarizing axis, known as *plane polarized light*. The plane polarized light is converted to circularly polarized light by a

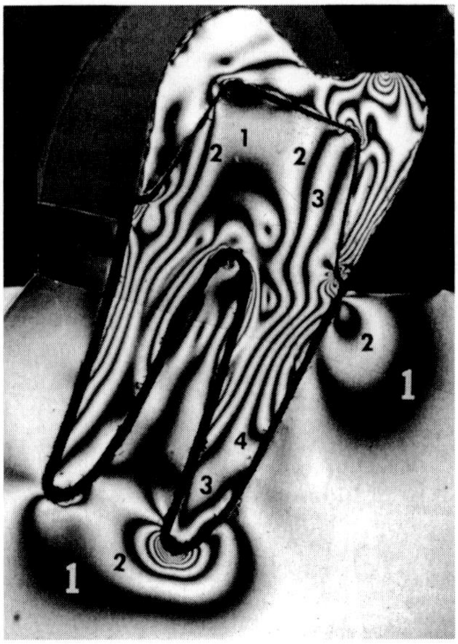

Fig. 4-36 Isochromatic fringes in a two-dimensional photoelastic model of a molar with a full crown under a concentrated force of 266 N; the numbers represent the fringe order of the isochromatic fringes. (From Hood JAA, Farah JW, Craig RG: *J Prosthet Dent* 34:415, 1975.)

quarter-wave plate, and this polarized beam is split into two components traveling along the directions of principal stress in the model. Depending on the state of stress in the model, the two beams travel at different rates. After the light emerges from the model, it passes through a second quarter-wave plate, which is crossed with respect to the first, and an analyzer that is usually perpendicular to the polarizer. The interference pattern may be recorded photographically as shown in Fig. 4-36, which is an isochromatic fringe pattern. These isochromatic fringes, or dark lines, represent locations where the difference in the principal stresses is a constant. The magnitude of the stress can be determined by identifying the order of the isochromatic fringes. Some of the fringe orders (numbers) are indicated on Fig. 4-36. The fringe order multiplied by a constant and divided by the thickness of the model gives the value of the differences in the principal stresses. Areas in the model where the fringes are close together are under higher stress gradients than areas where there are fewer fringes, and areas containing fringes of higher order are under higher stress than those having fringes of lower order.

The advantages of using photoelasticity are that it can quantify stresses throughout a three-dimensional structure and determine stress gradients. However, a birefringent material is needed and the technique is more difficult with complex geometries.

FINITE ELEMENT ANALYSIS

The finite element method is a numerical method and offers considerable advantages over photoelasticity. The method is valuable for analyzing complex geometries, and it can determine stresses and strains throughout a three-dimensional component. In this method, a finite number of discrete structural elements are interconnected at a finite number of points or nodes. These finite elements are formed when the original structure is divided into a number of appropriately shaped sections, with the sections retaining the actual properties of the real materials. The information needed to calculate the stresses and displacements in a finite element model is (1) the total number of nodal points and elements, (2) a numbering system for identifying each nodal point and element, (3) the elastic moduli and Poisson's ratio for the materials associated with each element, (4) the coordinates of each nodal point, (5) the type of boundary constraints, and (6) the evaluation of the forces applied to the external nodes. Note that finite element methods are purely numerical, are based on many limiting assumptions, and are potentially costly. Much more research is needed in this area before the numerical values can be accepted without question. In general, the finite element method is best suited for predicting trends and performing parametric analyses. There is an increased awareness that detailed knowledge of anisotropic material properties and constitutive relations is important in building a valid finite element model. There is also an increased emphasis on experimental validation of numerical results.

SUMMARY

The physical properties of oral restorations must adequately withstand the stresses of mastication. Several means may be used to ensure proper strength of a restoration. With a constant force, the stress is inversely proportional to the contact area; therefore stresses may be reduced by increasing the area over which the force is distributed. In areas of high stress, materials having high elastic moduli and strength properties should be used if possible. If a weaker material has desirable properties, such as esthetic qualities, one may minimize the stress by increasing the bulk of the material when possible.

As an example, consider cement bases used under amalgam restorations. Occlusal forces on the amalgam restoration create tensile stresses in the amalgam adjacent to the cement base. The tensile strength of amalgam is low, and if the cement base has a low modulus, it allows deflection of the amalgam adjacent to the cement base resulting in tensile stresses that are sufficient to initiate fracture of the amalgam. The use of zinc phosphate cement as a base rather than zinc oxide–eugenol cement reduces the probability of fracture of the amalgam because the zinc phosphate cement has a higher modulus. If zinc oxide–eugenol cement is necessary to protect the pulp, a minimum amount should be used, followed by the use of a zinc phosphate cement base to provide resistance to deflection.

Restorations and appliances should be designed so the resulting forces of mastication are distributed as uniformly as possible. Also, sharp line angles, nonuniform areas, and notched, scratched, or pitted surfaces should be avoided to minimize stress concentrations. For example, in the construction of a complete maxillary denture, the midline notch between the central incisors should remain at a minimum. This area is under repetitive stress during mastication as a result of the transverse bending of the denture. If a sharp notch is present in this area, the denture will be less resistant to fatigue or impact forces.

The maximum tensile stress in a metal partial-denture circumferential clasp is near the midpoint of the inside surface. Because brittle materials are generally weak in tension, this is a likely area of failure when a force is applied to the tip of the clasp. Other factors, such as the uniformity of the taper of the clasp, porosity in the clasp, or notches and scratches on the surface of the metal, may alter the stress pattern. If a thin or porous area exists between the junction and the tip of the clasp, failure may occur at this site rather than at the midpoint. Notched or scratched areas are especially subject to fracture from fatigue or impact. Because a partial denture clasp is flexed a great number of times at values well below the yield point, failure by fatigue is particularly significant.

The dentist is often concerned not so much with the fracture of an appliance as with the deflection that occurs when a force is applied. This is the case with a fixed bridge, which may be cast as a single unit or may consist of soldered units. As discussed earlier in this chapter, the deflection of a beam, or in this case a bridge, supported on each end with a concentrated load in the center depends directly on the cube of the beam length and indirectly on the cube of the beam thickness. Doubling the length of the beam, therefore, increases the deflection by eight times. This also indicates that decreasing the thickness of the beam by one half increases the deflection by eight times. If too much bulk is required to develop the stiffness desired, changing to a material with a higher elastic modulus would be beneficial. This is one advantage that nickel-chromium or cobalt-chromium alloys have over gold, because the elastic modulus is greater than 200 GPa, whereas the modulus of gold alloys is less than 100 GPa.

These isolated examples of applied knowledge of biting forces and stresses in dental structures indicate why an understanding of this subject is necessary to the practicing dentist.

In summary, three interrelated factors are important in the long-term function of dental restorative materials: (1) material choice, (2) component geometry (e.g., to minimize stress concentrations), and (3) component design (e.g., to distribute stresses as uniformly as possible). It should be noted that failures can and do occur. In such instances, several questions should be asked: (1) Why did it fail? (2) How did it fail? (3) Whose fault is it? and (4) Can such failures be prevented in the future? Lastly, remember that dental material behavior is dependent on interrelated physical, chemical, optical, mechanical, thermal, electrical, and biological properties, and improvement of one specific property often leads to a reduction in another property.

SPECIFICATIONS FOR RESTORATIVE MATERIALS

The properties described in this and other chapters serve as the basis for a series of specifications that have been developed for restorative materials, instruments, and equipment. One group is the American National Standards Institute/American Dental Association Standards Committee on Dental Products. Standards developed and approved by this committee are reviewed by the Council on Scientific Affairs of the ADA, which has responsibility for adopting specifications. Presently, 59 specifications have been adopted and another 27 are being developed. A larger group called Federal Specifications and Standards is designed to regulate requirements of federal government service agencies for the purchase and use of materials. Specifications of this type have been available for the past quarter of a century, and additional specifications continue to be added in each group. A series of similar specifications is available for products in Australia, Japan, and several other countries. In 1963, a program for international specifications was established that combined the efforts of the Fédération Dentaire Internationale and the International Organization for Standardization. The practice of using physical test controls through methods of applied specifications is well established and will likely continue. Both the dental student and the practitioner must not only recognize that specifications for certain materials are available, but learn to some extent the qualities that are controlled by each specification. Through the specifications the quality of each product is maintained and improved.

AMERICAN DENTAL ASSOCIATION SPECIFICATIONS

The first of the American Dental Association Specifications was for amalgam alloy, formulated and reported in 1930. Since that time other specifications have been or are being formulated, as indicated in Table 4-21.

Copies of the specifications and worksheets to assist in the recording of the required data are available from the Council on Scientific Affairs of the American Dental Association in Chicago. The website of the Council lists the trade names and manufacturers of accepted dental products. This publication can also be obtained from the American Dental Association.

An examination of each specification reveals a general pattern of standardization common to each material.

1. These features include an item on the scope and classification of the material, which defines the application and general nature of each material.
2. Each specification includes information on other applicable specifications.
3. The requirements of each material consider such factors as uniformity, color, or general working characteristics of the material, as well as the general limitations of test values.
4. The methods of sampling, inspection, and testing procedures include details of specimen preparation and physical tests to be performed.
5. Each specification includes information on preparation for delivery, with instructions concerning packaging, instructions for use, and marking with lot numbers and the date of manufacture.
6. Each specification includes notes that provide additional information on intended uses, and references to the literature or other special items.

The important features of each of these specifications are described appropriately in later chapters.

TABLE 4-21 List of American National Standards Institute/American Dental Association Specifications on Dental Materials, Instruments, and Equipment

ANSI/ADA No.	ISO No.*	Title	Date†
1	1559	Alloy for dental amalgam	1993
2	7490	Gypsum-bonded casting investment for dental gold alloys	1995
4	1561	Dental inlay casting wax	2000
5	1562	Dental casting alloys	1997
6	1560	Dental mercury	1995
11	1564	Dental agar impression materials	1997
12	1567	Denture base resins	1999
13	—	Denture cold-curing repair resin	1999
14	6871	Dental base metal casting alloy	1998
15	3336	Acrylic resin teeth	1999
16	—	Dental impression paste—zinc oxide–eugenol type	1999
17	—	Denture base temporary relining resin	1999
18	1563	Dental alginate impression material	1992
19	4823	Elastomeric dental impression materials	1993
20	—	Dental duplicating material	1995
23	3823‡	Dental excavating burs	1999
24	12163	Dental baseplate wax	1997
25	6873	Dental gypsum products	2000
26		Dental radiographic equipment and accessory devices	1999
27	4049	Direct filling resins	1993
28	3630-1	Endodontic files and reamers	1996
30	3107	Zinc oxide–eugenol and noneugenol cements	2000
32	—	Orthodontic wire	2000
33	1942	Dental terminology	1999
34	—	Dental aspirating syringes	2000
35	7785‡	High-speed, air-driven handpieces	NS
36	7711	Dental diamond rotary cutting instruments	NS
37	—	Dental abrasive powders	2000
38	9693	Metal-ceramic systems	2000
39	6874	Pit and fissure sealants	1999
40	5832-2‡	Dental implants	NS
41	7405	Biological evaluation of dental materials	2000
42	9694	Phosphate-bonded investments	NS
43	7488	Electrically powered dental amalgamators	1995
44	—	Dental electrosurgical equipment	1999
45	4824	Dental porcelain teeth	NS
46	6875	Dental patient chair	1997
47	7494	Dental units	1997
48	10650	Dental activator, disclosing, and transillumination devices	1989

*ISO number represents equivalent or similar specification or draft.
†Date of latest revision or reaffirmation of specification; *NS,* new standard under development.
‡Several ISO equivalent standards exist.

TABLE 4-21 List of American National Standards Institute/American Dental Association Specifications on Dental Materials, Instruments, and Equipment—cont'd

ANSI/ADA No.	ISO No.*	Title	Date†
53	10477	Crown and bridge plastics	2000
54	—	Dental needles	2000
57	6876	Endodontic sealing materials	2000
58	3630	Root canal files, type H (Hedstrom)	1997
59	—	Portable steam sterilizers	1992
62	—	Dental abrasive pastes	NS
63	3630-1	Rasps and barbed broaches	1999
65	—	Low-speed handpieces	NS
69	6872	Dental ceramic	1999
70	—	Dental radiographic protective aprons and accessory devices	1999
71	3630-3	Root canal filling condensers and spreaders	1995
73	7551	Dental absorbent points	1993
74	7493	Dental stools	NS
75	10139-1	Resilient denture liners	1997
76	—	Nonsterile latex gloves for dentistry	1999
77	8627	Stiffness of tufted area of toothbrushes	NS
78	6877	Dental obturating points	1994
79	—	Dental vacuum pumps	NS
80	7491	Color stability test methods	1997
82	13716	Combined reversible and irreversible hydrocolloid	1998
85	—	Prophy angles	NS
87	—	Impression trays	1995
88	9333	Dental brazing alloys	2000
89	9680	Dental operating lights	1999
90	—	Dental rubber dam	NS
91	11246	Ethyl silicate casting investment	1999
92	11245	Refractory die material	NS
93	11244	Soldering investments	2000
94	—	Dental compressed-air quality	1996
95	3630-2	Root canal enlargers	NS
96	9917	Dental water-based cements	2000
97	10271	Tarnish and corrosion testing	NS
98	—	Endodontic posts	NS
99	—	Mouth guards	NS
100	—	Orthodontic bracket and buccal tubes	NS
101	3630	Endodontic instruments—general requirements	NS
102	—	Non-sterile nitrile gloves for dentistry	1999
103	—	Non-sterile polyvinyl chloride gloves for dentistry	1999
104	—	Extraoral maxillofacial prosthesis elastomers	NS
105	—	Orthodontic elastomeric materials	NS

Continued

TABLE 4-21 List of American National Standards Institute/American Dental Association Specifications on Dental Materials, Instruments, and Equipment—cont'd

ANSI/ADA No.	ISO No.*	Title	Date†
106	13897	Dental amalgam capsules	NS
107	—	Antimicrobial agents and other chemicals for prevention, inactivation, and removal of biofilms in dental unit waterlines	NS
3950	3950	Designation system for teeth and areas of the oral cavity	1997

AMERICAN DENTAL ASSOCIATION ACCEPTANCE PROGRAM

The American Dental Association, through the Council on Scientific Affairs, maintains an acceptance program for dental materials, instruments, and equipment. If a specification exists, the manufacturer may provide evidence that the product complies with the appropriate specification. If the product complies, its name is placed on the Accepted List and the manufacturer is allowed to place the Seal of Acceptance of the American Dental Association on the product. If a specification is in preparation or one does not exist, the manufacturer may provide evidence that the product functions as claimed, and after review by the Council it may be placed on the Accepted List. Examples of such products are dental adhesives, denture adherents, dental floss, resilient reliners, and toothbrushes.

INDEX OF FEDERAL SPECIFICATIONS AND STANDARDS

The Index of Federal Specifications and Standards includes specifications for a number of restorative dental materials not described elsewhere. These specifications are used primarily by the federal services to maintain some quality control of dental products and are valuable for suppliers of these materials. In a few instances, reference is made to specific federal specifications and standards in later chapters.

SELECTED PROBLEMS

Problem 1

With an average biting force of 565 N on the first or second molar, how is it possible for a patient to fracture a gold alloy bridge in service when the alloy has a tensile strength of 690 MPa?

Solution

The stress produced by the biting force is a function of the cross section of the bridge and the size of the contact area over which the force is applied. When the contact area from the opposing tooth is very small and located near a portion of the bridge having a small cross section, bending produces tensile stresses that can exceed the tensile strength of the gold alloy. For example, in the above problem, relating the biting force of 565 N to the tensile strength of 690 MPa indicates that a minimum area of 0.82 mm^2 is necessary in this bridge:

$$\text{Area} = \text{Force/Stress} = 565\ \text{N}/690\ \text{MPa} = 8.2 \times 10^{-7}\ \text{m}^2 = 0.82\ \text{mm}^2$$

Problem 2

Why is the yield strength of a restorative material such an important property?

Solution

The yield strength defines the stress at the point at which the material changes from elastic to plastic behavior. In the elastic range, stresses and strains return to zero after biting forces are removed, whereas in the plastic range some permanent deformation results on removal of the force. Significant permanent deformation may result in a functional failure of a restoration even though fracture does not occur.

Problem 3

Why is the elongation value for a casting alloy not always an indication of the burnishability of the margins of the casting?

Solution

Although the elongation of an alloy gives an indication of its ductility, or ability to be drawn into a wire without fracturing, to burnish a margin of a casting, sufficient force must be applied to exceed the yield strength. Therefore alloys with high yield strengths are difficult to burnish even though they have high values for elongation.

Problem 4

Why does a mesial-occlusal-distal (MOD) amalgam fail in tension when compressive biting forces are applied from the opposing teeth?

Solution

The compressive load produces bending of the MOD amalgam, which results in compressive stress on the occlusal surface and tensile stresses at the base of the restoration. Amalgam is a brittle solid with much lower tensile than compressive strength, and therefore fails first at the base of the restoration, with the crack progressing to the occlusal surface of the amalgam.

Problem 5

Because the modulus of nickel-chromium alloys is about twice that of gold alloys, why is it not correct to reduce the thickness by one half and have the same deflection in bending?

Solution

Although the deflection in the bending equation is directly proportional to the modulus, it is inversely proportional to the cube of the thickness. Therefore only minimal reductions in thickness are possible for the nickel-chromium alloy to maintain the same deflection.

Problem 6

How is it possible to use a single elastomeric impression material and yet have the correct viscosity for use in the syringe and the tray?

Solution

Correct compounding of the polymer and filler produces a material that has the quality described as *shear thinning*. Such a material decreases in viscosity at high shear rates, such as during spatulation or syringing, and has a higher viscosity at low shear rates, as when it is placed and used as a tray material.

Problem 7

After an orthodontic latex band is extended and placed, the force applied decreases with time more than expected for the distance the tooth moves. Why?

Solution

Latex rubber bands behave elastically, viscoelastically, and viscously. It is principally the viscous deformation that is not recoverable that accounts for the greater than expected decrease in force as the band shortens from the movement of the tooth. This effect is even more pronounced when plastic rather than latex bands are used.

Problem 8

If dental manufacturers showed you the compliance versus time curve for their rubber impression material and pointed out that it had a high elastic compliance, moderate viscoelastic compliance, and a very low viscous compliance, how would you characterize the product?

Solution

The material would be highly flexible, should recover from deformation moderately rapidly, and the recovery from deformation should be nearly complete.

Problem 9

If you wished to measure the surface hardness of a material that had small isolated areas of widely varying hardnesses, which hardness test would be most appropriate and why?

Solution

Diamond pyramid hardness. Only the Knoop and diamond pyramid are appropriate for surface hardness and a wide range of hardness. The selection of the diamond pyramid over the Knoop test is based on the information that there were isolated areas of different hardness and the diamond pyramid indentation can be placed in smaller areas. Chose nano-indentation for the study of micro-phases.

Problem 10

Why is the selection of a cement base with a high modulus so important for an amalgam restoration, whereas the selection is not as critical for a composite restoration?

Solution

The cement base under an amalgam should have a high modulus (stiffness) to provide support and prevent bending, thus minimizing tensile stresses. Also, low-stress gradients occur across the amalgam-cement base interface when the modulus values are similar. The composite has greater tensile strength and a lower modulus than does amalgam, allowing the use of a cement base with a somewhat lower modulus.

BIBLIOGRAPHY

Forces on Dental Structures

Black GV: An investigation of the physical characters of the human teeth in relation to their diseases, and to practical dental operations, together with the physical characters of filling materials, *Dent Cosmos* 37:469, 1895.

Burstone CJ, Baldwin JJ, Lawless DT: The application of continuous forces in orthodontics, *Angle Orthod* 31:1, 1961.

Dechow PC, Carlson DS: A method of bite force measurement in primates, *J Biomech* 16:797, 1983.

Koolstra JH, van Euden TMGJ: Application and validation of a three-dimensional mathematical model of the human masticatory system in vivo, *J Biomech* 25:175, 1992.

Plesh O, Bishop B, McCall Jr WD: Kinematics of jaw movements during chewing at different frequencies, *J Biomech* 26:243, 1993.

Southard TE, Southard KA, Stiles RN: Factors influencing the anterior component of occlusal force, *J Biomech* 23:1199, 1990.

Stress Analysis and Design of Dental Structures

Chen J, Xu L: A finite element analysis of the human temporomandibular joint, *J Biomech Eng* 116:401, 1994.

Craig RG: Dental mechanics. In Kardestuncer H: *Finite element handbook,* New York, 1987, McGraw-Hill.

Craig RG, Farah JW: Stress analysis and design of single restorations and fixed bridges, *Oral Sci Rev* 10:45, 1977.

Craig RG, Farah JW: Stresses from loading distal-extension removable partial dentures, *J Prosthet Dent* 39:274, 1978.

Farah JW, Craig RG: Distribution of stresses in porcelain-fused-to-metal and porcelain jacket crowns, *J Dent Res* 54:255, 1975.

Farah JW, Craig RG, Sikarskie DL: Photoelastic and finite element stress analysis of a restored axisymmetric first molar, *J Biomech* 6:511, 1973.

Farah JW, Hood JAA, Craig RG: Effects of cement bases on the stresses in amalgam restorations, *J Dent Res* 54:10, 1975.

Farah JW, Powers JM, Dennison JB et al: Effects of cement bases on the stresses and deflections in composite restorations, *J Dent Res* 55:115, 1976.

Hart RT, Hennebel VV, Thonpreda N et al: Modeling the biomechanics of the mandible: a three-dimensional finite element study, *J Biomech* 25:261, 1992.

Hylander WL: Mandibular function in galago crassicaudatus and macaca fascicularis: an in vivo approach to stress analysis of the mandible, *J Morph* 159:253, 1979.

Kohn DH: Overview of factors important in implant design, *J Oral Implantol* 18:204, 1992.

Ko CC, Kohn DH, Hollister SJ: Micromechanics of implant/tissue interfaces, *J Oral Implantol* 18:220, 1992.

Koran A, Craig RG: Three-dimensional photoelastic stress analysis of maxillary and mandibular complete dentures, *J Oral Rehabil* 1:361, 1974.

Korioth TWP, Hannam AG: Deformation of the human mandible during simulated tooth clenching, *J Dent Res* 73:56, 1994.

Properties from Stress-Strain Curves

Flinn RA, Trojan PK: *Engineering materials and their applications,* ed 4, New York, 1995, Wiley.

Park, JB, Lakes, RS: *Biomaterials: An introduction,* New York, 1992, Plenum Press.

Titelman AS, McEvily AJ, Jr: *Fracture of structural materials,* New York, 1967, John Wiley & Sons.

von Recum AF, editor: *Handbook of biomaterials evaluation: scientific, technical, and clinical testing of implant materials,* Philadelphia, 1999, Taylor and Francis.

Fracture Toughness

Cruickshanks-Boyd DW, Lock WR: Fracture toughness of dental amalgams, *Biomaterials* 4:234, 1983.

de Groot R, Van Elst HC, Peters MCRB: Fracture mechanics parameters for failure prediction of composite resins, *J Dent Res* 67:919, 1988.

Dhuru VB, Lloyd CH: The fracture toughness of repaired composite, *J Oral Rehabil* 13:413, 1986.

El Mowafy OM, Watts DC: Fracture toughness of human dentin, *J Dent Res* 65:677, 1986.

Ferracane JL, Antonio RC, Matsumoto H: Variables affecting the fracture toughness of dental composites, *J Dent Res* 66:1140, 1987.

Ferracane JL, Berge HX: Fracture toughness of experimental dental composites aged in ethanol, *J Dent Res* 74:1418, 1995.

Ferracane JL, Marker VA: Solvent degradation and reduced fracture toughness in aged composites, *J Dent Res* 71:13, 1992.

Ferracane JL: Current trends in dental composites, *Crit Rev Oral Biol Med* 6:302, 1995.

Fujishima A. Ferracane JL: Comparison of four modes of fracture toughness testing for dental composites, *Dent Mater* 12:38, 1996.

Hassan R, Vaidyanathan TK, Schulman A: Fracture toughness determination of dental amalgams through microindentation, *J Biomed Mater Res* 20:135, 1986.

Hill RG, Bates JF, Lewis TT, Rees N: Fracture toughness of acrylic denture base, *Biomater* 4:112, 1983.

Kon M, Ishikawa K, Kuwayam N: Effects of zirconia addition on fracture toughness and bending strength of dental porcelains, *Dent Mater* J 9:181, 1990.

Lloyd CH: The fracture toughness of dental composites. II. The environmental and temperature dependence of the stress intensification factor (K_{IC}), *J Oral Rehabil* 9:133, 1982.

Lloyd CH: The fracture toughness of dental composites. III. The effect of environment upon the stress intensification factor (K_{IC}) after extended storage, *J Oral Rehabil* 11: 393, 1984.

Lloyd CH, Adamson M: The fracture toughness (K_{IC}) of amalgam, *J Oral Rehabil* 12:59, 1985.

Lloyd CH, Adamson M: The development of fracture toughness and fracture strength in posterior restorative materials, *Dent Mater* 3:225, 1987.

Lloyd CH, Iannetta RV: The fracture toughness of dental composites. I. The development of strength and fracture toughness. *J Oral Rehabil* 9:55, 1982.

Lloyd CH, Mitchell L: The fracture toughness of tooth coloured restorative materials, *J Oral Rehabil* 11:257, 1984.

Marcos Montes-G G, Draughn RA: Slow crack propagation in composite restorative materials, *J Biomed Mater Res* 21:629, 1987.

Morena R, Lockwood PE, Fairhurst CW: Fracture toughness of commercial dental porcelains, *Dent Mater* 2:58, 1986.

Mueller HJ: Fracture toughness and fractography of dental cements, lining, build-up, and filling materials, *Scanning Microsc* 4:297, 1990.

Neihart TR, Li SH, Flinton RJ: Measuring fracture toughness of high-impact poly (methyl methacrylate) with the short rod method, *J Prosthet Dent* 60:249, 1988.

Pilliar RM, Smith DC, Maric B: Fracture toughness of dental composites determined using the short-rod fracture toughness test, *J Dent Res* 65:1308, 1986.

Pilliar RM, Vowles R, Williams DF: The effect of environmental aging on the fracture toughness of dental composites, *J Dent Res* 66: 722, 1987.

Roberts JC, Powers JM, Craig RG: Fracture toughness of composite and unfilled restorative resins, *J Dent Res* 56:748, 1977.

Roberts JC, Powers JM, Craig RG: Fracture toughness and critical strain energy release rate of dental amalgam, *J Mater Sci* 13:965, 1978.

Rosenstiel SF, Porter SS: Apparent fracture toughness of metal ceramic restorations with different manipulative variables, *J Prosthet Dent* 61:185, 1989.

Rosenstiel SF, Porter SS: Apparent fracture toughness of all-ceramic crown systems, *J Prosthet Dent* 62:529, 1989.

Sih GC, Berman AT: Fracture toughness concept applied to methyl methacrylate, *J Biomed Mater Res* 14:311, 1980.

Taira M, Nomura Y, Wakasa K et al: Studies on fracture toughness of dental ceramics, *J Oral Rehabil* 17:551, 1990.

Uctasli S, Harrington E, Wilson HJ: The fracture resistance of dental materials, *J Oral Rehabil* 22:877, 1995.

Shear Strength

Black J: "Push-out" tests, *J Biomed Mater Res* 23:1243, 1989.

Johnston WM, O'Brien WJ: The shear strength of dental porcelain, *J Dent Res* 59:1409, 1980.

Bending and Torsion

Asgharnia MK, Brantley WA: Comparison of bending and torsion tests for orthodontic wires, *Am J Orthodont* 89:228, 1986.

Brantley WA, Augat WS, Myers CL et al: Bending deformation studies of orthodontic wires, *J Dent Res* 57:609, 1978.

Dolan DW, Craig RG: Bending and torsion of endodontic files with rhombus cross sections, *J Endodont* 8:260, 1982.

Ruyter IE, Svendsen SA: Flexural properties of denture base polymers, *J Prosthet Dent* 43: 95, 1980.

Viscosity

Combe EC, Moser JB: The rheological characteristics of elastomeric impression materials, *J Dent Res* 57:221, 1978.

Herfort TW, Gerberich WW, Macosko CW et al: Viscosity of elastomeric impression materials, *J Prosthet Dent* 38:396, 1977.

Koran A, Powers JM, Craig RG: Apparent viscosity of materials used for making edentulous impressions, *J Am Dent Assoc* 95:75, 1977.

Vermilyea SG, Huget EF, de Simon LB: Apparent viscosities of setting elastomers, *J Dent Res* 59:1149, 1980.

Vermilyea SG, Powers JM, Craig RG: Rotational viscometry of a zinc phosphate and a zinc polyacrylate cement, *J Dent Res* 56:762, 1977.

Vermilyea SG, Powers JM, Koran A: The rheological properties of fluid denture-base resins, *J Dent Res* 57:227, 1978.

Viscoelasticity

Bertolotti RL, Moffa JP: Creep rate of porcelain-bonding alloys as a function of temperature, *J Dent Res* 59:2062, 1980.

Cook WD: Permanent set and stress relaxation in elastomeric impression materials, *J Biomed Mater Res* 15:449, 1981.

Duran RL, Powers JM, Craig RG: Viscoelastic and dynamic properties of soft liners and tissue conditioners, *J Dent Res* 58:1801, 1979.

Ellis B, Al-Nabash S: The composition and rheology of denture adhesives, *J Dent* 8:109, 1980.

Ferracane JL, Moser JB, Greener EH: Rheology of composite restoratives, *J Dent Res* 60:1678, 1981.

Goldberg AJ: Viscoelastic properties of silicone, polysulfide, and polyether impression materials, *J Dent Res* 53:1033, 1974.

McCabe JF, Bowman AJ: The rheological properties of dental impression materials, *Br Dent J* 151:179, 1981.

Morris HF, Asgar K, Tillitson EW: Stress-relaxation testing. Part I: A new approach to the testing of removable partial denture alloys, wrought wires, and clasp behavior, *J Prosthet Dent* 46:133, 1981.

Nikolai RJ, Crouthers RC: On the relaxation of orthodontic traction elements under interrupted loads, *J Dent Res* 59:1071, 1980.

Park, JB, Lakes, RS: *Biomaterials: An introduction,* New York, 1992, Plenum Press.

Ruyter IE, Espevik S: Compressive creep of denture base polymers, *Acta Odont Scand* 38:169, 1980.

Tolley LG, Craig RG: Viscoelastic properties of elastomeric impression materials: polysulphide, silicone and polyether rubbers, *J Oral Rehabil* 5:121, 1978.

Wills DJ, Manderson RD: Biomechanical aspects of the support of partial dentures, *J Dent* 5:310, 1977.

Xu HHK, Liao H, Eichmiller FC: Indentation creep behavior of a direct-filling silver alternative to amalgam, *J Dent Res* 77:1991, 1998.

Dynamic Properties

Impact resistance of plastics and electrical insulating material, D 256-92. In ASTM Standards 1993, Vol. 8.01, Philadelphia, American Society for Testing and Materials, 1993.

Koran A, Craig RG: Dynamic mechanical properties of maxillofacial materials, *J Dent Res* 54:1216, 1975.

Properties of Composite Materials

Bayne SC, Thompson JY, Swift EJ Jr et al: A characterization of first-generation flowable composites, *J Am Dent Assoc* 129:567, 1998.

Braem MJA, Davidson CL, Lambrechts P et al: In vitro flexural fatigue limits of dental composites, *J Biomed Mater Res* 28:1397, 1994.

Braem M, Van Doren VE, Lambrechts P et al: Determination of Young's modulus of dental composites: a phenomenological model *J Mater Sci* 22:2037, 1987.

Choi KK, Condon JR, Ferracane JL: The effects of adhesive thickness on polymerization contraction stress of composite, *J Dent Res* 79:812, 2000.

Condon JR, Ferracane JL: Reduction of composite contraction stress through non-bonded microfiller particles, *Dent Mater* 14:256, 1998.

Ferracane JL: Current trends in dental composites, *Crit Rev Oral Biol Med* 6:302, 1995.

Ferracane JL, Berge HX, Condon JR: In vitro aging of dental composites in water—effect of degree of conversion, filler volume, and filler/matrix coupling, *J Biomed Mater Res* 42:465, 1998.

Ferracane JL, Condon JR: In vitro evaluation of the marginal degradation of dental composites under simulated occlusal loading, *Dent Mater* 15:262, 1999.

Flinn RA, Trojan PK: *Engineering materials and their applications,* ed 4, New York, 1995, Wiley.

Goldberg AJ, Burstone CJ, Hadjinikolaou I et al: Screening of matrices and fibers for reinforced thermoplastics intended for dental applications, *J Biomed Mater Res* 28:167, 1994.

McCabe JF, Wang Y, Braem M: Surface contact fatigue and flexural fatigue of dental restorative materials, *J Biomed Mater Res* 50:375, 2000.

Peutzfeldt A: Resin composites in dentistry: the monomer systems, *Eur J Oral Sci* 105:97, 1997.

Sakaguchi RL, Ferracane JL: Stress transfer from polymerization shrinkage of a chemical-cured composite bonded to a pre-cast composite substrate, *Dent Mater* 14:106, 1998.

Urabe I, Nakajima M. Sano H et al: Physical properties of the dentin-enamel junction region, *Am J Dent* 13:129, 2000.

Van der Varst PGT, Brekelmans WAM, De Vree JHP et al: Mechanical performance of a dental composite: probabilistic failure prediction, *J Dent Res* 72:1249, 1993.

Willems G, Lambrechts P, Braem M et al: Composite resins in the 21st century, *Quint Internat* 24:641, 1993.

Tear Strength and Tear Energy

Herfort TW, Gerberich WW, Macosko CW et al: Tear strength of elastomeric impression materials, *J Prosthet Dent* 39:59, 1978.

MacPherson GW, Craig RG, Peyton FA: Mechanical properties of hydrocolloid and rubber impression materials, *J Dent Res* 46:714, 1967.

Strength of conventional vulcanized rubber and thermoplastic elastomers, D 624-91. In ASTM Standards 1994, Vol. 9.01, Philadelphia, American Society for Testing and Materials, 1994.

Webber RL, Ryge G: The determination of tear energy of extensible materials of dental interest, *J Biomed Mater Res* 2:231, 1968.

Hardness

DeBellis A: Fundamentals of Rockwell hardness testing. In Hardness Testing Reprints, WD-673, Wilson Instrument Division, Bridgeport, Conn, 1967.

Doerner MF, Nix WD: A method for interpreting the data from depth-sensing indentation measurements, *J Mater Res* 1:601, 1986.

Flinn RA, Trojan PK: *Engineering materials and their applications,* ed 4, New York, 1995, Wiley.

Lysaght VE: How to make and interpret hardness tests on plastics. In Hardness Testing Reprints, WD-673, Wilson Instrument Division, Bridgeport, Conn, 1967.

Lysaght VE: *Indentation hardness testing,* New York, 1949, Reinhold.

Lysaght VE, DeBellis A: Microhardness testing. In Hardness Testing Reprints, WD-673, Wilson Instrument Division, Bridgeport, Conn, 1967.

Tirtha R, Fan PL, Dennison JB, Powers JM: In vitro depth of cure of photo-activated composites. *J Dent Res* 61:1184, 1982.

Van Meerbeek B, Willems G, Celis JP et al: Assessment by nano-indentation of the hardness and elasticity of resin-dentin bonding area, *J Dent Res* 72:1434, 1993.

Willems G, Celis JP, Lambrechts P et al: Hardness and young's modulus determined by nanoindentation technique of filler particles of dental restorative materials compared with human enamel, *J Biomed Mater Res* 27:747, 1993.

Xu HHK et al: Indentation damage and mechanical properties of human enamel and dentin, *J Dent Res* 77:472, 1998.

Specifications

Council on Scientific Affairs: Clinical products in dentistry; a desktop reference, Chicago, 1996, American Dental Association.

United States General Services Administration: Index of Federal Specifications and Standards, Washington, DC, 1994, Superintendent of Documents, U.S. Government Printing Office.

Wear

Abe Y, Sato Y. Akagawa Y. Ohkawa S. An in vitro study of high-strength resin posterior denture tooth wear. *Int J Prosthodont* 10:28, 1997.

Barbakow F, Lutz F, Imfeld T: A review of methods to determine the relative abrasion of dentifrices and prophylaxis pastes, *Quint Internat* 18:23, 1987.

Condon JR. Ferracane JL: Factors effecting dental composite wear in vitro. *J Biomed Mater Res* 38:303, 1997.

Condon JR, Ferracane JL: In vitro wear of composite with varied cure, filler level, and filler treatment. *J Dent Res* 76:1405, 1997.

Draughn RA, Harrison A: Relationship between abrasive wear and microstructure of composite resins, *J Prosthet Dent* 40:220, 1978.

Ferracane JL, Mitchem JC, Condon JR, Todd R: Wear and marginal breakdown of composites with various degrees of cure, *J Dent Res* 76:1508, 1997.

Hu X, Harrington E, Marquis PM et al: The influence of cyclic loading on the wear of a dental composite, *Biomat* 20:907, 1999.

Hu X, Marquis PM, Shortall AC: Two-body in vitro wear study of some current dental composites and amalgams, *J Prosthet Dent* 82:214, 1999.

Knibbs PJ: Methods of clinical evaluation of dental restorative materials, *J Oral Rehabil* 24:109, 1997.

Koczorowski R, Wloch S: Evaluation of wear of selected prosthetic materials in contact with enamel and dentin. *J Prosthet Dent* 81:453, 1999.

Powers JM, Craig RG: Wear of dental tissues and restorative materials. In proceedings of national symposium on wear and corrosion, June 4-6, 1979, Washington, DC, 1979, American Chemical Society.

Powers JM, Fan PL, Craig RG: Wear of dental restorative resins. In Gebelein CG, Koblitz FF, editors: *Biomedical and dental applications of polymers: Polymer science and technology,* vol 14, New York, 1981, Plenum Press.

Roberts JC, Powers JM, Craig RG: Wear of dental amalgam, *J Biomed Mater Res* 11:513, 1977.

Teoh SH, Ong LF, Yap AU et al: Bruxing-type dental wear simulator for ranking of dental restorative materials, *J Biomed Mater Res* 43:175, 1998.

Wu W, McKinney JE: Influence of chemicals on wear of dental composites, *J Dent Res* 61: 1180, 1982.

Yap AU, Ong LF, Teoh SH et al: Comparative wear ranking of dental restoratives with the BIOMAT wear simulator, *J Oral Rehabil* 26:228, 1999.

WEB SITES

Academy of Dental Materials: www.academydentalmaterials.org
American Dental Association Council on Scientific Affairs: www.ada.org
Biomaterials Database (University of Michigan): www.lib.umich.edu/dentlib/dental_tables
Biomaterials Journal Sites: www.bioforma.com
Dental Biomaterials Science Home Page: www.umds.ac.uk
Houston Biomaterials Research Center: www.db.uth.tmc.edu/biomaterials
International/American Association for Dental Research: www.iadr.org
Links for Dental Biomaterials: www.dental.uab.edu
NESAC/BIO: www.nb.engr.washington.edu
Society for Biomaterials: www.biomaterials.org
Surfaces in Biomaterials Foundation: www.surfaces.org

Chapter 5

Biocompatibility of Dental Materials

Biocompatibility is formally defined as the ability of a material to elicit an appropriate biological response in a given application in the body. Inherent in this definition is the idea that a single material may not be biologically acceptable in all applications. For example, a material that is acceptable as a full cast crown may not be acceptable as a dental implant. Also implicit in this definition is an expectation for the biological performance of the material. In a bone implant, the expectation is that the material will allow the bone to integrate with the implant. Thus an appropriate biological response for the implant is osseointegration. In a full cast crown, the expectation is that the material will not cause inflammation of pulpal or periodontal tissues, but osseointegration is not an expectation. Whether a material is biocompatible is therefore dependent on what physical function we ask of the material and what biological response we require from it. Using this definition, it makes little sense to say that any given material is or is not biocompatible, because we need to define how the material will be used before we can assess this. In this sense, biocompatibility is much like color. Color is a property of a material interacting with its environment (light), and the color of a material depends on the light source and the observer of the light. Similarly, biocompatibility is a property of a material interacting with its environment. The biological response may change if the host, the application of the material, or the material itself are changed (Fig. 5-1).

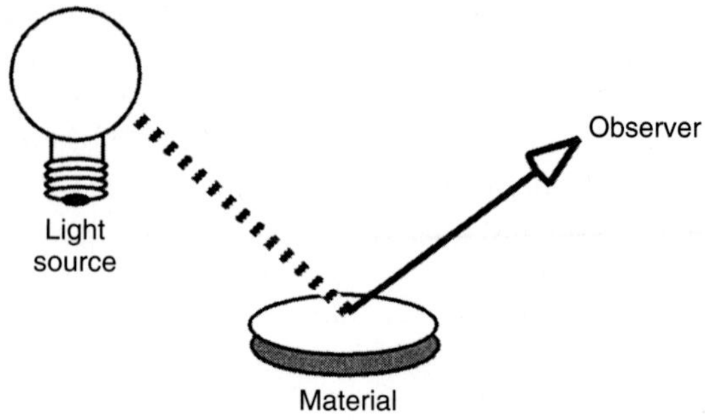

Fig. 5-1 Like color, biocompatibility is not a property of just a material, but rather a property of how a material interacts with its environment. A material's color depends on the character of the light source, how the light interacts with the material, and how the observer interprets the reflected light. In this sense, the material's color depends on its environment. The biocompatibility of a material is similar in the sense that it depends on its environment.

Dentistry shares concerns about biocompatibility with other fields of medicine, such as orthopedics, cardiology, and vascular biology, among others. Today, in the development of any biomaterial, one must consider not only the strength, esthetics, or functional aspects of the material, but its biocompatibility as well. Furthermore, demands for appropriate biological responses are increasing as we ask materials to perform more sophisticated functions in the body for longer periods. Thus considerations of biocompatibility are important to manufacturers, practitioners, scientists, and patients. The field of biocompatibility is interdisciplinary, and draws knowledge from materials science, bioengineering, biochemistry, molecular biology, and others.

This chapter surveys the tests used for evaluating the biocompatibility of dental materials, the specifications that govern such testing, and the strengths and weaknesses of the testing methods. In addition, the biocompatibility of various materials used in dentistry are discussed within a framework of principles. Because an understanding biocompatibility requires an understanding of the biological system into which materials are placed, this chapter will first summarize the anatomical and pathological aspects of the oral tissues relevant to dental materials.

ANATOMICAL AND PATHOLOGICAL ASPECTS OF ORAL TISSUES

THE TOOTH

Enamel Mature human enamel is highly mineralized (96% by weight), with only 1% of its weight being organic molecules and 3% being water. The organic matrix of enamel consists of at least two types of glycoproteins: amelogenins and enamelins. After synthesis by ameloblasts, the calcified organic matrix of enamel does not appear to be maintained in any way by cellular synthetic mechanisms, contrary to other calcified tissues such as dentin, bone, and cementum. Enamel rods have a specific orientation with each other, and this orientation provides maximal strength. Because of its high mineral (hydroxyapatite) content, enamel is much more brittle than dentin and is solubilized to a greater extent by acid solutions. This property is used to advantage with bonding agents, where acids are used to etch the enamel to provide micromechanical retention of resin composite materials. The differential etching that occurs is a consequence of the different orientation of enamel rods on the enamel surface. The permeability of enamel to most oral molecules is quite low, and in this sense enamel "seals" the tooth to outside agents. However, recent evidence indicates that enamel is not impermeable. Peroxides in bleaching agents have been shown to permeate intact enamel in just a few seconds.

Dentin and Pulp Because of their close anatomical relationship, most researchers consider the dentin and pulp to be a single organ. The dentinal matrix (both calcified and uncalcified) forms the greatest bulk of the tooth. Calcified dentin is about 20% organic, 70% inorganic, and 10% aqueous by weight. Collagen constitutes approximately 85% of the organic portion of dentin, and hydroxyapatite is the main inorganic compound. The dentinal matrix also contains many proteins, including collagenous proteins (mainly type I collagen with smaller amounts of type V and type I trimer collagens), noncollagenous dentin-specific proteins (phosphophoryns, dentin sialoprotein, and dentin matrix protein-1), and several nonspecific proteins associated with mineralized tissues (e.g., osteocalcin and osteopontin).

The dentinal matrix surrounds dentinal tubules that are filled with the odontoblastic processes. These processes stem from odontoblasts that reside in the pulp of the tooth. The tubules traverse the region between the dentoenamel junction (DEJ) and the pulp. The numbers of tubules per cross-sectional area range from about 20,000/mm^2 near the DEJ to 50,000/mm^2 near the pulp. The tubule diameter varies from about 0.5 μm at the DEJ to about 2.5 μm near the pulp (Fig. 5-2). Some odontoblastic processes extend through the dentin tubules to the DEJ. The percentage of processes that reach the DEJ is a matter of some conjecture.

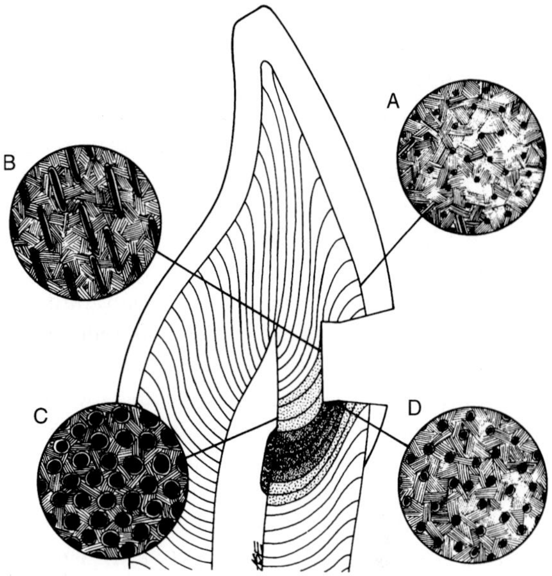

Fig. 5-2 Diagram of dentinal tubules. Dentinal tubules occur throughout the dentin, but their size and number vary as a function of proximity to the pulp of the tooth. Near the dentin-enamel junction *(A)*, the tubules are small in diameter and relatively few in number per centimeter squared. As the depth approaches the pulp *(B, D)*, the tubules become larger in diameter and are more dense in number. At the pulp *(C)*, the tubules are very dense and have the largest diameters. Furthermore, the tubules do not follow a straight path from the pulp to the enamel, but curve as a function of the shape of the tooth. Thus a cavity preparation may section the tubules in either a cross-section *(D)* or a longitudinal section *(B)*. The tubular structure of dentin is critical to biocompatibility because components of materials may use the tubules as conduits to pulpal tissues.

(Courtesy Avery JK: Ann Arbor, 1987, University of Michigan School of Dentistry.)

A serum-like fluid fills the dentinal tubules. This fluid has continuity with the extracellular fluid of the pulp tissue. The pulpal circulation maintains an intercellular hydraulic pressure of about 24 mm Hg (32.5 cm H_2O), which causes fluid flow in the tubules to be directed from the pulp outward toward the DEJ when enamel is removed. External hydrostatic and osmotic pressures can also cause fluid movement toward or away from the pulp. The positive or negative displacement of this fluid through exposed dentinal tubules is capable of affecting either odontoblasts or pulpal nerve endings. These effects are the basis of the hydrodynamic theory of hyperalgesia (pulpal hypersensitivity).

During cavity preparation by the dentist, a "smear layer" is formed by the action of the bur or hand instruments on the calcified dentin matrix (Fig. 5-3). This mat of organic and inorganic particles occludes the dentinal tubules to some extent. The smear layer is quite effective in reducing hydrostatic pressures, but less effective in reducing diffusion, especially if the layer is interrupted or defective. The smear layer can be removed by acid etching, which also demineralizes the openings of the tubules (Fig. 5-4). The dentinal tubules establish continuity with the pulpal fluid to facilitate the diffusion of molecules, both natural or from materials, into and out of the pulp. The smear layer, dentinal tubules, and dentinal matrix are all important in the application of dentinal bonding agents and the ability of components of the bonding agents to reach and affect pulpal tissues.

Moderately deep cavity preparation will damage odontoblasts by severing the odontoblastic processes. Deep cavity preparation may destroy most of the dentin and kill the primary odontoblasts. A number of investigators think that the extracellular matrix (ECM) of dentin and pulp is largely responsible for the differentiation of secondary odontoblasts that form reparative dentin. The source of secondary odontoblasts is not known, but much of the proliferative activity of granulation tissue following pulpal insult is found in perivascular areas proximal to the core of the pulp. In monkeys, the minimal amount of time between pulp injury and replacement odontoblast differentiation is about 5 days. Nerves and blood vessels, which arborize from the core of the pulp as they approach the odontoblastic layer, may influence the extent of the inflammatory response and the amount of new dentinal matrix formed during dentin repair.

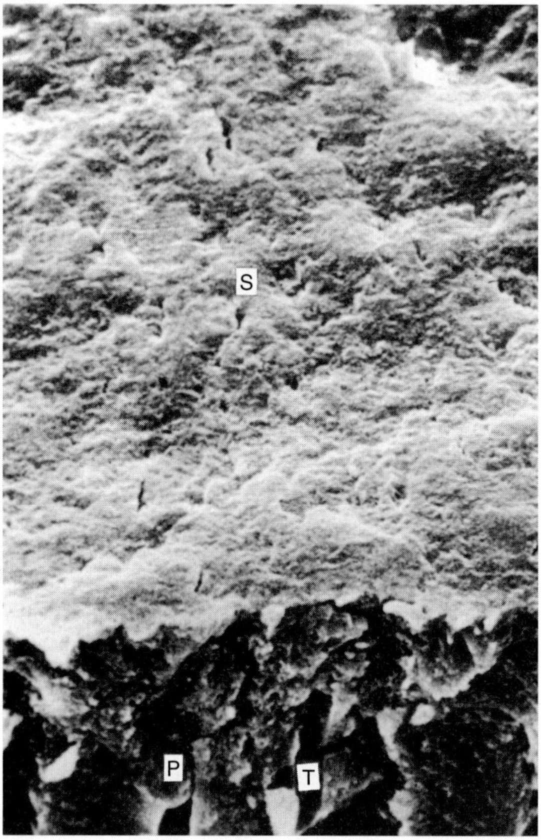

Fig. 5-3 Scanning electron micrograph of cut dentin. When a dentin surface is cut with a bur, a layer of debris, called the *smear layer (S),* remains on the surface. The smear layer consists of organic and inorganic debris that covers the dentinal surface and the tubules *(T).* Often, the debris fills the distal part of the tubules in a smear plug *(P).*

(From Brännström M: *Dentin and pulp in restorative dentistry,* Stockholm, 1981, Dental Therapeutics AB.)

In the absence of a smear layer, components of materials or bacterial products diffuse toward the pulp against the pressure gradient (diffusional permeability, see later discussion). Bacteria can sometimes be seen within tubules below a carious lesion or at the base of a prepared cavity, with or without a restoration (Fig. 5-5). When toxic bacterial or chemical products traverse the dentin, odontoblasts and the pulpal connective tissue usually respond first by focal necrosis (0 to 12 hours), which may be followed by an acute,

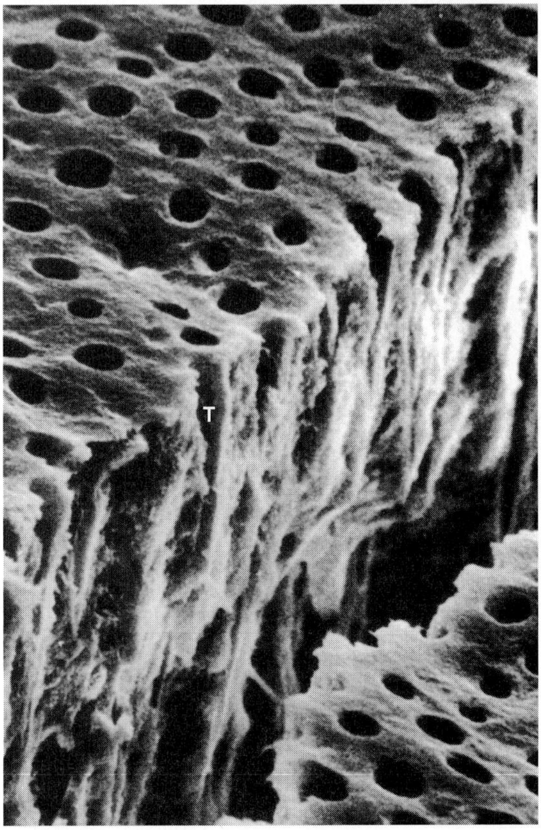

Fig. 5-4 Scanning electron micrograph of acid-etched dentin. When a smear layer (as seen in Fig. 5-3) is etched with an acid, the smear debris is removed. The rate of etching depends on the acid and the character of the dentin. The layer shown above was etched for 5 seconds with 37% phosphoric acid. The smear layer is completely gone and the tubules (*T*) are open. Further etching will open the tubules even further.
(From Brännström M: *Dentin and pulp in restorative dentistry,* Stockholm, 1981, Dental Therapeutics AB.)

but more widespread, pulpitis (12 hours to several days). This response may resolve naturally if the injurious agent is removed or the tubules are blocked. If the pulpitis does not resolve, it may spread to more completely involve the pulp in liquefaction necrosis (especially if the pulpitis results from bacterial products) or in chronic inflammation. Finally, both acute complete pulpitis and acute exacerbation of chronic pulpitis may lead to sequelae such as dental periapical lesions and osteomyelitis, which may be reviewed in oral pathology textbooks.

Dentin Permeability Much has been learned about dentin permeability in the last three decades. In practical terms, two types of dentin permeability occur. The first is fluid convection; that is, movement of fluid through the dentinal tubules. Fluid convection toward the pulp will occur under positive hydraulic pressure when a crown or inlay is being seated. If the dentinal tubules are open, this produces a sharp, localized pain in the pulp from stimulation of A-fibers. Fluid convection away from the pulp will occur with negative osmotic pressures when concentrated solutions, such as sucrose or saturated calcium chloride, are exposed to open dentinal tubules. Clinically, this situation occurs with cervical abrasion or carious lesions. Convection of fluids across dentin varies with the fourth power of the radius of the dentinal tubule (r^4), and thus is very sensitive to the diameter of the tubules. In general, coronal dentin exhibits greater convective permeability than root dentin. Axial wall dentin is more permeable than dentin in the floor of cavities, and dentin near pulp horns (where tubule diameter is greatest) is more permeable than dentin at a distance from the pulp horns. The presence of a smear layer or of cavity liners, sealers, crystals such as calcium oxalate, and even debris and bacteria in the dentinal tubules can dramatically reduce fluid convection.

The second type of dentin permeability is diffusion. Patent dentinal tubules, no matter how small the diameter, establish a diffusion gradient through which ions and molecules can move, even against positive hydraulic pressure. Diffusion is proportional to the length of the dentinal tubules and thus, roughly, to the thickness of the dentin between cavity preparation and the pulp. Smear layers created in cavity preparation are better than cavity liners and sealers at limiting diffusional permeability. However, if the smear layer is incomplete, interrupted, or removed, or if there is a disruption in a cavity liner, sealer, or base, then diffusion of molecules toward the pulp will occur.

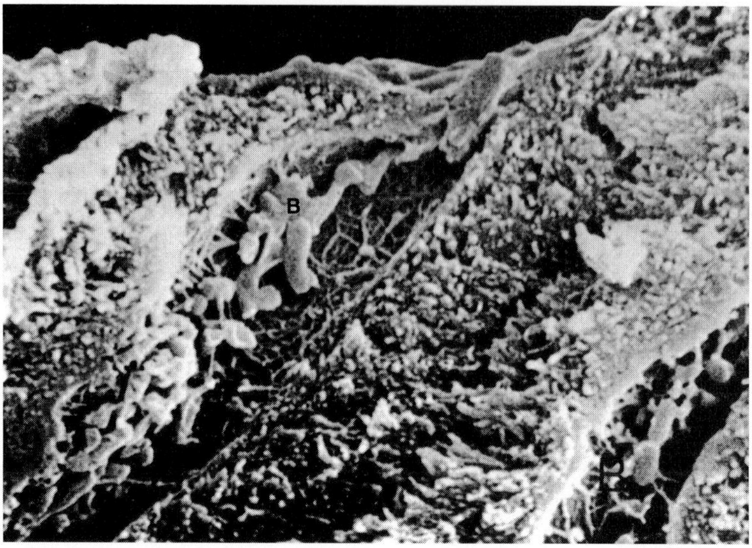

Fig. 5-5 Scanning electron micrograph of bacteria in dentinal tubules. The dentinal tubules may form a conduit for bacteria and bacterial products to reach the pulp of the tooth. Bacteria *(B)* are visible in the tubules under the smear layer, which is visible in cross-section at the top of the picture.

(From Brännström M: *Dentin and pulp in restorative dentistry,* Stockholm, 1981, Dental Therapeutics AB, and London, 1982, Wolfe Medical.)

Diffusion of natural and synthetic molecules through dentin has been studied. In general, diffusion through a given thickness of dentin is proportional to the molecular size of the molecule. Consequently, molecules the size (molecular weight [mw]) of urea (mw 60), phenol (mw 94), and glucose (mw 180) diffuse more easily than molecules the size of dextran (mw 20,000) and albumin (bovine serum albumin, mw 68,000). Through diffusion, small or globular molecules such as albumin, gamma globulin, and the bis-glycidyldimethacrylate (Bis-GMA, an oligomer of dental composites) are diluted 2000 to 10,000 times on the pulpal side of the dentin by 0.3 to 0.4 mm of dentin. Large, fibrous molecules such as fibrinogen are diluted 25,000 to 125,000 times by the same dentin thickness. Most molecules are probably adsorbed to some extent by dentin. Some molecules and atoms or ions, such as tetracycline, zinc, H_2O_2, and fluorescein, are adsorbed to a greater extent than the biological molecules and resin monomers mentioned above. Finally, the capillary beds and vascular dynamics in most healthy pulps are probably capable of removing relatively large amounts of cytotoxic chemicals and bacterial products once they diffuse through the dentin. However, if the pulp is already damaged (inflamed because of caries or trauma), edema and sluggish circulation probably compromise the removal of these materials. Much still needs to be learned about the dynamics and significance of diffusion and adsorption of both host and foreign molecules through dentin.

BONE

Bone is an extracellular matrix (ECM) with accompanying cells and tissue. The ECM of bone is a mineralized tissue composed of about 23% organic substances and about 77% hydroxyapatite. Like dentin, most (86%) of this organic matrix is type I collagen, which gives elastic and viscoelastic qualities to bone. The hydroxyapatite crystals are smaller and less well formed than those in dentin. Because of the vascularity of bone, the mineral phase serves as a major reservoir of calcium and phosphate ions for the body's metabolic processes.

The ECM of bone (osteoid) is synthesized by osteoblasts that constitute the innermost layer of the periosteum and endosteum. The osteoblasts also initiate mineralization of this ECM. As bone is formed, osteoblasts are trapped within the ECM and become osteocytes that reside in lacunae, communicate with cells in other lacunae through canaliculi, and maintain the vitality of bone. These cells die if surgical manipulation destroys the vascular supply or heats the bone above 45° C for more than a few minutes. Another bone-cell type, the osteoclast, decalcifies the ECM and resorbs the organic portion of bone. It also responds to both physiological stimuli and injury. The coupling of osteoblastic and osteoclastic activity directs remodeling and occurs almost continuously throughout life.

Bone has an excellent capacity for self-repair. In bony defects caused by tooth extraction or bone fracture, the site initially fills with blood. The fibrin cascade results in a blood clot that fills this site and attaches to the walls of the alveolar bony socket. Subsequently, mesenchymal cells and endothelial cells grow into the blood clot from the surrounding connective tissue of the alveolar bone and create a young, vascular granulation tissue. With succeeding weeks and months, new osteoblasts differentiate from the granulation tissue and elaborate an ECM that gradually mineralizes. Through osteoblastic and osteoclastic influence, the new bone subsequently remodels itself to the general shape and architecture of the surrounding bone. Alveolar bony mass and height are gradually lost, however, because of the lack of tensile forces from teeth and functional periodontal ligament.

Osseointegration and Biointegration

An issue that faces dentists, and particularly implantologists, is the development of materials for implants that are physically and biologically compatible with alveolar bone. Ideally, bone does not respond to the material as a foreign substance by forming a fibrous tissue capsule around it, but rather should integrate the material, substance, or device into the remodeled bone structure. Under optimum circumstances, bone differentiation should occur directly adjacent to the material (osseointegration). Ideally, osseointegration provides a stable bone-implant connection that can support a dental prosthesis.

Osseointegration is defined as the close approximation of bone to an implant material (Fig. 5-6). To achieve osseointegration, the bone must be viable, the space between the bone and implant must be less than 100 Å and contain no fibrous tissue, and the bone-implant interface must be able to survive loading by a dental prosthesis. In current practice, osseointegration is an absolute requirement for the successful implant-supported dental prosthesis. To achieve osseointegration between an implant and bone, a number of factors must be correct. The bone must be prepared in a way that does not cause necrosis or inflammation (see previous discussion, this section). The implant must be allowed to heal for a time without a load. Finally, the proper material must be placed, because not all materials will promote osseointegration. For reasons that are not completely clear, titanium alloys are by far the most successful materials in promoting osseointegration and are therefore widely used as dental implants. The physical properties of titanium alloys are discussed in Chapter 16.

In recent years there has been a trend to coat titanium alloys with a calcium-phosphate ceramic to better promote an implant bone connection. If successful, the ceramic coating becomes completely fused with the surrounding bone. In this case, the interface is called *biointegration* rather than osseointegration and there is no intervening space between the bone and the implant (see Fig. 5-6). A number of ceramic coatings have been used in this manner, including tricalcium phosphate, hydroxyapatite, and Bioglass. The long-term integrity of the ceramic coating in vivo is not known, but some evidence indicates that these coatings will resorb over time.

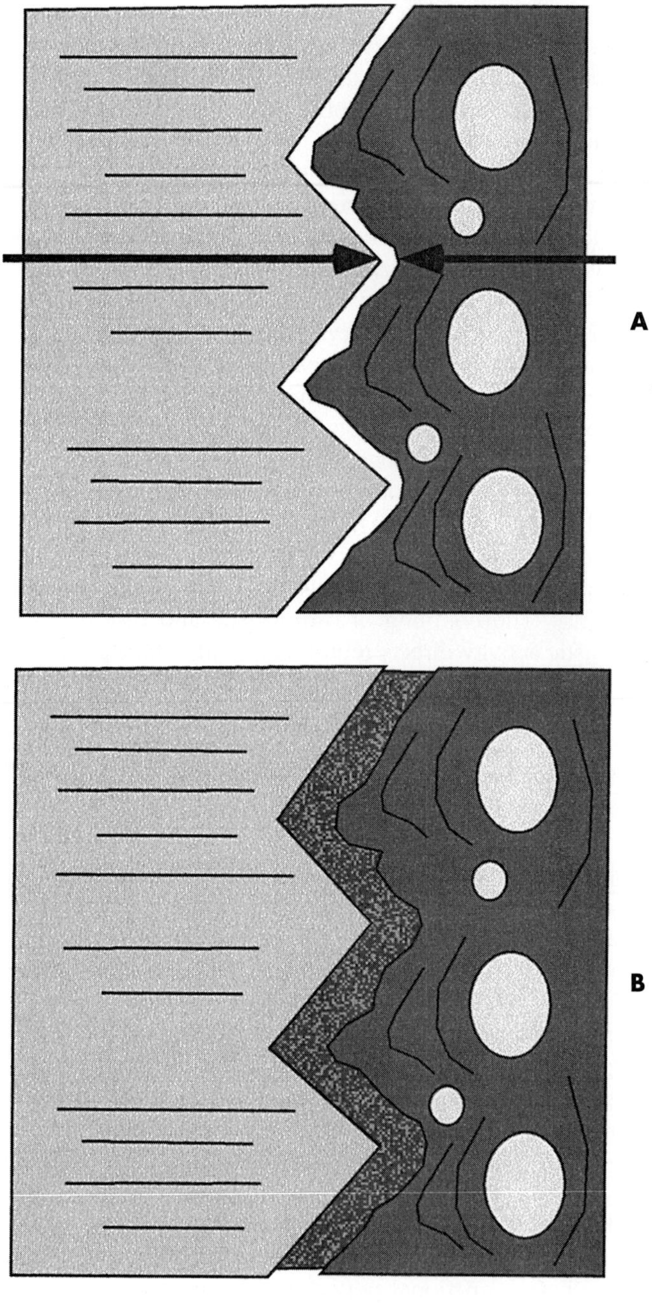

Fig. 5-6 Diagram illustrating the concepts of osseointegration and biointegration. **A,** In osseointegration, the implant material *(left)* and the bone *(right)* closely approximate one another. This approximation must be <100 Å *(arrows)*. In the intervening space, there can be no fibrous tissue. **B,** In biointegration, the implant and bone are fused and continuous with one another. Osseointegration commonly occurs with titanium alloys, whereas biointegration occurs with ceramics and ceramic-coated metallic implants.

PERIODONTIUM

The periodontium is a combination of tissues, including the periodontal ligament (PDL), cementum, and alveolar bone. The cementum and alveolar bone are mineralized extracellular matrices with the associated cells that are responsible for generating and maintaining them.

Collagenous fibers of the PDL extend from cementum to fibrous connective tissue above the alveolar crest, to alveolar cortical bone, or to the cementum of adjacent teeth. The ends of these collagenous fibers are anchored in a calcified ECM synthesized by cementoblasts (cementoid) or osteoblasts (osteoid). The orientation of the fibers translates compressive forces of mastication to tensile forces on the cementum and alveolar bone. The tensile stress stimulates low-grade cementogenesis and osteogenesis and maintains fairly constant alveolar bone heights, cementum thicknesses, and PDL widths. The exact mechanisms involved in these processes remain largely unknown and are of great interest in the fields of periodontology, implantology, and orthopedic surgery. In contrast, direct pressure (compression) on alveolar bone and cementum (e.g., in orthodontic movement) results in PDL and alveolar bone necrosis and an active biological resorption that removes portions of alveolar bone, cementum, and dentin from the tooth root. The necrosis is caused by ischemia of PDL and alveolar bone.

The PDL and its attachments to alveolar bone and teeth are maintained by cellular synthetic processes. At least in some animal species, there appears to be some compartmentalization of differentiated cells within the PDL, with fibroblasts in the tooth half of the PDL moving mesially with the constantly erupting incisor. Thus specific populations of differentiated, predifferentiated, or precursor cells probably give rise to and maintain the matrices of cementum, alveolar bone, and PDL. When cells that maintain the PDL are destroyed during injury and have no source of progenitor cells, ankylosis may result between tooth and bone (e.g., after tooth transplantation or placement of dental implant).

Regeneration of PDL, epithelial attachment, and alveolar bone around periodontally diseased teeth is an important issue in dentistry. In an attempt at regeneration, gingival epithelium replaces crevicular epithelium, which was originally responsible for the epithelial attachment of the tooth. Following scaling and curettage of periodontal pockets, this gingival epithelium proliferates faster than the PDL fibers can reattach in newly formed cementum. Although fibrous reattachment to alveolar bone appears to occur quite readily, the original orientation of fiber to the tooth surface seems quite difficult to achieve. This results in epithelial-lined subcrestal pockets in the PDL space between alveolar bone and tooth surface. When this process advances, it has the effect of exfoliating the tooth. Investigators have made efforts to limit epithelial downgrowth of the gingiva, to enhance PDL reattachment to tooth and bone surfaces by chemical and surgical means, and to use implant materials that maximize epithelial and connective tissue cell attachment and limit the apical migration of epithelial cells.

GINGIVA AND MUCOSA

The linings of the oral cavity are composed of gingiva and oral mucosa. The gingiva is a connective tissue with an epithelial surface that covers the alveolar ridge, surrounds the cervices of the teeth, and fills interproximal spaces between teeth. Gingiva is divided into attached and free gingiva. The attached gingiva forms a junction with the alveolar oral mucosa toward the vestibule of the mouth and with the free gingival margin toward the crowns of the teeth. The free gingiva fuses with the attachment epithelium, which surrounds the tooth at its cervix in the young, healthy tooth. Some of the crevicular epithelium and all the attachment epithelium, at least in the young individual, are derived embryologically from reduced enamel epithelium. The oral mucosa is composed of a loose fibroelastic connective tissue with a well-vascularized and innervated lamina propria and submucosa and is covered mainly by a parakeratinized stratified squamous epithelium.

The oral mucous membrane can be injured chemically or physically by dental materials. If the injury is short-term (acute) and leads to loss of tissue but does not involve infection by pathogenic microorganisms, the connective tissue defect is filled in with granulation tissue within 3 to 4 days and epithelium regenerates over the surface within a week. The tissue is remodeled to nearly normal by the end of 2 to 3 weeks. As with other body tissues, the ability to heal depends on the metabolic status of the patient and the removal of external irritating factors. Occasionally, immune hypersensitivity to materials or pharmaceutical agents may delay the healing response. The presence of microorganisms or immune hypersensitivity reactions results in an infiltration of acute or chronic inflammatory cells and delay of healing.

The gingival response to injury may be complicated by its association with the tooth. Calculus deposition on the tooth, malocclusion, and faulty restorations may enhance the destructive effects of microorganisms. The crevicular epithelium then becomes vulnerable to endotoxin and various exogenous and endogenous chemicals. The resulting breakdown of tissue leads to an acute inflammatory response by the gingival connective tissue called *acute gingivitis.* This condition is often reversible if the injurious agent is removed and the reaction is limited to the connective tissue above the alveolar bony crest. If the insult continues, the inflammatory infiltrate becomes mixed and then predominantly mononuclear. Inflamed epithelial-lined granulation tissue gradually spreads apically to and below the alveolar bony crest. At this point the condition is described as *chronic periodontal disease,* a progressive disease process that is probably reinforced by immune mechanisms. The relationship between periodontal disease and dental materials that are in close contact with the gingiva is not known but is an active area of research.

The reaction of gingival tissues to oral implants is also an important area of research. Permucosal implants present special problems, including epithelial ingrowth, encystification, and exfoliation of the implant. There is also the problem of maintaining a close epithelial attachment between the implant and soft tissue to exclude bacteria. Thus the implant material should ideally encourage firm attachment of epithelial cells on its surface, but only limited growth and migration of these cells. An inflammatory disease around implants, called *peri-implantitis,* has been described and is probably similar in etiology and progression to periodontal disease. Peri-implantitis occurs in response to bacteria that attach to implants and exist near the gingiva. The role of materials in altering the peri-implantitis process is not currently known.

Dental materials that are antigenic can cause immune hypersensitivity reactions in oral mucosa and gingiva. Local binding of antigens to membranes of white blood cells (i.e., lymphocytes, macrophages, basophils, mast cells) or Langerhans' cells of skin and oral mucosal epithelium plays a role in activating these various reactions. Although a few of the mucosal reactions are documented as Type I reactions (wherein vasoactive substances are released from mast cells because of antigen-IgE reactions), most reactions to dental materials are classified as Type IV (T-cell–mediated) reactions. This type of reaction is sometimes called *contact mucositis.* Skin testing can be used to help document Type I and Type IV reactions to environmental antigens, metallic elements used in alloys, and byproducts from polymers. In vitro tests for cell-mediated hyperimmunity are occasionally performed and include transformation of the patient's lymphocytes and production of a migration-inhibition factor by these cells in response to the antigenic stimulus.

MEASURING BIOCOMPATIBILITY

Measuring the biocompatibility of a material is not simple, and the methods of measurement are evolving rapidly as more is known about the interactions between dental materials and oral tissues and as technologies for testing improve. Historically, new materials were simply tried in humans to see if they were biocompatible. However, this practice has not been acceptable for many years, and current materials must be extensively screened for biocompatibility before they are ever used in humans. Several varieties of tests are currently used to try to ensure that new materials are biologically acceptable. These tests are classified as in vitro, animal, and usage tests. These three testing types include the clinical trial, which is really a special case of a usage test in humans. The remainder of this section will discuss several of each type of test, their advantages and disadvantages, how the tests are used together, and standards that rely on these tests to regulate the use of materials in dentistry.

IN VITRO TESTS

In vitro tests for biocompatibility are done in a test tube, cell-culture dish, or otherwise outside of a living organism. These tests require placement of a material or a component of a material in contact with a cell, enzyme, or some other isolated biological system. The contact can be either direct, where the material contacts the cell system without barriers, or indirect, where there is a barrier of some sort between the material and the cell system. Direct tests can be further subdivided into those in which the material is physically present with the cells and those in which some extract from the material contacts the cell system. In vitro tests can be roughly subdivided into those that measure cytotoxicity or cell growth, those that measure some metabolic or other cell function, and those that measure the effect on the genetic material in a cell (mutagenesis assays). Often there is some overlap in what a test measures. In vitro tests have a number of significant advantages over other types of biocompatibility tests (Table 5-1). They are relatively quick to perform, generally cost much less than animal or usage tests, can be standardized, are well suited to large scale screening, and can be tightly controlled to address specific scientific questions. The overriding disadvantage of in vitro tests is their questionable relevance to the final in vivo use of the material (see later section on correlation between tests). Other disadvantages include the lack of inflammatory and other tissue-protective mechanisms in the in vitro environment. It should be emphasized that in vitro tests alone cannot usually predict the overall biocompatibility of a material.

Standardization of in vitro tests is a primary concern of those trying to evaluate materials.

TABLE 5-1 Advantages and Disadvantages of Biocompatibility Tests

Test	Advantages	Disadvantages
In vitro tests	Quick to perform Least expensive Can be standardized Large-scale screening Good experimental control Excellence for mechanisms of interactions	Relevance to in vivo is questionable
In vivo tests	Allows complex systemic interactions Response more comprehensive than in vitro tests More relevant than in vitro tests?	Relevance to use of material questionable Expensive Time consuming Legal/ethical concerns Difficult to control Difficult to interpret and quantify
Usage tests	Relevance to use of material is assured	Very expensive Very time consuming Major legal/ethical issues Can be difficult to control Difficult to interpret and quantify

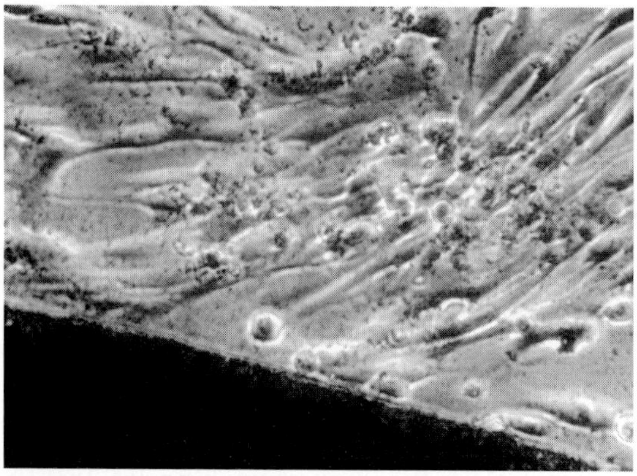

Fig. 5-7 Light microscopic view of a noncytotoxic interaction between a material (dark image at bottom of the picture) and periodontal ligament fibroblasts in a cell-culture (in vitro) test. The morphology of the fibroblasts indicates that they are alive and are not suffering from a toxic response (see Fig. 5-8 for contrast). The material in this case was a calcium hydroxide pulp-capping agent.

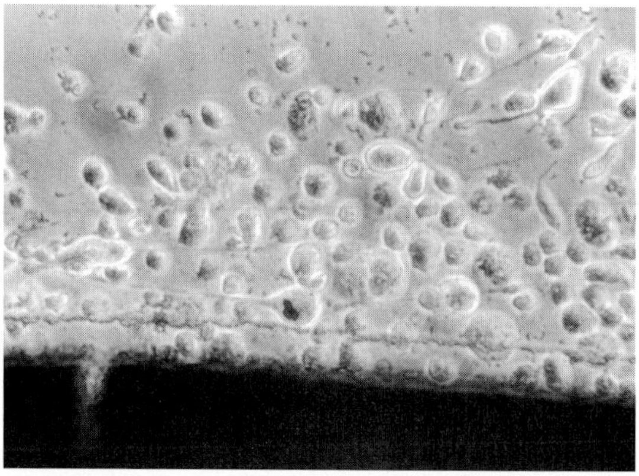

Fig. 5-8 Light microscopic view of a cytotoxic interaction between a material (dark image at the bottom of the picture) and periodontal ligament fibroblasts in a cell-culture test. The fibroblasts are rounded and detached (see Fig 5-7 for contrast), indicating that they are either dead or dying. The material is a type of calcium hydroxide pulp-capping agent, different from the one shown in Fig. 5-7.

Two types of cells can be used for in vitro assays. *Primary cells* are cells taken directly from an animal into culture. These cells will grow for only a limited time in culture but may retain many of the characteristics of cells in vivo. *Continuous cells* are primary cells that have been transformed to allow them to grow more or less indefinitely in culture. Because of their transformation, these cells may not retain all in vivo characteristics, but they consistently exhibit any features that they do retain. Primary cell cultures would seemingly be more relevant than continuous cell lines for measuring cytotoxicity of materials. However, primary cells have the problems of being from a single individual, possibly harboring viral or bacterial agents that alter their behavior, and often rapidly losing their in vivo functionality once placed in a cell culture. Furthermore, the genetic and metabolic stability of continuous cell lines contributes significantly toward standardizing assay methods. In the end, both primary and continuous cells play an important role in in vitro testing; both should be used to assess a material.

Cytotoxicity Tests Cytotoxicity tests assess the cytotoxicity of a material by measuring cell number or growth after exposure to a material. Cells are plated in a well of a cell-culture dish where they attach. The material is then placed in the test system. If the material is not cytotoxic, the cells will remain attached to the well and will proliferate with time. If the material is cytotoxic, the cells may stop growing, exhibit cytopathic features (Figs. 5-7 and 5-8), or detach from the well. If the material is a solid, then the density (number of cells per unit area) of cells may be assessed at different distances from the material, and a "zone" of inhibited cell growth may be described (Fig. 5-9). Cell density can be assessed either qualitatively, semi-quantitatively, or quantitatively. Substances such as Teflon can be used as negative (non-cytotoxic) controls, whereas materials such as plasticized polyvinyl chloride can be used as positive (cytotoxic) controls. Control materials should be well defined and commercially available to facilitate comparisons among testing laboratories.

Another group of tests is used to measure cytotoxicity by a change in membrane permeability (Fig. 5-10). *Membrane permeability* is the ease with which a dye can pass through a cell membrane. This test is used on the basis that a

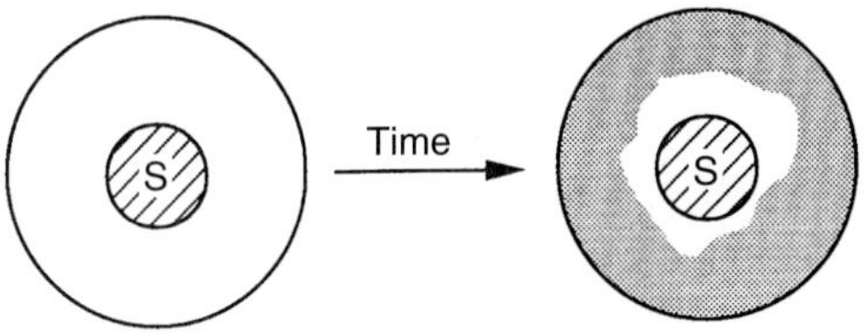

Fig. 5-9 A material sample *(S)* is placed in the center of a cell-culture well, and cells and medium are added. After 1 to 3 days, the cells have multiplied in areas where the material has not inhibited their growth. The area devoid of growth is often referred to as a *ring of inhibition*. Several methods are available to assess the amount of cellular growth around the samples.

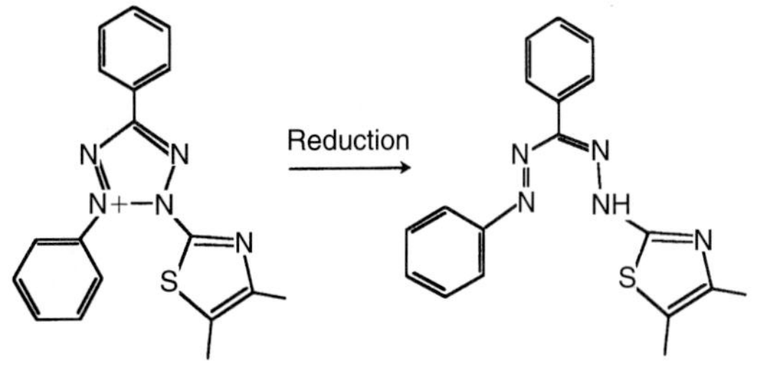

Fig. 5-11 MTT is a yellow, soluble molecule that can be used to assess cellular enzymatic activity. If the cell is able to reduce the MTT, the resulting formazan is blue and insoluble and deposits in the cell. The amount of formazan formed is proportional to the enzymatic activity. The activity of a number of cellular enzymes can be assessed in this manner.

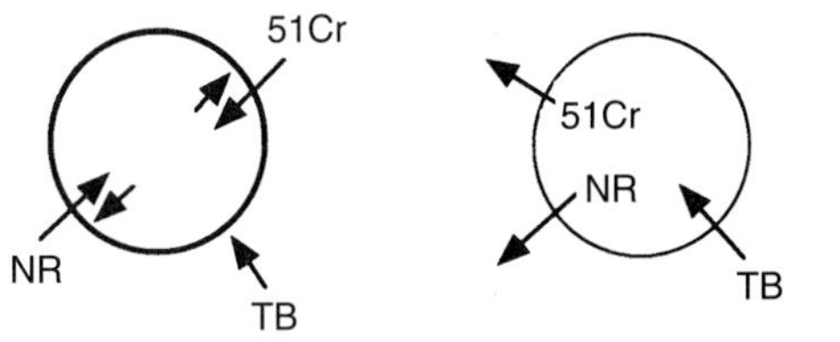

Fig. 5-10 The selective permeability of cell membranes is the basis for several cytotoxicity tests. Compounds such as $Na^{51}CrO_4$ *(^{51}Cr)*, and neutral red *(NR)* are actively sequestered by healthy cells. These compounds will leach out of the cell if the cell is injured and cannot maintain its membrane integrity. Other compounds such as trypan blue *(TB)* are excluded by a healthy cell, but can diffuse through the membrane of an injured cell.

loss in membrane permeability is equivalent to or very nearly equivalent to cell death. The advantage of the membrane permeability test is that it identifies cells that are alive (or dead) under the microscope. This feature is important because it is possible for cells to be physically present, but dead (when materials fix the cells). There are two basic types of dyes used. Vital dyes are actively transported into viable cells, where they are retained unless cytotoxic effects increase the permeability of the membrane. It is important to establish that the dye itself does not exhibit cytotoxicity during the time frame of the test. Nonvital dyes are not actively transported, and are only taken up if membrane permeability has been compromised by cytotoxicity. Many types of vital dyes have been used, including neutral red and $Na_2{}^{51}CrO_4$. The use of neutral red and $Na_2{}^{51}CrO_4$ are particularly advantageous because they are neither synthesized nor metabolized by the cell. Examples of nonvital dyes include trypan blue and propidium iodide.

Tests for Cell Metabolism or Cell Function Some in vitro tests for biocompatibility use the biosynthetic or enzymatic activity of cells to assess cytotoxic response. Tests that measure deoxyribonucleic acid (DNA) synthesis or protein synthesis are common examples of this type of test. The synthesis of DNA or protein by cells is usually analyzed by adding radioisotope-labeled precursors to the medium and quantifying the radioisotope (e.g., ^{3}H-thymidine or ^{3}H-leucine) incorporated into DNA or protein. A commonly used enzymatic test for cytotoxicity is the MTT test. This test measures the activity of cellular dehydrogenases, which convert a chemical called MTT, via several cellular reducing agents, to a blue, insoluble formazan compound (Fig. 5-11). If the dehydrogenases are not active because of cytotoxic effects, the formazan will not form. The production of formazan can be quantified by dissolving it and measuring the optical density of the resulting solution. Alternatively, the formazan can be localized around the test sample by light or electron microscopy. Other formazan-generating chemicals have been used, including NBT, XTT, and WST. Furthermore, many other activities of cells can be followed qualitatively or quantitatively in vitro. Recently, in vitro tests to measure gene activation, gene expression, cellular oxidative stress, and other specific cell functions have been proposed. However, these types of tests are not yet routinely used to assess the biocompatibility of materials.

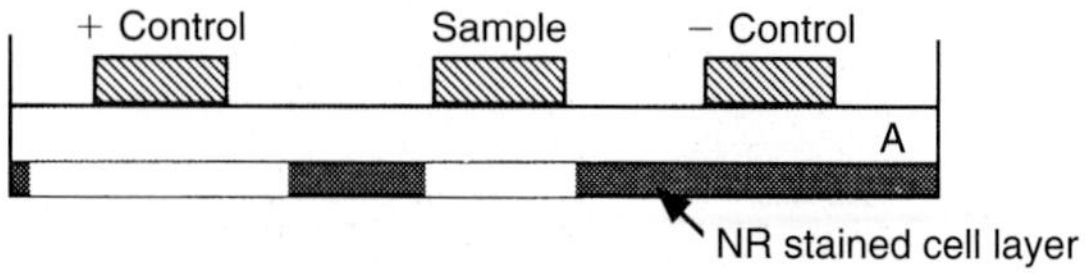

Fig. 5-12 The agar overlay method has been used to evaluate the cytotoxicity of dental materials. The cell layer, which has been previously stained with neutral red *(NR)*, is covered with a thin layer of agar *(A)*. Samples are placed on top of the agar for a time. If the material is cytotoxic, it will injure the cells and the neutral red will be released, leaving a zone of inhibition.

Tests That Use Barriers (Indirect Tests)

Most of the cytotoxicity tests presented thus far are performed with the material in direct contact with the cell culture. Researchers have long recognized that in vivo, direct contact often does not exist between cells and the materials. Separation of cells and materials may occur from keratinized epithelium, dentin, or extracellular matrix. Thus several in vitro barrier tests have been developed to mimic in vivo conditions. One such test is the agar overlay method (Fig. 5-12) in which a monolayer of cultured cells is established before adding 1% agar or agarose (low melting temperature) plus a vital stain, such as neutral red, to fresh culture media. The agar forms a barrier between the cells and the material, which is placed on top of the agar. Nutrients, gas, and soluble toxic substances can diffuse through the agar. Solid test samples or liquid samples adsorbed onto filter paper can be tested with this assay for up to 24 hours. This assay correlates positively with the direct-contact assays described above and the intramuscular implantation test in rabbits. However, the agar may not adequately represent barriers that occur in vivo. Furthermore, because of variability of the agar's diffusion properties, it is difficult to correlate the intensity of color or width of the zone around a material with the concentration of leachable toxic products.

A second barrier assay is the Millipore filter assay. This technique establishes a monolayer of cells on filters made of cellulose esters. The culture medium is then replaced with medium containing about 1% agar, and this mixture is allowed to gel over the cells. Finally, the filter-monolayer-gel is detached and turned over so that the filter is on top for placement of solid or soluble test samples for 2 or more hours. After exposure to the test samples, the filter is removed and an assay is used to determine the effect of the sample on a cellular metabolic activity. The succinyl dehydrogenase assay described previously can be used with this test. Like the agar overlay test and the cell contact tests, toxicity in the Millipore filter test is assessed by the width of the cytotoxic zone around each test sample. This test also has the drawback of arbitrarily influencing the diffusion of leachable products from the test material. The agar diffusion and Millipore filter tests can provide, at best, a cytotoxic ranking among materials.

Dentin barrier tests have shown improved correlation with the cytotoxicity of dental materials in usage tests in teeth, and are gradually being developed for screening purposes (Fig. 5-13). A number of studies have shown that dentin forms a barrier through which toxic materials must diffuse to reach pulpal tissue. Thus pulpal reaction to zinc oxide-eugenol is relatively mild as compared with the more severe reactions to the same material in direct contact with cells in in vitro assays and tissue in implantation tests. The thickness of the dentin correlates directly with the protection offered to the pulp. Thus

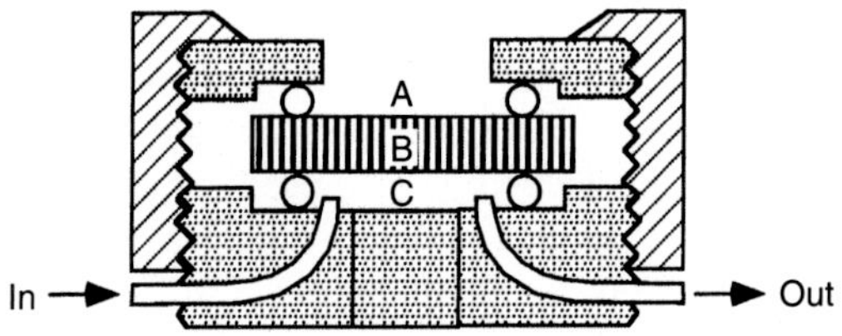

Fig. 5-13 A dentin disk used as a barrier in cytotoxicity tests that attempt to predict the toxicity of materials placed on dentin in vivo. The material is placed on one side *(A)* of the dentin disk *(B)* in the device used to hold the dentin disk. Collection fluid (cell culture medium or saline) is on the other side of the disk *(C)*. Cells can also be grown in the collection side. Components of the material may diffuse through the dentin and the effect of the medium on cell metabolism can then be measured. To assess the rate of diffusion, the collection fluid can be circulated into and out of the collection chamber *(C)*.

assays have been developed that incorporate dentin disks between the test sample and the cell assay system. The use of dentin disks offers the added advantage of directional diffusion between the restorative material and the culture medium.

Other Assays for Cell Function In vitro assays to measure immune function or other tissue reactions have also been used. The in vivo significance of these assays is yet to be ascertained, but many show promise for being able to reduce the number of animal tests required to assess the biocompatibility of a material. These assays measure cytokine production by lymphocytes and macrophages, lymphocyte proliferation, chemotaxis, or T-cell rosetting to sheep red blood cells. Other tests measure the ability of a material to alter the cell cycle or activate complement. The activation of complement is of particular concern to researchers working on artificial or "engineered" blood vessels and other tissues in direct contact with blood. Materials that activate complement may generate inflammation or thrombi, and may propagate a chronic inflammatory response. Whereas concerns about complement activation by dental materials are fewer, it is possible that activation of complement by resins or metals or their corrosion products may prolong inflammation in the gingiva or pulp.

Mutagenesis Assays Mutagenesis assays assess the effect of materials on a cell's genetic material. There is a wide range of mechanisms by which materials can affect the genetic material of the cell. Genotoxic mutagens directly alter the DNA of the cell through various types of mutations. Each chemical may be associated with a specific type of DNA mutation. Genotoxic chemicals may be mutagens in their native states, or may require activation or biotransformation to be mutagens, in which case they are called *promutagens*. Epigenetic mutagens do not alter the DNA themselves, but support tumor growth by altering the cell's biochemistry, altering the immune system, acting as hormones, or other mechanisms. *Carcinogenesis* is the ability to cause cancer in vivo. Mutagens may or may not be carcinogens, and carcinogens may or may not be mutagens. Thus the quantification and relevance of tests that attempt to measure mutagenesis and carcinogenesis are extremely complex. A number of government-sponsored programs evaluate the ability of in vitro mutagenesis assays to predict carcinogenicity.

The Ames' test is the most widely used short-term mutagenesis test and the only short-term test that is considered thoroughly validated. It uses mutant stocks of *Salmonella typhimurium* that require exogenous histidine. Native stocks of bacteria do not require exogenous histidine. Exclusion of histidine from the culture medium allows a chemical to be tested for its ability to convert the mutant strain to a native strain. Chemicals that significantly increase the frequency of reversion back to the native state have a reportedly high probability of being carcinogenic in mammals because they significantly alter genetic material. Performance of this test requires experience in the field and special strains of *Salmonella* to produce meaningful results. Several stains of *Salmonella* are used, each to detect a different type of mutation transformation. Furthermore, chemicals can be "metabolized" in vitro using homogenates of liver enzymes to simulate the body's action on chemicals before testing for mutagenicity.

A second test for mutagenesis is the Styles' Cell Transformation test. This test on mammalian cells was developed to offer an alternative to bacterial tests (Ames test), which may not be relevant to mammalian systems. This assay quantifies the ability of potential carcinogens to transform standardized cell lines so they will grow in soft agar. Untransformed fibroblasts normally will not grow within an agar gel, whereas genetically transformed cells will grow below the gel surface. This characteristic of transformed fibroblasts is the only characteristic that correlates with the ability of cells to produce tumors in vivo. At least four different continuous cell lines (Chang, BHK, HeLa, WI-38) have been used. In 1978, Styles claimed 94% "accuracy in determining carcinogenic or noncarcinogenic activity" when testing 120 compounds in two cell lines. However, there has been some difficulty in reproducing these results.

In a recent report, four short-term tests (STTs) for gene toxicity were compared (Table 5-2). The Ames test was the most specific (86% of noncarcinogens yielding a negative result). The Ames test also had the highest positive predictability (83% of positives were actually carcinogens) and displayed negative predictability equal to that of other STTs (i.e., 51% of all Ames test negatives were noncarcinogenic). However, the results were in agreement (concordance) with rodent carcinogenicity tests for only 62% of the chemicals. Also, the Ames test was sensitive to only 45% of the carcinogens; that is, it missed over half of the known carcinogens. The other three STTs were assays for chromosomal aberration, sister chromatid exchange in CHO cells, and the mouse lymphoma L5178Y cell mutagenesis assay. The sister chromatid exchange method, the mouse lymphoma mutagenesis assay, and the Ames test had 73%, 70%, and 45% sensitivity, respectively. However, because the Ames test is widely used, extensively described in the literature, and technically easier to conduct in a testing laboratory than the other tests, it is most often conducted in a screening program. These studies suggest that not all carcinogens are genotoxic (mutagenic) and not all mutagens are carcinogenic. Thus, although STTs for mutagenesis are

TABLE 5-2 Comparison of In Vitro Mutagenesis Tests

Test Parameter	Parameter Description	Test Results (Average %)			
		Ames	SCE	MOLY	ABS
Specificity	Known noncarcinogenic material gives negative test result	86	45	45	69
Sensitivity	Known carcinogenic material gives positive test result	45	73	70	55
Positive predictability	Positive test accurately predicts a carcinogen	83	67	66	73
Negative predictability	Negative test accurately predicts a noncarcinogen	51	52	50	50
Concordance	Percent of qualitative agreements between STT and rodent carcinogenicity tests	62	62	60	60

Adapted from Tennant RW, Margolin BH, Shelby MD, et al: *Science* 236:933, 1987.
SCE, Sister chromatid exchange test; *MOLY,* mouse lymphoma assay; *ABS,* chromosome aberration test; *STT,* short-term test.

helpful for predicting some carcinogens, STTs cannot predict all of them.

ANIMAL TESTS

Animal tests for biocompatibility are usually used in mammals such as mice, rats, hamsters, or guinea pigs, although many types of animals have been used. Animal tests are distinct from usage tests (which are also often done in animals) in that the material is not placed in the animal with regard to its final use. The use of an animal allows many complex interactions between the material and a functioning, complete biological system to occur. For example, an immune response may occur or complement may be activated in an animal system in a way that would be difficult to mimic in a cell-culture system. Thus the biological responses in animal tests are more comprehensive and may be more relevant than in vitro tests, and these are the major advantages of these tests (see Table 5-1). The main disadvantages of animal tests are that they can be difficult to interpret and control, are expensive, may be time consuming, and often involve significant ethical concerns and paperwork. Furthermore, the relevance of the test to the in vivo use of a material can be quite unclear, especially in estimating the appropriateness of an animal species to represent a human. A variety of animal tests have been used to assess biocompatibility, and a few are discussed in detail below.

The *mucous membrane irritation test* determines if a material causes inflammation to mucous membranes or abraded skin. This test is conducted by placing the test materials and positive and negative controls into contact with hamster cheek-pouch tissue or rabbit oral tissue. After several weeks of contact, the controls and test sites are examined, and the gross tissue reactions in the living animals are recorded and photographed in color. The animals are then sacrificed, and biopsy specimens are prepared for histological evaluation of inflammatory changes.

In the *skin sensitization test* in guinea pigs (guinea pig maximization test), the materials are injected intradermally to test for development of skin hypersensitivity reactions. Freund's adjuvant can be used to augment the reaction. This injection is followed by secondary treatment with adhesive patches containing the test substance. If hypersensitivity developed from the initial injection, the patch will elicit an inflammatory response. The skin-patch test can result in a spectrum from no reaction to intense redness and swelling. The degree of reaction in the patch test and the percentage of animals that show a reaction are the bases for estimating the allergenicity of the material.

Animal tests that measure the mutagenic and carcinogenic properties of materials have been developed by toxicologists. These tests are employed with a strategy called the *decision-point approach*. Using this strategy, tests are applied in a specific order, and testing is stopped when any one indicates mutagenic potential of the material or chemical. The validity of any of these tests may be affected by issues of species, tissue, gender, and other factors. Tests are generally divided into limited-term in vivo tests and long-term or lifetime tests. Limited-term in vivo tests measure altered liver function or increased tumor induction when animals are exposed to the chemicals for a fraction of their lifetimes. Long-term in vivo tests are performed by keeping the chemical in contact with the animal over the majority of its lifetime.

Implantation tests are used to evaluate materials that will contact subcutaneous tissue or bone. The location of the implant site is determined by the use of the material, and may include connective tissue, bone, or muscle. Although amalgams and alloys are tested because the margins of the restorative materials contact the gingiva, most subcutaneous tests are used for materials that will directly contact soft tissue during implantation, endodontic, or periodontal treatment. Short-term implantation is studied by aseptically placing the compounds in small, open-ended, polyethylene tubes into the tissue. The test samples and controls are placed at separate sites, and allowed to remain for 1 to 11 weeks. Alternatively, an empty tube is embedded first, and the inflammatory reaction from surgery is allowed to subside. The implant site is then reopened, and the test material is placed into this healed site or is packed into the tube that was placed previously. At the appropriate time, the areas are excised and prepared for microscopic examination and interpretation. The tissue response can be evaluated by normal histological, histochemical, or immunohistochemical methods. Implantation tests of longer duration, for identification of either chronic inflammation or tumor formation, are performed in a manner similar to that of short-term tests except the materials remain in place for 1 to 2 years before examination.

USAGE TESTS

Usage tests may be done in animals or in human volunteers. They are distinct from other animal tests because they require that the material be placed in a situation identical to its intended clinical use. The usefulness of a usage test for predicting biocompatibility is directly proportional to the fidelity with which the test mimics the clinical use of the material in every regard, including time, location, environment, and placement technique. For this reason, usage tests in animals usually employ larger animals that have similar oral environments to humans, such as dogs or monkeys. If humans are used, the usage test is identical to a clinical trial. The overwhelming advantage for a usage test is its relevance (see Table 5-1). These tests are the gold standard of tests in that they give the ultimate answer to whether a material will be biocompatible. One might ask, then, why bother with in vitro or animal tests at all. The answer is in the significant disadvantages of the usage test. These tests are extremely expensive, last for long periods, involve many ethical and often legal concerns, and are exceptionally difficult to control and interpret accurately. The statistical analysis of these tests is often a daunting process. In dentistry, dental pulp, periodontium, and gingival or mucosal tissues are generally the targets of usage tests.

Dental Pulp Irritation Tests Generally, materials to be tested on the dental pulp are placed in class-5 cavity preparations in intact, noncarious teeth of monkeys or other suitable animals. Care is taken to prepare uniformly sized cavities. After anesthesia and a thorough prophylaxis of teeth, cavities are prepared under sterile conditions with an efficient water-spray coolant to ensure minimal trauma to the pulp. The compounds are placed in an equal number of anterior and posterior teeth of the maxilla and mandible to ensure uniform distribution in all types of teeth. The materials are left in place from 1 to 8 weeks. Zinc oxide–eugenol and silicate cement have been used as negative and positive control materials, respectively.

At the conclusion of the study, the teeth are removed and sectioned for microscopic examination. The tissue sections are evaluated by the investigators without knowledge of the identity of the materials, and necrotic and inflammatory reactions are classified according to the intensity of the response. The thicknesses of the remaining dentin and reparative dentin for each histological specimen is measured with a photomicrometer and recorded. The response of the pulp is evaluated based on its appearance after treatment. The severity of the lesions is based on disruption of the structure of the tissue and the number of inflammatory cells (usually both acute and chronic) present. Pulpal response is classified as either slight (mild hyperemia, few inflammatory cells, slight hemorrhage in odontoblastic zone), moderate (definite increase in number of inflammatory cells, hyperemia, and slight disruption of odontoblastic zone), or severe (decided inflammatory infiltrate, hyperemia, total disruption of odontoblastic layer in the zone of cavity preparation, reduction or absence of predentin, and perhaps even localized abscesses). As with dental caries, the mononuclear cells are usually most prominent in the inflammatory response. If neutrophils are present, the presence of bacteria or bacterial products must be suspected. Some investigators now use zinc oxide–eugenol (ZOE) cements to "surface-seal" the restorations to eliminate the effects of microleakage on the pulp.

Until recently, most dental-pulp irritation tests have involved intact, noncarious teeth, without inflamed pulps. There has been increased concern that inflamed dental pulp tissue may respond differently than normal pulps to liners, cements, and restorative agents. Efforts have been made to develop techniques that identify bacterial insults to the pulp. Usage tests that study teeth with induced pulpitis allows evaluation of types and amount of reparative dentin formed and will probably continue to be developed.

Dental Implants into Bone At present, the best estimations of the success and failure of implants are gained from three tests: (1) penetration of a periodontal probe along the side of the implant, (2) mobility of the implant, and (3) radiographs indicating either osseous integration or radiolucency around the implant. Currently, an implant is considered successful if it exhibits no mobility, no radiographic evidence of peri-implant radiolucency, minimal vertical bone loss, and absence of persistent peri-implant soft tissue complications. Previously, investigators argued that formation of a fibrous connective tissue capsule around a subperiosteal implant or root cylinder was the natural reaction of the body to a material. They argued that this was actually an attachment similar to the periodontal ligament and should be considered a sign of an acceptable material. However, in most cases it resembled the wall of a cyst, which is the body's attempt to isolate the implanted material as the material slowly degrades and leaches its components into tissue. Currently, for implants in bone, implants should be completely encased in bone, the most differentiated state of that tissue. Fibrous capsule formation is a sign of irritation and chronic inflammation.

Mucosa and Gingival Usage Tests Because various dental materials contact gingival and mucosal tissues, the tissue response to these materials must be measured. Materials are placed in cavity preparations with subgingival extensions. The materials' effects on gingival tissues are observed at 7 days and again after 30 days. Responses are categorized as slight, moderate, or severe. A slight response is characterized by a few mononuclear inflammatory cells (mainly lymphocytes) in the epithelium and adjacent connective tissue. A moderate response is indicated by numerous mononuclear cells in the connective tissue and a few neutrophils in the epithelium. A severe reaction evokes a significant mononuclear and neutrophilic infiltrate and thinned or absent epithelium.

A difficulty with this type of study is the frequent presence of some degree of preexisting inflammation in gingival tissue. Bacterial plaque is the most important factor in causing this inflammation. Secondary factors are the surface roughness of the restorative material, open or overhanging margins, and overcontouring or undercontouring of the restoration. One way to reduce the interference of inflammation caused by plaque is to perform dental prophylaxis before preparing the cavity and placing the material. However, the prophylaxis and cavity preparation will themselves cause some inflammation of the soft tissues. Thus, if margins are placed subgingivally, time for healing (typically 8 to 14 days) must be allowed before assessing the effects of the restorative agents.

CORRELATION AMONG IN VITRO, ANIMAL, AND USAGE TESTS

In the field of biocompatibility, some scientists question the usefulness of in vitro and animal tests in light of the apparent lack of correlation with usage tests and the clinical history of materials. However, the lack of correlation is not surprising in light of the differences among these tests. In vitro and animal tests often measure aspects of the biological response that are more subtle or less prominent than in a material's clinical usage. Furthermore, barriers between the material and tissues may exist in usage tests or clinical use that may not exist in in vitro or animal tests. Thus it is important to remember that each type of test has been designed to measure different aspects of the biological response to materials, and correlation may not always be expected.

The best example of a barrier that occurs in use but not in vitro is the dentin barrier. When restorative materials are placed in teeth, dentin will generally be interposed between the material and the pulp. The dentin barrier, although possibly only a fraction of a millimeter thick, is effective in modulating the effects of dental materials. The effect of the dentin barrier is illustrated by the following classic study (Table 5-3). Three methods were used to evaluate the following materials: a ZOE cement, a composite material, and a silicate cement. The evaluation methods included (1) four different cell culture tests, (2) an implantation test, and (3) a usage test in class 5 cavity preparations in monkey teeth. The results of the four cell culture tests were relatively consistent, with silicate having only a slight effect on cultured cells, composite a moderate effect, and ZOE a severe effect. These three materials were also embedded subcutaneously in connective tissue in polyethylene tubes (secondary test), and observations were made at 7, 30, and 90 days. Reactions at 7 days could not be determined because of inflammation caused by the operative procedure. At 30 days, ZOE appeared to cause a more severe reaction than silicate cement. The inflammatory reactions at 90 days caused by ZOE and silicate were slight, and the reaction to composite materials was moderate. When the three materials were evaluated in class 5 cavity preparations under prescribed conditions of cavity size and depth (usage test), the results were quite different from those obtained by the screening methods. The silicate was found to have the most severe inflammatory reaction, the composite had a moderate to slight reaction, and the ZOE had little or no effect.

The apparent contradictions in this study may be explained by considering the components that were released from the materials and the environments into which they were released. The silicate cement released hydrogen ions that were probably buffered in the cell culture and implantation tests but may not have been adequately buffered by the dentin in the usage tests. Microleakage of bacteria or bacterial products may have added to the inflammatory reaction in the usage test. Thus this material appeared most toxic in the usage test. The composites released low-molecular-weight resins, and the ZOE released eugenol and zinc ions. In the cell-culture tests, these compounds had direct access to cells and probably caused the moderate to severe cytotoxicity. In the implantation tests, the released components may have caused some cytotoxicity, but the severity may have been reduced because of the capacity of the surrounding tissue to disperse the toxins. In usage tests, these materials probably were less toxic because the diffusion gradient of the dentin barrier reduced concentrations of the released molecules to low levels. The slight reaction observed with the composites also may also have been caused in part by microleakage around these restorations. The ZOE did not show this reaction, however, because the eugenol and zinc probably killed bacteria in the cavity, and the ZOE may have somewhat reduced microleakage.

Another example of the lack of correlation of usage tests with implantation tests is the inflammatory response of the gingiva at the gingival and interproximal margins of restorations that accumulate bacterial plaque and calculus. Plaque and calculus cannot accumulate on implanted materials and therefore the implantation test cannot hope to duplicate the usage test. However, connective tissue implantation tests are of great value in demonstrating the cytotoxic effects of materials and evaluating materials that will be used in contact with alveolar bone and apical periodontal connective tissues. In these cases, the implant site and the usage sites are suffi-

TABLE 5-3 Comparison of Reactions of Three Materials by Screening and Usage Tests

Material	Cell Culture	Implantation in Connective Tissue	Pulp Response
Silicate	+	+	++
Composite	++	++	+
ZOE	+++	+	0

From Mjör IA, Hensten-Pettersen A, Skogedal O: *Int Dent J* 27:127, 1977.
+++ = Severe; ++ = Moderate; + = Slight; 0 = No reaction; *ZOE,* zinc oxide-eugenol.

ciently similar to compare the test results of the two sites.

USING IN VITRO, ANIMAL, AND USAGE TESTS TOGETHER

For about 20 years, scientists, industry, and the government have recognized that the most accurate and cost-effective means to assess the biocompatibility of a new material is a combination of in vitro, animal, and usage tests. Implicit in this philosophy is the idea that no single test will be adequate to completely characterize the biocompatibility of a material. The ways by which these tests are used together, however, are controversial and have evolved over the years as knowledge has increased and new technologies developed (see Figs. 5-1 and 5-14). This evolution can be expected to continue as we ask materials to perform more-sophisticated functions for longer periods.

Early combination schemes proposed a pyramid testing protocol, in which all materials were tested at the bottom of the pyramid and materials were "weeded out" as the testing continued toward the top of the pyramid (Fig. 5-14). Tests at the bottom of the pyramid were "unspecific toxicity" tests of any type (in vitro or animal) with conditions that did not necessarily reflect those of the material's use. The next tier shows specific toxicity tests that presumably dealt with conditions more relevant to the use of the material. The final tier was a clinical trial of the material. Later, another pyramid scheme was proposed that divided tests into initial, secondary, and usage tests. The philosophy was similar to the first scheme,

A

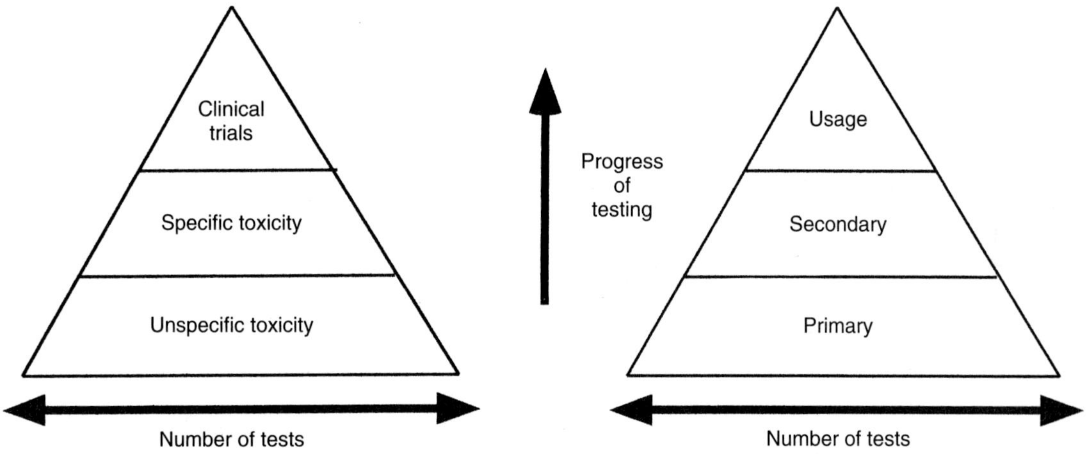

B

Fig. 5-14 Early and contemporary strategies for the use of biocompatibility tests to assess the safety of materials. Testing begins at the bottom of the pyramid and works up. The number of tests needed decreases with the progress of testing because unacceptable materials are theoretically eliminated in the early testing stages. **A,** The earliest strategy, in which the testing strategy is focused on toxicity only. *Unspecific toxicity* were tests not necessarily related to the use of the material, whereas the *specific toxicity* were more relevant. Clinical trials are equivalent to usage tests in this scheme. **B,** The contemporary strategy used in most standards documents. Primary tests are in vitro and in vivo tests, but not necessarily related to the use of the material. Secondary tests are more advanced biological tests that may be partly related to the use of the material. Usage tests are either clinical trials in humans or a close model of the use of a material in higher animals. In both of these testing strategies, the major problem is the inability of the early tests to accurately predict problems with the materials. Thus good materials might be screened out and poor materials might be advanced.

except the types of tests were broadened to encompass biological reactions other than toxicity, such as immunogenicity and mutagenicity. The concept of a usage test in an animal was also added (vs. a clinical trial in a human). There are several important features of these early schemes. First, only materials that "passed" the first tier of tests were graduated to the second tier, and only those that passed the second tier were graduated to the clinical trials.

Presumably, then, this scheme fed safer materials into the clinical trials area and eliminated unsafe materials. This strategy was welcomed because clinical trials are the most expensive and time-consuming aspect of biocompatibility tests. Second, any material that survived all three tiers of tests were deemed acceptable for clinical use. Third, each tier of the system put a great deal of onus on the tests use to accurately screen in or out a material. Although still used in principle today, the inability of in vitro and animal tests to unequivocally screen materials in or out has led to the development of newer schemes in biocompatibility testing.

Two newer testing schemes have evolved in the past 5 years with regard to using combinations of biocompatibility tests to evaluate materials (Fig. 5-15). Both of these newer schemes accommodate several important ideas. First, all tests (in vitro, animal, and usage) continue to be of value in assessing the biocompatibility of a material during its development and even in its clinical service. For example, tests in animals for inflammation may be useful during the development of a material, but may also be useful after a problem is noted with the material after it has been on the market for a time. Second, the newer schemes recognize the inability of current testing methods to accurately and absolutely screen in or out a material. Third, these newer schemes incorporate the philosophy that assessing the biocompatibility of a material is an ongoing process.

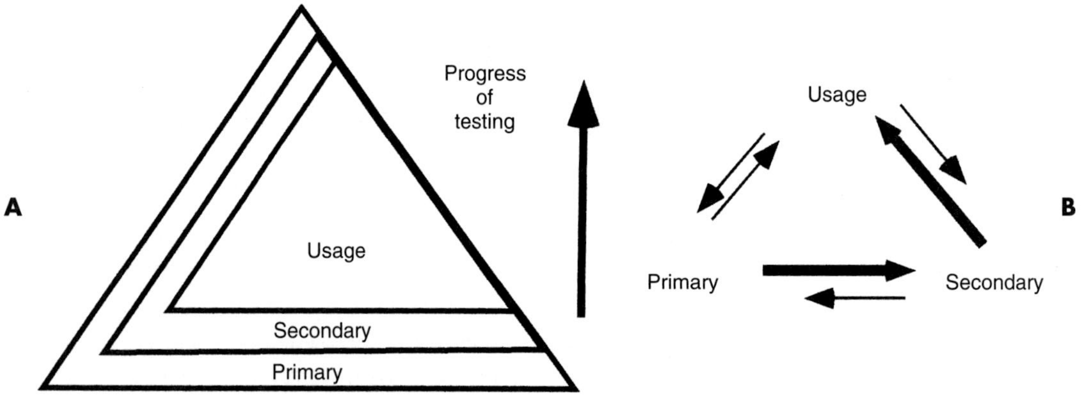

Fig. 5-15 Two suggested future strategies for biocompatibility testing of materials. **A,** The pyramid scheme of Fig. 5-14 is retained, but it is acknowledged that primary and secondary tests will play a continuing (but decreased) role as the progress of the testing continues. **B,** The usage test has the most stature and the most common progression of tests is from primary to secondary to usage, but the need to go through several iterations between testing types is acknowledged. Furthermore, the ongoing nature of biocompatibility is recognized by the need to use primary and secondary tests after clinical evaluation of a material. In this scheme the order of testing is ultimately determined as the testing and clinical use of the material continue to provide new data.

Undoubtedly, we will see still newer strategies in the use of combinations of biocompatibility tests as the roles of materials change and the technologies for testing improve.

STANDARDS THAT REGULATE THE MEASUREMENT OF BIOCOMPATIBILITY

The first efforts of the ADA to establish guidelines for dental materials came in 1926 when scientists at the National Bureau of Standards, now the National Institute of Science and Technology, developed specifications for dental amalgam. Unfortunately, recommendations on materials and conditions for biological compatibility have not kept pace with the technological development of dental materials. Reasons for this are (1) the fast advance of cellular and molecular biology, (2) the variety of tests available for assessing biocompatibility of materials, and (3) the lack of standardization of these tests.

Standardization is a difficult and lengthy process, made more difficult by disagreement on the appropriateness and significance of particular tests. One of the early attempts to develop a uniform test for all materials was the study by Dixon and Rickert in 1933, in which the toxicity of most dental materials in use at that time was investigated by implanting the materials into pockets in subdermal tissue. Small, standard-sized pieces of gold, amalgam, gutta-percha, silicates, and copper amalgam were sterilized and placed in uniformly sized pockets within skeletal muscle tissue. Biopsy specimens were evaluated microscopically after 6 months. Other early attempts to standardize techniques were carried out by Mitchell (1959) on connective tissue and by Massler (1958) on tooth pulp. Not until the passage of the Medical Device Bill by Congress in 1976 was biological testing for all medical devices (including dental materials) given a high priority. In 1972 the Council on Dental Materials, Instruments, and Equipment of ANSI/ADA approved Document No. 41 for Recommended Standard Practices for Biological Evaluation of Dental Materials. The committee that developed this document recognized the need for standardized methods of testing and for sequential testing of materials to reduce the number of compounds that would need to be tested clinically. In 1982, an addendum was made to this document, including an update of the Ames test for mutagenic activity.

ANSI/ADA Document 41 Three categories of tests are described in the 1982 ANSI/ADA document: initial, secondary, and usage tests. This document uses the testing scheme shown in Fig. 5-14, *B*. The initial tests include in vitro assays for cytotoxicity, red blood cell membrane lysis (hemolysis), mutagenesis and carcinogenesis at the cellular level, and in vivo acute physiological distress and death at the level of the whole organism. Based on the results of these initial tests, promising materials are tested by one or more secondary tests in small animals (in vivo) for inflammatory or immunogenic potential (e.g., dermal irritation, subcutaneous and bony implantation, and hypersensitivity tests). Finally, materials that pass secondary tests and still hold potential are subjected to one or more in vivo usage tests (placement of the materials in their intended contexts, first in larger animals, often primates, and finally, with Food and Drug Administration approval, in humans). The ANSI/ADA Doc. 41, 1982 Addendum, has two assays for mutagenesis, the Ames test and the Styles cell transformation test.

ISO 10993 In the past decade, an international effort was initiated by several standards organizations to develop international standards for biomedical materials and devices. Several multinational working groups, including scientists from ANSI and the International Standards Organization (ISO) were formed to develop these standards. The final document (ISO 10993) was published in 1992 and is the most recent standard available for biological testing. ISO 10993 contains 12 parts, each dealing with a different aspect of biological testing. For example, part 2 addresses animal welfare requirements, part 3 addresses tests for genotoxicity, carcinogenicity, and reproductive toxicity, and part 4 deals with tests for interactions with blood. The standard divides tests into "initial" and "supplementary" tests to assess the biological reaction to materials. Initial tests are tests for cytotoxicity, sensitization, and systemic toxicity. Some of these tests are done in vitro, others in animals in nonusage situations. Supplementary tests are tests such as chronic toxicity, carcinogenicity, and biodegradation. Most of the supplementary tests are done in animal systems, many in usage situations. The selection of tests for a specific material is left up to the manufacturer, who must present and defend the testing results. Guidelines for the selection of tests are given in part 1 of the standard and are based on how long the material will be present, whether it will contact body surface only, blood, or bone, and whether the device communicates externally from the body.

The current working version of the ISO standard is available from the International Organization for Standardization (www.iso.ch), Case Postale 56, CH-1211 Geneva 20, Switzerland, with reference to document ISO 10993-1: 1992(E). ANSI/ADA Document No. 41 is also being revised to conform to the ISO 10993 standard, but is not completed. Unlike the ISO standard, which covers all biomedical devices, the ANSI/ADA document is limited to dental devices. The new version will probably contain special emphasis on dental applications that are absent from ISO 10993, such as the dentin diffusion test. However, there will be many similarities between the two standards in both philosophy and application. The 1982 version of the ANSI/ADA document, which governs biocompatibility testing in the United States, is available from the Council on Dental Materials, Instruments and Equipment, American Dental Association (www.ada.org), 211 E. Chicago Avenue, Chicago, IL 60611, or the American National Standards Institute (www.ansi.org), 1819 L Street NW, Washington, DC 20036.

BIOCOMPATIBILITY OF DENTAL MATERIALS

REACTIONS OF PULP

Microleakage There is evidence that restorative materials may not bond to enamel or dentin with sufficient strength to resist the forces of contraction on polymerization, wear, or thermal cycling, although improvement in this area continues. If a bond does not form or debonding occurs, bacteria, food debris, or saliva may be drawn into the gap between the restoration and the tooth by capillary action. This effect has been termed *microleakage*. The importance of microleakage in pulpal irritation has been extensively studied. Early studies reported that various dental restorative materials irritated pulpal tissue in animal tests. However, other studies hypothesized that it was often the products of microleakage, not the restorative materials, which caused the pulpal irritation. Subsequently, numerous studies showed that bacteria present under restorations and in dentinal tubules might be responsible for pulpal irritation. Other studies showed that bacteria or bacterial products such as lipopolysaccharides could cause pulpal irritation within hours of being applied to dentin.

Finally, a classic animal study shed light on the roles of restorative materials and microleakage on pulpal irritation. Amalgam, composite, zinc-phosphate cement, and silicate cement were used as restorative materials in class 5 cavity preparations in monkey teeth. The materials were placed directly on pulpal tissues. Half of the restorations were surface-sealed with ZOE cement. Although some pulpal irritation was evident in all restorations at 7 days, after 21 days, the sealed restorations showed less pulpal irritation than those not sealed, presumably because microleakage had been eliminated. Only zinc phosphate cement elicited a long-term inflammatory response. Furthermore, the sealed teeth exhibited a much higher rate of dentin bridging under the material. Only amalgam seemed to prevent bridging. This study suggests that microleakage plays a significant role in pulpal irritation, but that the materials can also alter normal pulpal and dentinal repair.

Recently, the new concept of *nanoleakage* has been put forward. Like microleakage, nanoleakage refers to the leakage of saliva, bacteria, or material components through the interface between a material and tooth structure. However, nanoleakage refers specifically to dentin bonding, and may occur between mineralized dentin and a bonded material in the very small spaces of demineralized collagen matrix into which the bonded material did not penetrate. Thus nanoleakage can occur even when the bond between the material and dentin is intact. It is not known how significant a role nanoleakage plays in the biological response to materials, but it is thought to play at least some role and it is suspected of contributing to the hydrolytic degradation of the dentin-material bond, leading ultimately much more serious microleakage.

The full biological effects of restorative materials on the pulp are still not clear. Restorative materials may directly affect pulpal tissues, or may play an auxiliary role by causing sublethal changes in pulpal cells that make them more susceptible to bacteria or neutrophils. It is clear, however, that the design of tests measuring pulpal irritation *to materials* must include provisions for eliminating bacteria, bacterial products, and other microleakage. Furthermore, the role of dentin in mitigating the effects of microleakage remains to be fully revealed. Recent research has focused on the effects that resin components have on the ability of odontoblasts to form secondary dentin. Other research has established the rates at which these components traverse the dentin (see the next section on dentin bonding).

Dentin Bonding Traditionally, the strength of bonds to enamel have been higher than those to dentin, although dentin bonding has improved markedly in recent years. Bonding to dentin has proven more difficult because of its composition (being both organic and inorganic), wetness, and lower mineral content. The wettability of demineralized dentin collagen matrix has also been problematic. Because the dentinal tubules and their resident odontoblasts are extensions of the pulp, bonding to dentin also involves biocompatibility issues.

When the dentin surface is cut, such as in a cavity preparation, the surface that remains is covered by a 1- to 2-μm layer of organic and inorganic debris. This layer has been named the *smear layer* (see Fig. 5-3). In addition to covering the surface of the dentin, the smear layer debris is also deposited into the tubules to form dentinal plugs. The smear layer and dentinal plugs, which appear impermeable when viewed by electron microscopy, reduce the flow of fluid (convective transport) significantly. However, research has shown that diffusion of molecules as large as albumin (66 kDa) will occur through a smear layer. The presence of the smear layer is important to the strength of bonds of restorative materials and to the biocompatibility of those bonded materials.

Numerous studies have shown that removing the smear layer improves the strength of the bond between dentin and restorative materials with contemporary dentin bonding agents, although earlier research with older bonding agents showed the opposite. A variety of agents have been used to remove the smear layer, including acids, chelating agents such as ethylenediaminetetraacetic acid (EDTA), sodium hypochlorite, and proteolytic enzymes. Removing the smear layer increases the wetness of the dentin and requires that the bonding agent be able to wet dentin and displace dentinal fluid. The mechanism by which bonding occurs remains unclear, but it appears that the most successful bonding agents are able to penetrate into the layer of collagen that remains after acid etching, creating a "hybrid layer" of resin and collagen in intimate contact with dentin and dentinal tubules. The strength of the collagen itself has also been shown important to bond strengths.

From the standpoint of biocompatibility, the removal of the smear layer may pose a threat to the pulpal tissues for three reasons. First, its removal juxtaposes resin materials and dentin without a barrier, and therefore increases the risk that these materials can diffuse and cause pulpal irritation. Second, the removal of the smear layer makes any microleakage more significant because a significant barrier to the diffusion of bacteria or bacterial products toward the pulp is removed. Third, the acids used to remove the smear layer are a potential source of irritation themselves. Nevertheless, removal of the smear layer is now routine because of the superior bond strengths that can be achieved. Some recent techniques that etch and "bond" direct pulp exposures make the biocompatibility of the bonding agents even more critical, because the dentinal barrier between the materials and the pulp is totally absent.

The biocompatibility of acids used to remove the smear layer has been extensively studied. Numerous acids have been used to remove the smear layer, including phosphoric, hydrochloric, citric, and lactic acids. The effect of the acids on pulpal tissues depends on a number of factors, including the thickness of dentin between the restoration and the pulp, the strength of the acid, and the degree of etching. Most studies have shown that dentin is a very efficient buffer of protons, and most of the acid may never reach the pulp if sufficient dentin remains. A dentin thickness of 0.5 mm has proven adequate in this regard. Citric or lactic acids are less well buffered, probably because these weaker acids do not dissociate as efficiently. Usage tests that have studied the effects of acids have shown that phosphoric, pyruvic, and citric acids produce moderate pulpal inflammatory responses, which resolve after 8 weeks. Recent research has shown that in most cases the penetration of acids into the dentin is probably less than 100 μm. However, the possibility of adverse effects of these acids cannot be ruled out, because odontoblastic processes in the tubules may be affected even though the acids do not reach the pulp itself.

Dentin Bonding Agents A variety of dentin bonding agents have been developed and are applied to cut dentin during restoration of the tooth. There have been a number of studies on the biocompatibility of dentin bonding systems. Many of these reagents are cytotoxic to cells in vitro if tested alone. However, when placed on dentin and rinsed with tap water between applications of subsequent reagents as prescribed, cytotoxicity is often reduced. Longer-term in vitro studies suggest, however, that sufficient components of many bonding agents permeate up to 0.5 mm of dentin to cause significant suppression of cellular metabolism for up to 4 weeks after their application. This suggests that residual unbound reagents may cause adverse reactions.

Several studies have measured the biological effects of other resin-based dentin bonding agents. Hydroxyethyl methacrylate (HEMA), a hydrophilic resin contained in several bonding systems, is at least 100 times less cytotoxic in tissue culture than Bis-GMA. Studies using long-term in vitro systems have shown, however, that adverse effects of resins occur at much lower concentrations (by a factor of 100 or more) when exposure times are increased to 4 to 6 weeks. Many cytotoxic effects of resin components are reduced significantly by the presence of a dentin barrier. However, if the dentin in the floor of the cavity preparation is thin (<0.1 mm), there is some evidence that HEMA may be cytotoxic in vivo. Other studies have established the cytotoxicity in vitro of most of the common resins in dentin bonding agents, such as Bis-GMA, triethylene glycol dimethacrylate, urethane dimethacrylate (UDMA), and others. Other studies have shown that combinations of HEMA and other resins found in dentin bonding agents may act synergistically to cause cytotoxic effects in vitro. There have been very few clinical studies on the diffusion of hydrophilic and hydrophobic resin components through dentin. These studies indicate that at least some diffusion of these components occur in vivo as well. Interestingly, there is at least one report that some resin components enhance the growth of oral bacteria. If substantiated, this result would cause concern about the ability of resin-based materials to increase plaque formation.

Resin-Based Materials For tooth restorations, resin-based materials have been used as cements and restorative materials. Because they are a combination of organic and inorganic phases, these materials are called *resin composites*. In vitro, freshly set chemically cured and light-cured resins often cause moderate cytotoxic reactions in cultured cells over 24 to 72 hours of exposure, although several newer systems seem to have minimal toxicity. The cytotoxicity is significantly reduced 24 to 48 hours after setting and by the presence of a dentin barrier. Several studies have shown that some materials are persistently cytotoxic in vitro even up to 4 weeks, whereas others gradually improve, and a few newer systems show little toxicity even initially. In all cases, cytotoxicity is thought to be mediated by resin components released from the materials. Evidence indicates that the light-cured resins are less cytotoxic than chemically cured systems, but this effect is highly dependent on the curing efficiency of the light and the type of resin system. In vivo, usage tests have been used to assess the biological response to resin composites. The pulpal inflammatory response to hemically cured and light-cured resin composites is low to moderate after 3 days when they were placed in cavities with approximately 0.5 mm of remaining dentin. Any reaction diminished as the postoperative periods increased to 5 to 8 weeks and was accompanied by an increase in reparative dentin (Fig. 5-16). With a protective liner or a bonding agent, the reaction of the pulp to resin composite materials is minimal. The longer-term effects of resins placed directly on pulpal tissue are not known, but are suspected to be less favorable.

Amalgams and Casting Alloys Amalgams have been used extensively for dental restorations. The biocompatibility of amalgams is thought determined largely by corrosion products released while in service. Corrosion depends on the type of amalgam, whether it contains the γ_2 phase, and the composition of the amalgam. In cell-culture screening tests, free or unreacted mercury from amalgam is toxic, but low-copper amalgam that has set for 24 hours does not inhibit cell growth. With the addition of copper, amal-

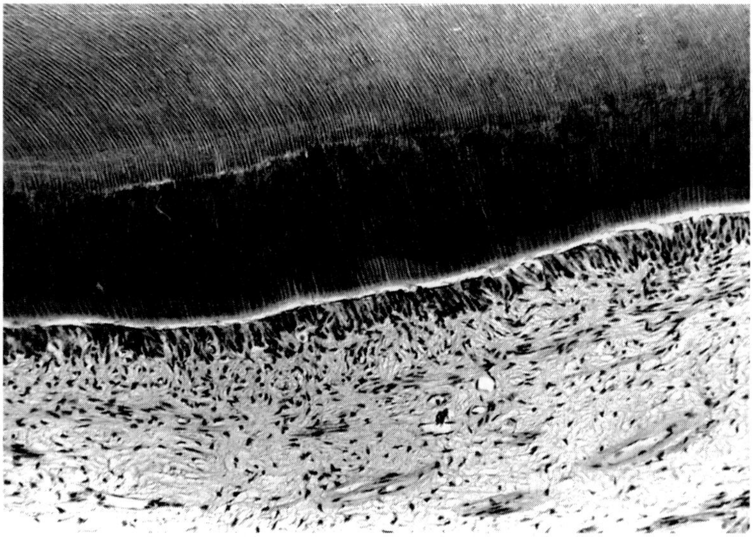

Fig. 5-16 Light micrograph of the dentinal and pulpal response to unlined composite at 5 to 8 weeks in a monkey. The primary dentin is the lighter layer seen at the top. The tubules are evident. Secondary dentin is occurring (the dark, wide middle layer), and it is closely approximated by intact odontoblasts in the pulp. Few inflammatory cells are present. The response seen in this micrograph is indicative of a favorable response to the material.
(Courtesy Avery JK: Ann Arbor, 1987, University of Michigan School of Dentistry.)

gams become toxic to cells in culture. Implantation tests show that low-copper amalgams are well tolerated, but high-copper amalgams cause severe reactions when in direct contact with tissue. In usage tests, the response of the pulp to amalgam in shallow cavities or in deeper but lined cavities is minimal. In deep cavities (0.5 mm or less of remaining dentin), pain results from using amalgams in unlined cavity preparations. An inflammatory response is seen after 3 days and after 5 weeks. In cavities with 0.5 to 1.0 mm of dentin remaining in the floor, the cavity preparation should be lined for two other reasons. First, thermal conductivity with amalgam is significant and can be a problem clinically. Second, margins of newly placed amalgam restorations show significant microleakage. Marginal leakage of corrosion and microbial products is probably enhanced by the daily natural thermal cycle in the oral cavity. The short-term pulpal response is significantly reduced when the cavity is lined, and amalgam rarely causes irreversible damage to the pulp. Long-term sealing of the margins occurs through the buildup of corrosion products.

A number of high-copper amalgams are in clinical use. Usage tests reported that at 3 days the pulpal responses elicited by these materials appear similar to those elicited by low-copper amalgams in deep, unlined cavities. At 5 weeks they elicited only slight pulpal response. At 8 weeks the inflammatory response was reduced. Bacterial tests on the high-copper amalgam pellets have revealed little inhibitory effect on serotypes of *Streptococcus mutans,* thus suggesting that the elements were not released in amounts necessary to kill these microorganisms. Although the high-copper amalgams seem biologically acceptable in usage tests, liners are suggested for all deep cavities.

Amalgams based on gallium rather than mercury have been developed to provide direct restorative materials that are free of mercury, although their use is not common. In cell culture, these alloys appear to be no more cytotoxic than traditional high-copper amalgams. These restorations release significant amounts of gallium in vitro, but the importance of this release is not known. In implantation tests, gallium alloys caused a significant foreign body reaction. Clinically, these materials show much higher corrosion rates than standard amalgams, leading to roughness and discoloration. There are few reports of pulpal responses to these materials.

Cast alloys have been used for single restorations, bridges, porcelain-fused-to-metal crowns, and partial dentures. The gold content in these alloys ranges from 0% to 85% (percentage by weight). These alloys contain several other noble and non-noble metals that may have an adverse effect on cells if they are released from the alloys. However, released metals are most likely to contact gingival and mucosal tissues, and the pulp is more likely to be affected by the cement retaining the restoration.

Glass Ionomers Glass ionomers are another type of material that have been used both as a cement (luting agent) and as a restorative material. Light-cured ionomer systems have also been introduced; these systems use Bis-GMA or other oligomers as pendant chains on the polyacrylate main chain. In screening tests, freshly prepared ionomer is mildly cytotoxic, but this effect is reduced with increased times after setting. The fluoride release from these materials, which is probably of some therapeutic value, may cause cytotoxicity in in vitro tests. Some researchers have reported that some systems are more cytotoxic than others, but the reasons for this observation are not clear. The overall pulpal biocompatibility of these materials has been attributed to the weak nature of the polyacrylic acid, which is unable to diffuse through dentin because of its high molecular weight. In usage tests the pulp reaction to glass ionomer cements is mild. Histological studies in usage tests show that any inflammatory infiltrate from ionomer is minimal or absent after 1 month. There have been several reports of pulpal hyperalgesia for short periods (days) after placing glass ionomers in cervical cavities. This effect is probably the result of increased dentin permeability after acid etching.

Liners, Varnishes, and Nonresin Cements *Calcium hydroxide* cavity liners come in many forms, ranging from saline suspensions with a very alkaline pH (above 12) to modified forms containing zinc oxide, titanium dioxide, and resins. Resin-containing preparations can be polymerized chemically, but light-activated systems have also been introduced. The high pH of calcium hydroxide in suspension leads to extreme cytotoxicity in screening tests. Calcium hydroxide cements containing resins cause mild-to-moderate cytotoxic effects in tissue culture in both the freshly set and long-term set conditions. The inhibition of cell metabolism is reversible in tissue culture by high levels of serum proteins, suggesting that protein binding or buffering in inflamed pulpal tissue may play an important role in detoxifying these materials in vivo. The initial response of exposed pulpal tissue to the highly alkaline aqueous pulp-capping agents is necrosis to a depth of 1 mm or more. The alkaline pH also helps to coagulate any hemorrhagic exudate of the superficial pulp. Shortly after necrosis occurs, neutrophils infiltrate into the subnecrotic zone. Eventually, after 5 to 8 weeks, only a slight inflammatory response remains. Within weeks to months, the necrotic zone undergoes dystrophic calcification, which appears to be a stimulus for dentin bridge formation. When resins are incorporated into the formulae, these calcium hydroxide compounds become less irritating and are able to stimulate reparative dentin bridge formation more quickly than the $Ca(OH)_2$ suspensions, and with no zone of necrosis. Therefore reparative dentin is laid down adjacent to the liner (Fig. 5-17), an indication that the replacement odontoblasts form the dentin bridge in contact with the liner. However, some of these materials evidently break down with time and create a gap between the restoration and the cavity wall. Resin-containing calcium hydroxide pulp capping agents are the most effective liners now available for treating pulp exposures. After pulp exposure, the uninfected pulp undergoes a relatively uncomplicated wound-healing process.

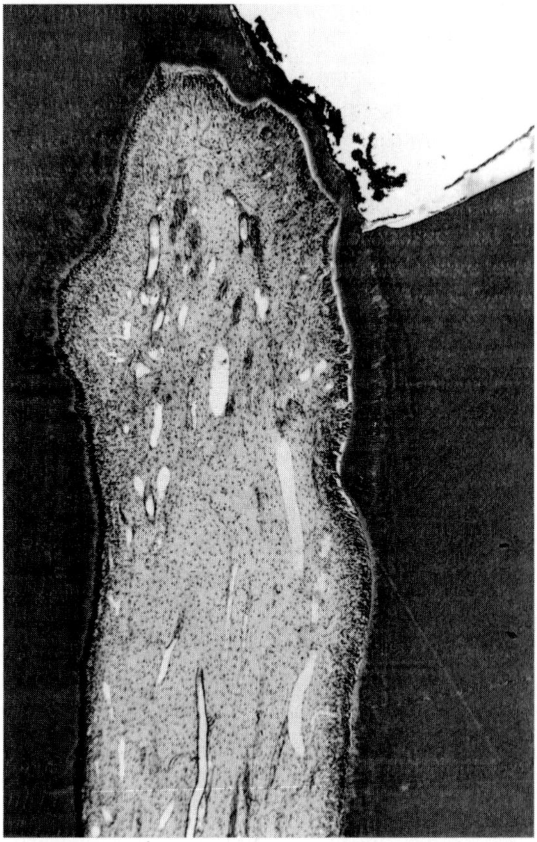

Fig. 5-17 Light micrograph of a dentin bridge that has formed between a material and the pulp in a monkey. Initially, the pulp of the tooth was purposely exposed *(top right)* with a bur. The exposure was covered with a calcium hydroxide pulp-capping agent for 5 weeks before histological evaluation. A layer of secondary dentin has formed at the site of the pulp exposure, forming a dentin bridge. Some inflammatory cells are evident under the bridge, but the pulpal response is generally favorable.

(Courtesy Heys DR: Ann Arbor, 1987, University of Michigan School of Dentistry.)

Numerous investigators have analyzed the effects of applying thin liners such as copal *varnishes* and polystyrenes under restorations. These materials are not generally used under resin-based materials, because resin components dissolve the thin film of varnish. Because liners are used in such thin layers, they do not provide thermal insulation, but they initially isolate the dentinal tubule contents from the cavity preparation. They may also reduce penetration of bacteria or chemical substances for a time. However, because of the thinness of the film and formation of pinpoint holes, the integrity of these materials is not as reliable as that of other cavity liners.

Zinc phosphate has been a widely used dental cement for castings, orthodontic bands and to base cavity preparations. Because the thermal conductivity of this cement is approximately equal to that of enamel and considerably less than that of metals, it has also been used to build up the remaining tooth structure. In vitro screening tests indicate that zinc-phosphate cement elicits strong-to-moderate cytotoxic reactions that decrease with increased time after setting. Leaching of zinc ions and a low pH may explain these effects. The dilution of leached cement products by dentin filtration has been shown to protect the pulp from most of these cytotoxic effects. Focal necrosis, observed in implantation tests with zinc phosphate cements injected into rat pulp, confirm the cytotoxic effects of this cement where it contacts tissue. In usage tests in deep cavity preparations, moderate-to-severe localized pulpal damage is produced within the first 3 days, probably because of the initial low pH on setting (4.2 at 3 minutes). The pH of the set cement approaches neutrality after 48 hours. By 5 to 8 weeks, only mild chronic inflammation is present, and reparative dentin has usually formed. Because of the initially painful and damaging effects on the pulp of this cement when placed in deep cavity preparations, the placement of a protective layer of a dentin bonding agent, ZOE, varnish, or calcium hydroxide is recommended under the cement. Other formulae have included calcium hydroxide in the powder, lowering the concentrations of phosphoric acid in the liquid, or included materials such as copper and fluoride ions that may function as antimicrobial agents. However, copper ions have proven extremely toxic to cells in culture and in implantation tests.

Zinc polyacrylate cements (polycarboxylate cements) were developed to combine the strength of zinc phosphate cements with the adhesiveness and biocompatibility of zinc oxide eugenol (ZOE). In short-term tissue culture tests, cytotoxicity of freshly set and completely set cements has correlated both with the release of zinc and fluorides into the culture medium and with a reduced pH. Some researchers suggest that this cytotoxicity is an artifact of tissue culture because the phosphate buffers in the culture medium encourage zinc ions to leach from the cement. Supporting this theory, cell growth inhibition can be reversed if EDTA (which chelates zinc) is added to the culture medium. Furthermore, inhibition of cells decreases as the cement sets. In addition, concentrations of polyacrylic acid above 1% appear to be cytotoxic in tissue culture tests. On the other hand, subcutaneous and bone implant tests over a 1-year period have not indicated long-term cytotoxicity of these cements. Thus other mechanisms such as buffering and protein-binding of these materials may neutralize these effects in vivo over time. Polyacrylic cements cause a pulpal response similar to that caused by ZOE, with a slight-to-moderate response after 3 days and only mild, chronic inflammation after 5 weeks. Reparative dentin formation is minimal with these cements, and thus they are recommended only in cavities with intact dentin in the floors of the cavity preparations.

Zinc oxide eugenol cements (ZOE) have been used in dentistry for many years. In vitro, eugenol from ZOE fixes cells, depresses cell respiration, and reduces nerve transmission with direct contact. Surprisingly, it is relatively innocuous in usage tests in class 5 cavity preparations. This is not contradictory for a number of reasons. The effects of eugenol are dose dependent and diffusion through dentin dilutes eugenol by several orders of magnitude. Thus, although the concentration of eugenol in the cavity preparations just below the ZOE has been reported to be 10^{-2} M (bactericidal), the concentration on the pulpal side of the dentin may be 10^{-4} M or less. This lower concentration reportedly suppresses nerve transmission and inhibits synthesis of prostaglandins and leukotrienes (anti-inflammatory). In addition and as described before, ZOE may form a temporary seal against bacterial invasion. In cavity preparations in primate teeth (usage tests), ZOE caused only a slight-to-moderate inflammatory reaction within the first week, and this was reduced to a mild, chronic inflammatory reaction, with some reparative dentin formation when cavities were deep, within 5 to 8 weeks. For this reason, it has been used as a negative control substance for comparison with restorative procedures in usage tests.

Bleaching Agents Bleaching agents have been used on nonvital and vital teeth for many years, but their use on vital teeth has increased astronomically in recent years. These agents usually contain some form of peroxide (generally carbamide peroxide) in a gel that can be applied to the teeth either by the dentist or at home by the patient. The agents may be in contact with teeth for several minutes to several hours depending on the formulation of the material. Home bleaching agents may be applied for weeks to even months in some cases. In vitro studies have shown that peroxides can rapidly (within minutes) traverse the dentin in sufficient concentrations to be cytotoxic. The cytotoxicity depends to a large extent on the concentration of the peroxide in the bleaching agent. Other studies have further shown that the peroxides rapidly even penetrate intact enamel and reach the pulp in a few minutes. In vivo studies have demonstrated adverse pulpal effects from bleaching, and most reports agree that a legitimate concern exists about the long-term use of these products on vital teeth. In clinical studies, the occurrence of tooth sensitivity is very common with the use of these agents, although the cause of these reactions are not known. Bleaching agents will also chemically burn the gingiva if the agent is not sequestered adequately in the bleaching tray, although this is not a problem with a properly constructed tray. Long-term, low-dose effects of peroxides on the gingival and periodontal tissues are not currently known.

REACTION OF OTHER ORAL SOFT TISSUES TO RESTORATIVE MATERIALS

Restorative materials may cause reactions in the oral soft tissues such as gingiva. At present, it is not clear how much of the in vivo cytotoxicity observed is caused by the restorative materials and how much is caused by products of bacterial plaque that accumulate on teeth and restorations. In general, conditions that promote retention of plaque, such as rough surfaces or open margins, increase inflammatory reactions in gingiva around these materials. However, released products of restorative materials also contribute either directly or indirectly to this inflammation, particularly in areas where the washing effects of saliva are less, such as in interproximal areas, in deep gingival pockets, or under removable appliances. Several studies have documented increased inflammation or recession of gingiva adjacent to restorations where plaque indexes are low. In these studies, released products from materials could cause inflammation in the absence of plaque or could inhibit formation of plaque and cause inflammation in gingiva. Some basic research has been done in vitro that shows, in principle, that components from dental materials and plaque may synergize to enhance inflammatory reactions.

Cements exhibit some cytotoxicity in the freshly set state, but this decreases substantially with time. The buffering and protein-binding effects of saliva appear to mitigate against the cytotoxic effects.

Composites are initially very cytotoxic in in vitro tests of direct contact with fibroblasts. The cytotoxicity is most probably primarily from unpolymerized components in the air-inhibited layer that leach out from the materials. Other in vitro studies, which have 'aged' the composites in artificial saliva for up to six weeks, have shown that the toxicity diminishes in some materials but remains high for others. Some of the newer composites with non-BisGMA non-UDMA matrices have significantly lower cytotoxicity in vitro, presumably because of lower amounts of leached components. Polished composites show markedly less cytotoxicity in vitro, although some materials are persistently toxic even in the polished state. Recently, there has been significant controversy about the ability of bis-phenol A and bis-phenol A dimethacrylate to cause estrogen-like responses in vitro. These compounds are basic components of many commercial composites. However, there is no evidence that xenoestrogenic effects are a concern in vivo from any commercially available resin. Relatively little is known about other in vivo effects of released components of composites on the soft tissues, although the concerns are similar to those regarding denture base resin and soft liners (see later discussion, this section). There is some evidence that methacrylate-based composite components may cause significant rates of hypersensitivity, although few clinical trials exist.

Amalgam restorations carried into the gingival crevice may cause inflammation of the gingiva because of products of corrosion or bacterial plaque. Seven days after placing an amalgam, a few inflammatory cells appear in the gingival connective tissue, and hydropic degeneration of some epithelial cells may be seen. Some proliferation of epithelial cells into the connective tissue may also occur by 30 days, and chronic mononuclear cell infiltration of connective tissue is evident. Increased vascularity persists, with more epithelial cells invaginating into the connective tissue. Some of these changes may be a chronic response of gingiva to plaque on the margins of the amalgams. Nevertheless, corrosion products from amalgam cannot be ruled out at this time because implanted amalgams produce similar responses in connective tissues in animals. In addition, although copper enhances the physical properties of amalgam and is bactericidal, it is also toxic to host cells and causes severe tissue reactions in implantation tests. Animal implantation studies have also shown severe reactions to gallium-based alloys that have been used as amalgam replacements.

There is a report in the literature in which amalgam and resin composite restorations were placed in cavity preparations in monkey central incisors that had been extracted for less than one hour. The cavities, with depths of about 2 mm, were placed halfway between the cemento-enamel junction and the root tip. The teeth were immediately reimplanted after restoration, and the animals were sacrificed at intervals up to 6 months. Repair of the PDL took place in a normal fashion except for the presence of an intense inflammatory infiltrate in the PDL adjacent to the amalgams through 2 weeks, but to the resin composites through 3 to 6 months. This result suggests that resin composites and amalgam release cytotoxic materials that cause tissue responses, at least at sites of implantation. For materials placed where they are rinsed in saliva, these cytotoxic agents are probably washed away before they harm the gingiva. However, rough surfaces on these types of restorations have been associated with increased inflammation in vivo. Usage tests in which restorations were extended into the gingival crevice have shown that finished materials gave a much milder inflammatory response than unfinished materials. The detrimental effect of surface roughness has been attributed to the increased plaque retention on these surfaces. However, rough surfaces on alloy restorations also caused increased cytotoxic effects in in vitro experiments where plaque was absent. This and other in vitro studies again would suggest that the cytotoxic response to alloys may be associated with release of elements from the alloys. The increased surface area of a rough surface may enhance release of these elements.

Casting alloys have a long history of in vivo use with a generally good record of biocompatibility. Some questions about the biological liability of elemental release from many of the formulations developed in the past 10 years have arisen, but there is no clinical evidence that elemental release is a problem, aside from hypersensitivity. Nickel allergy is a relatively common problem, occurring in 10% to 20% of females, and is a significant risk from nickel-based alloys because release of nickel ions from these alloys is generally higher than for high-noble or noble alloys. Palladium sensitivity has also been a concern in some countries, although the incidence of true palladium allergy is one third that of nickel allergy. However, it has been clinically documented that patients with palladium allergy are virtually always allergic to nickel. The converse is not true however. In vitro, there have been numerous articles published on the effects of metal ions on cells in the gingival tissues, such as epithelial cells, fibroblasts, and macrophages. For the most part, the concentrations of metal ions required to cause problems with these cells in vitro are greater than those released from most casting alloys. However, the most recent research has shown that extended exposures to low doses of metal ions may also have biological liabilities. These new data are noteworthy because the low-dose concentrations approach those known to be released from some alloys. The clinical significance of this research is not known, however.

Denture base materials, especially methacrylates, have been associated with immune hypersensitivity reactions of gingiva and mucosa probably more than any other dental material. The greatest potential for hypersensitization is for dental and laboratory personnel who are exposed repeatedly to a variety of unreacted components. Hypersensitivity has been documented to the acrylic and diacrylic monomers, certain curing agents, antioxidants, amines, and formaldehyde. For the patient, however, most of these materials have reacted in the polymerization reaction, and the incidence of hypersensitization is quite low. Screening tests for sensitization potential include testing of unreacted ingredients, the polymeric substance after reaction, and oil, saline, or aqueous extracts of the polymer in in vitro tests described previously and in skin tests in animals. In addition to hypersensitivity, visible light–cured denture base resins and denture base resin sealants have been shown to be cytotoxic to epithelial cells in culture.

Soft tissue responses to *soft denture liners and adhesives* are of concern because of the intimate contact between these materials and the gingiva. Plasticizers, which are incorporated into some materials to make them soft and flexible, are released in vivo and in vitro. Cell culture tests have shown that some of these materials are extremely cytotoxic and affect a number cellular metabolic reactions. In animal tests, several of these materials have caused significant epithelial changes, presumably from the released plasticizers. In usage, the effects of the released plasticizers are probably often masked by the inflammation already present in the tissues onto which these materials are placed. Denture adhesives have been evaluated in vitro and show severe cytotoxic reactions. Several had substantial formaldehyde content. The adhesives also allowed significant microbial growth. Newer formulations that add antifungal or antibacterial agents have not yet been shown to be clinically efficacious.

REACTION OF BONE AND SOFT TISSUES TO IMPLANT MATERIALS

There are four basic materials used in implant fabrication: ceramics, carbon, metals, and polymers (and combinations of the above). Interest in the biocompatibility of implant materials has grown as the use of implants in clinical practice has increased dramatically in the past 10 years. Most successful dental implant materials either promote osseointegration (an approximation of bone on the implant within 100 Å of the implant) or biointegration (a continuous fusion of bone with the implant).

Reactions to Ceramic Implant Materials

Most ceramic implant materials have very low toxic effects on tissues, either because they are in an oxidized state or are corrosion resistant. As a group, they have low toxicity, and are nonimmunogenic and noncarcinogenic. However, they are brittle and lack impact and shear strength, and therefore have been used as porous or dense coatings on metals or other materials. If the root surface porosities are more than 150 μm in diameter, the implants often become firmly bound to bone (through ankylosis or biointegration), especially if they are taken out of occlusion for a time. If the porosities are smaller, the tissue usually forms only fibrous ingrowth. Dense ceramics are also used as root replicas or bone screws. Made of either single crystal (sapphire) or polycrystalline aluminum oxide, they become biointegrated and provide excellent stability if left unloaded for a time. In one study, 60% of the restorations still performed adequately after 6 years in place.

Hydroxyapatite, a relatively nonresorbable form of calcium phosphate, has been used with some success as a coating material for titanium implants and as a ridge augmentation material. Studies indicate that the hydroxyapatite increases the rate of bony ingrowth toward the implant. However, the long-term corrosion of these coatings and the stability of the bond of the coating to the substrate are still controversial. Retrieval evidence indicates that even these "nonresorbable" coatings are resorbed over the long-term. Beta-tricalcium phosphate, another form of calcium phosphate, has been used in situations where resorption of the material is desirable, such as repair of bony defects. Carbon has been used as a coating and in bulk forms for implants. Although the biologic response to carbon coatings can be favorable, they have been supplanted by titanium, aluminum oxide bulk materials, and hydroxyapatite coatings. Finally, Bioglass forms a surface gel that reacts favorably with connective tissue, allowing bone formation adjacent to it.

Reactions to Pure Metals and Alloys

Pure metals and alloys are the oldest type of oral implant materials. All metal implants share the quality of strength. Initially, metallic materials were selected on the basis of ease of fabrication. Over time, however, biocompatibility with bone and soft tissue and the longevity of the implant have become more important. A variety of implant materials has been used, including stainless steel, chromium-cobalt-molybdenum, and titanium and its alloys. These materials have been used in a variety of forms, including root forms and subperiosteal and transosteal implants. In dentistry, the only metallic implant materials in common use today are titanium alloys.

Titanium is a pure metal, at least when first cast. In less than a second the surface forms a thin film of various titanium oxides, which is corrosion resistant and allows bone to osseointegrate. The major disadvantage of this metal is that it is difficult to cast. It has been wrought into endosteal blades and root forms, but this process introduces metallic impurities into the surface that may adversely effect bony response unless extreme care is taken during manufacturing. Titanium implants have been used with success as root forms that are left unloaded under the mucosa for several months before they are used to support a prosthesis. With frequent recall and good oral hygiene, the implants have been maintained in healthy tissue for up to 2 decades. Titanium-aluminum-vanadium alloys (Ti6Al4V) have been used successfully in this regard as well, but questions remain about the liability of released aluminum and vanadium. Clinical studies have been positive. Although titanium and titanium alloy implants have corrosion rates that are markedly less than other metallic implants, they do release titanium into the body. Currently there is no evidence that these released elements are a problem locally or systemically. The issue remains unresolved.

In the soft tissue, the bond epithelium forms with titanium is morphologically similar to that formed with the tooth, but this interface has not been fully characterized. Connective tissue apparently does not bond to the titanium, but does form a tight seal that seems to limit ingress of bacteria and bacterial products. Techniques are being developed to limit downgrowth of the epithelium and loss of bone height around the implant, which ultimately cause implant failure. Peri-implantitis is now a documented disease around implants and involves many of the same bacteria as periodontitis. The role of the implant material or its released components in the progression of peri-implantitis is not known.

SUMMARY

The biocompatibility of a dental material depends on its composition, location, and interactions with the oral cavity. Metal, ceramic, and polymer materials elicit different biological responses because of their differences in composition. Furthermore, diverse biological responses to these materials depend on whether they release their components and whether those components are toxic, immunogenic, or mutagenic at the released concentrations. The location of a material in the oral cavity partially determines its biocompatibility. Materials that appear biocompatible when in contact with the oral mucosal surface may cause adverse reactions if they are implanted beneath it. Materials that are toxic when in direct contact with the pulp may be essentially innocuous if placed on dentin or enamel. Finally, interactions between the material and the body influence the biocompatibility of the material. The material's response to changes in pH, the application of force, or the degradative effects of biological fluids can alter its biocompatibility. Features of a material's surface that promote or discourage the attachment of bacteria, host cells, or biological molecules determine whether the material will promote plaque retention, integrate with bone, or adhere to dentin.

SELECTED PROBLEMS

Problem 1

You have a group of six materials, all of which can be classified as posterior composites, but each of which has a slightly different formula. How would you determine which of these freshly set materials is the least toxic using the least expensive, least time-consuming tests?

Solution

You may choose a direct in vitro cell-culture test. The materials would be formed into disks of equal dimensions. The disks should be stabilized on the bottoms of cell-culture wells. Cells are then placed into the wells with the materials and are incubated in an appropriate incubation medium and environment for 24 hours or more. Then the disks and wells are observed and photographed under phase-contrast microscopy, taking special note of cytopathic effects around each disk for semi-quantitative results.

Problem 2

If you have the same situation as in Problem 1, but you want to quantify your results, what are your options?

Solution

You may choose the same test model as in the solution for Problem 1, but you would measure the cellular response quantitatively rather then by visual observation. There are two primary options: (1) measure the membrane permeability of the cells that remain around the disks using neutral red or ^{51}Cr (see Fig. 5-10); or (2) measure some aspect of cellular biosynthesis or metabolism (MTT test, DNA synthesis, protein synthesis, total protein). You might also choose another model, such as extracting the sample for 1 to 3 days in given volumes of solvent and then treating the cells with serial dilutions of the elutants.

Problem 3

With the same situation as in Problem 1, you want to know the effect of the setting reaction or time on the toxicity of the material. What would you do?

Solution

Usually the material is made into disks and allowed to set for varying periods (from 1 to several days). Then, for each period, the set disks are placed into tissue culture wells or are extracted with a solvent that is placed into tissue culture wells. Then your options are the same as those in the solutions for Problems 1 or 2.

Problem 4

You read a research paper on the in vitro cytotoxicity of composites that shows that some composites are initially very cytotoxic but improve with time of elution into artificial saliva, whereas others continue to be toxic. How can you interpret these results in terms of clinical use of the composites?

Solution

Extrapolation of in vitro tests to clinical situations is always difficult, but one interpretation could be that the composites that improve with time in vitro pose lower long-term risks clinically than those which continue to be cytotoxic. This line of reasoning may be dangerous, however, if the material is designed to release a substance that is cytotoxic in vitro but therapeutic in vivo. Such is the case for fluoride release from some composites and glass ionomer cements.

Problem 5

If you have a series of composites and you want to rank them according to the toxicity they may have specifically for pulpal tissues, what would you do?

Solution

You should choose a test model in which dentin is interspaced between material and cell test system. The dentin barrier may alter the effects of released components from the material and change the response of pulpal cells. Without such a barrier, the composites may appear more cytotoxic in vitro than they would be clinically.

Problem 6

One of your six composite materials is associated fairly consistently with pulpitis when used by you and your fellow clinicians. The cytotoxicity test that you chose indicates that this material is not much more toxic than the other materials. How can you better understand what is causing the pulpitis?

Solution

The pulpitis may be caused by microleakage of bacteria or by the material's ability to cause a chronic inflammatory (vs. toxicity) response. If the facilities are available, you may do in vitro chemotaxis tests, using human peripheral leukocytes with the test sample to determine which materials might be responsible for the inflammation. Tests on monocytes could also be done, using materials or material components at nontoxic concentrations. If the material does not show an inflammatory response in these tests, then usage tests in animals could be used to verify the pulpitis in vivo in a more controlled environment. Then, if usage tests in animals substantiate the pulpitis, you should be highly suspicious of microleakage of environmental materials or bacteria products. To confirm this suspicion, additional usage tests could be used where the margins of the restoration are surface-sealed to prevent microleakage.

Problem 7

You have a new polymeric substance that you believe might function well as a root cylinder implant. What kinds of tests should you conduct to answer questions of safety according to FDA standards, and how long will this take?

Solution

Initial tests should include cytotoxicity tests, a hemolysis test, some test for mutagenesis or gene toxicity, and probably an oral LD_{50} test. (All tests except mutagenesis can be performed and analyzed in about 2 to 3 weeks if run concurrently. The mutagenesis tests may require between 1 and 3 months for performance analysis.) Secondary tests might include implantation into bone and soft tissue of small animals, tests for mucous membrane irritation, and hypersensitivity tests. If done concurrently, this will take about 1 month before histological preparation of tissue is begun. Time required for histology and reading of slides may vary, depending on the size of the project. Usage tests (percutaneous implants) in jaws of larger animals may require that the implants remain in place for 1 to 2 years, followed by histological processing and evaluation.

Problem 8

You are a dentist who has been practicing for 20 years, and you like to do a lot of your own laboratory work. You have noticed that when you handle methacrylate denture base and monomer, you develop a rash on your hands. What is the problem, and what can you do about it?

Solution

You are probably hypersensitive to the monomer and should wear rubber gloves around monomer and freshly polymerized methacrylate. Try to avoid contact because monomer can penetrate latex rubber.

Problem 9

You have a patient who has an endosteal blade that had been implanted by her previous prosthodontist before she moved to town. The implant has been in place 1 year and appears to be somewhat mobile. What are your options for analyzing the problem?

Solution

Radiographs of the implant and tissue in the region should be done to look for areas of radiolucencies, both at the cervix and at the mesial and distal tips of the blade. A periodontal probe may be used gently to determine if there is tissue attachment around the implant. However, if the implant is mobile at all, failure is probably imminent.

Problem 10

A dental patient comes to you with concerns about the estrogenicity of dental composites you have placed. What will you tell her?

Solution

First, it is true that some starting components (bis-phenol A and its dimethacrylate) show estrogenic types of reactions in in vitro tests. However, the concentrations of these compounds in today's commercially available resins are *very* low. Second, there is no verifiable clinical evidence that these compounds or others are released in sufficient concentrations to cause estrogenic reactions. For example, the concentration of bis-phenol A required to cause an estrogenic response is 1000 times greater than that of the naturally occurring hormone estradiol. Finally, there are no documented cases of these materials having any estrogenic-type of reactions in dental patients, despite the placement of millions of these restorations.

BIBLIOGRAPHY

AAMI Standards and Recommended Practices: *Biological Evaluation of Medical Devices,* vol 4, Arlington, VA, Association for the Advancement of Medical Instrumentation, 1994.

American Dental Association: Addendum to American National Standards/American Dental Association Document No. 41 for recommended standard practices for biological evaluation for dental materials, Chicago, 1982, American Dental Association.

American Dental Association: American National Standards Institute/American Dental Association Document No. 41 for recommended standard practices for biological evaluation of dental materials, *J Am Dent Assoc* 99:697, 1979.

Barile FA: *In vitro cytotoxicity: mechanisms and methods.* CRC Press, Boca Raton, 1994.

Bergenholtz G: In vivo pulp response to bonding of dental restorations, *Trans Acad Dent Mater* November:123, 1998.

Bouillaguet S, Ciucchi B, Holz J: Potential risks for pulpal irritation with contemporary adhesive restorations: an overview, *Acta Med Dent Helv* 1:235, 1996.

Brännström M: *Dentin and pulp in restorative dentistry,* London, 1982, Wolfe Medical.

Cox CF, Keall CL, Keall HJ, Ostro EO: Biocompatibility of surface-sealed dental materials against exposed pulps, *J Prosthet Dent* 57:1, 1987.

deSouza Costa CA, Beling J, Hanks CT: Current status of pulp capping with dentin adhesive systems: a review, *Dent Mater* 16:188, 2000.

Ecobichon DJ: *The basis of toxicity testing,* Boca Raton, 1992, CRC Press.

Geurtsen W: Substances released from dental resin composites and glass ionomer cements, Eur J Oral Sci 106:687, 1998.

Geursten W: Biocompatibility of resin-modified filling materials, *Crit Rev Oral Biol Med* 11:333, 2000.

Geurtsen W, Leyhausen G: Biological aspects of root canal filling materials—histocompatibility, cytotoxicity, and mutagenicity, *Clin Oral Invest* 1:5, 1997.

Hanks CT, Wataha JC, Sun ZL: In vitro models of biocompatibility: a review, *Dent Mater* 12:186, 1996.

Hensten-Pettersen A: Skin and mucosal reactions associated with dental materials, *Eur J Oral Sci* 106:707, 1998.

Hodgson E, Levi PE, eds: *A textbook of modern toxicology,* New York, 1987, Elsevier Science.

Hume WR: A new technique for screening chemical toxicity to the pulp from dental restorative materials and procedures, *J Dent Res* 64:1322, 1985.

International Standards Organization: *Biological evaluation of medical devices,* ISO 10993, ed 1, Geneva, Switzerland, 1992, ISO.

Jontell M, Okiji T, Dahlgren U, Bergenholtz G: Immune defense mechanisms of the dental pulp, *Crit Rev oral Biol Med* 9:179, 1998.

Kawahara H, Yamagami A, Nakamura M: Biological testing of dental materials by means of tissue culture, *Int Dent J* 18:443, 1968.

Mackert JR: Dental amalgam and mercury, *J Am Dent Assoc* 122:54, 1991.

Mackert JR, Bergland A: Mercury exposure from dental amalgam filling: absorbed dose and the potential for adverse health effects, *Crit Rev Oral Biol Med* 8:410, 1997.

Meryon SD: The influence of dentine on the in vitro cytotoxicity testing of dental restorative materials, *J Biomed Mater Res* 18:771, 1984.

Mjör IA, Hensten-Pettersen A, Skogedal O: Biologic evaluation of filling materials: a comparison of results using cell culture techniques, implantation tests and pulp studies, *Int Dent J* 27:124, 1977.

National Institutes of Health: Consensus development statement on dental implants, June 13-15, 1988, *J Dent Educ* 52:824, 1988.

Pashley DH: The effects of acid etching on the pulpodentin complex, *Oper Dent* 17:229, 1992.

Pashley DH: Dynamic of the pulp-dentin complex, *Crit Rev Oral Biol Med* 7:104, 1996.

Schmalz G: Modern concepts in biocompatibility testing of restorative materials, *Trans Acad Dent Mater* 9:170, 1996.

Schmalz G: Concepts in biocompatibility testing of dental restorative materials, *Clin Oral Invest* 1:154, 1997.

Schmalz G: The biocompatibility of nonamalgam dental filling materials, *Eur J Oral Sci* 106:696, 1998.

Schuster GS, Lefebvre CA, Wataha JC, White SN: Biocompatibility of posterior restorative materials, *Calif Dent J* 24:17, 1996.

Tennant RW, Margolin BH, Shelby MD, Zeigler E, Haseman JK, Spalding J, Caspary W, Resnick M, Stasiewicz S, Anderson B, Minor R: Prediction of chemical carcinogenicity in rodents from in vitro genetic toxicity assays, *Science* 236:933, 1987.

Wataha JC: Biocompatibility of dental casting alloys: a review, *J Prosthet Dent* 83:223, 2000.

Wataha JC: Materials for endosseous dental implants, *J Oral Rehabil* 23:79, 1996.

Wataha JC, Hanks CT: Biological effects of palladium and risk of using palladium in dental casting alloys, *J Oral Rehabil* 23:309, 1996.

Wataha JC, Hanks CT, Craig RG: Precision of and new methods for testing in vitro alloy cytotoxicity, *Dent Mater* 8:65-71, 1992.

Williams DF: Toxicology of ceramics. In Williams DF, editor: *Fundamental aspects of biocompatibility,* vol 2, Boca Raton, Fla, 1981, CRC Press.

Chapter 6

Nature of Metals and Alloys

Metals and alloys play a prominent and important role in dentistry. These materials are used in almost all aspects of dental practice, including the dental laboratory, direct and indirect dental restorations, and instruments used to prepare and manipulate teeth. Metals and alloys have optical, physical, chemical, thermal, and electrical properties that are exploited to advantage in dentistry and are unique among the basic types of materials (metals, polymers, and ceramics). Although popular press dental journals have occasionally promoted "metal-free" dentistry as desirable, the metals remain the only clinically proven materials for many long-term dental applications. This chapter will summarize the aspects of metals and alloys that are relevant to dentistry. The concepts of crystallization, phase diagrams, alloy microstructure, and alloy strengthening will be described and related to the clinical practice of dentistry. Finally, this chapter will present a foundation for understanding the major classes of alloys used in dentistry: amalgam (see Chapter 11); noble alloys and solders (see Chapter 15); base metal alloys (see Chapter 16), and ceramic-metal restorations (see Chapter 19).

CHEMICAL AND ATOMIC STRUCTURE OF METALS

A metal is any element that ionizes positively in solution; metals constitute nearly two thirds of the periodic table (Fig. 6-1). During ionization,

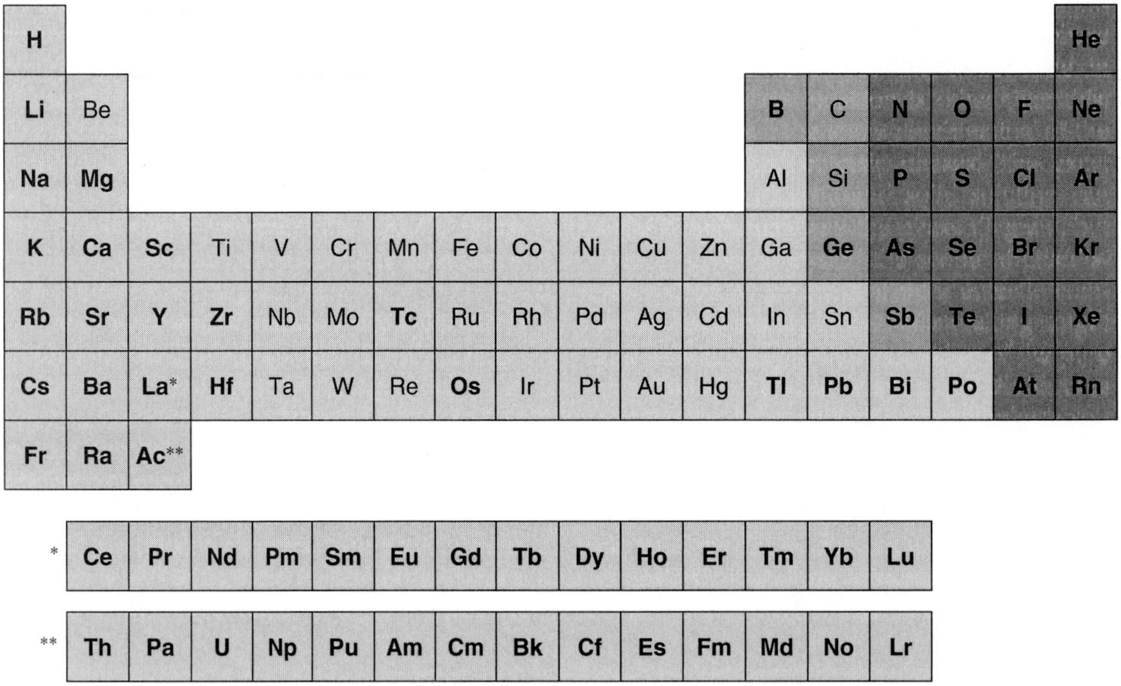

Fig. 6-1 The periodic table of the elements can be subdivided into metals *(lightly shaded backgrounds)*, metalloids *(intermediately shaded backgrounds)* and nonmetals *(darkly shaded backgrounds)*. Elements in outline type are used in dental alloys or as pure metals. The metals are elements that ionize positively in solution, and comprise the majority of elements in the periodic table. Note that not all elements are shown. The single-asterisk indicates the insertion point in the table for the lanthanide series of elements, whereas the double-asterisk indicates the insertion point for the actinide series of elements.

metals release electrons. This ability to exist as free, positively charged, stable ions is a key factor in the behavior of metals and is responsible for many metallic properties that are important in dentistry. Another important group of elements in Fig. 6-1 are the metalloids, including carbon, silicon, and boron. Although metalloids do not always form free positive ions, their conductive and electronic properties make them important components of many alloys.

ATOMIC STRUCTURE

At the atomic level, pure metals exist as crystalline arrays (Fig. 6-2) that extend for many repetitions in three dimensions. In these arrays, the nuclei and core electrons occupy the atomic centers, whereas the ionizable electrons float freely among the atomic positions. The mobility of the valence electrons are responsible for many properties of metals, such as electrical conductivity. It is important to note that the positively charged atomic centers are held together by the electrons and their charge is simultaneously neutralized by the electrons; thus pure metals have no net charge.

The relationships between the atomic centers in a metallic crystalline array are not always uniform in all directions. The distances in the x, y (horizontal), and z (vertical) axes may be the same or different, and the angles between these axes may or may not be 90 degrees. In all, there are six crystal systems that occur (Fig. 6-3), and these can be further divided into 14 crystalline arrays. Metallic nuclei may occur at the center of faces or vertices of the crystal. Within each array, the smallest repeating unit that captures all of the relationships among atomic centers is called a *unit cell* (see Fig. 6-2). The unit cells for the most common arrays in dental metals are shown in Fig. 6-4. In the body-centered cubic (BCC) array, all angles are 90 degrees and all atoms are equidistant from one another in the horizontal and vertical directions. Metallic atoms are located at the corners of the unit cell, and one atom is at the center of the unit cell (hence the name

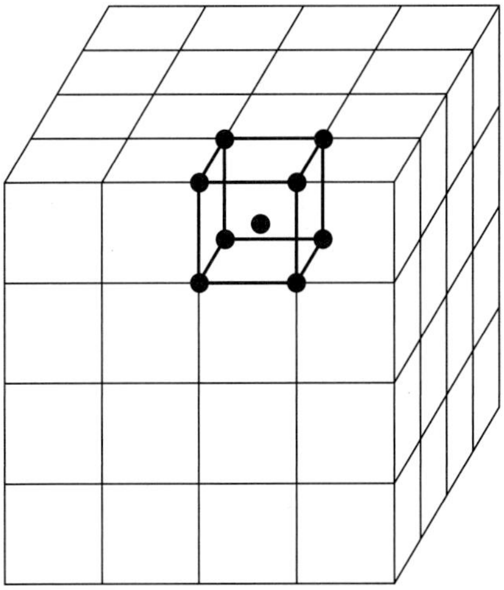

Fig. 6-2 A typical metallic crystal lattice, in this case a body centered cubic lattice. Every lattice has a unit cell *(shown in bold)* that extends (repeats) in three dimensions for large distances. Electrons are only relatively loosely bound to atomic nuclei and core electrons. The nuclei occupy specific sites *(shown as dots in the unit cell)* in the lattice, whereas the electrons are relatively free to move about the lattice. In reality, the metal atoms are large enough to touch each other.

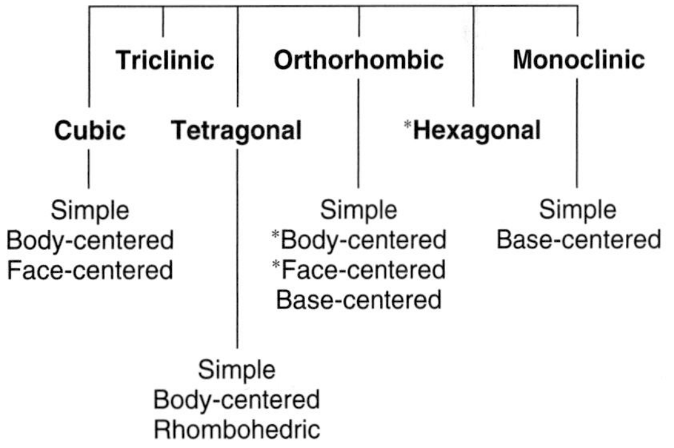

Fig. 6-3 All metals occur in one of the lattice structures shown. There are six families of lattices, four of which can be subdivided. Each family is defined by the distances between vertices and the angles at the vertices. The body-centered cubic, face-centered cubic, and hexagonal lattices *(asterisks)* are the most common in dental alloys and pure metals.

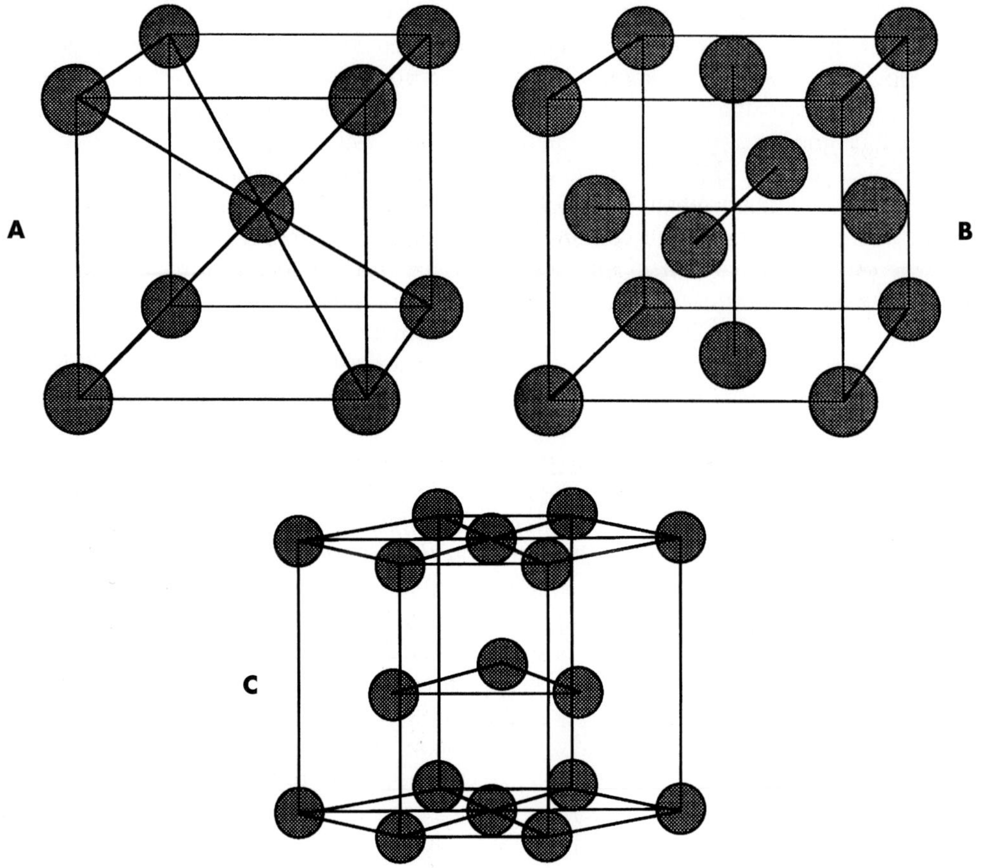

Fig. 6-4 The three most common crystal lattice unit cells in dental metals and alloys: **A,** body-centered cubic cell; **B,** face-centered cubic cell; and **C,** hexagonal close-packed cell. The atoms *(circles)* in all three cases would be larger and touching each other. They were drawn smaller to make the structures easier to visualize.

body-centered cubic). This is the crystal structure of iron and is common for many iron alloys. The face-centered cubic (FCC) array has 90-degree angles and atomic centers that are equidistant horizontally and vertically (as does the BCC), but atoms are located in the centers of the faces with no atom in the center of the unit cell (hence the name *face-centered cubic*). Most pure metals and alloys of gold, palladium, cobalt, and nickel have the FCC array. The more complex hexagonal close-pack array occurs with titanium. In this array, the atoms are equidistant from each other in the horizontal plane, but not in the vertical direction.

In a metallic crystal, the atomic centers are positively charged because the valence electrons have been released to float about the crystal. At first glance, it seems unlikely that these positively charge atoms could exist so close together. Rather, a repulsion between these centers would seem more likely. The metallic bond is a fundamentally important type of primary bond that holds the atomic centers together in a metal lattice. The freely floating electrons bind the atomic centers together and, although it is not directed between specific centers, this metallic bond has a formidable force between atomic centers. The metallic bond is fundamentally different from other primary bonds, such as covalent bonds, which occur in organic compounds, and ionic bonds, which occur in ceramics.

PHYSICAL PROPERTIES OF METALS

All properties of metals result from the metallic crystal structure and metallic bonds described previously. In general, metals have higher densities resulting from the efficient packing of atomic centers in the crystal lattice. The good electrical and thermal conductivity of metals occurs because of the mobility of the valence electrons in the crystal lattice. The opacity and reflective nature of metals result from the ability of the valence electrons to absorb and re-emit light. The melting points occur as the metallic bond energies are overcome by the applied heat. Interestingly, the number of valence electrons per atomic center influences the melting point somewhat. As the number of valence electrons increases, the metallic bond develops some covalent character that contributes to higher melting points. This phenomenon occurs for iron (Fe^{3+}) and nickel (Ni^{2+}).

The corrosion properties of metals depend on the ability of atomic centers and electrons to be released in exchange for energy. The amount of energy required depends on the strength of the metallic force (related to the freedom of the valence electrons) and the energy that the released ion can gain by solvating in solution. For metals like sodium or potassium, the metallic bond is weaker as the valence electrons are loosely held, and the energy of solvation is high. Thus these metals corrode into water with explosive energy release. For metals like gold or platinum, the metallic bond is stronger, valence electrons are more tightly held, and solvation energies are relatively low. Thus gold and platinum are far less likely to corrode. The corrosion of metals always involves oxidation and reduction. The released ion is oxidized because the electrons are given up, and the electrons (which cannot exist alone) are gained by some molecules in the solution (which is therefore reduced). Further explanation can be obtained in numerous chemistry texts.

Because the distances between metal atoms in a crystal lattice may be different in the horizontal and vertical directions (see Fig. 6-4), properties such as conductivity of electricity and heat, magnetism, and strength may also vary by direction if a single crystal is observed. These directional properties of metals and metalloids have been exploited in the semiconductor industry to manufacture of microchips for computers. However, in dentistry, a single crystal is rarely observed. Rather, a collection of randomly oriented crystals, each called a *grain,* generally make up a dental alloy. In this case, the directional properties are averaged out across the material. In general, a fine-grained structure (see discussion of grains later in this chapter) is desirable to encourage alloys with uniform properties in any direction. Such uniformity of directional properties is termed anisotropy.

Like the physical properties, the mechanical properties of metals are also a result of the metallic crystal structure and metallic bonds. Metals generally have good ductility (ability to be drawn into a wire) and malleability (ability to be pounded into a thin sheet) relative to polymers and ceramics. To a large extent, these properties result from the ability of the atomic centers to slide against each other into new positions within the same crystal lattice. Because the metallic bonds are essentially nondirectional, such sliding is possible.

If the metallic crystals were perfect, calculations have shown that the force required to slide the atoms in the lattice would be hundreds of times greater than experience shows is necessary. Less force is necessary because the crystals are not perfect, but have flaws called *dislocations.* Dislocations allow the atomic centers to slide past each other one plane at a time (Fig. 6-5). Because movement can occur one plane at a time, the force required is much less than if the forces of all the planes have to be overcome simultaneously. An analogy is moving a large heavy rug by forming a small fold or kink in the rug and pushing the fold from one end of the rug to the other. Dislocations are of several types, but all serve to allow the relatively easy deformation of metals. All methods for increasing the strength

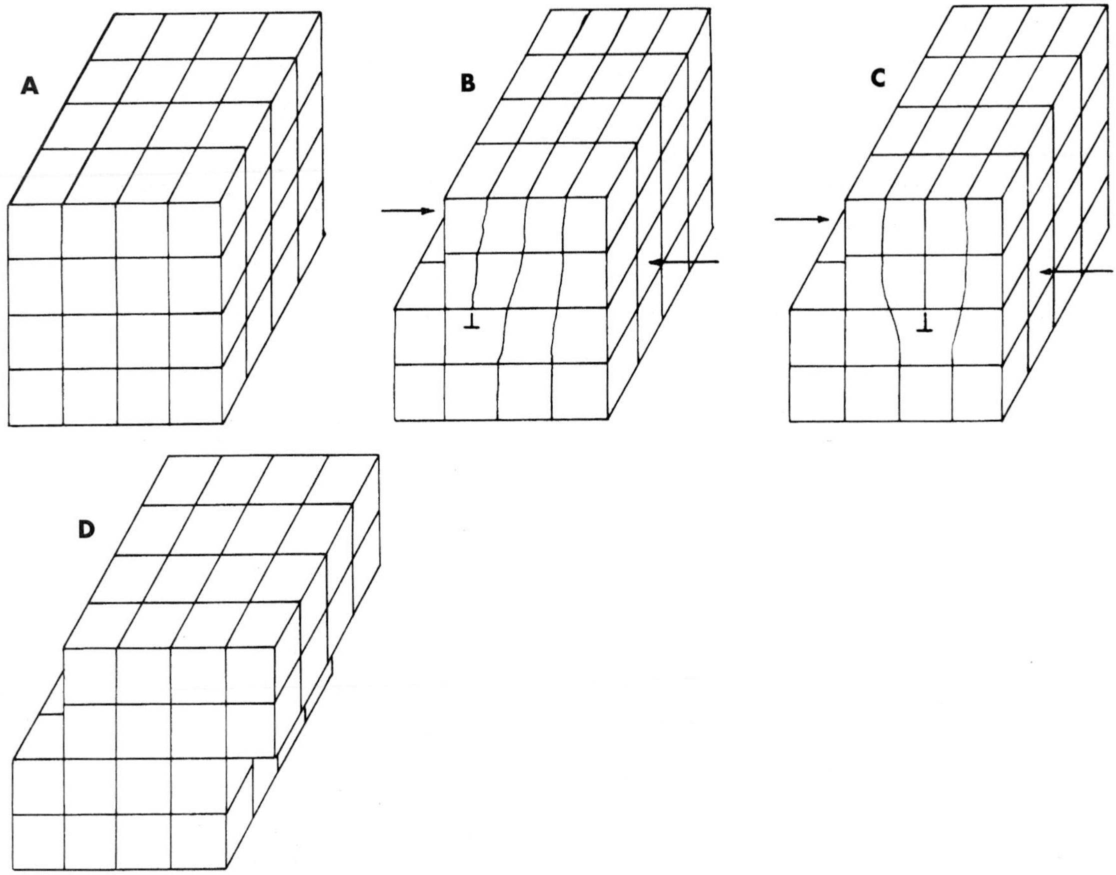

Fig. 6-5 Sketches representing a crystal and slip mechanisms resulting from movement of a dislocation. By the dislocation moving through the metal one plane at a time (**A** to **B** to **C** to **D**), far less energy is necessary to deform the metal. Furthermore, the movement occurs without fracture or failure of the crystal lattice.

of metals act by impeding the movement of dislocations. These methods will be discussed later in the chapter.

The fracture of metals occurs when the atomic centers cannot slide past one another freely. For example, this can happen when impurities block the flow of dislocations (Fig. 6-6). The inability of the dislocation to be moved through the solid results in the lattice rupturing locally. Once this small crack is started, it takes little force to propagate the crack through the lattice. An example illustrates this idea. Consider a plate of steel 15 cm wide and 6 mm thick. Suppose it has a 5-cm crack running into one side. The force required to make the crack run the remaining 10 cm would be about 180 kg. Without the aid of the crack, 230,000 kg would be required if the steel were the best grade commercially available. If the steel were a single, flawless crystal, 4.5 million kg would be necessary! The fracture of metals depends heavily on dislocations and the local rupture of the crystal lattice.

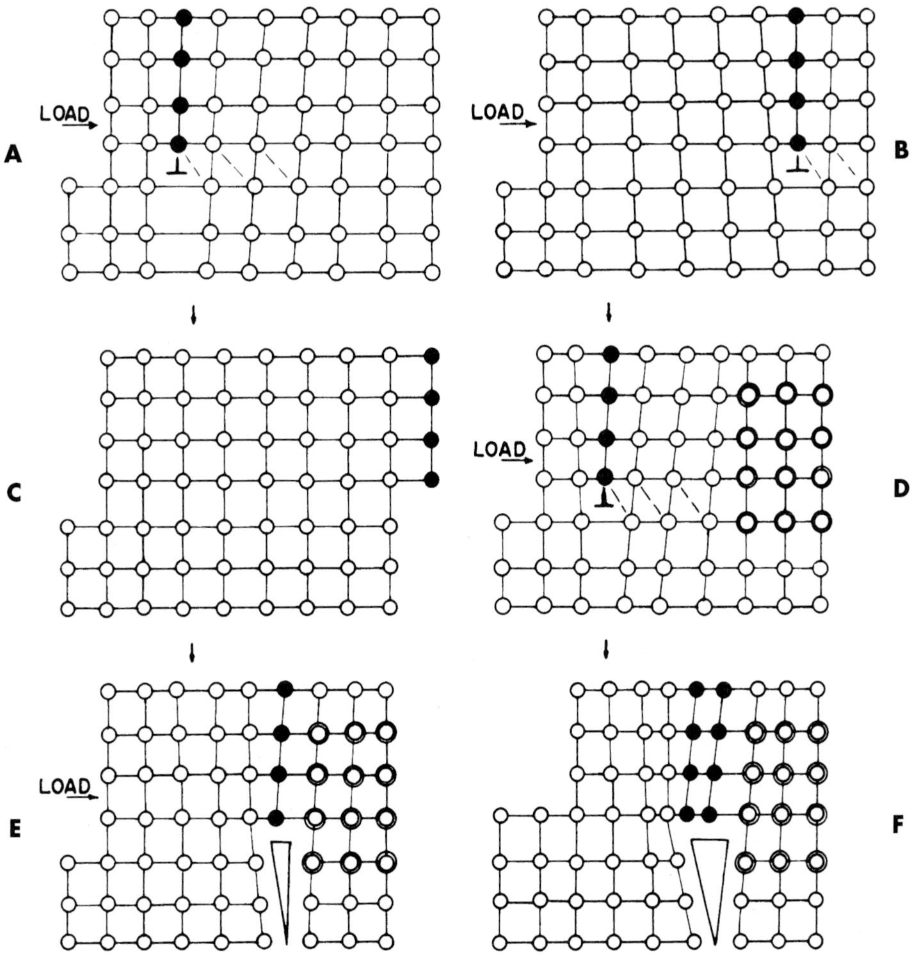

Fig. 6-6 Sketches showing plastic shearing with crack formation at the site of an impurity *(dark, open circles)*. Without the impurity **(A, B, C)**, the load forces the dislocations completely through the lattice without fracture (note the progression of solid dark circles from left to right). However, when the impurity is present **(D, E, F)**, it stops the progress of the dislocation. As other dislocations build up, the lattice below them cannot accommodate and a crack forms in the lattice **(E)**. In **E**, note the broken bonds between atoms. Once formed, a crack can rapidly and relatively easily grow and lead to catastrophic failure.

ALLOYS AND PRINCIPLES OF METALLURGY

Metals can be mixed together much as liquids are. A mixture of metals is called an *alloy*, and the study of metals and alloys is called *metallurgy*. Alloys may be a mixture of as few as two or (in the case of dental casting alloys) as many as nine or more different metals. As with liquids, not all metals will dissolve in one another freely; some metals will not dissolve at all into other metals. The concept of phases and phase diagrams was developed to help understand the nature of alloys and metal solubility. Alloys may have crystal structures like the pure metals previously discussed, or they may have other atomic structures, such as eutectics or intermetallic compounds.

These concepts will be discussed later in this chapter.

PHASE DIAGRAMS AND DENTAL ALLOYS

A *phase* is a state of matter that is distinct in some way from the matter around it. In a mixture of ice and water there are two phases because although ice and water are the same chemically, they each have distinct arrangements of atoms. Ice has the crystalline arrangement of a solid whereas water has the random atomic arrangement of a liquid. A solid dental alloy may also have one phase if the composition of the alloy is essentially homogeneous throughout. If the alloy has areas where compositions are different, it is called a *multiple-phase alloy*. The distinction between single- and multiple-phase alloys is important to the strength, corrosion, biocompatibility, and other alloy properties.

Phase diagrams are "maps" of the phases that occur when metals are mixed together. If there are two metals in an alloy, a binary phase diagram is used. If three metals are in the alloy, a ternary phase diagram may be used. Phase diagrams describing alloys with more than three metals are not used because they are too complex; the vast majority of phase diagrams describe only binary alloys. For dental alloys that contain four or more metals, the binary phase diagram of the two most abundant metals in the alloy typically describe the alloy. In practice, phase diagrams are determined by meticulous examination of a series of binary alloys cooled slowly and monitored for composition.

A typical phase diagram for a theoretical binary alloy *AB* is shown in Figure 6-7. The x-axis describes the composition of the elements in either weight percent or atomic percent (see Chapter 15). The y-axis is the temperature of the alloy system. It is important to remember that a phase diagram shows the composition and types of phases at a given temperature *and* at equilibrium. Every phase diagram divides an alloy system into at least three areas: the liquid phase, the liquid + solid phases, and the solid phase. For example, everything above the temperatures shown by line *ACB* in Fig. 6-7 is liquid. This line is therefore called the *liquidus*. Everything below line *ADB* is solid. This line is thus called the *solidus*. The area between these two lines contains some liquid and some solid. At 0% *B*, a single phase exists (100% *A*) that has a single melting point (800° C). At 100% *B*, a single phase exists that has a melting point (210° C). At any composition between these extremes, the melting range is defined as the temperature difference between the liquidus *(ACB)* and solidus *(ADB)*.

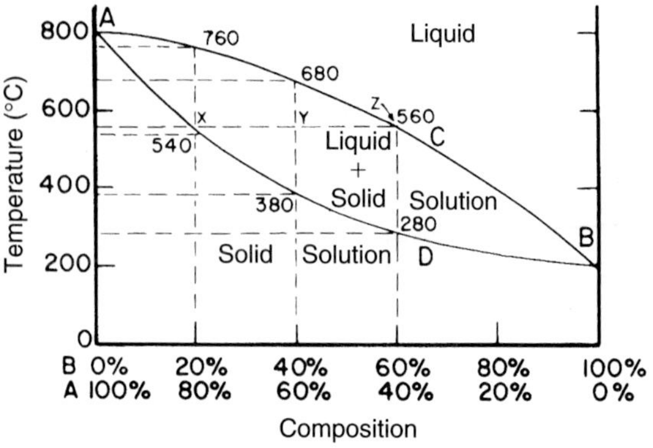

Fig. 6-7 A phase diagram for two theoretical components *A* and *B*. The liquidus for this system follows the line *ACB*. The solidus follows *ADB*. The melting points for each pure metal occur at *A* and *B*.

The phase diagram can also be used to find the composition of liquid and solid between the liquidus and solidus (see Fig. 6-7). Consider an alloy that is 20% *B* (and 80% *A*) at a temperature of 800° C. This alloy is all liquid. When the temperature drops to 700° C and the system equilibrates, there will be some liquid and some solid. If a line parallel to the x-axis is projected at 700° C to the liquidus, the composition of the liquid can be determined by projecting down to the x-axis. In this case, the liquid will be 60% *A* (and 40% *B*). By projecting at 700° C to the solidus then to the x-axis, the composition of the solid is 10% *B* (and 90% *A*). Below about 540° C, the alloy is 80% *A* and (20% *B*), or all solid. Thus the phase diagram can map the types and compositions of phases at any temperature and over any alloy composition.

When metals are mixed together in the molten state, then cooled to the solid state, there are

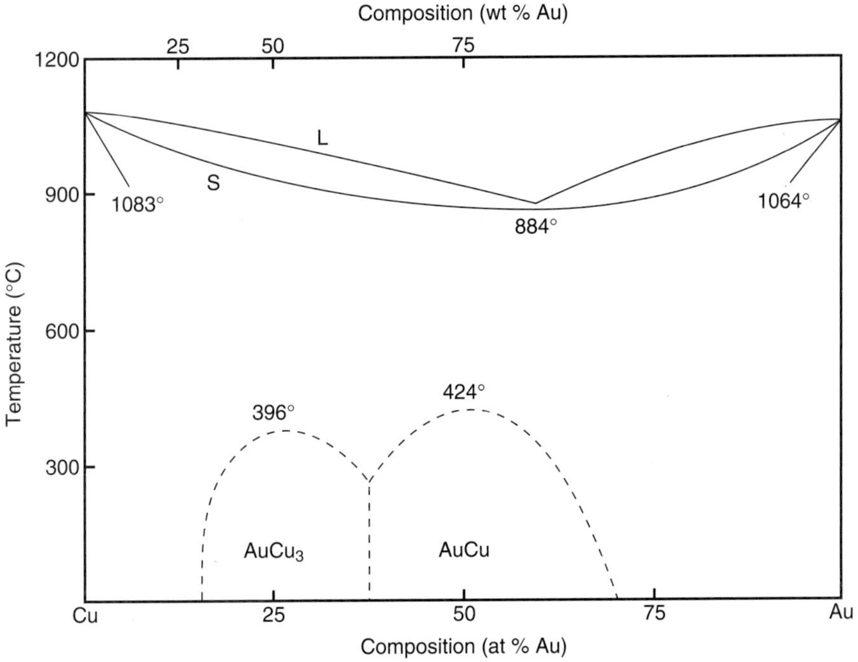

Fig. 6-8 The Au-Cu binary phase diagram illustrates well the principles of a solid solution alloy system. The Au and Cu are miscible (completely soluble in one another), thus there is only one solid phase for any composition of Au and Cu. The liquidus is indicated by *L*, the solidus by *S*. Au and Cu occupy random positions in the crystal lattice at all compositions except under the dotted lines. Within the dotted lines, there are specific patterns to the Au and Cu atoms in the lattice, hence the name *ordered solution.*

several outcomes depending on the solubility of the metals in each other. If the metals remain soluble in one another, the result is a solid solution. If the metals are not soluble in the solid state, then a eutectic may form. Sometimes, the elements react to form a specific compound, called an *intermetallic compound*. The phase diagrams that describe these outcomes will be presented in the following paragraphs.

Solid Solution Alloys Figure 6-8 shows a series of binary alloys of Au and Cu. Because there is only a single phase below the solidus *(S)*, this is a solid solution alloy system, common in dental casting alloys. Au and Cu are miscible; that is, they are soluble in any combination. If one were to examine the crystal structure of this alloy, the Au atoms would occupy some the positions of the face-centered cubic structure and the Cu atoms would occupy others. The relative positions of the Au and Cu atoms would be random, however. The solid solution system (see Fig. 6-8) is also characterized by a series of melting ranges that are more or less a smooth transition between the two melting points of the pure elements. The temperature distance between the liquidus and solidus determines the melting range; it is characteristic for each alloy system and varies with the composition within a system.

The Au-Cu system (see Fig. 6-8) also has several dotted lines below the solidus for alloy compositions between 20 and 70 atomic percent Au. These lines indicate the formation of ordered solutions. In ordered solutions, the Au and Cu atoms still occupy the face-centered cubic positions, but in a specific pattern that depends on the composition. Ordered solutions impart higher hardness and strengths to alloys (see Chapter 15).

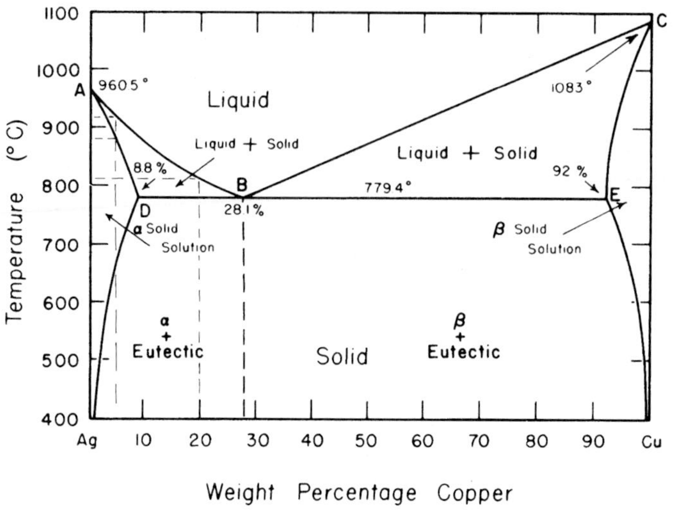

Fig. 6-9 A eutectic alloy system occurs when two metals are soluble as liquids but nearly insoluble as solids. These systems have a single composition (the eutectic composition) with a melting point that is lower than either component metal. These principles are illustrated well by the Ag-Cu eutectic system. The liquidus *(ABC)* and solidus *(ADBEC)* meet at the eutectic composition *(B)*, which is 28.1 wt% Cu with a melting point of 779.4° C. At other compositions, the solid contains two phases: a solid solution (either α or β) plus the eutectic. Note that below 400° C, almost no composition will support a single-phase composition, because the Ag and Cu are not soluble in each other below this temperature.

Eutectic Alloys Fig. 6-9 shows a series of binary Ag-Cu alloys. In this phase diagram, the liquidus and solidus meet at a mid-range composition and the solidus is lower (at 779.4° C) than either pure Ag (960.5° C) or Cu (1083° C). This liquidus-solidus configuration is characteristic of an eutectic alloy system. The Ag-Cu system is especially important in high-Cu dental amalgam, but is also important in the formulation of some dental casting alloys.

The eutectic system shown in Fig. 6-9 contains a pure solid solution below 400° C only at either extreme of composition (<1% Ag or <1% Cu) because the Ag and Cu are essentially insoluble in one another in the solid state. At all other equilibrium conditions below the solidus, a mixture of a solid solution (either α or β) and the eutectic composition occurs. The eutectic composition is 28.1% Cu (and 71.9% Ag) and has a layered appearance under a light microscope (Fig. 6-10). If the alloy is at the eutectic composition, all of the alloy will be in the eutectic phase at room temperature (see the dotted line in Fig. 6-9). If the composition is other than this, then the alloy will be some combination of the solid solution and eutectic phases. The exact proportions of eutectic and solid solution can also be determined from the phase diagram, but this calculation is beyond the scope of this discussion. Finally, note that a pure eutectic composition has a melting point (vs. a melting range) that is substantially lower than either of the pure components. The eutectic system of Pb-Sn uses the eutectic alloy composition as plumber's solder because of its low melting point.

Intermetallic Compounds If two metals react to form a new compound with a specific composition, the phase diagram reflects an intermetallic compound. Fig. 11-2 shows the for-

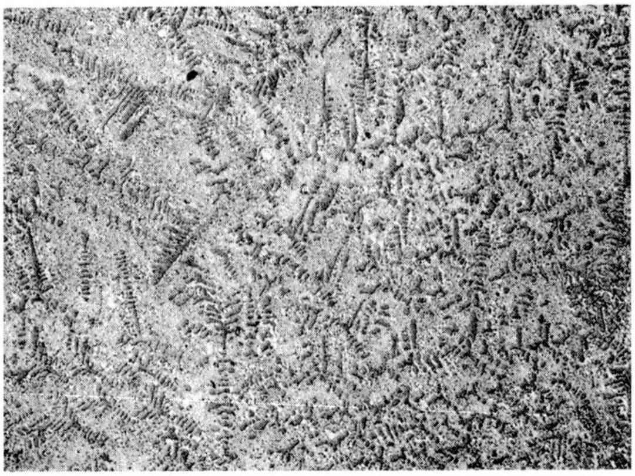

Fig. 6-10 A microscopic view of a Ag-Cu eutectic mixture (28.1 wt% Cu and 71.9 wt% Ag) magnified 50x. The eutectic composition is a fine layering between Ag and Cu. This layering is a result of the insolubility of Ag and Cu in the solid condition. This eutectic has a melting point rather than a melting range, as indicated on the phase diagram shown in Fig. 6-9.

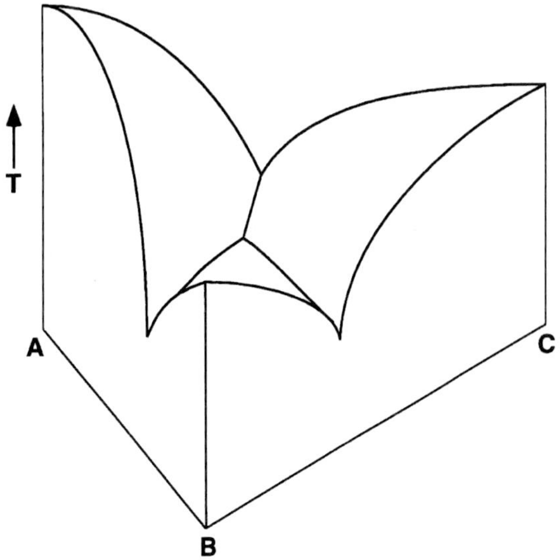

Fig. 6-11 Ternary phase diagram showing the liquid-solid surface formed between components *A*, *B*, and *C*. The vertical axis represents increasing temperature (*T*). The *AB*, *AC*, and *BC* axes reflect concentrations of the components. The three-dimensional surface that is visible represents the liquidus for this system. Other features of the phase diagram below the liquidus require a two-dimensional cross section parallel to the *ABC* plane. The shape of the liquidus indicates that this is a eutectic system.

mation of the intermetallic compound Ag_3Sn in the Ag-Sn alloy system. Ag_3Sn is a fundamentally important intermetallic compound in dental amalgam. The Ag-Sn phase diagram is extremely complex and its complete description is beyond the scope of this discussion. However, the intermetallic compound is seen in Fig. 11-2 at 26.8 wt% of Sn as a solid vertical line extending to room temperature.

Ternary Phase Diagrams It is possible to construct a phase diagram for a ternary alloy (with three components). These phase diagrams are three-dimensional, as shown in Fig. 6-11. Two dimensional representations in the shape of an equilateral triangle are also used to represent the three-dimensional structure. The ternary phase diagrams are difficult to prepare and interpret; their detailed description can be found in engineering and metallurgy texts.

Alloy Microstructure The internal appearance of alloys under light and electron microscopy has been extensively used to describe alloys and interpret alloy behavior. Atomic structure can be determined by x-ray diffraction or high-resolution electron microscopy. Alloy microstructure is viewed by polishing the alloy surface, then etching with an acid to bring out relevant features. The microstructure of any alloy is a consequence of the chemistry and thermodynamics governing the elements involved.

Grains, Grain Boundaries, and Dendrites When a molten alloy is cooled, the first solid alloy particles form as the temperature

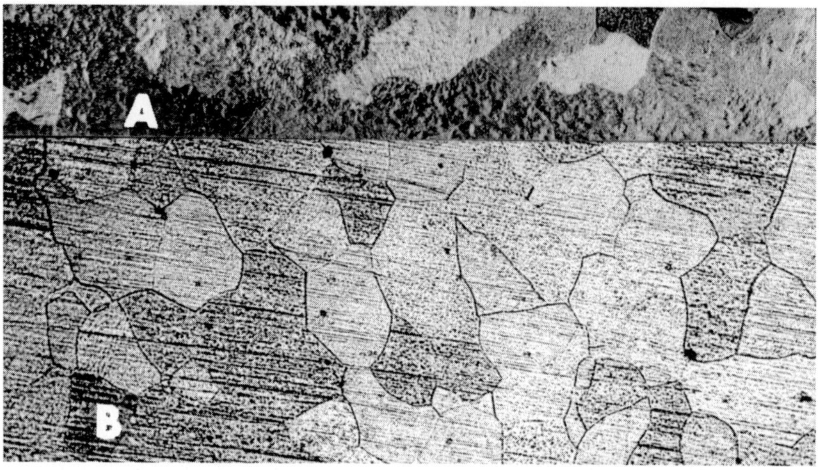

Fig. 6-12 Typical grain structure of pure gold *(A)* and 22-carat Au-Cu alloy *(B)* viewed at low magnification. Each grain is separated from other grains by grain boundaries *(dark lines),* and is a single metallic crystal. The grains have different shades because each crystal has a different orientation and therefore reflects light differently. Several inclusions *(small dark dots)* are also visible. These may represent impurities or voids.

reaches the liquidus. This process is called *nucleation*. In some alloys, fine particles of a high–melting point element such are Ir are added to encourage even nucleation throughout the alloy. These particles, used in this manner, are called *grain refiners*. As cooling continues, the nuclei grow into crystals called *grains,* and the grains enlarge until all of the liquid is gone and the grains meet and form boundaries between each other (at the solidus temperature). At this point, the grains are visible under a light microscope (Fig. 6-12) and are sometimes large enough to be seen with the unaided eye. The size of the grains depends on the cooling rate, alloy composition, presence of grain refiners, and other factors. Grain size may influence an alloy's strength, workability, and even susceptibility to corrosion (see Chapter 15). The junctions between grains are called *grain boundaries*. Grain boundaries are important because they often contain impurities such as oxides and are a site of corrosive attack. The grain boundaries are clearly visible in light microscopic views of alloys (see Fig. 6-12).

Dendrites result from grains that grow along major axes of the crystal lattice (Fig. 6-13) early in the freezing process. The dendritic skeleton structure persists to room temperature if the cooling rate of the alloy is too fast to allow equilibrium to occur. The dendritic structure is common in dental alloys and can be seen after etching and polishing the alloy (Fig. 6-14). Dendritic structure indicates that the alloy is not at equilibrium and its presence can increase the corrosion of the alloy.

Cast Microstructure Cast alloy microstructures have several distinguishing characteristics. Grains are usually visible and take on the appearance in Fig. 6-12. The size of the grains may be large or small depending on the cooling rate and other factors mentioned previously. A slow cooling rate and few impurities generally lead to large grains. Faster cooling rates or the presence of grain refiners lead to smaller grains. Grains that are uniform in size and shape throughout the alloy are described as *equiaxed*. Fine-grained (equiaxed) alloys are generally more desirable for dental applications because they have more-uniform properties (see Chapter 15). Different phases of a multiple-phase alloy may also be seen in cast microstructure.

Other factors may influence cast microstruc-

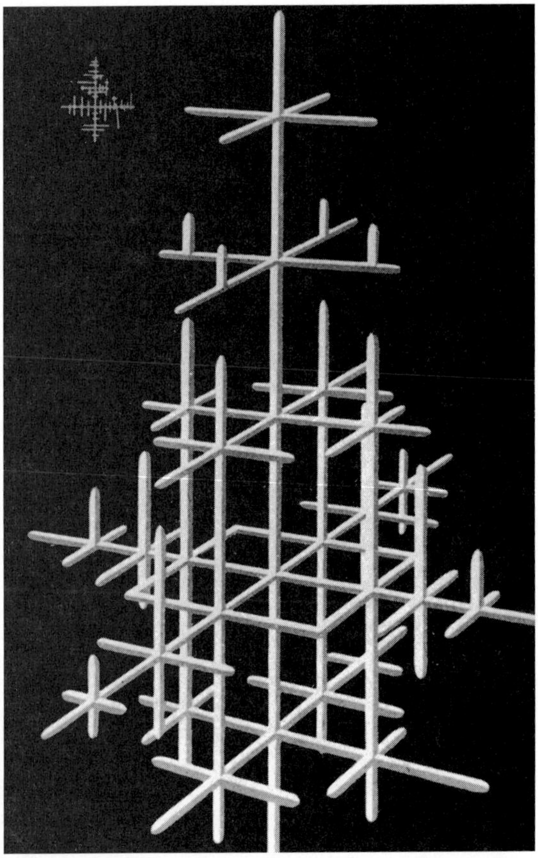

Fig. 6-13 Sketch of a dentritic structure of a crystal. The crystal grows preferentially in the x, y, or z axis due to the cooling of the alloy mass. If the cooling rate is fast enough, the dendrites will have a composition slightly different from the rest of the alloy because the equilibrium concentration specified by the phase diagram will not have had time to occur.

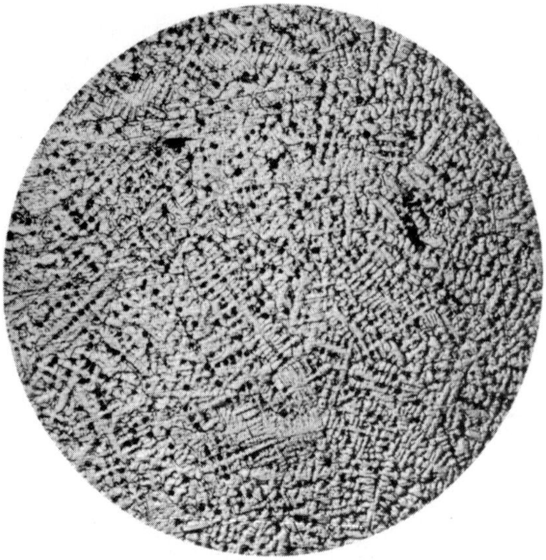

Fig. 6-14 Dendritic structure visible in a low-power light microscopic view of a gold alloy (polished, acid-etched). The treelike branching is similar to that sketched in Fig. 6-13.

ture. Insoluble impurities in an alloy may be detected at grain boundaries. Defects such as gas inclusions may cause small pits in the bulk of an alloy or at the surface. In the body of an alloy, pits may concentrate the stress and contribute to restoration failure. At the surface, pits may enhance corrosion, tarnish, or discoloration from the accumulation of organic debris. Voids in an alloy may result from improper cooling or improper investing (see Chapter 17 on Casting).

When a mass of molten metal is cast into a cold mold, the metal at the mold wall freezes first, and grains form and grow from the walls of the mold to the center of the mass. This type of grain growth is called *columnar growth* and can lead to alloy weakness from interference boundaries between the converging grains (Fig. 6-15). In general, it is more desirable to have the alloy freeze in a less ordered fashion. Sharp corners in any casting mold can enhance columnar grain growth and are generally undesirable.

Cold-Worked (Wrought) Microstructure

Metals and alloys are cast for two quite different purposes. In one instance, the casting serves as the final structure. In the second, it serves as an object that is further manipulated to form wires, sheets, bars, or similar fabricated structures. A typical cast structure in dentistry is an inlay or bridge restoration, which is not given further mechanical treatment except for polishing or marginal adaptation by hand operations. This limited treatment does not significantly modify the microstructure of the casting. Such a casting is designed to form to precision measurements, and the properties of the structure are those displayed by the cast metal or alloy.

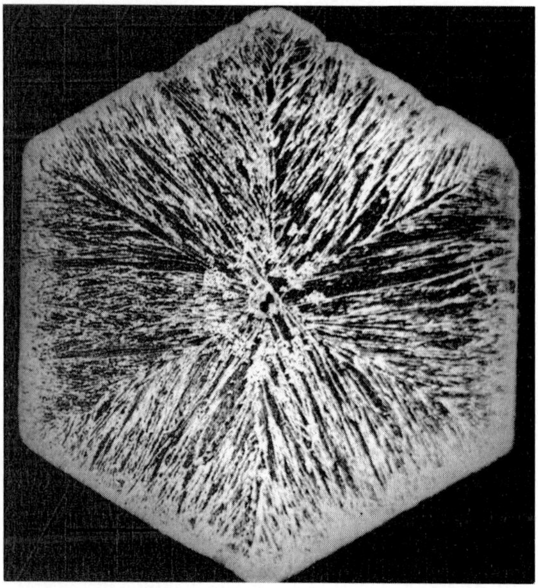

Fig. 6-15 Interference grain boundaries developed by an alloy poured into a hexagon-shaped mold (5×). The sharp corners of the mold cause the dendrites to "clash" and form the interference boundaries.

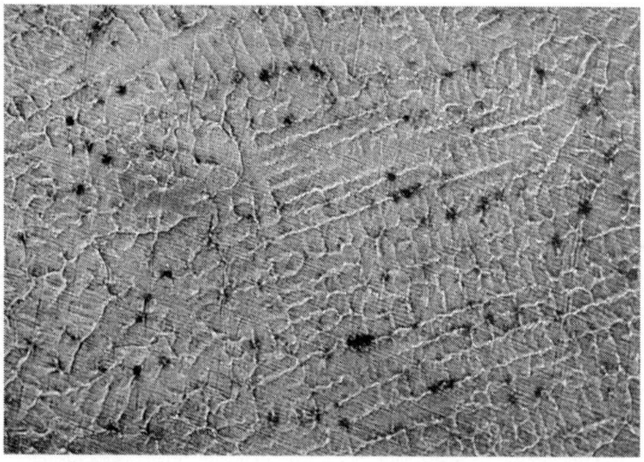

Fig. 6-16 Low-power light microscopic view of the typical grain structure of a cast gold alloy. Compare this grain structure to the same alloy after it has been pulled into wire form (see Fig. 6-17).

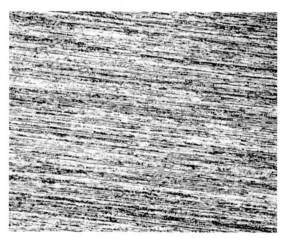

Fig. 6-17 Low-power light microscopic view of a wrought wire microstructure. The grains visible in Fig. 6-16 have been broken apart and tangled among one another. The entangled grains are lined up along the axis of the wire. This type of microstructure is called a *fibrous structure* for obvious reasons.

When the metal is to be used for wires, bands, bars, or other types of wrought structures, it is first cast into ingots that are then subjected to rolling, swaging, or wire-drawing operations that produce severe mechanical deformation of the metal. Such operations are described as *hot* or *cold working* of the metal, depending on the temperature at which the operation is performed. Many dental structures, such as orthodontic wires and bands, are formed by cold-working operations. The finished product is often described as a *wrought structure* to denote that it has been formed by severe working or shaping operations. The properties of wrought structures are quite different from those of cast structures in both internal appearance and mechanical characteristics.

The microscopic appearance of a cast metal is crystalline and sometimes has dendritic structure, as shown in Fig. 6-16. When this metal is subjected to cold-working operations, such as drawing into a wire, the grains are broken down, entangled in each other, and elongated to develop a fibrous structure or appearance that is characteristic of wrought forms, as shown in Fig. 6-17. This change in internal appearance is accompanied by a change in mechanical properties. In general, mechanical properties of the wrought structure are superior to those of a

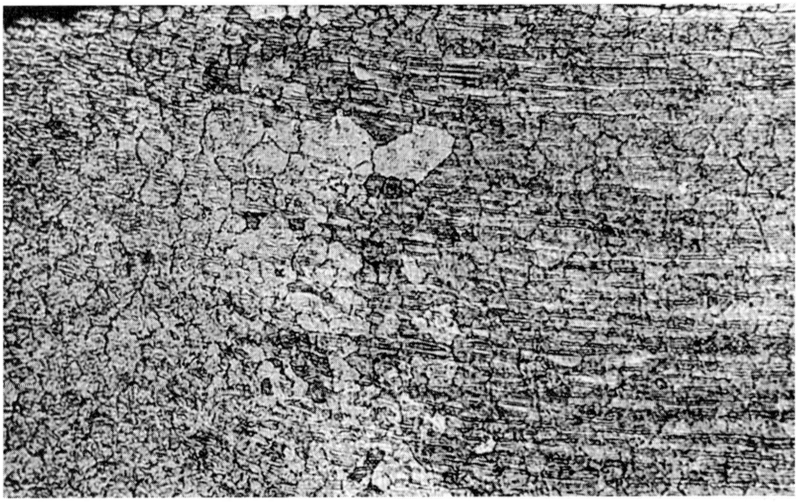

Fig. 6-18 The right side of this light microscopic view shows the fibrous microstructure typical of a wrought wire. Heat was applied to this wire from the left side, perhaps in a soldering operation, and the fibrous structure has been lost and replaced with the typical grain pattern of a cast structure. If more heat were applied, then the entire wire would revert to the cast structure. Such a conversion will cause the wire to be weaker but it will have a higher ductility. Because the wrought form was selected for its strength properties, the recrystallization shown here is not clinically desirable.

casting prepared from the same melt or alloy. It should be emphasized that in cast dental structures such as inlays, the mechanical properties of strength and hardness are not modified appreciably by simple polishing or marginal adaptation operations.

Recrystallization and Grain Growth

Metals or alloys that have been cold worked in the process of forming wires or bands change their internal structure and properties when heated or annealed. The characteristic fibrous structure of the wrought mass is gradually lost, and the grain or crystalline structure reappears. The process is known as *recrystallization* or *grain growth*. The degree of recrystallization is related not only to the alloy composition and mechanical treatment or strain hardening received during fabrication, but also to the temperature and the duration of the heating operation. High temperatures and long heating periods produce the greatest amount of recrystallization. It is not uncommon to find that during a soldering or annealing operation of a practical appliance, the temperature applied to the wire or band materials was sufficient to cause recrystallization of the wrought structure. Recrystallization of a segment of wire adjacent to a solder joint is shown in Fig. 6-18. Because the strength is usually reduced in recrystallized wrought structure (ductility often increases), it is necessary to guard against excessive heating during the assembly of a wrought metal appliance. Although the tendency for crystallization is more prevalent in some wires than others, it can be kept to a minimum when the time and temperature of heating are kept as low as possible.

Although there is probably some tendency for cast metal structures to recrystallize when heated after casting, grain growth does not become evident when the structure is heated within the range of practical operations. Under excessive conditions of heating there is some evidence of recrystallization in cast alloys, but the significance is not so pronounced as in the case of wrought forms. Within practical limits of operation, therefore, this characteristic of recrystallization and grain growth is limited to wrought structures.

The cause for grain growth in the wrought structure is related to the tendency for metals to maintain a crystalline internal orientation of the component atoms. During the formation of the wrought structure, the original grains produced during the crystallization of the original casting were deformed and broken into small units. The deformation of the metal mass occurred by slippage of one portion past another along definite crystallization planes. The deformation and slippage occurred in various directions to distort the grain boundaries. The greater the degree of cold working, the greater the degree of grain boundary deformation. This deformed structure is unstable in nature, with greater internal energy than one that is in the cast condition. Accordingly, it possesses modified physical properties and the tendency to recrystallize when heated.

Stress relieving, annealing, recrystallization, and grain growth can be illustrated by the series of sketches shown in Fig. 6-19. A wrought wire that has been bent beyond the proportional limit and that contains tensile and compressive stresses at the upper and lower boundaries is shown in Fig. 6-19, *A;* the wire has the typical fibrous structure and a deformed crystal lattice. Moderate temperatures cause the release of these stresses, as shown in Fig. 6-19, *B,* without other changes. Higher heating at annealing temperatures (Fig. 6-19, *C*) causes the disrupted crystal structure to contain sufficient energy to return to its normal crystal structure, but the fibrous wrought structure is still evident; under this condition the corrosion resistance is increased. Further increases in temperature or time, or both, as seen in Fig. 6-19, *D,* permit recrystallization with grains appearing and the fibrous structure disappearing. Finally, in Fig. 6-19. *E,* grain growth occurs, and the cast condition again dominates the microstructure.

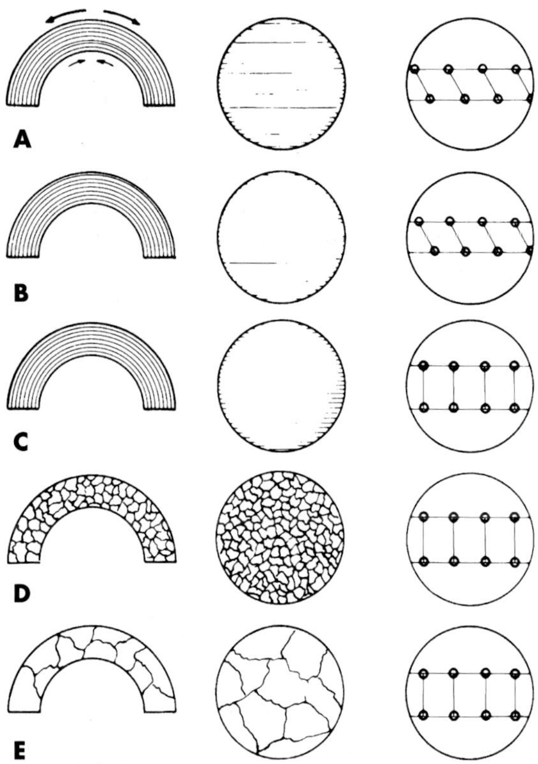

Fig. 6-19 Sketches depicting the gross view *(left column)*, microstructure *(middle column)*, and crystal view *(right column)* of wrought wire that has been bent. **A,** The fibrous microstructure is present and arrows indicate residual stresses. **B,** Minimal heat leaves the fibrous structure intact but relieves the stresses. However, the lattice remains distorted. **C,** Annealing with more heat allows the lattice deformation to be relieved. The fibrous microstructure remains. **D** and **E,** Further heating causes a loss of the fibrous structure and growth of the grains, which increase in size with increasing application of heat.

PROPERTIES OF ALLOYS

Dental alloys are diverse and use a wide variety of metallic elements and some of the metalloids (see Fig. 6-1). The compositions of dental alloys are dependent on the clinical use and environment for an alloy. Thus a carbide bur needs to be very hard to cut tooth structure, but its intraoral corrosion is of little concern. A dental crown must have excellent corrosion resistance and must not deform permanently. Endodontic files need to have moderate moduli and resist torsional failure. In each case, the alloys comprise elements that optimize the specific properties that are needed most for clinical success. In dentistry, solid solutions, eutectics, and intermetallic compounds and wrought alloys are used. It is the diversity of possible properties that makes alloys suitable for many clinical dental applications.

ALLOY-STRENGTHENING MECHANISMS

Alloys generally require high strength and hardness to be useful in dental applications. Several metallurgical strategies are used to strengthen alloys to appropriate levels. Nearly all of these strategies share the goal of impeding the deformation of the alloy by the dislocation mechanism (see previous discussion, this chapter).

Solid solutions are generally stronger and harder than either component pure metal. The presence of atoms of unequal size makes it more difficult for atomic planes to slide by each other. Even small differences in atomic size can strengthen alloys by the solid solution mechanism. Ordered solutions act to further strengthen a solid solution by providing a pattern of dissimilar sizes throughout the alloy's crystal structure. Solid and ordered-solution strengthening are very common in dental casting alloys.

Precipitation hardening is another strategy used to strengthen dental alloys. By heating some cast alloys carefully, a second phase can be made to appear in the body of the alloy. The new phase blocks the movement of dislocations, thereby increasing strength and hardness. The effectiveness of precipitation hardening is greater if the precipitate is still part of the normal crystal lattice. This type of precipitation is called *coherent precipitation*. Overheating may reduce alloy properties by allowing the second phase to grow outside of the original lattice structure. Fig. 6-20 shows the character of a casting alloy that was strengthened by the addition of as little as 0.08 wt% iron to a gold-platinum alloy. The iron formed an $FePt_3$ precipitate and the hardness of the alloy tripled under appropriate conditions.

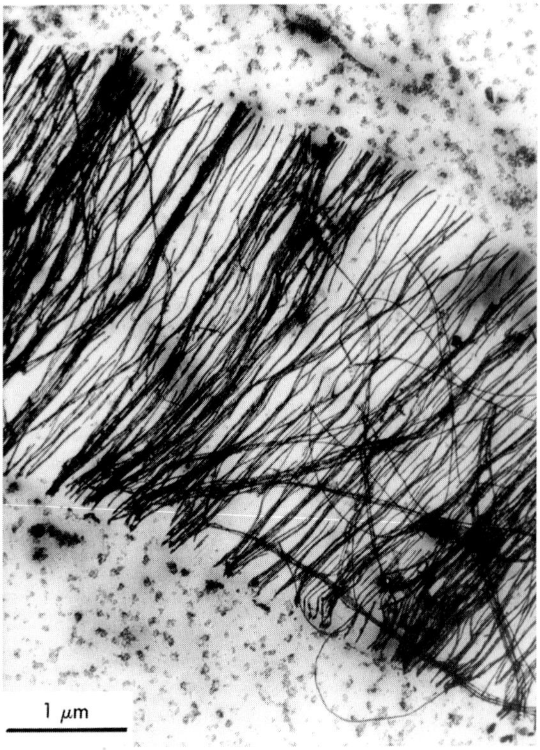

Fig. 6-20 Electron micrograph of $FePt_3$ (black, hairlike structures) formed in a gold-platinum alloy containing 0.08 wt% iron.

(From Sims JR Jr., Blumenthal RN, O'Brien WJ: *J Biomed Mater Res* 7:497, 1973.)

Other factors may increase alloy strength and hardness. Grain refiners such as Ir, Rh, and Ru improve the strength of alloys by several times. Moreover, strength and hardness are generally improved without sacrificing ductility. Fine-grained alloys have grain sizes below 70 μm in diameter. Cold working an alloy will significantly strengthen it. Cold working works out the dislocations, thereby making further deformation more difficult. However, cold working will also embrittle an alloy by making it less ductile.

PROPERTIES OF CASTING ALLOYS

In general, the properties of the solid solutions resemble those of the metals forming the alloy, with certain exceptions. Solid solution alloys often have higher strength and hardness and lower ductility than either pure metal. This is the basis of solid-solution strengthening. Solid solutions also possess melting ranges rather than melting points and always melt below the melting point of the highest points of both metals. These alloys are commonly used in dentistry because they have higher corrosion resistance than multiple-phase alloys. Also, in a few cases, solid solutions have higher corrosion resistance than the pure metals. A notable example is the addition of chromium to iron in solid solution to make the corrosion-resistant alloy "stainless steel." However, in the case of gold, adding other elements reduces the corrosion resistance.

Eutectic mixtures are usually harder and stronger than the metals used to form the alloy and are often quite brittle. They possess a melting point at the eutectic composition, not a melting range, and any other combination of the alloy system has a higher fusion temperature than the melting point of the eutectic mixture. Eutectic mixtures, along with other multiple-phase microstructures, often have poor corrosion resistance. Galvanic action between the two phases at a microscopic level can accelerate corrosion, as described in Chapter 3.

The intermetallic compounds formed in some alloy systems are usually very hard and brittle. Their properties rarely resemble those of the metals making the alloy. For example, Ag_2Hg_3 is an intermetallic compound formed in dental amalgam that has properties completely different from those of pure silver or mercury.

PROPERTIES OF WROUGHT ALLOYS

Compared with their cast counterparts, wrought alloys generally have high strengths and hardness. Ductility, on the other hand, decreases with cold work. Clinically, this loss of ductility can be a problem. For example, cast clasps on removable partial dentures may fail if multiple adjustments are made to a clasp. Cast properties can be regained by heating the wrought form sufficiently to allow recrystallization and grain growth.

SELECTED PROBLEMS

Problem 1

In the metallic crystal lattice, the valence electrons are relatively unbound to their atomic centers. What properties of metals result from this configuration?

Solution

The loose valence electrons are mobile and allow metals to readily conduct heat and electricity. The electrons can also accommodate shifts of the nuclear centers that often make the metals malleable and ductile. The high reflectivity (mirror-like surface) of a polished metallic surface occurs because the valence electrons reflect light that hits the surface.

Problem 2

A person hands you two samples of the same metal. In the first sample *(A)*, she tells you that there are absolutely no flaws in the crystal structure of the metal. In the second sample *(B)*, there are numerous crystal flaws. How do the strengths of *A* and *B* compare, and why?

Solution

A will be stronger by at least one order of magnitude. Without flaws, no dislocation-mediated sliding can take place and the total of the metallic bonds must be overcome at once. With flaws present, the metal can deform one row of atoms at a time, and thus the deformation occurs at a lower stress (see Fig. 6-5).

Problem 3

If you are given a single crystal of a pure metal with a hexagonal close-packed lattice in the shape of a cube 3 mm on a side, and you test the compressive strength in the horizontal and vertical directions, will the strengths be the same? If you take a sample, the same size, which is a collection of microscopic crystals, what will the result be?

Solution

For the single crystal, the strengths will not be the same because the distribution of the atoms in a crystal lattice are not anisotropic (independent of direction). Because the metal sample is a pure single crystal, the strength in the horizontal and vertical directions will depend on the conformation of atoms in those directions. Because the conformation of atoms in the hexagonal close-packed lattice is different in the horizontal and vertical directions, the horizontal and vertical strength will vary. For the sample with many smaller crystals, the strength will be the same (at least theoretically). This occurs because the different crystals are oriented at random with respect to one another, and any directional difference in properties is averaged out over the sample.

Problem 4

You are given a binary alloy of known composition and the phase diagram for that alloy. Using the phase diagram and knowing the composition of the alloy, can you predict the phases present in your alloy at room temperature?

Solution

No, certain prediction is probably not possible because you do not know if the alloy is at equilibrium or not. Phase diagrams give the phase structure of an alloy at equilibrium. If your alloy was cooled from the molten state such that equilibrium did not have time to occur, then you cannot know where along the temperature axis the alloy was frozen. Furthermore, formation of dendrites and other non-equilibrium anomalies may be present.

Problem 5

You are given two wires, the same diameter and length. One is wrought and the other is cast. Which will have the greatest percentage elongation?

Solution

Chances are that the cast wire will have the greatest elongation. By mechanically working a wire to its wrought form, the dislocations that allow elongation are "used up" and therefore further stress will result in fracture, not elongation. On the other hand, the tensile strength of the wrought wire is probably greater because it resists the deformation leading to fracture.

Problem 6

If a second element is added to pure gold to form an alloy, one finds that the ability of the second element to form a solid solution with the gold depends on the diameter of the second element versus that of the gold atoms. Why might this be true?

Solution

For the second element to be able to substitute at random into the gold crystal lattice, its diameter must be within a certain range of the gold atoms. If the diameter is too large or too small, it cannot substitute without disrupting the lattice. If its diameter is too small, the second element cannot interact properly with the gold atoms. The ability to form solid solutions sometimes also depends on the relative numbers of the two elements. A host crystal lattice can sometimes accommodate a second element only up to a certain concentration, above which the host lattice is overly disrupted.

Problem 7

You are constructing an orthodontic appliance that requires that a wrought wire be soldered to an orthodontic band. What variables in the soldering operation must be controlled to ensure that the fibrous microstructure of the wire is maintained during the soldering?

Solution

The two critical variables are the time it takes to do the soldering and the temperature of the soldering operation. If either variable is inappropriate (too much time or too high a temperature), then the fibrous wire structure will revert to a grain-based structure. The limit on each variables is dependent on the composition of the wire. Each alloy has different tolerances before recrystallization and grain growth occur.

Problem 8

Of the three types of alloys (solid solutions, eutectics, and intermetallic compounds), which is most likely appropriate for long-term dental applications and why?

Solution

Although all three types of alloys occur in dentistry, solid solutions are generally the most useful because they possess high strength, relatively high ductility, and low corrosion relative to eutectics and intermetallic compounds. Solid-solution alloys also offer a flexibility in composition that is not possible with eutectics and intermetallic compounds.

Problem 9

What methods can be used to improve the mechanical properties of a dental casting alloy?

Solution

Perhaps the best approach is to add grain-refining elements to the alloy. Fine grain size generally improves all mechanical properties, including ductility. Another method that can be used is solid-solution strengthening. Strength and hardness can be dramatically improved by small additions of alloying metals, which go into solution. However, with solid-solution strengthening the ductility may be reduced. Other techniques, such as alloying to form second phases to produce eutectic structure or precipitation hardening, are less desirable for use in dentistry because of increased susceptibility to corrosion. Finally, cold working a casting is generally impractical because the shape would be affected.

BIBLIOGRAPHY

Anusavice KJ: *Phillips' science of dental materials,* ed 10, Philadelphia, 1996, WB Saunders.

Council on Dental Materials, Instruments, and Equipment: Classification system for cast alloys, *J Am Dent Assoc* 109:766, 1984.

Council on Dental Materials, Instruments, and Equipment: Revised ANSI/ADA specification No. 5 for dental casting alloys, *J Am Dent Assoc* 118:379, 1989.

Craig RG, Powers JM, Wataha JC: *Dental materials: properties and manipulations,* ed 7, St Louis, 2000, Mosby.

Dieter G: *Mechanical metallurgy,* ed 3, New York, 1986, McGraw-Hill, Inc.

Flinn RA, Trojan PK: *Engineering materials and their applications,* ed 4, New York, 1994 John Wiley & Sons.

Fontana MG: *Corrosion engineering,* ed 3, New York, 1986, McGraw-Hill, Inc.

Gettleman L: Noble alloys in dentistry, *Current Opinion Dent* 2:218, 1991.

Leinfelder KF: An evaluation of casting alloys used for restorative procedures, *J Am Dent Assoc* 128:37, 1997.

Malhotra ML: Dental gold casting alloys: a review, *Trends Tech Contemp Dent Lab* 8:73, 1991.

Malhotra ML: New generation of palladium-indium-silver dental cast alloys: a review, *Trends Tech Contemp Dent Lab* 9:65, 1992.

Mezger PR, Stolls ALH, Vrijhoef MMA et al: Metallurgical aspects and corrosion behavior of yellow low-gold alloys, *Dent Mater* 5:350, 1989.

Moffa J: Alternative dental casting alloys, *Dent Clin North Am* 27:733, 1983.

Morris HF, Manz M, Stoffer W et al: Casting alloys: the materials and the 'clinical effects,' *Adv Dent Res* 6:28, 1992.

O'Brien WJ: *Dental materials and their selection,* ed 2, Carol Stream, IL, 1997, Quintessence.

Pourbauix M: Electrochemical corrosion of metallic biomaterials, *Biomaterials* 5:122, 1984.

Vermilyea SG, Cai Z, Brantley WA et al: Metallurgical structure and microhardness of four new palladium-based alloys, *J Prosthodont* 5:288, 1996.

Wendt SL: Nonprecious cast-metal alloys in dentistry, *Current Opinion Dent* 1:222, 1991.

Chapter 7

Polymers and Polymerization

Before the introduction of acrylic polymers to dentistry in 1937, the principal polymer used was vulcanized rubber for denture bases. Polymers introduced since then have included vinyl acrylics, polystyrene, epoxies, polycarbonates, polyvinylacetate-polyethylene, *cis*- and *trans*-polyisoprene, polysulfides, silicones, polyethers, and polyacrylic acids. In addition, oligomers from bisphenol A and glycidyl methacrylate (such as dimethacrylates) and urethane dimethacrylates have been applied.

In terms of quantity, the primary use of polymers has been in the construction of prosthetic appliances such as denture bases. However, they have also been used for highly important applications such as artificial teeth, tooth restoratives, cements, orthodontic space maintainers and elastics, crown and bridge facings, obturators for cleft palates, inlay patterns, implants, impressions, dies, temporary crowns, endodontic fillings, and athletic mouth protectors.

BASIC NATURE OF POLYMERS

CHEMICAL COMPOSITION

The term *polymer* denotes a molecule that is made up of many (poly) parts (mers). The *mer* ending represents the simplest repeating chemical structural unit from which the polymer is composed. Thus poly(methyl methacrylate) is a polymer having chemical structural units derived from methyl methacrylate, as indicated by the simplified reaction and structural formula I.

The molecules from which the polymer is constructed are called *monomers* (one part). Polymer molecules may be prepared from a mixture of different types of monomers. They are called *copolymers* if they contain two or more different chemical units and *terpolymers* if they contain three different units, as indicated by the structural formulas II and III.

As a convenience in expressing the structural formulas of polymers, the mer units are enclosed in brackets, and subscripts such as n, m, and p represent the average number of the various mer units that make up the polymer molecules. Notice that in normal polymers the mer units are spaced in a random orientation along the polymer chain. It is possible, however, to produce copolymers with mer units arranged so that a large number of one mer type are connected to a large number of another mer type. This special type of polymer is called a *block polymer*. It also is possible to produce polymers having mer units with a special spatial arrangement with respect to the adjacent units; these are called *stereospecific polymers*.

MOLECULAR WEIGHT

The molecular weight of the polymer molecule, which equals the molecular weight of the various mers multiplied by the number of the mers, may range from thousands to millions of molecular weight units, depending on the preparation conditions. The higher the molecular weight of the polymer made from a single monomer, the higher

I

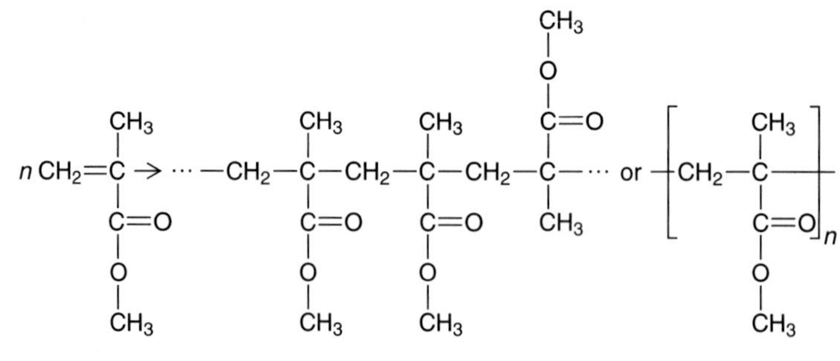

Methyl methacrylate

Poly (methyl methacrylate)

the degree of polymerization. The term *polymerization* is often used in a qualitative sense, but the *degree of polymerization* is defined as the total number of mers in a polymer molecule. In general, the molecular weight of a polymer is reported as the average molecular weight because the number of repeating units may vary greatly from one molecule to another. As would be expected, the fraction of low-, medium-, and high-molecular-weight molecules in a material or, in other words, the molecular weight distribution, has as pronounced an effect on the physical properties as the average molecular weight does. Therefore two poly(methyl methacrylate) samples can have the same chemical composition but greatly different physical properties because one of the samples has a high percentage of low-molecular-weight molecules, whereas the other has a high percentage of high-molecular weight molecules. Variation in the molecular weight distribution may be obtained by altering the polymerization procedure. These materials therefore do not possess any precise physical constants, such as melting point, as ordinary small molecules do. For example, the higher the molecular weight, the higher the softening and melting points and the stiffer the plastic.

SPATIAL STRUCTURE

In addition to chemical composition and molecular weight, the physical or spatial structure of the polymer molecules is also important in determining the properties of the polymer. There are three basic types of structures: linear, branched, and cross-linked. They are illustrated in Fig. 7-1 as segments of linear, branched, and cross-linked polymers. The linear homopolymer has mer units of the same type, and the random copolymer of the linear type has the two mer units randomly distributed along the chain. The linear block copolymer has segments, or blocks, along the chain where the mer units are the same. The branched homopolymer again consists of the same mer units, whereas the graft-branched copolymer consists of one type of mer unit on the main chain and another mer for the branches. The cross-linked polymer shown is made up of a homopolymer cross-linked with a single crosslinking agent.

II

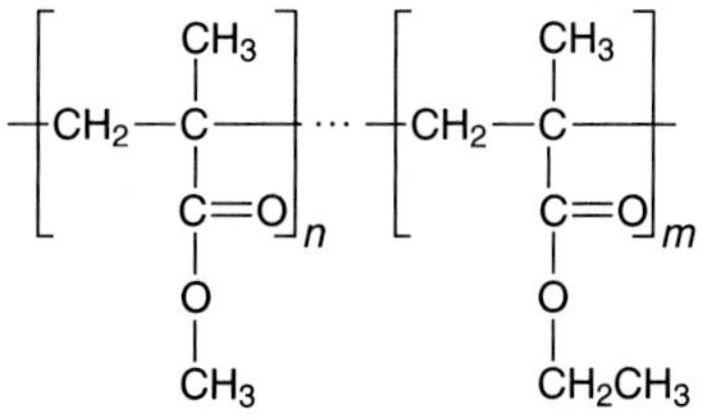

Methyl methacrylate–ethyl methacrylate copolymer

III

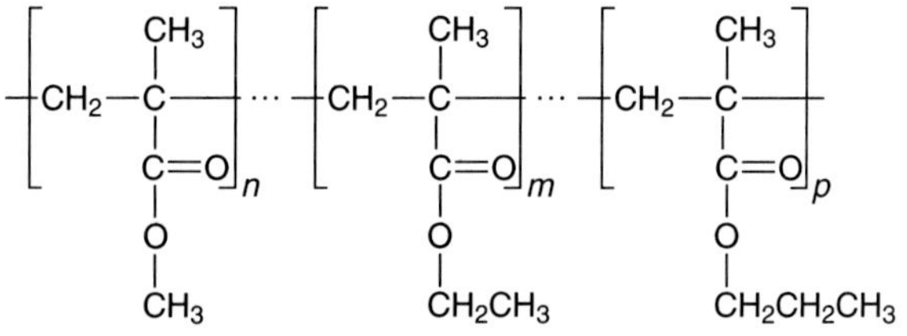

Methyl-, ethyl-, propyl methacrylate copolymer or terpolymer

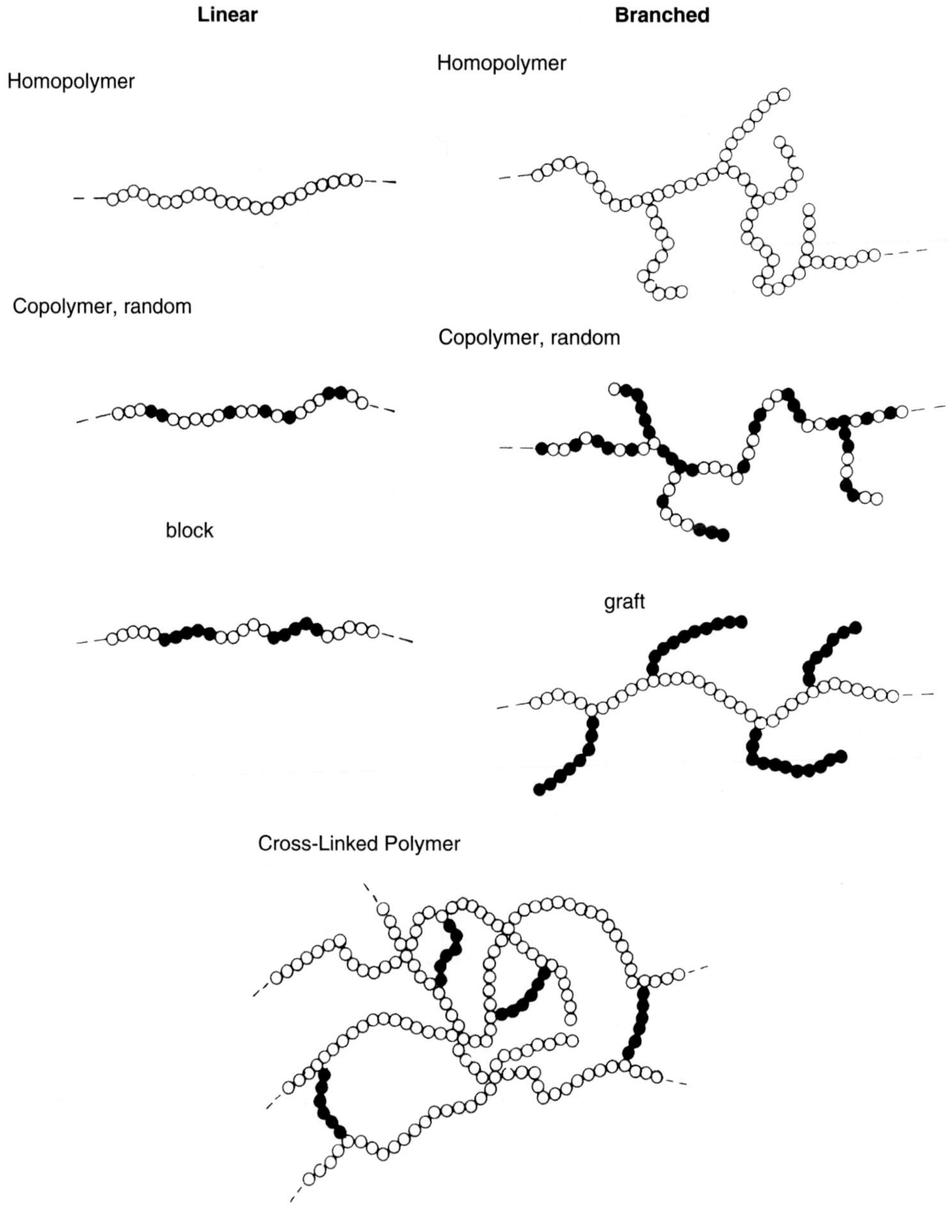

Fig. 7-1 Linear, branched, and cross-linked homopolymers and copolymers. *Open circles,* one type of mer unit; *solid circles,* another type of mer unit; *dashed lines,* only a segment of the polymer.

The linear and branched molecules are separate and discrete, whereas the cross-linked molecules are a network structure that may result in the polymer's becoming one giant molecule. The spatial structure of polymers affects their flow properties, but generalizations are difficult to make because either the interaction between linear polymer molecules or the length of the branches on the branched molecules may be more important in a particular example. In general, however, the cross-linked polymers flow at higher temperatures than linear or branched polymers. Another distinguishing feature of some cross-linked polymers is that they do not absorb liquids as readily as either the linear or branched materials.

An additional method of classifying polymers other than by their spatial structure is according to whether they are thermoplastic or thermosetting. The term *thermoplastic* refers to polymers that may be softened by heating and solidify on cooling, the process being repeatable. Typical examples of polymers of this type are poly(methyl methacrylate), polyethylene-polyvinylacetate, and polystyrene. The term *thermosetting* refers to plastics that solidify during fabrication but cannot be softened by reheating. These polymers generally become nonfusible because of a crosslinking reaction and the formation of a spacial structure. Typical dental examples are cross-linked poly(methyl methacrylate), silicones, *cis*-polyisoprene, and bisphenol A–diacrylates.

Polymers as a class have unique properties, and by varying the chemical composition, molecular weight, molecular-weight distribution, or spatial arrangement of the mer units, the physical and mechanical properties of polymers may be altered.

PREPARATION OF POLYMERS

Polymers are prepared by a process called *polymerization,* which consists of the monomer units becoming chemically linked together to form high-molecular-weight molecules. The polymerization process may take place by several different mechanisms, but most polymerization reactions fall into two basic types: addition polymerization and condensation polymerization. Important addition polymerization reactions are free-radical, ring-opening, and ionic reactions.

ADDITION POLYMERIZATION

Free-Radical Polymerization Free-radical polymerization reactions usually occur with unsaturated molecules containing double bonds, as indicated by the following equation, where *R* represents any organic group, chlorine, or hydrogen.

$$n\,CH_2{=}\underset{\substack{|\\R}}{CH} \xrightarrow[\text{Initiator}]{} \left[CH_2{-}\overset{\substack{H\\|}}{\underset{\substack{|\\R}}{C}} \right]_n$$

In this type of reaction, no byproduct is obtained. The reaction takes place in three stages, called the *initiation, propagation,* and *termination* stages. The reaction may be accelerated by heat, light, and traces of peroxides, as well as trialkyl borane and other chemicals. In any case, the reaction is initiated by a free radical, which may be produced by any of the methods mentioned, as shown in the equation on p. 190.

Sufficient free radicals for polymerization may be produced at room temperatures by the reaction of a chemical accelerator such as a tertiary amine or a sulfinic acid with the organic peroxide. *N,N*-dihydroxyethyl-para-toluidine,

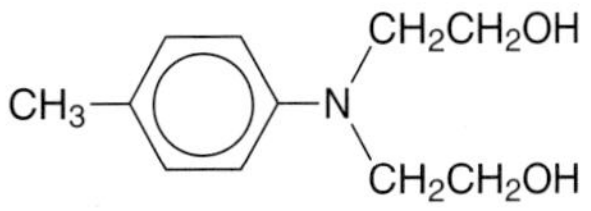

has commonly been used as an accelerator in dental products.

The initiation stage is followed by the rapid addition of other monomer molecules to the free radical and the shifting of the free electron to the end of the growing chain (see reactions below), which describes the propagation stage.

This propagation reaction continues until the growing free radical is terminated. The termination stage may take place in several ways, as indicated, where M represents the mer unit and n and m represent the number of mer units.

A study of these termination reactions reveals how branched and cross-linked polymer molecules may be obtained.

Free-radical polymerization reactions can be inhibited by the presence of any material that will react with a free radical, thus decreasing the rate of initiation or increasing the rate of termination. Decreasing the rate of initiation retards the polymerization reaction, and increasing the rate of termination decreases the degree of polymerization or the molecular weight of the final polymer. Such materials as hydroquinone, eugenol, or large amounts of oxygen will inhibit or retard the polymerization. Small amounts of hydroquinone are used to protect the methyl methacrylate monomer from premature polymerization, which prolongs the shelf life of the monomer.

Another important free-radical polymerization reaction is responsible for the setting of resin restorative composites. The manufacturer prepares a compound from one molecule of bisphenol A and two molecules of glycidyl methacrylate, called 2,2-*bis*[4(2-hydroxy-3 methacryloyloxy-propyloxy)-phenyl]propane. The acronym Bis-GMA has been used to identify this compound. Because it is not, strictly speaking, a monomer, it

Initiation stage

$$R'-\overset{\overset{O}{\|}}{C}-O-O-\overset{\overset{O}{\|}}{C}-R' \rightarrow 2R'\overset{\overset{O}{\|}}{C}-O\cdot \rightarrow 2R'\cdot + 2CO_2$$

Organic peroxide   Free radical

$$R'\cdot + CH_2=\underset{R}{CH} \rightarrow R'CH_2\underset{R}{CH}\cdot$$

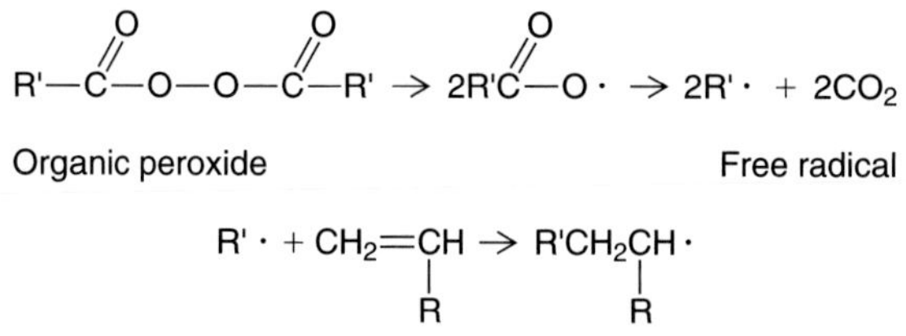

Propagation stage

$$R'CH_2\underset{R}{CH}\cdot + CH_2=\underset{R}{CH} \rightarrow R'CH_2\underset{R}{CH}-CH_2-\underset{R}{CH}\cdot \rightarrow \text{etc.}$$

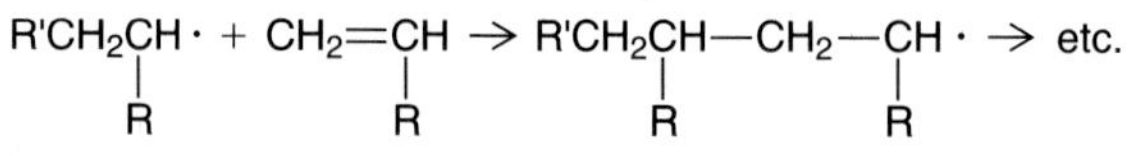

Termination stage

$$R'M_n\cdot + \cdot M_mR \rightarrow R'M_nM_mR$$

Annihilation reaction

$$R'CH_2\underset{R}{CH}\cdot + \cdot \underset{R}{HC}-CH_2R' \rightarrow R'\underset{R}{CH}=CH + H_2\underset{R}{C}-CH_2R'$$

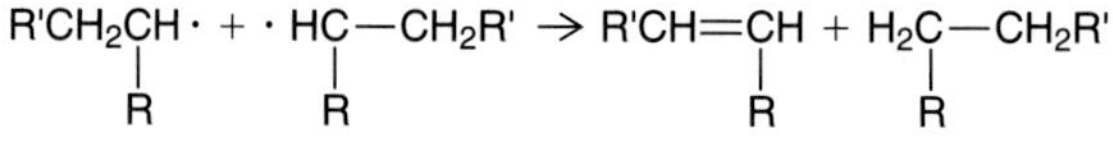

Disproportionation reaction

$$R'CH_2\underset{R}{CH}\cdot + CH_2=\underset{R}{CH} \rightarrow R'\underset{R}{CH}=CH + CH_3\underset{R}{CH}\cdot$$

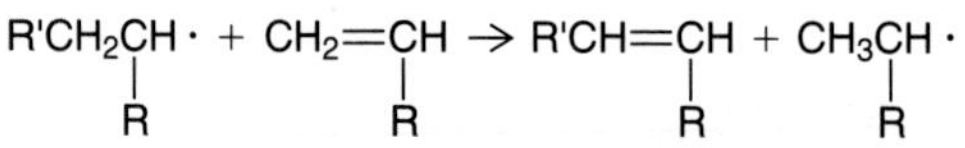

Transfer reaction

is called an *oligomer.* A simplified structural formula is shown in formula IV.

Lower-molecular-weight difunctional monomers such as triethyleneglycol dimethacrylate are added to reduce the viscosity, and polymerization is accomplished using free radicals. Because the Bis-GMA has reactive double bonds at each end of the molecule, just as the added lower-molecular-weight monomers do, a highly cross-linked polymer is obtained.

Free radicals needed to initiate the reaction are produced in composites by one of the two methods shown below.

Some composites contain oligomers that are urethane dimethacrylates, such as that shown in formula V below.

Polymerization is accomplished by free-radical initiation with a peroxide-amine system or a diketone-amine system and exposure to blue visible light.

The free-radical polymerization of monomers or oligomers with unsaturated double bonds does not result in all the double bonds reacting. The term *degree of conversion* describes the percentage of double bonds that react; depending on the conditions, the value may vary from 35% at the air-inhibited layer to 80% in the bulk.

Photo-initiation polymerization has become highly popular in dentistry; it has been shown that the degree of conversion with photo-initiation ranges from about 65% to 80%, whereas chemical initiation results in values from 60% to

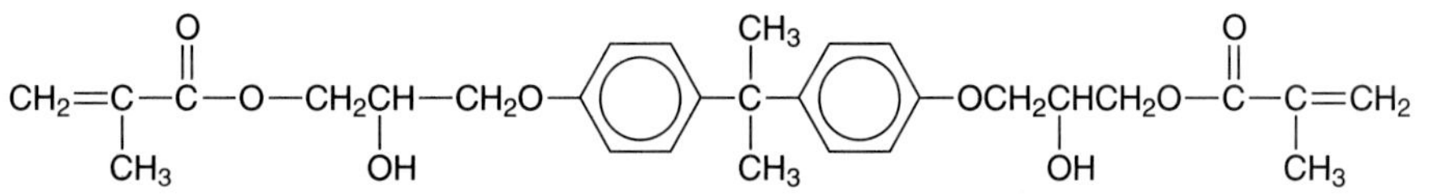

IV

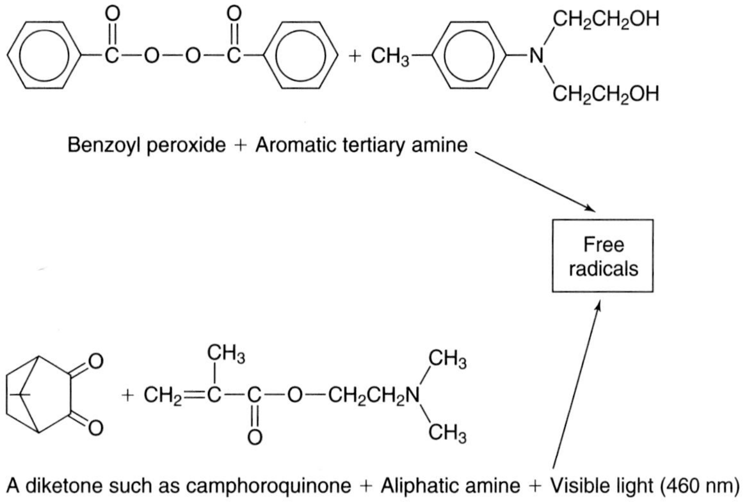

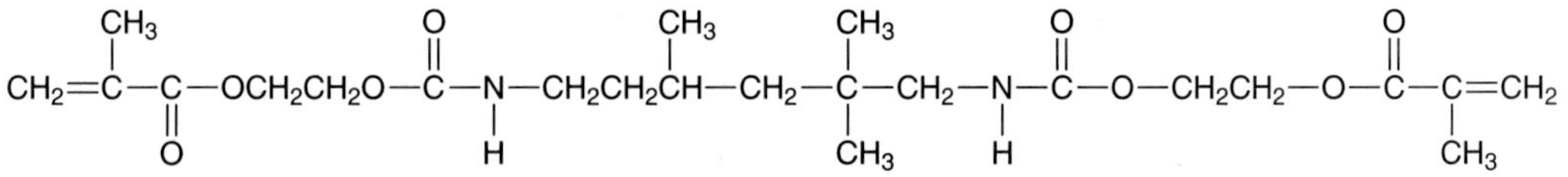

V

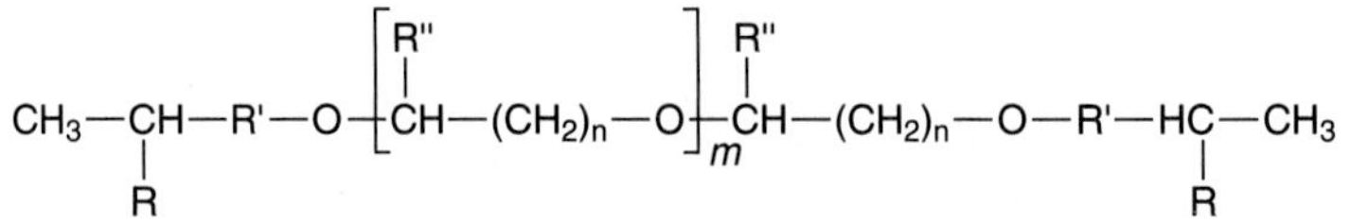

$$CH_3-CH-R'-O \left[CH-(CH_2)_n-O \right]_m CH-(CH_2)_n-O-R'-HC-CH_3$$

Polyether copolymer

$$CH_2=CH-\overset{CH_3}{\underset{CH_3}{Si}}-O \left[\overset{CH_3}{\underset{CH_3}{Si}}-O \right]_x \overset{CH_3}{\underset{CH_3}{Si}}-CH=CH_2 + \left[\overset{H}{\underset{CH_3}{Si}}-O \right]_y \cdots \left[\overset{CH_3}{\underset{CH_3}{Si}}-O \right]_z + \text{Pt catalyst} \rightarrow$$

Vinyl-terminated siloxane   Silane-containing siloxane   **VI**

$$\cdots \overset{CH_3}{\underset{CH_3}{Si}}-CH_2CH_2-\overset{CH_3}{\underset{O}{Si}}-\cdots, \text{etc.} \rightarrow \text{Silicone rubber}$$

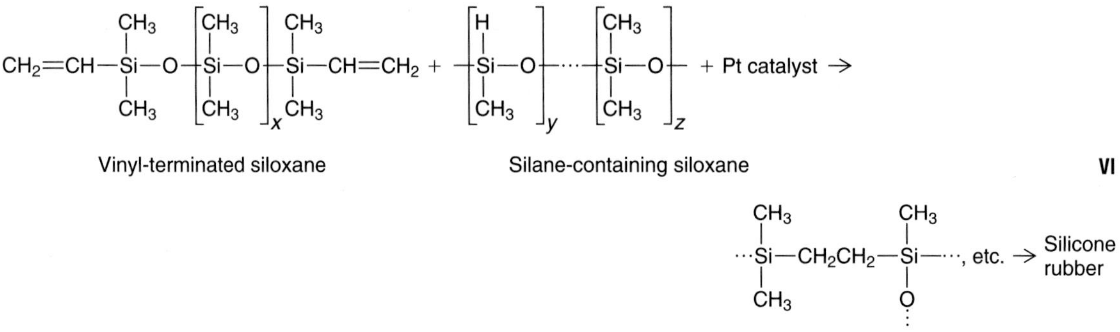

75%. Systems used to cement restorations often use both photo- and chemical-initiation (dual curing) because it is often difficult to expose regions of the material to sufficient light to reach the maximum degree of conversion and thus maximum strength. With these dual-curing materials, maximum degrees of conversion of 80% have been reported.

Ring-Opening Polymerization Two important ring-opening polymerizations in dentistry are the epoxy and ethylene imine reactions. The former is used to produce dies from rubber impressions, and the latter is used in the setting reaction of polyether rubber impression materials.

The reactants for the epoxy system are a difunctional epoxide oligomer and a difunctional amine, as shown in the following simplified equation:

$$H_2C-CH-R-HC-CH_2 + H_2N-R'-NH_2 \rightarrow$$

$$H_2C-CH-R-\overset{}{\underset{OH}{CH}}-CH_2-\overset{H}{\underset{}{N}}-R'-NH_2, \text{etc.} \rightarrow$$

Polymer

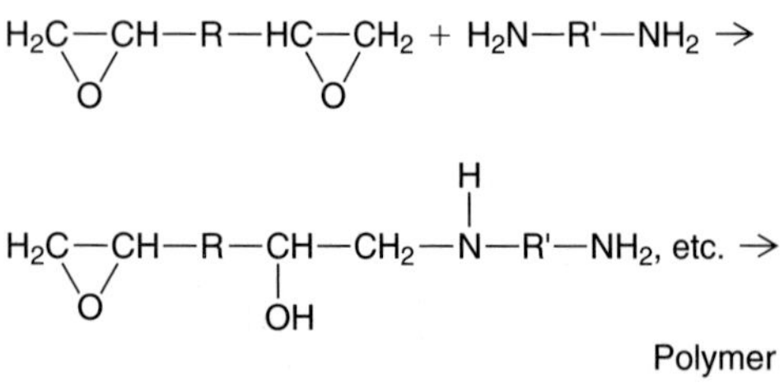

The amine opens the ring and crosslinking results in a rigid polymer. Water interferes with the setting reaction because it reacts with the epoxide. Therefore agar and alginate impressions are incompatible with this die material.

The polyether oligomer has a three-membered ring containing nitrogen shown as R in formula VI above. The ring is opened by the sulfonium fluoborate catalyst, and polymerization results in a cross-linked rubber. The oligomer and setting reaction are further discussed in Chapter 12, Impression Materials.

Hydrosilylation One final example of an addition reaction is with a vinyl-terminated silicone and a silane (–H)-containing siloxane, as shown above. In this instance the platinum catalyst attacks the hydrogen in the silane-containing dimethyl siloxane, and this complex reacts with the vinyl-terminated dimethyl siloxane to form a cross-linked silicone rubber. Compounds used in the vulcanization of latex surgical gloves interfere in the polymerization of addition silicones, and thus contact should be avoided.

CONDENSATION POLYMERIZATION

Condensation reactions result in polymerization plus the production of low-molecular-weight

$$HS{-}R{-}SH + PbO_2 \rightarrow HS{-}R{-}SS{-}R{-}SH + PbO + H_2O, \text{ etc.}$$
$$HS{-}R{-}SH + PbO \rightarrow HS{-}R{-}S{-}Pb{-}S{-}R{-}SH + H_2O$$
$$HS{-}R{-}S{-}Pb{-}S{-}R{-}SH + S \rightarrow HS{-}R{-}SS{-}R{-}SH + PbS, \text{ etc.} \rightarrow \text{Rubber}$$

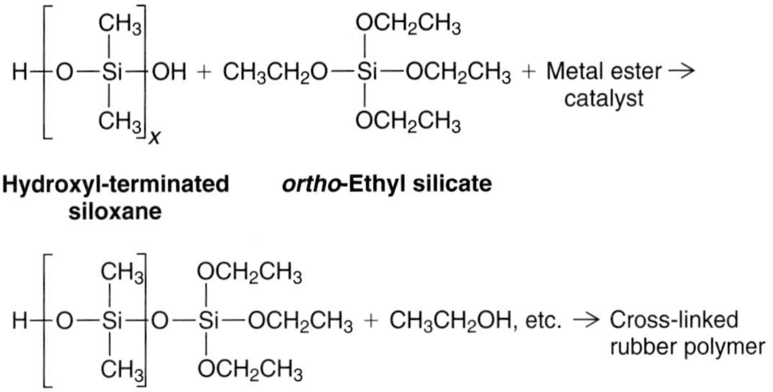

byproducts. Polysulfide rubbers are formed by a condensation reaction, the most general reaction being between low-molecular-weight polysulfide polymers having mercaptan (–SH) groups and lead dioxide, as shown above by the simplified reactions.

Water and lead sulfide are byproducts of the reaction. Mercaptan groups are also along the chain and thus crosslinking occurs. The rate of the reaction is proportional to –SH, PbO_2, and H_2O.

Condensation polymerization of the mercaptan groups can also be accomplished by use of a $Cu(OH)_2$, as shown by the following simplified reaction:

$$HS{-}R{-}SH + Cu(OH)_2 \rightarrow HS{-}R{-}S{-}Cu{-}S{-}R{-}SH + H_2O$$

$$HS{-}R{-}S{-}Cu{-}S{-}R{-}SH \rightarrow CuS + HS{-}R{-}SS{-}R{-}SH, \text{ etc.}$$

and

$$HS{-}R{-}SH + R'{-}OOH \rightarrow HS{-}R{-}SS{-}R + R'{-}OH + H_2O, \text{ etc.}$$

The polymerization with $Cu(OH)_2$ avoids the dark color of PbO_2 and the staining of fabric by the PbO_2-containing polysulfide impression materials.

Silicones may be polymerized by a condensation reaction if they contain terminal hydroxy groups, as shown by the reaction above.

Metal esters used have been stannous octoate and dibutyl tin dilaurate. The ortho-ethyl silicate is used as a crosslinking agent and is more stable if not combined with the metal ester. Ethyl alcohol is the byproduct, and its evaporation from the set rubber accounts for a significant portion of the shrinkage of condensation silicones after setting. Organosilicon compounds with only two ethoxy groups can be substituted for the ortho-ethyl silicate, thus reducing the byproduct and shrinkage on setting.

Polymer acids are used successfully in dentistry to react with hydrated metal ions such as Zn^{+2}, Ca^{+2}, or Al^{+3}. A copolymer of acrylic acid and itaconic acid in water is reacted with zinc oxide in an acid-base reaction to form a cement called *zinc polyacrylate,* as outlined:

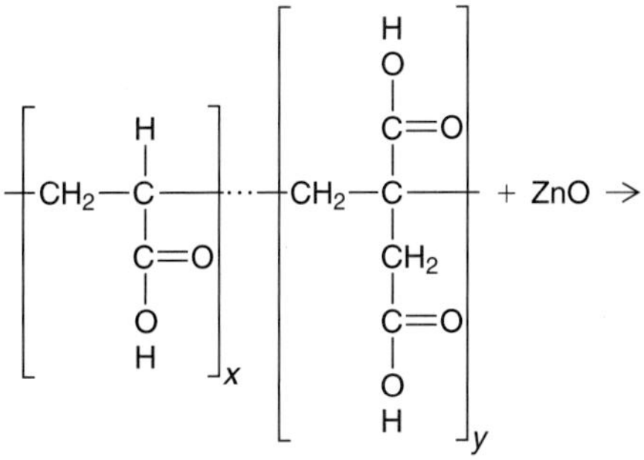

Acrylic acid mer unit　　Itaconic acid mer unit

or simplified:

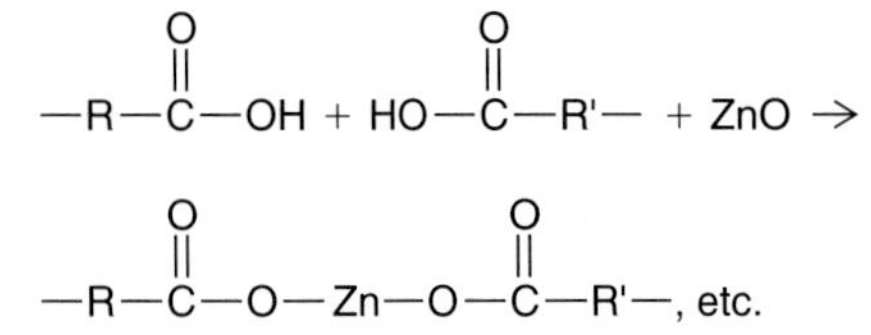

The copolymer acid can also be freeze-dried and included with the ZnO powder, and then only water is mixed with the powder.

A similar reaction with a copolymer of acrylic and itaconic acid in water solution is used with an aluminosilicate glass to form a glass ionomer. The copolymer is used rather than polyacrylic acid because the presence of itaconic acid prevents thickening of the water solution observed when only polyacrylic acid is used. Tartaric acid is also present in the formulation to increase the strength of the set ionomer by crosslinking from the difunctional acid groups.

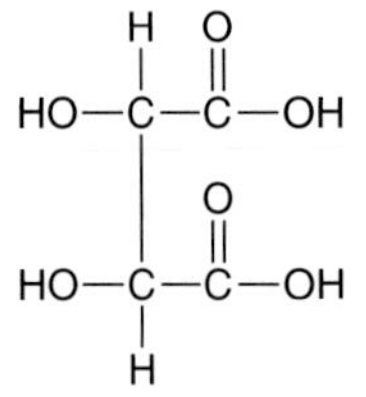

Tartaric acid

A stronger diacid, maleic acid, has been used to increase the rate of reaction, resulting in a higher early strength and allowing finishing at the placement appointment.

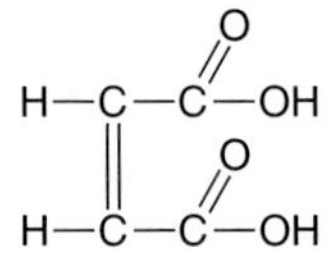

Maleic acid

The copolymer acid reacts first with Ca^{+2} and then Al^{+3} dissolved out of the glass by an ionic reaction to form metal esters. The material is called an *ionomer* and is used as both a restorative and a cement.

Materials called *compomers* use a combination of the ionomer reaction and free-radical polymerization. The polyacrylic acid molecules containing pendant methacrylate groups are dissolved in water along with 2-hydroxyethylmethacrylate and tartaric acid. The powder contains a glass and microencapsulated potassium persulfate and ascorbic acid catalyst. On mixing the powder and liquid, an acid-base ionomer reaction accompanied by a free-radical methacrylate reaction occurs.

Some compomers are made by reacting a polyfunctional organic acid with hydroxyethyl-

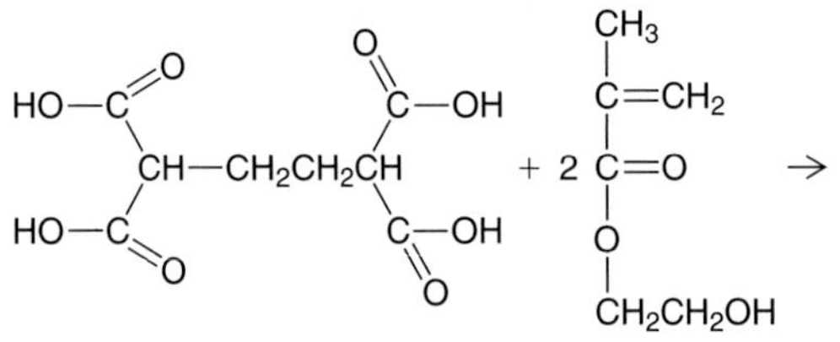

Tetra functional organic acid

2-Hydroxyethyl methacrylate

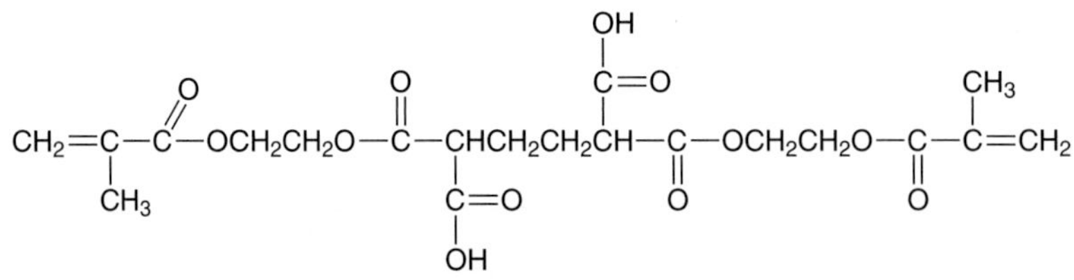

methacrylate to form a compound that will undergo both a free-radical and an acid-base reaction (see bottom of p. 194).

As a result, compomers of the resin-modified ionomer type and ionomer-modified composites type are available. Also, some products are polymerized by chemical and light initiation and by an acid-base reaction; these products are called *triple-cured materials*. The greater the number polyacid groups, the more the material is like a glass ionomer; the fewer the number of polyacid groups, the more it is like a resin composite.

OTHER POLYMERS

A variety of polymers are used in fully polymerized form without any polymerization reaction carried out by the dentist or laboratory technician. Polyisoprene is available in two forms, *cis* and *trans,* and both are natural rubbers. These structures are shown as follows:

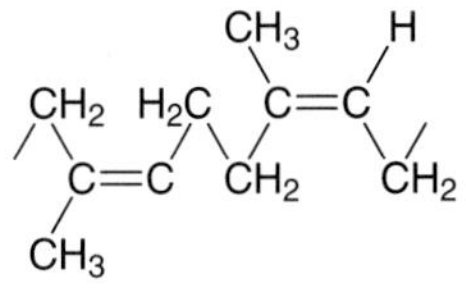

***cis*-Polyisoprene**

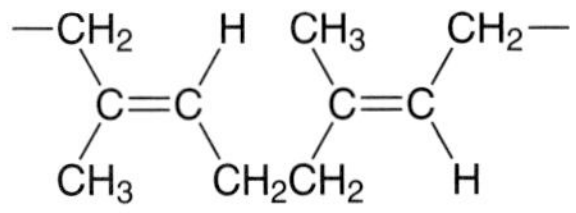

***trans*-Polyisoprene**

Notice that for the *cis* type the CH_3 and H are on the same (*cis*) side, whereas for the *trans* type they are on opposite (*trans*) sides. *cis*-Polyisoprene is cross-linked by the process of vulcanization with sulfur or other chemicals such as peroxides. In the vulcanized form it is very flexible and is used in surgical gloves, rubber dams for restorative procedures, and elastics for orthodontic applications. *trans*-Polyisoprene is rigid; it is compounded mainly with zinc oxide (but also with some waxes and zinc silicate) and is used for endodontic points as part of the filling material for root canals. For this application it is called *gutta-percha*.

A copolymer of ethylene and vinyl acetate has the following structural formula:

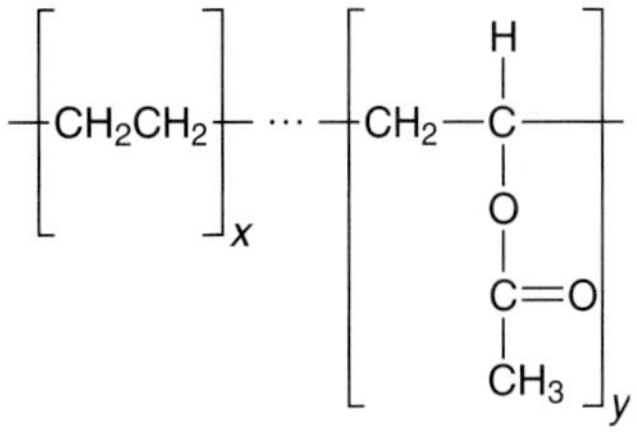

Copolymers containing 18% to 33% vinyl acetate are sold in fully polymerized sheets, which are heated to about 90° C and vacuum- or hand-formed over gypsum dental models to produce athletic mouth protectors. The higher the percentage of vinyl acetate, the softer the copolymer. The manufacturer uses a free-radical polymerization method to produce the polymer, which is then molded into sheets. No polymerization occurs in the dental processing of the mouth protector; they are processed as thermoplastics.

SELECTED PROBLEMS

Problem 1

Two samples of poly(methyl methacrylate) were listed by the manufacturer to be 100% pure, which was true, yet one had a significantly lower softening temperature than the other. Why?

Solution

The two samples could have had different average molecular weights, different molecular-weight distributions, or different spatial structures (linear, branched, or cross-linked).

Problem 2

The hardness and stiffness of two samples of ethylene-vinyl acetate copolymer used to fabricate athletic mouth protectors were found to be substantially different at body temperature. What is the most likely cause of the difference?

Solution

It is probable that the ratio of ethylene to vinyl acetate in the samples was different, with the softer and less stiff sample containing more vinyl acetate. It is also possible that the average molecular weights or their distributions were different.

Problem 3

Two denture-base poly(methyl methacrylate) products were heated. It was found that one sample softened and flowed, whereas the second decomposed rather than melted. What is the most likely reason for this observation?

Solution

The first poly(methyl methacrylate) sample was most likely a linear polymer and thus thermoplastic, whereas the second was a cross-linked poly (methyl methacrylate) that was not thermoplastic.

Problem 4

An experimenter determined the degree of polymerization of a poly(methyl methacrylate) material and used this information to calculate the degree of conversion. Would this procedure give a correct result?

Solution

No. The degree of polymerization measures the number of mer units in the polymer molecule, whereas the degree of conversion measures the number of unreacted carbon double bonds.

Problem 5

The dimensional change during polymerization of condensation-silicone rubber-impression material is significantly greater than during polymerization of addition-silicone rubber-impression materials. Why?

Solution

During the polymerization of condensation silicones and the rearrangement of chemical bonds, ethyl alcohol is released as a byproduct, but during the polymerization of addition silicones, the hydrogen of one silicone polymer adds to the carbon double bond of the second silicone polymer and no byproduct is formed.

Problem 6

Polyisoprene is available in two forms, one highly elastic and the other brittle. Why?

Solution

The *cis*-form has a spatial structure, with the methyl and hydrogen on the same side of the carbon double bond, that allows less intramolecular attraction than the *trans*-form, with the methyl carbon and the hydrogen on opposite sides of the carbon double bond.

Problem 7

What is the function of (1) itaconic acid, (2) tartaric acid, and (3) maleic acid in glass ionomer restorations?

Solution

(1) Itaconic acid is used to make a copolymer with acrylic acid, which prevents the water solution from becoming more viscous on storage by interfacing with the inter polymer chain attraction.

(2) Tartaric acid, being difunctional, provides crosslinking and improved strength.

(3) The setting reaction, first with Ca^{+2} and then Al^{+3}, takes several days to reach completion; final finishing of the ionomer restoration should not take place at the first appointment. The addition of maleic acid, a stronger acid that is also difunctional, results in faster setting and allows finishing at the first appointment.

Problem 8

Why should epoxy die materials not be used with alginate impressions but may be used with addition-silicone impressions?

Solution

The epoxide group is very reactive; it will react with water in the alginate impression, thus interfering with the reaction with the amine. The addition-silicone impression is a highly cross-linked rubber and does not contain molecules that interfere with the epoxide-amine reaction.

BIBLIOGRAPHY

Allen JG, Dart EC, Jones E et al: Photochemistry. In Jones DG: *ICI Corporate Laboratory, Chemistry and Industry,* no 3, p 79, Feb 7, 1976, p 86.

Asmussen E: NMR—analysis of monomers in restorative resins, *Acta Odontol Scand* 33:129, 1975.

Braden M: Characterization of the setting process in dental polysulfide rubbers, *J Dent Res* 45:1065, 1966.

Braden M, Elliott JC: Characterization of the setting process of silicone dental rubbers, *J Dent Res* 45:1016, 1966.

Braden M, Causton B, Clarke RL: A polyether impression rubber, *J Dent Res* 51:889, 1972.

Brauer GM, Antonucci JM: Dental applications. In *Encyclopedia of polymer science and engineering,* vol 4, ed 2, New York, 1986, Wiley.

Cook WD: Rheological studies of the polymerization of elastomeric impression materials. I. Network structure of the set state, *J Biomed Mater Res* 16:315, 1982.

Cook WD: Rheological studies of the polymerization of elastomeric impression materials. II. Viscosity measurements, *J Biomed Mater Res* 16:331, 1982.

Cook WD: Rheological studies of the polymerization of elastomeric impression materials. III. Dynamic stress relaxation modulus, *J Biomed Mater Res* 16:345, 1982.

Cook WD: Photopolymerization kinetics of dimethacrylates using camphoroquinone/amine initiator system, *Polymer* 33:600, 1992.

Craig RG: Chemistry, composition, and properties of composite resins, *Dent Clin North Am* 25:219, 1981.

Craig RG: Photopolymerization of dental composite systems. In Leinfelder KF, Taylor DF, editors: *Posterior composites: Proceedings of the International Symposium on Posterior Composite Resins,* Chapel Hill, NC, 1984, Taylor DF.

Darr AN, Jacobsen PH: Conversion of dual cure luting cements, *J Oral Rehabil* 22:43, 1995.

Harashima I, Nomata T, Hirasawa T: Degree of conversion of dual cured composite luting agents, *Dent Mater* 10:8, 1991.

Higashi S, Yasuda S, Horie K et al: Studies on rubber base impression materials. Discussions on the setting mechanism of polysulfide rubber as the dental impression material, chiefly viewed from variations of viscosity and molecular weight, *J Nihon Univ Sch Dent* 13:33, 1971.

Joos RW, McCue EC, Nachtsheim HG: Polymerization kinetics of two paste resin composites, *Int Assoc Dent Res Program and Abstracts* 160, 1971.

Kitian RJ: The application of photochemistry to dental materials. In Gebelein CG, Koblitz FF, editors: *Polymer science and technology,* vol 14, Biochemical and dental applications of polymers, New York, 1981, Plenum.

McCabe JR, Wilson HJ: Addition curing silicone rubber impression materials, *Br Dent J* 145:17, 1978.

Phillips D: Polymer photochemistry. In Bryce-Smith D, editor: *Photochemistry,* vol 1, London, 1970, The Chemical Society, Burlington House.

Ruyter IE: Monomer systems and polymerization. In Vanherle G, Smith DC, eds: *International Symposium on Posterior Composite Resin Dental Restorative Materials,* Peter Szulc Publ 6:109, Netherlands, 1985.

Ullmann's Encyclopedia of Industrial Chemistry, ed 6, 2000, Chapter 6.1.2 Elastomers, electronic release.

Williams JR, Craig RG: Physical properties of addition silicones as a function of composition, *J Oral Rehabil* 15:639, 1988.

Chapter 8

Preventive Materials

Ever since fluoride was documented as a chemotherapeutic measure providing resistance in tooth enamel to in vivo demineralization and the development of active carious lesions, prevention has been the foundation for clinical restorative dentistry. The first major advance came with the administration of low-level fluorides into urban water supplies to ensure systemic ingestion during early life, when tooth structure is forming. Fluoride can also be provided systemically as a dietary supplement to inhibit caries where drinking water is not intentionally fluoridated. For patients who are at high risk for the development of caries in spite of systemic fluoride administration, various means of topical application have been developed to increase caries protection, such as toothpastes, mouthrinses, gels, and varnishes. For effective application of the fluoride ion and uptake by the enamel surface, a vehicle material must be used to carry the active ingredient in the right concentration and place it in apposition to the tooth surface. It must then be held there for a sufficient, yet clinically practical period, to allow a high absorption rate. The vehicle must be nontoxic and easily disposed from the oral cavity after the therapy is completed. With the combination of systemic and topical fluoride applications, the prevalence of smooth surface caries has greatly diminished over the past 50 years. Pits and fissures on the occlusal surfaces of posterior teeth are more resistant to fluoride uptake because the morphology of the surface structure is irregular and there is opportunity for food retention and caries initiation. These surfaces can be dealt with by applying an adhesive resin coating to obtund the irregularities and create a non-retentive smooth surface that is less likely to decay.

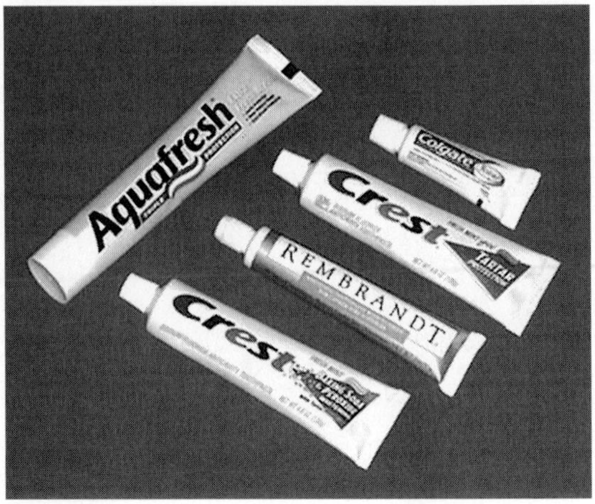

Fig. 8-1 A selection of toothpastes with a variety of active ingredients, including whitening agents, tartar control, total protection, and baking soda.

CHEMOTHERAPEUTIC AGENTS

TOOTHPASTE

The major function of a toothpaste (Fig. 8-1) is to enhance cleaning of the exposed tooth surfaces and removal of pellicle, plaque, and debris left from salivary deposits and the mastication of food. As a secondary function, toothpaste can be used as a carrier for fluorides, detergents, abrasives, and whitening agents to improve the quality and esthetics of erupted teeth. The use of toothpaste is a continually growing, vital part of home health care throughout the world, resulting in a multi-billion dollar industry. A practicing dentist should have a sound knowledge of the ingredients in most toothpastes and the therapeutic value, if any, in recommending them to patients for general and specific needs.

The general composition of most toothpastes includes the following:

- *Colloidal binding agent.* This agent acts as a carrier for the more active ingredients. Sodium alginate or methylcellulose will thicken the vehicle and prevent separation of the components in the tube during storage.
- *Humectants.* An example is glycerin, which is used to stabilize the composition and reduce water loss by evaporation.
- *Preservatives.* Preservatives are used to inhibit bacterial growth within the material.

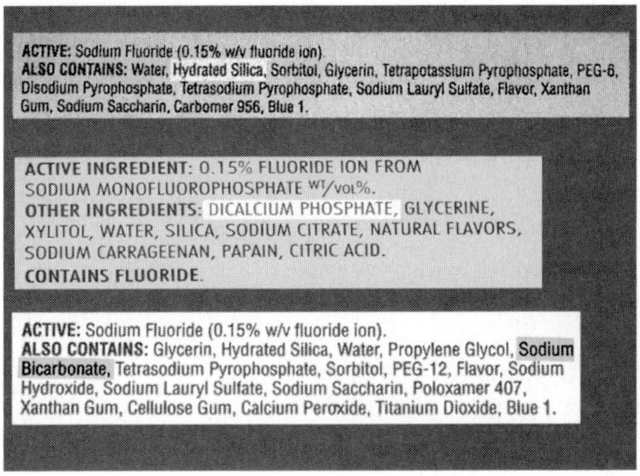

ACTIVE: Sodium Fluoride (0.15% w/v fluoride ion).
ALSO CONTAINS: Water, Hydrated Silica, Sorbitol, Glycerin, Tetrapotassium Pyrophosphate, PEG-6, Disodium Pyrophosphate, Tetrasodium Pyrophosphate, Sodium Lauryl Sulfate, Flavor, Xanthan Gum, Sodium Saccharin, Carbomer 956, Blue 1.
ACTIVE INGREDIENT: 0.15% FLUORIDE ION FROM SODIUM MONOFLUOROPHOSPHATE WT/VOL%.
OTHER INGREDIENTS: DICALCIUM PHOSPHATE, GLYCERINE, XYLITOL, WATER, SILICA, SODIUM CITRATE, NATURAL FLAVORS, SODIUM CARRAGEENAN, PAPAIN, CITRIC ACID.
CONTAINS FLUORIDE.
ACTIVE: Sodium Fluoride (0.15% w/v fluoride ion).
ALSO CONTAINS: Glycerin, Hydrated Silica, Water, Propylene Glycol, Sodium Bicarbonate, Tetrasodium Pyrophosphate, Sorbitol, PEG-12, Flavor, Sodium Hydroxide, Sodium Lauryl Sulfate, Sodium Saccharin, Poloxamer 407, Xanthan Gum, Cellulose Gum, Calcium Peroxide, Titanium Dioxide, Blue 1.

Fig. 8-2 A variety of toothpaste labels highlighting the abrasive material in each paste; *(top)* hydrated silica, *(center)* dicalcium phosphate, *(bottom)* sodium bicarbonate.

- *Flavoring agents*. Peppermint, wintergreen, and cinnamon are added to enhance consumer appeal and to combat oral malodors.
- *Abrasives*. Abrasives are incorporated into all pastes to aid in the removal of heavy plaque, adhered stains, and calculus deposits. Calcium pyrophosphate, dicalcium phosphate, calcium carbonate, hydrated silica, and sodium bicarbonate are used in varying amounts to obtain this effect (Fig. 8-2).
- *Detergents*. An example is sodium lauryl sulfate, which is used to reduce surface tension and enhance the removal of debris from the tooth surface.
- *Therapeutic agents*. Therapeutic agents are added to most toothpastes marketed in North America and Europe. The use of stannous fluorides has been demonstrated effective in the uptake of the fluoride ion and improved resistance of fluorapatite to acid demineralization in the initiation of carious lesions.
- *Other chemicals*. Minor miscellaneous ingredients are included to reduce tube corrosion, stabilize viscosity, and provide pleasing coloration. Minor amounts of peroxides are included in some pastes, with marketing claims that they will remove innate discolorations and improve esthetics.

From a materials standpoint, abrasivity is one of the most important characteristics of toothpaste. Abrasion is a very important functional property that can have widespread destructive effects in the oral environment. Toothbrushing introduces three-body abrasion in areas of the mouth that are not normally subject to that type of stress. The toothbrush bristle is one factor, as it is moved across the softer dentin surface of the root in teeth with gingival recession, and the paste becomes the third body, with its abrasive particles interposed.

Abrasivity of toothpaste has been measured with two different methods. One method is to use a radioactive surface as the substrate and to measure the loss of substance after brushing by measuring radioactivity in the abraded material. The second method uses a profilometer to measure the substrate before and after a brushing experiment; the loss of contour is measured and compared. Studies have generally confirmed that the radiotracer methods are similar and more reliable. The ADA, British Standards Institute, and ISO have standardized tests for abrasivity that differ slightly in methodology. The factors that have been associated with increased abrasion are larger particle sizes, more-irregular particle shapes, harder mineral composition of the particles, amount of particles in a given volume of the paste, and toothbrush bristle stiffness. Fig. 8-3 illustrates the various abrasive particle sizes and shapes incorporated into common commercial toothpastes.

Chemical agents have been placed in various toothpastes to control tartar formation, reduce caries risk, and whiten tooth surfaces. A new group of pastes have been marketed in recent years to control calculus deposition (Fig. 8-4). These pastes incorporate tetrasodium or tetrapotassium pyrophosphates, which act as inhibitors to hydroxyapatite crystal growth. Their efficacy

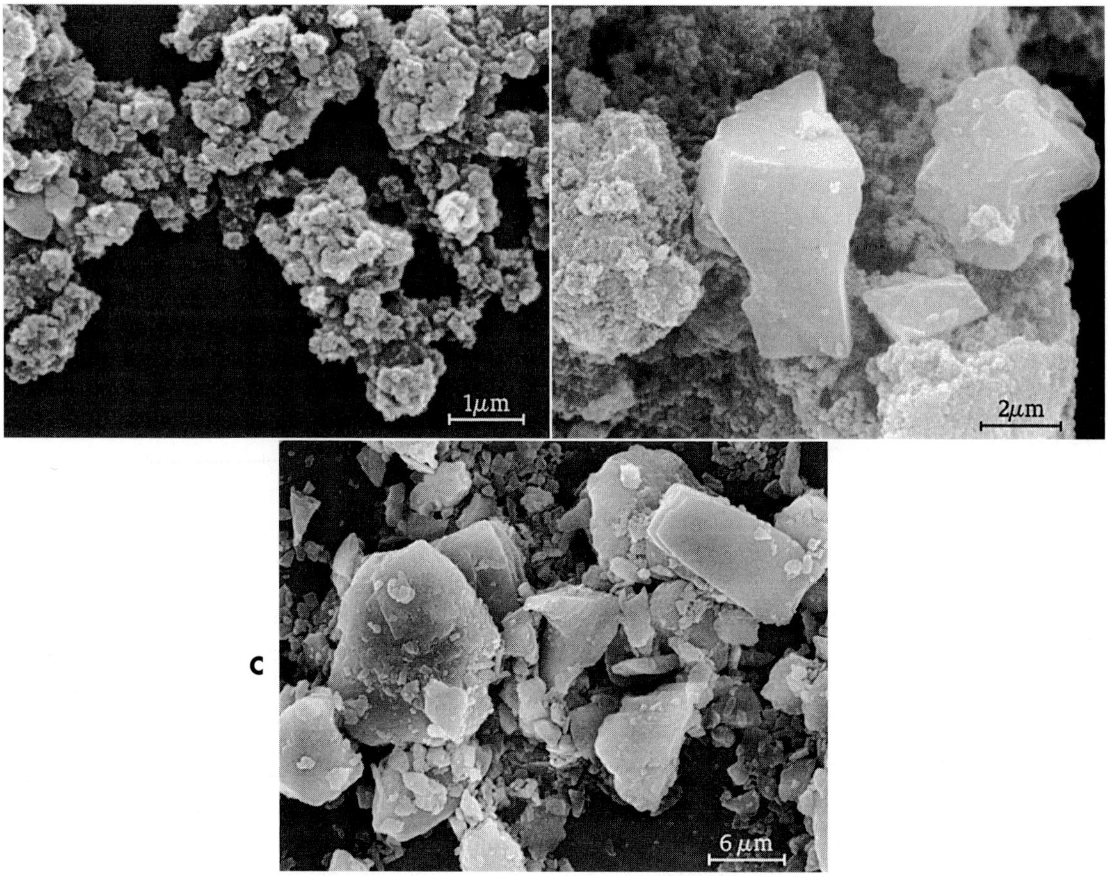
A
1μm
B
2μm
C
6 μm

Fig. 8-3 Scanning electron micrographs of abrasive particles taken from commercial toothpastes. **A,** hydrated silica, **B,** calcium carbonate, **C,** dicalcium phosphate.

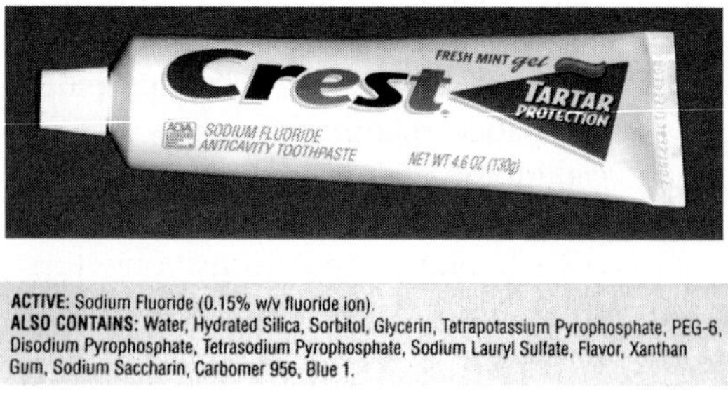
Crest
FRESH MINT gel
TARTAR PROTECTION
SODIUM FLUORIDE ANTICAVITY TOOTHPASTE
NET WT 4.6 OZ (130g)
ACTIVE: Sodium Fluoride (0.15% w/v fluoride ion).
ALSO CONTAINS: Water, Hydrated Silica, Sorbitol, Glycerin, Tetrapotassium Pyrophosphate, PEG-6, Disodium Pyrophosphate, Tetrasodium Pyrophosphate, Sodium Lauryl Sulfate, Flavor, Xanthan Gum, Sodium Saccharin, Carbomer 956, Blue 1.

Fig. 8-4 A typical anti-tartar toothpaste with contents noted on the label, including several pyrophosphates.

in reducing calculus formation and the control of periodontal problems is well documented, but they do have some side effects that prohibit their use in certain individuals. They create a slightly more alkaline environment as part of the active prevention mechanism, and this can lead to soft-tissue sensitivity reactions such as burning sensations, tissue sloughing, erythema, ulceration, or migratory glossitis. Because the pyrophosphates have a bitter taste, such pastes also have an increased concentration of flavoring agents and detergents, both of which can increase the

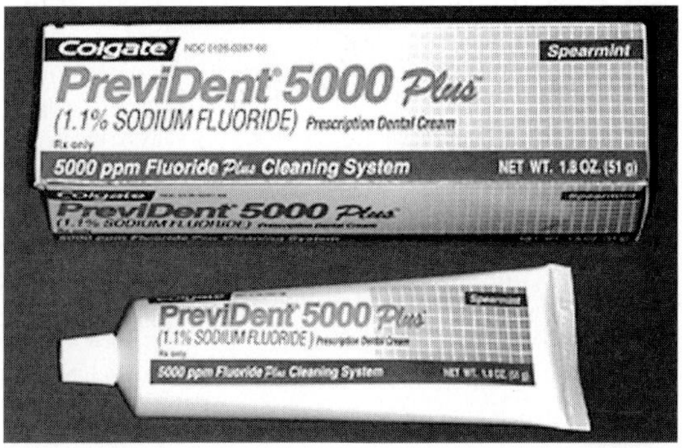

Fig. 8-5 A high–fluoride content toothpaste (1.1%) currently under prescription drug regulation.

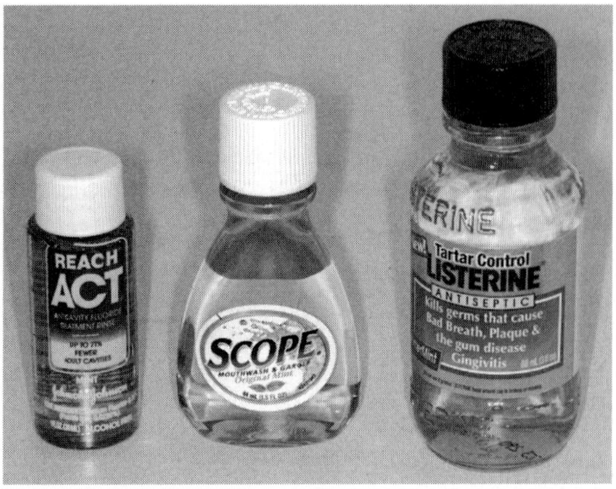

Fig. 8-6 A variety of typical commercial mouthwashes.

possibility of an adverse tissue response. The concentrations of fluoride in toothpastes range from 0.025% to 0.15%, with great variations among brands. The effectiveness of fluoride-containing toothpastes in preventing caries is highly dependent on fluoride concentration. Prescription pastes are also available with concentrations around 0.5% for use in professionally managed programs for patients at high risk for caries (Fig. 8-5). Bleaching toothpastes based on low-level peroxide formulations are also available to whiten teeth for esthetic purposes. They are effective in whitening teeth when used daily.

MOUTHWASH

Another vehicle for delivering active agents with desirable effects to the surfaces of the teeth and gingiva is mouthwash. Mouthwash is a liquid solution that is applied as a rinse on a regular basis to enhance oral health, esthetics, and breath freshness (Fig. 8-6). Mouthwashes are most effective when applied in the morning or the evening following mechanical cleansing of the tooth surfaces with a brush and toothpaste. The usual purpose is to deliver an active ingredient to the clean surface of teeth or tissues in a manner that will produce the greatest treatment effect.

Mouthwashes are composed of three main ingredients. An active agent is selected for a specific health care benefit, such as anticaries activity, antimicrobial effect, fluoride delivery, or reduction of plaque adhesion. The active agent is then delivered in a solution of water and/or alcohol. Alcohol is used to dissolve some active ingredients, enhance flavor, and act as a preservative to prolong shelf life. Surfactants are also added to most mouthwashes to help remove debris from the teeth and dissolve other ingredients. Surfactants can be nonionic block copolymers, anionic chemicals like sodium lauryl sulfate, or cetyl pyridinium chloride, which is cationic with antibacterial properties. Flavoring agents added for breath freshening include eucalyptol, menthol, thymol, and methyl salicylate. In formulating a mouthwash, it is extremely critical to guard against the use of additives that diminish the main effect of the active ingredient.

Two factors that should be considered in evaluating a mouthwash are its acidity and the ethanol content of the final solution. In measuring 12 proprietary mouthwashes in the United Kingdom, most were acidic, ranging from a pH of 3.4 to 6.6, one was almost neutral (6.9), and one was basic (8.3). For the same mouthwashes, the ethanol content ranged from a high of 27% to 0%, with little correlation between acidity and

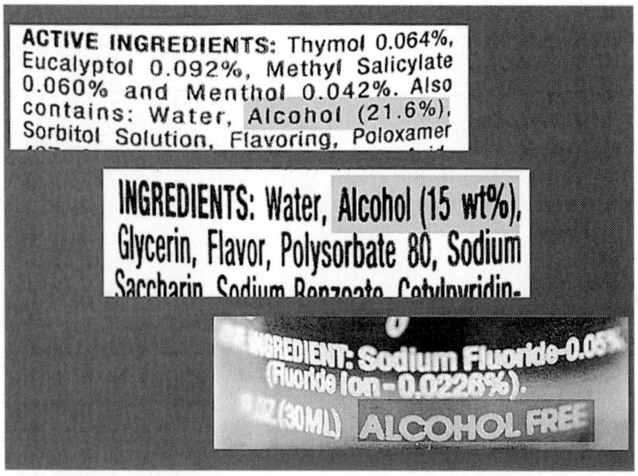

Fig. 8-7 Labels for the mouthwashes shown in Fig. 8-6, highlighting the alcohol content of each material: Listerine *(top)*, 21.6%; Scope *(center)*, 15%; ACT *(bottom)*, 0%.

ethanol content. In evaluating a similar group of rinses on the U.S. market, the ethanol content showed a similar range from 27% to 0% (Fig. 8-7). To compare with alcoholic beverages, beer contains about 4% and wine about 11% ethanol. Although these mouthwashes are not ingested as alcoholic beverages are, there are topical effects to be avoided by using solutions with such high ethanol content.

The two main active ingredients in mouthwashes with a positive treatment effect are chlorhexidine and fluoride. Chlorhexidine is a strong antibacterial agent that is used primarily in patients with soft-tissue or gum infections, such as gingivitis or pericoronitis (Fig. 8-8). Acceptable concentrations are between 0.1% and 0.2%. Chlorhexidine gluconate has been shown to reduce the aerosol associated with dental operations when it is used as a preoperative rinse. It is also effective in reducing soft-tissue inflammation associated with periodontal disease, but patient acceptance is compromised by a rather bitter taste and a tendency to stain tooth surfaces.

The anticaries effect of fluoride mouthwashes are also well documented. It would appear to result from a two-stage reaction. Initially, a layer of calcium fluoride–like material is deposited on the surfaces of exposed teeth. In time, this surface layer is absorbed and the underlying mineral structure is converted from hydroxyapatite to

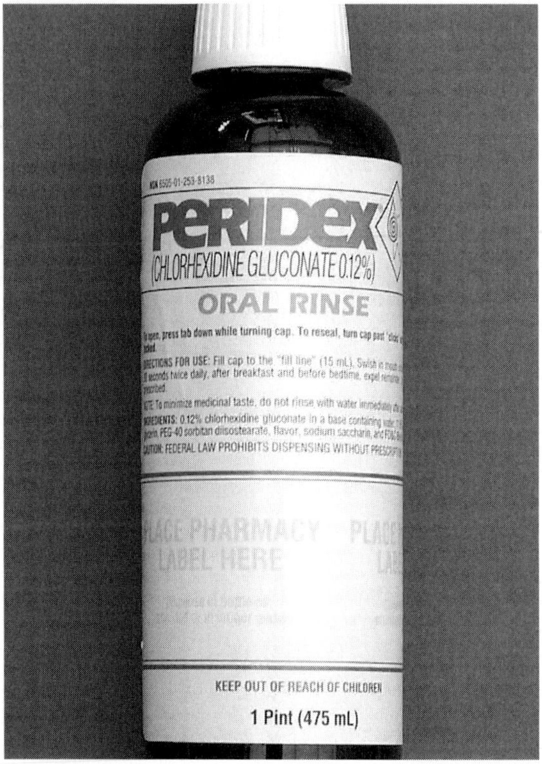

Fig. 8-8 A standard solution of chlorhexidene antibacterial oral rinse (Peridex).

fluorapatite, which is harder and more resistant to demineralization. The fluoride uptake was found to be dependent on concentration, with 0.2% NaF having a greater uptake than 0.05%. Uptake was also time dependent, with longer exposure times producing a greater treatment effect.

Mouthwashes can also have an effect upon restorative materials. Those with a higher ethanol content can produce softening of the surfaces of resin materials, such as resin composites, compomers, and sealants. Although more significant in light-cured resin materials, the softening effect, as demonstrated by an increased water sorption rate, was also found in laboratory-processed composites. A residual staining effect was also found using one popular rinsing material that also contained eugenol. The staining effect of chlorhexidine is dependent on concentration, so it is imperative to find an effective mid-range

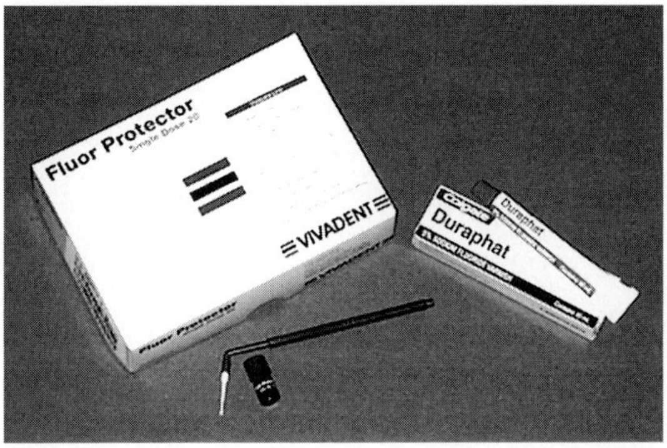

Fig. 8-9 Fluoride-containing cavity varnishes for professional application, supplied in a tube (Duraphat) or as a solution in unit doses (Fluor Protector).

concentration that will produce only minimal staining.

There is also a question about toxicity or biocompatibility in prescribing the routine use of mouthwashes, particularly those with a high ethanol content. Carcinogenic risks seem to go up with increased duration of exposure and frequency of use. The risk factor is similar to that resulting from increased ingestion of alcoholic beverages. Although there are mixed results among the various clinical studies, the association seems to be present only when the ethanol content of the rinse is high and the use is excessive.

FLUORIDE VARNISHES

Fluoride-containing varnishes provide an additional means of delivering fluoride topically to the surfaces of teeth in patients at risk for caries. Research has established their routine use in Europe for this purpose; however, the FDA has refused to approve them as anticariogenic agents. They are approved as cavity varnishes to be used under restorations and along the root surfaces of sensitive teeth with gingival recession. There are three products used routinely for topical application, usually after a prophylaxis. Two of these products contain 5% sodium fluoride (2.26% F^- or 22,600 ppm) and one contains 1% difluorsilane (0.1% F^- or 1,000 ppm) (Fig. 8-9). The fluoride is dissolved in an organic solvent that evaporates when applied or sets when exposed to moisture, leaving a thin film of material covering all exposed tooth surfaces. The mechanism of action for a fluoride varnish is similar to that described for a fluoride mouthwash; calcium fluoride is deposited on the tooth surface and later converted through a remineralization reaction to fluorapatite.

The one advantage of the varnish mode of application is the extended time of exposure for the active fluoride ingredient against the tooth surface. Instead of seconds, as with a mouthwash, it may be hours before a varnish wears off. Clinical trials have documented the efficacy of varnish in treating young children at risk for caries, with reductions reported as high as 70%. Another potential use for this type of material is in the prevention of root caries in an older population, which has increasing risk as aging occurs. Semiannual application of fluoride varnishes seems to provide optimum efficacy. The only negative aspect of using cavity varnishes is a slightly bitter taste, which is transient, and tooth discoloration, which lasts less than 24 hours. More research is necessary to fully document the value of using these materials in specific clinical situations with moderate to high caries risk.

PIT AND FISSURE SEALANTS

Pits and fissures in the occlusal surfaces of permanent teeth are particularly susceptible to decay, and fluoride treatments have been least effective in preventing caries in these areas. The susceptibility of occlusal pits and fissures to caries is related to the physical size and morphology of the individual pit or fissure, which can provide shelter for organisms and obstruct oral hygiene procedures. Cross-sectional views of typical fissure morphology, varying from a wide V shape to a bottleneck shape, are shown in Fig. 8-10.

A technique termed *occlusal sealing* was introduced in 1965. This procedure involved the use of methyl-2-cyanoacrylate, which was mixed with poly(methyl methacrylate) and inorganic powder and then placed in the pits and fissures. The cyanoacrylate polymerized on exposure to

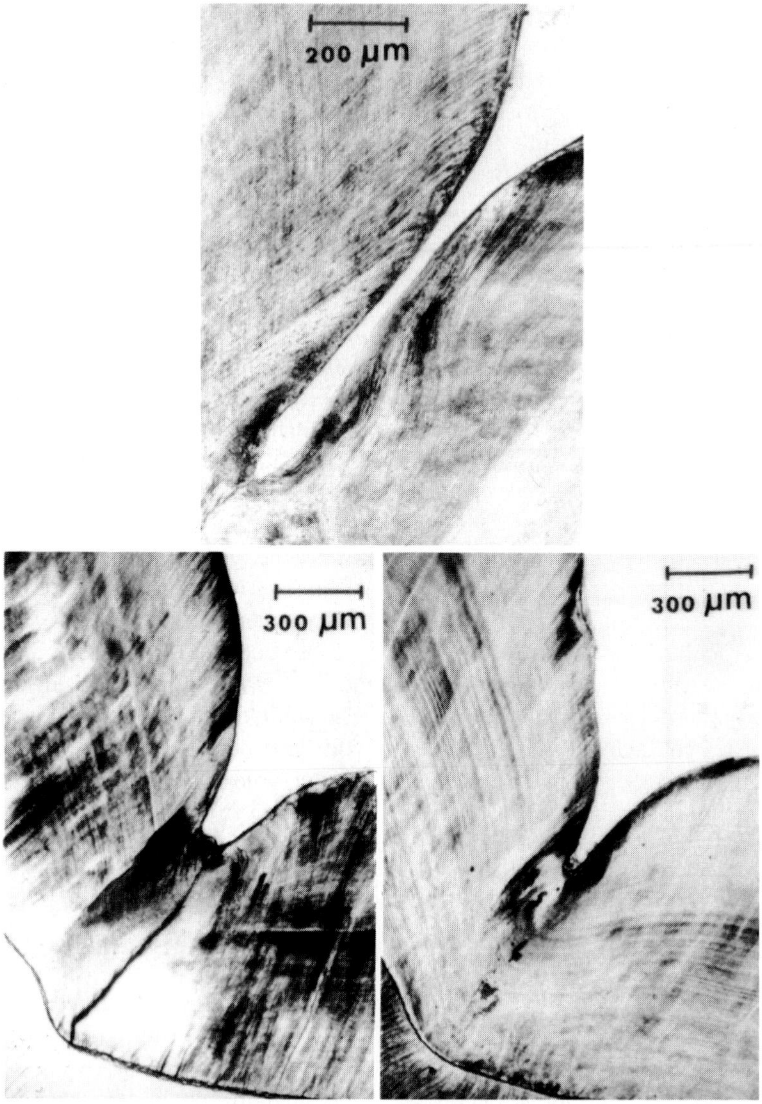

Fig. 8-10 Sections of teeth illustrating shapes of fissures.
(From Gwinnett AJ: *J Am Soc Prevent Dent* 3:21, 1973.)

moisture. Since that time, sealant systems have included the Bis-GMA resins (polymerized either by chemical means or by visible light), a polyurethane sealant containing inorganic fluoride compounds, and glass ionomers. The use of sealant materials that exhibit a slow release of the fluoride ion has been advocated as a way to maintain a high surface concentration of fluoride for a longer period of time than is possible with the usual topical gel treatments.

RESIN SEALANTS

The most common sealants are based on Bis-GMA resin and are light cured, although some self-cured products are still available. The full name for Bis-GMA is 2,2-bis[4(2-hydroxy-3-methacryloyloxy-propyloxy)-phenyl] propane. The chemistry of Bis-GMA sealants is the same as that described for composites in Chapters 7 and 9. The principal difference is that the Bis-GMA sealants must be much more fluid to penetrate into the pits, fissures, and etched areas produced on the enamel, which provide for retention of the sealant. Three parts of the viscous Bis-GMA are mixed with one part of diluent, such as methyl methacrylate or triethylene glycol dimethacrylate, to obtain a reasonably low-viscosity sealant. An alternative but similar oligomer base is urethane dimethacrylate; some materials are formulated from a combination of the two base resins. To provide stiffness to the material and improve wear resistance, filler particles of fumed silica or silanated inorganic glasses can be added to form low-viscosity composites.

Light-Cured Sealants Today, most sealants are light cured, activated by a diketone and an aliphatic amine. The complete reactions for composites are given in Chapter 7. Bis-GMA–light-cured sealant is supplied in a light-tight container and should be usable for a 12-month period. The sealant is applied to the pit and fissure area with an appropriate applicator and, when polymerization is desired, the end of the light source is held 1 to 2 mm from the surface and the sealant is exposed to light for 20 seconds. Sealants are applied in such thin sections that depth of cure should be adequate with minimal exposure times, even for opaque materials. The advantage in using a light-cured sealant is that the working time can be completely controlled by the operator and integrated with patient behavior. This control is particularly valuable when sealant is applied to very young patients or when cooperation is a problem.

Self-Cured Sealants The first generation of chemically-initiated Bis-GMA sealants was polymerized by an organic amine accelerator; commercial self-cured sealants are still available. The material is supplied as a two-component system: one component contains Bis-GMA resin and benzoyl peroxide initiator, and the other contains Bis-GMA resin with 5% organic amine accelerator. The two components are dispensed as viscous drops onto a suitable mixing surface (e.g., dappen dish, paper pad), and, after adequate mixing, they are applied directly to the tooth surface. The polymerization is an addition reaction in response to the formation of radicals, although somewhat less cross-linked than those of the composite restorative materials. The reaction is exothermic, but the clinical effect is minimal because the material is placed in limited bulk. The rate of reaction for all materials is sensitive to temperature, and the material sets more quickly in the mouth (typically 3 to 5 minutes) than on the mixing surface. Because quantities are usually small, use caution to include all material in the mixing and use a gentle motion to minimize air incorporation. Air inclusions during mixing and insertion can be manifested clinically as surface voids, which can discolor and retain plaque. To ensure optimum penetration, apply the self-cured sealant quickly after mixing. Manipulation late in the setting reaction can disrupt the polymerization and induce bond failure.

Air Inhibition of Polymerization During polymerization there is a surface layer of air inhibition that varies in depth with different commercial products. Sufficient material must be applied to completely coat all pits and fissures with a layer thick enough to ensure complete polymerization after removal of the tacky surface layer. This chemically active surface layer of unpolymerized resin is considered a source of potential biotoxicity. One of the components in the raw resin reaction is Bisphenol A (BPA), which has recently been related to estrogenic activity because of the similarity of its chemical structure to estrogen. The measurement of BPA in saliva is time dependent and material specific. For some materials, it has been detected in small quantities immediately after sealant placement but not after 1 or 24 hours post-placement. To remove this layer as soon as possible after curing, use an abrasive slurry of pumice, applied on a cotton pellet or with a prophylaxis cup in a rotary handpiece; this method is more effective than wiping or rinsing procedures. Premature contamination with moisture during insertion and the early application of biting forces can disrupt the setting and affect its strength and clinical durability.

Properties of Sealants Reports of the physical properties of sealants have been scarce because specimen preparation with such low-viscosity materials is difficult. The relationship between properties and clinical service is even more speculative than for most restorative materials. Typical properties obtained for an unfilled sealant and a filled sealant are given in Table 8-1. By adding about 40% by weight of finely divided filler particles, as in the composite systems, all properties except tensile strength show improvement. The specimens are usually tested for tensile failure by the diametral method, and the high deformation before fracture affects the reliability of the data. The modulus of elasticity shows the most dramatic improvement, and the increased rigidity makes the filled material less subject to deflection under occlusal stress. Filler is also added with the hope of improving wear resistance and making the material more visible on clinical inspection (Fig. 8-11).

TABLE 8-1 Physical Properties of Bis-GMA Resin Sealants

Property	Unfilled Amine-Accelerated	Filled Amine-Accelerated
Compressive strength (MPa)	130	170
Tensile strength (MPa)	24	31
Modulus of elasticity (GPa)	2.1	5.2
Hardness, Knoop (kg/mm^2)	20	25
Water sorption at 7 days (mg/cm^2)	2.0	1.3

Penetration studies on closed capillary tubes, which are somewhat analogous to pits and fissures, have indicated that a sealant will adapt more closely to the enamel surface if it possesses a high coefficient of penetration. Optimal penetration will occur when the sealant has a high surface tension, good wetting, and a low viscosity, thus permitting it to flow readily along the enamel surface. The surface wettability is demonstrated by the contact angle of a drop of liquid on the enamel surface. A drop that spreads readily has a low contact angle and is indicative of a highly wetted surface that is most conducive to a strong bond. Polymer tags that form in direct apposition to the surface irregularities created by acid etching are responsible for the mechanical bond that retains the sealant to enamel. Functional durability of the sealant bond can be related to stresses induced by initial polymer shrinkage, thermal cycling, deflection under occlusal forces, water sorption, and abrasion, with total failure manifested by the clinical loss of material.

Sealant materials have a variety of features that must be selected carefully by the health care provider. As previously stated, there are filled sealants that behave more like composite resins, and unfilled materials that are pure resins. Most current materials are light cured rather than self-cured because of the ease and speed of application. Tooth-colored or clear resins are available that are very natural looking on the tooth surface, but they are also available in opaque or tinted materials to make the recall examination process easier (Fig. 8-12). An increasing number of sealants are marketed as vehicles for the slow release of fluoride, which has been documented in vitro in water solutions for a number of products. The release is highest in the first 24 hours after placement and then tapers to a low maintenance level, which may or may not be sufficient to provide extended clinical protection against caries.

Clinical Studies Many clinical studies have been reported using the Bis-GMA systems. In earlier studies on effectiveness of treatment with sealant in newly erupting teeth, a light-cured sealant demonstrated a retention rate of

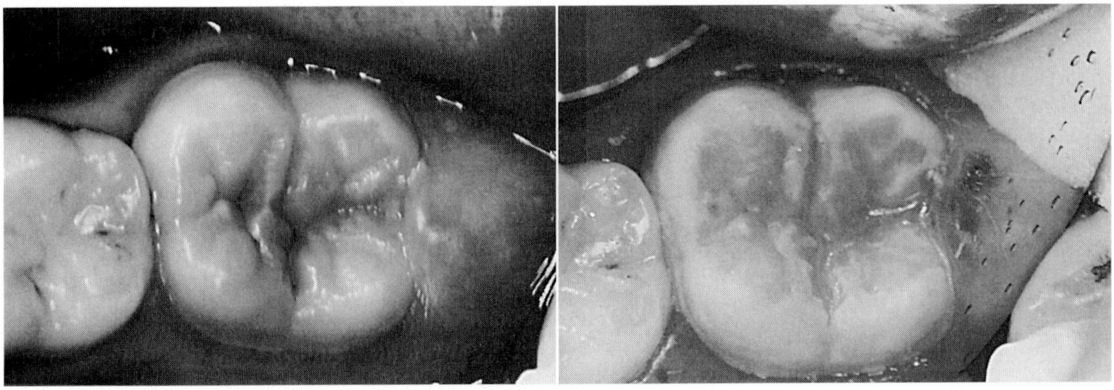

Fig. 8-11 A typical molar with stained fissures and no diagnosable caries. **A,** Before sealing, and **B,** after sealing with a natural-colored sealant material.

42% and an effectiveness of 35% in caries reduction after 5 years. In a similar study, a filled resin sealant showed a retention rate of 53% and a clinical effectiveness of 54% after 4 years. Results involving a quicker-setting unfilled resin sealant with very good penetration showed a retention rate of 80% and an effectiveness of 69% after 3 years. The longest published study on sealant effectiveness is a 15-year evaluation of a self-cured unfilled material, which showed 27.6% complete retention and 35.4% partial retention.

In pairwise comparisons, the treated first molars had 31.3 dfs and the untreated controls had 82.8 dfs. In a more current 4-year study comparing a fluoride-releasing sealant with one that did not have fluoride, retention rates were 91% for the fluoride material (77% complete and 14% partial) and 95% for the non-fluoride sealant (89% complete and 6% partial). Although the retention was somewhat lower in the fluoride-containing sealant, the caries incidence for both groups was identical (10%). In a study conducted in private practice, the 2-year retention rates for two newer fluoride-containing resins were greater than 90%, and no caries was detected on the test teeth. In a continuing study with retreatment of all defective sealant surfaces at 6-month recalls, the teeth were maintained caries free for a 5-year period. The retreatment rate

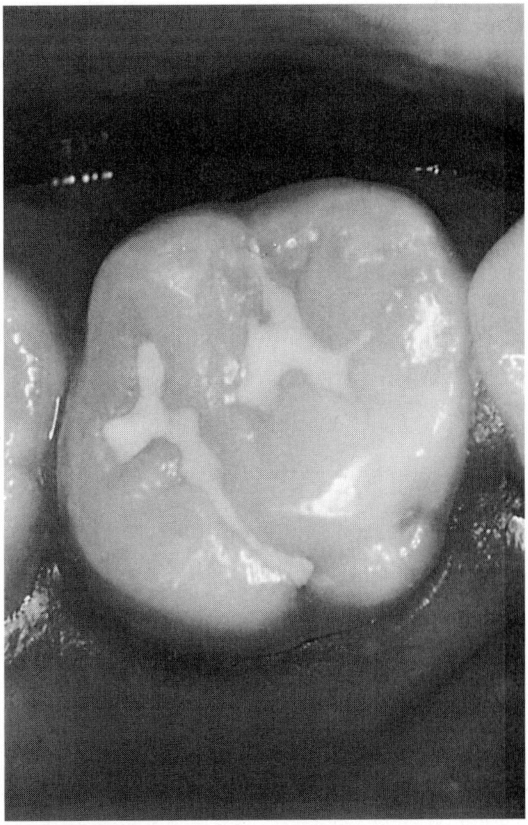

Fig. 8-12 A maxillary molar tooth with opaque sealant that has been in place for five years.

was highest (18%) at 6 months, and then diminished as time progressed, but at each recall period at least two teeth (about 4%) required reapplication.

Almost all studies show a direct correlation between sealant retention and caries protection. Therefore it is important to develop materials that are retentive to enamel, resistant against occlusal wear, and easily applied with minimal opportunities for surface contamination. Current evidence indicates that sealants are most effective on occlusal surfaces where pits and fissures are well defined and retentive to food and in patients with a demonstrated risk for pit and fissure caries.

Manipulation of Sealants The handling characteristics of a sealant are dependent on the composition of the material and the nature of the surface to which it is applied. Optimal preparation of both aspects will lead to close adaptation of the sealant to the tooth enamel, a strong seal against the ingress of oral fluids and debris, and long-term material retention.

Enamel Surface Preparation The penetration of any of the sealants to the bottom of the pit is important. The wettability of the enamel by the sealant is improved by etching, and some advocate pretreatment with silanes in a volatile solvent. The problem of filling the fissure is real; air is often trapped in the bottom of the fissure, or the accumulation of debris at the base of the fissure prevents it from being completely filled, as shown in Fig. 8-13. Control of the viscosity of the sealant is important to obtain optimum results. The viscosity determines the penetration of resin into the etched areas of enamel to provide adequate retention of the sealant. Penetration of sealant, forming tags, to a depth of 25 to 50 μm is shown in Fig. 8-14.

Etch the pit and fissure surface for a specified time (15 to 30 seconds is adequate for enamel with a normal mineral and fluoride content) with a solution or a gel of 35% to 40% phosphoric acid. Flush the acid thoroughly with water, and dry the area with warm air. Inadequate rinsing permits phosphate salts to remain on the surface as a contaminant, interfering with bond formation. Avoid rubbing the etched surface during etching and drying because the roughness developed can easily be destroyed. Isolation of the site is imperative throughout the procedure to achieve optimum tag formation and clinical success. If salivary contamination occurs during the treatment, rinse and dry the surface and repeat the acid etching. On clinical inspection, acid-etched enamel should appear white and dull with an obviously rough texture. If this appearance is not uniform, perform an additional 30 seconds of etching. The etched area should extend be-

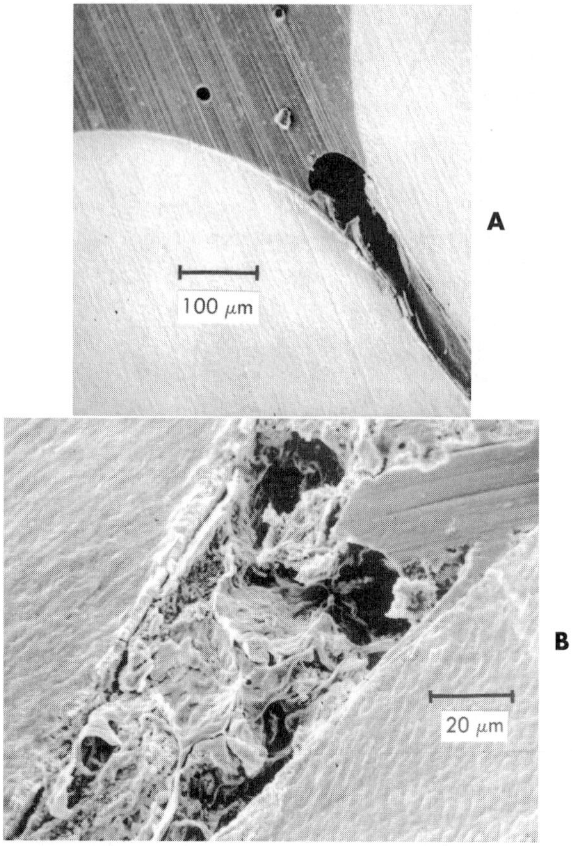

Fig. 8-13 Section showing a fissure incompletely filled with sealant as a result of air, **A**, and debris, **B.** (From Gwinnett AJ: *J Am Soc Prevent Dent* 3:21, 1973.)

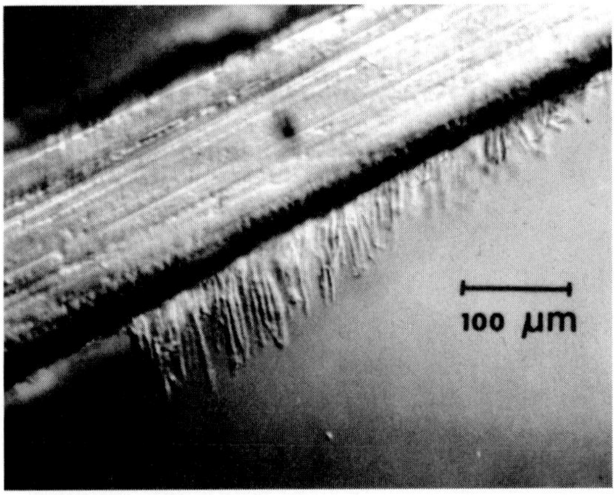

Fig. 8-14 Penetration of sealant into etched enamel; these tags are responsible for the bonding to enamel. (From Gwinnett AJ: *J Am Soc Prevent Dent* 3:21, 1973.)

yond the anticipated area for sealant application to secure optimum bonding along the margin and reduce the potential for early leakage. Clinical studies have shown that the use of a light-cured bonding agent (see Chapter 10) against the freshly etched enamel before placing the sealant will improve retention, especially when there appears to be minor moisture or salivary contamination.

Sealant Application Depending on its viscosity and setting time, the sealant may best be applied with a thin brush, a ball applicator, or a syringe. Take care to avoid the buildup of excess material that could interfere with developing occlusion, but apply sufficient material to completely cover all exposed pits and provide a smooth transition along the inclines of the enamel cusps. Over-working of even the light-cured sealants on the tooth surface during application can introduce air voids that appear later as surface defects.

Wipe away the air-inhibited surface layer immediately after curing and inspect the coating carefully for voids or areas of incomplete coverage. Cover defects at this time by repeating the entire reapplication procedure, including the acid etch, and applying fresh sealant only to those areas with insufficient coverage. After the sealant is applied and fully cured, check and adjust the occlusion, if necessary, to eliminate functional prematurities that can result in hypersensitivity.

Glass Ionomer Sealants Because of their demonstrated ability to release fluoride and provide some caries protection on tooth surfaces at risk, glass ionomers have been suggested and tested for their ability to function as a fissure sealant. Glass ionomers are generally more viscous, and it is difficult to gain penetration to the depth of a fissure. Their lack of penetration also makes it difficult to obtain mechanical retention to the enamel surface to the same degree as Bis-GMA resins. They are also more brittle and less resistant to occlusal wear. Clinical studies using various formulations of glass ionomers have shown significantly lower retention rates, but greater fluoride deposition in the enamel surfaces.

In areas where high-risk children cannot afford dental care, a conservative holding technique has been advocated to seal remaining caries in a fluoride-rich environment and establish some degree of remineralization. Atraumatic restorative treatments involve opening a lesion, removing soft surface decay, and filling or sealing the surface with high-filled glass ionomer with a fast setting time. Future studies in this area may produce a new generation of sealant materials noted for their fluoride deposition rather than their mechanical obturation.

FLOWABLE COMPOSITES

Low-viscosity, high-flow composites marketed as flowable composites are advocated for a wide variety of applications, such as preventive resin restorations, cavity liners, restoration repairs, and cervical restorations. These applications are not well supported with data, but their clinical use is widespread. The properties of flowable composites are described in Chapter 9.

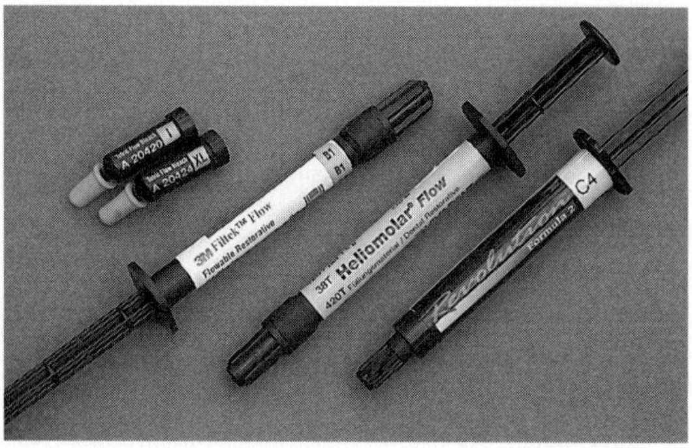

Fig. 8-15 A selection of flowable composite resins in syringe and compule delivery systems.

MANIPULATION

Flowable composites are usually packaged in syringes or in compules (Fig. 8-15). These can be used for direct application to the cavity or the tooth surface; however, it is easy to exert a little pressure on the syringe and express an excessive amount of material. These materials can also be deposited from the syringe to a paper pad surface and then applied to the tooth using a ball-tipped applicator or a microbrush. In dispensing the material, care must be exercised to avoid introducing air bubbles, which eventually become surface voids. Depth of cure after light activation should be slightly better than that of highly filled composites.

Because the physical properties of flowable composites are lower than the restorative composites, it is generally considered that these materials should be reserved for nonfunctional tooth surface restorations. However, they provide an advantage when used as the sealant portion of a preventive resin restoration. A bonding agent should be applied to the etched enamel and light cured to provide the basic adhesion for retention. The flowable composite can then be used to cover the restored area and the exposed pits and fissures on the occlusal surface of molars and premolars. The high flow characteristics also work well in restoring minimal cavity preparations involving fissures that are cleaned or prepared with air abrasion techniques (Fig. 8-16). Because they have a higher filler content than most resin sealants, flowable composites should have better wear resistance in this clinical situation. A current clinical study has verified good retention and caries resistance after 24 months. Long-term clinical efficacy of preventive resin restoration using a flowable composite is yet to be established.

GLASS IONOMERS

The final materials that need to be considered for caries prevention are glass ionomers and hybrid ionomers (resin-modified glass ionomers). Because of their documented slow release of fluoride, glass ionomers are used in cervical and Class 5 restorations in adults where esthetics is not critical. They are specifically recommended for patients with high caries risk (Table 8-2).

COMPOSITION AND REACTION

Glass ionomers are supplied as powders of various shades and a liquid. The powder is an ion-leachable aluminosilicate glass, and the liquid is a water solution of polymers and copolymers of acrylic acid. The material sets as a result of the metallic salt bridges between the Al^{+++} and Ca^{++} ions leached from the glass and the acid groups on the polymers. The reaction goes to completion slowly, with the formation of a crosslinked gel matrix in the initial set and an aluminum ion exchange strengthening the crosslinking in the final set. A chelation effect takes place with the calcium on the exposed tooth surface, creating an adhesive bond. The surfaces of new restorations should be protected from saliva during the initial set with a heavy varnish or light-cured bonding agent.

PROPERTIES

The handling characteristics and physical properties of glass ionomers can be varied to suit various clinical applications by altering the glass composition and or polyacid formulation. The properties of glass ionomers are compared qual-

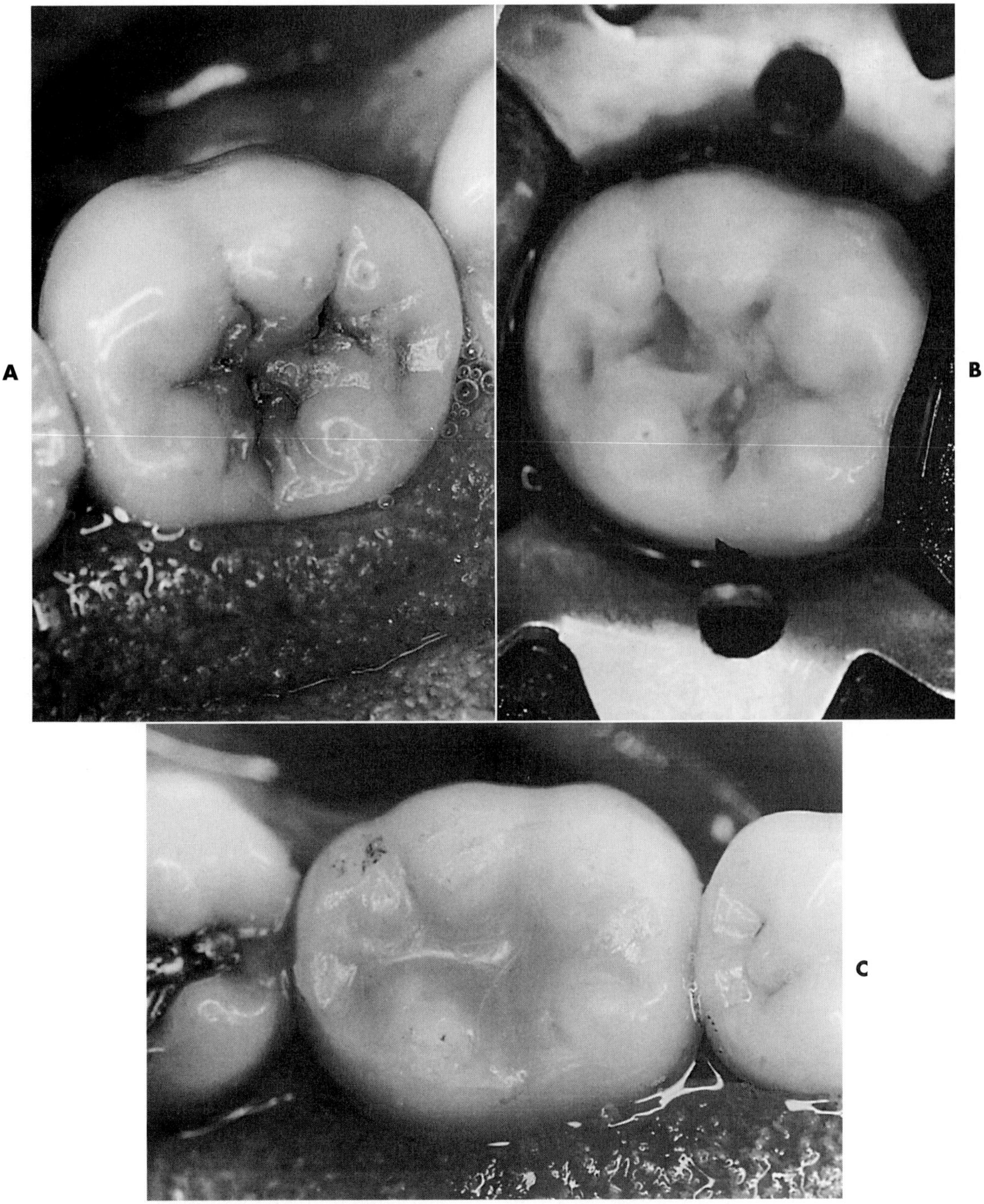

Fig. 8-16 Air abrasion application for a preventive resin restoration. **A,** Preoperative view of carious fissures in a mandibular molar; **B,** cavity preparation with air abrasion; **C,** restoration with flowable resin composite.

TABLE 8-2 Uses of Composites, Compomers, Hybrid Ionomers, and Glass Ionomers

Type	Uses
Hybrid/microfilled composite	Class 1, 2, 3, 4, 5, low caries-risk patients Class 1, 3, 4, medium caries-risk patients
Compomer	Primary teeth, Class 1, 2 restorations in children Cervical lesions, Class 3, 5, medium caries-risk patients
Hybrid ionomer	Cervical lesions, Class 3, 5, primary teeth, sandwich technique, Class 5, high caries-risk patients, root caries
Glass ionomer	Cervical lesions, Class 5 restorations in adults where esthetics are less important, root caries

TABLE 8-3 Ranking of Selected Properties of Hybrid Ionomers and Glass Ionomers

Property	Hybrid Ionomer	Glass Ionomer
Compressive strength	Med	Low-Med
Flexural strength	Med	Low-Med
Flexural modulus	Med	Med-High
Wear resistance	Med	Low
Fluoride release	Med-High	High
Fluoride rechargability	Med-High	High
Esthetics	Good	Acceptable

itatively with other restorative materials in Table 8-3. Properties especially noteworthy are a modulus that is similar to dentin, a bond strength to dentin of 2 to 3 MPa, an expansion coefficient comparable to tooth structure, low solubility, and fairly high opacity. The flux used in fusion of the glass contains fluoride that is released slowly to provide an anticariogenic effect on adjacent tooth structure.

Although the bond strength of glass ionomers to dentin is lower than that of composites, clinical studies have shown that the retention of glass ionomers in areas of cervical erosion are considerably better than for composites. When the dentin is conditioned (etched) using a dilute solution (15% to 25%) of polyacrylic acid, the glass ionomer may be applied without a cavity preparation. Four-year clinical data showed a retention rate for glass ionomer cervical restorations of 75%. The surfaces of the restorations seen in the studies were noticeably rough, and some shade mismatches were present. Pulp reaction to glass ionomers is mild; if the thickness of dentin is less than 1 mm, use a calcium hydroxide liner. Although the surface remains slightly rough, cervical restorations did not contribute to inflammation of gingival tissues. Less *Streptococcus mutans* exists in plaque adjacent to glass ionomer restorations.

MANIPULATION

Glass ionomers are packaged in bottles and in vacuum capsules for mechanical mixing in an amalgamator. In bulk dispensing, the powder and liquid are dispensed in proper amounts on the paper pad, and half the powder is incorporated to produce a homogeneous milky consistency. The remainder of the powder is added, and a total mixing time of 30 to 40 seconds is used with a typical initial setting time of 4 minutes. After placing the restorative and developing the correct contour, protect the surface from saliva by applying varnish or bonding agent. Trimming and finishing are done, if possible, after 24 hours.

The liquid in the unit-dose capsule is forced into the powder by a press and is mixed by a mechanical mixer. The mixture is injected directly into the cavity preparation with a special syringe. Working time is short and critical, so it is

A 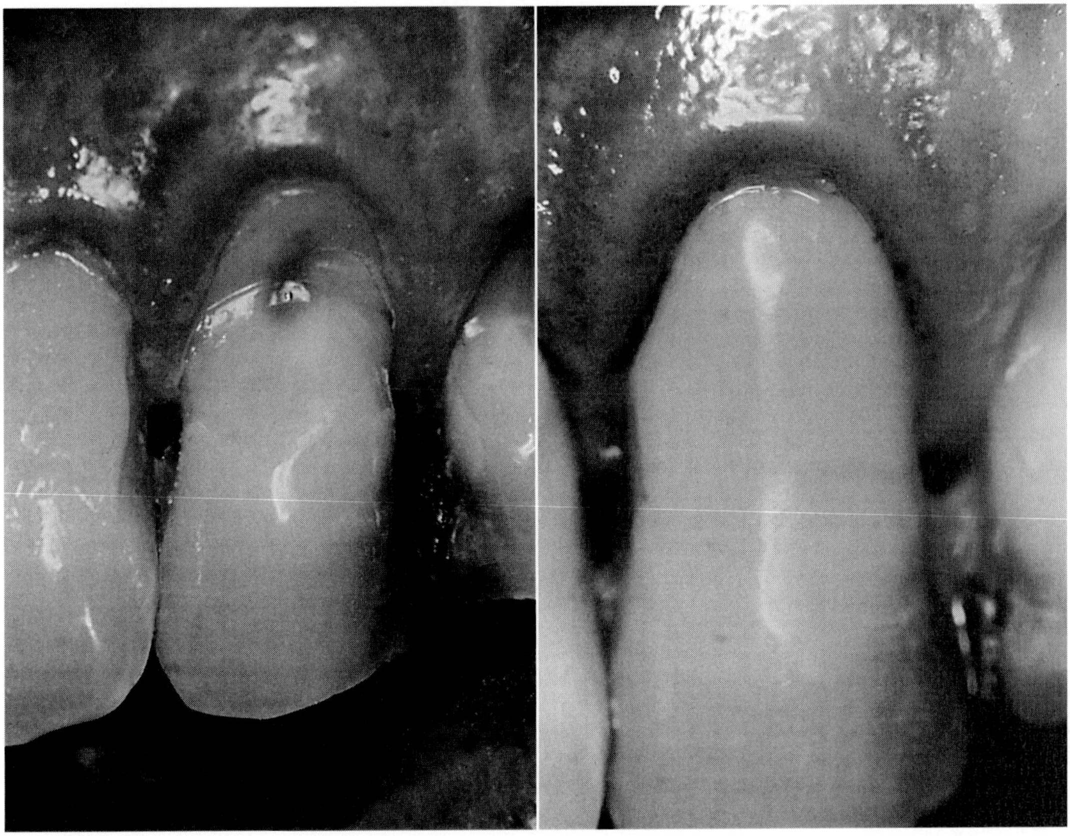 B

Fig. 8-17 Restoration of a root surface lesion. **A,** Abrasion/erosion lesion on the facial surface of a maxillary cuspid. **B,** Restoration with a resin-modified glass ionomer cement.

imperative to place the material with a minimum of manipulation. If the gel stage of the reaction is disrupted during the early phase of the reaction, the physical properties will be very low and adhesion can be lost.

Adhere rigidly to clinical techniques for glass ionomers, maintaining isolation, using adequate etching procedures, protecting the restoration from saliva after placement, and delaying final finishing for 1 day or longer if possible.

HYBRID IONOMERS

Hybrid ionomers or resin-modified glass ionomers are used for restorations in low stress–bearing areas and are recommended for patients with high caries risk (see Table 8-3). These restorations are more esthetic than glass ionomers because of their resin content. Examples of cervically eroded teeth and hybrid ionomer restorations are shown in Fig. 8-17.

COMPOSITION AND REACTION

The powder of hybrid ionomers is similar to that of glass ionomers. The liquid contains monomers, polyacids and water. Hybrid ionomers set by a combined acid-base ionomer reaction and light-cured resin polymerization of 2-hydroxyethyl methacrylate. Placing a dentin bonding agent before inserting a hybrid ionomer is contraindicated, because it decreases fluoride release.

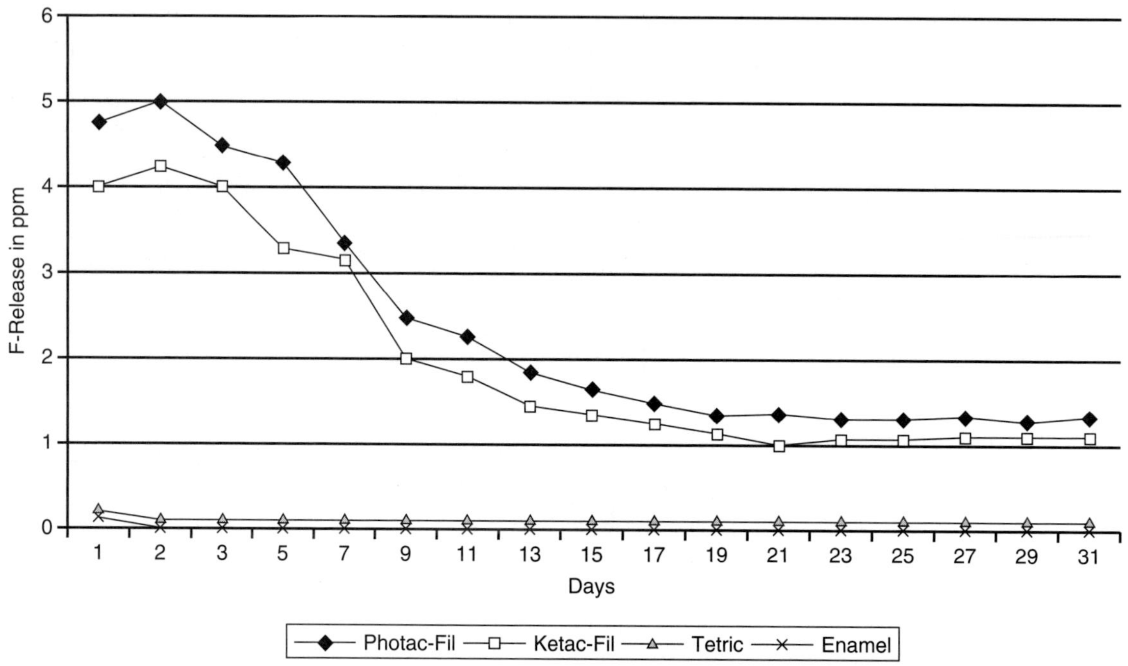

Fig. 8-18 Fluoride release from glass ionomer cements and composite resin in distilled water over 30 days.

(Adapted from Strothers JM, Kohn DH, Dennison JB, Clarkson BH: *Dent Mater* 14:129, 1998.)

PROPERTIES

Hybrid ionomers bond to tooth structure without the use of a dentin bonding agent. Typically, the tooth is conditioned (etched) with polyacrylic acid or a primer before placing the hybrid ionomer. The transverse strength of a hybrid ionomer is almost double that of a standard glass ionomer. Hybrid ionomers release more fluoride than compomers and composites but almost the same as glass ionomers. Fig. 8-18 illustrates the release of fluoride ions from a standard glass ionomer and resin-modified glass ionomer over a 30-day period. There is an early period of high release, which tapers after about 10 days to 1 ppm. Glass ionomers and hybrid ionomers recharge when exposed to fluoride treatments or fluoride dentifrices. Fig. 8-19 illustrates this recharge capability with a similar time-dependent release curve. In evaluating the effectiveness of this release, fluoride has been measured in plaque samples immediately adjacent to glass ionomer–based restorations (Fig. 8-20). For these two materials from the same manufacturer, plaque adjacent to the resin-modified glass ionomer had a significantly higher fluoride content than plaque adjacent to compomer restorations at 2 days and 21 days after insertion of the restorations.

MANIPULATION

An example of a hybrid ionomer packaged in capsules is shown in Fig. 8-21. Hybrid ionomers are also packaged as powder-liquids; their manipulation is like that of standard glass ionomers. Mechanical mixing of the unit-dose capsules provides a uniform mix that has much fewer of the larger air voids that can be introduced during hand spatulation. Optimum powder/liquid ratio is critical to the long-term maintenance of physical properties and the clinical success of restorations. Unlike glass ionomer restorations, hybrid ionomers set immediately when light-cured and can be finished soon after. Glass ionomer–based

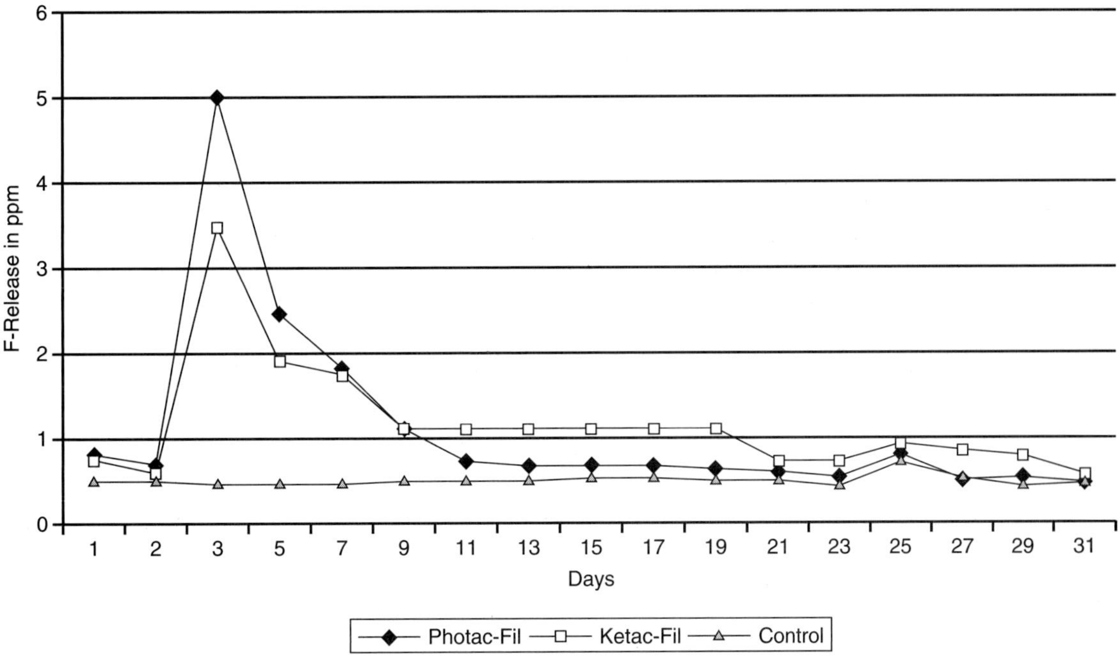

Fig. 8-19 Fluoride re-uptake and re-release from glass ionomer cements after recharging the material with 1.1% neutral sodium fluoride gel.

(Adapted from Strothers JM, Kohn DH, Dennison JB, Clarkson BH: *Dent Mater* 14:129, 1998.)

materials are an increasingly important part of operative dentistry for both an aging population with high incidence of root caries and children who have minimal dental care but high caries-risk factors.

ATHLETIC MOUTH PROTECTORS

The use of athletic mouth protectors in contact sports has increased rapidly; they are routinely used in football, soccer, ice hockey, basketball, wrestling, field hockey, softball, and other sports. This increased use is justified by studies that showed that 38% of participants in sports sustained orofacial injuries and only 15% of those injured were wearing a mouth protector at the time of injury. A survey found that 62% of injuries occurred in unorganized sports.

Injuries to teeth from trauma caused by athletic activity have involved pulpitis, pulpal necrosis, resorption, replacement resorption, inter-

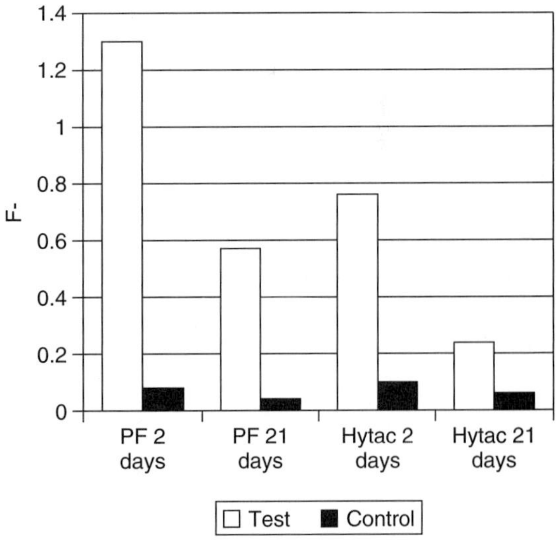

Fig. 8-20 Total fluoride concentration in plaque (μg fluoride per mg plaque) adjacent to resin-modified glass ionomer and compomer restorations over 21 days; restored test teeth vs. nonrestored control teeth.

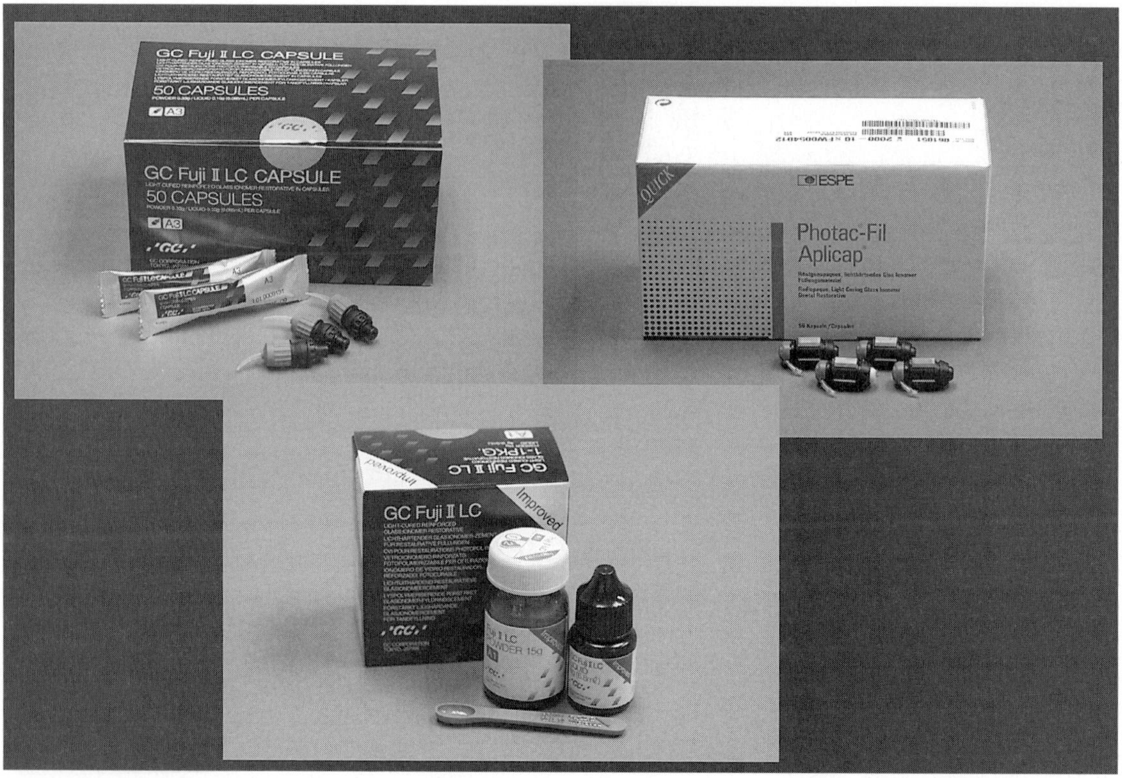

Fig. 8-21 Resin-modified glass ionomer materials available for hand mixing or encapsulated for mechanical mixing.

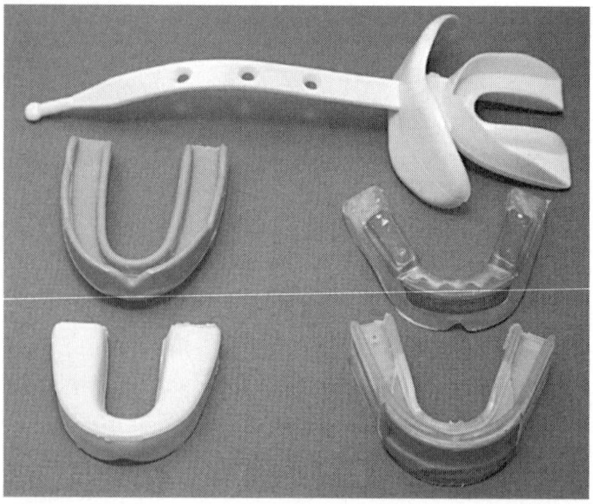

Fig. 8-22 Examples of stock and mouth-formed mouth protectors. Note the protector on the *top* is a mouth and lip protector and those on the *left* and *right center* have had the straps cut off to allow testing of the percentage of impact absorbed.

nal hemorrhage, pulp canal obliteration, and inflammatory resorption.

As a result of the possibilities of orofacial injury, high school athletes are required to wear internal mouth protectors, and the National Collegiate Athletic Association has adopted a mouth-protector rule. As a result of these actions, more professional athletes are wearing mouth protectors. Because of the increased use of mouth protectors, it is estimated that 50,000 orofacial injuries are prevented each year.

Stock, mouth-formed (boil-and-bite), and custom mouth protectors are the three types available and all provide some protection to the athlete. A few examples of stock and mouth-formed protectors are shown in Fig. 8-22. Custom-made mouth protectors are usually vacuum-formed from sheets of flexible, thermoplastic polymers about 14 cm square and 1.6 to 3 mm

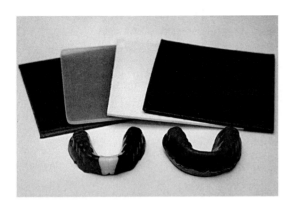

Fig. 8-23 Thermoplastic sheets for fabricating mouth protectors and fabricated mouth protectors. The one on the right is on a dental stone model; the one on the left was fabricated from a tricolored sheet.

in thickness; they may be clear or colored. Examples of these sheets and fabricated mouth protectors are shown in Fig. 8-23. In most instances the sheets are of a single material, but they may be laminates of two thermoplastic polymers. Laminated mouth protectors are fabricated so that the softer of the two layers contacts the teeth and soft tissue.

Most sheets for custom mouth protectors are vinyl acetate–ethylene copolymers (PVAc-PE). Manufacturers use several different hardnesses of the material, with copolymers containing more ethylene being harder.

The advantages of custom-made mouth protectors are (1) excellent fit, (2) comfort, (3) ease of speaking, and (4) durability; these qualities are poor for stock protectors and poor to good for mouth-formed protectors. In spite of the advantages of custom-made protectors, they are not as common as stock or mouth-formed protectors because of their higher cost.

PROPERTIES

Selected properties of thermoplastic sheets and fabricated custom-made, mouth-formed, and stock protectors are listed in Table 8-4. The Shore "A" hardness of the materials for all types of mouth protectors ranges from 70 to 80, and all have low values of water sorption and solubility. The tear strength of the laminate is somewhat lower than single material sheets; it is not possible to test the values of the fabricated mouth protectors. With an impact of 113 N/cm, the percentage absorbed by thermoplastic sheets and custom mouth protectors placed on high-strength stone models in the area of the central incisors is essentially the same, with values of 80% to 90%. A wider range of impact absorption, 76% to 93%, is found for mouth-formed and stock protectors. These results confirm clinical studies that demonstrate no difference in the incidence of oral injuries of athletes wearing custom-made, mouth-formed, or stock protectors. Thus the main advantages of the custom-made mouth protectors are those previously mentioned—fit, comfort, and ease of speaking—which should increase the probability that the protector will be tried in.

FABRICATION OF CUSTOM-MADE PROTECTORS

The fabrication of a custom-made mouth protector involves the following general steps: (1) making an alginate impression of the maxillary arch; (2) pouring a dental stone or high-strength stone model into the impression, minus the palate; (3) vacuum-forming a heated sheet of PVAc-PE over the model; (4) trimming the excess PVAc-PE around the model; and (5) smoothing the edges of the mouth protector.

A commercial dental vacuum machine used to fabricate mouth protectors is shown in Fig. 8-24, *A*. The procedure involves clamping the PVAc-PE sheet in the frame and raising the frame to the top position, shown in the sketch in Fig. 8-24, *B*, and centering the model on the perforated metal platform. Turn the heater on and heat the sheet until it sags about 3 cm at the center, at which point turn the vacuum on and push the frame down to its lower position using the plastic handles. Swing the heater out of the way and turn it off, but leave the vacuum on for 30 seconds. Allow the thermoplastic sheet to cool to room temperature before removing it from the model. A thermoplastic sheet vacuum-formed over a model is shown in Fig. 8-25. Trim the excess of

TABLE 8-4 Properties of PVAc-PE Sheets and Custom-Made, Mouth-Formed, and Stock Mouth Protectors at Mouth Temperature

	Hardness Shore "A"	Water Sorption* (wt %)	Tear Strength (N/cm)	Impact Absorbed (%)
PVAc-PE sheets	75-80	0.14-0.25	410	81-89
PVAc-PE laminated sheets	75-76†	0.15	330	87
PVAc-PE custom-made protectors	75-80	0.14-0.25	-	86-90
Mouth-formed and stock mouth protectors	71-78	0.16-0.24	-	76-93

*Water solubility was an average of 0.003 wt %.
†Tongue side was softer (75).

A

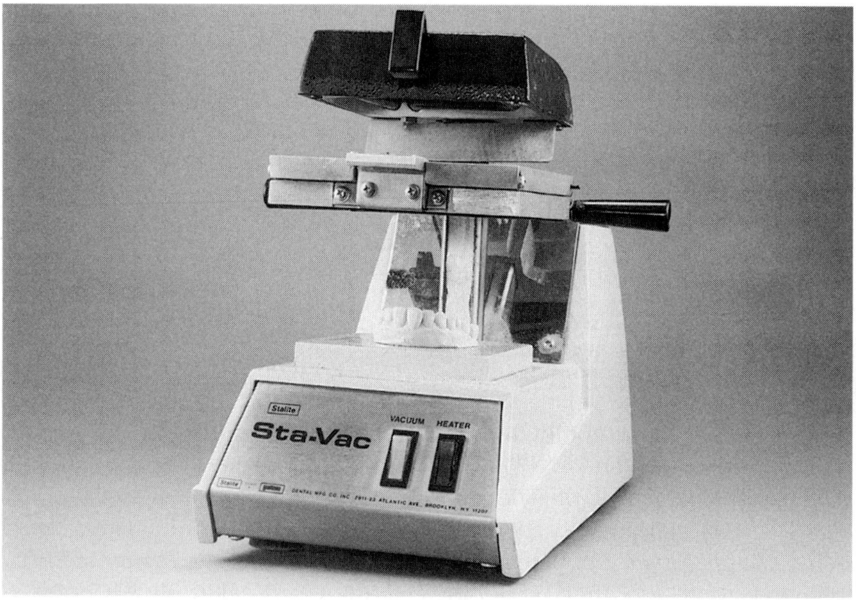

Fig. 8-24 A, Typical vacuum-forming machine.

(**A,** From Craig RG, Powers, JM, Wataha JC: *Dental materials: properties and manipulation,* ed. 7, St Louis, 2000, Mosby.)

Continued

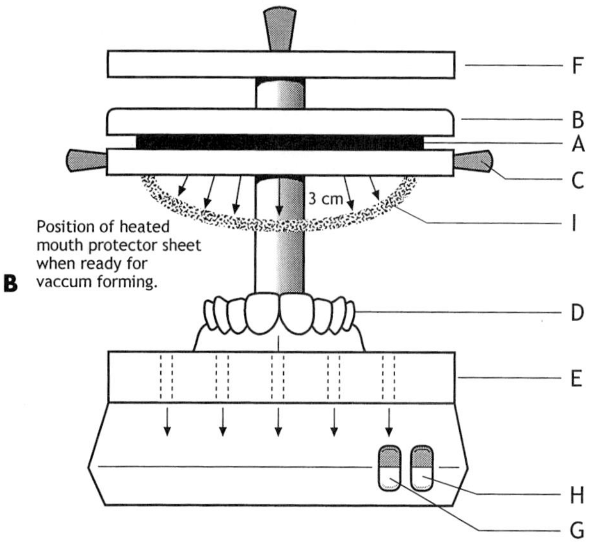

Fig. 8-24, cont'd B, Illustration showing the essential parts. The sheet of mouth protector material, *A*, is held between the upper, *B*, and lower clamp, *C*. The model, *D*, is centered on the perforated support plate, *E*, and the heater, *F*, is turned on by switch *H*. Heating continues until the sheet sags about 3 cm (shown as *I*), and then the vacuum switch, *G*, is turned on. The heated sheet is quickly lowered over the model using the attached plastic handles, *C*. The sheet is vacuum-sealed to the support plate via the perforations and is then vacuum-formed over the model. The heater is turned off and swung away 90 degrees using the attached handle on *F*; the vacuum is turned off after 30 to 60 seconds. The vacuum-formed mouth protector remains on the model until cool and then trimming and finishing can begin.

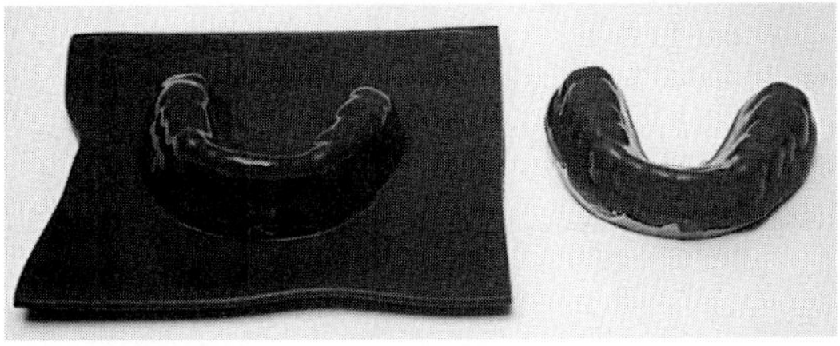

Fig. 8-25 A mouth protector sheet vacuum-formed over a model is shown on the left, and a trimmed and finished protector is shown on a model at the right.

the thermoplastic sheet 3 mm short of the labial fold using a curved pair of scissors, making sure to provide clearance for the buccal and labial frenum. Smooth the edges with a wheel such as a Moore's Satin Buff Wheel or, if one is not available, with the flame from an alcohol torch, followed by adaptation with wet fingers.

Several considerations should be taken into account related to making impressions and preparing models used to fabricate mouth protectors. Remove removable appliances before making the alginate impression. If the athlete is wearing a fixed orthodontic appliance, block it out on the model with dental stone before fabricating the mouth protector. Also, if permanent teeth are still erupting, block out that space on the model.

In the absence of a vacuum, soften the thermoplastic sheet in hot water and adapt to the model using a wet sponge and wet fingers. Significantly better adaptation results from vacuum-forming the protector.

If it is found necessary to equalize the occlusion when the mouth protector is worn, make the following adjustment. Gently heat the contacting surfaces of the mouth protector using an alcohol torch, just enough to barely soften the material. Dip the mouth protector in warm water and place it in the athlete's mouth. Ask the athlete to close until all the opposing teeth contact the mouth protector.

PREPARING A MOUTH-FORMED MOUTH PROTECTOR

Manufacturers supply instructions for the boil-and-bite mouth protector; in general, the procedure is as follows. Place the protector in a pan of boiling water, just removed from the heat, for 10 to 35 seconds, based on the manufacturer's directions. Remove the protector from the hot water, immerse it in a pan of cold water for 1 second and then place it in the mouth, centering it around the maxillary teeth. Ask the athlete to bite down gently and suck out any air and water by pressing the tongue against the back of the maxillary teeth. Leave the protector in the mouth for 30 seconds before removal. If a good fit is not obtained, the procedure can be repeated. Also, if the mouth protector is too large, cut off the ends to the appropriate length before placing it in the hot water.

CARE OF ATHLETIC MOUTH PROTECTORS

Give the following recommendations to the athlete:

1. After each use, rinse the mouth protector under cold water.
2. Periodically clean the mouth protector using a solution of soap in cold water.
3. Don't use abrasive dentifrices to clean the protector.
4. Don't use alcoholic solutions or denture cleaners to clean the protector.
5. Store the mouth protector stress-free in a container provided, or better yet on the model on which it was fabricated. Also, retain the model to allow a replacement to be made in case the mouth protector is lost or damaged.

OTHER APPLICATIONS FOR VACUUM-FORMING

In addition to athletic mouth protectors, vacuum-forming is used to prepare trays for impression materials, fluoride treatments, bleaching procedures, and surgical splints.

SELECTED PROBLEMS

Problem 1

What are the functions of humectants and detergents in toothpaste?

Solution

Humectants such as glycerin are added to stabilize the composition and reduce evaporation of water, whereas detergents such as sodium lauryl sulfate are added to reduce the surface tension and improve removal of debris from the teeth.

Problem 2

What factors are related to increased abrasion of toothpaste?

Solution

Larger and more irregular shapes of the abrasive increase abrasion, as do harder abrasive minerals and a higher volume fraction of the abrasive.

Problem 3

What chemicals have been added to toothpastes to control calculus deposits?

Solution

Tetrasodium or tetrapotassium pyrophosphates are added to inhibit growth of hydroxyapatite crystals.

Problem 4

Cite two active ingredients in mouthwashes and state their function.

Solution

Chlorhexidine is an antibacterial agent used to control soft tissue or gum infections. Sodium fluoride is added for its anticaries effect.

Problem 5

What is the advantage of a fluoride varnish versus other means of applying fluoride to teeth?

Solution

The main advantage is the extended time of exposure of the teeth to the active fluoride ingredient compared with mouthwashes.

Problem 6

Why are pit-and-fissure sealants needed to control caries on occlusal surfaces of permanent teeth?

Solution

Pits and fissures in the occlusal surfaces of permanent teeth are susceptible to caries because their physical size and morphology provide shelter for organisms and obstruct oral hygiene procedures. As a result, fluoride treatments have not been effective in reducing caries in occlusal pits and fissures.

Problem 7

When selecting a material as a pit and fissure sealant, what are the relevant characteristics of a filled resin sealant?

Solution

The relevant characteristics are: better physical properties and improved abrasion resistance (but with occlusal prematurities that should be adjusted after insertion); a slightly higher viscosity than an unfilled sealant but a much lower viscosity than a composite; and better control in application procedures.

Problem 8

When selecting a sealant material, what are the relevant characteristics of an unfilled resin sealant?

Solution

The relevant characteristics are: lower viscosity; less wear resistance but with occlusal prematurities that will wear down readily; and less control in application procedures.

Problem 9

Postoperative evaluation of a freshly placed sealant revealed subsurface air voids, some communicating with the external surface. What manipulative variables can be controlled to minimize this problem?

Solution

The problem can be minimized by controlling the following variables: avoid mixing or stirring the sealant if at all possible after it is dispensed for application, or use a photoinitiated resin; avoid using a brush for application, which tends to carry excess material and incorporate air; use a ball-tipped applicator, which permits the application of smaller increments of material to specific sites on the tooth surface with only minimal manipulation of the setting sealant; avoid moisture contamination during application because it can produce subsurface voids after equilibrium is reached through water sorption; avoid the use of a material beyond its shelf life or one that has been stored in a warm environment because the increase in viscosity results in air entrapment during application; and avoid application of the sealant to a nonwettable or inadequately etched enamel surface.

Problem 10

Six months after sealant application, a first molar was clinically evaluated at recall and found to have no sealant present. What are the possible causes for this early failure?

Solution a

One cause might be inadequately prepared enamel surface, possibly caused by (1) failure to remove pellicle and debris from the surface during preoperative prophylaxis cleaning; (2) inadequate acid etching by using concentrated or diluted etchant, exposure to etchant for insufficient time, or the presence of acid-resistant enamel with a high fluoride composition; (3) insufficient rinsing of the acid etchant solution or gel, leaving contaminating salts present to reduce surface energy; (4) moisture or salivary contamination during sealant application; or (5) contamination of the etched enamel site by oil or by water in the compressed air used for drying.

Solution b

A second causative factor might be inadequately cured photoinitiated sealant, possibly caused by (1) the light wand being held too high above the tooth surface; (2) failure to make multiple light applications to completely expose the entire surface; (3) inadequate exposure time to the light source; (4) use of a sealant that has previously been exposed to light or has been used beyond its shelf life; or (5) use of an opaque or deeply colored sealant without increasing the exposure time.

Problem 11

At recall evaluations, sealants may have an orange-brown stain along specific marginal areas, which is indicative of bond failure and marginal leakage. What are the causative factors for this failure?

Solution

The causative factors are inadequate enamel preparation at the failure site or contamination of the etched enamel; overextension of sealant beyond the periphery of adequately etched enamel; and functional occlusal forces, placed directly over thin extensions of sealant, producing stresses that exceed the bond strength of sealant to enamel.

Problem 12

Although the bond strength of glass ionomers to dentin is lower than that of composites, clinical experience has shown that the retention of glass ionomers to areas of cervical erosion are better. Why?

Solution

Although the bond strength of glass ionomers to dentin is only 2 to 3 MPa in the setting reaction, chelation occurs with the calcium on the tooth surface, producing an adhesive bond, whereas the bond of composites to tooth structure is essentially micromechanical.

Problem 13

Compared with glass ionomers and composites, what are the advantages of hybrid ionomers for low stress–bearing restorations?

Solution

The transverse strength of hybrid ionomers is about twice that of glass ionomers. They release more fluoride than composites and are more esthetic than glass ionomers.

Problem 14

During the vacuum-forming of a mouth protector, bubbles appeared in the PVAc-PE sheet at the tip of the cusps in some teeth. What precautions should be taken during the remake to prevent this problem?

Solution

The most likely cause was overheating of the PVAc-PE sheet. When vacuum-forming occurred, the material became excessively thin in the region of the cusps. The hot sheet released air from the model, causing the bubble. The problem would be accentuated if the model was poured in dental plaster rather than high-strength stone, which is less porous, and if the model were in dry rather than wet condition.

Problem 15

During the vacuum-forming of a mouth protector, it was observed that the occlusal anatomy lacked detail and the protector when worn lacked retention. What could have caused these problems?

Solution a

In all probability, the thermoplastic sheet was not heated enough and did not flow well under vacuum.

Solution b

It is also possible that the frame holding the heated PVAc-PE sheet was lowered over the model before turning on the vacuum. The sequence should be: (1) turn on the vacuum, (2) lower the frame holding the heated PVAc-PE sheet, (3) swing the heater away, and (4) maintain the vacuum for 30 seconds.

Problem 16

After vacuum-forming, trimming, and finishing a mouth protector, it fit poorly. What might have caused this result?

Solution a

After vacuum-forming, the model may have been removed from the PVAc-PE sheet while it was still warm. The stresses during removal resulted in permanent distortion of the protector.

Solution b

After trimming the mouth protector, the edges may have been flamed to make them smooth; released stresses in the material may have caused distortion of the protector.

Solution c

If it were necessary to equalize the occlusion, too much heat may have been applied to the occlusal surface, resulting in distortion of the protector.

Problem 17

The athlete stored the protector by squeezing it between the face guard and a football helmet. At the next use the mouth protector fit poorly. Explain.

Solution

The mouth protector is made of a thermoplastic material, which can permanently deform under pressure even at room temperature, resulting in loss of fit. The higher the room temperature the worse the problem. The best storage for the protector is on the model; next best is in the box provided by the laboratory.

Problem 18

The athlete diligently cleaned the protector after each use in water but figured the hotter the water the better. Why did the protector fit poorly after cleaning?

Solution

The PVAc-PE is thermoplastic and, if heated, release of processing stresses causes warpage of the mouth protector. Therefore, wash the mouth protector in cold water.

BIBLIOGRAPHY

Toothpastes

Allen CE, Nunez LJ: A look at toothpaste ingredients, *Gen Dent* 33:58, 1985.

De Boer P, Duinkerke ASH, Arends J: Influence of tooth paste particle size and tooth brush stiffness on dentine abrasion in vitro, *Caries Res* 19:232, 1985.

DeLattre VF: Factors contributing to adverse soft tissue reactions due to the use of tartar control toothpastes: Report of a case and literature review, *J Periodontol* 70:803, 1999.

Dyer D, Addy M, Newcombe RG: Studies in vitro of abrasion by different manual toothbrush heads and a standard toothpaste, *J Clin Periodontol* 27:99, 2000.

Hefferren JJ, Kingman A, Stookey GK et al: An international collaborative study of laboratory methods for assessing abrasivity to dentin, *J Dent Res* 63:1176, 1984.

Sainio EL, Kanerva L: Contact allergens in toothpastes and a review of their hypersensitivity, *Contact Derm* 33:100, 1995.

Mouthwashes

Addy M, Wade W, Goodfield S: Staining and antimicrobial properties in vitro of some chlorhexidine formulations, *Clin Prevent Dent* 12:13, 1991.

Bhatti SA, Walsh TF, Douglas CWI: Ethanol and pH levels of proprietary mouthrinses, *Community Dent Health* 11:71, 1994.

Cruz R, Rolla G, Ogaard B: Formation of fluoride on enamel in vitro after exposure to fluoridated mouthrinses, *Acta Odontol Scand* 49:329, 1991.

Forward GC, James AH, Barnett P et al: Gum health product formulations: what is in them and why? *Periodontol 2000* 15:32, 1997.

Gurgan S, Onen A, Koprulu H: In vitro effects of alcohol-containing and alcohol-free mouthrinses on microhardness of some restorative materials, *J Oral Rehabil* 24:244, 1997.

Logothetis DD, Martinez-Welles JM: Reducing bacterial aerosol contamination with a chlorhexidine gluconate pre-rinse, *J Am Dent Assoc* 126:1634, 1995.

Penugonda B, Settembrini L, Scherer W et al: Alcohol-containing mouthwashes: effect on composite hardness, *J Clin Dent* 5:60, 1994.

Settembrini L, Penugonda B, Scherer W et al: Alcohol-containing mouthwashes: effect on composite color, *Oper Dent* 20:14, 1995.

Weiner R, Millstein P, Hoang E et al: The effect of alcoholic and nonalcoholic mouthwashes on heat-treated composite resin, *Oper Dent* 22:249, 1997.

Winn DM, Blot WJ, McLaughlin JK et al: Mouthwash use and oral conditions in the risk of oral and pharyngeal cancer, *Cancer Res* 51:3044, 1991.

Fluoride Varnishes

Beltran-Aguilar ED, Goldstein JW: Fluoride varnishes: a review of their clinical use, cariostatic mechanism, efficacy and safety, *J Am Dent Assoc* 131:589, 2000.

Petersson LG, Twetman S, Pakhomov GN: The efficiency of semiannual silane fluoride varnish applications: a two-year clinical study in preschool children, *J Public Health Dent* 58:57, 1998.

Skold L, Sundquist B, Eriksson B et al: Four-year study of caries inhibition of intensive Duraphat application in 11-15 year-old children, *Community Dent Oral Epidemiol* 22:8, 1994.

Sealants

Arenholt-Bindslev D, Breinholt V, Preiss A et al: Time-related bisphenol-A content and estrogenic activity in saliva samples collected in relation to placement of fissure sealants, *Clinical Oral Invest* 3:120, 1999.

Boksman L, Carson B: Two-year retention and caries rates of UltraSeal XT and FluoroShield light-cured pit and fissure sealants, *General Dent* 46:184, 1998.

Buonocore MG: Adhesive sealing of pits and fissures for caries prevention, with use of ultraviolet light, *J Am Dent Assoc* 80:324, 1970.

Charbeneau GT, Dennison JB: Clinical success and potential failure after single application of a pit and fissure sealant: a four-year report, *J Am Dent Assoc* 98:559, 1979.

Dennison JB, Powers JM: Physical properties of pit and fissure sealants (annot), *J Dent Res* 58:1430, 1979.

Dennison JB, Straffon, LH: Clinical evaluation comparing sealant and amalgam after 7 years: final report, *J Am Dent Assoc* 117:751, 1988.

Feigal RJ, Hitt J, Splieth C: Retaining sealant on salivary contaminated enamel, *J Am Dent Assoc* 124:88, 1993.

Frencken JE, Makoni F, Sithole WD: Atraumatic restorative treatment and glass-ionomer sealants in a school oral health programme in Zimbabwe, *Caries Res* 30:429, 1996.

Garcia-Gordoy F, Abarzua I, De Goes MF et al: Fluoride release from fissure sealants, *J Clin Pediatr Dent* 22:45, 1997.

Handleman SL, Buonocore MG, Heseck DJ: A preliminary report on the effect of fissure sealant on bacteria in dental caries, *J Prosthet Dent* 27:390, 1972.

Horowitz HS, Heifetz SB, Poulsen S: Retention and effectiveness of a single application of an adhesive sealant in preventing occlusal caries: final report after five years of a study in Kalispell, Montana, *J Am Dent Assoc* 95:1133, 1977.

Lygidakis NA, Oulis KI: A comparison of Fluroshield with Delton fissure sealant: four year results, *Pediatric Dent* 21:429, 1999.

Myers CL, Rossi F, Cartz F: Adhesive taglike extensions into acid-etched tooth enamel, *J Dent Res* 53:435, 1974.

O'Brien WJ, Fan PL, Apostolidis A: Penetrativity of sealants and glazes, *Oper Dent* 3:51, 1978.

Pahlavan A, Dennison JB, Charbeneau GT: Penetration of restorative resins into acid-etched human enamel, *J Am Dent Assoc* 93:1170, 1976.

Rueggeberg FA, Dlugokinski M, Ergle JW: Minimizing patient's exposure to uncured components in a dental sealant, *J Am Dent Assoc* 130:1751, 1999.

Simonsen RJ: Retention and effectiveness of dental sealant after 15 years, *J Am Dent Assoc* 122:34, 1991.

Steinmetz MJ, Pruhs RJ, Brooks JC et al: Rechargeability of fluoride releasing pit and fissure sealants and restorative resin composites, *Am J Dent* 10:36, 1997.

Straffon LH, Dennison JB, More FG: Three-year evaluation of sealant: effect of isolation on efficacy, *J Am Dent Assoc* 110:714, 1985.

Symons AL, Chu CY, Meyers IA: The effect of fissure morphology and pretreatment of the enamel surface on penetration and adhesion of fissure sealants, *J Oral Rehabil* 23:791, 1996.

Taylor CL, Gwinnett AJ: A study of the penetration of sealants into pits and fissures, *J Am Dent Assoc* 87:1181, 1973.

Williams B, Laxton L, Holt RD et al: Tissue sealants: a 4-year clinical trial comparing an experimental glass polyalkenoate cement with a bis glycidyl methacrylate resin used as fissure sealants, *Br Dent J* 180:104, 1996.

Flowable Composites

Behle C: Flowable composites: properties and applications, *Pract Periodont Aesthet Dent* 10:347, 1998.

Fortin D, Vargas MA: The spectrum of composites: new techniques and materials, *J Am Dent Assoc* 131:26S, 2000.

Houpt M, Fuks A, Eidelman E: The preventive resin (composite resin/sealant) restoration: nine-year results, *Quint Int* 25:155, 1994.

Unterbrink GL, Liebenberg WH: Flowable resin composites as "filled adhesives": literature review and clinical recommendations, *Quint Int* 30:249, 1999.

Glass Ionomers and Hybrid Ionomers

Bapna MS, Mueller HJ: Leaching from glass ionomer cements, *J Oral Rehabil* 21:577, 1994.

Berry EA III, Powers JM: Bond strength of glass ionomers to coronal and radicular dentin, *Oper Dent* 19:122, 1994.

Braundau HE, Ziemiecki TZ, Charbeneau GT: Restoration of cervical contours on nonprepared teeth using glass ionomer cement: a 4½ year report, *J Am Dent Assoc* 104:782, 1984.

Cattani-Lorente MA, Dupuis V, Moya F et al: Comparative study of the physical properties of a polyacid-modified composite resin and a resin-modified glass ionomer, *Dent Mater* 15:21, 1999.

Council on Dental Materials, Instruments, and Equipment: Using glass ionomers, *J Am Dent Assoc* 121:181, 1990.

Croll TP: Glass ionomers in esthetic dentistry, *J Am Dent Assoc* 123:51, 1992.

El-Kalla IH, Garcia-Godoy F: Mechanical properties of compomer restorative materials, *Oper Dent* 24:2, 1999.

Farah JW, Powers JM, editors: Fluoride-releasing restorative materials, *Dent Advis* 15:2, 1998.

Forss H: Release of fluoride and other elements from light-cured glass ionomer in neutral and acidic conditions, *J Dent Res* 72:1257, 1993.

Garcia R, Caffesse RG, Charbeneau GT: Gingival tissue response to restoration of deficient cervical contours using a glass-ionomer material, a 12-month report, *J Prosthet Dent* 46:393, 1981.

Heys RJ, Fitzgerald M, Heys DR et al: An evaluation of a glass ionomer luting agent: pulpal histological response, *J Am Dent Assoc* 114:607, 1987.

Hotta M, Hirukawa H, Aono M: The effect of glaze on restorative glass-ionomer cements: evaluation of environmental durability in lactic acid solution, *J Oral Rehabil* 22:685, 1995.

Kent BE, Lewis BG, Wilson AD: The properties of a glass ionomer cement, *Br Dent J* 135:322, 1973.

Maldonado A, Swartz ML, Phillips RW: An in vitro study of certain properties of a glass ionomer cement, *J Am Dent Assoc* 96:785, 1978.

McLean JW, Wilson AD: The clinical development of the glass-ionomer cements, *Aust Dent J* 22:31, 1977.

Mitchell CA, Douglas WH: Comparison of the porosity of hand-mixed and capsulated glass-ionomer luting cements, *Biomat* 18:1127, 1997.

Mount GJ: The role of glass ionomer cements in esthetic dentistry: a review, *Esthet Dent Update* 4:7, 1993.

Müller J, Brucker G, Kraft E et al: Reaction of cultured pulp cells to eight different cements based on glass ionomers, *Dent Mater* 6:172, 1990.

Quackenbush BM, Donly KJ, Croll TP: Solubility of a resin-modified glass ionomer cement, *J Dent Child* 65:310, 1998.

Strother JM, Kohn DH, Dennison JB et al: Fluoride release and re-uptake in direct tooth colored restorative materials, *Dent Mater* 14:129, 1998.

Ribeiro AP, Serra MC, Paulillo LA et al: Effectiveness of surface protection for resin-modified glass-ionomer materials, *Quint Int* 30:427, 1999.

Sidhu S, Watson TF: Resin-modified glass ionomer materials: a status report for the American Journal of Dentistry, *Am J Dent* 8:59, 1995.

Wellbury RR, Shaw AJ, Murray JJ et al: Clinical evaluation of paired compomer and glass ionomer restorations in primary teeth, *Br Dent J* 189:93, 2000.

Wilder AD, Boghosian AA, Bayne SC et al: Effect of powder/liquid ratio on the clinical and laboratory performance of resin-modified glass ionomers, *J Dent* 26:369, 1998.

Ylp HK, Smales RJ: Fluoride release and uptake by aged resin-modified glass ionomers and a polyacid-modified resin composite, *Int Dent J* 49:217, 1999.

Athletic Mouth Protectors

Craig RG, Godwin WC: Physical properties of materials for custom-made mouth protectors, *Mich Dent Assoc J* 49:34, 1967.

Craig RG, Godwin WC: Properties of athletic mouth protectors and materials, *J Oral Rehabil,* in press 2000.

DeYoung AK, Robinson E, Godwin WC: Comparing comfort and wearability: custom-made vs. self-adapted mouthguards, *J Am Dent Assoc* 125:1112, 1994.

Godwin WC, Craig RG, Koran A et al: Mouth protectors in junior football players, *Phys Sportsmed* 10:41, 1982.

Soporowski NJ: Fabricating custom athletic mouthguards, *Mass Dent Soc J* 43:25, 1994.

Westerman B, Stringfellow PM, Eccleston JA: The effect on energy absorption of hard inserts in laminated EVA mouthguards, *Aust Dent J* 45:1, 2000.

Wilkinson EE, Powers JM: Properties of stock and mouth-formed mouth protectors, *J Mich Dent Assoc* 68:83, 1986.

Wilkinson EE, Powers JM: Properties of custom-made mouth protector materials, *Phys Sportsmed* 14:77, 1986.

Chapter 9

Composite Restorative Materials

Resin composites are used to replace missing tooth structure and modify tooth color and contour, thus enhancing facial esthetics. Composites discussed in this chapter include all-purpose, microfilled, packable, flowable, and laboratory types. In addition, core composites, provisional composites, and compomers are described. Direct filling materials such as glass and hybrid ionomers, used primarily because of their fluoride release, are discussed in Chapter 8. Light-curing units are also discussed in this chapter, because most composites and compomers are light activated.

Of the direct restorative materials, silicates were developed first, followed by acrylic resins, then resin composites. Silicates were introduced in 1871 and were prepared from alumina-silica glass powder and phosphoric acid liquid. Although silicates provided an anticariogenic feature, early clinical failure was noted and was most frequently related to dissolution in oral fluids, loss of translucency, surface crazing, and a lack of adequate mechanical properties. These deficiencies caused the demise of silicates in the 1960s.

Acrylic restorative resins were unfilled, low–molecular weight polymers and lacked the reinforcement provided by the ceramic filler particles used in composites. Early clinical failure of acrylics was related directly to dimensional instability, resulting in unsightly stains and often recurrent caries.

The development of composites about 1960 has resulted in higher mechanical properties, lower thermal coefficient of expansion, lower dimensional change on setting, and higher resistance to wear, thereby improving clinical performance. Later development of bonding agents for bonding composites to tooth structure (see Chapter 10) has also improved the quality of composite restorations.

Compomers were introduced in 1995 to provide improved handling and fluoride release as compared to composites.

ALL-PURPOSE COMPOSITES

Composites were initially developed for anterior Class 3 to Class 5 restorations, in which esthetics were crucial, and for Class 1 restorations, in which moderate occlusal stresses occur. In the 1990s, modifications of materials and techniques extended their application to Class 2 and Class 6 (MOD) posterior restorations. Laboratory-

TABLE 9-1 Types of Restorations and Recommended Composites

Type of Restoration	Recommended Composite
Class 1	All-purpose, packable microfilled (posterior),* compomer (posterior)*
Class 2	All-purpose, packable, laboratory, microfilled (posterior),* compomer (posterior)*
Class 3	All-purpose, microfilled, compomer
Class 4	All-purpose
Class 5	All-purpose, microfilled, compomer
Class 6 (MOD)	Packable
Cervical lesions	Flowable, compomer
Pediatric restorations	Flowable, compomer
3-unit bridge or crown	Laboratory (with fiber reinforcement)
Alloy substructure	Laboratory (bonded)
Core build-up	Core
Temporary restoration	Provisional
High caries-risk patients	Glass ionomers, hybrid ionomers (see Chapter 8)

*Special microfilled composites and compomers are available for posterior use.
MOD, Mesial-occlusal-distal.

processed composites are used for crowns and even bridges, when reinforced with fibers, and can be bonded to an alloy substructure. Types of restorations and recommended composites are listed in Table 9-1. Characteristics of these composites are summarized in Table 9-2.

COMPOSITION

Overview A resin composite is composed of four major components: organic polymer matrix, inorganic filler particles, coupling agent, and the initiator-accelerator system. The organic polymer matrix in most composites is either an aromatic or urethane diacrylate oligomer. Oligomers are viscous liquids, the viscosity of which is reduced to a useful clinical level by the addition of a diluent monomer.

The dispersed inorganic particles may consist of several inorganic materials such as glass or quartz (fine particles) or colloidal silica (microfine particles). Two-dimensional diagrams of fine and microfine particles surrounded by polymer matrix are shown in Fig. 9-1.

The coupling agent, an organosilane (silane), is applied to the inorganic particles by the manufacturer before being mixed with the unreacted oligomer. The silane contains functional groups (such as methoxy), which hydrolyze and react with the inorganic filler, as well as unsaturated organic groups that react with the oligomer during polymerization. Silanes are called *coupling agents,* because they form a bond between the inorganic and organic phases of the composite.

Composites are formulated to contain accelerators and initiators that allow self-curing, light curing, and dual curing. ISO 4049 for polymer-based filling, restorative, and luting materials

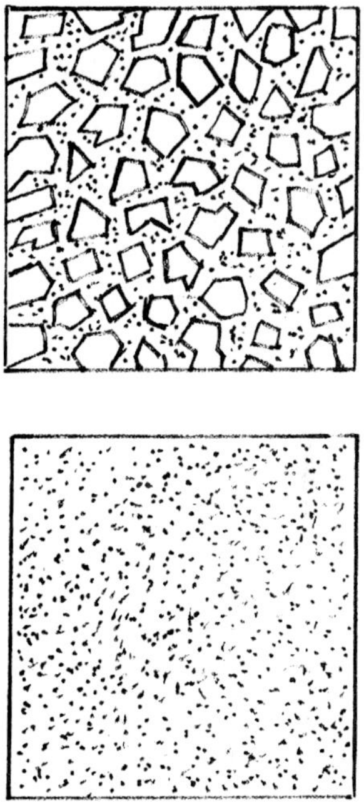

Fig. 9-1 Two-dimensional diagrams of composites with, **A,** fine and microfine, and, **B,** microfine particles. (From Craig RG, Powers JM, Wataha JC: *Dental materials: properties and manipulation,* ed 7, St Louis, 2000, Mosby.)

TABLE 9-2 Characteristics of Various Types of Composites

Type of Composite	Size of Filler Particles (μm)	Volume of Inorganic Filler (%)	Handling Characteristics and Properties: Advantages	Disadvantages
All-purpose	0.04, 0.2-3.0	60-70	High strength, high modulus	
Microfilled	0.04	32-50	Best polish, best esthetics	Higher shrinkage
Packable	0.04, 0.2-20	59-80	Packable, less shrinkage, lower wear	
Flowable	0.04, 0.2-3.0	42-62	Syringeable, lower modulus	Higher wear
Laboratory	0.04, 0.2-3.0	60-70	Best anatomy and contacts, lower wear	Lab cost, special equipment, requires resin cement

(ANSI/ADA No. 27) describes two types and three classes of composites, as shown by the following:

Type 1: Polymer-based materials suitable for restorations involving occlusal surfaces
Type 2: Other polymer-based materials
- Class 1: Self-cured materials
- Class 2: Light-cured materials
  - Group 1: Energy applied intra-orally
  - Group 2: Energy applied extra-orally
- Class 3: Dual-cured materials

Oligomers The two most common oligomers that have been used in dental composites are dimethacrylates (Bis-GMA) 2,2-*bis*[4(2-hydroxy-3 methacryloyloxy-propyloxy)-phenyl] propane and urethane dimethacrylate (UDMA). These oligomers were described in Chapter 7. Both contain reactive carbon double bonds at each end that can undergo addition polymerization. A few products use both Bis-GMA and UDMA oligomers.

The viscosity of the oligomers, especially Bis-GMA, is so high that diluents must be added, so a clinical consistency can be reached when they are compounded with the filler. Low–molecular weight compounds with difunctional carbon double bonds, usually triethylene glycol dimethacrylate (TEGDMA), shown below, are added by the manufacturer to reduce and control the viscosity of the compounded composite.

New monomers are being developed to reduce shrinkage and internal stress build-up resulting from polymerization in an effort to improve clinical durability.

Fillers A helpful method of classifying dental composites is by the particle size, shape, and distribution of filler. Early composites contained large (20 to 30 μm) spherical particles, followed by products containing large irregularly shaped particles, microfine particles (0.04 to 0.2 μm), fine particles (0.4 to 3 μm), and finally blends (microhybrids) containing mostly fine particles with some microfine particles. Based on the type of filler particles, composites are currently classified as *microhybrid* and *microfilled* products.

Microhybrid composites contain irregularly shaped glass (borosilicate glass; lithium or barium aluminum silicate; strontium or zinc glass) or quartz particles of fairly uniform diameter. Typically, composites have a distribution of two or more sizes of fine particles plus microfine filler (5% to 15%). This distribution permits more efficient packing, whereby the smaller particles fill the spaces between the larger particles. Microhybrid composites may contain 60% to 70% filler by volume, which, depending on the density of the filler, translates into 77% to 84% by weight in the composite. Most manufacturers report filler concentration in weight percent (wt %). A micrograph of a typical, fine glass filler is shown in Fig. 9-2, *A*.

Microfilled composites contain silica with a very high surface area (100 to 300 m^2/g) having particle diameters of 0.04 to 0.2 μm. Because of the high surface area, only 25% by volume or 38% by weight can be added to the oligomer to keep the consistency of the paste sufficiently low for clinical applications. Fillers consisting of microfine silica in polymerized oligomers are prepared and ground into particles 10 to 20 μm in diameter. These reinforced fillers may be added to the oligomer in concentrations, so the inorganic content can be increased to 32% to 50% by

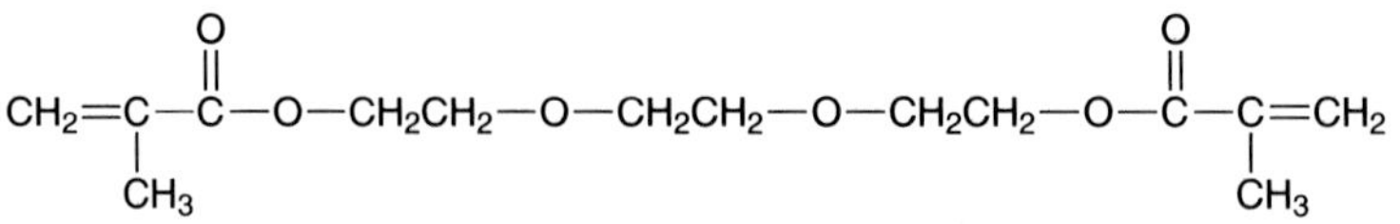

volume or about 50% to 60% by weight. A variation of this modification is used in which most of the filler is reinforced filler, with smaller amounts of silica added to the oligomer. Another modification (homogeneous microfill) has no reinforced filler, but rather microfine silica dispersed in the oligomer. A typical microfine silica filler is shown in Fig. 9-2, *B*, and a reinforced filler containing microfine silica is shown in Fig. 9-2, *C*.

Coupling Agents For a composite to have successful properties, a good bond must form between the inorganic filler and the organic oligomer during setting. Bonding is accomplished by the manufacturer, who treats the surface of the filler with a coupling agent before mixing it with the oligomer. The most common coupling agents are organic silicon compounds called *silanes*. A typical silane is shown in the following equation:

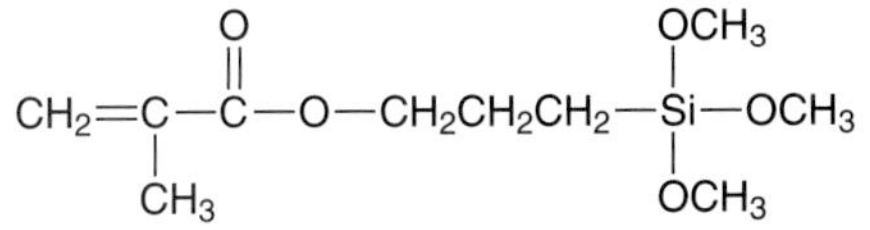

3-methacryloxypropyltrimethoxysilane

During the deposition of the silane on the filler, the methoxy groups hydrolyze to hydroxy groups that react with adsorbed moisture or –OH groups on the filler. They can also condense with –OH groups on an adjacent hydrolyzed silane to form a homopolymer film on the surface of the filler. During the setting reaction of the oligomer, the carbon double bonds of the silane react with the oligomer, thus forming a bond from the filler through the coupling agent to the polymer matrix (see the schematic sketch on p. 236). This coupling reaction binds the filler and the oligomer, so when a stress is applied to a composite, the stress can be transferred from one strong filler particle to another through the rather low-strength polymer. As a result, the strength of the composite is intermediate to that of the filler and the polymer separately. This bond can be degraded by water absorbed by the composite during clinical use.

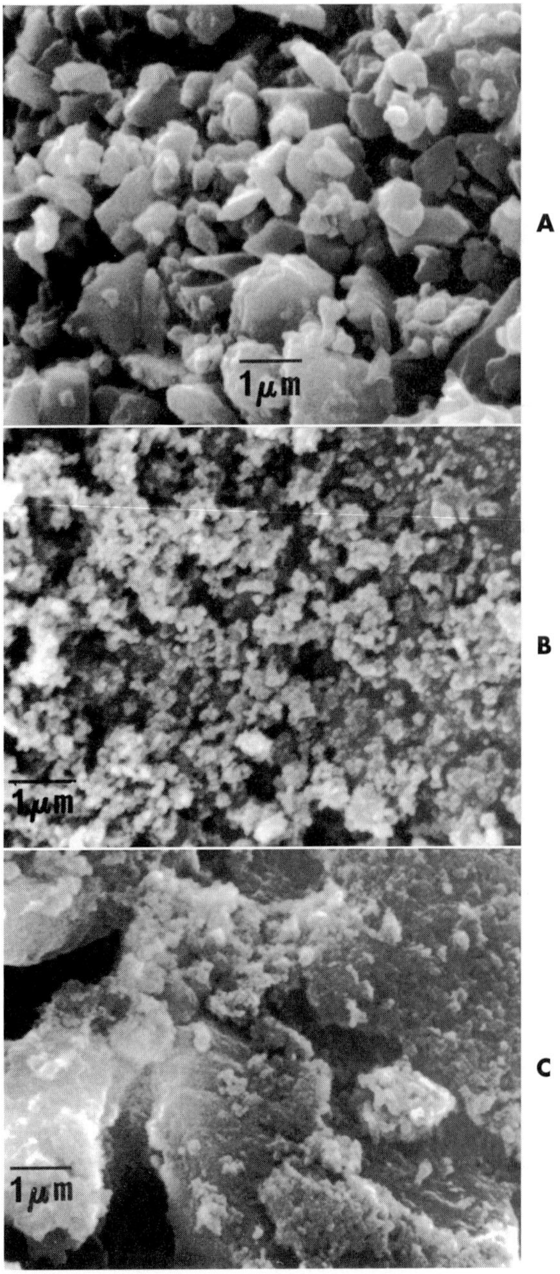

Fig. 9-2 Scanning electron micrographs of types of filler. **A,** Fine inorganic filler; **B,** microfine silica filler; **C,** microfine silica in organic polymer filler.

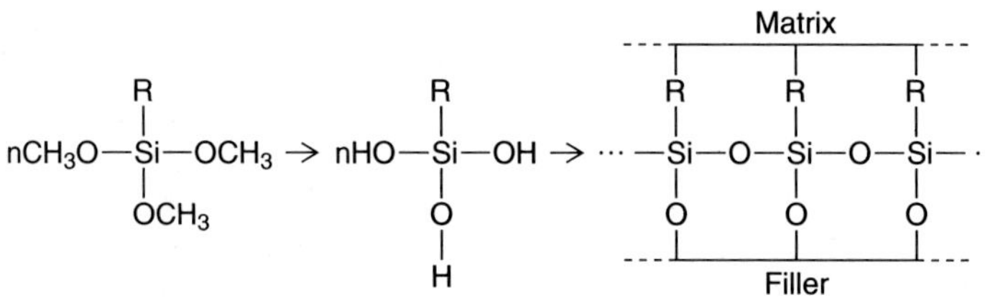

$$nCH_3O-\underset{\underset{OCH_3}{|}}{\overset{\overset{R}{|}}{Si}}-OCH_3 \rightarrow nHO-\underset{\underset{\underset{H}{|}}{\overset{|}{O}}}{\overset{\overset{R}{|}}{Si}}-OH \rightarrow \cdots -\underset{\underset{O}{|}}{\overset{\overset{R}{|}}{Si}}-O-\underset{\underset{O}{|}}{\overset{\overset{R}{|}}{Si}}-O-\underset{\underset{O}{|}}{\overset{\overset{R}{|}}{Si}}-\cdots$$

Matrix / Filler

Initiators and Accelerators   Composites are light cured or self-cured, with the former being more common. Light activation is accomplished with blue light with a peak wavelength of about 470 nm, which is absorbed usually by a photo-activator, such as camphoroquinone, added by the manufacturer in amounts varying from 0.2% to 1.0%. The reaction is accelerated by the presence of an organic amine containing a carbon double bond (see Chapter 7). The amine and the camphoroquinone are stable in the presence of the oligomer at room temperature, as long as the composite is not exposed to light. Although camphoroquinone is the most common photo-activator, others are sometimes used to accommodate special curing conditions, such as the use of plasma-arc lights with rapid-cured composites.

Chemical activation is accomplished at room temperature by an organic amine (catalyst paste) reacting with an organic peroxide (universal paste) to produce free radicals, which in turn attack the carbon double bonds, causing polymerization. Once the two pastes are mixed, the polymerization reaction proceeds rapidly.

Some composites, such as core and provisional products, are dual cured. These formulations contain initiators and accelerators that allow light activation followed by self-curing or self-curing alone.

Pigments and Other Components   Inorganic oxides are usually added in small amounts to provide shades that match the majority of tooth shades. Numerous shades are supplied, ranging from white bleaching shades to yellow to gray. An ultraviolet (UV) absorber may be added to minimize color changes caused by oxidation.

SETTING REACTION

The basic chemistry and general setting reactions for free-radical addition polymerization are presented in Chapter 7. The polymerization reaction of self-cured composites is chemically initiated with a peroxide initiator and an amine accelerator. Polymerization of light-cured composites is initiated by visible blue light. Dual-cured products use a combination of chemical and light activation to carry out the polymerization reaction. Light-curing units are described in detail later in this chapter.

The polymerized resin is highly cross-linked because of the presence of the difunctional carbon double bonds. The degree of polymerization varies, depending on whether it is in the bulk or in the air-inhibited layer of the restoration. The polymerization of light-cured composites varies according to the distance from the composite to the light and the duration of light exposure. The percentage of the double bonds that react may vary from 35% to 80%. The degree of polymerization is higher for laboratory composites that are post-cured at elevated temperatures.

PACKAGING OF COMPOSITES

Light-Cured Composites   These composites are supplied in various shades in spills, syringes, and compules, examples of which are shown in Fig. 9-3. The syringes are made of opaque plastic to protect the material from exposure to light and thus provide adequate shelf life. If packaged as a compule, the compule is placed on the end of a syringe, and the paste is extruded after removal of the protective tip. The advantages of compules are ease of placement of the composite paste, decrease in cross infection,

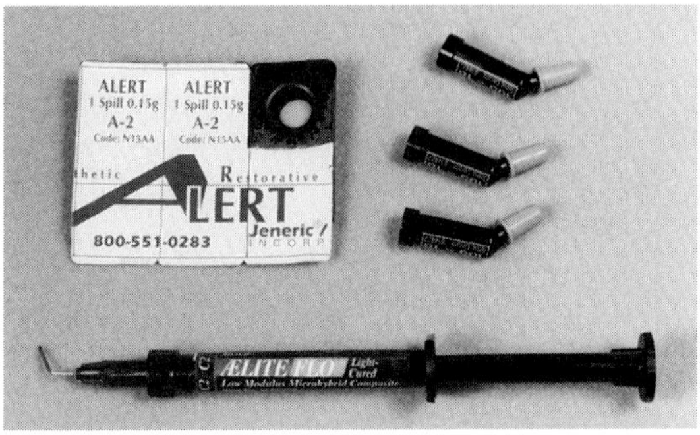

Fig. 9-3 Single-paste, visible light–initiated composite.

(From Craig RG, Powers JM, Wataha JC: *Dental materials: properties and manipulation,* ed 7, St Louis, 2000, Mosby.)

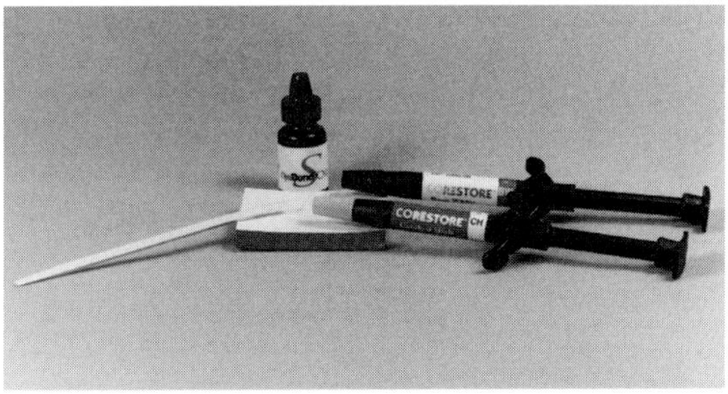

Fig. 9-4 Self-cured, two-paste core composite with single-bottle bonding agent.

(From Craig RG, Powers JM, Wataha JC: *Dental materials: properties and manipulation,* ed 7, St Louis, 2000, Mosby.)

and protection of the paste from exposure to ambient light.

Self-Cured/Dual-Cured Composites

Self- and dual-cured composites are typically packaged in syringes or tubs of paste and catalyst and require mixing. An example of a two-paste core composite is shown in Fig. 9-4.

PROPERTIES OF COMPOSITES

OVERVIEW

Important properties of composites include working and setting times, polymerization shrinkage, thermal properties, water sorption and solubility, mechanical properties, color stability, and radiopacity. Selected properties of all-purpose, microfilled, packable, flowable, laboratory, and core composites plus compomers are listed in Table 9-3. Values of properties for polymer-based filling and restorative materials based on ISO 4049 (ANSI/ADA No. 27) are summarized in Table 9-4.

PHYSICAL PROPERTIES

Working and Setting Times For light-cured composites, initiation of polymerization is related specifically to the application of the light beam to the material; about 75% of the polymerization takes place during the first 10 minutes. The curing reaction continues for a period of 24 hours. Not all of the available unsaturated carbon double bonds react; studies report that about 25% remain unreacted in the bulk of the restoration. If the surface of the restoration is not protected from air by a transparent matrix, polymerization is inhibited; the number of unreacted carbon double bonds may be as high as 75% in the tacky surface layer. Although the restoration can be finished with abrasives and is functional after 10 minutes, the optimum physical properties are not reached until about 24 hours after the reaction is initiated.

For most composites that are initiated by visible light, there is a critical time period after dispensing of the paste onto a paper pad during which fresh composite flows against tooth structure at an optimum level. Within 60 to 90 seconds after exposure to ambient light, the surface of the composite may lose its capability to flow readily against tooth structure, and further work with the material becomes difficult. Fluorescent lights labeled "gold" can be substituted to provide unlimited working time for light-cured composites.

The setting times for chemically activated composites range from 3 to 5 minutes. These short setting times have been accomplished by controlling the concentration of initiator and accelerator.

Polymerization Shrinkage The linear polymerization shrinkage of typical composites are listed in Table 9-3. Free volumetric polymer-

TABLE 9-3 Properties of Various Types of Composites and Compomers

Property	All-Purpose Composite	Microfilled Composite	Packable Composite	Flowable Composite	Laboratory Composite	Core Composite	Compomer
Flexural strength (MPa)	80-160	60-120	85-110	70-120	90-150†	—	65-125
Flexural modulus (GPa)	8.8-13	4.0-6.9	9.0-12	2.6-5.6	4.7-15†	—	4.5-14
Flexural fatigue limit (MPa)	60-110	—	—	—	—	—	70
Compressive strength (MPa)	240-290	240-300	220-300	210-300	210-280†	210-250	180-250
Compressive modulus (GPa)	5.5-8.3	2.6-4.8	5.8-9.0	2.6-5.9	—	7.5-22	6-7
Diametral tensile strength (MPa)	30-55	25-40	—	33-48	—	40-50	25-40
Linear polymerization shrinkage (%)	0.7-1.4	2-3	0.6-0.9	—	—	—	—
Color stability, accelerated aging—450 kJ/m^2 (ΔE^*)‡	1.5	—	—	1.5	1.1-2.3	—	2.1
Color stability, stained by juice/tea (ΔE^*)‡	4.3	—	—	—	1.7-3.9	—	5.7

†Without fiber reinforcement.
‡ΔE^* <3.3 is considered not clinically perceptible.

TABLE 9-4 Requirements for Polymer-based Filling and Restorative Materials Based on ISO 4049

Property	Class 1	Class 2	Class 3
Working time (min, sec)	90	—	90
Setting time (max, min)	5	—	10
Depth of cure (min, mm)			
Opaque shades	—	1.0	—
Other shades	—	1.5	—
Water sorption (max, μg/mm³)	40	40	40
Solubility (max, μg/mm³)	7.5	7.5	7.5
Flexural strength (MPa)			
Type 1	80	80* 100†	80
Type 2	50	50*	50

*Group 1: cured intraorally.
†Group 2: cured extraorally.

ization shrinkage is a direct function of the amount of oligomer and diluent, and thus microhybrid composites shrink only 0.6% to 1.4%, compared with shrinkage of microfilled composites of 2% to 3%. This shrinkage creates polymerization stresses as high as 13 MPa between the composite and tooth structure. These stresses severely strain the interfacial bond between the composite and the tooth, leading to a very small gap that can allow marginal leakage of saliva. This stress can exceed the tensile strength of enamel and result in stress cracking and enamel fractures along the interfaces. The potential for this type of failure is even greater with microfilled composites, in which there is a much higher volume percent of polymer present, and polymerization shrinkage is greater. The net effect of polymerization shrinkage can be reduced by incrementally adding a light-cured composite and polymerizing each increment independently, which allows for some contraction within each increment before successive additions.

Thermal Properties The thermal expansion coefficient of composites ranges from 25 to $38 \times 10^{-6}/° C$ for composites with fine particles to 55 to $68 \times 10^{-6}/° C$ for composites with microfine particles. The values for composites are considerably less than the average of the values for the polymer matrix and the inorganic phase, however, the values are higher than those for dentin ($8.3 \times 10^{-6}/° C$) and enamel ($11.4 \times 10^{-6}/° C$). The higher values for the microfilled composites are related mostly to the greater amount of polymer present. Certain glasses may be more effective in reducing the effect of thermal change than are others, and some resins have more than one type of filler to compensate for differential rates.

Thermal stresses place an additional strain on the bond to tooth structure, which further compounds the detrimental effect of the polymerization shrinkage. Thermal changes are also cyclic in nature, and although the entire restoration may never reach thermal equilibrium during the application of either hot or cold stimuli, the cyclic effect can lead to material fatigue and early bond failure. If a gap were formed, the difference between the thermal coefficient of expansion of composites and teeth could allow for the percolation of oral fluids.

The thermal conductivity of composites with fine particles (25 to 30 × 10^{-4} cal/sec/cm^2 [° C/cm]) is greater than that of composites with microfine particles (12 to 15 × 10^{-4} cal/sec/cm^2 [° C/cm]) because of the higher conductivity of the inorganic fillers compared with the polymer matrix. However, for highly transient temperatures the composites do not change temperature as fast as tooth structure and this difference does not present a clinical problem.

Water Sorption The water sorption of composites with fine particles (0.3 to 0.6 mg/cm^2) is greater than that of composites with microfine particles (1.2 to 2.2 mg/cm^2), because of the lower volume fraction of polymer in the composites with fine particles. The quality and stability of the silane coupling agent are important in minimizing the deterioration of the bond between the filler and polymer and the amount of water sorption. It has been postulated that the corresponding expansion associated with the uptake of water from oral fluids could relieve polymerization stresses. In the measurement of hygroscopic expansion starting 15 minutes after the initial polymerization, most resins required 7 days to reach equilibrium and about 4 days to show the majority of expansion. Because composites with fine particles have lower values of water sorption than composites with microfine particles, they exhibit less expansion when exposed to water.

Solubility The water solubility of composites varies from 0.01 to 0.06 mg/cm^2. Adequate exposure to the light source is critical in light-cured composites. Inadequate polymerization can readily occur at a depth from the surface if insufficient light penetrates. Inadequately polymerized resin has greater water sorption and solubility, possibly manifested clinically with early color instability.

During the storage of microhybrid composites in water, the leaching of inorganic ions can be detected; such ions are associated with a breakdown in interfacial bonding. Silicon leaches into the water bath in the greatest quantity (15 to 17 μg/ml) during the first 30 days of storage and decreases with time of exposure. Microfilled composites leach silicon more slowly and show a 100% increase in amount during the second 30-day period (14.2 μg/ml). Boron, barium, strontium, and lead, which are present in glass fillers, are leached to various degrees (6 to 19 μg/ml) from the various resin-filler systems. Breakdown and leakage can be a contributing factor to the reduced resistance to wear and abrasion of composites.

Color and Color Stability The color and blending of shades for the clinical match of esthetic restorations are important. The characteristics of color are discussed in Chapter 3, and these principles can be applied specifically to composites for determining appropriate shades for clinical use. Universal shades vary in color among currently marketed products.

Change of color and loss of shade-match with surrounding tooth structure are reasons for replacing restorations. Stress cracks within the polymer matrix and partial debonding of the filler to the resin as a result of hydrolysis tend to increase opacity and alter appearance. Discoloration can also occur by oxidation and result from water exchange within the polymer matrix and its interaction with unreacted polymer sites and unused initiator or accelerator.

Color stability of current composites has been studied by artificial aging in a weathering chamber (exposure to UV light and elevated temperatures of 70 °C) and by immersion in various stains (coffee/tea, cranberry/grape juice, red wine, sesame oil). As shown in Table 9-3, composites are resistant to color changes caused by oxidation but are susceptible to staining.

MECHANICAL PROPERTIES

Flexural Strength and Modulus Values of flexural strength and modulus for composites are listed in Table 9-3. The flexural strengths of the various composites are similar. The flexural moduli of microfilled and flowable composites are about 50% lower than values for all-purpose and packable composites, which reflects the lower volume percent filler present in the microfilled and flowable composites (see Table 9-2).

Compressive Strength and Modulus

Values of compressive strength and modulus for composites are listed in Table 9-3. The compressive strengths of the various composites are similar. The flexural moduli of microfilled and flowable composites are typically lower than values for all-purpose and packable composites, which reflects the lower volume percent filler present in the microfilled and flowable composites (see Table 9-2). For comparison, the modulus of elasticity in compression is 62 GPa for amalgam, 19 GPa for dentin, and 83 GPa for enamel.

Knoop Hardness Values of Knoop hardness for composites (22 to 80 kg/mm^2) are low compared with values of 343 kg/mm^2 for human enamel and 110 kg/mm^2 for dental amalgam. The Knoop hardness of composites with fine particles is somewhat greater than values for composites with microfine particles because of the hardness and volume fraction of the filler particles. These values indicate a moderate resistance to indentation under functional stresses for the more highly filled composites, but this difference does not appear to be a major factor in resisting functional wear.

A microhardness measurement such as Knoop can be misleading on composites with large filler particles (>10 μm in diameter), in which the small indentation could be made solely on the organic or the inorganic phase. However, with most current products, filler particle sizes have become much smaller (<1 μm), and the microhardness values appear more reliable.

Bond Strength to Dental Substrates

Bonding of composites to tooth structure and other dental substrates is discussed in detail in Chapter 10.

Enamel and Dentin The bond strength of composites to etched enamel and dentin is typically between 20 and 30 MPa. Bonding is principally a result of micromechanical retention of the bonding agent into the etched surfaces of enamel and dentin. In dentin, a hybrid layer of bonding resin and collagen is often formed, and the bonding adhesive penetrates the dentinal tubules (Fig. 9-5).

Other Substrates Composite can be bonded to existing composite restorations, ceramics, and alloys when the substrate is roughened and primed appropriately (see Chapter 10). In general, the surface to be bonded is sandblasted (microetched) with 50-μm alumina and then treated with a resin-silane primer for composite, a silane primer for ceramic, or a special alloy primer. Bond strengths to treated surfaces are typically greater than 20 MPa.

CLINICAL PROPERTIES

Clinical requirements for composites accepted for unrestricted use, including cuspal replacement in posterior teeth as defined by American Dental Association (Proposed) Guidelines for Resin-based Composites for Posterior Restorations, are listed in Table 9-5.

Depth of Cure (Light-cured Composites)

Maximum intensity of the light radiation beam is concentrated near the surface of a light-cured composite. As the light penetrates the material, it is scattered and reflected and loses intensity. A number of factors influence the degree of polymerization at given depths from the surface after light curing. The concentration of photoinitiator or light absorber in the composite must be such that it will react at the proper wavelength and be present in sufficient concentration. Both filler content and particle size are critical to dispersion of the light beam. For this reason, microfilled composites with smaller and more numerous particles scatter more light than microhybrid composites with larger and fewer glass particles. Longer exposure times are needed to obtain adequate depth of cure of microfilled composites.

The light intensity at the resin surface is a

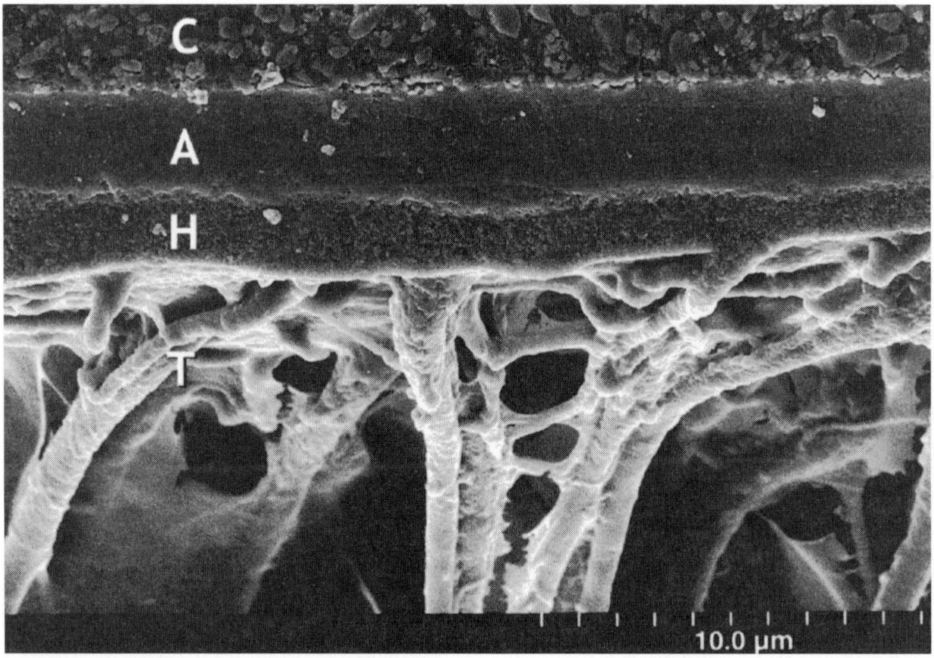

Fig. 9-5 Transverse section of composite bonded to dentin showing composite *(C)*, adhesive layer *(A)*, hybrid layer *(H)*, and resin tags *(T)*.
(Courtesy Dr. Jorge Perdigao, University of Minnesota.)

TABLE 9-5 Clinical Requirements for Composites Accepted for Unrestricted Use, Including Cuspal Replacement, in Posterior Teeth*

Property	Criteria
Maintenance of color (18 mo)	No more than 10% Charlie
Marginal discoloration (18 mo)	No more than 10% Charlie
Marginal integrity (18 mo)	No more than 5% Charlie
Caries—recurrent or marginal (18 mo)	No more than 5% Charlie
Maintenance of interproximal contact (18 mo)	95% showing no observable broadening of contacts
Postoperative sensitivity	Thorough history of adverse sensitivity to hot, cold, and biting stimuli
Failure (18 mo)	No more than 5%
Wear between 6 and 18 mo	No more than 50 μm

*Proposed American Dental Association guidelines for resin-based composites for posterior restorations.
A = alpha, *B* = bravo, *C* = charlie

critical factor in completeness of cure at the surface and within the material. The tip of the light source must be held within 1 mm of the surface to gain optimum penetration. More-opaque shades reduce light transmission and cure only to minimal depths (1 mm). A standard exposure time using most visible lights is 20 seconds. In general, this is sufficient to cure a light shade of resin to a depth of 2 or 2.5 mm. A 40-second exposure improves the degree of cure at all depths, but it is required to obtain sufficient cure with the darker shades. Application of the light beam through 1 mm or less thickness of tooth structure produces a sufficient cure at shallower depths, but the hardness values obtained are not consistent. Because the light beam does not spread sufficiently beyond the diameter of the tip at the emitting surface, it is necessary to "step" the light across the surface of large restorations so the entire surface receives a complete exposure. Larger tips have been manufactured for placement on most light-curing units. However, as the light beam is distributed over a larger surface area, the intensity at a given point is reduced. Use a longer exposure time of up to 60 seconds when larger emitting tips are used.

To evaluate the effective depth of cure of a specific light-curing unit, cut a small section of 5 to 10 mm from a clear straw and place it on a glass slide. Pack the section with composite. Apply the light directly to the top surface for 20 to 40 seconds according to the recommended technique. Cut off the straw, and scrape uncured composite from the bottom of the specimen with a sharp knife. Measure the length of the apparently cured specimen and divide in half to estimate the effective depth of cure.

Radiopacity Modern composites include glasses having atoms with high atomic numbers, such as barium, strontium, and zirconium. Some fillers, such as quartz, lithium-aluminum glasses, and silica, are not radiopaque and must be blended with other fillers to produce a radiopaque composite. Even at their highest volume fraction of filler, the amount of radiopacity seen in composites is noticeably less than that exhibited by a metallic restorative like amalgam. The microhybrid composites achieve some radiopacity by incorporating very finely divided heavy-metal glass particles.

Aluminum is used as a standard reference for radiopacity. A 2-mm thickness of dentin is equivalent in radiopacity to 2.5 mm of aluminum, and enamel is equivalent to 4 mm of aluminum. To be effective, a composite should exceed the radiopacity of enamel, but international standards accept radiopacity equivalent to 2 mm of aluminum. Amalgam has a radiopacity greater than 10 mm of aluminum, which exceeds all the composite materials available.

Wear Rates Clinical studies have shown that composites are superior materials for anterior restorations in which esthetics are essential and occlusal forces are low. One problem with composites is the loss of surface contour of composite restorations in the mouth, which results from a combination of abrasive wear from chewing and toothbrushing and erosive wear from degradation of the composite in the oral environment (Fig. 9-6).

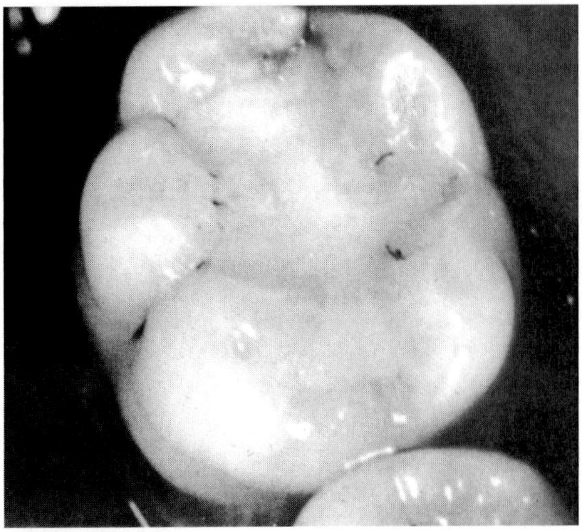

Fig. 9-6 A posterior composite resin restoration exhibiting excessive occlusal wear and marginal discoloration.

Wear of posterior composite restorations is observed at the contact area where stresses are the highest. Interproximal wear has also been observed. Ditching at the margins within the composite is observed for posterior composites, probably resulting from inadequate bonding and polymerization stresses. Currently accepted composites for posterior applications require clinical studies that demonstrate, over a 5-year period, a loss of surface contour less than 250 μm or an average of 50 μm per year of clinical service. Products developed as packable or laboratory composites usually have better wear resistance than microfilled or flowable composites.

Biocompatibility Details about the biocompatibility of composites are discussed in Chapter 5, but some of the central issues are mentioned here. Nearly all of the major components of composites (Bis-GMA, TEGDMA, and UDMA, among others) have been found cytotoxic *in vitro* if used in pure form, but the biological liability of a cured composite depends on the release of these components from the composite. Although composites release some levels of components for weeks after curing, there is considerable controversy about the biological effects of these components. The amount of release depends on the type of composite and the method and efficiency of the cure of the composite. A dentin barrier markedly reduces the ability of components to reach pulpal tissues, but these components can traverse dentin barriers, albeit at reduced concentrations. The effects of low-dose, long-term exposures of cells to resin components is not generally known. On the other hand, the use of composite materials as direct pulp-capping agents poses a higher risk for adverse biological responses, because no dentin barrier exists to limit exposure of the pulp to the released components.

The effects of released components from composites on oral or other tissues is not known with certainty, although no studies have documented any adverse biological effects. The tissue at highest risk from this type of release would appear to be gingiva in close, long-term contact with composites. Components of composites are known allergens, and there has been some documentation of contact allergy to composites. Most of these reactions occur with dentists or dental personnel who regularly handle uncured composite and, therefore, have the greatest exposure. There are no good studies documenting the frequency of allergy to composites in the general population.

Finally, there has been some controversy about the ability of components of composites to act as xenoestrogens. Studies have proven that Bis-phenol A and its dimethacrylate are estrogenic in *in vitro* tests that measure this effect using breast cancer cell growth. Trace levels of these components have been identified in some commercial composites; however, estrogencity from cured commercial composites has not been demonstrated. Furthermore, there is considerable controversy about the accuracy and utility of *in vitro* tests using breast cancer cells to measure a true estrogenic effect. An early study in this area, which claimed that dental sealants and composites were estrogenic in children, has since been largely discredited.

MANIPULATION OF COMPOSITES

PULPAL PROTECTION

If a deep cavity exists after preparation, protect the pulp with a calcium hydroxide cavity liner or glass ionomer, hybrid ionomer, or compomer base. Liners and bases are described in Chapter 20.

ETCHING AND BONDING

To provide a bond between composite and tooth structure, etch the enamel and dentin of the cavity preparation with acid for 30 seconds with an etchant supplied by the manufacturer, often a 34% to 37% phosphoric acid solution or gel. Flush the acid away with water, and gently dry the surface with a stream of air. The etched enamel will appear dull. The bonding agent penetrates the etched enamel and dentin surfaces and provides micromechanical retention of the restoration. Recently, self-etching primers have been developed that do not require etching with phosphoric acid or rinsing. Bonding agents and their interactions with tooth structure are discussed in Chapter 10.

DISPENSING

Light-Cured Composites Dispense small increments of composite onto a paper pad and pack into the cavity preparation as described subsequently. A controlled setting time allows for the individual polymerization of small increments of composite, thus permitting the use of multiple shades of composite within a single restoration and accommodating polymerization shrinkage within each increment as opposed to the total shrinkage in a bulk-cure method.

Self- and Dual-Cured Composites An example of a self-cured, core composite supplied as two pastes is shown in Fig. 9-4. One syringe contains the peroxide initiator or catalyst and the other syringe includes the amine accelerator. Mix equal amounts of universal and catalyst pastes thoroughly for 20 to 30 seconds. Use plastic or wooden spatulas, but avoid metal spatulas, because the inorganic filler particles are abrasive and small amounts of the metal can be abraded and discolor the composite.

INSERTION

The composite can be inserted into the cavity preparation by several methods. Place it with a plastic instrument, such as one of those shown in Fig. 9-7, *A*, which does not stick to the composite during insertion. The composite may also be placed in the plastic tip of a syringe, such as shown in Fig. 9-7, *B*, and then injected into the cavity preparation. The syringe or compule allows the use of small mixes, reduces the problem of incorporating voids in the composite during insertion, and facilitates placement of the material in the areas of retention.

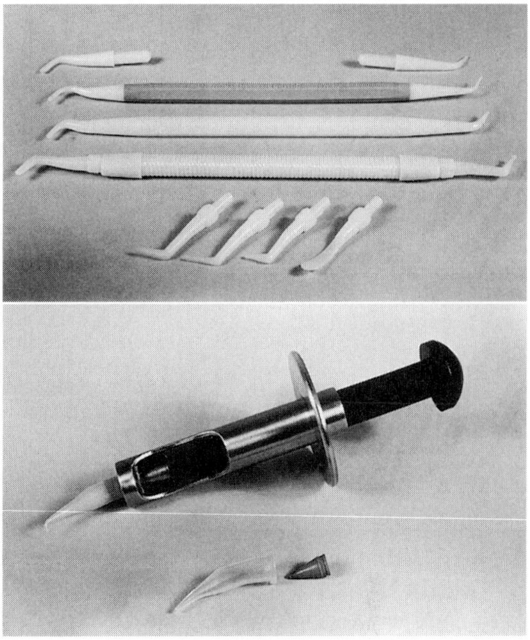

A

B

Fig. 9-7 **A,** Instruments for placing composites. **B,** Syringe for injecting composites.

(From Craig RG, Powers JM, Wataha JC: *Dental materials: properties and manipulation,* ed 7, St Louis, 2000, Mosby.)

POLYMERIZATION

Light-Cured Composites Exposure times for polymerization vary depending on the type of light-curing unit and the type, depth, and shade of the composite. Times may vary from 20 to 60 seconds for a restoration 2 mm thick. Microfilled composites require longer exposure than microhybrid composites because the small filler particles scatter the light more. Darker shades or more opaque composites require longer exposure times (up to 60 seconds longer) than lighter shades or more translucent composites. In deep restorations, add and polymerize the composite in layers. One layer bonds to another without any loss of strength.

TABLE 9-6 Surface Roughness (μm) of Various Types of Composites

Finisher/Polisher	All-purpose Composite	Microfilled Composite	Packable Composite	Laboratory Composite
Mylar surface	0.03-0.07	0.03-0.08	0.08-0.18	0.02-0.04
Diamond finishing bur	1.20-1.60	—	1.10-2.10	0.67-0.80
Carbide bur (16-fluted)	0.29-0.52	0.38-0.57	0.51-0.74	0.21-0.26
Composite polishers*	0.20-0.37	0.12-0.17	0.37	0.11-0.17
Aluminum oxide, xfine*	0.09-0.15	0.07-0.11	0.14-0.17	0.08-0.09

*After finishing with 16-fluted carbide bur.

The setting time of light-cured composite and the depth of cure within a given mass depend on the intensity and penetration of the light. A material with a low absorption coefficient cures to the greatest depth. The presence of ultraviolet absorbers for color stabilization, fluorescent dyes for esthetics, or excessive initiator concentration has a detrimental effect on completeness of cure.

Light-curing units are discussed in detail later in this chapter.

Self- and Dual-Cured Composites After mixing, the self-cured composite has a working (or insertion) time of 1 to 1½ minutes. The mix will begin to harden, and the material should not be disturbed until the setting time of about 4 to 5 minutes from the start of the mix.

Dual-cured composites contain chemical accelerators and light activators, so polymerization can be initiated by light and then continued by the self-cured mechanism.

FINISHING AND POLISHING

For gross reduction, use diamonds, carbide finishing burs, finishing disks, or strips of alumina. For final finishing of either microhybrid or microfilled composites, use abrasive-impregnated rubber rotary instruments or a rubber cup with various polishing pastes. Finishing should be done in a wet field with a water-soluble lubricant. Final finishing of light-cured composites can be started immediately after light curing.

Polishing is the final step of finishing and is usually performed with aluminum oxide abrasives with progressively finer grit sizes. Polishing of composites is important, because a smooth surface is desired to prevent retention of plaque and is needed to maintain good oral hygiene.

A measure of the quality of polishing is surface roughness. A comparison of surface roughness of various composites is listed in Table 9-6. The smoothest surface is achieved by use of a Mylar matrix. Carbide burs produce smoother surfaces than diamond burs, but after polishing the surface roughness is similar.

COMPOSITES FOR SPECIAL APPLICATIONS

MICROFILLED COMPOSITES

These composites are recommended for use in Class 3 and Class 5 restorations, where a high polish and esthetics are most important. One product has been used successfully in posterior restorations. They are composed of light-activated, dimethacrylate resins with 0.04-μm colloidal silica fillers with a filler loading of 32-50% by volume (see Table 9-2).

Typical properties of microfilled composites are listed in Table 9-3. Because they are less highly filled, microfilled composites have higher values of polymerization shrinkage, water sorption and thermal expansion as compared with microhybrid composites.

PACKABLE COMPOSITES

These composites (see Table 9-1) are recommended for use in Classes 1, 2, and 6 (MOD) cavity preparations. They are composed of light-activated, dimethacrylate resins with fillers (fibers or porous or irregular particles) that have a filler loading of 66% to 70% by volume (see Table 9-2). The interaction of the filler particles and modifications of the resin cause these composites to be packable.

Typical properties of packable composites are listed in Table 9-3. Important properties include high depth of cure, low polymerization shrinkage, radiopacity, and low wear rate (3.5 μm/year), which is similar to that of amalgam. Several packable composites are packaged in unit-dose compules. A bulk-fill technique is recommended by manufacturers but has not yet been demonstrated effective in clinical studies. Use single-bottle bonding agents with these composites.

FLOWABLE COMPOSITES

These light-cured, low-viscosity composites are recommended for cervical lesions, pediatric restorations, and other small, low stress–bearing restorations (see Table 9-1). They contain dimethacrylate resin and inorganic fillers with a particle size of 0.7 to 3.0 μm and filler loading of 42% to 53% by volume (see Table 9-2).

Typical properties of flowable composites are listed in Table 9-3. Flowable composites have a low modulus of elasticity, which may make them useful in cervical abfraction areas. Because of their lower filler content, they exhibit higher polymerization shrinkage and lower wear resistance than microhybrid composites. The viscosity of these composites allows them to be dispensed by a syringe for easy handling.

LABORATORY COMPOSITES

Crowns, inlays, veneers bonded to metal substructures, and metal-free bridges are prepared indirectly on dies from composites processed in the laboratory (see Table 9-1), using various combinations of light, heat, pressure, and vacuum to increase the degree of polymerization and the wear resistance.

Typical properties of laboratory composites are listed in Table 9-3. For increased strength and rigidity, laboratory composites can be combined with fiber reinforcement. Restorations are usually bonded with composite cements. Cavity preparations for indirect composites must be nonretentive rather than retentive, as typically prepared for direct placement.

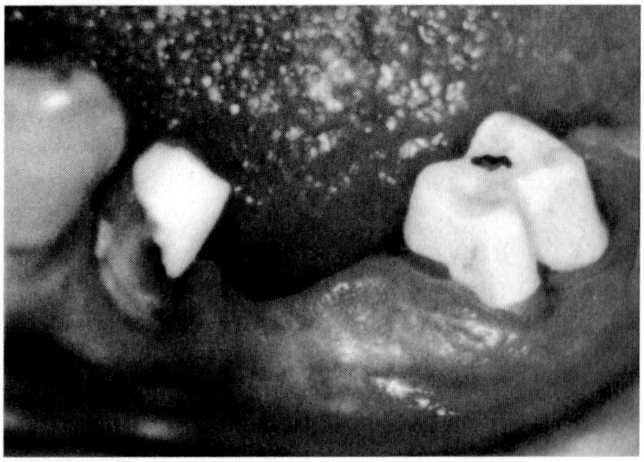

Fig. 9-8 A reconstructed composite resin core prepared for a cast metal crown.

CORE COMPOSITES

At times, so much tooth structure is lost from caries that the crown of the tooth must be built up to receive a crown. Amalgam is the most common core material, but composite is becoming popular. Composite core materials are typically two-paste, self-cured composites (see Fig. 9-4), although light-cured and dual-cured products are available. Core composites are usually tinted (blue, white, or opaque) to provide a contrasting color with the tooth structure. Some products release fluoride. An example of a composite core build-up is shown in Fig. 9-8. Typical properties of core composites are listed in Table 9-3.

Composite cores have the following advantages as compared with amalgam: can be bonded to dentin, can be finished immediately, are easy to contour, have high rigidity, and have good color under ceramic restorations. Composite cores are bonded to remaining enamel and dentin using bonding agents. Be careful to use a bonding agent recommended by the manufacturer of the core material, because some self-cured composite core materials are incompatible with some light-cured bonding agents.

TABLE 9-7 Properties of Provisional Composites and Acrylics

Property	Provisional Composite	Provisional Acrylic
Flexural strength (MPa)	35-70	45-80
Flexural modulus (GPa)	0.8-2.5	0.8-2.6
Compressive strength (MPa)	130-260	—
Linear polymerization shrinkage (%)	2.5-3.3	2.7-7.0
Color stability, accelerated aging—60 kJ/m^2 (ΔE)*†	0.5-9.5	2.0-8.0
Color stability, staining (ΔE)*†	4.9-11	1.2-3.6

†ΔE* <3.3 is considered not clinically perceptible.

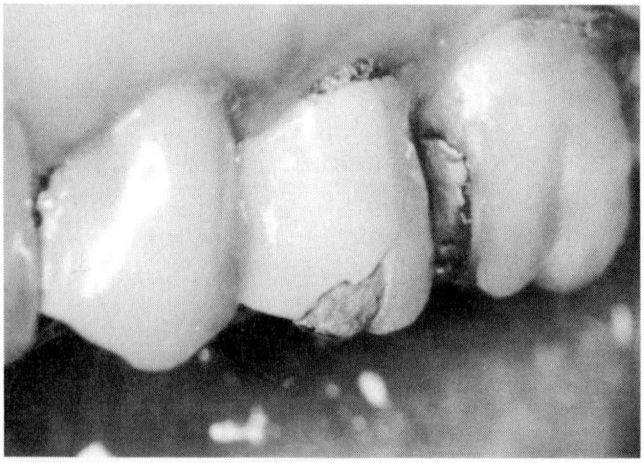

Fig. 9-9 A fractured porcelain-fused-to-metal restoration that could be repaired with composite resin.

PROVISIONAL COMPOSITES

Temporary inlays, crowns, and long-span bridges are usually fabricated from composite or acrylic resins. The purposes of provisional restorations are to maintain the position of the prepared tooth, seal and insulate the preparation and protect the margins, establish proper vertical dimension, aid in diagnosis and treatment planning, and evaluate esthetic replacements. The properties of acrylic and composite provisional materials are compared in Table 9-7.

REPAIR OF CERAMIC OR COMPOSITE

A fractured porcelain-fused-to-metal restoration, as shown in Fig. 9-9, may be repaired using an all-purpose or flowable composite. These repairs require adequate bond strength between the remaining ceramic and alloy and the added composite. To achieve the maximum bond strength, the remaining ceramic/alloy surface is cleaned and treated with a silane, resin, or silane-resin primer supplied in a liquid form. The primer is supplied separately, and a composite of choice is used with it.

The repair of composites is accomplished by abrading the surface of the remaining composite with 50-μm alumina, then keeping the surface well isolated from saliva and moisture. Treat the surface of the composite with primer, and add the new composite. Repair bond-strength is about 60% to 80% of the cohesive strength of the original composite.

COMPOMERS

Compomers or poly acid–modified composites are used for restorations in low stress–bearing areas, although a recent product is recommended by the manufacturer for Class 1 and Class 2 restorations in adults (see Table 9-1). Compomers are recommended for patients at medium risk of developing caries.

COMPOSITION AND SETTING REACTION

Compomers contain poly acid–modified monomers with fluoride-releasing silicate glasses and are formulated without water. Some compomers have modified monomers that provide additional fluoride release. The volume percent filler ranges from 42% to 67% and the average filler particle size ranges from 0.8 to 5.0 μm. Compomers are packaged as single-paste formula-

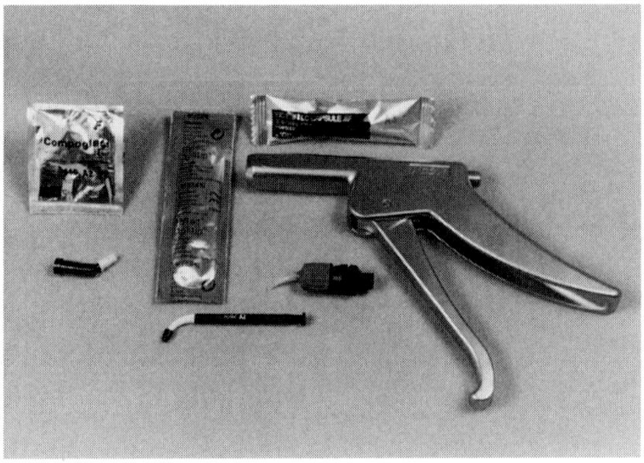

Fig. 9-10 Examples of compomers (packaged in compules and syringes) and a hybrid ionomer (packaged in capsules with applier) for restoring cervically eroded teeth.

(From Craig RG, Powers JM, Wataha JC: *Dental materials: properties and manipulation,* ed 7, St Louis, 2000, Mosby.)

tions in compules and syringes, as shown in Fig. 9-10.

Setting occurs primarily by light-cured polymerization, but an acid-base reaction also occurs as the compomer absorbs water after placement and upon contact with saliva. Water uptake is also important for fluoride transfer.

PROPERTIES

Typical properties of compomers are listed in Table 9-3. Compomers release fluoride by a mechanism similar to that of glass and hybrid ionomers. Because of the lower amount of glass ionomer present in compomers, the amount of fluoride release and its duration are lower than those of glass and hybrid ionomers. Also, compomers do not recharge from fluoride treatments or brushing with fluoride dentifrices as much as glass and hybrid ionomers.

MANIPULATION

Compomers are formulated as a single-paste packaged in unit-dose compules. Because of their resin content, compomers require a bonding agent to bond to tooth structure. Some compomers are used with single-bottle bonding agents that contain acidic primers. Acidic primers bond to enamel and dentin without the need for additional etching with phosphoric acid. However, most manufacturers recommend phosphoric acid etching before priming to improve bond strength.

LIGHT-CURING UNITS

OVERVIEW

The most common light-curing source used in dentistry is the quartz-tungsten-halogen light. In the mid-1990s, high-intensity, plasma-arc lights were introduced. In 2000, blue light–emitting diodes became available. Definitions of terms used to describe light sources used to polymerize dental resins are listed in Table 9-8.

QUARTZ-TUNGSTEN-HALOGEN LIGHT-CURING UNITS

An example of a quartz-tungsten-halogen (QTH) light-curing unit used to activate polymerization of composites is shown in Fig. 9-11. The peak wavelength varies among units from about 450 to 490 nm. Typically, the intensity (power density) ranges from 400 to 800 mW/cm^2, but high-intensity QTH units are available. Some units provide energy at two or three different intensities (step cure) or at a continuously increasing (ramp cure) intensity. A typical resin composite requires an energy density of 16 J/cm^2 (400 $mW/cm^2 \times 40\ s = 16{,}000\ mW\ s/cm^2$) for polymerization.

A decrease in line voltage of 6% shows a corresponding reduction in output of about 25% in intensity in some lamps, but only 10% in lamps with voltage regulators in their circuitry. In general, the output from the various lamps decreases with continuous use and the intensity is not uniform for all areas of the light tip, being greatest at the center. Also, the intensity of the light decreases with distance from the source nearly linearly to the log of the intensity divided by the distance. Although the intensity is important with respect to the depth of cure, it has been shown for some products that a threefold dif-

TABLE 9-8 Definitions of Terms Used to Describe Light Sources for Polymerization of Dental Resins

Term	Unit	Definition
Spectral emission	nm	Effective bandwidth of wavelengths emitted by light source
Spectral requirement	nm	Bandwidth of wavelengths required to activate photo-initiator(s) of dental resin
Power	mW	Number of photons per second emitted by light source
Power density (intensity)	mW/cm^2	Number of photons per second emitted by light source per unit area of curing tip
Energy	J*	Power × time
Energy density	J/cm^2	Power density × time

*Joule (J) = 1000 mW × s.

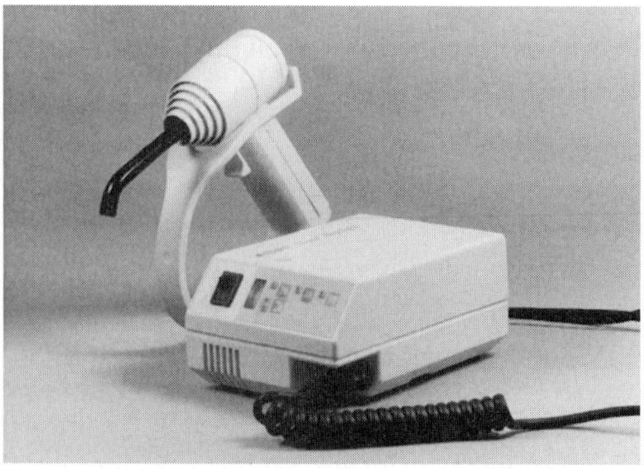

Fig. 9-11 Visible-light sources for photo-initiation of composition.

(From Craig RG, Powers JM, Wataha JC: *Dental materials: properties and manipulation*, ed 7, St Louis, 2000, Mosby.)

ference in intensity had only a 15% difference in the depth of cure. Bulb life ranges from 50 to 75 hours.

Although there is minimal potential for radiation damage to surrounding soft tissue inadvertently exposed to visible light, use caution to prevent retinal damage to the eyes. Because of the high intensity of the light, do not look directly at the tip or the reflected light from the teeth. A number of devices are marketed to filter the visible-light beam so the operator can directly observe the curing procedure and to protect the patient and staff. These devices are eyeglasses, flat shields that can be held over the field of vision, and curved shields that attach directly to the handpiece delivering the light beam (Fig. 9-12).

Some lamps produce considerable heat at the curing tip, which can produce pulpal irritation. Too much heat is being generated if one cannot hold a finger 2 to 3 mm from the tip for 20 seconds.

Maintenance of QTH lights must be provided on a regular basis, as summarized in Table 9-9.

PLASMA-ARC LIGHT-CURING UNITS

Plasma-arc (PAC) lights are high-intensity light-curing units. Light is obtained from an electrically conductive gas (plasma) that forms between two tungsten electrodes under pressure. The output is filtered to minimize transmission of infrared and ultraviolet energy. The energy transmitted is in the visible range between 380 and 500 nm, with an output peak near 480 nm. Because of the high intensity of light available at lower wavelengths, PAC lights are able to

TABLE 9-9 Factors Causing Decrease in Intensity of Light from Quartz-tungsten-halogen (QTH) Light-curing Units and Maintenance Hints

Factors	Maintenance Hints
Dust or deterioration of reflector Burn-out of bulb filament	Clean or replace reflector Replace bulb
Darkening/frosting of bulb Age of components	Replace bulb Monitor intensity, replace unit
Chipping of light tip Resin deposit on light tip	Replace light tip Clean or replace light tip
Change in line voltage Lack of uniformity across light tip	Get built-in voltage regulator Overlap curing on larger surface
Increased distance of tip from material to be cured	Keep light tip close to material

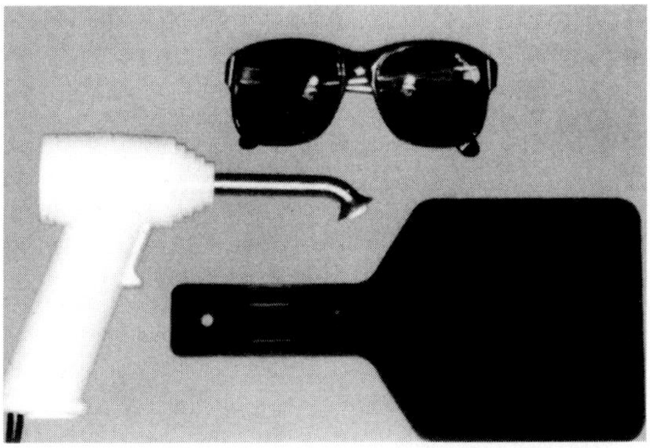

Fig. 9-12 Eye protection devices that can be used with a polymerizing visible-light device. *Top to bottom:* glasses, an instrument shield, and a flat plate.

cure composites with photo-initiators other than camphoroquinone.

PAC lights save time during procedures requiring multiple exposures, such as incremental build-ups, quadrant restorations, veneers, and bonding of orthodontic brackets. Typically, an exposure of 10 seconds from a PAC light is equivalent to 40 seconds from a QTH light. Use of 2-mm increments is still required.

Properties of composites cured with PAC lights depend on the composite and light-curing unit. In general, PAC lights produce equal or lower degrees of conversion, depths of cure, and flexural moduli, but flexural strengths equal to QTH light-curing units. Wall-to-wall polymerization shrinkages are equal or less with PAC lights.

LIGHT-EMITTING DIODES

Solid state light-emitting diodes (LEDs) use junctions of doped semiconductors (p-n junctions) based on gallium nitride to emit blue light. The spectral output of blue LEDs falls between 450 and 490 nm, so these units are effective for curing materials with camphoroquinone photo-initiators. LED units do not require a filter, have a long life span, and do not emit significant heat. Recently, a hybrid, light-curing unit that combines LED and QTH sources was introduced. With this unit, polymerization is initiated by the LED source and then completed by the combination of light from both sources.

Composites cured with LED units have flexural properties similar to those cured with QTH units. Depth of cure with LED units is higher.

SELECTED PROBLEMS

Problem 1

In selecting a composite for placing a large Class 4 restoration, what are several advantages of a light-cured composite?

Solution

Contour can be more adequately achieved through incremental addition; fewer air voids should be incorporated, because mixing of two pastes is not necessary; shade development can more readily be accomplished through the increments of different-colored composites; and less excess material should exist after insertion and curing of the restoration, thus finishing should be facilitated.

Problem 2

An extensive posterior core buildup is required on a lower molar. Why is a self-cured, core composite is the material of choice?

Solution

Uniform curing takes place under a crown form, lower-viscosity resin adapts better to pins or posts, and opaque, colored composites can be used to differentiate core from tooth structure during crown preparation.

Problem 3

When small air voids appear on the surface of a self-cured composite restoration during finishing, what are the causative manipulative factors?

Solution

The problem may be caused by exposing the dispensed composite to operatory light before incremental insertion; extended working of each increment to the point that voids are incorporated between layers; mixing of increments of two different shades of pastes on a pad before insertion; or excessive use of alcohol as a lubricant on the insertion instrument.

Problem 4

Is there reason to expect that the color of a large Class 4 restoration will be more stable when a light-cured composite is used instead of a self-cured composite? Why?

Solution

Yes. A self-cured composite contains an aromatic amine accelerator that is more susceptible to breakdown by oxidation than the aliphatic amine in a light-cured system.

Problem 5

When a thin composite anterior veneer is being placed to modify tooth color, what are the advantages of a microfilled composite?

Solution

The advantages are the following: greater translucency improves vitality in the final shade; smoother surface texture provides a glossy surface with light-reflective patterns similar to enamel; in a thin layer supported by the bond to enamel, high physical and mechanical properties are not as important as in a free-standing Class 4 restoration.

Problem 6

In polymerizing a large, light-cured, resin composite restoration, what manipulative variables can be controlled to improve the depth of cure?

Solution

The following variables can be controlled: the exposure time of the light can be increased for darker shades and thicker increments (beyond 2 mm); the light source can be maintained within 1 mm of the resin surface; the light tip can be drawn across the composite surface in steps, with multiple exposures ensuring uniformity of cure.

Problem 7

In selecting a composite for a large, Class 4 anterior restoration with significant incisal function, what are the enhanced properties of microhybrid composite that make it the material of choice?

Solution

The beneficial properties are greater strength and elastic modulus, lower polymerization shrinkage, lower thermal coefficient of expansion, lower water sorption, and greater wear resistance.

Problem 8

In the clinical evaluation of a 2-year-old composite restoration, penetrating marginal discoloration is noted. What factors contribute to this bond failure?

Solution

Contributing factors are residual stress from polymerization shrinkage; fatigue stresses on the bond from thermal cycling; contamination at the bond site during material insertion; deflection stress at the restoration margins caused by intermittent functional loading of the restoration; and hydrolytic breakdown of the bond at the tooth interface (particularly if it is dentin).

Problem 9

When repairing an anterior veneer restoration with a small area of severe marginal leakage, the discolored composite is removed and the deficient area is rebonded with new material. What is the character of the bond between old cured composite and new?

Solution

The bond is primarily micromechanical and is formed against the roughened surface of the original composite. A weak chemical bond may be formed between exposed unreacted bonds in the old material and the new bonding agent/composite. The repaired composite has less cohesive strength than the original composite and is more durable if an adjacent fresh enamel area can also be prepared by acid etching.

Problem 10

In assessing the use of composites in posterior teeth, what are the factors that contribute to early wear and failure?

Solution

These factors are the loss of substance as a result of deterioration of the silane coupling agent that bonds the filler particles to the matrix; excessive polymerization shrinkage from the relatively large volume of such restorations; stress-crack propagation across filler-polymer interfaces; and the low abrasion resistance of a relatively large volume of polymer matrix.

BIBLIOGRAPHY

Composites

Asmussen E: Clinical relevance of physical, chemical, and bonding properties of composite resins, *Oper Dent* 10:61, 1985.

Bailey SJ, Swift EJ Jr: Effects of home bleaching products on composite resins, *Quint Int* 23:489, 1992.

Bayne SC, Thompson JY, Swift EJ Jr et al: A characterization of first-generation flowable composites, *J Am Dent Assoc* 129:567, 1998.

Boyer DB, Chan KC, Reinhardt JW: Build-up and repair of light-cured composites: bond strength, *J Dent Res* 63:1241, 1984.

Braem M, Davidson CL, Lambrechts P et al: In vitro flexural fatigue limits of dental composites, *J Biomed Mater Res* 28:1397, 1994.

Braem M, Finger W, Van Doren VE et al: Mechanical properties and filler fraction of dental composites, *Dent Mater* 5:346, 1989.

Chantler PM, Hu X, Boyd NM: An extension of a phenomenological model for dental composites, *Dent Mater* 15:144, 1999.

Choi KK, Condon JR, Ferracane JL: The effects of adhesive thickness on polymerization contraction stress of composite, *J Dent Res* 79:812, 2000.

Condon JR. Ferracane JL: Factors effecting dental composite wear in vitro, *J Biomed Mater Res* 38:303, 1997.

Condon JR. Ferracane JL: In vitro wear of composite with varied cure, filler level, and filler treatment, *J Dent Res* 76:1405, 1997.

Condon JR, Ferracane JL: Reduction of composite contraction stress through non-bonded microfiller particles, *Dent Mater* 14:256, 1998.

Cook WD: Spectral distributions of dental photopolymerization sources, *J Dent Res* 61:1436, 1982.

Council on Scientific Affairs: Posterior resin-based composites, *J Am Dent Assoc* 129:1627, 1998.

Cross M, Douglas WH, Fields RP: The relationship between filler loading and particle-size distribution in composite resin technology, *J Dent Res* 62:850, 1983.

Dauvillier BS, Feilzer AJ, de Gee AJ et al: Visco-elastic parameters of dental restorative materials during setting, *J Dent Res* 79:818, 2000.

Dennison JB, Powers JM, Koran A: Color of dental restorative resins, *J Dent Res* 57:557, 1978.

DeWald J, Ferracane JL: A comparison of four modes of evaluating depth of cure of light-activated composites, *J Dent Res* 66:727, 1987.

Dietschi D, Holy J: A clinical trial of four light-curing posterior composite resins: two-year report, *Quint Int* 21:965, 1990.

Doray PG, Wang X, Powers JM et al: Accelerated aging affects color stability of provisional restorative materials, *J Prosthodont* 6:183, 1997.

El Hejazi AA, Watts DC: Creep and visco-elastic recovery of cured and secondary-cured composites and resin-modified glass-ionomers, *Dent Mater* 15:138, 1999.

Eldiwany M, Friedl K-H, Powers JM: Color stability of light-cured and post-cured composites, *Am J Dent* 8:179, 1995.

Eldiway M, Powers JM, George LA: Mechanical properties of direct and post-cured composites, *Am J Dent* 6:222, 1993.

Fan PL, Edahl A, Leung RL et al: Alternative interpretations of water sorption values of composite resins, *J Dent Res* 64:74, 1985.

Farah JW, Powers JM, editors: Laboratory composites, *Dent Advis* 16:1, 1999.

Farah JW, Powers JM, editors: Core materials, *Dent Advis* 16:1, 1999.

Farah JW, Powers JM, editors: Packable composites, *Dent Advis* 16:1, 1999.

Farah JW, Powers JM, editors: Provisional materials, *Dent Advis* 17:1, 2000.

Farah JW, Powers JM, editors: Microhybrid composites, *Dent Advis* 17:1, 2000.

Farah JW, Powers JM, editors: Flowable composites, *Dent Advis* 17:4, 2000.

Farah JW, Powers JM, editors: PAC lights, *Dent Advis* 18:5, 2001.

Fay R-M, Servos T, Powers JM: Color of restorative materials after staining and bleaching, *Oper Dent* 24:292, 1999.

Feilzer AJ, de Gee AJ, Davidson CL: Setting stress in composite resin in relation to configuration of the restoratives, *J Dent Res* 66:1636, 1987.

Feilzer AJ, de Gee AJ, Davidson CL: Quantitative determination of stress reduction by flow in composite restorations, *Dent Mater* 6:167, 1990.

Ferracane JL: Elution of leachable components from composites, *J Oral Rehabil* 21:441, 1994.

Ferracane JL: Current trends in dental composites, *Crit Rev Oral Biol Med* 6:302, 1995.

Ferracane JL, Mitchem JC, Condon JR et al: Wear and marginal breakdown of composites with various degrees of cure, *J Dent Res* 76:1508, 1997.

Ferracane JL, Moser JB, Greener EH: Rheology of composite restoratives, *J Dent Res* 60:1678, 1981.

Gerzina TM, Hume WR: Effect of dentine on release of TEGDMA from resin composite *in vitro, J Oral Rehabil* 21:463, 1994.

Geurtsen W: Biocompatibility of resin-modified filling materials, *Crit Rev Oral Biol Med* 11:333, 2000.

Hanks CT, Craig RG, Diehl ML et al: Cytotoxicity of dental composites and other dental materials in a new *in vitro* device, *J Oral Path* 17:396, 1988.

Hanks CT, Strawn SE, Wataha JC et al: Cytotoxic effects of composite resin components on cultured mammalian fibroblasts, *J Dent Res* 70:1450, 1991.

Hanks CT, Wataha JC, Parsell RR et al: Permeability of biological and synthetic molecules through dentine, *J Oral Rehabil* 21:475, 1994.

Hirasawa T, Hirano S, Hirabayashi S et al: Initial dimensional change of composites in dry and wet conditions, *J Dent Res* 62:28, 1983.

Hu X, Harrington E, Marquis PM et al: The influence of cyclic loading on the wear of a dental composite, *Biomater* 20:907, 1999.

Hu X, Marquis PM, Shortall AC: Two-body in vitro wear study of some current dental composites and amalgams, *J Prosthet Dent* 82:214, 1999.

Inohoshi S, Willems G, Van Meerbeek B et al: Dual-cure luting composites, Part I filler particle distribution, *J Oral Rehabil* 20:133, 1993.

Johnson GH, Bales DJ, Gordon GE et al: Clinical performance of posterior composite resin restorations, *Quint Int* 23:705, 1992.

Johnson GH, Gordon GE, Bales DJ: Postoperative sensitivity associated with posterior composite and amalgam restorations, *Oper Dent* 13:66, 1988.

Jones DW: Composite restorative materials, *J Canad Dent Assoc* 56:851, 1990.

Kalachandra S: Influence of fillers on the water sorption of composites, *Dent Mater* 5:283, 1989.

Kim K-H, Park J-H, Imai Y et al: Fracture toughness and acoustic emission behavior of dental composite resins, *Engin Fract Mech* 40:811, 1991.

Labella R, Lambrechts P, Van Meerbeek B et al: Polymerization shrinkage and elasticity of flowable composites and filled adhesives, *Dent Mater* 15:128, 1999.

Lee Y-K, El Zawahry M, Noaman KM et al: Effect of mouthwash and accelerated aging on the color stability of esthetic restorative materials, *Am J Dent* 13:159, 2000.

Leinfelder KF: Posterior composite resins: the materials and their clinical performance, *J Am Dent Assoc* 126:663, 1995.

Letzel H: Survival rates and reasons for failure of posterior composite restorations in multicentre clinical trial, *J Dent* 17:S10, 1989.

Leung RL, Fan PL, Johnston WM: Post-irradiation polymerization of visible light-activated composite resin, *J Dent Res* 62:363, 1983.

Manhart J, Kunzelmann K-H, Chen HY et al: Mechanical properties and wear behavior of light-cured packable composite resins, *Dent Mater* 16:33, 2000.

Mitchem JC, Gronas DG: The continued in vivo evaluation of the wear of restorative resins, *J Am Dent Assoc* 111:961, 1985.

Neo JC, Denehy GE, Boyer DB: Effects of polymerization techniques on uniformity of cure of large-diameter, photo-initiated composite resin restorations, *J Am Dent Assoc* 113:905, 1986.

Oysaed H, Ruyter IE: Water sorption and filler characteristics of composites for use in posterior teeth, *J Dent Res* 65:1315, 1986.

Pallav P, DeGee AJ, Davidson CL et al: The influence of admixing microfiller to small-particle composite resin on wear, tensile strength, hardness, and surface roughness, *J Dent Res* 68:489, 1989.

Park Y-J, Chae K-H, Rawls HR: Development of a new photoinitiation system for dental light-cure composite resins, *Dent Mater* 15:120, 1999.

Perry R, Kugel G, Kunzelmann K-H, et al: Composite restoration wear analysis: conventional methods vs. three-dimensional laser digitizer, *J Am Dent Assoc* 131:1472, 2000.

Powers JM: Lifetime prediction of dental materials: an engineering approach, *J Oral Rehabil* 22:491, 1995.

Powers JM, Burgess JO: Performance standards for competitive dental restorative materials, *Trans Acad Dent Mater* 9:68, 1996.

Powers JM, Dennison JB, Koran A: Color stability of restorative resins under accelerated aging, *J Dent Res* 57:964, 1978.

Powers JM, Dennison JB, Lepeak PJ: Parameters that affect the color of direct restorative resins, *J Dent Res* 57:876, 1978.

Powers JM, Hostetler RW, Dennison JB: Thermal expansion of composite resins and sealants, *J Dent Res* 58:584, 1979.

Powers JM, Smith LT, Eldiwany M et al: Effects of post-curing on mechanical properties of a composite, *Am J Dent* 6:232, 1993.

Pratten DH, Johnson GH: An evaluation of finishing instruments for an anterior and a posterior composite, *J Prosthet Dent* 60:154, 1988.

Rathbun MA, Craig RG, Hanks CT et al: Cytotoxicity of a BIS-GMA dental composite before and after leaching in organic solvents, *J Biomed Mater Res* 25:443, 1991.

Sakaguchi RL, Berge HX: Reduced light energy density decreases post-gel contraction while maintaining degree of conversion in composites, *J Dent* 26:695, 1998.

Sakaguchi RL, Peters MCRB, Nelson SR, Douglas WH: Effects of polymerization contraction in composite restorations, *J Dent* 20:178, 1992.

Soderholm K-JM: Leaking of fillers in dental composites, *J Dent Res* 62:126, 1983.

Soderholm K-J, Zigan M, Ragan M et al: Hydrolytic degradation of dental composites, *J Dent Res* 63:1248, 1984.

Stanford CM, Fan PL, Schoenfeld CM et al: Radiopacity of light-cured posterior composite resins, *J Am Dent Assoc* 115:722, 1987.

Suh BI, Ferber C, Baez R: Optimization of hybrid composite properties, *J Esthetic Dent* 2:44, 1990.

Tate WH, Friedl K-H, Powers JM: Bond strength of composites to hybrid ionomers, *Oper Dent* 21:147, 1996.

Tate WH, Powers JM: Surface roughness of composites and hybrid ionomers, *Oper Dent* 21:53, 1996.

Tirtha R, Fan PL, Dennison JB et al: In vitro depth of cure of photo-activated composites, *J Dent Res* 61:1184, 1982.

Van Dijken JWV: A clinical evaluation of anterior conventional, microfiller, and hybrid composite resin fillings: a 6-year follow-up study, *Acta Odontol Scand* 44:357, 1986.

Van Dijken JWV, Ruyter IE, Holland RI: Porosity in posterior composite resins, *Scand J Dent Res* 94:471, 1986.

Van Dijken JWV, Sjöström S, Wing K: The effect of different types of composite resin fillings on marginal gingiva, *J Clin Periodont* 14:185, 1987.

Wataha JC, Hanks CT, Strawn SE et al: Cytotoxicity of components of resin and other dental restorative materials, *J Oral Rehabil* 21:453, 1994.

Watts DC, Haywood CM, Smith R: Thermal diffusion through composite restorative materials, *Br Dent J* 154:101, 1983.

Wendt SL Jr: The effect of heat used as a secondary cure upon the physical properties of three composite resins. I. Diametral tensile strength, compressive strength, and a marginal dimensional stability, *Quint Int* 18:265, 1987.

Wendt SL Jr: Microleakage and cusp fracture resistance of heat-treated composite resin inlays, *Am J Dent* 4:10, 1991.

Wendt SL Jr, Leinfilder KF: The clinical evaluation of heat-treated composite resin inlays, *J Am Dent Assoc* 120:177, 1990.

Xu HHK: Whisker-reinforced heat-cured dental resin composites: effects of filler level and heat-cure temperature and time, *J Dent Res* 79:1392, 2000.

Compomers

Cattani-Lorente MA, Dupuis V, Moya F et al: Comparative study of the physical properties of a polyacid-modified composite resin and a resin-modified glass ionomer cement, *Dent Mater* 15:21, 1999.

Farah JW, Powers JM, editors: Compomers, *Dent Advis* 15:1, 1998.

Light-Curing Units

Albers HF: Resin polymerization, *Adept Report* 6:1, 2000.

Fan PL, Wozniak WT, Reyes WD et al: Irradiance of visible light-curing units and voltage variation effects, *J Am Dent Assoc* 115:442, 1987.

Farah JW, Powers JM, editors: Light-curing units, *Dent Advis* 16:1, 1999.

Harrington E, Wilson HJ: Determination of radiation energy emitted by light activation, *J Oral Rehabil* 22:377, 1995.

Jandt KD, Mills RW, Blackwell GB et al: Depth of cure and compressive strength of dental composites cured with blue light emitting diodes (LEDs), *Dent Mater* 16:41, 2000.

Mills RW, Jandt KD, Ashworth SH: Dental composite depth of cure with halogen and blue light emitting diode technology, *Br Dent J* 186:388, 1999.

Peutzfeldt A, Sahafi A, Asmussen E: Characterization of resin composites polymerized with plasma arc curing units, *Dent Mater* 16:330, 2000.

Sakaguchi RL, Berge HX: Reduced light energy density decreases postgel contraction while maintaining degree of conversion in composites, *J Dent* 26:695, 1998.

Satrom KD, Morris MA, Crigger LP: Potential retinal hazards of visible light photopolymerization units, *J Dent Res* 66:731, 1987.

Stahl F, Ashworth SH, Jandt KD et al: Light emitting diodes (LED) polymerisation of dental composites: flexural properties and polymerisation potential, *Biomater* 21:1379, 2000.

Watts DC, Al Hindi A: Intrinsic 'soft-start' polymerisation shrinkage-kinetics in an acrylic-based resin-composite, *Dent Mater* 15:39, 1999.

Chapter 10

Bonding to Dental Substrates

Every dental restoration requires retention by some system of connection or attachment. Dentures are held in place by the combination of tissue irregularities, saliva, and adhesives. Crowns are held in place by luting cement that mates with minor irregularities along the crown and dentin surfaces. Partial dentures are held in place by clasps. Undercut regions in the cavity preparation retain dental amalgam. All of these methods of retention rely predominantly on macroscopic mechanisms. Even so, there has always been a strong desire to develop a dental adhesive that could provide a bonded and sealed interface. The scientific beginnings of dental adhesion originated in the early 1950s with studies of bonding to enamel and dentin. Now, 50 years later, bonding agents are used routinely in restorative and preventive dentistry. This chapter focuses on the science, systems, and success of bonding systems for dental substrates with emphasis on bonding resin composites to tooth structure.

PRINCIPLES OF ADHESION

ADHESIVE JOINTS

Adhesion or bonding is the process of forming an adhesive joint. The initial substrate is called the *adherend,* whereas the material producing the interface is generally called the *adhesive.* If two substrates are being joined, the adhesive produces two interfaces as part of the adhesive joint, as illustrated in Fig. 10-1. In dentistry, most adhesive joints involve two interfaces. A dental sealant attached to enamel is a simple adhesive joint with one interface. A bonded composite restoration is a more complex joint. In dentistry, there may be several steps in creating the adhesive layer, and these stages may involve separate components. These components are called a *bonding agent.*

ADHESION VERSUS BOND STRENGTH

Dentistry is interested in the process of forming a joint and the resistance of the joint to failure. The

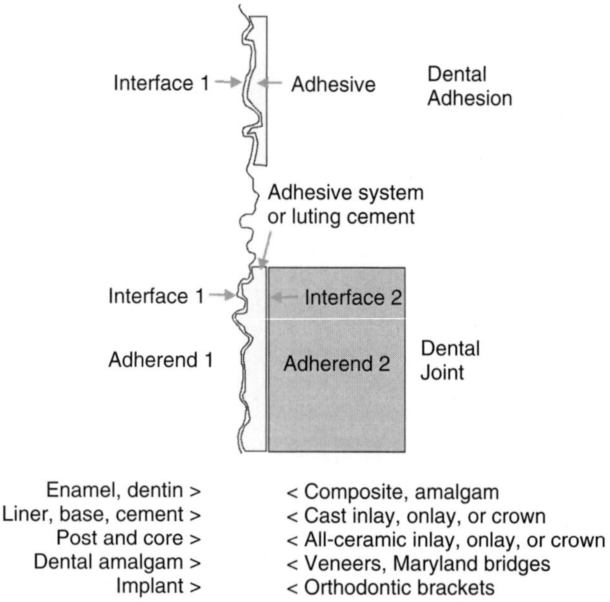

Fig. 10-1 Definitions of the terminology associated with adhesive systems (adhesives, adherends or substrates, and interfaces). Most dental joints involve at least one adhesive, two substrates, and two interfaces.

science of adhesion studies the formation of an adhesive joint. There is a specific energy of adhesion determined by the chemical, physical, and mechanical attributes of the substrate and adhesive. Once formed, the joint's resistance to failure depends on the extent of defects along the interface that allow cracks to form, grow, and rupture the joint. Failure processes depend on the bulk properties of the adherend and adhesive, the environment of the bond, and time. Strengths of the bonded system are measured by bond tests.

INTERFACE FORMATION FOR ADHESION

Formation of an optimally bonded interface requires that (1) the surface of the substrate be clean; (2) the adhesive wet the substrate well, have a low contact angle, and spread onto the surface; (3) adaptation to the substrate produce intimate approximation of the materials without entrapped air or other intervening materials; (4) the interface include the sufficient physical, chemical and/or mechanical strength to resist intraoral forces of debonding; and (5) the adhesive be well cured under the conditions recommended for use. These events are schematically summarized in Fig. 10-2.

Cleaning the surface of the substrate and then keeping it clean until the adhesive is applied are technical problems within a patient's mouth. Dental surfaces exposed to the oral environment contain a pellicle of adsorbed materials from saliva. The pellicle may be contaminated by the formation of plaque or the deposition of components of food, such as stains. This material must be removed before bonding. Once a surface is cleaned, its surface energy is higher, and it is more likely to adsorb material from the surrounding air, such as moisture or saliva droplets, to decrease its energy. Therefore the surface must be protected and the next step in a bonding procedure should proceed promptly.

Enamel and dentin prepared with rotary instruments contain a debris layer that is smeared onto their surfaces, called the *smear layer*. This layer is usually a few micrometers thick and adheres weakly to the substrate. Thus it is essential to either remove this layer or penetrate it with adhesives. The most common approach to removing a smear layer is to chemically dissolve part or all of it.

When adhesive is applied to a substrate, it must wet the surface well. Good wetting is evidenced by a small contact angle and spreading of the adhesive onto the substrate (see Chapter 2). Clean dentin is hydrophilic and will be wet best by an adhesive that is also hydrophilic. In addition, the adhesive must flow in a practical time. Adding solvent to the adhesive promotes lower viscosity and good flow. However, it is not always possible to apply adhesive materials carefully in poorly accessible areas and in thin films.

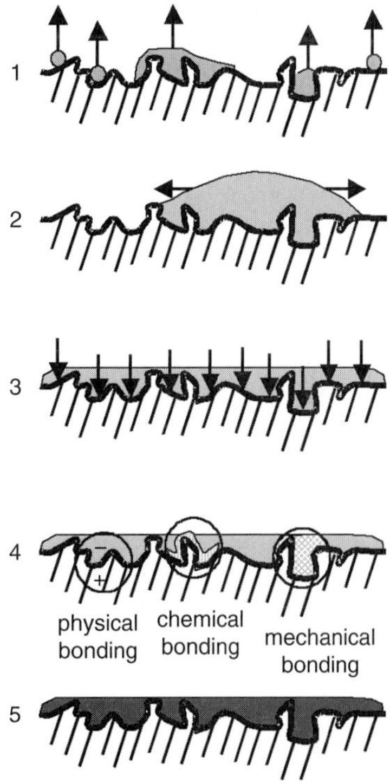

Fig. 10-2 Examples of the microscopic steps involved in the formation of an adhesive joint. *1,* Good adherend; *2,* good wetting; *3,* intimate adaptation; *4,* bonding; *5,* good curing.

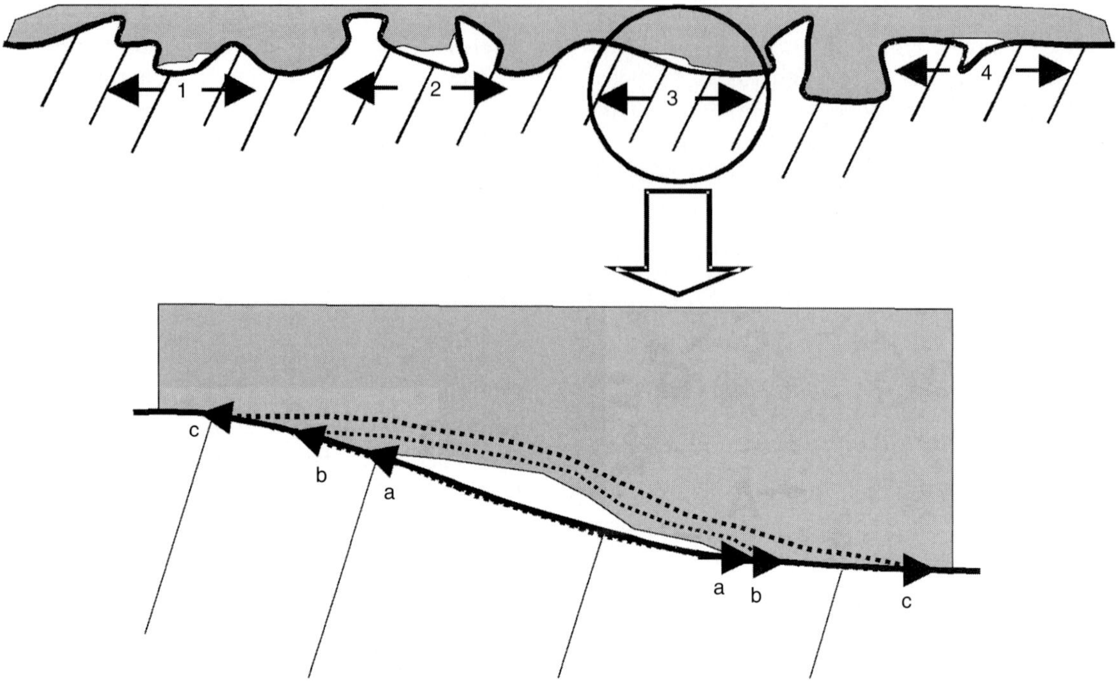

Fig. 10-3 Defects in dental joints caused by *(1)* poor wetting, *(2)* poor adaptation, *(3)* inadequate bonding, and *(4)* inadequate curing. Polymerization shrinkage may cause an inadequately bonded area to debond further *(a-c)* as shown in the enlargement of *3*.

Once good wetting is achieved, the adhesive should intimately contact the substrate to produce physical, chemical, or mechanical bonding. For effective chemical bonding, the distance between the adhesive and substrate must be less than a few Angstroms and a high density of new bonds must form along the interface. Because this is rarely the case, bonding of restorative materials involves mostly mechanical bonding. Mechanical bonds (gross mechanical retention and micro-mechanical retention) involve adhesive interlocking with surface irregularities. Cavity preparation produces some irregularities. In other cases, surface roughness is increased by sandblasting or etching.

The final practical consideration for bonding is the method of curing (polymerizing) the adhesive. Most contemporary bonding agents harden by chemical reactions initiated by visible light, although self-cured and dual-cured systems are also available. If curing does not continue to a sufficient degree, the under-cured adhesive may not provide good retention and sealing.

MECHANISMS OF INTERFACIAL DEBONDING

Debonding of dental joints occurs by a process of crack formation and propagation and subsequent joint failure. Cracks form at defects along the interface. Examples of defects include sites of interfacial contamination, excess moisture, trapped air bubbles, voids formed during solvent evaporation, places of poor wetting, bubbles within the adhesive, and curing shrinkage pores (Fig. 10-3). The bonded system includes the outermost layers of the substrate, which may have been altered during bonding techniques, the adhesive layer, and the restorative material interface. For all practical purposes, the bulk properties of the tooth substrates (enamel, dentin) and restorative substrates (composites, ceramics) are much stronger than the bond strength of

TABLE 10-1 Examples of Bulk Shear Strengths Versus Shear Bond Strengths of Materials Involved in Dental Bonding

Material	Bulk Shear Strength (MPa)	Shear Bond Strength (MPa)
Amalgam	185	
Human dentin	140-165	
Composite	140	
Dentin-adhesive-amalgam		4-8
Dentin-adhesive-composite		20
Enamel-adhesive-composite		20

the restorations (Table 10-1). Therefore cracks that form generally remain in the bonded interface zone.

As cracks grow, they contribute to stress concentrations or stress redistributions within the substrates. The final failure may often extend for short distances through portions of tooth structure or restorative material. The amount of substrate fractured is often indicative of the relative strength of the joint. Failed surfaces should be examined carefully with moderate magnification to identify the origin of the critical crack, although this crack may not be readily apparent. Therefore failures are reported as being within the substrate (cohesive), between the adhesive and substrate (adhesive), within the restorative material (cohesive), or mixed. Generally, this information is not very useful to understanding why the failure occurred.

MEASUREMENTS OF BOND STRENGTH

Bond strength testing is one of most popular analyses conducted in evaluations of dental materials. Available tests accommodate differences in specimen size, test configurations for loading, and patterns of loading. There is no absolute bond strength; rather the measured bond strength is influenced by the concentrations of defects created in forming the interface and experimental testing variables, which may or may not be controlled. Different research investigators and different testing designs produce different values. Although the ADA and ISO have attempted to standardize the procedures, different values of bond strength are measured in different laboratories. It is therefore critical to include a control along with test results. Generally, the control for bond strength to dentin is the bond strength to enamel.

Bond strength can be studied using prospective or retrospective clinical models, or with in vitro using simulated clinical models or bonding to a standardized substrate. In a simulated clinical model, for example, a ceramic restoration is bonded with resin cement to extracted human or bovine teeth, and in vitro bond strength is tested in shear or tension. The advantage of this model is that both the tooth and ceramic restoration are present, so the test appears to be clinically relevant. The disadvantage is that often bond failures occur at both interfaces, so it is difficult to isolate the weak link in the tooth-resin cement-ceramic system. A more fundamental test is the isolated interface model, in which, for example, bonding of the tooth-resin cement interface is studied separately from the ceramic-resin cement interface.

Shear bond strength is the most prevalent bond test (Fig. 10-4). It is difficult to control the position of the knife edge in this test, so there is some bending involved that causes variability. A reproducible tensile bond test for the isolated interface model is the inverted, truncated cone test (Fig. 10-5). Diameters of bonded test interfaces typically range from 3.0 to 4.5 mm. It appears that tests that use 3-mm joints produce less variation in bond strength. Shear and tensile tests report bond strengths of clinically successful composites bonded to human enamel and dentin to be in the range of 15 to 35 MPa. Coefficients of

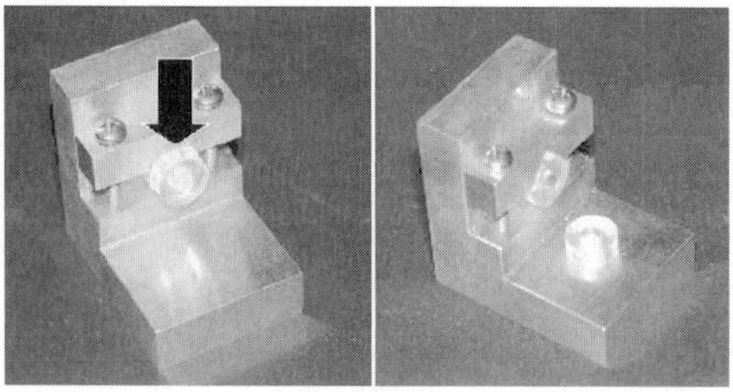

Fig. 10-4 Composite bonded to dentin within plastic rings and debonded by shear bond strength (SBS) testing along the interface.

(Courtesy SC Bayne, University of North Carolina School of Dentistry, Chapel Hill, NC.)

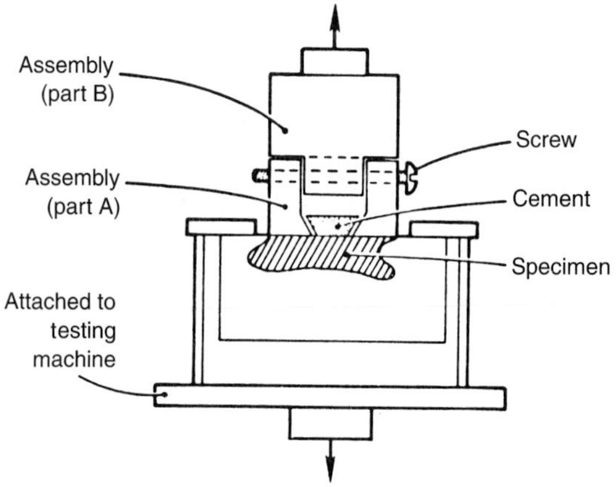

Fig. 10-5 Tensile bond strength test using inverted, truncated cone in an isolated interface test model.

(Adapted from Barakat MM, Powers JM: *Aust Dent J* 31:415, 1986.)

variation for shear bond tests range from 20% to 60%, whereas those for tensile bond strength tests range from 20% to 40%.

During the mid 1990s, there were numerous attempts to minimize the problems of in vitro bond strength testing and allow testing with fewer numbers of extracted teeth. The microtensile bond strength test (Fig. 10-6) was devised to be a more clinically relevant test. It is claimed that the test reduces the probability of crack initiation and propagation within individual specimens because of the small bonded area (1 mm^2).

TABLE 10-2 Composition of Human Enamel and Dentin in Weight and Volume Percent

	Enamel		Dentin	
Constituents	**Wt%**	**Vol%**	**Wt%**	**Vol%**
Water	3	11	10	21
Noncollagenous proteins, lipids, ions	1	2	2	5
Collagen	—	—	18	27
Hydroxyapatite	95	87	70	47

Adapted from LeGeros RZ: Calcium phosphates in oral biology and medicine, *Monogr Oral Sci* 15:108-113, 1991.

For all bond strength tests, faster loading rates tend to increase the observed bond strengths. Higher test temperatures may contribute to post-curing and strengthen the adhesive. Wet specimens are generally weaker than dry ones, as a result of the plasticizing effect of absorbed water. Fig. 10-7 demonstrates the variability reported by different laboratories attempting to test the same bonding agent.

CHARACTERIZATION OF HUMAN ENAMEL AND DENTIN

Adhesion in dentistry involves a wide range of substrates, but most applications involve adhesion to enamel and dentin. Challenges for adhesive procedures are related directly to the structure of these tissues. The following information is therefore provided as background for bonding to enamel and dentin.

STRUCTURE AND MORPHOLOGY OF ENAMEL

Enamel prisms are filled with millions of hydroxyapatite crystals, which occupy about 89% by volume of the entire enamel structure. Between the crystals are small amounts or remnant

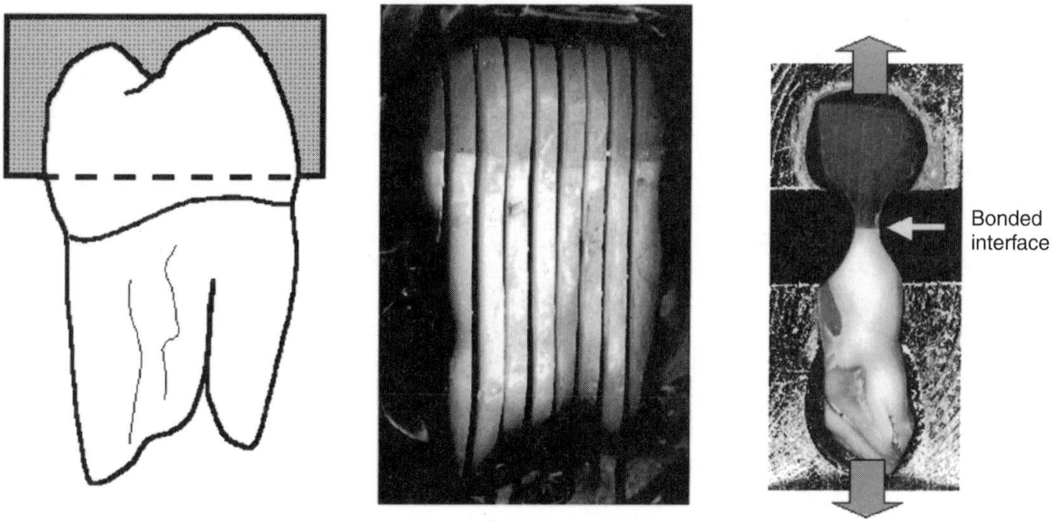

Fig. 10-6 Production and testing of micro-tensile bond strength specimens. An extracted tooth with the roots embedded in resin is flattened across the occlusal surface and attached to composite using a bonding agent. The tooth is sectioned parallel to the long axis. A longitudinal section in the region near the bonded interface is reduced in size with high-speed bur to generate a small dumbbell-shaped section for tensile testing. The ends of the section are cemented to the test equipment and then pulled in tension.

(Courtesy B Rosa, São Paulo, Brazil.)

protein structure and water. The general composition of enamel and dentin by weight and volume are reported in Table 10-2. Enamel crystals are packed with their long axes roughly aligned with the long axis of the enamel prism. Crystals are hexagonal in cross-section and elongated. Looking down along the long axis of the enamel prism, the crystals are perpendicular to the view in the center of the prism but are more tipped toward the periphery. The crystals in the tail are the least densely packed and tipped at perhaps as much as 30 degrees away from perpendicular. Chemical properties of the prism vary between the center and perimeter.

Enamel prisms are essentially parallel to each other and run from the dento-enamel junction (DEJ) outward in a radial pattern. In the neighborhood of enamel cusps, the prisms are perpendicular to the DEJ. Near the cemento-enamel junction, the prisms are highly tipped. It is crucial to avoid undermining enamel rods during cavity preparation, or bonding will tend to dislodge the

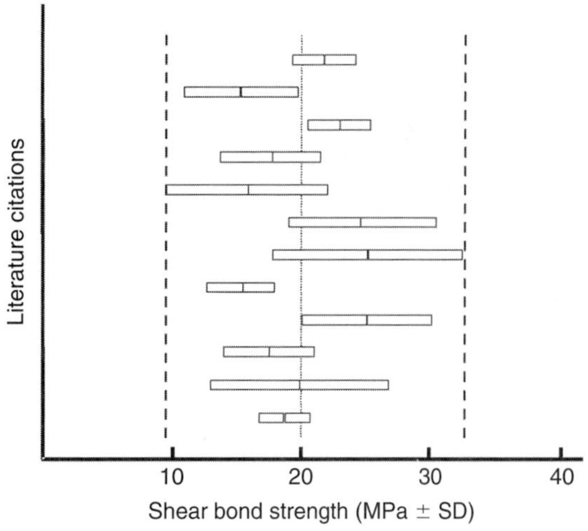

Fig. 10-7 Example of variability of shear bond strengths reported by 12 different laboratories performing the same test on 3M Single-Bond Adhesive and 3M Z100 Composite.

(Adapted from May KN Jr, Swift EJ Jr, Bayne SC: *Am J Dent* 10:195, 1997.)

enamel prisms in those regions during mechanical loading.

Etching of enamel with phosphoric acid eliminates smear layers associated with cavity preparation, dissolves persisting layers of prismless enamel in deciduous teeth, and differentially dissolves enamel crystals in each prism. The pattern of etching (Fig. 10-8) is categorized as Type 1 (preferential prism center etching), Type 2 (preferential prism periphery etching), and Type 3 (mixed). There appears to be no difference in micro-mechanical bonding of the different etching patterns. In a standard cavity preparation for a composite, the orientation of the enamel surfaces being etched could be perpendicular to enamel prisms (perimeter of the cavity outline), oblique cross-section of the prisms (beveled occlusal or proximal margins), and axial walls of the prisms (cavity preparation walls).

During the early stages of etching, when only a small amount of enamel crystal dissolution occurs, it may be difficult or impossible to detect the extent of the process. However, as the etching pattern begins to develop, the etched surface develops a frosty appearance (Fig. 10-9, *B*), which has been used as the traditional clinical landmark for sufficient etching.

STRUCTURE AND MORPHOLOGY OF DENTIN

Dentin's composition is much more rich in organic material than enamel. Only about 50% by volume of dentin is mineralized with hydroxyapatite crystals (see Table 10-2). A large proportion of the crystals is interspersed among collagen fibers. Within collagen fibers, individual fibrils contain crystals at their ends as well. The lower mineral content of dentin permits more elastic deformation during loading.

Dentin tubules are 0.5 to 1.5 μm in diameter and are formed at a slight angle to the DEJ and pulp chamber. There is a higher density of tubules along the inner or deep dentin (43,000 tubules/mm^2) than at the middle dentin (35,000 tubules/mm^2) or the outer, superficial dentin (15,000 tubules/mm^2). A labyrinth of secondary tubules among neighboring tubules often interconnects primary tubules. Fig. 10-10 is a scanning electron micrograph of dentin prepared for bonding. It reveals the primary tubule in the

A

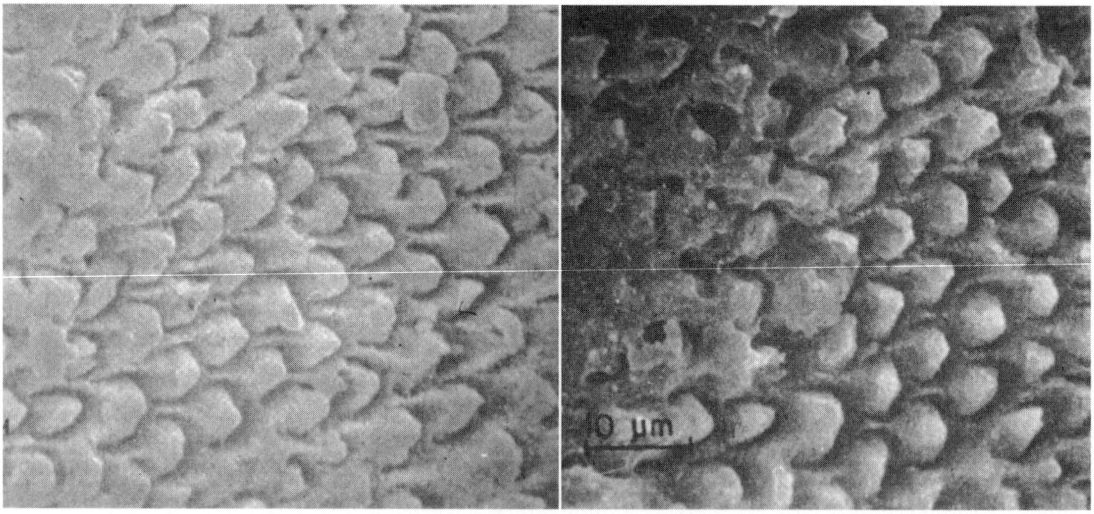

B

Fig. 10-8 Types of enamel etching patterns. **A,** Type 1, preferential prism core etching; **B,** Type 2, preferential prism periphery etching.

(Courtesy GW Marshall, UCSF School of Dentistry, San Francisco, CA.)

center with secondary (lateral) tubules branching off from the tubule. Intertubular dentin comprises collagen, hydroxyapatite, and water. Under normal circumstances, the tubule is filled with the odontoblastic process.

Etching of dentin surfaces primarily dissolves hydroxyapatite crystals within the surface of the intertubular dentin and along the surface of the outermost peritubular dentin. A smear layer exists from cavity preparation (Fig. 10-11, *A* and *B*) that is typically 1 to 2 μm thick with smear plugs within the ends of the tubules (Fig. 10-11, *C*). The smear layer is almost entirely hydroxyapatite debris from high-speed cutting during cavity preparation. High surface temperatures along the cutting interface pyrolize most of the organic material.

When the etchant first contacts the smear layer it begins to dissolve and penetrate it. Immediately the underlying intertubular dentin, peritubular dentin, and tubules come into contact with acid. Intertubular dentin contains

A B C D

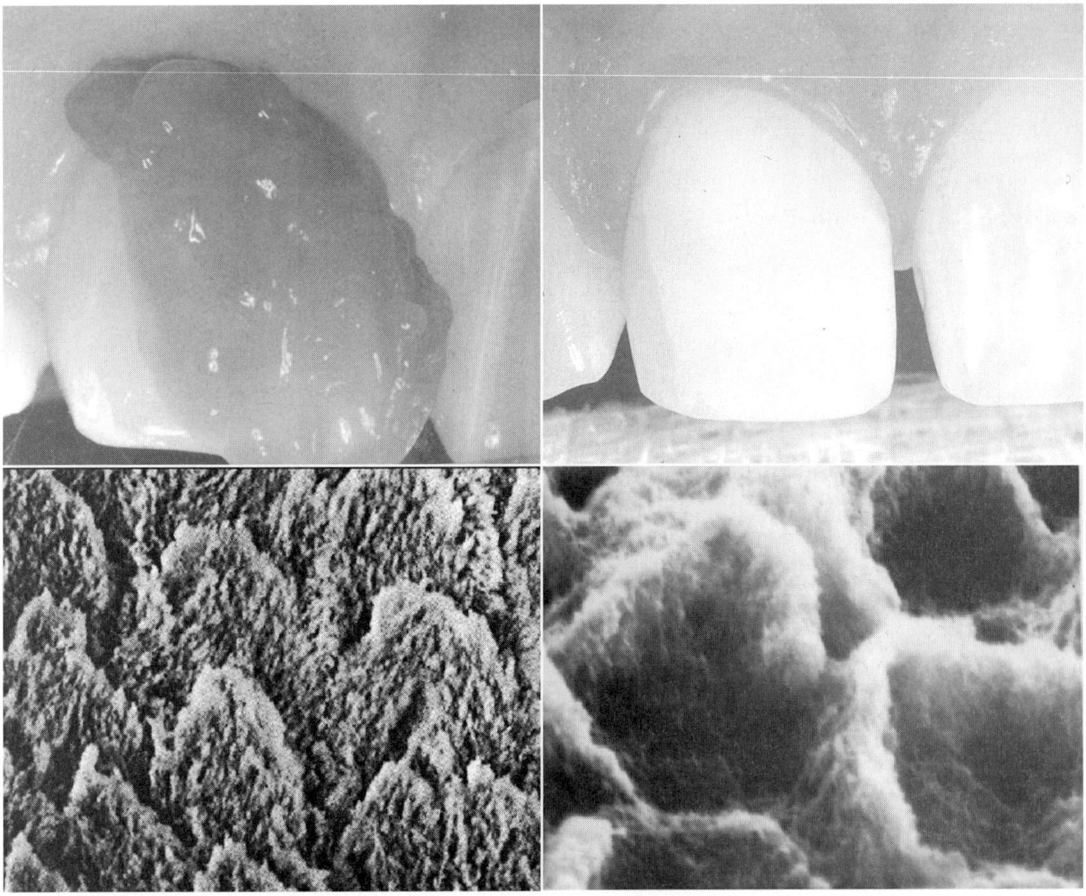

Fig. 10-9 Micro-mechanical retention to human enamel. **A,** Gel etchant dispensed from a syringe onto the enamel portion of the cavity preparation. **B,** Frosty or dull appearance of enamel after etching, rinsing, and drying. **C,** Magnified view of etched enamel with Type 2 relief. **D,** Magnified view of bonding agent revealed by dissolving enamel.
(Courtesy SC Bayne, University of North Carolina School of Dentistry, Chapel Hill, NC.)

Continued

E

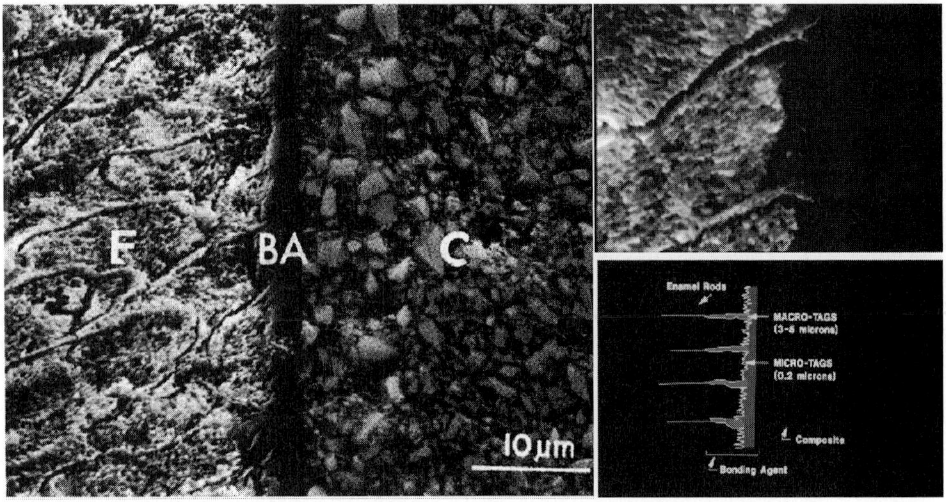

F

Fig. 10-9, cont'd E, Scanning electron photomicrograph of macrotags and microtags in enamel formed by bonding system. **F,** Schematic representation of macrotags and microtags.
(Courtesy SC Bayne, University of North Carolina School of Dentistry, Chapel Hill, NC.)

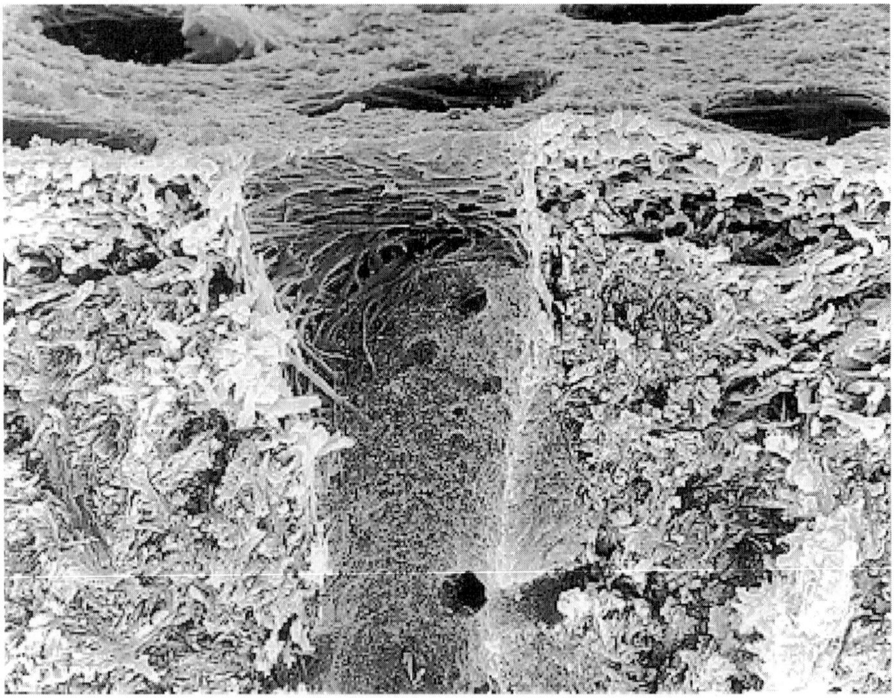

Fig. 10-10 Scanning electron photomicrograph of fractured human dentin revealing intertubular (collagen, hydroxyapatite, water), peritubular (collagen, hydroxyapatite), and tubular dentin. The surface has been etched with phosphoric acid to remove the smear layer and dissolve hydroxyapatite crystals in a superficial zone of about 2 μm. The lateral orientation of most collagen fibers is revealed along the top edge of the dentinal tubule. Smaller orifices of lateral tubules are seen easily within the primary dentinal tubule.
(Courtesy J Perdigão, University of Minnesota, Minneapolis, MN.)

A

B

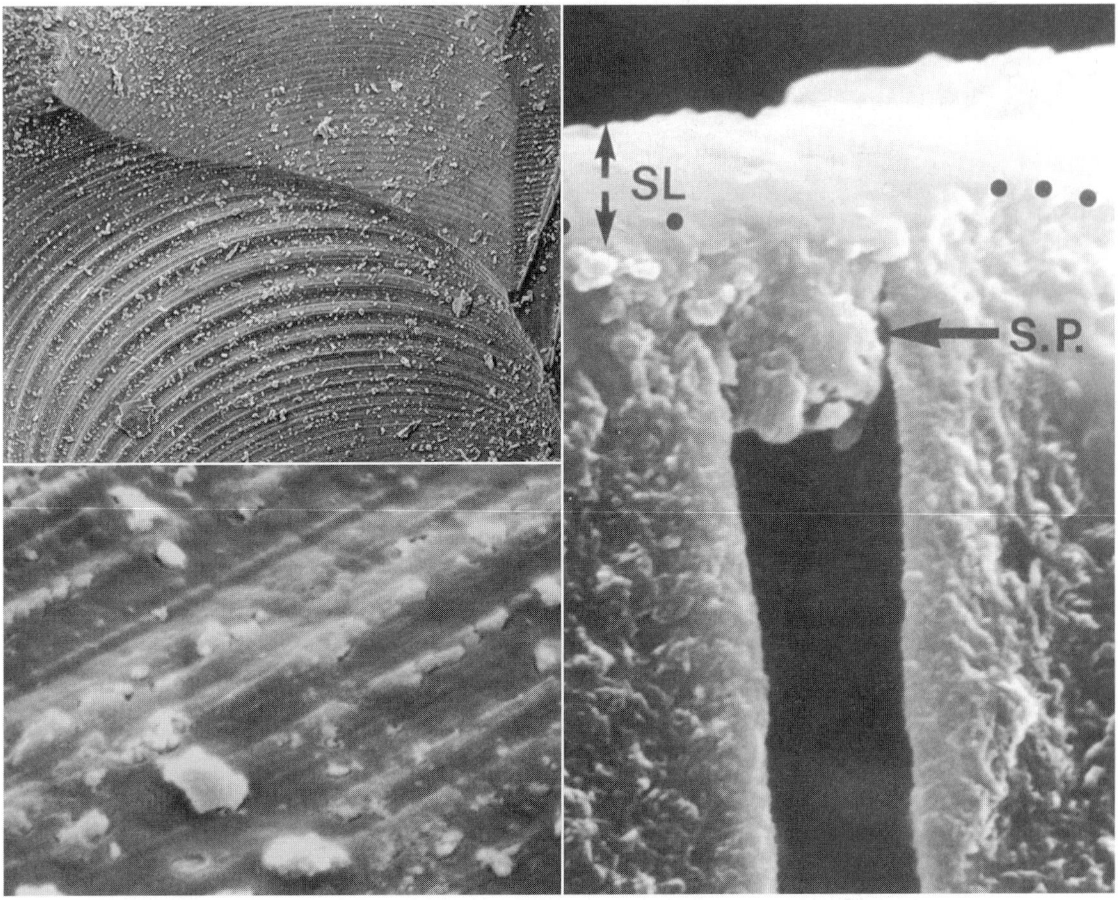

C

Fig. 10-11 Smear layer on dentin. **A,** Scanning electron photomicrograph of cavity preparation showing dentin smear layer with some loose debris on surface. **B,** High-magnification scanning electron microscopic (SEM) view of smear layer on same surface as *A* showing some cracks within the compacted debris layer. **C,** Cross-sectional view of smear layer (1 to 2 μm in thickness) with smear plugs compacted into dentinal tubule openings.

(**A** and **B,** Courtesy SC Bayne, University of North Carolina School of Dentistry, Chapel Hill, NC; **C,** courtesy D Pashley, Medical College of Georgia, Augusta, GA.)

about 50% hydroxyapatite crystals; these crystals are the same size as in enamel and are embedded within the spaces between collagen fibers. This material is relatively quickly dissolved. Peritubular dentin is about 80% to 90% hydroxyapatite crystals by volume and is readily dissolved in acid. The dentinal fluid is highly buffered. Therefore acid that mixes with dentinal fluid is quickly neutralized. Effects of acid etching are typically limited to 0.1 to 5 μm of the superficial region of intertubular dentin and about 2 to 10 μm along the walls of peritubular dentin (Fig. 10-12, *A*). The result of the etching process is the creation of a demineralized zone of dentin between the tubules and along the outer mouth of individual dentinal tubules. This surfacc is porous and allows primer penetration for tag formation. Fig. 10-12, *B*, is an atomic force microscope image of the etching sequence.

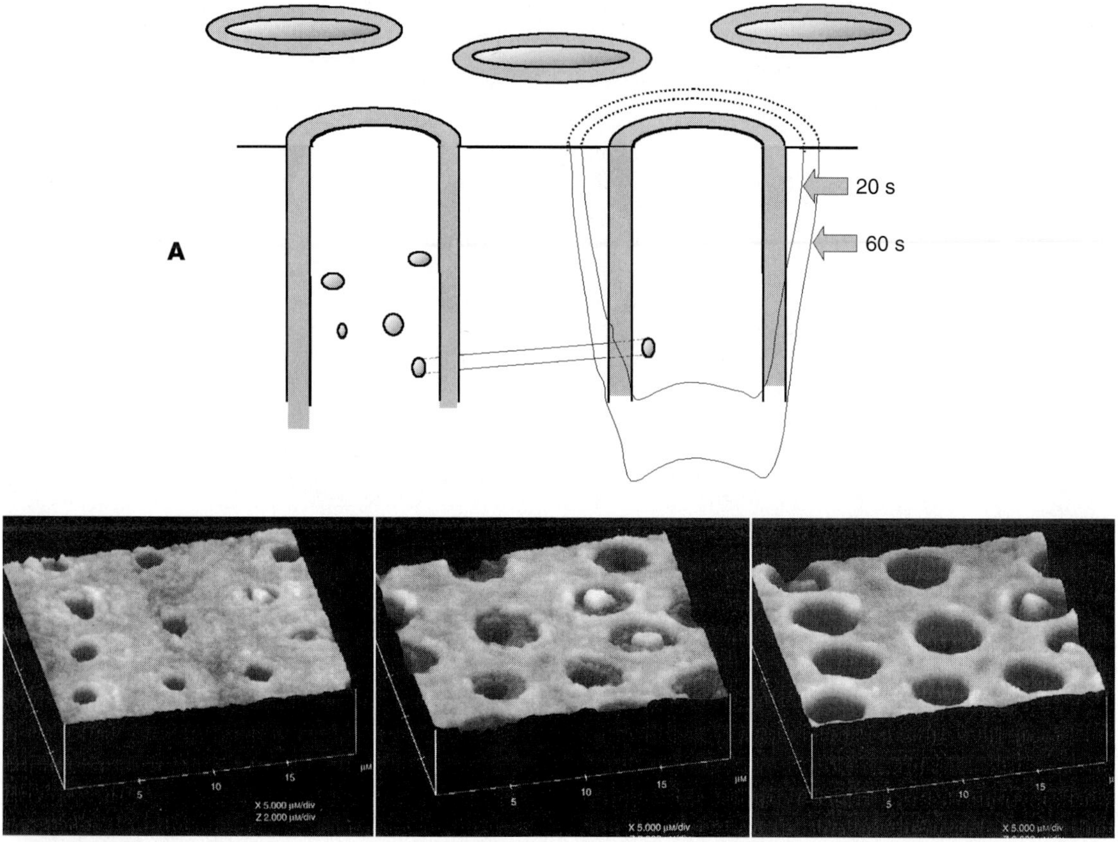

Fig. 10-12 Acid-etching effects on dentin. **A,** Schematic view of the progression of acid etching on dentin. **B,** Atomic force microscope image of the acid-etching effects of dentin, showing progress after 20s, 60s, and 100s, respectively, with citric acid etching.
(Courtesy GW Marshall, UCSF School of Dentistry, San Francisco, CA.)

ENAMEL AND DENTIN BONDING AGENTS FOR DIRECT COMPOSITES

OVERVIEW

A chronology of the development of bonding agents used to place direct composites is shown in Table 10-3. Modern bonding agents contain three major ingredients (etchant, primer, adhesive) that may be packaged separately or combined. Examples of commercial bonding agents are shown in Fig. 10-13. Table 10-4 presents a summary of the components of currently available fourth-, fifth-, and sixth-generation bonding agents. Typical compositions of these components are summarized in Table 10-5.

Etchants are relatively strong acid solutions that are mainly based on phosphoric acid. Primers contain hydrophilic monomers to produce good wetting. Adhesives include typical dimethacrylate oligomers that are found in composites. Most fourth- and fifth-generation bonding agents are remarkably similar.

TABLE 10-3 Chronology of Developments for Bonding of Direct Composites to Tooth Structure

Generation	Time Period	Development
	1950-1970	Experimentation with mineral acids for bonding acrylic to enamel; concern about etching of dentin; bonding agents not utilized with composites
	Early 1970s	Acid-etching of enamel; enamel bonding agents (self-cured)
	Late 1970s	Hydrophobic enamel bonding agents, hydrophilic dentin bonding agents, light-cured components
4	Mid to late 1980s	Removal of dentin smear layer; acidic monomers and acidic pretreatments; reduction of steps in bonding technique; multiuse bonding agents
5	Early 1990s	Etching to achieve hybrid layer in dentin; hydrophilic agents for both enamel and dentin; bonding to moist tooth structure; single-bottle primer-adhesives
6	Mid to late 1990s	Self-etching primers and primer-adhesives; light- and dual-cured options
	Future	Low-shrinkage, self-adhesive restorative materials?

COMPOSITION

Etchants A wide range of organic (maleic, tartaric, citric, EDTA, acidic monomers), polymeric (polyacrylic acid), and mineral (hydrochloric, nitric, hydrofluoric) acids have been investigated as etchants, but phosphoric acid solutions and gels (37%, 35%, 10%) have been shown to produce the most reliable etching patterns. Acid etchants are also called *conditioners* to disguise the fact that most are relatively strong acids (pH≅1.0).

Originally, etching solutions were free-flowing liquids and were difficult to control during placement. Gel etchants were developed by adding small amounts of microfiller or cellulose thickening agents. These gels flow under slight pressure but do not flow under their own weight.

Primers Primers are hydrophilic monomers (see Table 10-5) usually carried in a solvent. Acidic primers containing carboxylic acid groups are used in self-etching bonding agents. The solvents used in primers are acetone, ethanol-water, or primarily water. In some primers, the

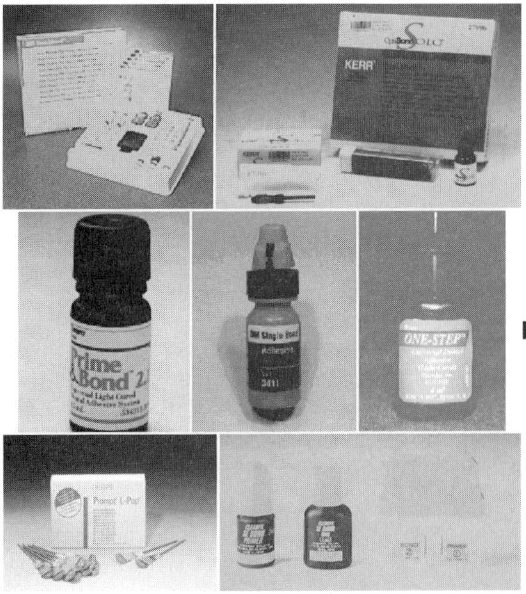

Fig. 10-13 Examples of dentin bonding agents (circa 2001). **A,** 4th-generation (Scotchbond Multi Purpose, *left*), 5th-generation (OptiBond Solo *right*). **B,** 5th-generation (Prime & Bond NT, Single Bond, One-Step). **C,** 6th-generation (Prompt L-Pop, Clearfil SE Bond).

TABLE 10-4 Components of 4th-, 5th- and 6th-Generation Bonding Agents

Generation	Number of Components	Description of Components
4th—light-cured*	3	Etchant, primer, adhesive
4th—dual-cured*	5	Etchant, primer and catalyst, adhesive and catalyst
5th—light-cured†	2	Etchant, primer-adhesive
5th—dual-cured†	3	Etchant, primer-adhesive, catalyst
6th—light-cured‡	1 or 2	Acidic primer-adhesive or acidic primer, adhesive
6th—dual-cured‡	3	Acidic primer and catalyst, adhesive

*Also called *multiuse bonding agent.*
†Also called *single-bottle bonding agent.*
‡Also called *self-etching primer.*

TABLE 10-5 Representative Compositions of Major Components of Bonding Agents

Component	Composition of Major Components
4TH-GENERATION	
Etchant	Phosphoric acid (32%-37%)
	Citric acid (10%)/calcium chloride (20%)
	Oxalic acid/aluminum nitrate
Primer	NTG-GMA/BPDM, HEMA/GPDM
	4-META/MMA, glutaraldehyde
Adhesive	Bis-GMA/TEGMA
Solvent	Acetone, ethanol/water
5TH-GENERATION	
Etchant	Phosphoric acid
Primer-adhesive	PENTA, methacrylated phosphonates
Solvent	Acetone, ethanol/water, solvent-free
6TH-GENERATION	
Acidic primer-adhesive	Methacrylated phosphates
Solvent	Water

4-META, 4-methacryloxyethyl trimellitic anhydride; *Bis-GMA,* 2,2-*bis*[4(2-hydroxy-3 methacryloyloxy-propyloxy)-phenyl]propane; *BPDM,* biphenyl dimethacrylate; *GPDM,* glycerophosphoric acid dimethacrylate; *HEMA,* 2-hydroxyethylmethacrylate; *MMA,* methyl methacrylate; *NTG-GMA,* N-tolylglycine-glycidyl methacrylate; *PENTA,* dipentaerythritol pentacrylate phosphoric acid ester; *TEGMA,* triethyleneglycoldimethacrylate.

solvent levels can be as high as 90%. A few fourth- and fifth-generation bonding agents are solvent-free. Therefore primers have different evaporation rates, drying patterns, and penetration characteristics, all of which can influence the resulting bond strength. Advantages and disadvantages of primers with various solvents are listed in Table 10-6.

Adhesives Adhesives are generally hydrophobic, dimethacrylate oligomers (see Table 10-5) that are compatible with monomers used

TABLE 10-6 Advantages and Disadvantages of Primers with Various Solvents

Solvent	Advantages	Disadvantages
Acetone	Dries quickly	Evaporates quickly after being dispensed; can evaporate from container; sensitive to wetness of dentin; multiple coats may be required; offensive odor
Ethanol/water	Evaporates less quickly, less sensitive to wetness of dentin	Extra drying time
Water	Slow evaporation, not sensitive to wetness of dentin	Long drying time; water can interfere with adhesive if not removed
Solvent-free	No drying, single coat	Higher film thickness

in the primer and composite. These oligomers are usually diluted with lower–molecular weight monomers.

Initiators and Accelerators Most bonding agents are light cured and contain an activator such as camphoroquinone and an organic amine. Dual-cured bonding agents include a catalyst to promote self-curing.

Fillers Although most bonding agents are unfilled, some products contain inorganic fillers ranging from 0.5% to 40% by weight. Filler particles include micro fillers, also called *nanofillers,* and sub-micron glass. Filled bonding agents tend to produce higher in vitro bond strengths.

Other Ingredients Bonding agents may contain fluoride or antimicrobial ingredients. One bonding agent contains glutaraldehyde as a desensitizer. The effectiveness of fluoride release from a bonding agent has not been demonstrated.

PROPERTIES

Laboratory Properties

Bond Strength Most bonding agents produce bond strengths to human enamel and superficial dentin of 15 to 35 MPa. Bond strengths determined for deep dentin tend to be lower than superficial dentin. A variety of clinical problems can reduce bond strength. Some clinical problems and suggested solutions are listed in Table 10-7.

Fatigue Strength Over long periods (>10 years), the bonded interface will undergo extensive fatigue cycling. Combinations of mechanical and thermal cycling stresses may produce as many as 1 million cycles of loading on the interfaces per year. Weak or compromised interfaces will debond and allow microleakage and fluid flow. The latter is detectable as pain. Only a limited number of low-cycle fatigue tests have been performed on dentin bonding systems in the laboratory. Fatigued systems failed at the bonded interface and displayed 50% reduction in bond strength even after only 1000 cycles of loading. To date there are no laboratory data that would strongly support long-term success of bonding agents.

Biological Properties Solvents and monomers in bonding agents are typically skin irritants. Certain material, such as 2-hydroxyethylmethacrylate (HEMA), is not considered biocompatible as a monomer. Bonding agents may produce local and systemic reactions in dentists and dental assistants sufficient to preclude their

TABLE 10-7 Clinical Problems That Can Decrease Bond Strength of Bonding Agents and Suggested Solutions

Problem	Solution
Dentin surface too dry	Use moist cotton pellet to rehydrate surface
Dentin surface too wet	Gently air dry to achieve glistening surface
Contamination with saliva or blood	Rinse, re-etch if contamination is moderate or greater
Contamination with caries detector, handpiece lubricant or hemostatic agent	Rinse and re-etch
Contamination by eugenol	Avoid eugenol-containing provisional materials and temporary cements
Remaining caries-affected dentin	Remove caries
Surface doesn't glisten after application of primer	Apply additional coats of primer
Self-cured composite or resin cement debonds from adhesive	Use dual-cured bonding agent with self-cured composite or resin cement
Bonding agent undercured	Cure recommended time with properly maintained light-curing unit, be sure bonding agent is compatible with light-curing unit
Recent bleaching procedure	Wait 1 week after bleaching

further use in the dental office. It is critical that dental personnel protect themselves from recurring exposure. Protective techniques include wearing gloves, immediately replacing contaminated gloves, using high-volume evacuation where the materials are being used, keeping all bottles tightly closed, and disposing of materials in such a way that the monomers cannot evaporate into the office air. Even with double gloves, contact with these aggressive solvents and monomers will produce actual skin contact in a few minutes. Follow all reasonable precautions, and if unwanted contact occurs, immediately flush affected areas with copious amounts of water and soap. Once the materials are polymerized, there is very little risk of side effects; although patients should be protected during bonding operations, properly polymerized materials have not been shown to create any subsequent patient hazard.

Clinical Properties Enamel bonding has a long history of success when enamel is etched appropriately, microtags are formed, and components are cured. Clinical evaluations of the performance of bonding agents were initiated in the late 1970s but were primarily focused on the ability of enamel bonding agents to suppress microleakage. There were no standardized clinical procedures for evaluating bonding systems until the ADA developed "Guidelines for Dental Adhesion" in 1994. These guidelines require the testing of adhesives for bonding restorations to non-retentive Class 5 lesions. The lesions, which may be saucer-shaped or notch-shaped, are found on enamel margins along the coronal mar-

A

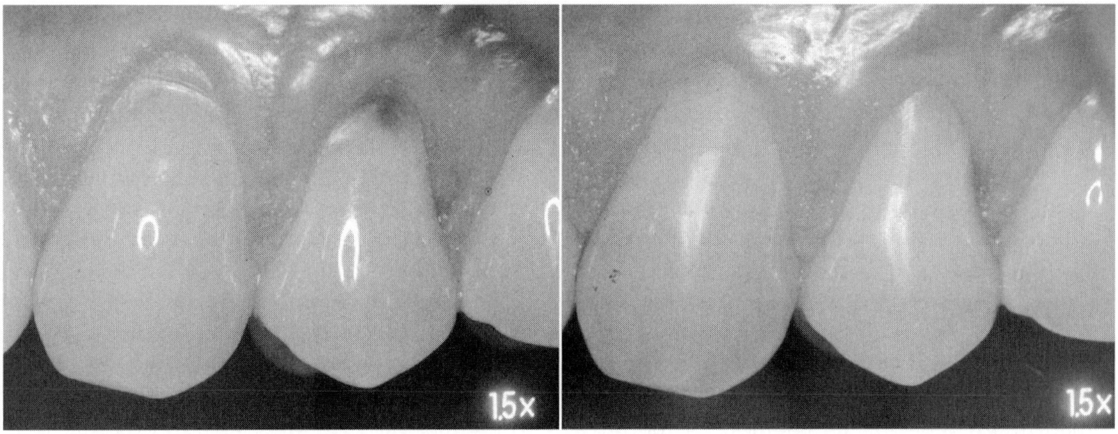

B

Fig. 10-14 Clinical testing of bonding systems by restoring non-retentive Class 5 lesions. **A,** Clinical examples of Class 5 lesions. **B,** Clinical examples of the same lesions restored with a bonding agent and composite restorations.

gin and dentin along the apical margin (Fig. 10-14, *A*). The success of a bonding agent is evaluated indirectly by examining the performance of the restorations for: (1) postoperative sensitivity, (2) interfacial staining, (3) secondary caries, and (4) retention or fracture from insertion to 18 months. These clinical trials test short-term retention and initial sealing.

Most commercial products for enamel and dentin bonding are successful in clinical trials. However, these clinical trials generally combine enamel and dentin bonding. There is no acceptable clinical regimen for critically testing dentin bonding only in retentive preparations. Because clinical trials are usually highly controlled, they are often not predictive of average clinical usage in general practice. Longevity of bonding in general practice may only be 40% that achieved in clinical trials, because of technique or other failures. Long-term clinical performance of bonding systems (>10 years) for a wide range of materials has not yet been reported.

Sites of failure for most bonded restorations occur along cervical margins where the bonding is primarily to dentin. Examination of bonded composites in Class 2 restorations demonstrates that 95% of all secondary caries associated with composite occurs interproximally. These margins are the most difficult to fabricate during placement of the restoration, are typically bonded to dentin and cementum rather than enamel, and are hard to access with visible light for adequate polymerization.

MANIPULATION

Enamel Bonding Bonding to enamel occurs primarily by micro-mechanical retention after acid etching is used to remove smear layers and preferentially dissolve hydroxyapatite crystals in the outer surface of the interface. Fluid adhesive constituents penetrate into the newly produced surface irregularities and become locked into place after polymerization of the adhesive.

Gel etchants are dispensed from a syringe onto tooth surfaces to be etched (see Fig. 10-9, *A*). Etching times for enamel vary depending on the type and quality of enamel. Generally, a 15-second etch with 37% phosphoric acid is sufficient to produce microtags. However, until macro-spaces are evident, the characteristic clinical endpoint of a frosty enamel appearance will not develop. Deciduous enamel generally contains some prismless enamel that has not yet worn away. It takes longer to etch through this outer layer and to reveal characteristic etch patterns on the underlying prism enamel. It is therefore commonplace to recommend 120 seconds of acid etching for primary enamel.

Some enamel may have been rendered more insoluble as a result of fluorosis. In those cases, extended etching times are required to ensure that sufficient micro-mechanical bonding can occur. It is not uncommon to extend etching times for several minutes to accomplish an adequate etch. The only caution is that dentin should be protected from exposure to acid for this long a time.

After the intended etching time, the materials are rinsed away and the tooth structure is maintained in a moist surface condition for the next stage of bonding. Then, primer can be flowed onto the surface to penetrate into the available surface irregularities. Primer and adhesive that flow into larger irregularities, such as the prism peripheries shown in Fig. 10-9, *D*, produce resin tags once the adhesive is cured. These tags are actually "macrotags." Inspection of the details of the surfaces for a single prism reveals that smaller tags, "microtags," form where adhesive flows into the spaces between partially dissolved individual hydroxyapatite crystals (see Fig. 10-9, *E* and *F*). Microtags are much more numerous and contribute to most of the micro-mechanical retention.

Dentin Bonding Dentin bonding involves three distinct processes—etching (conditioning), priming, and bonding. In contrast to enamel, dentin contains more water (see Table 10-2) and is strongly hydrophilic. To manage this problem, primers have hydrophilic components that wet dentin and penetrate the surface. The goal is to produce microtags for micro-mechanical adhesion.

Modern bonding agents are applied to moist dentin surfaces. Any drying must be done cautiously. Once the hydroxyapatite component of the outer layer of dentin is removed, dentin contains about 50% unfilled space and about 20% remaining water. Even a short air blast from an air-water spray can inadvertently dehydrate the outer surface and cause the remaining collagen sponge to collapse onto itself. Once this happens, the collagen mesh readily excludes the penetration of primer and bonding will fail. It is then necessary to rehydrate the dentin surface before priming. Hold a cotton pellet moistened with water against the surface for about 10 to 15 seconds or apply a rewetting agent (surfactant solutions in water). Do not bond to dentin unless the surface looks glistening. This is the critical clinical clue that the surface is sufficiently hydrated. An overly moist condition is equally bad. Excess moisture tends to dilute the primer and interfere with resin interpenetration. Generally, etch enamel and dentin simultaneously. Apply etchant to enamel first and then to dentin. Rinse excess material from the surfaces. Use gentle air-drying to check the enamel for a frosty appearance, but guard against over-drying etched dentin as you do so. If necessary, rehydrate the dentin to a glistening appearance before applying primer.

The process of resin impregnation of etched dentin by the primer is called *hybrid layer formation*, as described in Fig. 10-15. The result of this process has been called the *resin-interpenetration zone* or *resin-interdiffusion zone*. This layer is critical to bonding and creates the necessary microtags. The hybrid layer is revealed to be quite variable in thickness (see Fig. 10-15, *D*). Concurrent with hybrid layer formation is the penetration of primer into the fluid-filled and/or open dentinal tubules. This generates quite large macrotags. However, these appear to be of little value to overall bonding at the present time. This material is generally undercured and behaves as soft flexible tags. If dentin is dehydrated before priming and bonding, these macrotags are more likely to be quite extensive.

The thickness of a hybrid layer is not a critical requirement for success. Dentin bond strength is probably proportional only to the number of microtags, not the length of the microtags. Effective etching and priming of dentin does not require long times to produce acceptable dentin bond strengths. Inadequate etching or priming, however, is a concern; therefore the tendency is to err routinely on the side of longer-than-needed etching times. If the etched zone is too

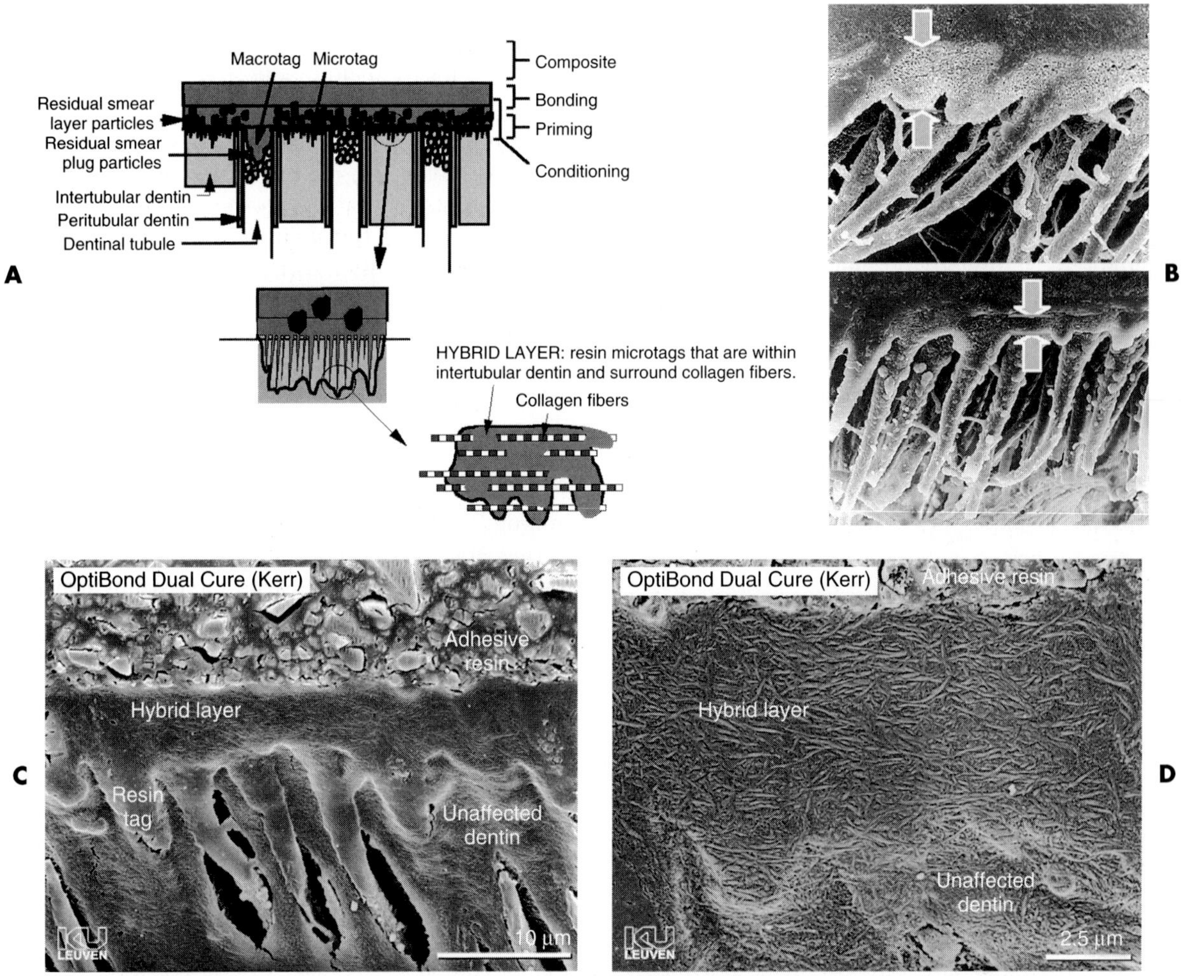

Fig. 10-15 Hybrid layer formation. **A,** Etching removes hydroxyapatite crystals within intertubular dentin and along peritubular dentin. Primer penetrates intertubular spaces and fluid-filled tubular spaces. Cured primer forms microtags within intertubular dentin and macrotags within tubules. **B,** Scanning electron photomicrographs indicating the varying thickness of the hybrid layer. **C,** SEM of restoration and hybrid layer after removal of dentin structure. **D,** Higher magnification of region of hybrid layer showing interpenetration of polymerized primer and collagen.

(**B,** Courtesy J Perdigão, University of Minnesota, Minneapolis, MN; **C** and **D,** courtesy B van Meerbeek, Catholic University of Leuven, Belgium.)

deep, it is more challenging to fill the zone with primer. A potential problem presents if decalcified dentin is not fully impregnated. The etched but not impregnated space may reside as a mechanically weak zone and promote nanoleakage. While this zone has been detected in laboratory experiments, the clinical results of this process have never been demonstrated to be a problem.

Primers contain solvents to enhance their wetting and to co-solubilize the range of monomers involved. During application of the primer, most of the solvent evaporates quickly. Very little of the original primer that is applied actually remains as polymerizable material to produce dentin impregnation. Thus several layers usually must be applied. The rule of thumb is that one should apply as many layers as are necessary to produce a persisting glistening appearance on dentin.

Once the primer is applied adequately, an adhesive is applied and light cured. Surfaces of the cured bonding agents are initially air inhibited and do not immediately react. However, as composite is placed against the surface, the air is displaced and copolymerization occurs.

BONDING SYSTEMS FOR OTHER SUBSTRATES

AMALGAM

For bonding to dental amalgam, the objective is to cause the unset bonding agent and unset amalgam to intermingle before they set. Because dental amalgam is opaque, the bonding system must be chemically cured.

A bonding agent is applied to the cavity preparation. Dental amalgam is condensed against the unset bonding system. The thickness of the bonding layer must be increased by using multiple layers of bonding agent or by adding thickening agents to the bonding agent. One bonding agent uses an admixture of small, polymethyl methacrylate powder particles in the bonding agent to thicken it. Generally, the thickness of the bonding layer is increased to 20 to 50 μm. Fig. 10-16, *A,* portrays this process schematically. Fig. 10-16, *B,* provides a scanning electron photomicrograph of the resulting interface. In the absence of suitable commingling, the bond strength might be only 4 to 8 MPa. However, with micro-mechanical interlocking at the interface, the bond strength may be 20 MPa. In most restorations, amalgam bonding agents simply seal the cavity against fluid flow and microleakage. Amalgam bonding agents provide little or no retention for set amalgams, even if they are roughened, because the bonding systems do not wet or adapt to the set amalgam surfaces very well.

LABORATORY COMPOSITES

Restorations made with laboratory composites (see Chapter 9), include inlays, onlays, veneers, or milled restorations, and are fabricated indirectly in a dental laboratory and then bonded into existing cavity preparations. Bonding requires agents for both the tooth structure and the undersurfaces of the indirect restoration. Resin composite cements are usually used to fill the space between the two surfaces. Bonding to the tooth structure and composite cement is straightforward and reliable.

Bonding to the indirect composite surfaces is difficult. The goal is to swell the outer surfaces of the resin matrix and allow new monomers from the bonding agent to penetrate spaces among existing polymer chains. At the time of curing, the new polymer chains become micromechanically intertwined with the existing polymer chains, producing relatively strong bonding. Bonding can be enhanced by blasting (microetching) with particles of aluminum oxide, etching with hydrofluoric acid gel, or treating with primers. Sandblasting roughens the surface. Etching removes smear layers and partially dissolves glass filler particles. Primers provide good wetting and potential chemical bonding to exposed glass filler particle surfaces. Commercial primers for laboratory composites contain silane, unfilled resin monomers, or silane-monomer combinations.

Bonding composite cement to laboratory composites generally produces bond strengths in the range of 20 to 35 MPa.

CERAMIC

Ceramic restorations bonded to enamel and dentin include a number of bonding interfaces. Enamel and dentin are treated with whatever bonding agent is desirable. The under-surface of the all-ceramic inlay, onlay, crown, bridge, or veneer is treated with 5% to 9% hydrofluoric acid gel. The pH of this gel is low and capable of removing any smear layers while etching the phase boundaries and the more soluble silicate glass phases. Although this process does not

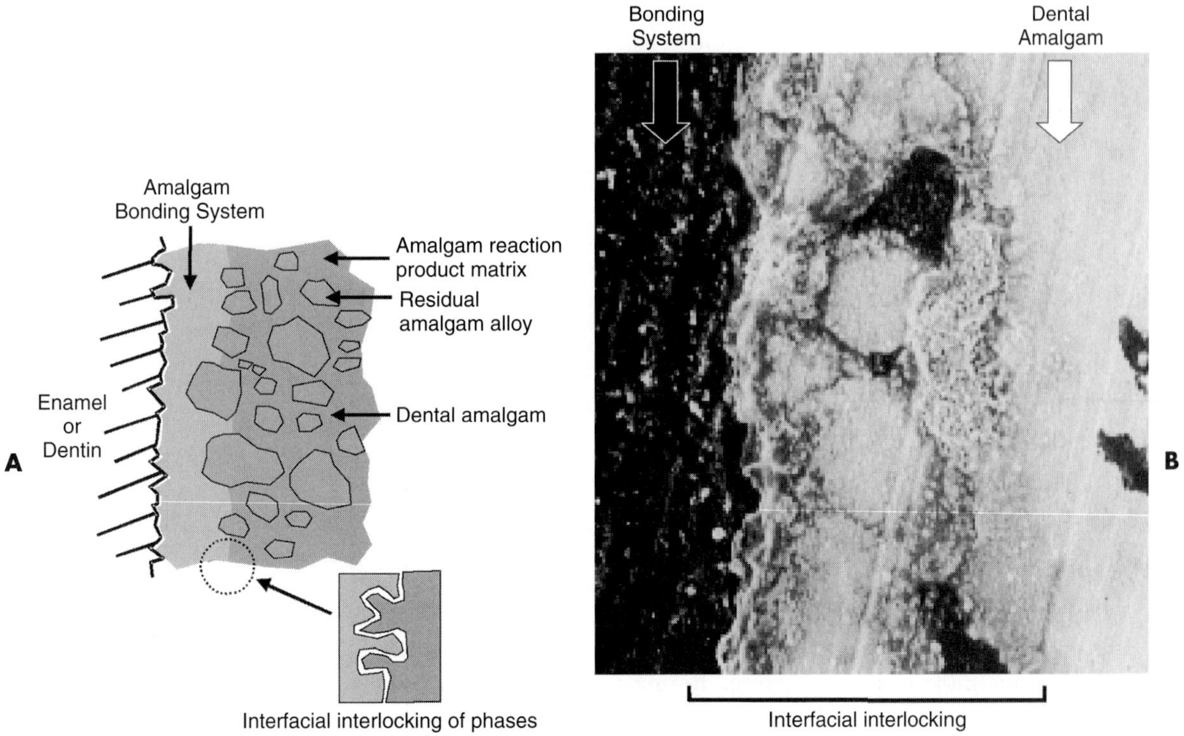

Fig. 10-16 Mechanism of bonding amalgam to tooth structure. **A,** Schematic of thickened layer of bonding agent to permit intermingling with fluid dental amalgam along the interface during amalgam placement and before setting. **B,** Scanning electron photomicrograph of interface between bonding agent and dental amalgam.
(**B,** Adapted from Ramos JC, Perdigão J, *Am J Dent* 10:152, 1997.)

work on alumina- or zirconia-based ceramics, it is effective for other ceramics. Another popular option is to blast (micro-etch) the surface with 50-μm aluminum oxide particles.

Once the ceramic surface is prepared, an aqueous and acidified solution of silane is applied to enhance wetting and potentially function as a chemical coupling agent. Silane is a difunctional molecule capable of reacting to the hydroxyls on the silicate phases along the treated surface's restoration. The other end of the silane is capable of copolymerizing with resin composite cement, which is used to attach the two treated surfaces and fill in the typically 100 μm of intervening space after seating (Fig. 10-17).

Bonding systems used with resin cements for all-ceramic systems can be light cured but are often dual cured or self cured. Bond strengths for a bonded ceramic restoration to tooth structure are generally in the range of 20 to 40 MPa.

COMPOSITE BONDED TO CAST ALLOYS

It is sometimes desirable to bond a resin composite to a cast alloy substrate rather than ceramic. Traditionally, resin bonding to metal substrates has relied on macro-mechanical retention (latticework, mesh, beads, or posts along the metal surface). Another approach to resin-metal adhesion was introduced in 1984 and trademarked "Silicoating." A silicon oxide coating is generated to create a surface that is capable of chemical bonding. This technique has been applied to gold, cobalt-chromium, silver-palladium,

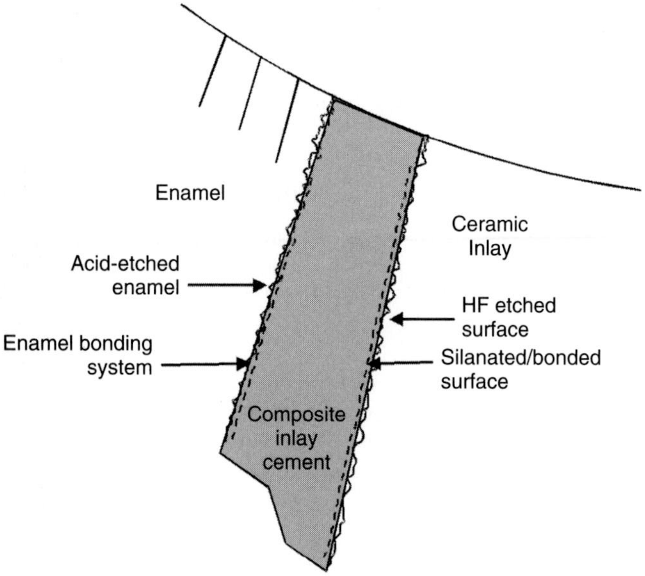

Fig. 10-17 Schematic of materials and interfaces involved in bonding all-ceramic restorations to tooth structure.

and titanium alloys. For Silicoating, a metal surface is roughened by sandblasting with 250-μm Al_2O_3, cleaned, silica coated, chemically silanated, primed, and the composite is bonded.

Other techniques for treating alloy surfaces to be bonded with composite include thermally applied silica and ceramic blasting (Table 10-8). Recently, liquid primers composed of thiophosphate monomers have become available. These techniques are equally effective in providing a relatively strong bond (18 to 30 MPa) of composites to alloy substrates.

TABLE 10-8 Systems for Bonding Composites to Noble and Base-Metal Alloys

System	Example
Pyrogenic silica	Silicoater
Thermally applied silica	Silicoater MD, Siloc
Ceramic blasting	Rocatec Junior, CoJet-Sand
Liquid primer	Thiophosphate monomer

REPAIR OF COMPOSITE, CERAMIC, AND PORCELAIN-FUSED-TO-METAL RESTORATIONS

It is quite common to encounter restorations that require repair because of long-term wear, unwanted color change, the appearance of small surface defects or chipping. These situations can be easily managed by veneering the surface with fresh composite. The damaged surface is removed to a depth of 1 to 1.5 mm below the final intended surface employing small burs, and the excavation is extended to neighboring enamel margins. The margins are roughened and etched to remove any smear layer and provide micromechanical retention. Priming produces tags into the enamel and diffusion into the surface of the old restoration. It is critical that the old composite is not over-dried because water in the old restoration tends to hold open the old polymer network and allow some hybrid layer formation. The bonding agent is cured. Restorative material is added, cured, and polished. Excellent repair bond strengths (20 to 35 MPa) are possible.

SELECTED PROBLEMS

Problem 1

The enamel portion of a tooth was etched for 15 seconds and rinsed. Upon observation, it did not appear frosty. What might explain the inadequate etch and what is a possible method to obtain a better etch?

Solution

The tooth may contain a higher than normal level of fluoride and thus may be resistant to normal etching. Apply the phosphoric acid for a longer period (up to 120 seconds) to obtain a frosty enamel appearance.

Problem 2

During removal of an impression of a first molar with a composite core build-up, the core material debonded. What might explain the failed bond and what is a possible solution to obtain an adequate bond of the composite core material to the tooth?

Solution a

Self-cured composite core materials are popular because they are esthetic and easy to use. However, some self-cured composite cores are incompatible with certain light-cured bonding agents. Be sure to pick compatible composite core materials and bonding agents for this application.

Solution b

Choose a dual-cured bonding agent or use a light-cured composite core material.

Problem 3

During fabrication of an all-ceramic crown, a dentist used a provisional composite cemented with eugenol-based temporary cement. Upon bonding the all-ceramic crown, there was a problem with setting of the bonding agent and resin cement. Explain the problem and offer a solution.

Solution a

The polymerization of most bonding agents and resin cements is severely hindered in the presence of eugenol. Take care to remove all remnants of the eugenol cement, then rinse and re-etch the tooth.

Solution b

In the future, use a resin-based provisional cement.

Problem 4

A dentist learned at a study club that her colleagues were etching tooth structure with phosphoric acid before applying a sixth-generation bonding agent. Is it desirable to etch with phosphoric acid before applying a self-etching primer-adhesive?

Solution

Current sixth-generation bonding agents bond effectively to enamel and dentin without prior etching with phosphoric acid. The additional etching achieved with phosphoric acid could result in over-etching of dentin and subsequent nanoleakage.

Problem 5

After etching, a dentist inadvertently over-dried the tooth. Explain the problem and offer a solution.

Solution

Most modern bonding agents bond best to a moist tooth. If dentin is over-dried, it is best to rehydrate it by applying a moist cotton pellet for 15 seconds before applying the primer of the bonding agent.

BIBLIOGRAPHY

General Reading

Cagle CV: *Handbook of adhesive bonding,* ed 1, New York, 1973, McGraw-Hill.

Bonding to Tooth Structure

Abdalla AI, Davidson CL: Bonding efficiency and interfacial morphology of one-bottle adhesives to contaminated dentin surfaces, *Am J Dent* 11:281, 1998.

Barakat MM, Powers JM: In vitro bond strength of cements to treated teeth, *Aust Dent J* 31:415, 1986.

Bayne SC, Fleming JE, Faison S: SEM-EDS analysis of macro and micro resin tags of laminates, *J Dent Res* 61A:304, 1982.

Bayne SC, Swift Jr EJ: Solvent analysis of three reduced-component dentin bonding systems, *Trans Acad Dent Mater* 1:156, 1997.

Boghosian A: Clinical evaluation of a filled adhesive system in Class 5 restorations, *Compend Contin Educ Dent* 17:750-752, 754, 1996.

Bouillaguet S, Wataha JC, Hanks CT et al: In vitro cytotoxicity and dentin permeability of HEMA, J Endodont 22:244, 1996.

Bouillaguet S, Wataha JC, Virgillito M et al: Effect of sub-lethal concentrations of HEMA (2-hydroxyethyl methacrylate) on THP-1 human monocyte-macrophages, in vitro, *Dent Mater* 16:213, 2000.

Bowen RL, Eick JD, Henderson DA et al: Smear layer: removal and bonding considerations, *Oper Dent Suppl* 3:30, 1984.

Bozalis WG, Marshall Jr GW, Cooley RO: Mechanical pretreatments and etching of primary-tooth enamel, *ASDC J Dent Child* 46:43, 1979.

Buonocore MG: Simple method of increasing the adhesion of acrylic filling materials to enamel surfaces, *J Dent Res* 34:849, 1955.

Choi KK, Condon JR, Ferracane JL: The effects of adhesive thickness on polymerization contraction stress of composite, *J Dent Res* 79:812, 2000.

Clemmensen S: Sensitizing potential of 2-hydroxyethylmethacrylate. *Contact Dermatitis* 12:203, 1985.

Costa CA, Teixeira HM, do Nascimento AB et al: Biocompatibility of an adhesive system and 2-hydroxyethylmethacrylate, *ASDC J Dent Child* 66:337, 1999.

Davidson CL, Feilzer AJ: Polymerization shrinkage and polymerization shrinkage stress in polymer-based restoratives, *J Dent* 25:435, 1997.

Drummond JL, Sakaguchi RL, Racean DC et al: Testing mode and surface treatment effects on dentin bonding, *J Biomed Mater Res* 32:533, 1996.

Eick JD, Wilko RA, Anderson CH et al: Scanning electron microscopy of cut tooth surfaces and identification of debris by use of the electron microprobe, *J Dent Res* 49 (Suppl):1359, 1970.

Eick JD: Smear layer—materials surface, *Proc Finn Dent Soc* 88 (Suppl 1):225, 1992.

el-Kalla IH, Garcia-Godoy F: Saliva contamination and bond strength of single-bottle adhesives to enamel and dentin, *Am J Dent* 10:83, 1997.

Farah JW, Powers JM, editors: Bonding agents, *Dent Advis* 17(9):1, 2000.

Fissore B, Nicholls JI, Yuodelis RA: Load fatigue of teeth restored by a dentin bonding agent and a posterior composite resin, *J Prosthet Dent* 65:80, 1991.

Frankenberger R, Kramer N, Petschelt A: Fatigue behaviour of different dentin adhesives, *Clin Oral Investig* 3:11, 1999.

Fritz UB, Finger WJ, Stean H: Salivary contamination during bonding procedures with a one-bottle adhesive system, *Quint Int* 29:567, 1998.

Fusayama T: [Cavity preparation for a new adhesive restorative resin], *Shikai Tenbo* 57:1223, 1981.

Fusayama T: A simple pain-free adhesive restorative system by minimal reduction and total etching, Tokyo, 1993, Ishiyaku EuroAmerica, Inc.

Garberoglio R, Brannstrom M: Scanning electron microscopic investigation of human dentinal tubules, *Arch Oral Biol* 21:355, 1976.

Hansen EK, Munksgaard EC: Saliva contamination vs. efficacy of dentin-bonding agents, *Dent Mater* 5:329, 1989.

Johnson ME, Burgess JO, Hermesch CB et al: Saliva contamination of dentin bonding agents, *Oper Dent* 19:205, 1994.

Katsuno K, Manabe A, Hasegawa T et al: Possibility of allergic reaction to dentin primer—application on the skin of guinea pigs, *Dent Mater J* 11:77, 1992.

LeGeros RZ: Calcium phosphates in oral biology and medicine, Monographs in Oral Science, Vol. 15, Basel, 1992, Karger.

Marshall GW Jr, Wu-Magidi IC, Watanabe LG et al: Effect of citric acid concentration on dentin demineralization, dehydration, and rehydration: atomic force microscopy study, *J Biomed Mater Res* 42:500, 1998.

May KN Jr, Swift EJ Jr, Bayne SC: Bond strengths of a new dentin adhesive system, *Am J Dent* 10:195, 1997.

Mjor IA: Frequency of secondary caries at various anatomical locations, *Oper Dent* 10:88, 1985.

Munksgaard EC: Permeability of protective gloves to (di)methacrylates in resinous dental materials, *Scand J Dent Res* 100:189, 1992.

Nakabayashi N, Ashizawa M, Nakamura M: Identification of a resin-dentin hybrid layer in vital human dentin created in vivo: durable bonding to vital dentin, *Quint Int* 23: 135, 1992.

Nakabayashi N, Nakamura M, Yasuda N: Hybrid layer as a dentin-bonding mechanism, *J Esthet Dent* 3:133, 1991.

Nakabayashi N. Dentinal bonding mechanisms, *Quintessence Int* 22:73, 1991.

Nakabayashi N: The hybrid layer: a resin-dentin composite, *Proc Finn Dent Soc* 88 (Suppl 1):321, 1992.

Pashley DH, Carvalho RM, Sano H et al: The microtensile bond test: a review, *J Adhes Dent* 1:299, 1999.

Pashley DH: Smear layer: overview of structure and function, *Proc Finn Dent Soc* 88 (Suppl 1):215, 1992.

Pashley DH: Smear layer: physiological considerations, *Oper Dent Suppl* 3:13, 1984.

Pashley DH: Dentin: a dynamic substrate—a review, *Scan Microsc* 3:161, 1989.

Perdigão J, Lambrechts P, van Meerbeek B et al: Morphological field emission-SEM study of the effect of six phosphoric acid etching agents on human dentin, *Dent Mater* 12:262, 1996.

Powers JM, Finger WJ, Xie, J: Bonding of composite resin to contaminated human enamel and dentin, *J Prosthodont* 4:28, 1995.

Roeder LB, Berry III EA, You C et al: Bond strength of composite to air-abraded enamel and dentin, *Oper Dent* 20:186, 1995.

Rose EE, Joginder L, Williams NB et al: The screening of materials for adhesion to human tooth structure, *J Dent Res* 34:577, 1955.

Sano H, Ciucchi B, Matthews WG et al: Tensile properties of mineralized and demineralized human and bovine dentin, *J Dent Res* 73:1205, 1994.

Sano H, Takatsu T, Ciucchi B et al: Nanoleakage: leakage within the hybrid layer, *Oper Dent* 20:18, 1995.

Sano H, Yoshiyama M, Ebisu S et al: Comparative SEM and TEM observations of nanoleakage within the hybrid layer, *Oper Dent* 20:160, 1995.

Silverstone LM, Saxton CA, Dogon IL et al: Variation in the pattern of acid etching of human dental enamel examined by scanning electron microscopy, *Caries Res* 9:373, 1975.

Swift EJ, Perdigão J, Heymann HO et al: Clinical evaluation of a filled and unfilled dentin adhesive, *J Dent,* in press, 2001.

Tate WH, You C, Powers JM: Bond strength of compomers to dentin using acidic primers, *Am J Dent* 12:235, 1999.

Tate WH, You C, Powers JM: Bond strength of compomers to human enamel, *Oper Dent* 25:283, 2000.

van Meerbeek B, Dhem A, Goret-Nicaise M et al: Comparative SEM and TEM examination of the ultrastructure of the resin-dentin interdiffusion zone, *J Dent Res* 72:495, 1993.

Xie J, Flaitz CM, Hicks MJ et al: In-vitro bond strength of composite to sound dentin and artificial carious lesions in dentin, *Am J Dent* 9:31, 1996.

Xie J, Powers JM, McGuckin RS: In vitro bond strength of two adhesives to enamel and dentin under normal and contaminated conditions, *Dent Mater* 9:295, 1993.

Yoshii E: Cytotoxic effects of acrylates and methacrylates: relationships of monomer structures and cytotoxicity, *J Biomed Mater Res* 37:517, 1997.

Bonding to Other Substrates

Crumpler DC, Bayne SC, Sockwell S et al: Bonding to re-surfaced posterior composites, *Dent Mater* 5:417, 1989.

DeSchepper EJ, Cailletea, JG, Roeder L et al: In vitro tensile bond strengths of amalgam to treated dentin, J Esthet Dent 3:117, 1991.

Hansson O, Moberg LE: Evaluation of three silicoating methods for resin-bonded prostheses, *Scand J Dent Res* 101:243, 1993.

Hero H, Ruyter IE, Waarli ML et al: Adhesion of resins to Ag-Pd alloys by means of the silicoating technique, *J Dent Res* 66:1380, 1987.

Hummel SK, Pace LL, Marker VA: A comparison of two silicoating techniques, *J Prosthodont* 3:108, 1994.

Masil R, Tiller HJ: The adhesion of dental resin to metal surfaces: the Kulzer Silicoater technique, Wehrbeim: Kulzer and Co., Gmbh, 1st ed, 9, 1984.

Mazurat RD, Pesun S: Resin-metal bonding systems: a review of the Silicoating and Kevloc systems, *J Can Dent Assoc* 64:503, 1998.

Miller BH, Nakajima H, Powers JM et al: Bond strength between cements and metals used for endodontic posts, *Dent Mater* 14:312, 1998.

Mukai M, Fukui H, Hasegawa J: Relationship between sandblasting and composite resin-alloy bond strength by a silica coating, *J Prosthet Dent* 74:151, 1995.

NaBadalung DP, Powers, JM, Connelly ME: Comparison of bond strengths of three denture base resins to treated nickel-chromium-beryllium alloy, *J Prosthet Dent* 80:354, 1998.

O'Keefe KL, Miller BH, Powers JM: In vitro tensile bond strength of adhesive cements to new post materials, *Int J Prosthodont* 13:47, 2000.

Pesun S, Mazurat RD: Bond strength of acrylic resin to cobalt-chromium alloy treated with the Silicoater MD and Kevloc systems, *J Can Dent Assoc* 64:798, 1998.

Ramos JC, Perdigão J: Shear bond strengths and SEM morphology of dentin-amalgam adhesives, *Am J Dent* 10:152, 1997.

Roulet JF, Soderholm KJ, Longmate J: Effects of treatment and storage conditions on ceramic/composite bond strength, *J Dent Res* 74:381, 1995.

Schneider W, Powers JM, Pierpont HP: Bond strength of composites to etched and silica-coated porcelain fusing alloys, *Dent Mater* 8:211, 1992.

Shahverdi S, Canay S, Sahin E et al: Effects of different surface treatment methods on the bond strength of composite resin to porcelain, *J Oral Rehabil* 25:699, 1998.

Stokes AN, Tay WM, Pereira BP: Shear bond of resin cement to post-cured hybrid composites, *Dent Mater* 9:370, 1993.

Sturdevant JR, Swift Jr EJ, Bayne SC: Cement bond strength to millable composite for CAD/CAM restorations, *J Dent Res* 79:453, 2000.

Suliman AH, Swift EJ Jr, Perdigão J: Effects of surface treatment and bonding agents on bond strength of composite resin to porcelain, *J Prosthet Dent* 70:118, 1993.

Tate WH, Friedl K-H, Powers JM: Bond strength of composites to hybrid ionomers, *Oper Dent* 21:147, 1996.

Thompson VP, Del Castillo E, Livaditis GJ: Resin-bonded retainers. Part I: resin bond to electrolytically etched nonprecious alloys, *J Prosthet Dent* 50:771, 1983.

Watanabe I, Kurtz KS, Kabcenell JL et al: Effect of sandblasting and silicoating on bond strength of polymer-glass composite to cast titanium, *J Prosthet Dent* 82:462, 1999.

Wolf DM, Powers JM, O'Keefe KL: Bond strength of composite to etched and sand-blasted porcelain, *Am J Dent* 6:155, 1993.

Chapter 11

Amalgam

An amalgam is an alloy of mercury and one or more other metals. Dental amalgam is produced by mixing liquid mercury with solid particles of an alloy of silver, tin, copper, and sometimes zinc, palladium, indium, and selenium. This combination of solid metals is known as the *amalgam alloy.* It is important to differentiate between dental amalgam and the amalgam alloy that is commercially produced and marketed as small filings, spheroid particles, or a combination of these, suitable for mixing with liquid mercury to produce the dental amalgam.

Once the amalgam is freshly mixed with liquid mercury, it has the plasticity that permits it to be conveniently packed or condensed into a prepared tooth cavity. After condensing, the dental amalgam is carved to generate the required anatomical features. Amalgam is used most commonly for direct, permanent, posterior restorations and for large foundation restorations, or cores, which are precursors to placing crowns. Dental amalgam restorations are reasonably easy to insert, are not overly technique sensitive, maintain anatomical form, have reasonably adequate resistance to fracture, prevent marginal leakage after a period of time in the mouth, can be used in stress bearing areas, and have a relatively long service life.

The principal disadvantage of dental amalgam is that the silver color does not match tooth structure. In addition, they are somewhat brittle; are subject to corrosion and galvanic action; may demonstrate a degree of marginal breakdown; and do not help retain weakened tooth structure. Finally, there are regulatory concerns about amalgam being disposed in the wastewater. In summary, dental amalgam is a highly successful material clinically and is very cost effective, but alternatives such as cast gold and esthetic restorative materials are now very competitive in terms of frequency of use. Many argue, however, that the use of amalgam must be strongly supported given its large public health benefit in the United States and many other countries.

In this chapter, the composition and morphology of the different dental amalgams are presented, followed by a discussion of low- and high-copper amalgams, the chemical reactions occurring during amalgamation, and the resultant microstructures. Various physical and mechanical properties are covered in the next section, as well as the factors related to the manipulation of amalgam. Finally, biological effects of amalgam and mercury are presented.

DENTAL AMALGAM ALLOYS

COMPOSITION AND MORPHOLOGY

ANSI/ADA Specification No. 1 for amalgam alloy (ISO 1559) includes a requirement for composition. This specification does not state precisely what the composition of alloys shall be; rather, it permits some variation in composition. The chemical composition must consist essentially of silver and tin. Copper, zinc, gold, palladium, indium, selenium, or mercury may be included in lesser amounts. Metals such as palladium, gold,

TABLE 11-1 Approximate Composition of Low- and High-Copper Amalgam Alloys

		Element (wt%)					
Alloy	**Particle Shape**	**Ag**	**Sn**	**Cu**	**Zn**	**In**	**Pd**
Low copper	Irregular or spherical	63-70	26-28	2-5	0-2	0	0
High copper							
Admixed regular	Irregular	40-70	26-30	2-30	0-2	0	0
	Spherical	40-65	0-30	20-40	0-1	0	0-1
Admixed unicomposition	Irregular	52-53	17-18	29-30	0	0	0.3
	Spherical	52-53	17-18	29-30	0	0	0.3
Unicompositional	Spherical	40-60	22-30	13-30	0	0-5	0-1

and indium in smaller quantities and copper in larger quantities have been included to alter the corrosion resistance and certain mechanical properties of the finished amalgam mass. These and other elements may be included, provided the manufacturer submits the alloy's composition and adequate clinical and biological data to the ADA's Council on Scientific Affairs to show that the alloy is safe to use as directed.

Alloys with more than 0.01% zinc are classified as zinc containing, and those with less than 0.01% as non-zinc alloys. Zinc has been included in amalgam alloys as an aid in manufacturing by helping to produce clean, sound castings of the ingots. However, improved manufacturing procedures have resulted in the elimination of zinc in most alloys. Recent studies have shown, however, that small amounts of zinc in high-copper dental amalgams improve clinical performance, presumably by reducing brittleness.

The approximate composition of commercial amalgam alloys is shown in Table 11-1, along with the shape of the particles. The alloys are broadly classified as low-copper (5% or less copper) and high-copper alloys (13% to 30% copper). Particles are irregularly shaped; microspheres of various sizes; or a combination of the two. Scanning electron micrographs of the particles are presented in Fig. 11-1. The low-copper alloys are either irregular or spherical. Both mor-

A

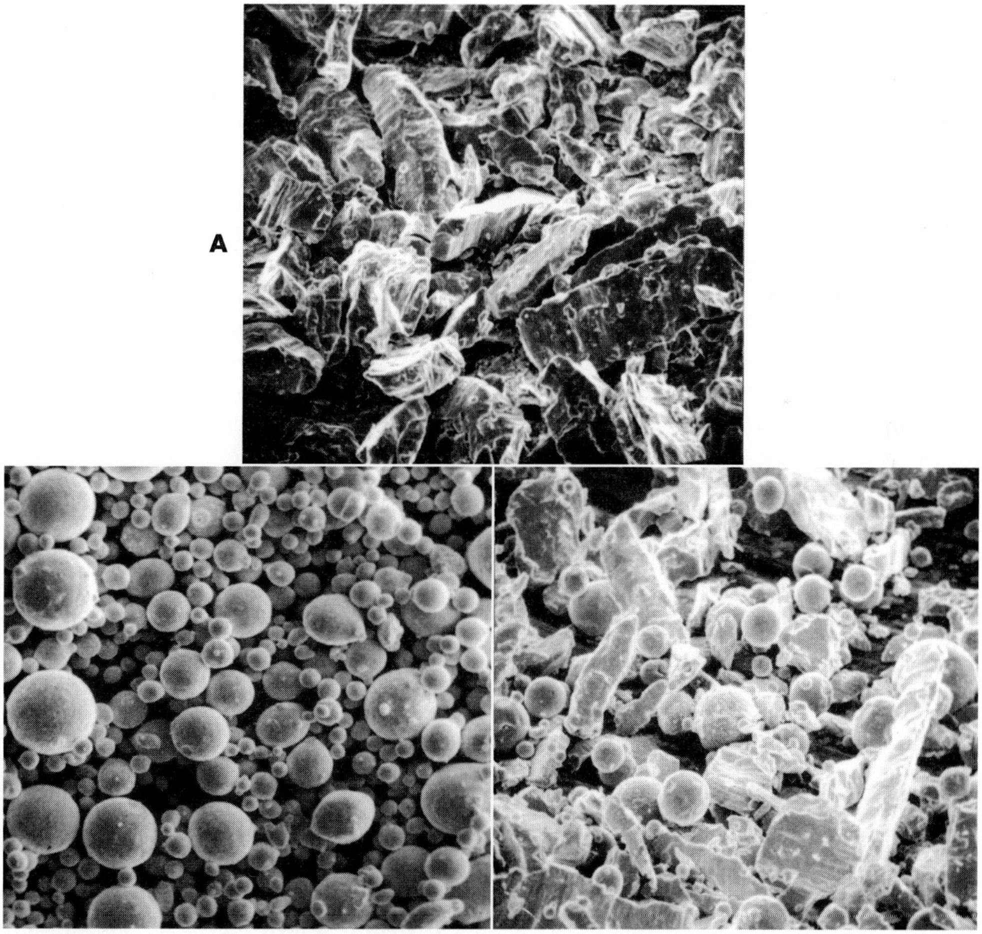

B

C

Fig. 11-1 Scanning electron micrographs. **A,** Lathe-cut; **B,** spherical; and **C,** admixed amalgam alloys.

phologies contain silver and tin in a ratio approximating the intermetallic compound Ag_3Sn. High-copper alloys contain either all spherical particles of the same composition (unicompositional) or a mixture of irregular and spherical particles of different or the same composition (admixed).

When the particles have different compositions, the admixed alloys are made by mixing particles of silver and tin with particles of silver and copper. The silver-tin particle is usually irregular, whereas the silver-copper particle is usually spherical in shape. The composition of the silver-tin particles in most commercial alloys is the same as that of the low-copper alloys. Different manufacturers, however, have somewhat different compositions for the silver-copper particle. The compositional ranges of the spherical silver-copper particles are shown in Table 11-1. The admixed regular alloy contains 33% to 60% spherical particles that have a composition close to the eutectic composition of Ag_3Cu_2 (see Fig. 6-9); the balance are irregular particles.

Like the admixed alloy, the unicompositional alloys have higher copper contents than the conventional lathe-cut or spherical low-copper alloys, but all the particles are spherical, as seen in Fig. 11-1. The silver content of the unicompositional alloys varies from 40% to 60%, copper content from 13% to 30%, and tin content varies only slightly.

A high-copper admixed alloy is also available, in which both spherical and irregular particles have the same composition and the copper content is between 29% and 30%. High-copper alloys are less commonly supplied as unicompositional, irregular particles. The lathe-cut, high-copper alloys contain more than 23% copper.

Interest has increased in admixed amalgams containing 10% to 15% indium (In) in the mercury. The addition of In to Hg decreases the amount of Hg needed, decreases the Hg vapor during and after setting, and increases the wetting. These amalgams have low creep and lower early-compressive strengths, but higher final strengths than comparable amalgams without indium. It is proposed that the lower levels of Hg vapor are due to oxides of In formed at the surface or the lower amount of Hg used in the mix.

It is estimated that more than 90% of the dental amalgams currently placed are high-copper alloys. Of the high-copper alloys, admixed are used more often than spherical types, and fewer irregularly shaped or lathe-cut types are selected. A high-copper alloy is selected to obtain a restoration with high early strength, low creep, good corrosion resistance, and good resistance to marginal fracture.

In general, alloy composition; particle size, shape, and distribution; and heat treatment control the characteristic properties of the amalgam.

PRODUCTION

Irregular Particles To produce lathe-cut alloys, the metal ingredients are heated and protected from oxidation until melted, then poured into a mold to form an ingot. The ingot is cooled relatively slowly, leading to the formation of mainly Ag_3Sn (γ) and some Cu_3Sn (ε), Cu_6Sn_5 (η') and Ag_4Sn (β). After the ingot is completely cooled, it is heated for various periods of time (often 6 to 8 hours) at 400° C to produce a more homogeneous distribution of Ag_3Sn. The ingot is then reduced to filings by being cut on a lathe and ball milled. The particles are passed through a fine sieve and then ball milled to form the proper particle size. The particles are typically 60 to 120 μm in length, 10 to 70 μm in width, and 10 to 35 μm in thickness. Most products are labeled as fine-cut. The particle size and shape of lathe-cut amalgam alloys are shown in Fig. 11-1, *A*.

In general, freshly cut alloys amalgamate and set more promptly than aged particles, and some aging of the alloy is desirable to improve the shelf life of the product. The aging is related to relief of stress in the particles produced during the cutting of the ingot. The alloy particles are aged by subjecting them to a controlled temperature of 60° to 100° C for 1 to 6 hours. Irregularly shaped high-copper particles are made by spraying the molten alloy into water under high pressure.

Spherical Particles Spherical particles of low- or high-copper alloys are produced when all the desired elements are melted together. In the molten stage the metallic ingredients form the desired alloy. The liquid alloy is then sprayed, under high pressure of an inert gas, through a fine crack in a crucible into a large chamber. Depending on the difference in surface energy of the molten alloy and the gas used in the spraying process, the shape of the sprayed particles may be spherical or somewhat irregular, as shown in Fig. 11-1, *B*. The size of the spheres varies from 2 to 43 μm.

SILVER-TIN ALLOY

Because two of the principal ingredients in the amalgam alloy are silver and tin, it is appropriate to consider the binary system and the equilibrium phase diagram for these two metals, as shown in Fig. 11-2.

The most important feature in this diagram concerning the silver-tin alloy is that, when an alloy containing approximately 27% tin is slowly cooled below a temperature of 480° C, an intermetallic compound (Ag_3Sn) known also as the *gamma* (γ) *phase* is produced. This Ag_3Sn compound is an important ingredient in the silver amalgam alloy and combines with mercury to produce a dental amalgam of desired mechanical properties and handling. This silver-tin compound is formed only over a narrow composition range. The silver content for such an alloy would be approximately 73%. Practically, the tin content is held between 26% and 30%, and the remainder of the alloy consists of silver, copper, and zinc. If the concentration of tin is less than 26%, the beta one (β_1) phase, which is a solid solution of silver and mercury, forms. In one product, 5%

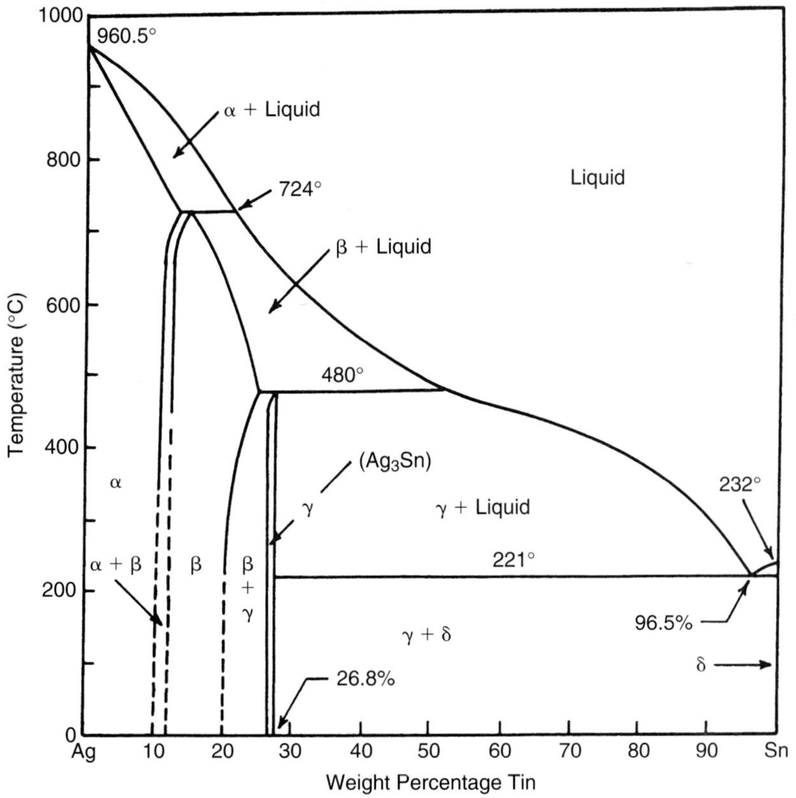

Fig. 11-2 Silver-tin phase diagram.
(Adapted from Murphy AJ: *Inst Metals J* 35:107, 1926.)

tin is replaced by 5% indium, whereas another product contains less than 1% palladium. Adding this small amount of palladium enhances the mechanical properties and corrosion resistance. The replacement of silver by an equal amount of copper produces a copper-tin compound (Cu_3Sn).

In general, larger (>30%) or smaller (<26%) quantities of tin in the alloy are detrimental to the final properties of the amalgam. The reason for this unfavorable shift in properties is generally considered related to the fact that the amount of Ag_3Sn is reduced as the percentage of tin is altered beyond the indicated limits. This is the basis for the rather narrow limits of the alloy compositions of current products with acceptable properties.

Silver-tin amalgam alloys compounded to produce largely Ag_3Sn react favorably with mercury to produce only slight dimensional setting changes when properly manipulated. The strength of the amalgam mass is greater from the Ag_3Sn compound than from an excess of tin. In addition, the setting time is shortened by increasing silver content. Creep resistance is also superior when an alloy of Ag_3Sn is used rather than one with higher tin content.

AMALGAMATION PROCESSES

LOW-COPPER ALLOYS

The amalgam alloy is intimately mixed with liquid mercury to wet the surface of the particles so the reaction between liquid mercury and alloy can proceed at a reasonable rate. This mixing is called *trituration*. During this process, mercury diffuses into the γ phase of the alloy particles and begins to react with the silver and tin portions of the particles, forming various compounds, predominantly silver-mercury and tin-mercury compounds, which depend on the exact composition of the alloy. The silver-mercury compound is Ag_2Hg_3 and is known as the *gamma one* (γ_1) *phase,* and the tin-mercury compound is $Sn_{7\text{-}8}Hg$ and is known as the *gamma two* (γ_2) *phase*. However, the silver-tin, silver-mercury, and tin-mercury phases are not pure. For example, Ag_3Sn always contains some copper and occasionally small amounts of zinc. The Ag_2Hg_3 dissolves small amounts (1% to 3%) of tin and Cu_6Sn_5 (η'), and, similarly, Cu_6Sn_5 could dissolve various elements present. Therefore γ, γ_1, and γ_2 are better descriptive terms of these three phases formed in dental amalgam than are the pure compounds.

While crystals of the γ_1 and γ_2 phases are being formed, the amalgam is relatively soft and easily condensable and carvable. As time progresses, more crystals of γ_1 and γ_2 are formed; the amalgam becomes harder and stronger, and is no longer condensable or carvable. The lapse of time between the end of the trituration and when the amalgam hardens and is no longer workable is called *working time.*

The amount of liquid mercury used to amalgamate the alloy particles is not sufficient to react with the particles completely. Therefore the set mass of amalgam contains unreacted particles. About 27% of the original Ag_3Sn compound remains as unreacted particles. A simplified reaction of a low-copper amalgam alloy with mercury can be summarized in the following manner:

$$\underset{\text{excess}}{\gamma\,(Ag_3Sn)} + Hg \rightarrow \underset{\text{unreacted}}{\gamma\,(Ag_3Sn)} + \gamma_1\,(Ag_2Hg_3) + \gamma_2\,(Sn_{7\text{-}8}Hg)$$

The dominating phase in a well-condensed, low-copper dental amalgam is the Ag_2Hg_3 (γ_1) phase, which is about 54% to 56% by volume. The percentages of the γ and γ_2 phases are 27% to 35% and 11% to 13%, respectively.

HIGH-COPPER ALLOYS

The main difference between the low- and high-copper amalgam alloys is not merely the percentage of copper but the effect that the higher copper content has on the amalgam reaction. The copper in these alloys is in either the silver-copper eutectic or ε (Cu_3Sn) form. The proper amount of copper causes most, if not all, of the γ_2 phase to be eliminated within a few hours after its formation, or prevents its formation entirely. The γ_2 phase in amalgam is the weakest and is the most susceptible to corrosion; therefore restorations using amalgam made with insufficient copper have a shorter period of serviceability, whereas high-copper amalgams tend to have superior physical and mechanical properties.

Reaction of Mercury in an Admixed High-Copper Amalgam Alloy During trituration, mercury diffuses into the amalgam particles and dissolves. The solubility of mercury in silver, tin, and copper differs considerably. Whereas 1 mg of mercury dissolves in copper, 10 mg can dissolve in silver and 170 mg in tin, all at the same temperature. Therefore particles composed mainly of silver and tin dissolve almost all the mercury, whereas very little mercury is dissolved by the silver-copper eutectic particles. The mercury dissolved in the silver-tin particles reacts as in low-copper alloys and forms the γ_1 and γ_2 phases, leaving some silver-tin particles unreacted. In a relatively short time, however, the newly formed γ_2 phase ($Sn_{7\text{-}8}Hg$) around the silver-tin particles reacts with silver-copper particles, forming Cu_6Sn_5, the eta prime (η') phase of the copper-tin system, along with some of the γ_1 phase (Ag_2Hg_3) around the silver-copper particles. The amalgamation reaction may be simplified as follows:

The initial reaction is the same as for low-copper dental amalgam,

$$\gamma\,(Ag_3Sn) + \text{Ag-Cu (eutectic)} + Hg \rightarrow \gamma\,(Ag_3Sn) + \gamma_1\,(Ag_2Hg_3) + \gamma_2\,(Sn_{7\text{-}8}Hg) + \underset{\text{excess}}{} \; \underset{\text{unreacted}}{\text{Ag-Cu (eutectic)}}$$

and the secondary, slow solid-state reaction is

$$\gamma_2\,(Sn_{7\text{-}8}Hg) + \text{Ag-Cu (eutectic)} \rightarrow \eta'\,(Cu_6Sn_5) + \gamma_1\,(Ag_2Hg_3) + \underset{\text{excess}}{\text{Ag-Cu (eutectic)}}$$

Reaction of Mercury in a Unicompositional Alloy In unicompositional alloys, too, the difference in solubility of mercury in tin, silver, and copper plays an important role. Because the solubility of mercury in tin is 170 times more than in copper and 17 times more than in silver, much more mercury dissolves and reacts with tin than with copper or silver. Thus tin in the periphery of the particle is depleted by the formation of the γ_2 phase, whereas the percentage of copper increases as a result of the limited reaction with mercury. As a result, particles of unicompositional alloys in the very early stages of setting are surrounded by γ_1 and γ_2 phases, whereas the periphery of a unicompositional alloy becomes an alloy of silver and copper. As with the admixed type of alloy, the γ_2 phase reacts with the silver-copper phase, forming Cu_6Sn_5 (η') and more Ag_2Hg_3 (γ_1).

The difference in the elimination of the γ_2 phase in an admixed and unicompositional alloy is that, in the admixed type, the γ_2 forms around the silver-tin particles and is eliminated around the silver-copper particles. In unicompositional alloys the particles at the beginning of the reaction function like silver-tin particles of the admixed type, providing proper working time and ease of manipulation. Later, the same particles function like the silver-copper particles of the admixed type, eliminating the γ_2 phase.

The unicompositional particle is composed of a very fine distribution of Ag_3Sn (γ) and Cu_3Sn (ε). The overall simplified reaction with Hg is

$$\gamma\,(Ag_3Sn) + \varepsilon\,(Cu_3Sn) + Hg \rightarrow \eta'\,(Cu_6Sn_5) + \gamma_1\,(Ag_2Hg_3)$$

Thus the reaction of mercury with either the high-copper admixed or the unicompositional alloys results in a final reaction, with Cu_6Sn_5 (η') being produced rather than $Sn_{7\text{-}8}Hg$ (γ_2).

In some high-copper alloys, there may be residual γ_2 of less than 1%. Note that there is no definitive proof that the γ_2 phase ever forms, even temporarily. By the time electron microprobe analyses can be performed, the reaction will have reached equilibrium, and the final reaction products of η' and γ_1 will have already formed.

MICROSTRUCTURE OF AMALGAM

In dental applications the amount of liquid mercury used to amalgamate with the alloy particles is less than that required to complete the reaction. Thus the set amalgam mass consists of unreacted particles surrounded by a matrix of the reaction products. The reaction is principally a surface reaction, and the matrix bonds the unreacted particles together. The initial diffusion and reaction of mercury and alloy are relatively rapid, and the mass changes rapidly from a plastic consistency to a hard mass. Completion of the reaction may take several days to several weeks, which is reflected by the change in mechanical properties over this time.

The microstructures of set amalgam of the low-copper, lathe-cut, and spherical types are shown in Fig. 11-3. The outlines of the unreacted alloy particles (γ) are visible *(A)*. The γ_1 and γ_2 phases in the matrix are identified by the letters

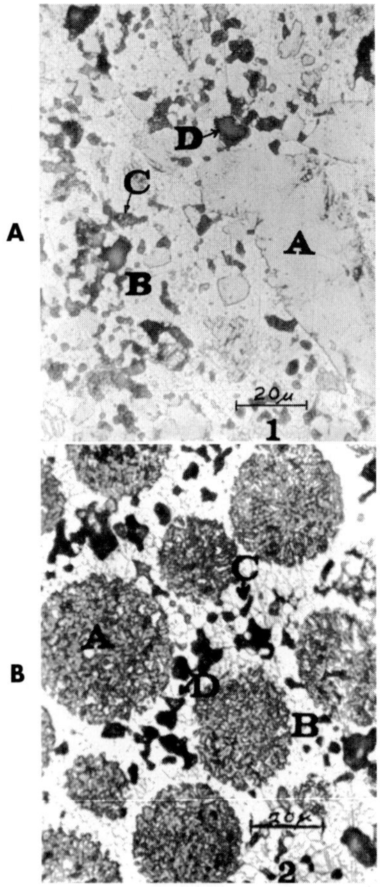

Fig. 11-3 Microstructure of set dental amalgam, etched with iodine etch. **A,** Lathe-cut particles: *A,* unreacted original particle, γ; *B,* γ_1; *C,* γ_2; *D,* void.
B, Spherical alloy particles: *A,* original particle; *B,* γ_1; *C,* γ_2; *D,* void.
(From Allen FC, Asgar K, Peyton FA: *J Dent Res* 44:1002, 1965.)

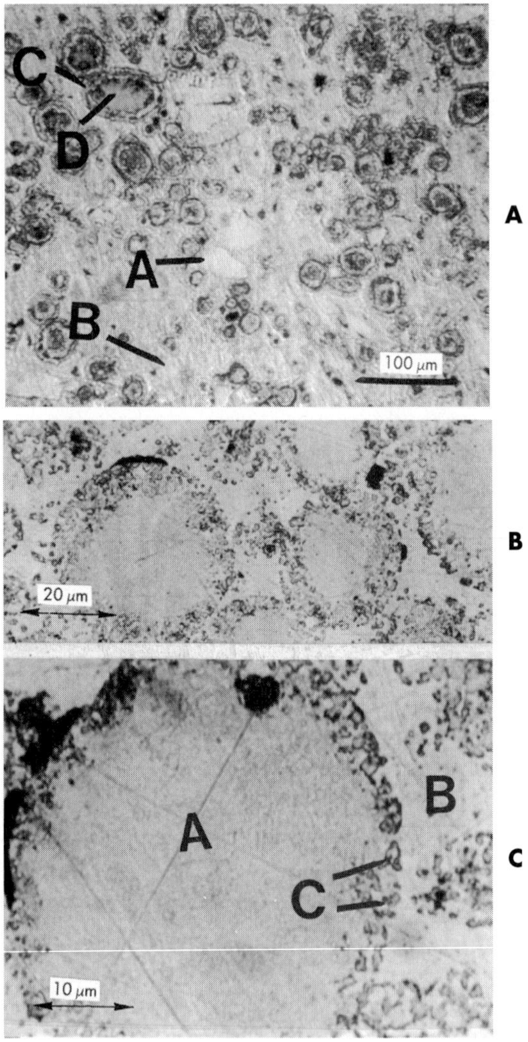

Fig. 11-4 Microstructure of high-copper admixed **(A)** and spherical unicompositional **(B, C)** alloys.
A, *A* is an unreacted portion of γ; *B* is the γ_1 phase; *C* is the reaction zone around the Ag-Cu eutectic particle; *D* is an unreacted portion of an Ag-Cu particle.
C, *A* is an unreacted portion of a spherical unicompositional Ag-Sn-Cu particle; *B* is the γ_1 phase; *C* is the reaction zone around an original particle.

B and *C*, respectively. Voids in each of the two samples are identified by the letter *D*. After the completion of the solid-state reaction in the high-copper admixed and unicompositional alloys, the microstructures show no γ_2 phase (Fig. 11-4).

PROPERTIES OF AMALGAM

Important properties for dental amalgam include dimensional changes, compressive strength, creep, and corrosion resistance. These properties may be explained in part by the composition, microstructure, and manipulation of the amalgam.

ANSI/ADA SPECIFICATION NO. 1 FOR AMALGAM ALLOY

ANSI/ADA Specification No. 1 for amalgam alloy contains requirements that help significantly control the qualities of dental amalgam. The specification lists three physical properties as a measure of amalgam quality: creep, compressive strength, and dimensional change. When a cylindrical specimen is 7 days old, a 36-MPa stress is applied in a 37° C environment. Creep is measured between 1 and 4 hours of stressing. The maximum allowable creep is 3%. The minimum allowable compressive strength 1 hour after setting, when a cylindrical specimen is compressed at a rate of 0.25 mm/minute, is 80 MPa. The dimensional change between 5 minutes and 24 hours must fall within the range of ±20 μm/cm.

PHYSICAL AND MECHANICAL PROPERTIES

Compressive Strength Resistance to compression forces is the most favorable strength characteristic of amalgam. Because amalgam is strongest in compression and much weaker in tension and shear, the prepared cavity design should maximize the compression forces in service and minimize tension or shear forces. The early-compressive strengths (after 1 hour of setting) for several low- and high-copper alloys are listed in Table 11-2. The percent mercury used in preparing the samples is also listed; the lathe-cut alloy requires the greatest amount of mercury, and the unicompositional alloy the least. Notice that amalgams are viscoelastic and the compressive strength is a function of the rate of loading. In general, the higher the rate of loading, the higher the compressive strength, although some studies have shown that compressive strength may decrease at very high strain rates. As a result, when comparing the compressive strength of amalgam samples, it is imperative that they be tested at the same rate of loading.

When subjected to a rapid application of stress either in tension or in compression, a dental amalgam does not exhibit significant deformation or elongation and, as a result, functions as a brittle material. Therefore a sudden application of excessive forces to amalgam tends to fracture the amalgam restoration.

The high-copper unicompositional materials have the highest early-compressive strengths of more than 250 MPa at 1 hour. The compressive strength at 1 hour was lowest for lathe-cut alloy (45 MPa), followed by one of the low-copper spherical alloys (88 MPa), and then two low-copper spherical alloys and the high-copper admixed alloy (118 to 141 MPa). These data indicate that only some of the older lathe-cut alloys would not meet the requirement for compressive strength at 1 hour of ANSI/ADA Specification No. 1. High values for early-compressive strength are an advantage for an amalgam, because they reduce the possibility of fracture by prematurely high contact stresses from the patient before the final strength is reached. The compressive strengths at 7 days and the final strengths are again highest for the high-copper unicompositional alloys, with only modest differences in the other alloys.

Tensile Strength The tensile strengths of various amalgams after 15 minutes and 7 days are listed in Table 11-3. The tensile strengths at 7 days for both non-γ_2 and γ_2-containing alloys are about the same. The tensile strengths are only a fraction of their compressive strengths; therefore cavity designs should be constructed to reduce tensile stresses resulting from biting forces.

The tensile strengths at 15 minutes for the

TABLE 11-2 Compressive Strength and Creep of Amalgams

Product	Mercury in Mix (%)	1-hr Compressive Strength (MPa) (0.5 mm/min)	7-Day Compressive Strength (MPa)		Creep (%)
			0.2 mm/min	0.05 mm/min	
LOW-COPPER ALLOYS					
Fine-cut					
Caulk 20th Century Micro Cut	53.7	45	302	227	6.3
Spherical					
Caulk Spherical	46.2	141	366	289	1.5
Kerr Spheraloy	48.5	88	380	299	1.3
Shofu Spherical	48.0	132	364	305	0.50
HIGH-COPPER ALLOYS					
Admixed					
Dispersalloy	50.0	118	387	340	0.45
Unicompositional					
Sybraloy	46.0	252	455	452	0.05
Tytin	43.0	292	516	443	0.09

Adapted from Malhotra ML, Asgar K: *J Am Dent Assoc* 96:446, 1978.

TABLE 11-3 Tensile Strength and Dimensional Change of Amalgams

Product	Tensile Strength at 0.5 mm/min (MPa)		Dimensional Change (μm/cm)
	15 min	7 days	
LOW-COPPER ALLOYS			
Fine-cut			
Caulk 20th Century Micro Cut	3.2	51	−19.7
Spherical			
Caulk Spherical	4.7	55	−10.6
Kerr Spheraloy	3.2	55	−14.8
Shofu Spherical	4.6	58	−9.6
HIGH-COPPER ALLOYS			
Admixed			
Dispersalloy	3.0	43	−1.9
Unicompositional			
Sybraloy	8.5	49	−8.8
Tytin	8.1	56	−8.1

Adapted from Malhotra ML, Asgar K: *J Am Dent Assoc* 96:447, 1978.

high-copper unicompositional alloys are 75% to 175% higher than for the other alloys. However, no correlation exists between the tensile strengths at 15 minutes and 7 days. The high early tensile strengths of the high-copper unicompositional alloys are important, because they resist fracture by premature biting stresses better than other amalgams.

Transverse Strength These values are sometimes referred to as the *modulus of rupture.* Because amalgams are brittle materials, they can withstand little deformation during transverse strength testing. The main factors related to the high values of deformation are (1) the slow rates of load application, (2) high creep of the specific amalgam, and (3) higher temperature of testing. Thus, high copper amalgams with low creep should be supported by bases with high moduli to minimize deformation and transverse failure.

Strength of Various Phases The relative strengths of the different amalgam phases are important. By studying the initiation and propagation of a crack in a set amalgam, the relative strength of the different phases can be observed. Fig. 11-5 shows the propagation of a crack in a dental amalgam specimen. It is possible to view the crack initiation and propagation of an amalgam specimen under a conventional metallographical microscope with a strain viewer. The propagation of the crack can be halted and the specimen etched to identify the various phases. Results of such studies have led to the following ranking, from strongest to weakest, of the different phases of a set low-copper amalgam: Ag_3Sn (γ), the silver-mercury phase (γ_1), the tin-mercury phase (γ_2), and the voids.

Silver-mercury and tin-mercury act as a matrix to hold the unreacted amalgam alloy together. When relatively smaller amounts of silver-mercury and tin-mercury phases form, up to a certain minimum required for bonding the unreacted particles, a set amalgam is stronger. When a higher percentage of mercury is left in the final mass, it reacts with more of the amalgam alloy, producing larger amounts of silver-mercury and tin-mercury phases and leaving relatively smaller amounts of unreacted particles. The result is a weaker mass. Therefore the effect of various manipulative conditions can be explained in this

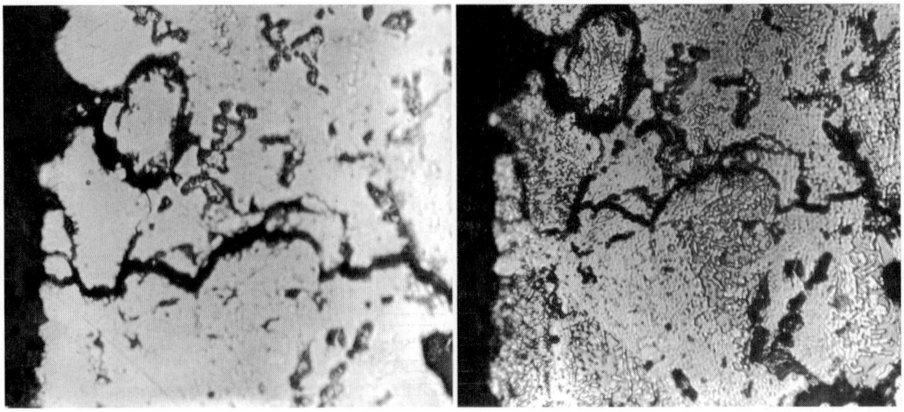

Fig. 11-5 Propagation of a crack in a dental amalgam. **A,** Unetched. **B,** After etching. (From Asgar K, Sutfin L: *J Dent Res* 44:985, 1965.)

manner. In high- copper amalgams, there is preferential crack propagation through the γ_1 phase and around copper-containing particles.

Elastic Modulus When the elastic modulus is determined at low rates of loading, such as 0.025 to 0.125 mm/min, values in the range of 11 to 20 GPa are obtained. High-copper alloys tend to be stiffer than low-copper alloys. If the rate of loading is increased so the viscoelastic property does not significantly influence the elastic modulus, values of approximately 62 GPa have been obtained.

Creep The viscoelastic properties of amalgam are also reflected by the creep or permanent deformation under static loads. Under a continued application of force in compression, an amalgam shows a continued deformation, even after the mass has completely set. Amalgam has no tendency for work hardening or for resisting deformation more effectively after the mass has been deformed, as may be experienced with the cast gold alloys.

Values for creep are determined in an instrument similar to that shown in Fig. 11-6. A cylindrical sample is placed in the position indicated by the arrow 7 days after preparation. A static stress of 36 MPa is applied by the spring. The change in length of the sample is determined at 37 ± 0.3° C by a calibrated differential transformer, the output of which is recorded on a chart. The change in length between 1 hour and 4 hours after placing the static stress is used to calculate the percentage creep.

Creep values for various amalgams are listed in Table 11-2. The highest value of 6.3% was found for the low-copper cut alloy, and the lowest values (0.05% to 0.09%) were determined for the high-copper unicompositional spherical alloys. The high-copper admixed alloy and one of the low-copper alloys had slightly higher creep values of 0.45% to 0.50%, and the remaining two low-copper spherical alloys had values of 1.3% to 1.5%.

Multiple regression analyses of creep data have shown that the most influential variables are volume percentage of the η' phase, grain size of the γ_1 phase, volume percentage of the γ and ε phases, number of very small η' crystals (less than 1.5 μm)/mm, and weight percentage of mercury. All of these values except weight percentage of mercury correlate negatively with creep. When γ_1 has a concentration of tin greater than 1%, creep is controlled more by the distribution of tin and tin-mercury intergranular precipitates than by grain size. After aging at oral temperature for 6 months, amalgam exhibits a decrease in creep. This decrease in creep is related to β_1 formation and not to changes in either γ_1 grain size or composition.

A direct relationship exists between γ_2 content

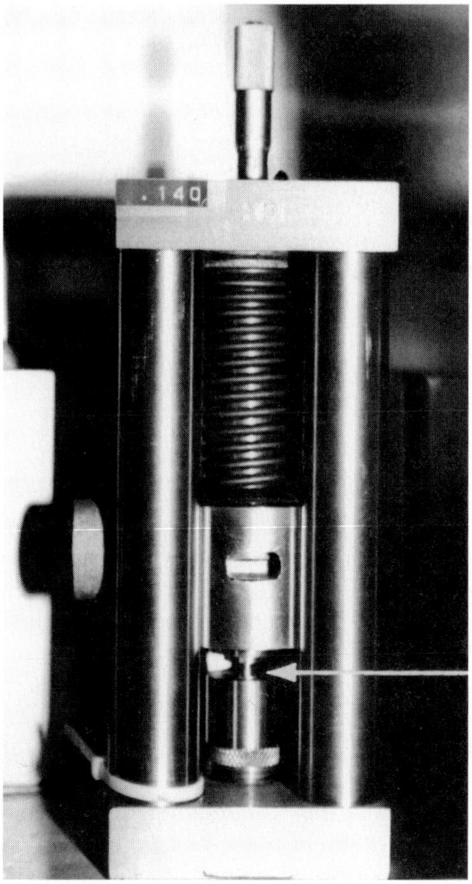

Fig. 11-6 An instrument for measuring creep of amalgam. Arrow points to specimen.

and a high incidence of marginal fracture of amalgam restorations. In addition, there is a general relationship between low static creep values and low marginal fracture in clinical service, which may be explained by the fact that the time to rupture under a constant load is inversely proportional to creep rate. Amalgams having higher compressive strengths at 7 days, determined at slow rates of loading, have demonstrated better marginal integrity. In general, amalgams having low values of creep *and* high 7-day compressive strength at slow rates of loading have better clinical performance.

Note that the low creep values of high-copper amalgams increase the brittleness of the amalgam and decrease the relief of stresses at contact areas under load. As a result, a high-modulus base under a high-copper amalgam is essential to minimize deformation and the development of tensile stresses at the amalgam-cement base interface.

Dimensional Change The dimensional change during the setting of amalgam is one of its most characteristic properties. Modern amalgams mixed with mechanical amalgamators usually have negative dimensional changes. The initial contraction after a short time (the first 20 minutes) is believed to be associated with the solution of mercury in the alloy particles. After this period an expansion occurs, although the total change remains negative, which is believed to be a result of the reaction of mercury with silver and tin and the formation of the intermetallic compounds. The dimensions become nearly constant after 6 to 8 hours, and thus the values after 24 hours are final values. The only exception to this statement is the excessive delayed dimensional change resulting from contamination of a zinc-containing alloy with water during trituration or condensation.

The dimensional change may be determined with an instrument such as the one shown in Fig. 11-7. The amalgam specimens identified by the arrows are placed in position 5 minutes after setting, and the probe is placed on top of them. The probe is mechanically attached to a differential transformer, and the electrical output is used to determine expansion or contraction. The change in length can be determined continuously, although ANSI/ADA Specification No. 1 requires only the value at 24 hours.

The dimensional changes in micrometers per centimeter for the various alloys are listed in Table 11-3. The largest dimensional change of −19.7 μm/cm occurred with the low-copper, lathe-cut alloy, and the lowest change of −1.9 μm/cm was for the high-copper admixed alloy. The remainder of the alloys had values ranging from −8.8 to −14.8 μm/cm. All the amalgams meet the requirements of ANSI/ADA Specification No. 1 of ±20 μm/cm. Notice that the ranking of the dimensional change does not correlate

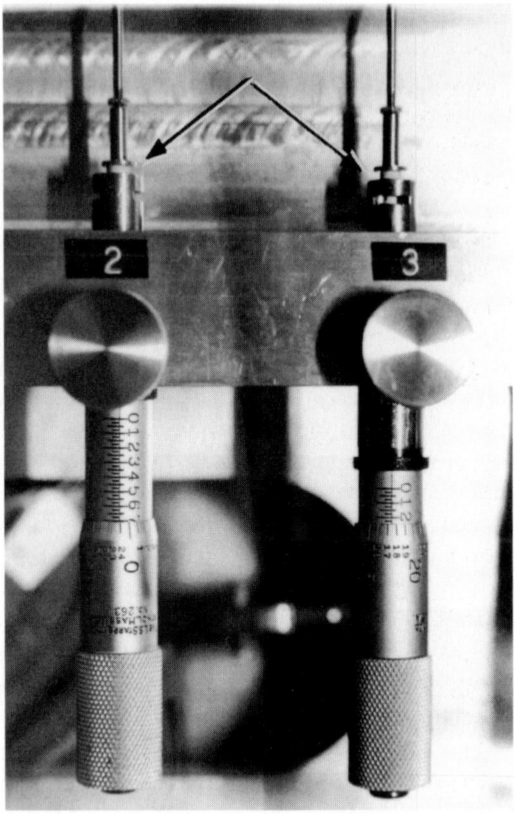

Fig. 11-7 An instrument for measuring dimensional change of amalgam. Arrows point to amalgam specimens.

with any of the other mechanical properties. The dimensional change is susceptible to influence from various manipulative factors, especially final mercury content. Higher mercury content results in less shrinkage but also in lower mechanical strength.

Some question remains concerning the significance of dimensional change with respect to clinical success. The belief was that if amalgam expanded during hardening, leakage around the margins of restorations would be eliminated. With current alloys and proper techniques of trituration, however, most alloys show some shrinkage. Evidently the detrimental effect of shrinkage occurs when the amalgam mass shrinks more than 50 μm. ANSI/ADA Specification No. 1 for dental amalgam allows up to 20 μm/cm shrinkage, and no correlation of clinical success with the magnitude of the shrinkage determined in the laboratory has been shown. Furthermore, the expansion of an amalgam mass may seem to have a beneficial effect for one-surface restorations such as Class 1 and 5, but offers hardly any advantage when Class 2 and 6 restorations are considered. The expanded amalgam around the cervical areas of Class 2 and 6 restorations would have to pull away from the preparation, and this may have as undesirable an effect as the shrinking of amalgams for one-surface restorations.

Corrosion In general, corrosion is the progressive destruction of a metal by chemical or electrochemical reaction with its environment. Excessive corrosion can lead to increased porosity, reduced marginal integrity, loss of strength, and the release of metallic products into the oral environment.

The following compounds have been identified on dental amalgams in patients: SnO, SnO_2, $Sn_4(OH)_6Cl_2$, Cu_2O, $CuCl_2 \cdot 3Cu(OH)_2$, $CuCl$, $CuSCN$, and $AgSCN$.

Because of their different chemical compositions, the different phases of an amalgam have different corrosion potentials. Electrochemical measurements on pure phases have shown that the Ag_2Hg_3 (γ_1) phase has the highest corrosion resistance, followed by Ag_3Sn (γ), Ag_3Cu_2, Cu_3Sn (ε), Cu_6Sn_5 (η'), and $Sn_{7\text{-}8}Hg$ (γ_2). However, the order of corrosion resistance assigned is true only if these phases are pure and they are not in the pure state in dental amalgam.

The presence of small amounts of tin, silver, and copper that may dissolve in various amalgam phases has a great influence on their corrosion resistance. The γ_1 phase has a composition close to Ag_2Hg_3 with 1% to 3% of dissolved tin. The higher the tin concentration of Ag_2Hg_3 (γ_1), the lower its corrosion resistance. In general, the tin content of the γ_1 phase is higher for low-copper alloys than for high-copper alloys. The presence of a relatively high percentage of tin in low-copper alloys reduces the corrosion resistance of their γ_1 phase so it is lower than their γ phase. This is not true for high-copper alloys. The average depth of corrosion for most amalgam alloys is 100 to 500 μm.

In the low-copper amalgam system, the most corrodible phase is the $Sn_{7-8}Hg$ or γ_2 phase. Although a relatively small portion (11% to 13%) of the amalgam mass consists of the γ_2 phase, in time and in an oral environment the structure of such an amalgam will contain a higher percentage of corroded phase. On the other hand, neither the γ nor the γ_1 phase is corroded as easily. Studies have shown that corrosion of the γ_2 phase occurs throughout the restoration, because it is a network structure. Corrosion results in the formation of tin oxychloride from the tin in the γ_2, and also liberates mercury, as shown in the following equation:

$$Sn_{7\text{-}8}Hg + \tfrac{1}{2}O_2 + H_2O + Cl^- \rightarrow Sn_4\,(OH)_6\,Cl_2 + Hg$$

The reaction of the liberated mercury with unreacted γ can produce additional γ_1 and γ_2. It is proposed that the dissolution of the tin oxide or tin chloride and the production of additional γ_1 and γ_2 result in porosity and lower strength.

The high-copper admixed and unicompositional alloys do not have any γ_2 phase in the final set mass. The Cu_6Sn_5 or η' phase formed with high-copper alloys is not an interconnected phase such as the γ_2 phase, and it has better corrosion resistance. However, η' is the least corrosion-resistant phase in high-copper amalgams; and a corrosion product, $CuCl_2 \cdot 3Cu(OH)_2$, has been associated with storage of amalgams in synthetic saliva, as shown below.

$$Cu_6\,Sn_5 + \tfrac{1}{2}O_2 + H_2O + Cl^- \rightarrow Cu\,Cl_2 \cdot 3\,Cu\,(OH)_2 + Sn\,O$$

Phosphate buffer solutions inhibit the corrosion process; thus saliva may provide some protection of dental amalgams from corrosion.

A study of amalgams that had been in service for 2 to 25 years revealed that the bulk elemental compositions were similar to newly prepared amalgams, except for the presence of a small amount of chloride and other contaminants. The compositions of the phases were also similar to new amalgams, except for internal amalgamation of the γ particles. The distribution of phases in the clinically aged amalgams, however, differed from that of new amalgams. The low-copper amalgams had decreased amounts of γ, γ_1, and γ_2 and increased β_1 and tin-chloride. High-copper admixed amalgams had decreased γ_1, increased β_1, and enlarged reaction rings of γ_1 and η'. There was also evidence of a conversion of γ_1 to β_1 and γ_2 to η'.

Note that the processes of corrosion and wear are frequently coupled and that wear can lower the corrosion potential and increase the corrosion rate by an order of magnitude.

Fig. 11-8 compares an amalgam restoration on the distal portion of a tooth prepared from a low-copper spherical alloy with one on the mesial portion prepared from high-copper admixed alloy. The restorations have been in service for 3 years, and the higher marginal fracture, presumably resulting from the corrosion of the γ_2 phase of the low-copper amalgam, is readily apparent.

Surface tarnish of low-copper amalgams is more associated with γ than γ_1, whereas in high-copper amalgams surface tarnish is related to the copper-rich phases, η' and silver-copper eutectic.

PROPERTIES OF MERCURY

ANSI/ADA Specification No. 6 for dental mercury requires that mercury have a clean reflecting surface that is free from surface film when agitated in air. It should have no visible evidence of surface contamination and contain less than 0.02% nonvolatile residue. Mercury that complies with the requirements of the United States Pharmacopoeia also meets requirements for purity in ANSI/ADA Specification No. 6. Mercury amalgamates with small amounts of many metals and is contaminated by sulfur gases in the atmosphere, which combine with mercury to form sulfides. Small quantities of these foreign materials in mercury destroy its bright, mirror-like surface and can be readily detected by visual inspection.

Mercury, which has a freezing point of

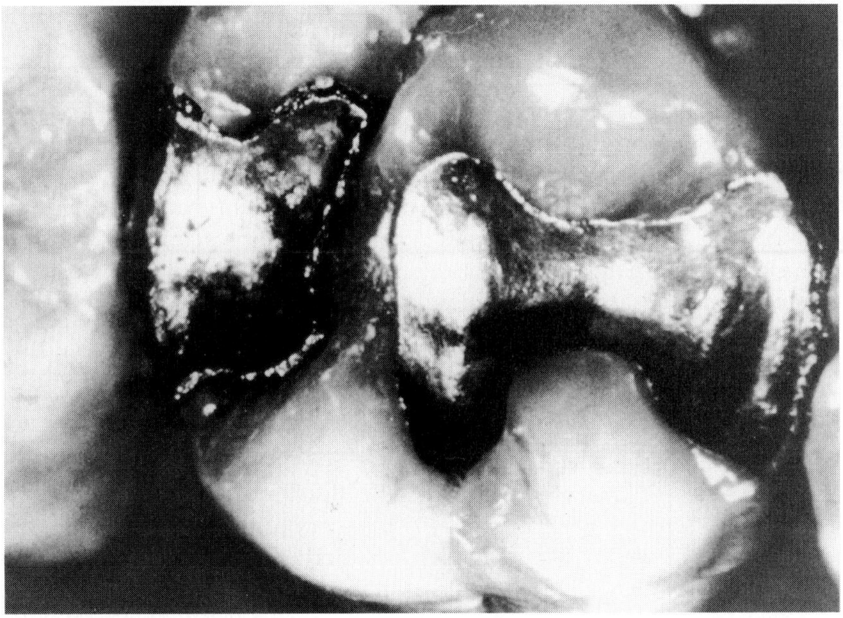

Fig. 11-8 Amalgam restoration from a low-copper spherical alloy *(left)* and an amalgam from a high-copper admixed alloy *(right)* after 3 years of service.
(Courtesy GT Charbeneau, Ann Arbor, 1979, University of Michigan School of Dentistry.)

−38.87° C, is the only metal that remains in the liquid state at room temperatures. It combines readily to form an amalgam with several metals such as gold, silver, copper, tin, and zinc, but does not combine under ordinary conditions with such metals as nickel, chromium, molybdenum, cobalt, and iron.

Mercury boils at 356.9° C, and, if pure, has a significant vapor pressure at room temperature. Extended inhalation can result in mercury poisoning. Globules dropped on a surface roll about freely without leaving a tail and retain their globular form. This tendency to form globules is related to the high surface tension of liquid mercury, which is 465 dynes/cm at 20° C, as compared with 72.8 dynes/cm for water. Mercury with a very high degree of purity exhibits a slight tarnish after a short time because impurities contaminate the metal and produce a dull surface appearance. Impurities in mercury can reduce the rate at which it combines with the silver alloy.

MANIPULATION OF AMALGAM

SELECTION OF ALLOY

The selection of an alloy involves a number of factors, including setting time, particle size and shape, and composition, particularly as it relates to the elimination of the γ_2 phase and the presence or absence of zinc. It is estimated that more than 90% of the dental amalgams currently placed are high-copper alloys. The majority of the alloys selected are high-copper unicompositional (spherical) and admixed types, with the admixed being favored slightly. A high-copper alloy is selected because the result is a restoration with no γ_2, high early strength, low creep, good corrosion resistance, and good resistance to marginal fracture.

Finer particle sizes are used for low-copper, irregular alloys because of improved properties and enhanced clinical convenience. Finer particles produce a smoother surface during carving and finishing. The clinical manipulation of dental amalgam alloys is influenced to a modest extent by the shape of the particles. Lathe-cut alloys exhibit rough, irregular surfaces having a large area/volume ratio to react with mercury, and generally require nearly 50% or more mercury to obtain adequate plasticity during trituration. Spherical alloys are smoother, consist of various sizes of spheres (2 to 43 μm), which is important in packing, have more-regular surfaces with a lower area/volume ratio, and generally require less mercury for trituration and suitable plasticity development. Mercury concentrations as low as 42% permit acceptable handling characteristics with certain products.

Lathe-cut and spherical alloys react differently to condensation forces. These differences result from frictional forces within the amalgam mass that offer higher resistance to the face of the condenser in lathe-cut alloys than in spherical alloys. Carving the excess amalgam from the overfilled cavity to restore morphological and functional anatomy presents further differences.

Because of improved manufacturing, few products contain zinc because the contamination of a zinc-containing alloy by moisture may result in excessive dimensional change. If an alloy contains more than 0.01% zinc, the package must carry a printed precaution that the amalgam made from the material will show excessive corrosion and expansion if moisture is introduced during mixing and condensation.

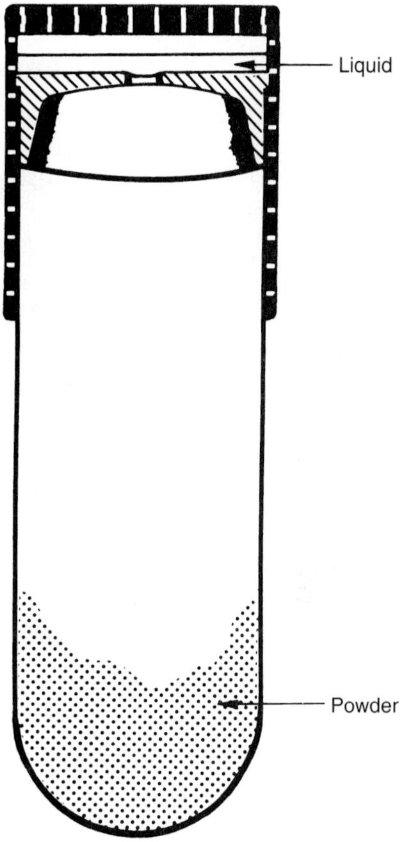

Fig. 11-9 Cross-sectional sketch of a disposable capsule containing amalgam alloy and mercury.

PROPORTIONS OF ALLOY TO MERCURY

Correct proportioning of alloy and mercury is essential for forming a suitable mass of amalgam for placement in a prepared cavity. Some alloys require mercury-alloy ratios in excess of 1:1, whereas others use ratios of less than 1:1; the percentage of mercury varies from 43% to 54%. Automatic mechanical dispensers for alloy and mercury have been used in the past and are described in previous editions of this textbook. With the recommendation for "no touch" procedures for handling mercury and amalgam, capsules with preproportioned amounts of alloy and mercury have been substituted for mercury and alloy dispensers. The correct amounts of alloy and mercury are kept separated in the capsule by a membrane, as shown in the sketch in Fig. 11-9. Just before the mix is triturated the membrane is ruptured by compression of the capsule, or it is automatically activated during trituration. Various manufacturers' amalgam alloys with their corresponding capsules are shown in Fig. 11-10. Some capsules contain a plastic pestle in the shape of a disk or rod, as illustrated in the disassembled capsules in Fig. 11-11. To prevent any escape of mercury from the friction-fitted capsule during trituration, some capsules are hermetically sealed; the mercury is contained in a small plastic film packet which ruptures during mixing.

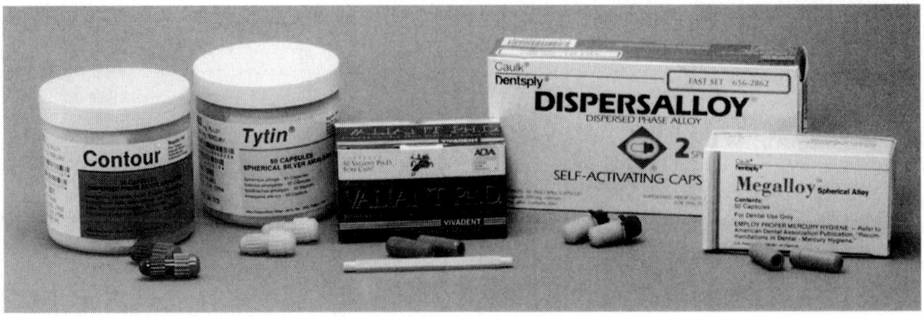

Fig. 11-10 Examples of spherical and admixed dental amalgam alloys in capsules.
(From Craig RG, Powers JM, Wataha JC: *Dental materials: properties and manipulation,* ed 7, St. Louis, 2000, Mosby.)

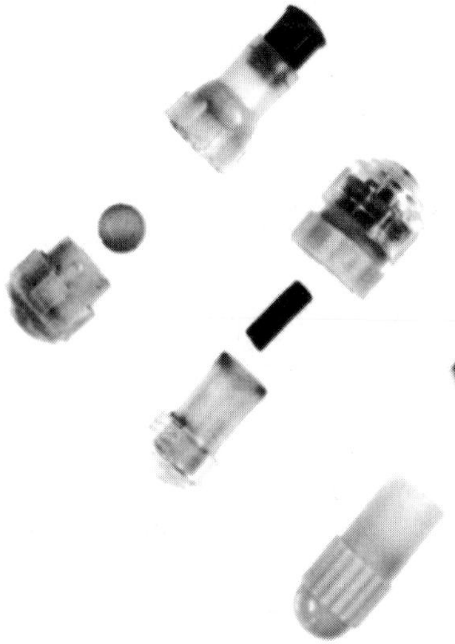

Fig. 11-11 Types of capsules with and without pestles.

Size of Mix Manufacturers commonly supply capsules containing 400, 600, or 800 mg of alloy and the appropriate amount of Hg, color coded for ease of identification. Clinical consensus is that these amounts are sufficient for most restorations. It is usually suggested that if larger amounts are required that several smaller mixes be made at staggered times so the consistency of the mixed amalgam remains reasonably constant during the preparation of the restoration. However capsules containing 1200 mg of alloy are available if a large amount of amalgam is needed to produce an amalgam core on a severely broken down tooth.

MIXING OF AMALGAM

Trituration of amalgam alloy and mercury is done with a mechanical mixing device called an *amalgamator* or *triturator.* The two amalgamators shown in Fig. 11-12 have controls for the speed and duration of trituration. The amalgamator shown on the left has a slot on the lower right for the insertion of plastic cards. There is a separate card for each size mix; insertion of the card automatically sets the correct mixing time and speed. Each of the amalgamators has a housing that is placed over the capsule area during trituration to confine any mercury lost from the capsule during mixing.

The capsule holder is attached to a motor that rotates the holder and capsule eccentrically. The trituration may be accomplished simply by the agitation of the alloy particles and mercury, or the manufacturer may have included a plastic pestle to aid in the mixing.

Spherical or irregular low-copper alloys may be triturated at low speed (low energy), but most high-copper alloys require high speed (high energy). Effective trituration depends on a combination of the duration and speed of mixing. Duration of amalgamation is the easiest factor

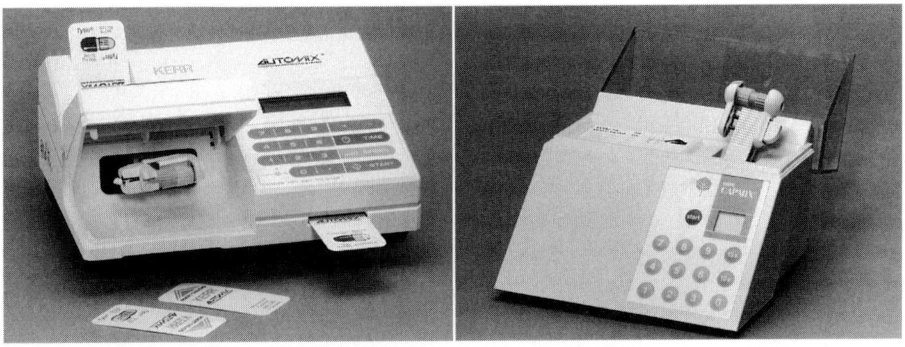

Fig. 11-12 A and **B,** Variable-speed mechanical amalgamators for triturating amalgam. Note that the Automix amalgamator, **A,** has plastic cards for particular alloys and size of mix, which, when inserted into the slot, set the amalgamator for the correct speed and time.

(From Craig RG, Powers JM, Wataha JC: *Dental materials: properties and manipulation,* ed 7, St. Louis, 2000, Mosby.)

to vary; however, it should be emphasized that variations of 2 to 3 seconds of mixing time may be enough to produce an amalgam that is undermixed or overmixed. Mechanical amalgamators allow some variation in speed to adjust to differing amounts of alloy and mercury in the capsules.

Low-, medium-, and high-speed amalgamators operate at about 3200 to 3400, 3700 to 3800, and 4000 to 4400 cycles per minute, respectively, at correct live voltage. However, an amalgamator set at la speed of 3300 cpm may actually be operating at 3000 cpm with a decrease in line voltage from 120 to 100 volts, and undermixed amalgams may result. This problem can be avoided by installing a voltage regulator between the line plug and the amalgamator. Using a parameter called the coherence time (t_c), defined as the minimum mixing time required for an amalgam to form a single coherent pellet, it has been found that the compressive strength, dimensional change, and creep are optimized if mixing is carried out for a time of $5t_c$. The value of t_c can be determined experimentally for a particular amalgam alloy, size of mix, and speed of the amalgamator. However, most packages of amalgam alloys will contain recommendations for times and speeds for a variety of amalgamators, and these guidelines should be followed.

With the introduction of disposable capsules containing premeasured amounts of amalgam alloy and mercury, mercury and alloy dispensers have become obsolete, as have reusable capsules; however, the discussion of their selection and use is described in the 9th and earlier editions of this textbook.

Mixing Variables Undermixing, normal mixing, or overmixing can result from variations in the condition of trituration of the alloy and mercury. The three mixes have a different appearance and respond differently to subsequent manipulation. The undermixed amalgam appears dull and is crumbly, the normal mix appears shiny and separates in a single mass from the capsule, and the overmixed amalgam appears soupy and tends to stick to the inside of the capsule. Examples of these mixes are shown in Fig. 11-13. The three types of mixes have characteristically different mechanical properties of dimensional change, strength, and creep. These three conditions can be developed from variations in the mixing variables described earlier. Therefore the type of mix contributes to the success or failure of the amalgam restoration.

Not all types of alloys respond in the same manner to overtrituration and undertrituration. Spherical and lathe-cut alloys respond differently. The effect of overtrituration and undertritu-

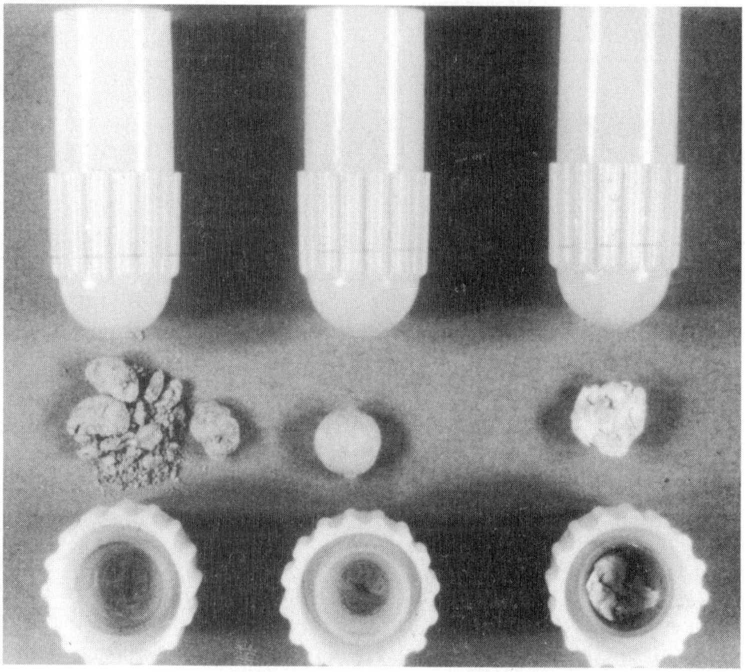

Fig. 11-13 Amalgam. *Left,* undermixed; *center,* normal mixed; *right,* overmixed. (Courtesy Dr. K Asgar, University of Michigan School of Dentistry, Ann Arbor, Mich.)

ration of amalgam on working time, dimensional change, compressive and tensile strengths, and creep is summarized as follows.

Working Time and Dimensional Change Working time of all types of amalgam, spherical or irregular, decreases with overtrituration. High- or low-copper alloys respond alike. Overtrituration results in slightly higher contraction for all types of alloys. High- and low-copper alloys show the same effect.

Compressive and Tensile Strengths Both compressive and tensile strengths of irregular shaped alloys increase by overtrituration. However, this is not true for spherical alloys. Compressive and tensile strengths of spherical alloys are greatest at normal trituration time. Both overtrituration and undertrituration reduce compressive and tensile strengths. The admixed high-copper alloys consist of both shapes of particles and behave like spherical alloys; normal trituration times produce the highest strength values, whereas overtrituration results in significant decreases in strength.

Creep Overtrituration increases creep, and undertrituration lowers it. As mentioned earlier in this chapter, two properties that are closely related to the clinical behavior of alloys are low creep and high compressive strength. By overtriturating irregular amalgams, a higher compressive strength can be obtained, which is beneficial. However, the amalgam has a higher creep, a property that is not desirable. If there is doubt about the correct trituration time, a slightly overtriturated amalgam is better than a slightly undertriturated one. This suggestion is particularly true for high-copper alloys.

Some manufacturers recommend altering the trituration time to obtain a longer or shorter working time. Altering the trituration time does change the working time of amalgam, but it also affects other properties. When amalgam is triturated for shorter than normal times, mercury does not completely wet the outer surface of amalgam particles. As a result, mercury does not react with the amalgam alloy over the entire surface of the particle. The mass remains soft for a longer period of time, producing an amalgam with a longer working time. Such an amalgam mass contains excessive amounts of porosity, has lower strength, and possesses poorer corrosion resistance.

Overtrituration reduces working time, causing the reaction rate to increase because the amalgamated mass becomes hot. When amalgams with longer or shorter working times are desired, one should use amalgam alloys that are designed to react faster or slower and not attempt to achieve the change by altering the trituration time.

CONDENSATION OF AMALGAM

During condensation, adaptation of the amalgam mass to the cavity walls is accomplished and the operator controls the amount of mercury that will remain in the finished restoration, which in turn influences the dimensional change, creep, and compressive strength. In general, the more mercury left in the mass after condensation, the weaker the alloy. With irregularly shaped alloys, in which a higher percentage of mercury is used initially, the operator should remove as much mercury as possible during condensation by using as great a force as possible on the condenser. With spherical alloys, the amount of mercury supplied in the capsules is lower, and it is not necessary to remove as much mercury as for the irregularly shaped alloys; however, increasing the condensation pressure from 3 to 7 MPa results in a significant increase in compressive strength. Further increase in condensation pressure to 14 MPa does not result in additional compressive strength.

Hand or Mechanical Condensation A large number of instruments designed for hand condensation of amalgam have been available to the dental profession for many years. The instruments and the techniques for their use have been described in textbooks of operative dentistry.

In general, a suitable instrument for hand condensation of amalgam would be shaped so that the operator could readily grasp it and exert a force of condensation by appropriately placing one finger on a finger rest of the instrument. Hand instruments that do not permit a convenient grasping may inhibit proper condensation practices and mercury removal. In many instances, circular condenser tips may prove adequate, whereas in other cavity areas and designs, the triangular, oval, crescent, or other shape of tip may be effective. In general, a condenser tip that is too small in cross section tends to be ineffective in condensing a reasonable quantity of amalgam. The size of the condenser tip and the direction and magnitude of the force placed on the condenser also depend on the type of amalgam alloy selected.

With irregularly shaped alloys, one should use condensers with a relatively small tip, 1 to 2 mm, and apply high condensation forces in a vertical direction. During condensation, as much mercury-rich mass as possible should be removed from the restoration.

When condensers with small tips are used with high condensation forces on spherical amalgams, the particles tend to roll over one another, the tip penetrates the amalgam, and the mass does not adapt well to the cavity walls. With spherical alloys one should use condensers with larger tips, almost as large as the cavity permits. For example, at the cervical margin of a Class 2 preparation with a small opening, a condenser with a very small tip should be used. As the cavity is filled and the opening toward the occlusal surface becomes larger, condensers with larger tips should be used. Because of the spherical shape of the particles, a lateral direction of condensation provides better adaptation of amalgam to cavity walls than of condensation toward the pulpal floor. With high-copper spherical amalgams, a vertical and lateral direction of condensation with vibration is recommended.

Small- to medium-diameter condensers are advocated with admixed high-copper alloys with a medium-to-high force and vertical and lateral directions of condensation.

Many mechanical devices are available for condensing amalgam. These devices are more popular and more useful for condensing irregularly shaped alloys when high condensation forces are required. With the development of spherical alloys, the need for mechanical condensers was eliminated. Ultrasonic condensers are not recommended because during condensation they increase the mercury vapor level to values above the safety standards for mercury in the dental office.

Effect of Delay in Condensation It is important that an amalgam be condensed into the tooth cavity promptly after the mercury and alloy are suitably mixed. Delay of the condensation operation permits the amalgam to set partially before being transferred to the cavity. A delay in the condensation operation with a partial reaction of the mercury and alloy makes it impossible to remove the mercury effectively during condensation. As a result, an amalgam mass that has remained uncondensed for any period of time will contain more mercury than one that is condensed promptly. The resulting amalgam with the additional mercury content will show less strength in compression and higher creep. Delay in the condensation operation reduces the plasticity of the mix, and amalgams with reduced plasticity do not adapt well to the cavity walls. In a large restoration involving considerable time to place the amalgam mass, condensation of the final portions of amalgam becomes a problem. In such cases, it is preferable to make two smaller mixes of amalgam rather than one excessively large mix and not to use the amalgam if more than 3 or 4 minutes have elapsed from the time of initial mixing.

Mercury Content of Amalgam Restorations Amalgam restorations containing greater amounts of mercury in the set mass demonstrate less favorable clinical characteristics. Having more mercury in the set amalgam produces a greater amount of Ag_2Hg_3 and $Sn_{7\text{-}8}Hg$, the γ_1 and γ_2 phases, thereby leaving less unreacted Ag_3Sn, the γ phase. As discussed earlier, both γ_1 and γ_2 have lower strength than the γ phase. Therefore, when amalgam specimens are subjected to compressive stress, those containing increasing quantities of mercury exhibit decreasing strength values. The compressive strength decreases 1% for each 1% increase in mercury above 60%.

The mercury content of an amalgam restoration is not uniform throughout. Higher concentrations of mercury are located around the margins of the restoration. As a result, cavities should be overfilled and then carved back to minimize this problem. When using alloys that require higher mercury/alloy ratios, as much mercury as possible should be removed from the amalgamated mass. Note that the maximum allowable amount of mercury remaining in a hardened amalgam mass depends on the original mercury/alloy ratio. In other words, for alloys requiring high mercury/alloy ratios for trituration, 50% mercury in the hardened amalgam might be acceptable; however, for alloys needing low mercury/alloy ratios for trituration, 50% mercury in the set amalgam would be detrimental.

Although the lower mercury/alloy ratios currently being used are favorable regarding the total quantity of mercury in the set mass, remember that condensation forces alter mercury content within the restoration. Because condensation brings mercury to the surface of the amalgam mass, such "plashy" material should be periodically removed when filling the cavity to prevent trapping high mercury concentrations within the restoration. Overfilling of the cavity is carried out for the same reason, that is, to remove the amalgam that contains higher mercury content from the restoration contour.

When alloys that permit lower mercury/alloy ratios are used to obtain a plastic mass suitable for condensation, the operator should expect a lesser volume of excess mercury to be brought to the surface for removal than was observed with older materials.

Moisture Contamination During Insertion Moisture contamination during the mixing and condensing operations is the factor that may produce excessive expansion. There is no evidence, however, that the presence of moisture on the surface will cause any serious damage once the condensation operation is completed and the restoration is finished, except for trimming and polishing.

Because moisture in the saliva is a potential source of contamination for the amalgam, the tooth cavity must remain dry and the amalgam must be free from saliva contamination. Techniques and procedures in operative dentistry provide for an isolated field of operation, and these techniques should be followed to gain the best properties of the set amalgam.

With zinc-containing amalgam, the presence of saliva on the amalgam during condensation probably was a principal source of excessive delayed expansion and other poor qualities in the restoration. Moisture contamination of a zinc-containing amalgam mass from any source results in an excessive delayed expansion of several hundred micrometers per centimeter after the restoration has been placed in the tooth for several hours or days. This excessive expansion results from the decomposition of moisture. The trapped hydrogen gas in the amalgam restoration continues to be developed until sufficient force is produced to cause the excessive expansion. This decomposition of moisture results from the presence of zinc in the amalgam alloy and can be overcome by the use of non-zinc alloys.

FACTORS RELATED TO FINISHING AMALGAM RESTORATIONS

When an amalgam restoration has been properly placed, with adequate condensation, and the excess mercury has been removed from the final surface layer of the restoration, it will be sufficiently hardened within a few minutes to permit careful carving. If the restoration is not well condensed, it will not harden promptly, and the carving operation must be delayed. Usually the amalgam is sufficiently well set and hardened that carving with sharp instruments can be started almost immediately after condensation.

Burnishing, or rubbing the newly condensed amalgam with a metal instrument having a broad surface contact, can be employed to smooth the surface, thereby making the amalgam more susceptible to finishing and polishing. Burnishing can produce a tenfold reduction in surface roughness.

If final finishing and polishing are to be done at a second appointment, the restoration should be left undisturbed for a period of at least 24 hours. The patient should be cautioned that the freshly inserted restoration is relatively weak and that heavy biting forces should be avoided for a few hours after the time of insertion. Occlusal contacts must be carefully established. However, current all-spherical high-copper alloys have a much higher early strength than other types and can withstand biting forces sooner than earlier amalgams. One-hour compressive strengths of spherical high-copper alloys are about twice as high as high-copper admixed types and are comparable with those of low-copper alloys at 6 to 7 hours.

High-copper unicompositional amalgams with high early strengths can be finished at the first appointment. After condensation the surface is burnished and carved for clear definition of the margins, and all excess amalgam is removed. A creamy paste of triple-x silex and water is applied gently with an unwebbed rubber cup and a slow-speed handpiece. Light pressure should be applied for no more than 30 seconds per surface, and polishing should be directed from the center toward the margins of the restoration.

This early finishing begins 8 to 10 minutes after the start of trituration, depending on the particular alloy. Results of a 3-year clinical study have shown that restorations polished 8 minutes after trituration and those polished after 24 hours had no difference in longevity. Also, as time in the mouth increased, it became difficult to determine which method had been used to finish the restoration. The 24-hour polishing procedure used in the study was that normally used for polishing amalgam restorations. The procedure used for the 8-minute polish was different; no polishing bur was used, and the amalgam was carved carefully. Because the 24-hour polishing technique requires a second appointment, many restorations go without polishing. The main advantage of the 8-minute polishing technique is the elimination of the second appointment. This technique is limited to those amalgams that have high early-compressive strengths.

A well-finished and well-polished restoration will retain its surface appearance and be easier to keep clean than one that is poorly finished, because a rough surface on the restoration contains microscopic pits in which acids and small food particles from the mouth accumulate. These pits tend to encourage galvanic action on the surface of the restoration, leading to tarnish and perhaps even a corroded appearance.

The final polish at a second appointment is developed through a series of final finishing and polishing steps after a careful carving operation. This final polish is accomplished through a sequence of operations that includes the use of fine stones and abrasive disks or strips. To develop the final polish, a rotating soft brush is used to apply a suitable polishing agent, such as extrafine silex, followed by a thin slurry of tin oxide.

During the final polishing operation, the restoration should remain moist to avoid overheating from the use of dry polishing surfaces. Because the amalgam is weak in tension and shear resistance, it should not be drawn over the margin by burnishing or drawing operations that tend to produce extensions that subsequently will be fractured from the amalgam mass. To avoid such overextensions, all recommended operative practices should be followed faithfully.

BONDING OF AMALGAM

Although amalgam has been a highly successful restorative material when used as an intracoronal restoration, it does not restore the strength of the clinical crown to its original strength. Additional features, such as pins, slots, holes and grooves to increase retention of the restoration, must be supplied with the preparations for large amalgam restorations, but they do not reinforce the amalgam or increase its strength.

With the development of adhesive systems for dental composites came the opportunity to attempt to bond amalgams to tooth structure. Adhesive plastics containing 4-META, an acronym for 4-methacryloxyethyl trimellitic anhydride (see Chapter 10), have been the most successful products. Shear bond strengths of amalgam to dentin as high as 10 MPa have been reported using these adhesives. Comparable values for the shear bond strength of microfilled composites to dentin using these same adhesives have been 20 to 22 MPa. The fracture resistance of teeth restored with amalgam-bonded MOD restorations was more than twice that of restorations containing unbonded amalgams. Also, in spite of the lower shear strength of amalgam-bonded-to-dentin test samples compared with composites, the fracture strength of MODs in teeth restored with bonded amalgams was as high as for composites, although neither were as high (45% to 80%) as values for the intact tooth. As expected, amalgam bonded MODs with narrow preparations had higher strengths than those with wide preparations. Other studies showed the retention of amalgam-bonded MODs with proximal boxes was as great as pin-retained amalgams. In addition, amalgam-bonded restorations decreased marginal leakage in Class 5 restorations compared with unbonded amalgams. Finally, the plastic bonding agents for amalgam have not been successful in increasing the amalgam-to-amalgam bond strength in the repair of amalgam restorations. Thus at this stage of development, adhesive bonding of amalgam restorations to tooth structures is an improvement over nonbonded amalgams.

MERCURY AND BIOCOMPATIBILITY ISSUES

Amalgams have been used for 150 years; about 200 million amalgams are inserted each year in the United States and Europe. In spite of its substantial history, however, periodically concern arises about the biocompatibility of amalgam. Allergic reactions to mercury in amalgam restorations do occur, albeit infrequently. This is not surprising, because there is no material that 100% of the population is immune to 100% of the time. However, such allergic responses usually disappear in a few days or, if not, on removal of the amalgam. Aside from varying reports of mercury accumulation, no other local or systemic effects from mercury contained in dental amalgam have been demonstrated. If amalgam is used correctly, biocompatibility should not be a problem.

Even in their passive condition, metals are not inert. In vitro and in vivo experiments have established that there is a passive dissolution from all metals. The following eight questions are linked to the issues of dissolution, corrosion, and potential allergic response and toxicity:

1. Is any material released into the mouth?
2. What material is released?
3. What is the form of the released material?
4. How much material is released?
5. In what subsequent reactions do the released products get involved?
6. What percentage of the released products is excreted and what percentage is retained?
7. Where does the retained percentage accumulate?
8. What biological responses will result from the retained fraction?

Therefore any analysis of the literature and discussion of mercury toxicity in amalgams must continually refer to these eight questions, particularly questions 3 and 4, relating to the dosage and form of the mercury to which the body is exposed.

SOURCES OF MERCURY

In addressing these eight questions, the sources of the potential toxins must be evaluated. Exposure to mercury can occur from many different sources, including diet, water, air, and occupational exposure (Table 11-4). The World Health Organization (WHO) has estimated that eating seafood once a week raises urine mercury levels to 5 to 20 μg/L, two to eight times the level of exposure from amalgam (1 μg/L = 1 mg/m^3 = 1 part per billion [ppb]). Thus the amount of mercury vapor released from amalgam is less than that received from eating many common fish. It has been estimated that a patient with 9 amalgam occlusal surfaces will inhale daily only about 1% of the amount the Occupational Safety and Health Administration (OSHA) allows to be inhaled in the workplace. Blood and urine mercury levels are easily influenced by other factors and cannot often be directly linked to amalgam. In general, elemental mercury from amalgam seems to make only a small contribution to the total body burden of mercury. On the basis of epidemiological studies, blood and serum mercury levels correlate highly with occupational exposure and diet, whereas urine mercury relates to amalgam burden. Urine mercury levels relate to methods of condensation and ventilation more than to the amalgam per se.

FORMS OF MERCURY

Mercury has many forms, including organic and inorganic compounds. The most toxic organic compounds are methyl and ethyl mercury, and the next most toxic form is mercury vapor. The least toxic forms of mercury are the inorganic

TABLE 11-4 Estimated Daily Intake of Mercury

Source	μg Hg Vapor	μg Inorganic Hg	μg Methyl Hg
Atmosphere	0.12	0.038	0.034
Drinking water	—	0.05	—
Food, fish	0.94	—	3.76
Food, nonfish	—	20.00	—

compounds. Liquid mercury reacts with silver to form an inorganic silver-mercury compound via a metallic bond. Reports of people and animals being poisoned by eating food high in mercury are traced to the contamination of these foods by methyl mercury.

Mercury vapor is released, in minute quantities, during all procedures involving amalgam, including mixing, setting, polishing, and removal. Mercury vapor has also been reported to be released during mastication and drinking of hot beverages. The amount of mercury on amalgam surfaces has correlated with the quantity of mercury used during trituration. However, measuring the flow and flow rate is difficult and not precise, especially when working with a small area such as the mouth. Furthermore, ambient mercury must be considered, especially if such readings are taken in a dentist's office. With good ventilation, mercury levels return to background levels 10 to 20 minutes after placing an amalgam, and a charcoal filter system decreases levels 25% during the operative procedure. Fresh amalgams release more mercury than 2-year-old amalgams even with a *Streptococcus mutans* biofilm, and it has been shown that most oral organisms can grow in dental plaque containing 2 μg of mercury. Under normal conditions amalgam is covered by saliva, tending to reduce vapor pressure. Amalgams can also be constrained with a sealant resin for the first several days after insertion. Adding indium (8% to 14%) also decreases the vapor pressure.

CONCENTRATIONS OF MERCURY

OSHA has set a Threshold Limit Value (TLV) of 0.05 mg/m^3 as the maximum amount of mercury vapor allowed in the workplace. Nearly all dental offices worldwide comply with this standard. As an example of the factor of safety in this boundary, the fetuses of pregnant rats exposed to atmospheres with mercury concentrations of 2 mg/m^3 showed no ill effects. Fetuses exposed to mercury concentrations of 5 mg/m^3, or 40 times the allowable concentration, were stillborn. The lowest dose of mercury that illicits a toxic reaction is 3 to 7 μg/kg body weight. Paresthesia (tingling of extremities) occurs at about 500 μg/kg of body weight, followed by ataxia at 1000 μg/kg of body weight, joint pain at 2000 μg/kg of body weight, and hearing loss and death at 4000 μg/kg of body weight. Therefore these values are much greater in magnitude than the exposure to mercury from amalgam or from a normal diet.

Mercury in Urine The body cannot retain metallic mercury, but passes it through the urine. By using radioactive mercury in amalgams, it is possible to monitor the mercury levels in urine caused only by dental amalgams. One study showed that urine mercury levels peak at 2.54 μg/L 4 days after placing amalgams and, after 7 days return to zero. On removal of amalgam, urine mercury levels reach a maximum value of 4 μg/L and return to zero after a week. Although mercury is readily cleared in both cases, peak urine levels of mercury are nearly twice as great when amalgam is removed rather than inserted. The same is true for mercury vapor, with higher levels recorded on removal of an amalgam than on insertion. Other studies, using more sensitive techniques such as atomic absorption spectroscopy, show conflicting findings. There are reports demonstrating no increase in urine mercury levels and reports showing higher levels. Even in those cases in which urine mercury is elevated, the concentrations are still less than 1 μg/L.

As a comparison, consider the WHO estimate that eating seafood once a week will raise urine mercury to 5 to 20 μg/L, or two to eight times the level of exposure from amalgam determined in the study just cited. Neurological changes are not detected until urine mercury levels exceed 500 μg/L, nearly 170 times the peak levels found on insertion of an amalgam.

Mercury in Blood The maximum allowable level of mercury in the blood is 3 μg/L. Several studies have shown that freshly placed amalgam restorations elevate blood mercury levels to 1 to 2 μg/L. Removal of amalgam decreases blood mercury levels, with a half time of approximately 1 to 2 months for elimination of mercury.

However, as with urine mercury levels, there is first an increase of around 1.5 μg/L, which decreases in about 3 days. One study monitored blood mercury levels for a year and showed that patients with amalgams had a lower than average blood mercury level (0.6 μg/L) than patients without amalgams (0.8 μg/L). Presumably the blood mercury level is easily influenced by other factors and therefore cannot be explicitly related to amalgam. Evidently, a relationship exists between plasma and urine mercury levels.

Another study showed that patients with and without amalgams do not differ in the mean number or percentage of lymphocytes. Some studies have shown the blood mercury levels of dentists to be normal, whereas others report an increase. For those studies that indicate higher blood mercury levels in dentists, results have varied regarding any correlation between mercury concentration and number of amalgams placed. Elevated blood mercury levels may relate to mercury spills in the office, a factor that can easily be controlled. Both blood and serum mercury levels seem to correlate best with occupational exposure and not with the number of amalgams or length of time with amalgams in place.

Release of Corrosion Products Mercury release into various media, including water, saline, buffered citric and phosphoric acid, and synthetic saliva, has been measured by a number of techniques, such as atomic emission spectroscopy and atomic absorption spectroscopy. Ion release tends to be greatest in the first 1 to 24 hours after trituration. Once the amalgam is fully set, ionic dissolution is very low. This reduction in ion flux with time probably results from a combination of the chemical reaction progressing further and the formation of a passive surface film. In general, low-copper alloys release more ions than high-copper alloys, because of their inferior corrosion resistance. Greater amounts of mercury and silver are released from unpolished specimens than from polished specimens.

The effect of electrolytic concentration on corrosion has been compared for conventional and high-copper admixed alloys following storage for 4 months. The main corrosion products were tin compounds at the surface of the amalgams. Low-copper amalgam showed surface corrosion only, whereas subsurface corrosion occurred with high-copper amalgam, especially following immersion in an NaCl solution without phosphate. For low-copper amalgam, the release of elements decreased with time, possibly indicating passivation. For high-copper amalgam, the release of elements increased with time, except for copper and tin in a solution with a high concentration of phosphate, indicating that phosphate inhibits corrosion of the copper-tin phases. Other studies have revealed a tendency for tin and copper to be preferentially released from amalgam. Presumably, tin release originates from surface corrosion, whereas copper release results from subsurface corrosion. Stronger galvanic influences enhance copper release and, to a lesser extent, zinc release. Tin tends to provide a passive layer and to suppress the dissolution of mercury. It is suspected that indium functions similarly. In zinc-free alloys, the tin oxide is mercury depleted.

Another recent study has shown that following 1 week of aging in 0.9% NaCl solution at 37° C, the amount of mercury released from γ_1 was 14 to 60 times that released from amalgam and 5 times that released from β_1. The γ_2 phase released the least amount of mercury.

ALLERGIC REACTIONS AND DISEASE

Allergic reactions to mercury in amalgam restorations are rare, although there are case reports of allergic contact dermatitis, gingivitis, stomatitis, and remote cutaneous reactions. Such responses usually disappear on removal of the amalgam. Other local or systemic effects from mercury contained in dental amalgam have not been demonstrated. No well-conducted scientific study has conclusively shown that dental amalgam produces any ill effects.

Random reports of various diseases, such as multiple sclerosis, cannot unequivocally link the diseases to amalgams and therefore must be interpreted with caution. Reports of multiple sclerosis patients being instantly cured when amalgam is removed cannot be upheld scientifically. Because a week must pass for all mercury to be cleared by the body, an instantaneous recovery after removing the potential source of the mercury is unlikely.

Local Reactions In patients with oral lesions near amalgam sites, positive patch tests have been reported. However, the appropriate patch test has still not been determined, and many of the materials used for patch testing contain excessive concentrations of mercury. There are also reports of inflammatory reactions of the dentin and pulp, similar to the reactions to many other restorative materials. Mercury has been found in the lysosomes of macrophages and fibroblasts in some patients with lesions. Inflammation can usually be alleviated with a cavity liner. With the increased use of more corrosion-resistant amalgams, the volume of corrosion products and subsequent reactions are reduced.

Macrophages play an important role in the removal of foreign particulate matter from tissue. A number of cell culture studies have assessed the potential cytotoxicity of amalgam and its constituents. Unreacted mercury or copper leaching out from high-copper alloys has usually been the constituent leading to adverse responses. An in vitro study of the effects of particulate amalgams and their individual phases on macrophages showed that all particles except the γ_2 are effectively phagocytized by macrophages. Cell damage was seen in treated cultures exposed to particulate γ_1.

Systemic Reactions Implantation studies have shown that amalgam is reasonably well tolerated by soft and hard tissue. In a rabbit muscle implantation model, biological reactions to amalgams were found to depend on the time of implantation. All amalgams were strongly toxic 1 hour after setting. After 7 days, only high-copper amalgam showed any reaction.

In another series of studies, low- and high-copper amalgam powders and various phases of amalgam were implanted subcutaneously in guinea pigs. The result was a mild, early inflammatory response, in which particles were taken up by macrophages and giant cells. After 1.5 to 3 months, chronic granulomas developed. With low-copper amalgam, early changes occurred in the intracellular material, associated with the rapid degradation of the γ_2 phase. Later, intracellular particles from both low- and high-copper amalgam underwent progressive degradation, producing fine secondary particles containing silver and tin, which were distributed throughout the lesions and gave rise to macroscopic tattooing of the skin. Secondary material and small, degrading, primary particles from both types of amalgam were detected in the submandibular lymph nodes.

Elevated mercury levels were detected in the blood, bile, kidneys, liver, spleen, and lungs, with the highest concentrations found in the renal cortex. Mercury was excreted in the urine and feces. Mercury levels in the blood, liver, renal cortex, and feces were lower with the high-copper amalgam.

Black, refractile particulate deposits approximately 1 to 3 μm in diameter were found in the cytoplasm and nuclei of kidney cells. The ratio of nuclear to cytoplasmic deposits was higher in animals receiving high-copper amalgam. The cytoplasmic deposits consisted of collections of fine particles within lysosomes. Both lysosomal and nuclear deposits contained mercury and selenium, which were present in the animals' diet at low levels. Neither this study nor others have demonstrated any changes in biochemical function of any of the laden organs.

Subcutaneous implantation of only the powdered γ_2 phase led to a limited initial release of mercury from extracellular material. Thereafter, chronic granulomas developed around the implants, and particles degraded slowly in macrophages and giant cells. Fine secondary particles containing tin were produced. Subcutaneous implantation of only the powdered γ_1 phase induced a severe initial tissue response, and the majority of the material was extruded from the healing wounds. This process was accompanied by the release of significant amounts of mercury, which appeared in the body organs and excreta. The small numbers of particles remaining in the tissues underwent a slow degradation in macrophages and giant cells in chronic granulomas. Minute secondary particles containing silver and sulfur were deposited in the tissues and gave rise to macroscopic tattooing of the skin above the implants.

In another study, primates received occlusal amalgam fillings or maxillary bone implants of amalgam for 1 year. Amalgam fillings caused deposition of mercury in the spinal ganglia, anterior pituitary, adrenal, medulla, liver, kidneys, lungs, and intestinal lymph glands. Maxillary amalgam implants released mercury into the same organs, except for the liver, lungs, and intestinal lymph glands. Organs from control animals were devoid of precipitate.

Note that studies on powders probably overestimate the amount of breakdown products, and therefore biological response, because the surface area of powders can be 5 to 10 times the surface area of a solid component. It must also be emphasized that any reaction to amalgam, whether in cell culture, local tissue response, or systemic response, does not necessarily imply a reaction to mercury. Such reactions could be in response to some other constituent of the amalgam or corrosion product. For example, in vitro cell culture testing that measured fibroblasts affected by various elements and phases of amalgams has shown that pure copper and zinc show greater cytotoxicity than pure silver and mercury. Pure tin has not been shown to be cytotoxic (Fig. 11-14). The γ_1 phase is moderately cytotoxic. Cytotoxicity is decreased by the addition of 1.5% and 5% tin (Fig. 11-15). However, the addition of 1.5% zinc to γ_1 containing 1.5% tin increases cytotoxicity to the same level as that of pure zinc. Whenever zinc is present, higher cytotoxicity is revealed. High-copper amalgams show the same cytotoxicity as a zinc-free, low-copper amalgam. The addition of selenium does not reduce amalgam cytotoxicity, and excessive additions of selenium increase cytotoxicity. The cytotoxicity of amalgams decreases after 24 hours, possibly from the combined effects of surface oxidation and further amalgamation. The results of this study suggest that the major contributor to the cytotoxicity of amalgam alloy powders is probably copper, whereas that for amalgam is zinc.

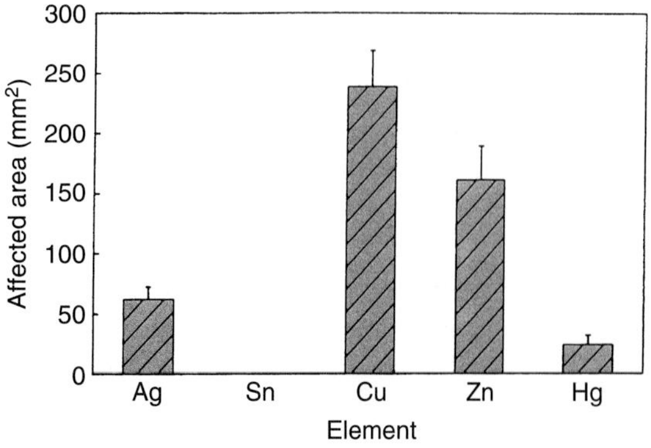

Fig. 11-14 Quantitative representation of the affected areas of fibroblasts, which reveals the magnitude of cytotoxicity of amalgam elements. Standard deviations are represented by vertical bars.

(From: Kaga M, Seale NS, Hanawa T et al: Cytotoxicity of amalgams, alloys, and their elements and phases, *Dent Mater* 7:68, 1991.)

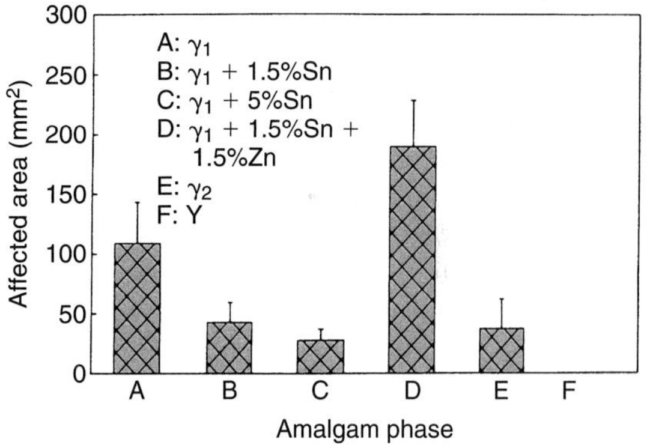

Fig. 11-15 Quantitative representation of the affected areas of fibroblasts, which reveals the magnitude of cytotoxicity of amalgam phases. Standard deviations are represented by vertical bars.

(From Kaga M, Seale NS, Hanawa T et al: Cytotoxicity of amalgams, alloys, and their elements and phases, *Dent Mater* 7:68, 1991.)

RISKS TO DENTISTS AND OFFICE PERSONNEL

Of the two groups of people (i.e., patients and dental office personnel) potentially at risk to mercury exposure with dental amalgam, the dental office personnel are at greater risk because of frequent handling of the freshly mixed material. The concern with the potential for mercury toxicity therefore centers primarily on dental office personnel. The blood mercury levels of dentists have been shown to be normal in several studies, especially when the following recommendations in mercury hygiene are followed:

1. Store mercury in unbreakable, tightly sealed containers.
2. To confine and facilitate the recovery of spilled mercury or amalgam, perform all operations involving mercury over areas that have impervious and suitably lipped surfaces.
3. Clean up any spilled mercury immediately. Droplets may be picked up with narrow-bore tubing connected (via a wash-bottle trap) to the low-volume aspirator of the dental unit.
4. Use tightly closed capsules during amalgamation.
5. Use a no-touch technique for handling the amalgam.
6. Salvage all amalgam scrap and store it under water that contains sodium thiosulfate (photographic fixer is convenient).
7. Work in well-ventilated spaces.
8. Avoid carpeting dental operatories; decontamination of carpeting is very difficult.
9. Eliminate the use of mercury-containing solutions.
10. Avoid heating mercury or amalgam.
11. Use water spray and suction when grinding dental amalgam.
12. Use conventional dental amalgam condensing procedures, manual and mechanical, but do not use ultrasonic amalgam condensers.
13. Perform yearly mercury determinations on all personnel regularly employed in dental offices.
14. Determine mercury vapor levels in operatories periodically.
15. Alert all personnel who handle mercury, especially during training or indoctrination periods, of the potential hazard of mercury vapor and the necessity for observing good mercury and amalgam hygiene practices.

SELECTED PROBLEMS

Problem 1

An amalgam mix is difficult to remove from the capsule and appears excessively wet. What can be done to obtain a better mix?

Solution a

The most common cause is related to overtrituration. Trituration time should be decreased by 1 or 2 seconds, and the mix should then be tested for plasticity.

Solution b

The speed of trituration may have been too fast; a slower speed should be selected for the next mix. Remember that the work of trituration is important in obtaining a normal mix and that the work is a function of the speed and the duration of trituration; increasing either increases the work of trituration.

Problem 2

Mixes of amalgam are consistently on the dry side and lack plasticity during condensation. What can cause a dry mix to occur, and how can it be corrected?

Solution a

In contrast to the previous case, a dry mix is often caused by undertrituration. Several mixes should be made at increased trituration times (an additional 1 to 2 seconds), and each one should be tested for plasticity. Listen for significant sound changes during trituration; the pestle can become wedged for the first few seconds, and the work-energy during that time is lost. Another choice would be to use a higher speed on the amalgamator.

Solution b

A dry mix can result from loss of mercury from the capsule during trituration. The two portions of most premeasured capsules are held together by a friction fit and occasionally some mercury can leak out during mixing. Check the inside of the housing covering the capsule area for small droplets of mercury, which also may appear like dust. If mercury is found follow the clean up procedures listed in the text at the end of this chapter. Changing to a hermetically sealed capsule is suggested if the problem persists with the product being used.

Problem 3

When larger restorative procedures are performed with amalgam, the amalgam is difficult to carve and seems to set before an adequate carving can be completed. What can cause this problem?

Solution a

The working time of an alloy can be influenced by the specific composition or particle size of an alloy and by the aging treatment during manufacturing. If the working characteristics of a particular alloy appear to change from those previously experienced, the cause may be an alteration made by the manufacturer. On the other hand, if the faster reaction rate occurs at initial trials with a new or unfamiliar alloy, this may simply indicate that the alloy has a short setting time and is unsuitable for use by certain operators or with specific techniques.

Solution b

The two most common manipulative variables that can accelerate the reaction and make carving difficult are overtrituration and decreased mercury/alloy ratios. An overtriturated mix is recognizable by its shiny and very wet appearance and by its high initial plasticity. A low mercury/alloy ratio appears quite dry during condensation and presents difficulty in handling.

Solution c

The increased rate of the reaction may be compensated for by making several smaller mixes as material is used. Do not try to complete large restorations from a single mix or continue to use a mix after it has exceeded the usable range for plasticity. Also, the technique should be evaluated; most carving problems can be remedied by obtaining assistance and improving operator speed.

Problem 4

When trying a new alloy, some amalgams may appear dry and brittle at the carving stage and tend to break away in large increments rather than to carve smoothly. What can cause this problem?

Solution a

A check should be made with a stopwatch to determine the point after initiating the mix at which this brittleness or loss of plasticity is first noticed. Prolonged condensation involves working the material beyond its limit of plasticity, and the loss of cohesiveness between increments complicates carving. Delayed condensation, in which there is a short, unavoidable interruption during the procedure, can also result in working the material after significant matrix has formed, causing the structure to break down. The result is a weak, friable surface that will not carve smoothly. It is very important to condense and carve an alloy in one continuous operation and within the time framework of the setting reaction for the alloy being used.

Solution b

The setting or working time of the alloy could be too short for the particular procedure being performed. Newer alloys appear to be faster setting and somewhat less consistent with respect to working time. The causes for a shortened setting time or an increased reaction rate are reviewed in the preceding problem.

Solution c

In certain instances a lack of condensation force can result in a restoration with a large number of air voids or poor cohesion between increments. This often occurs when the cavity preparation is not confining and an unstable matrix technique is used. It can also occur when moisture contamination interferes with cohesion between increments.

Problem 5

What factors are related to excessive tarnish and corrosion that appear several years after placement?

Solution a

A high residual mercury level in the final restoration can lead to increased corrosion as a result of an increase in the tin-mercury (γ_2) phase. This mercury can result from a mercury/alloy ratio that is too high in the initial mix or from inadequate condensation to remove excessive mercury.

Solution b

Patients on a high-sulfur diet or dietary supplement show increased tarnish on amalgam restorations. A well-polished surface is the best preventive measure to minimize tarnishing.

Solution c

Surface texture is also important in preventing corrosion. Small scratches and exposed voids develop concentration cells, with saliva as the electrolyte. Thus corrosion weakens the amalgam in critical areas such as the margin interface and begins the breakdown process. One of the major advantages of polishing amalgam surfaces to a smooth texture is that polishing minimizes the effects of corrosion and thus enhances clinical performance.

Solution d

Galvanic action can also develop in the mouth when two dissimilar metals come into contact. The most common cause of galvanic action is gold and amalgam placed in adjacent teeth. The effects can be seen in the darkened corrosion products appearing on the surface of the amalgam. This does not occur in every mouth, and the severity may relate to salivary composition and its function as an electrolyte.

Solution e

Moisture contamination during condensation causes air voids to develop throughout the mass of the restoration and corrosion to progress at a faster rate.

Problem 6

As amalgam restorations wear, the marginal integrity is usually the first area to show signs of failure. Small increments of amalgam or unsupported enamel fracture and crevices develop, thus leading to increased leakage and eventual secondary caries. What factors contribute to marginal deterioration of this type?

Solution a

Initially, every margin of a preparation should be examined for potential areas of enamel failure. Unsupported enamel rods and undercut walls are potential sites for fracture when subjected to occlusal forces. All cavosurface margins should be smooth-flowing curves and be free of unsupported enamel. Cavity walls should meet the external surface of the tooth at a 90-degree angle to provide optimum support for the tooth and sufficient bulk in the amalgam to resist fracture along the margin.

Solution b

Carving of the amalgam should be continuous with existing tooth form and should provide an accurate adaptation to the exposed cavity margin. Thin overextensions of amalgam beyond the margins and onto enamel can fracture readily into the bulk of amalgam and leave a crevice.

Solution c

Inadequate condensation of the amalgam in areas adjacent to the margins, especially in the areas of occlusal overpacking, causes a high residual mercury level to remain at the margin interface. The excessive γ_2 phase in that area leads to an increase in flow and corrosion and a decrease in strength that predisposes the restoration to fracture.

Solution d

Use of an alloy with a higher creep value, such as a microcut, results in evidence of early marginal fractures when subjected to occlusal function. The high-copper content alloys have less creep and demonstrate more durable marginal adaptation.

Problem 7

Small interproximal restorations often fail by fracturing across the occlusal isthmus. How can this type of failure be avoided?

Solution a

The major cause of gross fracture of amalgam restorations is usually found in the design of the cavity preparation. Sufficient bulk of material must be provided to support occlusal forces. This can best be accomplished by keeping the isthmus narrow and providing adequate cavity depth; however, on occasion the reverse might be necessary to avoid pulpal involvement. The axiopulpal line angle should be rounded to reduce stress concentration in that area.

Solution b

Occlusal contacts should be adjusted to avoid excessive contact on the marginal ridge. A torquing action places the isthmus under tension and results in fracture sooner.

Solution c

A smaller condenser must be used in the isthmus area so that adequate condensation can be accomplished. Inadequately condensed amalgam results in a weakening of the area and a predisposition to fracture.

Solution d

If enough dentin is removed during cavity preparation to require the placement of a cement base, a sufficiently rigid material must be selected for use. Zinc phosphate cement is the best material having a high enough modulus to minimize deflection of the amalgam. Other dental cements, particularly zinc oxide–eugenol types, have low moduli; under occlusal function they allow too much deflection and brittle failure is likely to occur in the amalgam. The axiopulpal line angle is a critical area and should be reconstructed in a supporting base of zinc phosphate cement.

Problem 8

A high-copper, fast-setting amalgam could not be finished by the early polishing procedure until 20 minutes after amalgamation and a satisfactory finish could not be obtained. What was the cause, and what would be the proper clinical procedure at this point?

Solution

For amalgams of this type to be polished at the first appointment, finishing should be started 8 to 10 minutes after trituration, depending on the alloy. If the finishing is delayed until

20 minutes after trituration, the setting of the amalgam has proceeded too far, and strength of the alloy is too great to complete the finishing with triple-x silex and water. If the finishing is delayed too long, attempts at early finishing should be stopped, and final finishing should be done in the standard manner at a second appointment.

Problem 9

A spherical amalgam mix was condensed with a 2-mm diameter condenser to obtain a high condensation pressure and a well-condensed restoration. However, a low-strength amalgam restoration and failure resulted. Why?

Solution

Spherical alloys triturated with mercury do not resist small condenser tips well, but allow them to penetrate the mass and thus reduce the condensation pressure. Larger diameter–tip condensers should be used that do not penetrate the mass as readily, thus allowing higher pressures and better condensation. These amalgams appear to condense easily and there is a tendency to use less than the desired condensation force. For optimum strength, a condensation pressure of 7 MPa should be used.

Problem 10

Why should scrap amalgam be stored in a sodium thiosulfate solution such as photographic fixer rather than just water?

Solution

Any mercury vapor released will react with the thiosulfate ions and lower the vapor pressure of mercury to levels below the instrument detection level of 0.01mg/m^3. If scrap amalgam is stored under water only, the amount of mercury in the air above the water increases with the log of time.

Problem 11

What assurances can you give a patient to dispel fears of mercury toxicity from dental amalgams?

Solution

Except for the rare allergic reaction there is no scientific documentation of local or systemic effects of dental amalgams. Patients with nine occlusal surfaces of amalgam will inhale less than 1% of the mercury that a person would inhale in a workplace having a level allowed by OSHA. Ingested mercury is eliminated through feces and urine. The daily intake of mercury from air, water, and food exceeds that from dental amalgams.

BIBLIOGRAPHY

Dental Amalgam—Review Articles

Allen EP, Bayne SC, Becker IM et al: Annual review of selected dental literature: report of the committee on scientific investigation of the American Academy of Restorative Dentistry, *J Prosthet Dent* 82:54, 1999.

Allen EP, Bayne SC, Donovan TE et al: Annual review of selected dental literature, *J Prosthet Dent* 76:82, 1996.

Bryant RW: γ_2 Phase in conventional dental amalgams—discrete clumps or continuous network? a review, *Aust Dent J* 29:163, 1984.

De Rossi SS, Greenberg MS: Intraoral contact allergy: a literature review and case reports, *J Am Dent Assoc* 129:1435, 1998.

Halbach S: Amalgam tooth fillings and man's mercury burden [Review]: *Human Exper Toxicol* 13:496, 1994.

Jendresen MD, Allen EP, Bayne SC et al: Annual review of selected dental literature: report of the committee on scientific investigation of the American Academy of Restorative Dentistry, *J Prosthet Dent* 80:109, 1998.

Jendresen MD, Allen EP, Bayne SC et al: Annual review of selected dental literature: report of the committee on scientific investigation of the American Academy of Restorative Dentistry, *J Prosthet Dent* 74:83, 1995.

Jendresen MD, Allen EP, Bayne SC et al: Annual review of selected dental literature: report of the committee on scientific investigation of the American Academy of Restorative Dentistry, *J Prosthet Dent* 78:82, 1997.

Lloyd CH, Scrimgeour SN, editors: Dental materials: 1994 literature review, *J Dent* 24:159, 1996.

Lloyd CH, Scrimgeour SN, editors: Dental materials: 1995 literature review, *J Dent* 25:180, 1997.

Mitchell RJ, Okabe T: Setting reactions in dental amalgam: part 1. Phases and microstructures between one hour and one week [Review], *Crit Rev in Oral Biol and Med* 7:12, 1996.

Okabe T, Mitchell RJ: Setting reactions in dental amalgam: part 2. The kinetics of amalgamation [Review], *Crit Review in Oral Biol and Med* 7:23, 1996.

Strang R, Whitters CJ, Brown D et al: Dental materials: 1996 literature review, *J Dent* 26:196, 1998.

Whitters CJ, Strang R, Brown D et al: Dental materials: 1997 literature review, *J Dent* 27:407, 1999.

Dental Amalgam—Reactions and Properties

Allan FC, Asgar K, Peyton FA: Microstructure of dental amalgam, *J Dent Res* 44:1002, 1965.

Asgar K: Amalgam alloy with a single composition behavior similar to Dispersalloy, *J Dent Res* 53:60, 1974.

Asgar K, Sutfin L: Brittle fracture of dental amalgam, *J Dent Res* 44:977, 1965.

Baran G, O'Brien WJ: Wetting of amalgam alloys by mercury, *J Am Dent Assoc* 94:898, 1977.

Boyer DB, Edie JW: Composition of clinically aged amalgam restorations, *Dent Mater* 6:146, 1990.

Brockhurst PJ, Culnane JT: Organization of the mixing time of dental amalgam using coherence time, *Aust Dent J* 32:28, 1987.

Brown IH, Maiolo C, Miller DR: Variation in condensation pressure during clinical packing of amalgam restorations, *Am J Dent* 6:255, 1993.

Brown IH, Miller DR: Alloy particle shape and sensitivity of high-copper amalgams to manipulative variables, *Am J Dent* 6:248, 1993.

Corpron R, Straffon L, Dennison J et al: Clinical evaluation of amalgams polished immediately after insertion: 5-year results, *J Dent Res* 63:178, 1984.

Council on Dental Materials, Instruments, and Equipment. Addendum to American National Standards Institute/American Dental Association, Specification No. 1 for alloy for dental amalgam, *J Am Dent Assoc* 100:246, 1980.

Dunne SM, Gainsford ID, Wilson NH: Current materials and techniques for direct restorations in posterior teeth. Part 1: silver amalgam, *Int Dent J* 47:123, 1997.

Farah JW, Hood JAA, Craig RG: Effects of cement bases on the stresses in amalgam restorations, *J Dent Res* 54:10, 1975.

Farah JW, Powers JM, editors:, High copper amalgams, *Dent Advis* 4(2):1, 1987.

Farah JW, Powers JM, editors: Dental amalgam and mercury, *Dental Advis* 8(2):1, 1991.

Gottlieb EW, Retief DH, Bradley EL: Microleakage of conventional and high copper amalgam restorations, *J Prosthet Dent* 53:355, 1985.

Hero, H: On creep mechanisms in amalgam, *J Dent Res* 62:44, 1983.

Jensen SJ, Jørgensen KD: Dimensional and phase changes of dental amalgam, *Scand J Dent Res* 93:351, 1985.

Johnson GH, Bales DJ, Powell LV: Clinical evaluation of high-copper dental amalgams with and without admixed indium, *Am J Dent* 5:39, 1992.

Johnson GH, Powell LV: Effect of admixed indium on properties of a dispersed phase high-copper dental amalgam, *Dent Mater* 8:366, 1992.

Jørgensen KD: The mechanism of marginal fracture of amalgam fillings, *Acta Odont Scand* 23:347, 1965.

Jørgensen KD, Esbensen AL, Borring-Moller G: The effect of porosity and mercury content upon the strength of silver amalgam, *Acta Odont Scand* 24:535, 1966.

Jørgensen KD, Wakumoto S: Occlusal amalgam fillings; marginal defects and secondary caries, *Odont Tskr* 76:43, 1968.

Katz JL, Grenoble DE: A composite model of the elastic behavior of dental amalgam, *J Biomed Mater Res* 5:515, 1971.

Kawakami M, Staninec M, Imazato S et al: Shear bond strength of amalgam adhesives to dentin, *Am J Dent* 7:53, 1994.

Leinfelder KF: Dental amalgam alloys, *Curr Opin Dent* 1:214, 1991.

Letzel H, Van 'T Hof MA, Marshall GW et al: The influence of the amalgam alloy on the survival of amalgam restorations: a secondary analysis of multiple controlled clinical trials, *J Dent Res* 76:1787, 1997.

Lloyd CH, Adamson M: Fracture toughness (KlC) of amalgam, *J Oral Rehabil* 12:59, 1985.

Mahler DB: Amalgam, International State-of-the-Art Conference on Restorative Dental Materials, Bethesda, Md, 1986.

Mahler, DB: Slow compressive strength of amalgam, *J Dent Res* 51:1394, 1972.

Mahler DB: The high-copper dental amalgam alloys, *J Dent Res* 76:537, 1997.

Mahler DB, Adey JD: Factors influencing the creep of dental amalgam, *J Dent Res* 70:1394, 1991.

Mahler DB, Adey JD, Marantz RL: Creep versus microstructure of gamma 2 containing amalgams, *J Dent Res* 56:1493, 1977.

Mahler DB, Adey JD, Marek M: Creep and corrosion of amalgam, *J Dent Res* 61:33, 1982.

Mahler DB, Adey JD, Marshall SJ: Effect of time at 37 degrees C on the creep and metallurgical characteristics of amalgam, *J Dent Res* 66:1146, 1987.

Mahler DB, Marantz RL, Engle JH: A predictive model for the clinical marginal fracture of amalgam, *J Dent Res* 59:1420, 1980.

Mahler DB, Nelson LW: Factors affecting the marginal leakage of amalgam, *J Am Dent Assoc* 108:50, 1984.

Mahler DB, Terkla LG, van Eysden J et al: Marginal fracture vs mechanical properties of amalgam, *J Dent Res* 49:1452, 1970.

Mahler DB, van Eysden J, Terkla LG: Relationship of creep to marginal fracture of amalgam, *J Dent Res* 54:183, 1975.

Malhotra ML, Asgar K: Physical properties of dental silver-tin amalgams with high and low copper contents, *J Am Dent Assoc* 96:444, 1978.

Martin JA, Bader JD: Five-year treatment outcomes for teeth with large amalgams and crowns, *Oper Dent* 22:72, 1997.

McCabe JF, Carrick TE: Dynamic creep of dental amalgam as a function of stress and number of applied cycles, *J Dent Res* 66:1346, 1987.

Meletis EI, Gibbs CA, Lian K: New dynamic corrosion test for dental materials, *Dent Mater* 5:411, 1989.

O'Brien WJ, Greener EH, Mahler DB: Dental amalgam. In Reese, JA, and Valega, TM, editors: *Restorative dental materials: an overview,* London, 1985, Quintessence.

Ogura H, Miyagawa Y, Nakamura K: Creep and rupture of dental amalgam under bending stress, *Dent Mater J* 8:65, 1989.

Osborne JW, Gale EN: Failure at the margin of amalgams as affected by cavity width, tooth position, and alloy selection, *J Dent Res* 60:681, 1981.

Papathanasiou AG, Curzon ME, Fairpo CG: The influence of restorative material on the survival rate of restorations in primary molars, *Paediatr Dent* 16:282, 1994.

Powers JM, Farah JW: Apparent modulus of elasticity of dental amalgams, *J Dent Res* 54:902, 1975.

Ryge G, Telford RF, Fairhurst CW: Strength and phase formation of dental amalgam, *J Dent Res* 36:986, 1957.

Sarkar NK, Eyer CS: The microstructural basis of creep of gamma 1 in dental amalgam, *J Oral Rehabil* 14:27, 1987.

Smales RJ, Hawthorne WS: Long-term survival of extensive amalgams and posterior crowns, *J Dent* 25:225, 1997.

Watkins JH, Nakajima H, Hanaoka K et al: Effect of zinc on strength and fatigue resistance of amalgam. *Dent Mater* 11:24, 1995.

Wilson NH, Wastell DC, Norman RD: Five-year performance of high-copper content amalgam restorations in a multiclinical trial of a posterior composite, *J Dent* 24:203, 1996.

Wing G, Ryge G: Setting reactions of spherical-particle amalgam, *J Dent Res* 44:1325, 1965.

Young FA, Jr Johnson, LB: Strength of mercury-tin phase in dental amalgam *J Dent Res* 46:457, 1967.

Zardiackas, LD, Anderson L, Jr: Crack propagation in conventional and high copper dental amalgam as a function of strain rate, *Biomater* 7:259, 1986.

Dental Amalgam—Retention and Bonding

Barkmeier WW, Gendusa NJ, Thurmond JW et al: Laboratory evaluation of Amalgambond and Amalgambond Plus, *Am J Dent* 7:239, 1994.

Ben-Amar A, Liberman R, Rothkoff Z et al: Long term sealing properties of Amalgambond under amalgam restorations, *Am J Dent* 7:141, 1994.

Boyer DB, Roth L: Fracture resistance of teeth with bonded amalgams, *Am J Dent* 7:91, 1994.

Eakle WS, Staninec M, Yip RL et al: Mechanical retention versus bonding of amalgam and gallium alloy restorations, *J Prosthet Dent* 72:351, 1994.

Edgren BN, Denehy GE: Microleakage of amalgam restorations using Amalgambond and Copalite, *Am J Dent* 5:296, 1992.

Fischer GM, Stewart GP, Panelli J: amalgam retention using pins, boxes, and Amalgambond, *Am J Dent* 6:173, 1993.

Hadavi R, Hey JH, Strasdin RB et al: Bonding amalgam to dentin by different methods, *J Prosthet Dent* 72:250, 1994.

Ianzano JA, Mastrodomenico J, Gwinnett AJ: Strength of amalgam restorations bonded with Amalgambond, *Am J Dent* 6:10, 1993.

Nuckles DB, Draughn RA, Smith TI: Evaluation of an adhesive system for amalgam repair: bond strength and porosity, *Quint Internat* 25:829, 1994.

Santos AC, Meiers JC: Fracture resistance of premolars with MOD amalgam restorations lined with Amalgambond, *Oper Dent* 19:2, 1994.

Staninec M, Holt M: Bonding of amalgam to tooth structure: tensile, adhesion and microleakage tests, *J Prosthet Dent* 59:397, 1988.

Staninec M: Retention of amalgam restorations: undercuts versus bonding, *Quint Internat* 20:347, 1989.

Dental Amalgam—Mercury and Biocompatibility Issues

Abraham JE, Svare EW: The effect of dental amalgam restorations on blood mercury levels, *J Dent Res* 63:71, 1984.

American Dental Association Council on Scientific Affairs: Dental amalgam—update on safety concerns, *J Am Dent Assoc* 129:494, 1998.

Arenholt-Bindslev D: Environmental aspects of dental filling materials, *Eur J Oral Sci* 106:713, 1998.

Bakir F, Damluji SF, Amin-Zaki L et al: Methyl mercury poisoning in Iraq, *Science* 181:230, 1973.

Berglund A: Estimation of the daily dose of intra-oral mercury vapor inhaled after release from dental amalgam, *J Dent Res* 69:1646, 1990.

Berglund A, Bergdahl J, Hansson Mild K: Influence of low frequency magnetic fields on the intra-oral release of mercury vapor from amalgam restorations, *Eur J Oral Sci* 106:671, 1998.

Berlin MH, Clarkston TW, Friberg LT et al: Maximum allowable concentrations of mercury vapor in air, *Lakartidningen* 64:3628, 1967.

Berry TG, Nicholson J, Troendle K. Almost two centuries with amalgam: where are we today? *J Am Dent Assoc* 125:392, 1994.

Berry TG, Summitt JB, Chung AKH et al: Amalgam at the new millennium, *J Am Dent Assoc* 129:1547, 1998.

Birke G, Johnels AG, Plantin L-O et al: Hg i livsmedel (3): Metylkvicksilverförgiftning genom förtaring av fisk? [Hg in food (3): Methyl mercury poisoning through eating fish?] *Lakartidningen* 64:3628, 1967.

Bolewska J, Holmstrup P, Moller-Madsen B et al: Amalgam-associated mercury accumulations in normal oral mucosa, oral mucosal lesions of lichen planus and contact lesions associated with amalgam, *J Oral Pathol Med* 19:19, 1990.

Brune D: Corrosion of amalgams, *Scand J Dent Res* 89:506, 1981.

Burrows D: Hypersensitivity to mercury, nickel and chromium in relation to dental materials, *Internat Dent J* 36:30, 1986.

Chang SB, Siew C, Gruninger SE: Factors affecting blood mercury concentrations in practicing dentists, *J Dent Res* 71:66, 1992.

Chew CL, Soh G, Lee AS et al: Comparison of release of mercury from three dental amalgams, *Dent Mater* 5:244, 1989.

Clarkson TW: The toxicology of mercury, *Crit Reviews in Clinical Lab Sci* 34:369, 1997.

Consumer Reports: The mercury in your mouth 56(5): 316, 1991.

Council on Dental Materials and Devices: Recommendations in mercury hygiene, *J Am Dent Assoc* 92:1217, 1976.

Council on Dental Materials, Instruments, and Equipment: Safety of dental amalgam, *J Am Dent Assoc* 106:519, 1983.

Corbin SB, Kohn WG: The benefits and risks of dental amalgam: current findings reviewed. *J Am Dent Assoc* 125:381, 1994.

Cox SW, Eley BM: Further investigations of the soft tissue reaction to the gamma 1 phase (Ag_2Hg_3) of dental amalgam, including measurements of mercury release and redistribution, *Biomater* 8:296, 1987.

Cox SW, Eley BM: Further investigations of the soft tissue reaction to the gamma 2 phase ($Sn_{7-8}Hg$) of dental amalgam, including measurements of mercury release and redistribution, *Biomater* 8:301, 1987.

Cox SW, Eley BM: Mercury release, distribution and excretion from subcutaneously implanted conventional and high-copper amalgam powders in the guinea pig, *Arch Oral Biol* 32:257, 1987.

Cox SW, Eley BM: Microscopy and x-ray microanalysis of subcutaneously implanted conventional and high-copper dental amalgam powders in the guinea pig, *Arch Oral Biol* 32:265, 1987.

Cox SW, Eley BM: The release, tissue distribution and excretion of mercury from experimental amalgam tattoos, *Br J Exp Pathol* 67:925, 1986.

Craig RG: Biocompatibility of mercury derivatives, *Dent Mater* 2:91, 1986.

Danscher G, Horsted-Bindslev P, Rungby J: Traces of mercury in organs from primates with amalgam fillings, *Exp Mol Pathol* 52:291, 1990.

Ekstrand J, Bjorkman L, Edlund C et al: Toxicological aspects on the release and systemic uptake of mercury from dental amalgam, *Eur J Oral Sci* 106:678, 1998.

Eley BM, Cox SW: Renal cortical mercury levels associated with experimental amalgam tattoos: effects of particle size and amount of implanted material, *Biomater* 8:401, 1987.

Eley BM, Cox SW: The development of mercury- and selenium-containing deposits in the kidneys following implantation of dental amalgams in guinea pigs, *Br J Exp Pathol* 67:937, 1986.

Ferracane JL, Adey JD, Nakajima H et al: Mercury vaporization from amalgams with varied alloy compositions, *J Dent Res* 74:1414, 1995.

Ferracane JL, Engle JH, Okabe T et al: Reduction in operatory mercury levels after contamination or amalgam removal, *Am J Dent* 7:103, 1994.

FDI Commission: Environmental issues in dentistry—mercury, *Internat Dent J* 47:105, 1997.

Forsell M, Larsson B, Ljungqvist A et al: Mercury content in amalgam tattoos of human oral mucosa and its relations to local tissue reactions, *Eur J Oral Sci* 106:582, 1998.

Gronka PA, Bobkoskie RL, Tomchick GJ et al: Mercury vapor exposures in dental offices, *J Am Dent Assoc* 81:923, 1970.

Guthrow CE, Johnson CB, Lawless KB: Corrosion of dental amalgam and its component phases, *J Dent Res* 46:1372, 1967.

Haikel Y, Gasser P, Salek P et al: Exposure to mercury vapor during setting, removing, and polishing amalgam restorations, *J Biomed Mater Res* 24:1551, 1990.

Heintze U, Edwardsson S, Derand T et al: Methylation of mercury from dental amalgam and mercuric chloride by oral streptococci in vitro, *Scand J Dent Res* 91:150, 1983.

Holland GA, Asgar K: Some effects of the phases of amalgam induced by corrosion, *J Dent Res* 53:1245, 1974.

Johansson C, Moberg LE: Area ratio effects on metal ion release from amalgam in contact with gold, *Scand J Dent Res* 99:246, 1991.

Kaaber S: Allergy to dental materials with special reference to the use of amalgam and polymethylmethacrylate, *Internat Dent J* 40:359 1990.

Kaga M, Seale NS, Hanawa T et al: Cytotoxicity of amalgams, *J Dent Res* 67:1221, 1988.

Kaga M, Seale NS, Hanawa T et al: Cytotoxicity of amalgams, alloys, and their elements and phases, *Dent Mater* 7:68, 1991.

Kingman A, Albertini T, Brown LJ: mercury concentrations in urine and whole blood associated with amalgam exposure in a US military population, *J Dent Res* 77:60, 1998.

Kuntz WD: Maternal and cord blood background mercury level, *Am J Obstet Gynecol* 143:440, 1982.

Kurland LT, Faro SN, Siedler H: Minamata disease, *World Neurol* 1:370, 1960.

Laine J, Kalimo K, Forssell H et al: Resolution of oral lichenoid lesions after replacement of amalgam restorations in patients allergic to mercury compounds, *Br J Dermatol* 126:10, 1992.

Langolf GD, Chaffin DB, Henderson R et al: Evaluation of workers exposed to elemental mercury using quantitative test of tremor and neuromuscular function, *Am Ind Hyg Assoc J* 39:976, 1978.

Langworth S, Elinder CG, Gothe CJ et al: Biological monitoring of environmental and occupational exposure to mercury, *Int Arch Occup Environ Health* 63:161, 1991.

Lyttle HA, Bowden GH: The level of mercury in human dental plaque an interaction in vitro between biofilms of Streptococcus mutans and dental amalgam, *J Dent Res* 72:1320, 1993.

Lyttle HA, Bowden GH: The resistance and adaptation of selected oral bacteria to mercury and its impact on their growth, *J Dent Res* 72:1325, 1993.

Mackert Jr JR: Dental amalgam and mercury, *J Am Dent Assoc* 122:54, 1991.

Mackert Jr JR, Berglund A: Mercury exposure from dental amalgam fillings: absorbed dose and the potential for adverse health effects, *Crit Reviews in Oral Biol and Med* 8:410, 1997.

Mackert JR, Jr, Leffell MS, Wagner DA et al: Lymphocyte levels in subjects with and without amalgam restorations, *J Am Dent Assoc* 122:49, 1991.

Mandel ID: Amalgam hazards: an assessment of research, *J Am Dent Assoc* 122:62, 1991.

Marek M: Acceleration of corrosion of dental amalgam by abrasion, *J Dent Res* 63:1010, 1984.

Marek M: Corrosion test for dental amalgam, *J Dent Res* 59:63, 1980.

Marek M: The effect of the electrode potential on the release of mercury from dental amalgam, *J Dent Res* 72:1315, 1993.

Marek M: The release of mercury from dental amalgam: the mechanism and in vitro testing, *J Dent Res* 69:1167, 1990.

Marek M, Hockman RF, Okabe T: In vitro corrosion of dental amalgam phases, *J Biomed Mater Res* 10:789, 1976.

Marshall SJ, Lin JHC, Marshall GW: Cu_2O and $CuCl_2 \cdot 3Cu(OH)_2$ corrosion products on copper rich dental amalgams, *J Biomed Mater Res* 16:81, 1982.

Martin MD, Naleway C, Chou H-N: Factors contributing to mercury exposure in dentists, *J Am Dent Assoc* 126:1502, 1995.

Mateer RS, Reitz CD: Galvanic degradation of amalgam restorations, *J Dent Res* 51:1546, 1972.

Miller JM, Chaffin DB, Smith RG: Subclinical psychomotor and neuromuscular changes exposed to inorganic mercury, *Am Ind Hyg Assoc J* 36(10):725, 1975.

Moberg LE, Johansson C: Release of corrosion products from amalgam in phosphate containing solutions, *Scand J Dent Res* 99:431, 1991.

Molin M, Marklund S, Bergman B et al: Plasma-selenium, glutathione peroxidase in erythrocytes and mercury in plasma in patients allegedly subject to oral galvanism, *Scand J Dent Res* 95:328 1987.

Molin M, Marklund SL, Bergman B et al: Mercury, selenium, and glutathione peroxidase in dental personnel, *Acta Odontol Scand* 47:383, 1989.

Mueller HJ, Bapna MS: Copper-, indium-, tin-, and calcium-fluoride admixed amalgams: release rates and selected properties, *Dent Mater* 6:256, 1990.

Okabe T, Ferracane J, Cooper C et al: Dissolution of mercury from amalgam into saline solution, *J Dent Res* 66:33, 1987.

Okabe T, Yomashita T, Nakajima H et al: Reduced mercury vapor release from dental amalgams prepared with binary Hg-In liquid alloys, *J Dent Res* 73:1711, 1994.

Olsson S, Bergman M: Daily dose calculations from measurements of intra-oral mercury vapor, *J Dent Res* 71:414, 1992.

Olsson S, Berhlund A, Bergman M: Release of elements due to electrochemical corrosion of dental amalgam, *J Dent Res* 73:33, 1994.

Olstad ML, Holland RI, Pettersen AH: Effect of placement of amalgam restorations on urinary mercury concentration, *J Dent Res* 69:1607, 1990.

Ott KH, Vogler J, Kroncke A et al: Mercury concentrations in blood and urine before and after placement of non-gamma 2 amalgam fillings, *Dtsch Zahnarztl Z* 44:551, 1989.

Palaghias, G: The role of phosphate and carbonic acid-bicarbonate buffers in the corrosion processes of the oral cavity, *Dent Mater* 1:139, 1985.

Pierce P, Thompson JF, Likosky WH et al: Alkyl mercury poisoning in humans, *J Am Med Assoc* 220:1439, 1972.

Pohl L, Bergman M: The dentist's exposure to elemental mercury vapour during clinical work wit amalgam, *Act Odont Scand* 53:1023, 1995.

Powell LV, Johnson GH, Bales DJ: Effect of admixed indium on mercury vapor release from dental amalgam, *J Dent Res* 68:1231, 1989.

Powell LV, Johnson GH, Yashar N et al: Mercury vapor release during insertion and removal of dental amalgam. *Oper Dent* 19:70, 1994.

Rao GS, Radchenko V, Tong YS: Reproductive effects of elemental mercury vapor in pregnant Wistar rats, Annual Session Program, American Association for Dental Research Abstracts, Cincinnati, 232, 1983.

Sandborough-Englund G, Elinder C-G, Landworth S et al: Mercury in biological fluids after mercury removal, *J Dent Res* 77:615, 1998.

Sarkar NK, Park JR: Mechanism of improved corrosion resistance of Zn-containing dental amalgams, *J Dent Res* 67:1312, 1988.

Saxe SR, Snowdon DA, Wekstein MW et al: Dental amalgam and cognitive function in older women: findings from the nun study, *J Am Dent Assoc* 126:1495, 1995.

Scarlett JM, Gutenmann WH, Lisk DJ: A study of mercury in the hair of dentists and dental-related professionals in 1985 and subcohort comparison of 1972 and 1985 mercury hair levels, *J Toxicol Environ Health* 25:373, 1988.

Schmalz G, Schmalz C: Toxicity tests on dental filling materials, *Int Dent J* 31:185, 1981.

Skare I, Engqvist A: Urinary mercury clearance of dental personnel after a long-term intermission in occupational exposure, *Swed Dent J* 14:255, 1990.

Snapp KR, Boyer DB, Peterson LC et al: The contribution of dental amalgam to mercury in blood, *J Dent Res* 68:780, 1989.

Syrjanen S, Hensten-Pettersen A, Nilner K: In vitro testing of dental materials by means of macrophage cultures. II. Effects of particulate dental amalgams and their constituent phases on cultured macrophages, *J Biomed Mater Res* 20:1125, 1986.

Takaku S: Studies of mercury concentration in saliva with particular reference to mercury dissolution from dental amalgam into saliva, *Gakho Shikwa* 82:285, 1982.

Veron C, Hildebrand HF, Martin P: Dental amalgams and allergy, *J Biol Buccale* 14:83, 1986.

von Mayenburg J, Rakoski J, Szliska C: Patch testing with amalgam at various concentrations, *Contact Dermatitis* 24:266, 1991.

Chapter 12

Impression Materials

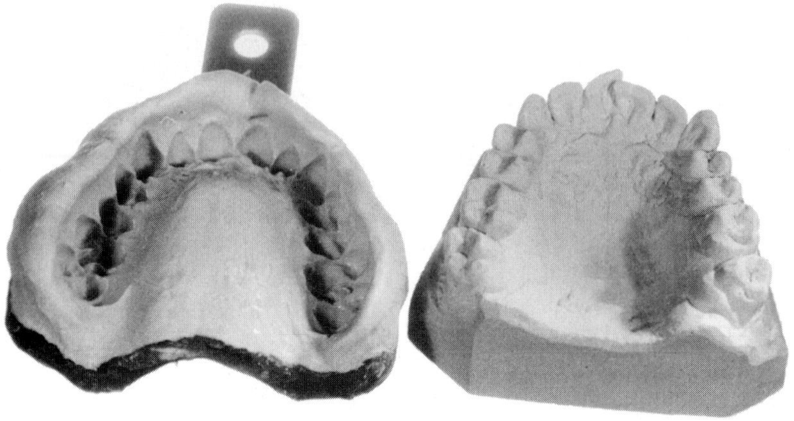

Fig. 12-1 An alginate impression and a stone cast removed from the impression.

Impression materials are used to register or reproduce the form and relationship of the teeth and oral tissues. Hydrocolloids and synthetic elastomeric polymers are among the materials most commonly used to make impressions of various areas of the dental arch, whereas zinc oxide–eugenol and modeling compound are used less frequently. Each of these classes of materials has certain advantages and disadvantages. An understanding of the physical characteristics and the limitations of each material is necessary for their successful use in clinical dentistry.

PURPOSE OF IMPRESSION MATERIALS

Impression materials are used to make an accurate replica of the hard and soft oral tissues. The area involved may vary from a single tooth to the whole dentition, or an impression may be made of an edentulous mouth. The impression gives a negative reproduction of the tissues, and by filling the impression with dental stone or other model material, a positive cast is made that can be removed after the model material has set. An impression and a stone cast made from it are shown in Fig. 12-1. Casts of the mouth are used to evaluate the dentition when orthodontic, occlusal, or other problems are involved, and in the fabrication of restorations and prostheses.

Usually the impression material is carried to the mouth in an unset (plastic) condition in a tray and applied to the area under treatment. When the impression material has set, it is removed from the mouth with the tray. The cast is made by filling the impression with dental stone or other model material. Sometimes the impression is electroformed with copper or silver to make a metal cast or model. The accuracy, detail, and quality of this final replica are of greatest importance. When the positive reproduction takes the form of the tissues of the upper or lower jaw and serves for the construction of dentures, crowns, bridges, and other restorations, it is described as a *cast*. The positive reproduction of the form of a prepared tooth constitutes a die for the preparation of inlays or bridge structures. When a positive likeness of the arch or certain teeth is reproduced for orthodontic treatment, it is sometimes described as a *model,* although the term *cast* is proper. On other occasions and in other branches of dentistry, these terms are used interchangeably. Sometimes impression materials are used to duplicate a cast or model that has been formed when more than one positive reproduction is required. Such impression materials are referred to as *duplicating materials*.

A variety of impression trays are used to make impressions. Examples of typical impression trays are shown in Fig. 12-2. The tray is placed so the material is brought into contact with the oral

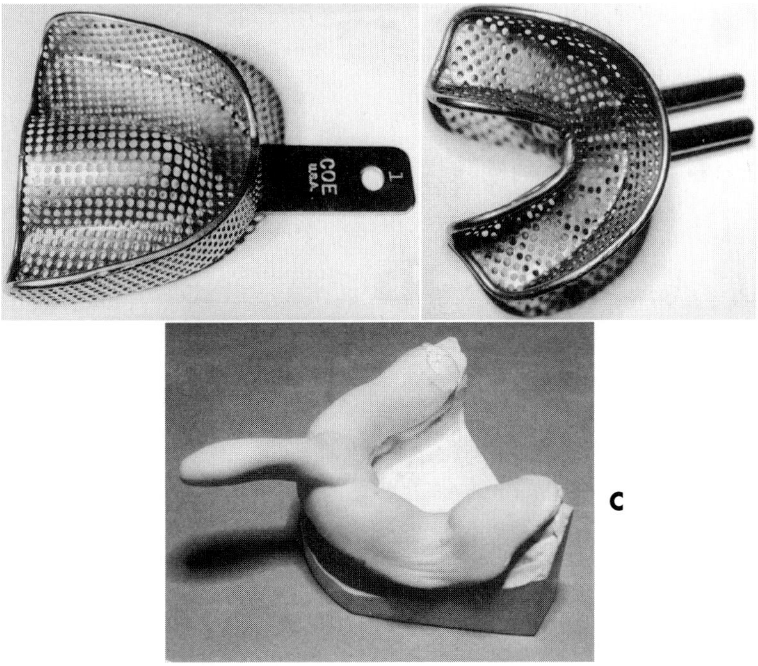

Fig. 12-2 Three types of impression trays. **A,** Perforated metal tray for use with alginate hydrocolloid impression materials. **B,** Water-cooled metal tray for use with agar hydrocolloid impression materials; water enters tubes on the occlusal surface of the tray through one of the projecting tubes and is conveyed away through the other projecting tube. **C,** Custom acrylic tray on a study cast for an elastomeric impression material.

tissues and held without movement until the impression material has set. The tray with the impression material is then removed from the mouth, and the impression is ready for making a positive replica. The clinical impression technique and the production of the cast vary with each impression material; details are described in appropriate textbooks.

DESIRABLE QUALITIES

Contact with living tissues in the mouth and the needs of clinical procedures dictate critical requirements for the physical properties of dental impression materials. No impression material fulfills all these requirements, and the selection of the material best suited for a particular clinical situation and technique rests with the dentist. The desirable properties of an impression can be summarized briefly as follows:

1. A pleasant odor, taste, and esthetic color
2. Absence of toxic or irritant constituents
3. Adequate shelf life for requirements of storage and distribution
4. Economically commensurate with the results obtained
5. Easy to use with the minimum of equipment
6. Setting characteristics that meet clinical requirements
7. Satisfactory consistency and texture
8. Readily wets oral tissues
9. Elastic properties with freedom from permanent deformation after strain
10. Adequate strength so it will not break or tear on removal from the mouth

11. Dimensional stability over temperature and humidity ranges normally found in clinical and laboratory procedures for a period long enough to permit the production of a cast or die
12. Compatibility with cast and die materials
13. Accuracy in clinical use
14. Readily disinfected without loss of accuracy
15. No release of gas during the setting of the impression or cast and die materials

TYPES OF IMPRESSION MATERIALS

The alginate hydrocolloid, agar hydrocolloid, and synthetic elastomeric impression materials are the most widely used today, and the properties of these are examined first. The zinc oxide–eugenol materials, gypsum, and compound impression materials are discussed later in this chapter for use as bite registration materials.

ALGINATE HYDROCOLLOIDS

Dental alginate impression materials change from the sol phase to the gel phase because of a chemical reaction. Once gelation is completed, the material cannot be reliquefied to a sol. These hydrocolloids are called *irreversible* to distinguish them from the agar reversible hydrocolloids described later. Alginate impressions are widely used to form study casts used to plan treatment, monitor changes, and create crowns, bridges, and removable prostheses.

Alginate impression products have acceptable elastic properties and compare well with agar materials. Preparation for use requires only the mixing of measured quantities of powder and

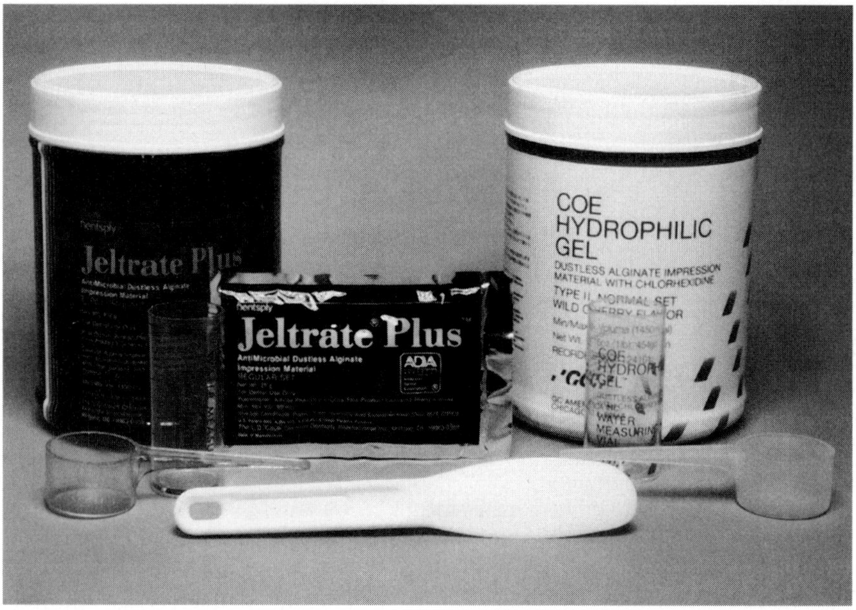

Fig. 12-3 Alginate impression products: in bulk in a can with a scoop for measuring powder, a measuring cylinder for water, and a preweighed alginate in a foil package. These products are dustless and contain disinfection agents.

(From Craig RG, Powers JM, Wataha JC: *Dental materials: properties and manipulation*, ed 7, St Louis, 2000, Mosby.)

water. The resulting paste flows well and registers acceptable anatomical detail. Gypsum casts or models are made by pouring dental plasters, stone, or investment into the impression; no separating medium is necessary. The powder is supplied in bulk containers along with suitable measures for dispensing the correct quantities of powder and water. The powder is also available in small sealed packets containing a quantity suitable for one impression and ready for mixing with a measured quantity of water. These methods of packaging, together with the measuring devices supplied by the manufacturer, are shown in Fig. 12-3.

COMPOSITION AND CHEMISTRY

Potassium and sodium salts of alginic acid have properties that make them suitable for compounding a dental impression material. Alginic acid, which is prepared from a marine plant, is a high–molecular weight block copolymer of anhydro-β-D-mannuronic acid and anhydro-β-D-guluronic acid, as shown in the top part of the formula for alginate on p. 334. The properties of alginate raw material depend largely on the degree of polymerization and the ratio of guluronan and mannuronan blocks in the polymeric molecules. The mannuronan regions are stretched and flat, whereas the guluronan regions contribute less flexibility. Also, mainly guluronan blocks bind with Ca^{+2}. Therefore, alginates rich in guluronan form strong, brittle gels, whereas those rich in mannuronan form weaker and more elastic gels.

Solutions of these soluble salts, when reacted with a calcium salt, produce an insoluble elastic gel commonly called *calcium alginate;* the structures are shown below. Upon mixing with water, the alginate impression material first forms a sol. Following the chemical reaction described on p. 334, a gel is formed to create the set impression material. The gel-forming ability of alginates is mainly related to the proportion of L-guluronan blocks. The concept of sols and gels is presented in the discussion of colloids in Chapter 2.

The nature of this chemical reaction is shown on p. 335 for the sodium salt. The equally common potassium salt reacts similarly. In an alginate impression compound, the calcium sulfate dihydrate, soluble alginate, and sodium phosphate are included in the powder. When water is added to the powder, compounds disassociate as shown. Calcium ions from the calcium sulfate dihydrate react preferentially with phosphate ions from the sodium phosphate and pyrophosphate to form insoluble calcium phosphate. Calcium phosphate is formed rather than calcium alginate because it has a lower solubility; thus the sodium phosphate is called a *retarder* and provides working time for the mixed alginate.

After the phosphate ions are depleted, the calcium ions react with the soluble alginate to form the insoluble calcium alginate, which together with water forms the irreversible calcium alginate gel. The calcium alginate is insoluble in water, and its formation causes the mixed material to gel. This reaction is irreversible; it is not possible to convert the calcium alginate to a sol after it has set.

To meet the critical requirements of a dental impression material, this reaction must be controlled to attain the desirable properties of consistency, working time, setting time, strength, elastic quality, and smooth, hard surfaces on gypsum casts. These requirements are achieved by adding agents to control the rate of the reaction, develop strength and elasticity in the gel, and counteract the delaying effect of alginate on the setting of gypsum products. The use of suitable fillers in correct quantities produces a consistency that is suitable for various clinical uses.

The composition of a typical alginate impression material and the function of its ingredients are shown in Table 12-1. Manufacturers adjust the concentration of sodium phosphate to produce regular- and fast-set alginates. They also adjust the concentration of filler to control the flexibility of the set impression material from soft-set to hard-set. Although alginate impressions are usually made in a tray, injection types are much more fluid after mixing and more

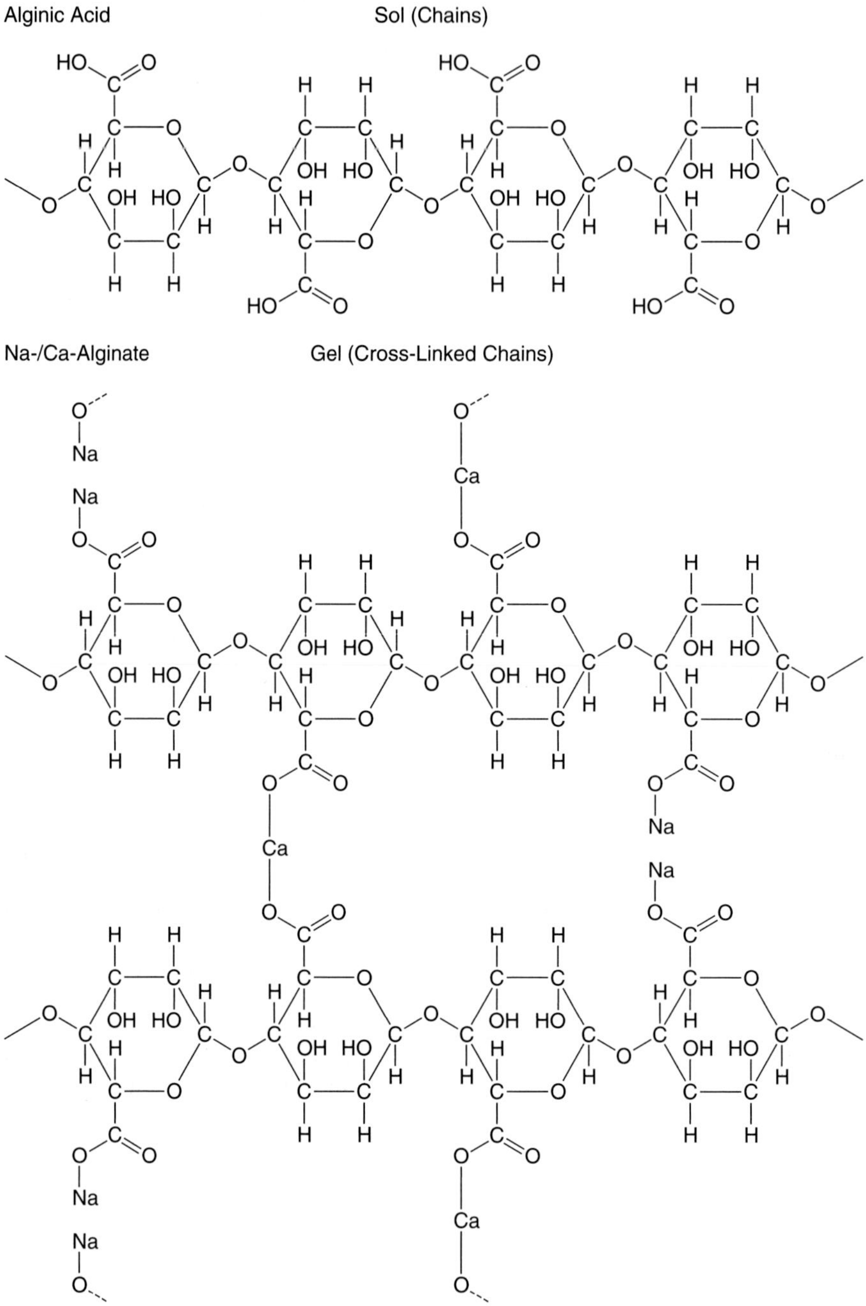
Alginic Acid
Sol (Chains)
Na-/Ca-Alginate
Gel (Cross-Linked Chains)

$$CaSO_4 - 2H_2O(s) \longrightarrow Ca^{2+}(aq) + SO_4^{2-}(aq)$$
$$Na - Alginate(s) \longrightarrow Na^{+}(aq) + Alginate^{-}(aq)$$
$$Na_4P_2O_7(s)\ (retarder) \longrightarrow 4Na^{+}(aq) + P_2O_7^{4-}(aq)$$
$$2Ca^{2+}(aq) + P_2O_7^{4-}(aq) \longrightarrow Ca_2P_2O_7(s)$$

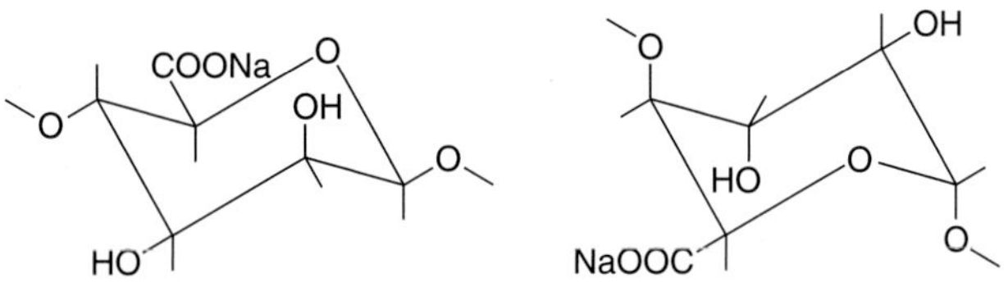

Mannuronate Guluronate

sol

$$Ca^{2+}(aq) + Alginate^{-}(aq) \longrightarrow Ca - Alginate^{+}$$

gel network

TABLE 12-1 Ingredients in an Alginate Impression Powder and Their Functions

Ingredient	Weight (%)	Function
Potassium alginate	18	To dissolve in water and react with calcium ions
Calcium sulfate dihydrate	14	To react with potassium alginate to form an insoluble calcium alginate gel
Potassium sulfate, potassium zinc fluoride, silicates, or borates	10	To counteract the inhibiting effect of the hydrocolloid on the setting of gypsum, giving a high-quality surface to the die
Sodium phosphate	2	To react preferentially with calcium ions to provide working time before gelation
Diatomaceous earth or silicate powder	56	To control the consistency of the mixed alginate and the flexibility of the set impression
Organic glycols	Small	To make the powder dustless
Wintergreen, peppermint, anise	Trace	To produce a pleasant taste
Pigments	Trace	To provide color
Disinfectants (e.g., quaternary ammonium salts and chlorhexidine)	1-2	To help in the disinfection of viable organisms

flexible after setting. The alginate powder is finely divided, and considerable dust may be involved during dispensing. The dimensions of 10% to 15% of the siliceous dust particles are similar to asbestos fibers that produce fibrogenesis and carcinogenesis; therefore inhalation of the dust should be avoided. Coating the powder with a glycol results in a dustless alginate, and no detectable levels of dust have been measured at the operator level for the dustless products. Alginates containing disinfectants reduce the viable organisms by up to 90%; however, additional disinfection by solutions or sprays should be carried out.

PROPORTIONING AND MIXING

The proportioning of the powder and water before mixing is critical to obtaining consistent results. Changes in the water/powder ratio will alter the consistency and setting times of the mixed material and also the strength and quality of the impression. Usually the manufacturers provide suitable containers for proportioning the powder and water by volume, and these are sufficiently accurate for clinical use.

The mixing time for regular alginate is 1 minute; the time should be carefully measured, because both undermixing and overmixing are detrimental to the strength of the set impression. Fast-set alginates should be mixed with water for 45 seconds. The powder and water are best mixed in a rubber bowl with an alginate spatula or a spatula of the type used for mixing plaster and stone.

Automatic mixing systems have been developed for paste/paste alginates. These systems consist of a mixing unit that mixes an aqueous base paste and an organic initiator paste in a 4:1 ratio. The base paste is believed to contain sodium alginate and polyacrylic acid as a viscosity modifier, the initiator paste contains calcium sulphate-hemihydrate and sodium phosphate. The mixer uses a dynamic mixing principal and is available in Japan.

PROPERTIES

Some typical properties of a tray-type alginate impression material are listed in Table 12-2, along with comparable values for agar impression material, which are discussed in the next major section.

Working Time The fast-set materials have working times of 1.25 to 2 minutes, whereas time of the regular-set materials is usually 3 minutes, but may be as long as 4.5 minutes. With a mixing time of 45 seconds for the fast-set types, 30 to 75 seconds of working time remain before the impression needs to be completely seated. For the regular-set materials, a mixing time of 60 seconds leaves 2 to 3.5 minutes of working time for materials that set at 3.5 to 5 minutes. In both cases, the mixed alginate must be loaded into the tray and the impression made promptly.

TABLE 12-2 Typical Properties of Alginate and Agar Hydrocolloid Tray Type of Impression Materials

	Working Time (min)	Setting Time (min)	Gelation (° C)	Recovery from Deformation* (%)	Flexibility† (%)	Compressive Strength‡ (g/cm^2)	Tear Strength§ (g/cm)
Alginate	1.25-4.5	1.5-5.0	—	98.2	8-15	5000-9000	380-700
Agar	—	—	37-45	99.0	4-15	8000	800-900

*At 10% compression for 30 sec.
†At a stress of 1000 g/cm^2.
‡At a loading rate of 10 kg/min.
§ASTM Tear Die C at 25 cm/min.

Setting Time Setting times range from 1 to 5 minutes. The ANSI/ADA Specification No. 18 (ISO 1563) requires that it be at least that value listed by the manufacturer and at least 15 seconds longer than the stated working time. Lengthening the setting time is better accomplished by reducing the temperature of the water used with the mix than by reducing the proportion of powder. Reducing the ratio of powder to water reduces the strength and accuracy of the alginate. Selecting an alginate with a different setting time should also be considered rather than changing the water/powder ratio.

The setting reaction is a typical chemical reaction, and the rate can be approximately doubled by a temperature increase of 10° C. However, using water that is cooler than 18° C or warmer than 24° C is not advisable. The clinical setting time is detected by a loss of surface tackiness. If possible, the impression should be left in place 2 to 3 minutes after the loss of tackiness, because the tear strength and resistance to permanent deformation increase significantly during this period.

Color-changing alginates provide a visual indication of working time and setting time. The mechanism of the color change is a pH-related change of a dye. One such alginate changes its color from light pink to white.

Permanent Deformation A typical alginate impression is compressed about 10% in areas of undercuts during removal. The actual magnitude depends on the extent of the undercuts and the space between the tray and the teeth. The ANSI/ADA Specification requires that the recovery from deformation be more than 95% (or a permanent deformation of less than 5%) when the material is compressed 20% for 5 seconds at the time it would normally be removed from the mouth. As indicated in Table 12-2, a typical value for recovery from deformation is 98.2%. The corresponding permanent deformation is 1.8%.

The permanent deformation, indicated as percent compression set, is a function of percent compression, time under compression, and time after removal of the compressive load, as illustrated in Fig. 12-4. Note that permanent deformation is a time-dependent property. Lower permanent deformation (higher accuracy) occurs (1) when the percent compression is lower, (2) when the impression is under compression a shorter time, and (3) when the recovery time is longer, up to about 8 minutes after the release of the load. Clinically these factors translate into requirements for a reasonable bulk of alginate between the tray and the teeth and a rapid or snap removal of the impression. The usual procedures followed to produce a gypsum model provide adequate time for any recovery that might occur.

Flexibility The ANSI/ADA Specification permits a range of 5% to 20% at a stress of 1000 g/cm^2, and most alginates have a typical value of 14%. However, some of the hard-set

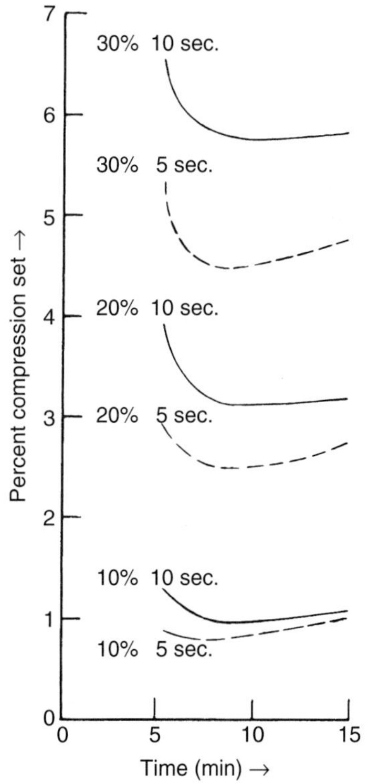

Fig. 12-4 Variation of compression set with time of an alginate impression material at strains of 10%, 20%, and 30% applied for 5 and 10 seconds.
(Adapted from Wilson HJ: *Br Dent J* 121:466, 1966.)

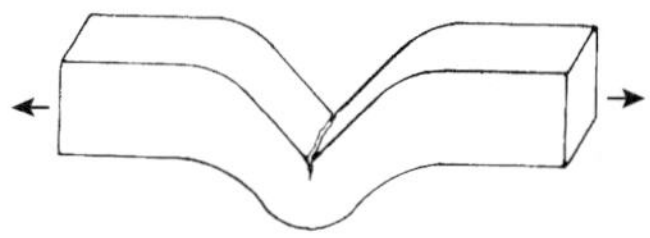

Fig. 12-5 Sketch of tear strength specimen with load applied in the directions of the arrows; the specimen tears at the V-notch.

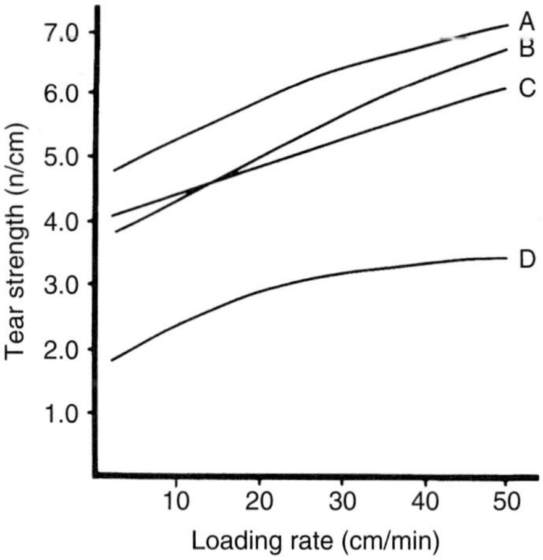

Fig. 12-6 Tear strength of alginate impression materials as a function of rate of loading; materials *A, B,* and *C* are designed to be used in a tray; *D* is a syringe material.

(Adapted from MacPherson GW, Craig RG, Peyton FA: *J Dent Res* 46:717, 1967.)

materials have values from 5% to 8%. A reasonable amount of flexibility is required for ease of removal of the impression.

Strength The compressive and tear strengths of alginates are listed in Table 12-2. Both properties are time dependent, with higher values obtained at higher rates of loading. Compressive strengths range from 5000 to 9000 g/cm^2. The ANSI/ADA Specification requires that certified products have a compressive strength of at least 3570 g/cm^2. Tear strengths vary from 380 to 700 g/cm, and this property is probably more important than the compressive strength. The tear strength is a measure of the force/thickness ratio needed to initiate and continue tearing and is often determined on a specimen of the shape shown in Fig. 12-5. Tearing occurs in the thin sections of the impression, and the probability of tearing decreases with increasing rates of removal. The effect of loading rate on the tear strength of several alginates is shown in Fig. 12-6. Values for tray materials range from 3.8 to 4.8 N/cm at 2 cm/min to 6 to 7 N/cm at 50 cm/min. The lower tear strength at corresponding rates for the syringe materials reflects the decreased alginate in the syringe material.

Compatibility with Gypsum The selection of an alginate-gypsum combination that produces good surface quality and detail is highly important. The surface quality and ability of alginate-gypsum combinations to reproduce fine V-shaped grooves are shown in Fig. 12-7, *A* and *B*. A Type III model plaster was poured against an alginate in Fig. 12-7, *A,* and Type IV dental stone was poured against the same alginate in Fig. 12-7, *B*. The finest groove was 0.025 mm wide in each instance. The combination in Fig. 12-7, *B,* was not as compatible as the one in Fig. 12-7, *A,* with respect to either surface quality or detail. For purposes of comparison, in Fig. 12-7, *C,* the same Type IV dental stone used in Fig. 12-7, *B,* was poured against polysulfide impression.

The impression must be rinsed well in cold water to remove saliva and any blood, and then disinfected. Next, all free surface water should be removed before preparing a gypsum model. Saliva and blood interfere with the setting of gypsum, and if free water accumulates, it tends to collect in the deeper parts of the impression and dilute the model material, yielding a soft, chalky surface. The excess surface water has been removed when the reflective surface becomes dull. If the alginate impression is stored for 30 minutes or more before preparing the model, it should be rinsed with cool water to remove any exudate on the surface caused by syneresis of the alginate gel; exudate will retard the setting of the gypsum. Thereafter it should be wrapped loosely in a

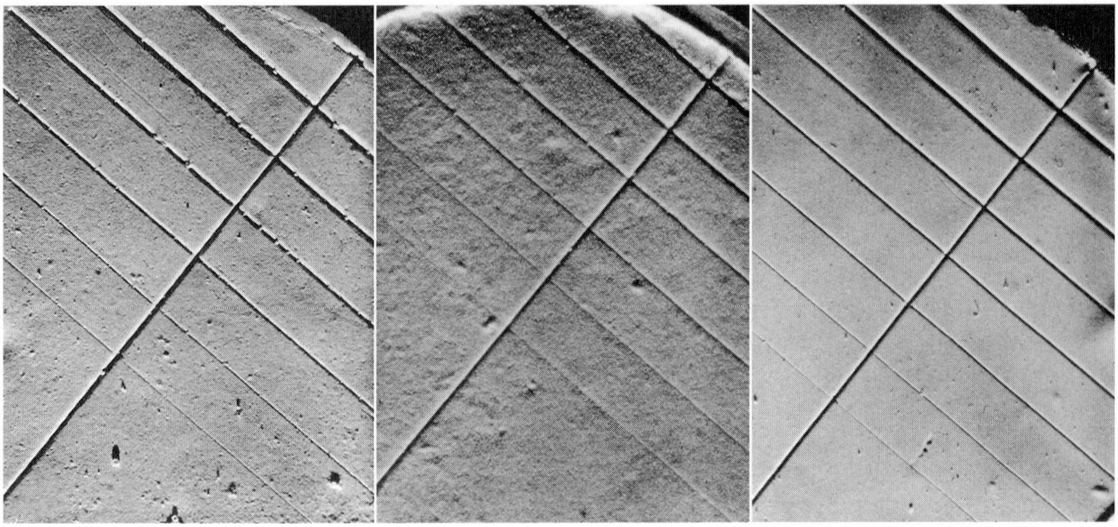

A B C

Fig. 12-7 Surface quality and reproduction of, **A,** model plaster poured against alginate; **B,** dental stone poured against the same alginate; and **C,** the same dental stone poured against polysulfide. It should be emphasized that another alginate with the same plaster and stone could yield opposite results.

(From Craig RG, MacPherson GW: Ann Arbor, 1965, University of Michigan School of Dentistry.)

moist paper towel and sealed in a plastic bag to avoid moisture loss.

The set gypsum model should not remain in contact with the alginate impression for periods of several hours because contact of the slightly soluble calcium sulfate dihydrate with the alginate gel containing a great deal of water is detrimental to the surface quality of the model.

Dimensional Stability Alginate impressions lose water by evaporation and shrink on standing in air. Impressions left on the bench for as short a time as 30 minutes may become inaccurate enough to require remaking the impression. Even if the impression stored for more than 30 minutes in air is immersed in water, it is not feasible to determine when the correct amount of water has been absorbed, and in any case the previous dimensions would not be reproduced. For maximum accuracy, the model material should be poured into the alginate impression as soon as possible. If for some reason the models cannot be prepared directly, the impressions should be stored in 100% relative humidity in a plastic bag or wrapped in a damp (but not wringing-wet) paper towel.

Storage of alginate impressions in 100% relative humidity is satisfactory for some materials for periods up to 2 hours, as indicated in Fig. 12-8 for material *A*. Materials *C* and *D* should not be stored in 100% relative humidity, even for short periods. However, some cases requiring less accuracy, such as study of orthodontic models, properly stored alginate impressions are sent to a laboratory where the model is prepared.

Disinfection Disinfection of impressions is a concern with respect to viral diseases such as hepatitis B, acquired immunodeficiency syndrome, and herpes simplex, because the viruses may be transferred to gypsum models and presents a risk to dental laboratory and operating personnel.

All alginate colloid impressions should be disinfected before pouring with gypsum to form a cast. The most common form of disinfection is by

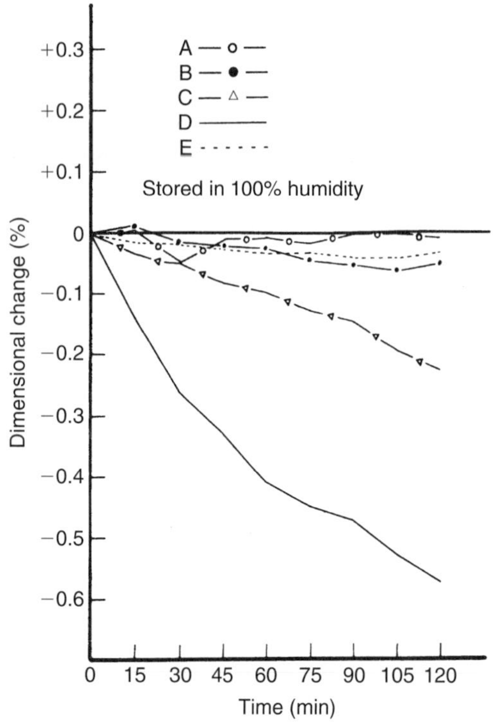

Fig. 12-8 Dimensional change of alginate impression materials stored in 100% relative humidity.
(From Craig RG, MacPherson GW: Ann Arbor, 1965, University of Michigan School of Dentistry.)

spray, but studies have shown that such impressions can be immersed in disinfectant also. The effect of disinfection in 1% sodium hypochlorite or 2% potentiated glutaraldehyde solutions on accuracy and surface quality has been measured after 10- to 30-minute immersion. Statistically significant dimensional changes were observed; however, the changes were in the order of 0.1% and the quality of the surface was not impaired. Such changes would be insignificant for clinical applications such as the preparation of study models and working casts. In another study, immersion disinfection of alginates demonstrated little effect on accuracy and surface quality, but it was shown that one alginate product was best immersed in iodophor and another brand in glyoxal glutalaldehyde. The effect of disinfection on agar impression materials has not been reported, but, considering the similarity of the two hydrocolloids, similar recommendations are reasonable.

AGAR HYDROCOLLOIDS

Agar hydrocolloid impression materials are compounded from reversible agar gels. When heated, they liquefy or go into the sol state, and on cooling they return to the gel state. Because this process can be repeated, a gel of this type is described as *reversible,* in contrast to the irreversible alginate gels.

The preparation of agar hydrocolloid for clinical use requires careful control and moderately expensive apparatus. Many dentists prefer a metal die for inlay and crown laboratory procedures, and no practical method has been developed to make a metal die from an agar hydrocolloid or alginate impression. Agar hydrocolloid impressions are dimensionally unstable on standing; thus models should be made as soon as possible after the impression is taken. The registration of the cervical areas of prepared teeth has presented difficulties when they are below the soft tissues of the gingiva. However, modern techniques of tissue control have largely eliminated this problem. Complaints sometimes arise from patients as a result of thermal shock to the teeth, producing pain and discomfort. This situation can arise from the heat from the impression material when introduced into the mouth or the comparatively low temperatures attained during cooling of the impression to obtain a set gel.

Provided the agar hydrocolloid type of impression material is used carefully with an understanding of its physical properties, it is an excellent, highly accurate elastic impression material and registers fine detail.

CHEMICAL INGREDIENTS

The main active constituent of a reversible hydrocolloid impression product is agar, often known commercially as agar-agar, which is a sulfuric ester of a galactan complex, having a complex structural formula, as shown on p. 341.

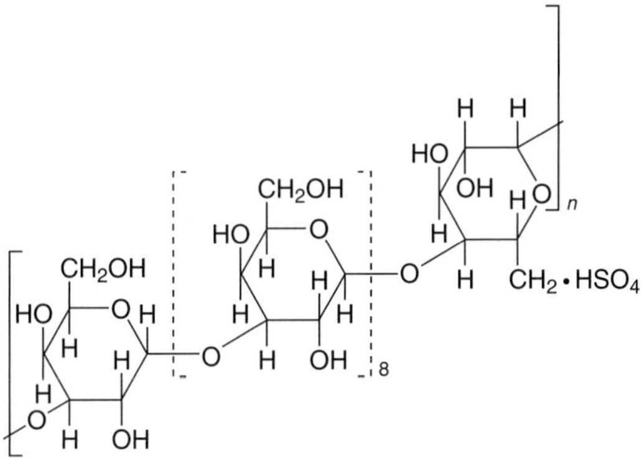

Agar
n = about 90, or for dental grade agar a molecular weight of about 150,000

TABLE 12-3 Typical Composition of Agar Impression Material and the Function of the Components

Ingredient	Weight (%)	Function
Agar	12.5	To provide the dispersed phase of the sol and the continuous fibril structure of the gel
Potassium sulfate	1.7	To counteract the inhibiting effect of borax and agar on the setting of gypsum model material
Borax	0.2	To produce intermolecular attraction in order to improve the strength of the gel
Alkyl benzoate	0.1	To prevent the growth of mold in the impression material during storage
Water	85.5	To provide the continuous phase in the sol and the second continuous phase in the gel; the amount controls the flow properties of the sol and the physical properties of the gel
Color and flavors	Trace	To improve the appearance and taste

Adapted from Preble B: US Patent No. 2,234,383, March 11, 1941.

This material forms a colloid with water, which liquefies between 71° and 100° C and sets to a gel again between 30° and 50° C, varying with the concentration of the agar.

A typical composition and the functions of the various ingredients are listed in Table 12-3. The material described is a tray type and is considerably stiffer at the time of making the impression than a syringe type. The agar content is reduced in the syringe type of material, so it is much more fluid at the time of injection than is the tray material at the time of insertion.

CLINICAL MANIPULATION OF THE SOL-GEL

Clinically, the tray type agar can be liquefied conveniently by immersion in boiling water, usually 8 to 12 minutes, depending on the bulk of material. If the material is to be used immediately after boiling, the tube is immersed in water at 43° to 49° C and manipulated to ensure even cooling. The tube is then opened and a tray filled. The filled tray is finally tempered for a minimum of 2 minutes in water at 46° C ± 1°. Before the tray is placed in the mouth, a thin layer of material that has been in direct contact with the water in the bath is removed with a suitable instrument.

When the material is liquefied, it can be stored for several hours and kept ready for use by immersing the container in water at 63° to 66° C. When needed, the material is taken from the storage bath and placed immediately in a warmed tray. The filled tray is then tempered at 46° C ± 1° for a minimum of 2 minutes before it is inserted into the mouth. Tempering is necessary to cool the material to a temperature that is compatible with the oral tissues, and this also serves to develop a heavier consistency.

A slightly more fluid agar hydrocolloid material is made for use in injection syringes for inlay, crown, and bridge impressions. The increased fluidity is achieved by decreasing the agar content and increasing the water content. Usually this material is supplied in small cylinders of the correct size to fit the syringe. The syringe, loaded with a cylinder, is placed in boiling water for 10 minutes and then stored at 63° C until needed. No tempering is required before use; the syringe is taken from the storage bath and the agar hydrocolloid injected directly into the tooth preparation. The thin strand of material passing down the needle rapidly cools to a temperature compatible with the oral tissues. These procedures may vary from one product to another; manufacturers' directions should be followed carefully.

After the impression is placed in the mouth, the agar is cooled to obtain a set condition. Cool tap water is circulated around tubes built into agar impression trays to hasten setting. After removal the impression is rinsed, disinfected, superficially dried, and poured in dental stone. After the initial setting of the stone, the gypsum model and impression should be stored in a humidor to prevent drying and shrinkage of the impression before the model is removed.

PROPERTIES

Typical properties of the tray type of agar hydrocolloid impression materials are listed in Table 12-2.

Gelation Temperature After boiling for 8 minutes, the material should be fluid enough to be extruded from the container. After tempering, the sol should be homogeneous and should set to a gel between 37° and 45° C when cooled, as required by ANSI/ADA Specification No. 11 (ISO 1564) for dental agar hydrocolloid impression material.

Permanent Deformation Permanent deformation is determined in the same manner as for alginates and at the time the material is removed from the mouth. The ANSI/ADA Specification requires that the recovery from deformation be greater than 96.5% (permanent deformation be less than 3.5%) after the material is compressed 20% for 1 second. Most tray types of agar hydrocolloid impression materials readily meet this requirement with recovery values of about 99%. However, a reasonable thickness of impression material should be present between the tray and the undercut areas so compressions higher than 10% do not occur, because higher compression results in higher permanent deformation. As for alginates, the magnitude of the permanent deformation depends on the time under compression, and impressions should be removed rapidly.

Flexibility The ANSI/ADA Specification requirement for flexibility allows a range of 4% to 15%; most agar hydrocolloid impression materials meet this requirement. Materials with low flexibility can be accommodated in areas of undercuts by providing somewhat more space for the impression material so it is subjected to a lower percentage of compression during removal.

Strength The compressive strength of a typical agar hydrocolloid impression material is 8000 g/cm^2. The tear strength of agar hydrocolloid impression materials is about 800 to 900 g/cm, which is higher than the ANSI/ADA Specification requirement of 765 g/cm. Because agar hydrocolloid impressions are viscoelastic, the strength properties are time dependent, and higher compressive and tear strengths occur at higher rates of loading. These properties again emphasize the importance of removing the impressions with a snap, because such a procedure minimizes the chances of rupture or tearing of the impression.

Compatibility with Gypsum Not all agar hydrocolloid impression materials are equally compatible with all gypsum products, and the manufacturer's suggestions should be followed. The ANSI/ADA specification requires manufacturers to list compatible model materials. Agar hydrocolloid impression materials are more compatible with gypsum model materials than alginates. The impression should be washed of saliva and any trace of blood, which retard the setting of gypsum. After the impression is rinsed with water and disinfected, the excess liquid should be carefully blown from the impression with an air syringe to avoid dehydrating the surface of the agar hydrocolloid impression.

If the agar hydrocolloid impression must be stored in a humidor, it should be rinsed with cool water to remove any exudate formed from syneresis before pouring up the gypsum model.

Dimensional Stability When stored in air, agar hydrocolloid gels lose water and contract. The extent of contraction varies from product to product, as shown in Fig. 12-9. After 1 hour in air, one product shrank only 0.15%, whereas another shrank about 1%. Replacing the agar in water resulted in absorption and swelling. After an hour the materials had almost retained their original dimensions, although one was

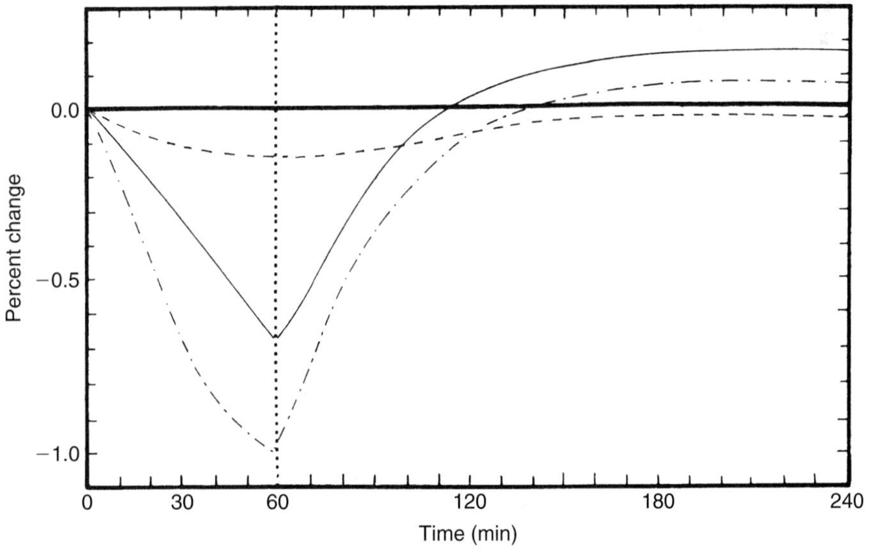

Fig. 12-9 Curves showing shrinkage of three agar hydrocolloids exposed to air over a period of 1 hour, and subsequent expansion when immersed in water.
(Adapted from Skinner EW, Cooper EN, Beck FE: *J Am Dent Assoc* 40:196, 1950.)

0.05% larger, and two were 0.1% smaller. Continued storage in water resulted in continued swelling.

As with alginate impressions, agar hydrocolloid impressions are best stored in 100% relative humidity if the gypsum models cannot be prepared immediately. Even in 100% humidity they can be stored for only limited times, such as 1 hour, without shrinkage of the impression material caused by *syneresis*. The best procedure is to pour up the impression immediately after removing, rinsing, disinfecting, and superficial drying.

The suggestions for disinfection of alginates should also be followed with agar hydrocolloid impressions.

AGAR-ALGINATE COMBINATION IMPRESSIONS

The equipment needed for taking an agar hydrocolloid impression can be minimized with an agar-alginate, syringe-tray combination impression. In this procedure, a syringe type of agar hydrocolloid in a cartridge is heated in boiling water for 6 minutes and stored in a 65° C water bath 10 minutes before use. Several products and a simple heater are shown in Fig. 12-10. The tray alginate of the regular set type is mixed and placed in a tray. The agar hydrocolloid is injected around the preparation, and the mixed alginate is promptly seated on top of the agar hydrocolloid. The alginate sets in about 3 minutes, and the agar gels within this time as a result of being cooled by

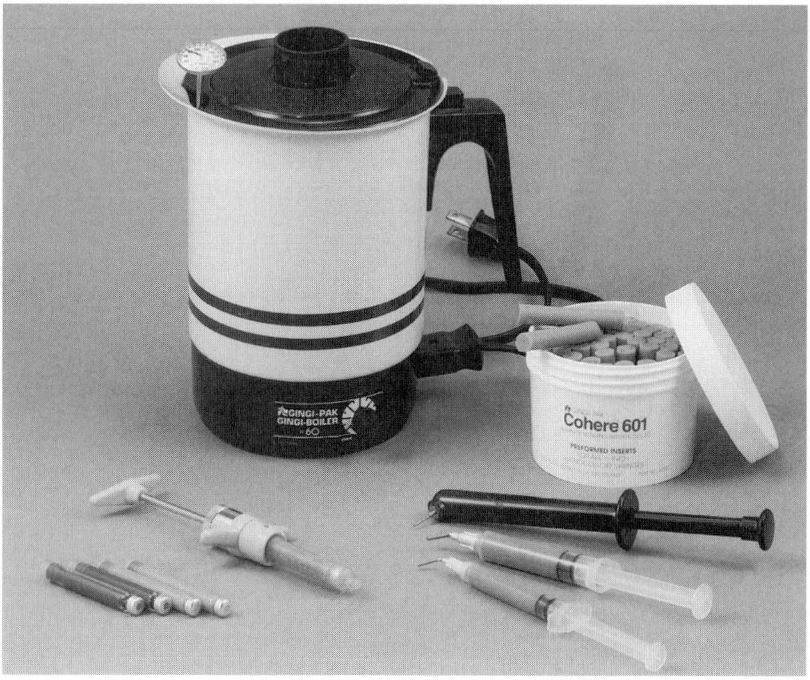

Fig. 12-10 Agar hydrocolloid supplied in glass cartridges, and sticks for use in reusable syringes and plastic disposable syringes, plus a simple heater for liquefying and storing agar for the agar-alginate combination technique.

(From Craig RG, Powers JM, Wataha JC: *Dental materials: properties and manipulation,* ed 7, St Louis, 2000, Mosby.)

the alginate. During the setting of the alginate and gelling of the agar hydrocolloid, a bond forms between them. The impression may be removed in about 4 minutes. Cross-sections of impressions of a laboratory model are shown in Fig. 12-11. The surface of the impression is in agar hydrocolloid backed by the alginate. The same precautions used in preparing stone models in alginate or agar hydrocolloid impressions should be observed.

For effective bonding between agar and alginate, the materials must be placed when both are in a flowable state; some combinations of agar hydrocolloid and alginate bond together better than others, with tensile bond strengths ranging from 600 to 1100 g/cm^2. Values at the high end of the range result in cohesive failure of the agar hydrocolloid, whereas those at the low end produce adhesive failure between the agar hydrocolloid and alginate. Therefore following the manufacturer's suggestions for appropriate combinations is important.

The accuracy of the agar-alginate impressions was determined with a laboratory model shown in Fig. 12-12. Impressions were taken, and models poured in high-strength stone. The accuracy of (1) the interpreparation distance, (2) buccolingual diameter, and (3) preparation height of the models was measured and compared with values obtained with polysulfide, condensation-silicone, polyether, and addition-silicone impression materials. These values are listed in Table 12-4. Except for the interpreparation distance, the agar-alginate system had the same

TABLE 12-4 Percent Deviations of Models Prepared with Various Impression Materials and the Master Die

	Impression Type				
Location	**Agar-Alginate**	**Polysulfide**	**Condensation Silicone**	**Polyether**	**Addition Silicone**
Interpreparation	+0.20	+0.05	−0.03	−0.02	0.00
Buccolingual diameter	+0.32	+0.04	+0.03	−0.14	+0.22
Height	−0.22	−0.23	−0.25	−0.17	−0.03

Adapted from Johnson GH, Craig RG: *J Prosthet Dent* 55:1, 1986.

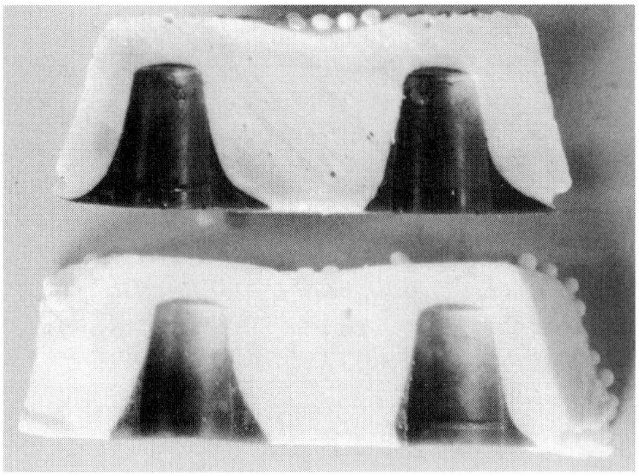

Fig. 12-11 Cross-section of agar-alginate combination impressions showing thickness of the agar in various positions.

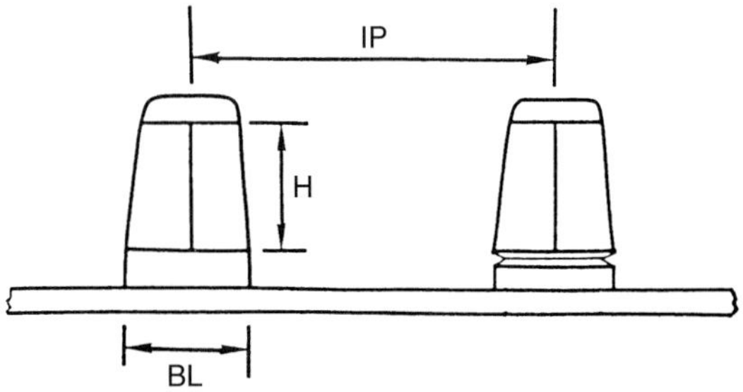

Fig. 12-12 Sketch of the model used to determine the accuracy of impressions. *IP,* Interpreparation; *H,* height; *BL,* buccal-lingual.

order of accuracy as the elastomeric impression materials.

In summary, the advantages of the agar-alginate combination impression compared with the agar hydrocolloid system alone are the simplification of heating equipment, the elimination of water-cooled impression trays, and the overall simplification of the procedure. In addition, the agar hydrocolloid is more compatible with gypsum model materials than alginates, making them useful for crown and bridge impressions; the accuracy is acceptable, and the cost of materials is low.

DUPLICATING IMPRESSION MATERIALS

In preparing partial dentures, a duplicate should be made of the plaster or stone cast of the patient's mouth. This duplicate is required for two reasons: (1) the cast on which the wax pattern of the metal framework is to be formed must be made from a refractory investment, because it must withstand the casting temperatures required for gold or base metal alloys; and (2) the original cast is needed for checking the accuracy of the metal framework and for processing the plastic portion of the partial denture.

A duplicate refractory cast is obtained by making an impression of the original cast in an elastic duplicating material. The most common duplicating materials are agar hydrocolloid compounds. Their composition is quite similar to the agar hydrocolloid impression compounds, but a greater proportion of water is used with the duplicating compounds. For example, an impression compound may be diluted with as much as one to three times its weight of water and used as a duplicating compound.

Agar hydrocolloid duplicating materials have many advantages. They are reversible, and the material may be reused a number of times. This is particularly important in duplication procedures, because 200 to 400 ml of the material may be needed for each duplication. The agar hydrocolloid duplicating materials may be continuously stored in the sol state at 54° to 66° C and used when needed without converting the material from the gel to the sol state each time it is required. After a duplication procedure, the gel is chopped up, reheated until in the sol condition, and added to the material being stored at 54° to 66° C. This procedure may be repeated about 20 times before the material is discarded. Of prime importance is that the agar hydrocolloid duplicating materials have adequate strength and elastic properties to duplicate undercut areas. The accuracy of the agar hydrocolloid duplication compounds is also quite satisfactory if proper techniques are followed.

The disadvantages of agar hydrocolloid duplicating materials are similar to those of agar hydrocolloid impression compounds. The set material is a gel and therefore is subject to dimensional changes if stored in air or water. Generally, the best storage condition is 100% relative humidity. The best procedure is to pour the duplicate refractory cast as soon as possible. The agar is a polysaccharide and gradually hydrolyzes at storage temperatures. Accompanying this hydrolysis is a loss of elasticity and strength, which eventually renders the agar hydrocolloid duplicating material useless. While in use, the duplicating material is contaminated by components of the stone, investment, hardening solutions, separators, and others. Indications are that some of these components accelerate the degradation of agar hydrocolloid.

Other types of materials, such as alginate hydrocolloids, reversible plastic gels, silicones, and polyethers, have been used as duplicating materials. Obviously, the major objection to the alginate type is that the material is irreversible. However, its use does not require heating and storage equipment, as do the reversible agar hydrocolloid and plastic duplicating compounds. The reversible plastic gel is a polyvinylchloride gel that is quite fluid at 99° to 104° C. The main advantages of this material are its high-strength properties and high chemical stability, which permit a large number of duplications before replacement. Silicones and polyethers that set at room temperatures are examples of the nonreversible non-aqueous type. The principal problem with them has been their cost, and numerous techniques have been developed to use minimum amounts in a duplicating procedure. At present, agar hydrocolloid duplicating materials are the most common type used in dental laboratories.

Properties ANSI/ADA Specification No. 20 for dental duplicating materials includes two types: thermoreversible and nonreversible. Within these two types are the hydrocolloid and non-aqueous classes.

The specification requires these materials to be free from foreign agents and impurities and to be suitable for taking impressions of plaster, stone, or investment casts of the oral tissues.

Pouring temperature and the temperature of gel formation are defined for the thermoreversible products. Working and setting times are specified for the nonreversible materials. Compatibility with at least one type of investment and the ability to reproduce detail satisfactorily are required. The duplicating material may be compatible with a silicate- or phosphate-bonded investment but not with a gypsum-bonded investment. Fig. 12-13 shows the surface reproduction and detail when a single agar hydrocolloid duplicating material was poured up in *A,* a silicate-bonded investment; *B,* a phosphate-bonded investment; and *C,* a gypsum-bonded investment. High-quality surfaces were obtained with silicate- and phosphate-bonded investments, but a poor-quality surface was found with gypsum-bonded investment. This incompatibility is often caused by the addition of glycerin or glycols to the duplicating material to reduce the loss of water from the gel; these compounds interfere with the setting of the gypsum matrix.

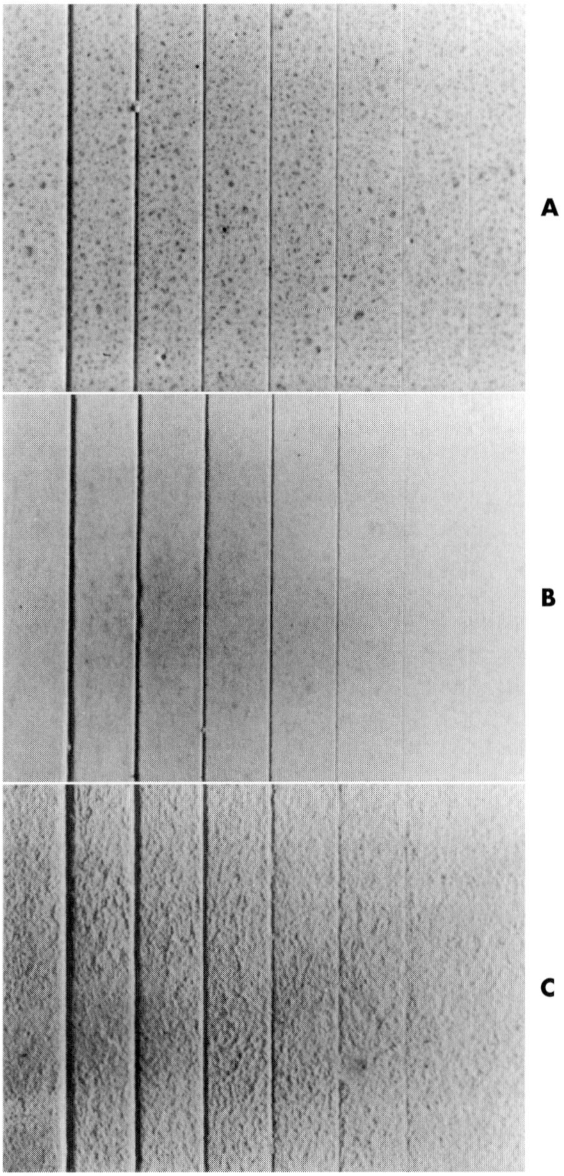

Fig. 12-13 Surface quality of, **A,** silicate-bonded, **B,** phosphate-bonded, and **C,** gypsum-bonded investments formed against the same agar duplicating material.

(From Craig RG, Dootz ER: Ann Arbor, 1965, University of Michigan School of Dentistry.)

Type I products are required to show no mold growth after inoculation under controlled conditions. Requirements for permanent deformation (or recovery from deformation), strain in compression, and resistance to tearing are described for each type and class; and the acceptable values and ranges are listed in Table 12-5. Aging tests are described, and permissible changes

TABLE 12-5 Specification Requirements of Some Properties of Dental Duplicating Materials

	Maximum Permanent Deformation (%)	Strain in Compression	Minimum Compressive Strength (g/cm^2)		Minimum Resistance to Tear (g/cm)	
			Original	Aged	Original	Aged
TYPE I (THERMOREVERSIBLE)						
Class I (hydrocolloidal)	3*	4-25	2200	2000	—	—
Class II (nonaqueous organic)	3*	4-25	—	—	900	700
TYPE II (NONREVERSIBLE)						
Class I (hydrocolloidal)	3*	4-25	2800	2600	—	—
Class II (nonaqueous organic)	3*	4-25	—	—	900	700

*Minimum elastic recovery of 97%.

in physical properties defined. Packaging must include instructions that indicate the type of investment that can be used with the material and, for Type I products, must also include (1) method of liquefying, (2) tempering or storing temperature, and (3) pouring temperature.

ELASTOMERIC IMPRESSION MATERIALS

Four types of synthetic elastomeric impression materials are available to record dental impressions: polysulfides, condensation silicones, addition silicones (polyvinylsiloxanes), and polyethers. Although polysulfides were the first synthetic elastomeric impression material introduced (1950), the latter three types form the vast majority of elastomeric impressions used worldwide today. Condensation silicones were made available to dentists in 1955, polyether in 1965, and addition silicones in 1975. Changes in recent years have provided greater choice of consistency and new mixing techniques.

CONSISTENCIES

Elastomeric impression materials are typically supplied in two to four consistencies (viscosities) to accommodate a range of impression techniques. Polysulfide impression materials are supplied in three consistencies: low (syringe or wash), medium (regular), and high (tray). Addition silicones are available in these three consistencies plus an extra-low and putty (very high) type, whereas condensation silicones are usually supplied in low and putty consistencies. The catalyst of the condensation silicone can be supplied as a putty or a liquid. The first polyether impression materials were medium consistency, but they are now available in low, medium, and high consistencies.

MIXING SYSTEMS

Three types of systems are available to mix the catalyst and base thoroughly before taking the impression: hand mixing, static automixing, and dynamic mechanical mixing. All three systems are illustrated Fig. 12-14 and are described below. Impression pastes are most commonly dispensed from collapsible tubes, as shown in Fig. 12-14, *A*. Equal lengths of catalyst and base are dispensed on a paper pad, as shown in Fig. 12-15, *A*. Initial mixing is accomplished with a circular motion, as shown in Fig. 12-15, *B*, and final mixing to produce a mix free from streaks is done with broad strokes of the spatula, as shown in Fig. 12-15, *C*. Mixing is readily accomplished within 45 seconds, although the low-consistency material is easier to mix than high-consistency mate-

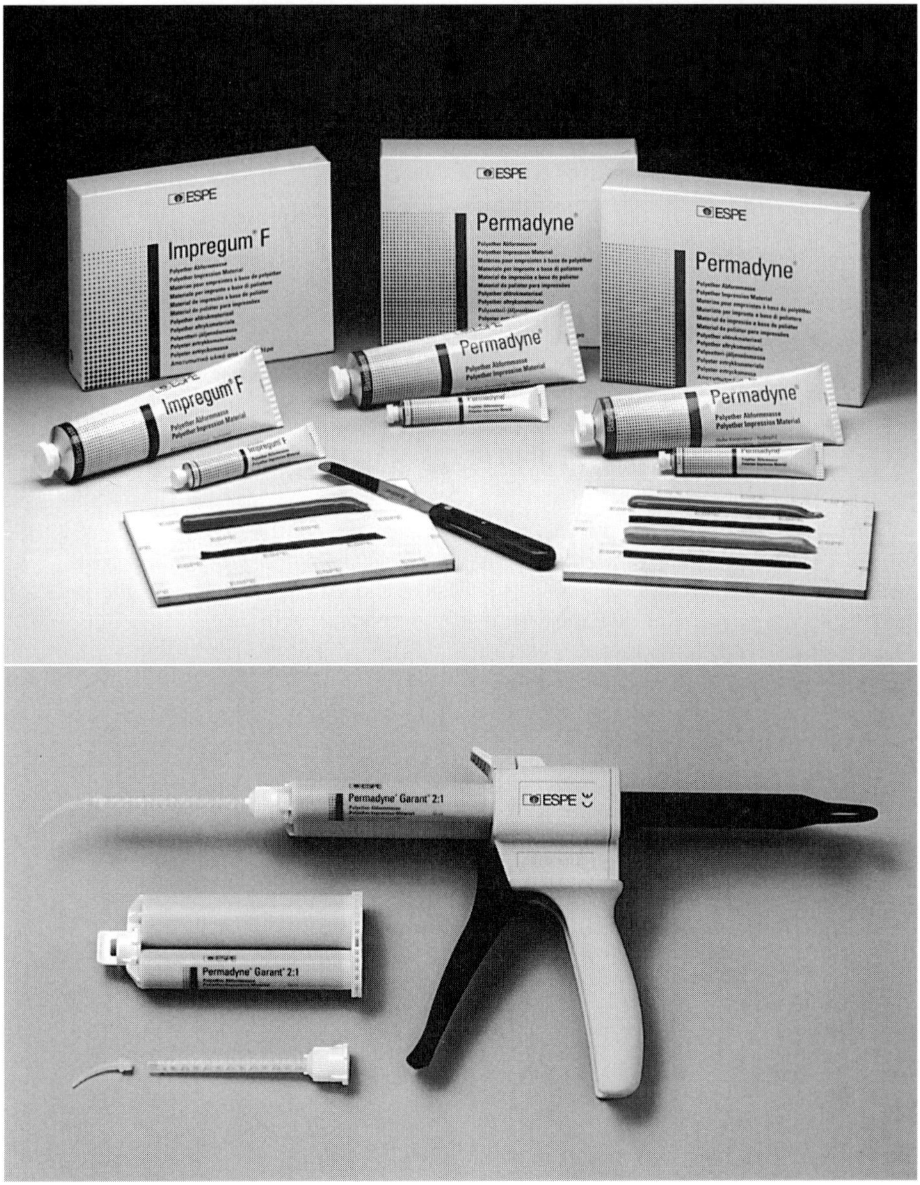

A

B

Fig. 12-14 Three different dispensing and mixing systems used for polyether impression materials. **A,** Tubes of two consistencies of polyether impression material. Each consistency contains a tube of catalyst and base paste, which are dispensed onto a mixing pad in equal lengths and mixed by hand. **B,** The assembled cartridge and static-mixing tip in the holder *(top).* A cartridge showing separate tubes of catalyst and base *(middle left).* The static-mixing tip and optional syringe tip for direct injection *(bottom left).*

Continued

C

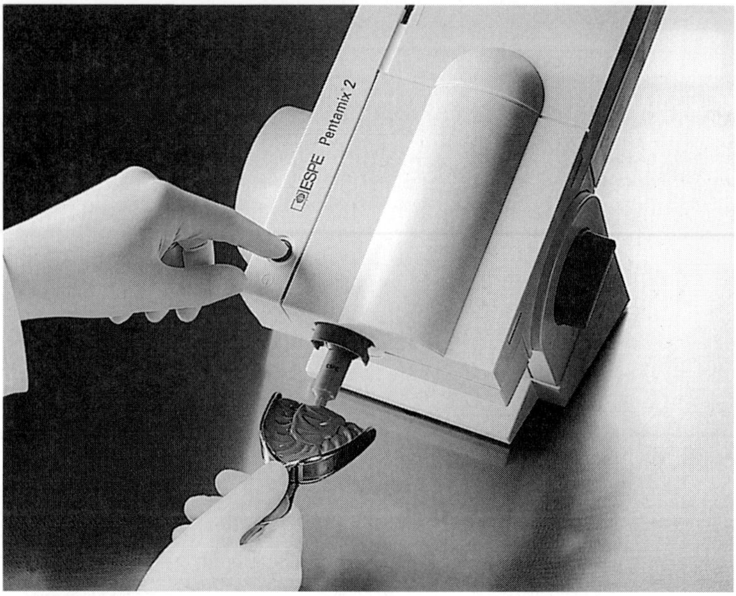

Fig. 12-14, cont'd C, Mechanical mixer with a dynamic-mixing tip. Once a new tip is placed, the machine is activated by the button shown and material is dispensed into the tray and syringe. The catalyst and base are in large foil bags within the mixer.

(Courtesy 3M ESPE, St. Paul, Minnesota)

A B C

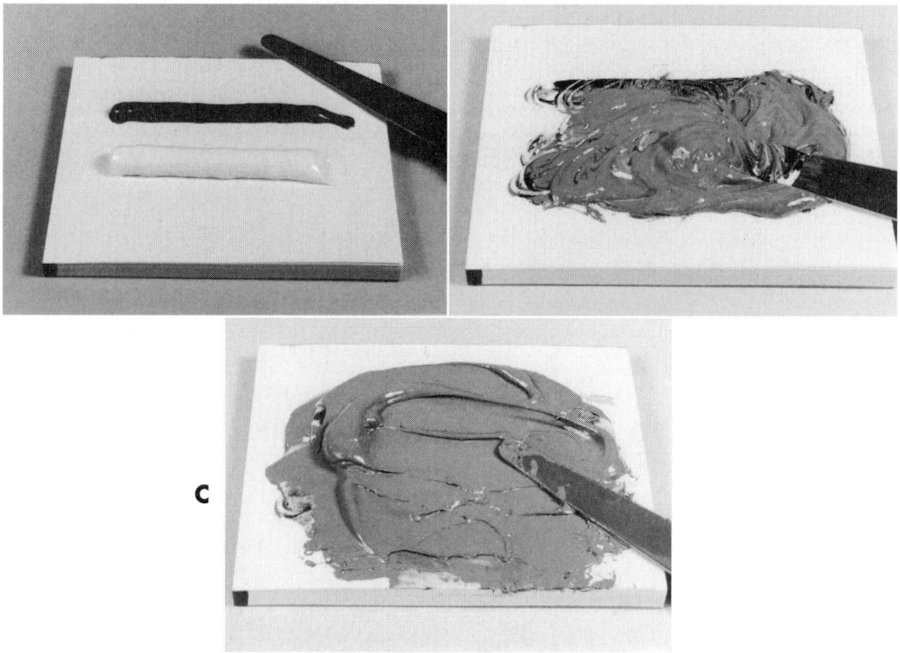

Fig. 12-15 Dispensing and mixing of a polysulfide impression material. **A,** Base and accelerator extruded onto a paper mixing pad. **B,** Initial mixing of base and accelerator. **C,** Final mixing of base and accelerator.

(From Craig RG, Powers JM, Wataha JC: *Dental materials: properties and manipulation,* ed 7, St Louis, 2000, Mosby.)

rials. When the catalyst is supplied as a liquid, a specified number of drops per unit of length is indicated in the instructions, and mixing is accomplished in a manner similar to that of the two-paste systems. All four types of impression materials are available for mixing in this fashion.

One variation in hand mixing is with the two-putty systems, offered both with condensation and addition silicones. Scoops are supplied by the manufacturer for dispensing, and the putties are most often kneaded with fingers until free from streaks. The putty materials that have a liquid catalyst are initially mixed with a spatula until the catalyst is reasonably incorporated, and mixing is completed by hand. It should be noted that latex gloves may interfere with setting of addition-silicone impression materials, as discussed later.

A very popular means of mixing the catalyst and base is with a so-called *automixing* system, as illustrated in Fig. 12-14, *B*. The base and catalyst are in separate cylinders of the plastic cartridge. The cartridge is placed in a mixing gun containing two plungers that are advanced by a ratchet mechanism to extrude equal quantities of base and catalyst. The base and catalyst are forced through the static-mixing tip containing a stationary plastic internal spiral; the two components are folded over each other many times as they are pushed through the spiral, generally resulting in a uniform mix at the tip end. Because one cylinder may be filled slightly more that the other, the first part of the mix from a new cartridge should be discarded.

The mixed material can be extruded directly into an injection syringe or into the impression tray. Intraoral delivery tips can be placed on the end of the static mixing tip, as shown in Fig. 12-14, *B,* and the mixed material can be injected into and around the cavity preparation. The tip can be removed, and additional mixed material can be extruded into the impression tray. The automixing systems have been shown to result in mixes with many fewer voids than hand mixes. Although for each mix the material left in the mixing tip is wasted, the average loss is only 1 to 2 ml, depending on the manufacturer's tip, whereas three to four times this much is wasted in a hand mix as a result of overestimating the amount needed. Initially, automixing was used for low consistencies, but new designs of guns and mixing tips allow all consistencies except putty to be used with this system. Addition silicones, condensation silicones, and polyethers are available with this means of mixing.

The third and newest system is a dynamic, mechanical mixer, illustrated in Fig. 12-14, *C*. The catalyst and base are supplied in large plastic bags housed in a cartridge, which is inserted into the top of the mixing machine. A new, plastic mixing tip is placed on the front of the machine, and when the button is depressed, as shown in the figure, parallel plungers push against the collapsible plastic bags, thereby opening the bags and forcing material into the dynamic mixing tip. This mixing tip differs from automixing in that the internal spiral is motor driven so it rotates. Thus mixing is accomplished by this rotation plus forward motion of the material through the spiral. In this manner, thorough mixing can be ensured and higher viscosity material can be mixed with ease. The advantage of this system is ease of use, speed, and thoroughness of mixing, but more must be invested in the purchase of the system compared with hand and automixing. In addition, there is slightly more material retained in the mixing tip than with automixing, but less than that wasted when mixed by hand. Polyether and addition-silicone impression materials are available for mixing with this system.

IMPRESSION TECHNIQUES

Three common methods for making crown and bridge impressions are a simultaneous, dual-viscosity technique, a single-viscosity or monophase technique, and a putty-wash technique. In nearly all cases, impression material is injected directly on and into the prepared teeth and a tray containing the bulk of the impression material is placed thereafter. After the impression is set, the tray is removed.

The simultaneous, dual-viscosity technique is one in which low-consistency material is injected with a syringe into critical areas and the high-consistency material is mixed and placed in an impression tray. After injecting the low-viscosity material, the tray containing the higher-viscosity material is placed in the mouth. In this manner, the more-viscous tray impression material forces the lower-viscosity material to flow into fine aspects of the areas of interest. Because they are both mixed at nearly the same time, the materials join, bond, and set together. After the materials have set, the tray and the impression are removed. An example of an impression for a bridge using this procedure is shown in Fig. 12-16.

In the single-viscosity or monophase technique, impressions are often taken with a medium-viscosity impression material. Addition-silicone and polyether impression materials are well suited for this technique because both have a capacity for shear thinning. As described in Chapter 4, pseudoplastic materials demonstrate a decreased viscosity when subjected to high shear rates such as occurs during mixing and syringing. When the medium viscosity material is forced through an impression syringe, the viscosity is reduced, whereas the viscosity of the same material residing in the tray is unaffected. In this manner, such materials can be used for syringing and for trays, as previously described for the simultaneous, dual-viscosity technique. The mechanism for shear thinning is discussed in the later section on the viscosity of impression materials.

The putty-wash technique is a two-step impression procedure whereby a preliminary impression is taken in high- or putty-consistency material before the cavity preparation is made. Space is provided for a low-consistency material by a variety of techniques, and after cavity preparation a low-consistency material is syringed into the area and the preliminary impression reinserted. The low- and high-consistency materials bond, and after the low-consistency material sets, the impression is removed. This procedure is sometimes called a *wash technique*. The putty-consistency material and this technique were developed for condensation silicones to minimize the effects of dimensional change during polymerization. Most of the shrinkage during polymerization takes place in the putty material when the preliminary impression is made, confining final shrinkage to the thin wash portion of the impression. Care must be taken so the wash material can freely escape via vents in the putty material when the wash impression is made. If not, the wash material can compress the putty in the second-stage impression, inducing permanent distortion and inaccuracies to the impression. The putty-wash technique was extended to addition silicones after their introduction, even though their polymerization shrinkage is significantly lower.

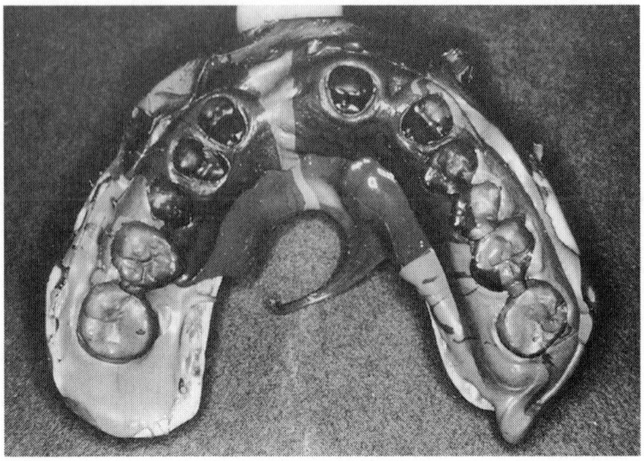

Fig. 12-16 A elastomeric impression of a maxillary anterior bridge case. Dark material is of a low or injection consistency, and light material of a high or tray consistency. Note that the palate is omitted from the tray to facilitate removal of the impression.

Manufacturers add coloring agents to the accelerator and/or base as an aid in determining the thoroughness of the mix. Normally a different color is used for each consistency of a particular product line so one can distinguish the wash (low) consistency from the tray consistency in the set impression. Retarders may be added as well to control working and setting time of the products.

COMPOSITION AND REACTIONS

The next four sections describe the general composition and setting reactions of polysulfide, condensation silicone, addition silicone, and polyether impression materials. The following section describes their physical properties, rather than presenting the information material by material.

TABLE 12-6 Ingredients of a Typical Polysulfide Rubber Impression Material

Ingredient	Weight (%)
BASE	
Polysulfide polymer	80-85
Titanium dioxide, zinc sulfate, copper carbonate, or silica	16-18
ACCELERATOR	
Lead dioxide	60-68
Dibutyl or dioctyl phthalate	30-35
Sulfur	3
Other substances such as magnesium stearate and deodorants	2

This approach permits a more direct comparison of the various types and their properties.

Polysulfide Polysulfide impression materials are supplied as two pastes in collapsible tubes, one labeled *base* and the other labeled *accelerator* or *catalyst.* A typical list of ingredients and their concentrations is given in Table 12-6. The polysulfide polymer has a molecular weight of 2000 to 4000 and terminal and pendant mercaptan groups (–SH). The terminal and pendant groups of adjacent molecules are oxidized by the accelerator to produce chain extension and cross-linking, respectively. This reaction can be represented diagrammatically as shown in the equation on p. 354. The reaction results in a rapid increase in molecular weight, and the mixed paste is converted to a polysulfide rubber. The reaction is only slightly exothermic, with a typical increase in temperature of 3° to 4° C. Although the mixes set to a rubber consistency in about 10 to 20 minutes, polymerization continues, and the properties change for a number of hours after the material sets. Cross-linking is used to reduce the permanent deformation (increase the elastic recovery) of the set material under compression or extension during removal from the mouth.

The ingredients and their weight percent may vary from one product to another. In general, the weight percent of the filler in the base paste increases from low to medium to high consistencies. The particle size of the fillers is about 0.3 μm. Although the most common active ingredient in the accelerator is lead dioxide, some magnesium oxide may also be present. Whitening agents cannot cover the dark color of the lead dioxide; thus these pastes range from dark brown to gray-brown. Other oxidizing agents such as hydrated copper oxide, $Cu(OH)_2$, have been used as a substitute for lead dioxide, producing a green mix.

Condensation Silicone Condensation silicones are supplied as a base and an accelerator. The base contains a linear silicone called a *polydimethylsiloxane,* which has reactive terminal hydroxyl groups. Fillers may be calcium carbonate or silica having particle sizes from 2 to 8 μm, and in concentrations from 35% for low consistencies to 75% for puttylike consistencies. The accelerator may be a liquid that consists of stannous octoate suspension and alkyl silicate, or it may be supplied as a paste by adding a thickening agent. The reaction proceeds as mentioned, producing a three-dimensional network with the liberation of ethyl alcohol and an exothermic temperature rise of about 1° C. The polymerization accompanied by the release of the byproduct causes a shrinkage that is greater in the low consistency than in the puttylike consistency. In the product shown in Fig. 12-17, the shrinkage has been reduced by having only two reactive groups on the cross-linking agent, thus only half the amount of byproduct is formed. The two-step putty-wash impression technique also reduces polymerization shrinkage. The accelerator does not have unlimited shelf life, because the stannous octoate may oxidize and the ortho-ethyl silicate is not entirely stable in the presence of the tin ester.

Addition Silicone The addition type is available in extra low, low, medium, heavy, and very heavy (putty) consistencies. A representative product line of addition silicones is shown in Fig. 12-18. The base paste of this class of impression materials contains a moderately low–

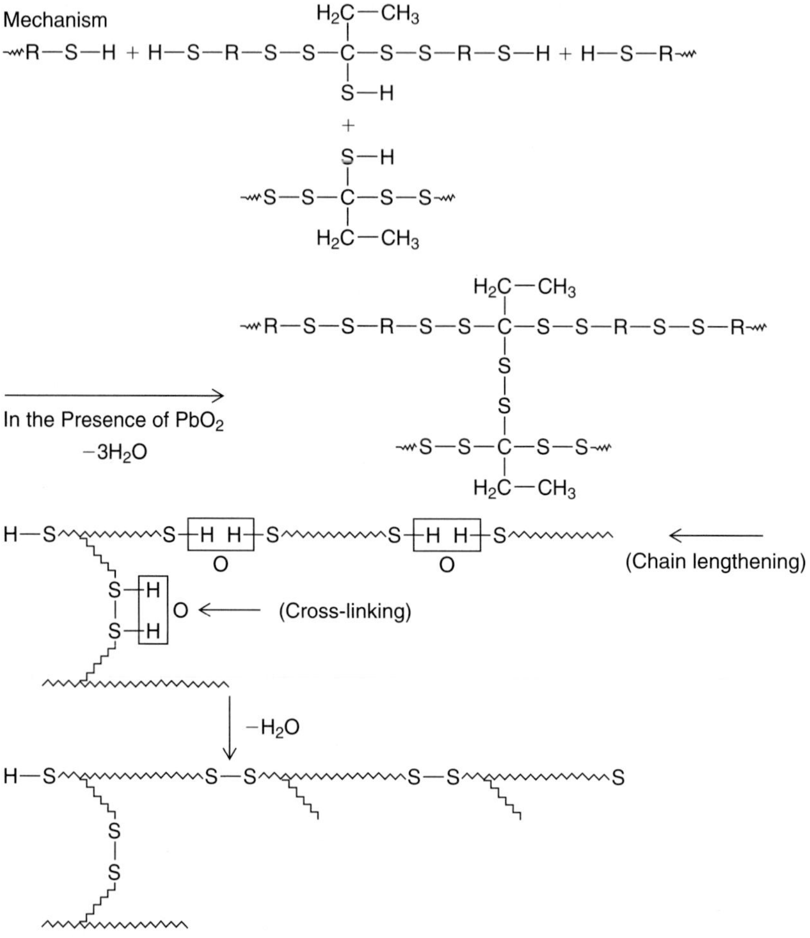

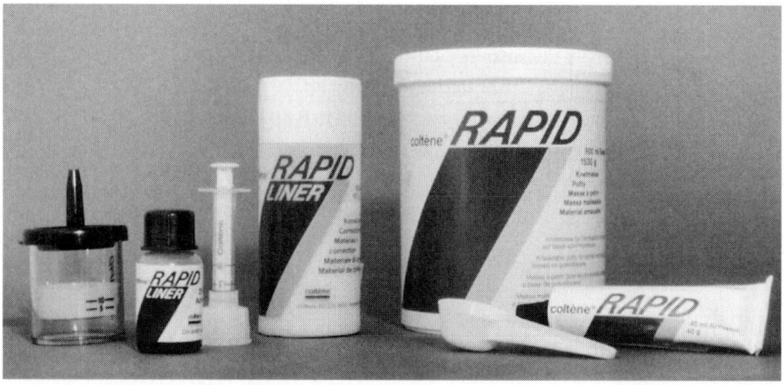

Fig. 12-17 Condensation silicone product having low consistencies and puttylike consistencies. The low-consistency wash and liquid accelerator are in the small container and bottle on the *left,* and the putty and paste accelerator are in the larger container and tube on the *right.* The liquid accelerator is dispensed with the syringe and mixed with the wash material in the container on the left. The putty is dispensed with the scoop.

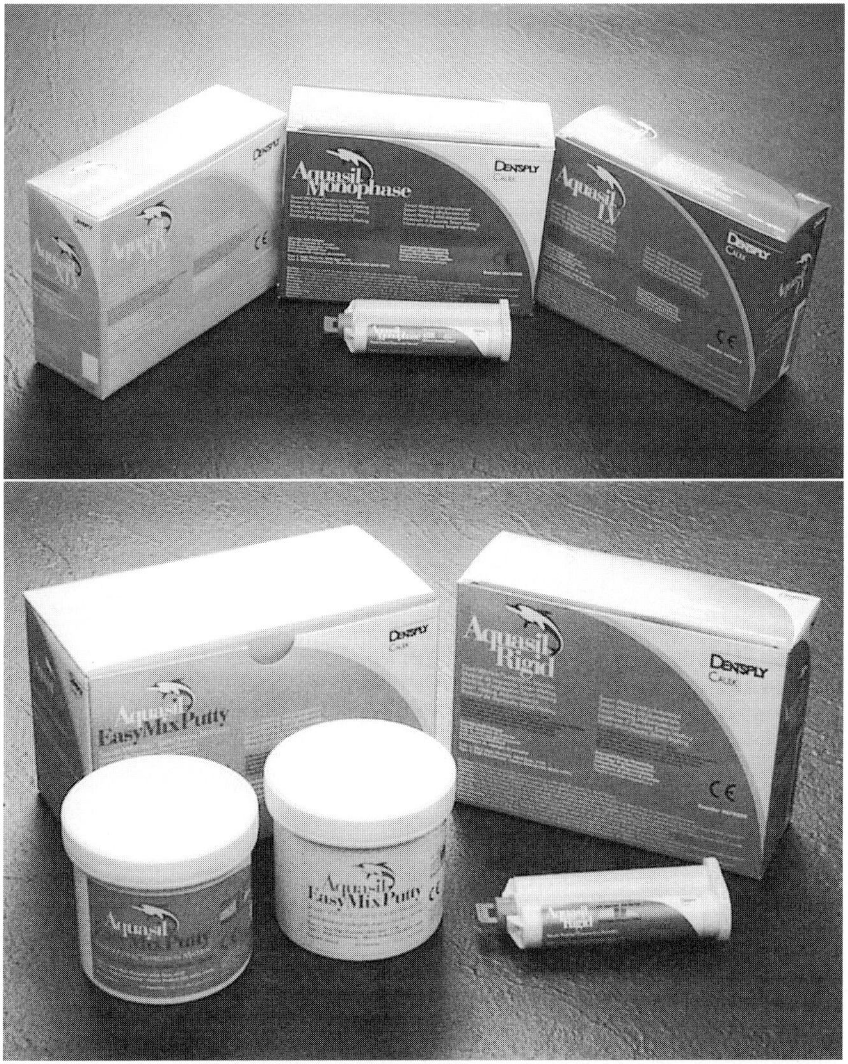

A

B

Fig. 12-18 A, Extra-low-viscosity *(XLV)*, low-viscosity *(LV)*, and monophase *(shear thinning)* addition-silicone impression materials supplied in automixing cartridges. **B,** A high-viscosity (rigid) addition silicone, also supplied in automixing cartridges, and a very high–viscosity (putty) material, supplied in tubs of catalyst and base pastes.

(Courtesy L.D. Caulk, Dentsply, York, Pa.)

molecular weight polymer (polymethylhydrosiloxane) with more than three and up to ten pendant or terminal hydrosilane groups per molecule (see formulas at top of p. 356 and AS1). The base also contains filler.

The accelerator (catalyst) and the base paste contain a dimethylsiloxane polymer with vinyl terminal groups, plus filler. The accelerator also contains a platinum catalyst of the so-called *Karstedt* type, which is a complex compound

Pendant hydrosilane groups

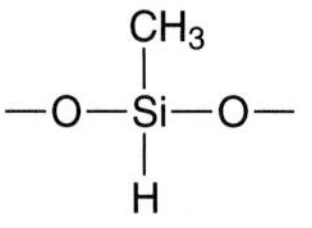

Terminal hydrosilane groups

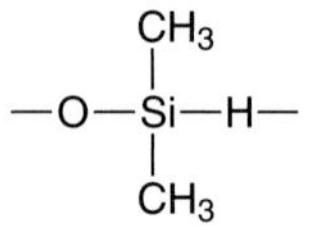

consisting of platinum and 1,3 divinyltetramethyldisiloxane. Unlike the condensation type, the addition reaction does not normally produce a low–molecular weight byproduct, as indicated in the reaction shown on p. 357 (AS2).

AS1

Polymethylhydrosiloxane

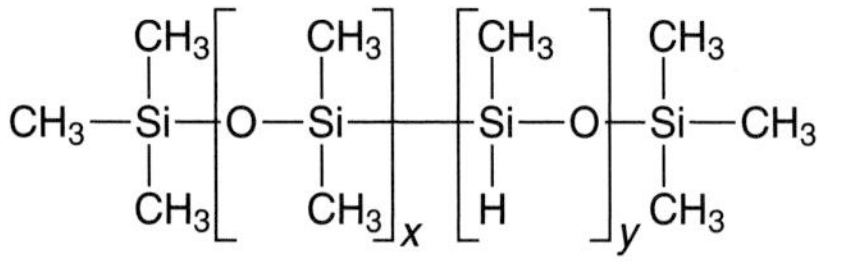

Vinylpolysiloxane

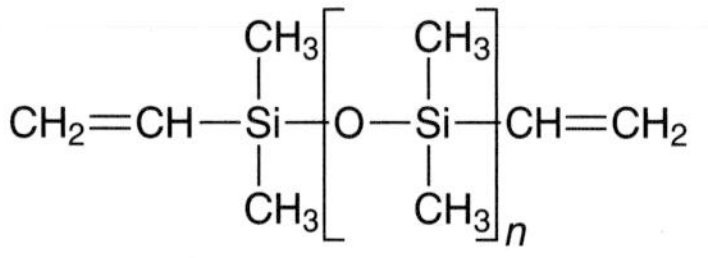

A secondary reaction can occur however with the production of hydrogen gas if –OH groups are present. The most important source of –OH groups is water (H–OH), the reaction of which under consumption of Si–H-units is illustrated on p. 357 (AS3). Another possible source of hydrogen gas is a side reaction of the Si–H units of the polymethylhydrosiloxane with each other, under the influence of the platinum catalyst, also shown on p. 357 (AS3).

Not all addition-silicone impression materials release hydrogen gas, and because it is not known which do, it is recommended that one wait at least 30 minutes for the setting reaction to be completed before the gypsum models and dies are poured. Epoxy dies should not be poured until the impression has stood overnight. The difference in the delay with gypsum and epoxy is that gypsum products have much shorter setting times than epoxy die materials. Some products contain a hydrogen absorber such as palladium, and gypsum and epoxy die materials can be poured against them as soon as practical. Examples of high-strength stone poured after 15 minutes against addition silicone, with and without a hydrogen absorber, are shown in Fig. 12-19.

Latex gloves have been shown to adversely affect the setting of addition-silicone impressions. Sulfur compounds that are used in the vulcanization of latex rubber gloves can migrate to the surface of stored gloves. These compounds can be transferred onto the prepared teeth and adjacent soft tissues during tooth preparation and when placing tissue retraction cord. They can also be incorporated directly into the impression material when mixing two putties by hand. These compounds can poison the platinum-containing catalyst, which results in retarded or no polymerization in the contaminated area of the impression. Thorough washing of the gloves with detergent and water just before mixing sometimes minimizes this effect, and some brands of gloves interfere with the setting more than others. Vinyl gloves do not have such an effect. The preparation and adjacent soft tissues can also be cleaned with 2% chlorhexidine to remove contaminants.

Polyether Polyethers are supplied in low, medium, and heavy-body consistency, and the three mixing systems previously described are available for polyethers. The base paste consists of a long-chain polyether copolymer with alternating oxygen atoms and methylene groups ($O–[CH_2]_n$) and reactive terminal groups (PE1, p. 358). Also incorporated are a silica filler, compatible plasticizers of a non-phthalate type, and triglycerides. In the catalyst paste, the former 2,5-dichlorobenzene sulfonate was replaced by an aliphatic cationic starter as a cross-linking agent.

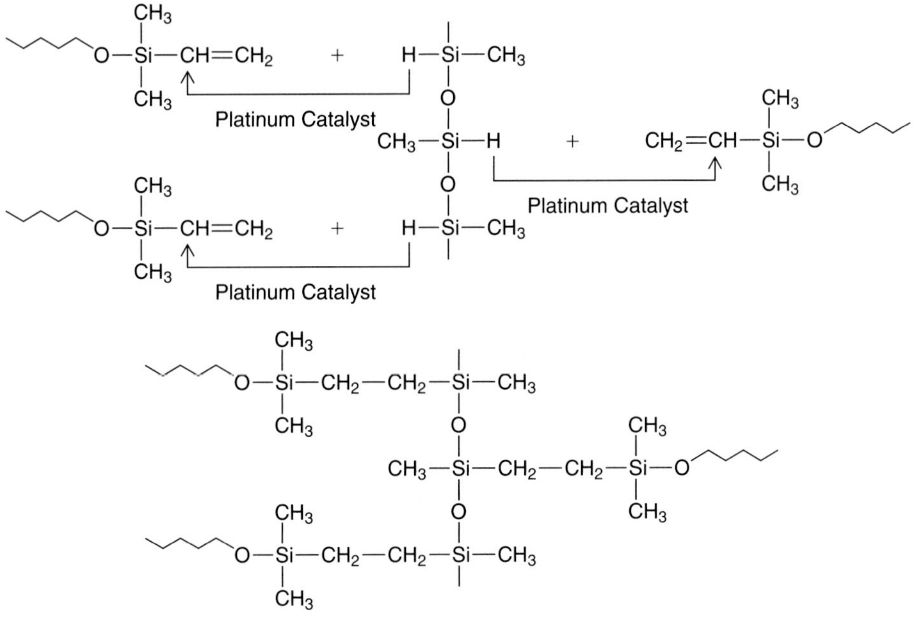

AS2

Platinum Catalyst

Platinum Catalyst

Platinum Catalyst

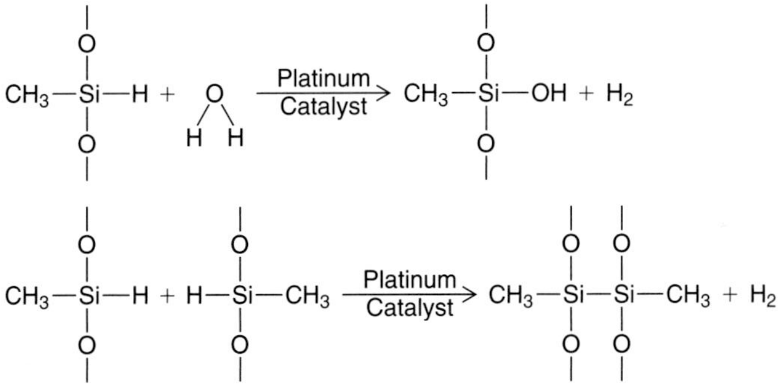

AS3

$$CH_3-Si-H + H_2O \xrightarrow{\text{Platinum Catalyst}} CH_3-Si-OH + H_2$$

$$CH_3-Si-H + H-Si-CH_3 \xrightarrow{\text{Platinum Catalyst}} CH_3-Si-Si-CH_3 + H_2$$

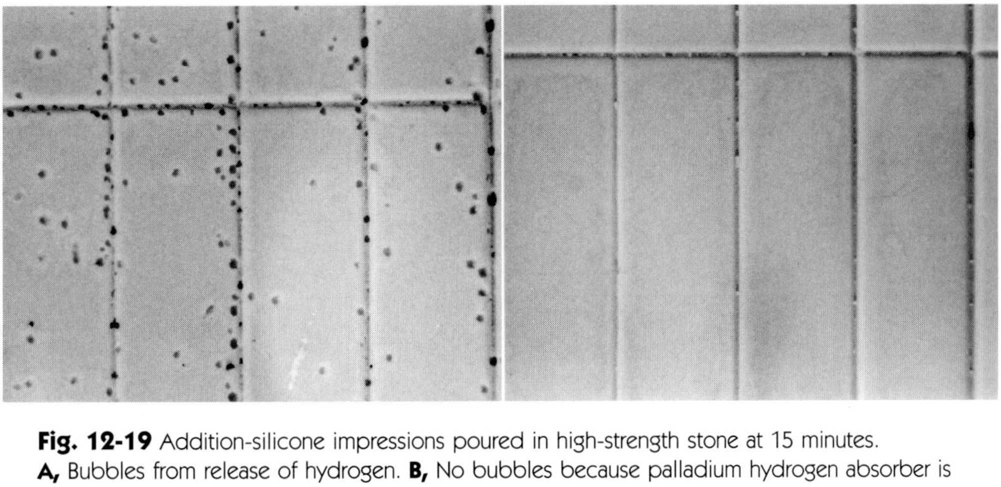

Fig. 12-19 Addition-silicone impressions poured in high-strength stone at 15 minutes. **A,** Bubbles from release of hydrogen. **B,** No bubbles because palladium hydrogen absorber is included in the impression material.

PE1

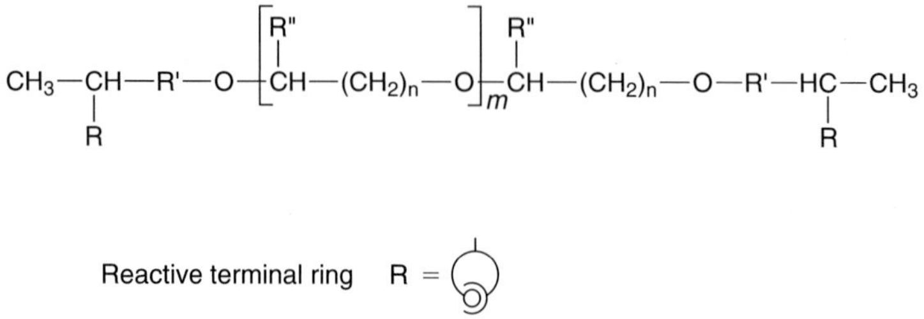

PE2

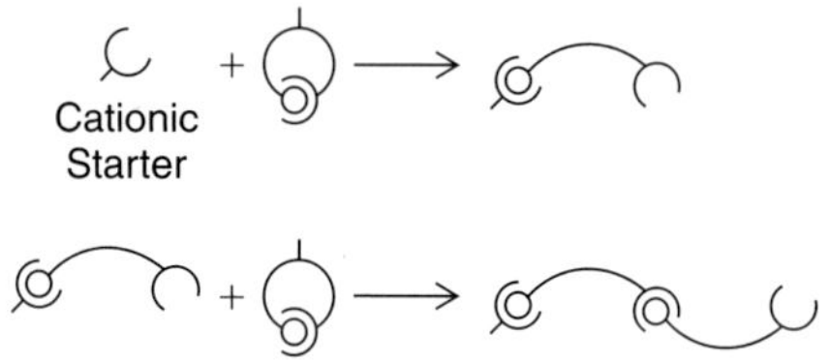

The catalyst also includes a silica filler and plasticizers. Coloring agents are added to base and catalyst to aid in the recognition of different material types. Examples of polyether impression materials are shown in Fig. 12-14.

The reaction mechanism is shown above (PE2) in a simplified form. The elastomer is formed by cationic polymerization by opening of the reactive terminal rings. The backbone of the polymer is believed to be a copolymer of ethylene oxide and tetramethylene oxide units. The reactive terminal rings open under the influence of the cationic initiator of the catalyst paste and can then, as a cation itself, attack and open additional rings. Whenever a ring is opened, the cation function remains attached, thus lengthening the chain (PE3). Because of the identical chemical base, all polyether consistencies can be freely combined with each other. A chemical bond between all materials develops during curing.

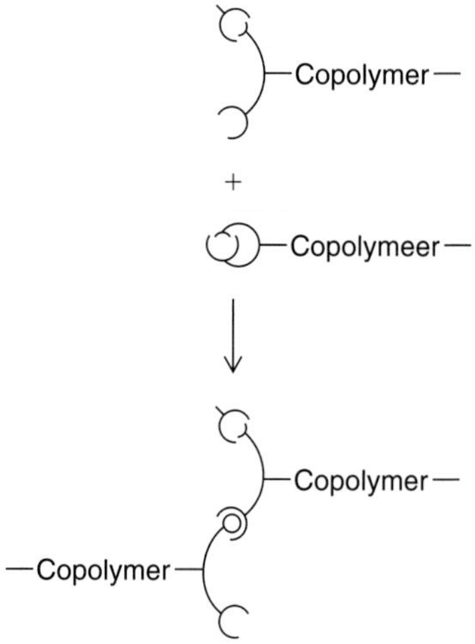

PE3

SETTING PROPERTIES

Typical values of the setting properties of elastomeric impression materials are presented in Table 12-7. The temperature rise in typical mixes of impression materials was pointed out in the previous section, but Table 12-7 illustrates that the temperature rise is small and of no clinical concern.

Viscosity The viscosity of materials 45 seconds after mixing is listed in Table 12-7. As expected, the viscosity increases for the same type of material from low to high consistencies. Viscosity as a function of time after the start of mixing is shown in Fig. 12-20 for mixes stored at 25° C. The most rapid increase in viscosity with time occurred with silicones and polyether materials, with the latter increasing slightly more rapidly than the former.

Attention must be paid to proper mixing times and times of insertion of the impression material into the mouth if the materials are to be used

TABLE 12-7 Setting Properties of Rubber Impression Materials

Material	Consistency	Temperature Rise (° C)	Viscosity 45 sec after Mixing (cp)	Working Time (min)	Setting Time (min)	Dimensional Change at 24 hr (%)
POLYSULFIDES						
	Low	3.4	60,000	4-7	7-10	−0.40
	Medium		110,000	3-6	6-8	−0.45
	High		450,000	3-6	6-8	−0.44
SILICONES						
Condensation	Low	1.1	70,000	2.5-4	6-8	−0.60
	Very high			2-2.5	3-6	−0.38
Addition	Low			2-4	4-6.5	−0.15
	Medium		150,000	2-4	4-6.5	−0.17
	High			2.5-4	4-6.5	−0.15
	Very high			1-4	3-5	−0.14
POLYETHERS						
	Low	4.2		3	6	−0.23
	Medium		130,000	2.5-3	6	−0.24
	High			2.5	5.5	−0.19

to their best advantage. For example, low-consistency polysulfide injected or placed in the mouth at 5.5 minutes would have the same viscosity as medium-consistency polysulfide at 3 minutes. Similarly, a medium-consistency polysulfide at 4 minutes would have the same viscosity as a high-consistency material at 2 minutes.

A shearing force can affect the viscosity of polyether and silicone impression materials, as was mentioned in the section on impression techniques. This effect is called *shear thinning* or *pseudoplasticity*. For impression materials possessing this characteristic, the viscosity of the unset material diminishes with an increasing outside force or shearing speed. When the influence is discontinued, the viscosity immediately increases. This property is very important for the use of monophase impression materials, and is illustrated for polyether in Fig. 12-21. In the case of polyether, shear-thinning properties are influenced by a weak network of triglyceride crystals. The crystals align when the impression material is sheared, as occurs when mixed or flowing

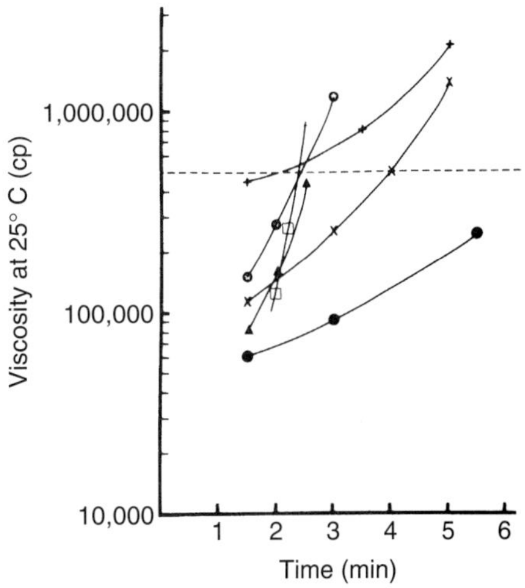

Fig. 12-20 Viscosity of elastomeric impression materials after mixing at 25° C. Polysulfide light, •; polysulfide regular, ×; polysulfide heavy, +; condensation silicone, ▲; addition silicone, ✪; polyether, □. (Adapted from Herfort TW, Gerberich WW, Macosko CW et al: *J Prosthet Dent* 38:396, 1977.)

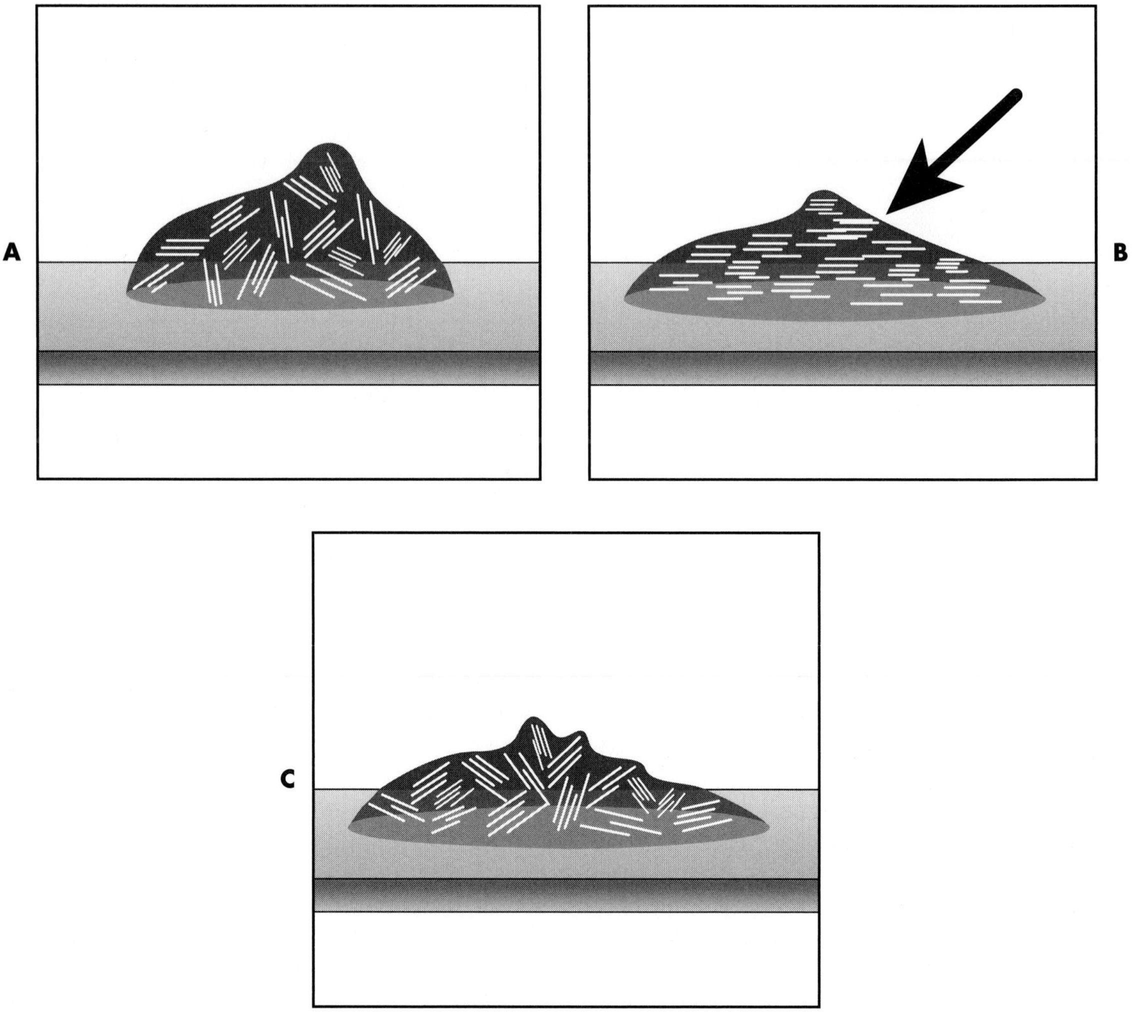

Fig. 12-21 Demonstration of the mechanism for the property of shear thinning or pseudoplasticity in polyethers. The trigliceride network, **A,** within the impression material aligns when sheared as with syringing, **B,** to achieve a lower viscosity. Once the shear force is removed, the viscosity increases with randomization of the triglyceride network, **C.**

through a syringe tip. The microcrystalline triglyceride network ensures that the polyether remains viscous in the tray or on the tooth but flows under pressure. This allows a single or monophase material to be used as a low- and medium-consistency material. Cooling of the pastes results in substantial viscosity increase. Before using, pastes have to be brought to room temperature.

The effect of shear rate (rotational speed of the viscometer) on the viscosity of single-consistency (monophase) addition silicones is shown in Fig. 12-22. Although all products showed a decrease in viscosity with increasing shear rate, the effect was much more pronounced for two products, Ba and Hy, with about an eightfold to elevenfold decrease from the lowest to the highest shear rate. The substantial decrease in viscosity at high shear stress, which is comparable with the decrease during syringing, permits the use of a single mix of material, with a portion to be

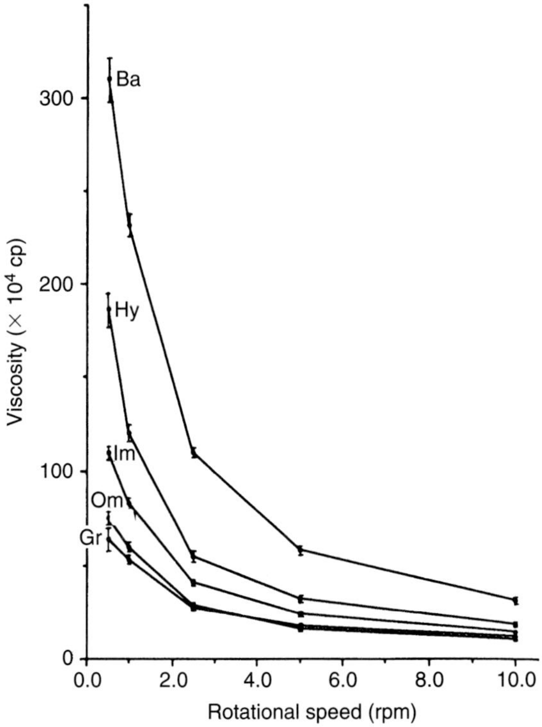

Fig. 12-22 Viscosity in centipoise as a function of shear rate (rotational speed of the viscometer) for five single-consistency addition-silicone impression materials. A rotational speed of 0.5 rpm would represent a shear rate comparable with that observed when placing the material in a tray, and a speed of 10 rpm would represent a shear rate comparable with that experienced when syringing the material.

(From Kim KN, Craig RG, Koran A, III: *J Prosthet Dent* 67:794, 1992.)

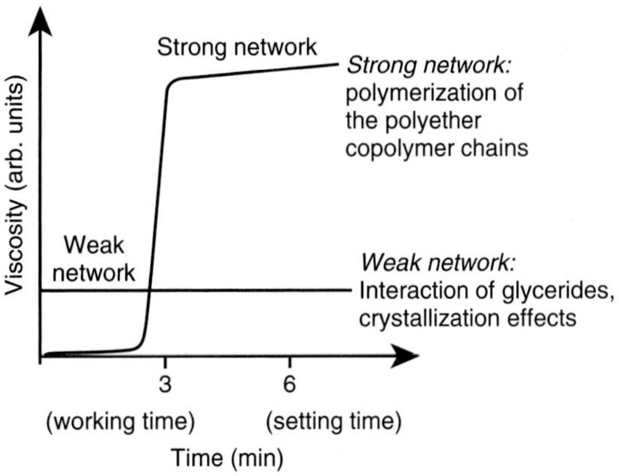

Fig. 12-23 Illustration of the snap-set of polyether. The initial viscosity of the unset material is influenced by the structural triglycerides, whereas the polymerization of copolymer chains thereafter provides the quick increase in viscosity as the material sets.

used as syringe material and another portion to be used as tray material in the syringe-tray technique.

Working and Setting Times The working and setting times of elastomeric impression materials are listed in Table 12-7. Polysulfides have the longest times, followed by silicones and polyethers. In general, for a given class of elastomeric impression materials by a specific manufacturer, the working and setting times decrease as the viscosity increases from low to high. Polyethers show a clearly defined working time with a sharp transition into the setting phase. This behavior is often called *snap-set*. This transition from plastic condition into elastic properties is rather short compared with addition silicones, which was shown in investigations of rheological properties of setting materials (Fig. 12-23).

Note that the working and setting times of the elastomeric impression materials are shortened by increases in temperature and humidity; on hot, humid days this effect should be considered in the clinical application of these materials.

The initial (or working) and final setting times can be determined fairly accurately by using a penetrometer with a needle and weight selected to suit these materials. The Vicat penetrometer, as shown in Fig. 12-24, with a 3-mm diameter needle and a total weight of 300 g, has been used by a number of investigators. A metal ring, 8 mm high and 16 mm in diameter, is filled with freshly mixed material and placed on the penetrometer base. The needle is applied to the surface of the impression material for 10 seconds, and a reading is taken. This is repeated every 30 seconds. The initial set is that time at which the needle no longer completely penetrates the specimen to the bottom of the ring. The final set is the time of the first of three identical non-maximum penetration readings. When the material has set, the elasticity

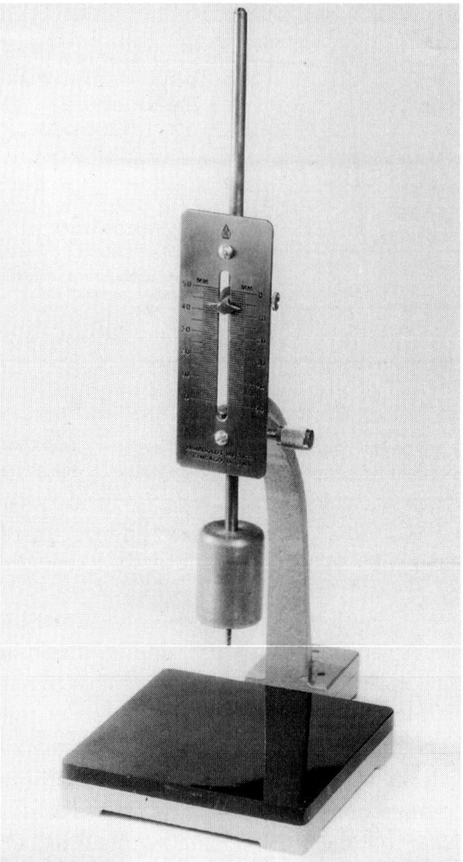

Fig. 12-24 Vicat penetrometer used to determine setting time of impression materials and other restorative materials.

still allows penetration of the needle, but it is the same at each application.

Dimensional Change on Setting The impression material undergoes a dimensional change on setting. The major factor for contraction during setting is cross-linking and rearrangement of bonds within and between polymer chains. Additional shrinkage can arise from the loss of volatile components such as water in polysulfides and ethanol in condensation silicones. Impressions can expand if water sorption takes place and an impression can be distorted if seated after the material has set to any degree. Finally, distortion or creep will occur if the material does not recover elastically when the set impression is removed from undercuts. Imbibition is discussed in the section on disinfecting impressions, and creep-induced distortion is discussed under permanent deformation.

All types of elastomeric impression materials undergo shrinkage due to polymerization, and those with reaction byproducts undergo additional contraction. The linear dimensional change between a die and the impression after 24 hours is listed in Table 12-7. The polysulfides and condensation silicones have the largest dimensional change during setting, in the range of –0.4 to –0.6%. The shrinkage is a result of the evaporation of volatile byproducts and the rearrangement of the bonds with polymerization. The addition silicones have the smallest change, about –0.15%, followed by the polyethers at about –0.2%. The contraction is lower for these two products because there is not loss of byproducts.

The rate of shrinkage of elastomeric impression materials is not uniform during the 24 hours after removal from the mouth. In general, about half the shrinkage observed at 24 hours occurs during the first hour after removal; for greatest accuracy, therefore, the models and dies should be prepared promptly, although the elastomeric impression materials are much more stable in air than hydrocolloid products.

MECHANICAL PROPERTIES

Typical mechanical properties of elastomeric impression materials are listed in Table 12-8. The permanent deformation (in the current specification, elastic recovery, which is 100% minus the permanent deformation), strain in compression, and dimensional change are properties used in ANSI/ADA Specification No. 19 (ISO 4823) to classify elastomeric impression materials as low, medium, high, or very high viscosity types. The requirements for these properties are given in Table 12-9. Further requirements of the specification for rubber impression materials are indicated in Table 12-10. The consistency diameter is used to classify viscosity by measuring the diameter of the disk formed when 0.5 ml of mixed material is subjected to a 575-g weight at 1.5 min-

TABLE 12-8 Mechanical Properties of Elastomeric Impression Materials

Material	Consistency	Permanent Deformation* (%)	Strain in Compression (%)	Flow (%)	Shore A Hardness	Tear Strength (g/cm)
POLYSULFIDES						
	Low	3-4	14-17	0.5-2	20	2500-7000
	Medium	3-5	11-15	0.5-1	30	3000-7000
	High	3-6	9-12	0.5-1	35	—
SILICONES						
Condensation	Low	1-2	4-9	0.05-0.1	15-30	2300-2600
	Very high	2-3	2-5	0.02-0.05	50-65	—
Addition	Low	0.05-0.4	3-6	0.01-0.03	35-55	1500-3000
	Medium	0.05-0.3	2-5	0.01-0.03	50-60	2200-3500
	High	0.1-0.3	2-3	0.01-0.03	60-70	2500-4300
	Very high	0.2-0.5	1-2	0.01-0.1	50-75	—
POLYETHERS						
	Low	1.5	3	0.03	35-40	1800
	Medium	1-2	2-3	0.02	40-60	2800-4800
	High	2	3	0.02	40-50	3000

*Elastic recovery from deformation is 100% minus the percent permanent deformation.

TABLE 12-9 Elastic Recovery, Strain in Compression, and Dimensional Change Requirements for Elastic Impression Materials

Viscosity Type	Minimum Elastic Recovery (%)	Strain in Compression (%)		Maximum Dimensional Change in 24 hr (%)
		Min	Max	
Low	96.5	2.0	20	1.5
Medium	96.5	2.0	20	1.5
High	96.5	0.8	20	1.5
Very high	96.5	0.8	20	1.5

Adapted from ISO Specification 4823.

utes after mixing for 12 minutes. Because the setting times of elastomeric impression materials vary, the consistency diameter is affected not only by the viscosity but also by the setting time. The classification of a material by the consistency diameter may be different from that by a true viscosity measurement.

Permanent Deformation The order in which the permanent deformation of the elastomeric impression materials is listed in Table 12-8 demonstrates that addition silicones have the best elastic recovery during removal from the mouth, followed by condensation silicones and polyethers, and then polysulfides.

The trend is to report the elastic recovery rather than the permanent deformation. Thus a material with a permanent deformation of 1% has an elastic recovery of 99%.

Strain The strain in compression under a stress of 1000 g/cm^2 is a measure of the flexibility of the material. Table 12-8 illustrates that, in general, the low-consistency materials of each

TABLE 12-10 Requirements by ANSI/ADA Specification No. 19 (ISO 4823) for the Various Viscosities of Rubber Impression Materials

Viscosity	Maximum Mixing Time (min)	Minimum Working Time (min)	Diameter of Consistency Disk (mm)		Reproduction of Detail	
			Min	Max	Line Width in Impression (mm)	Line Width in Gypsum (mm)
Low	1	2	36	—	0.020	0.020
Medium	1	2	31	41	0.020	0.020
High	1	2	—	35	0.050	0.050
Very High	1	2	—	35	0.075	0.075

Adapted from ISO Specification 4823.

type are more flexible than the high-consistency elastomeric impressions. For a given consistency, polyethers are generally the stiffest followed by addition silicones, condensation silicones, and polysulfides.

Flow Flow is measured on a cylindrical specimen 1 hour old, and the percent flow is determined 15 minutes after a load of 100 g is applied. As seen in Table 12-8, silicones and polyethers have the lowest values of flow, and polysulfides have the highest values.

Typical elastomeric impression materials apparently have no difficulty meeting the mechanical property requirements of ANSI/ADA Specification No. 19 (see Table 12-9). Although the flow, hardness and the tear strengths of elastomeric impression materials are not mentioned in the specification, these are important properties; they are also listed in Table 12-8.

Hardness The Shore A hardness increases from low to high consistency. When two numbers are given, the first represents the hardness 1.5 minutes after removal from the mouth, and the second number is the hardness after 2 hours. The polysulfides and the low-, medium-, and high-viscosity addition silicones do not change hardness significantly with time, whereas the hardness of condensation silicones, addition-silicone putties, and polyethers does increase with time. In addition, the hardness and strain affect the force necessary to remove the impression from the mouth. Low flexibility and high hardness can be compensated for clinically by producing more space for the impression material between the tray and the teeth. This can be accomplished with additional block-out for custom trays or by selecting a larger tray when using disposable trays.

A new variation in polyether provides less resistance to deformation during removal of the impression from the mouth and the gypsum cast from the impression. To achieve this, the filler content was reduced from 14 to 6 parts per unit, thereby reducing the Shore A hardness from 46 to 40 after 15 minutes, and from 61 to 50 after 24 hours. The ratio of high-viscous softener to low-viscous softener was changed to achieve a consistency similar to that of the conventional monophase polyether.

Tear Strength Tear strength is important because it indicates the ability of a material to withstand tearing in thin interproximal areas. The tear strengths listed in Table 12-8 are a measure of the force needed to initiate and continue tearing a specimen of unit thickness. A few polysulfides have high tear strengths of 7000 g/cm, but the majority have lower values in the 2500 to 3000 g/cm range. As the consistency of the impression type increases, tear strength undergoes a small increase, but most of the values are between 2000 and 4000 g/cm. Values for very high consistency types are not listed because this property is not important for these materials. Higher tear strengths for elastomeric impression

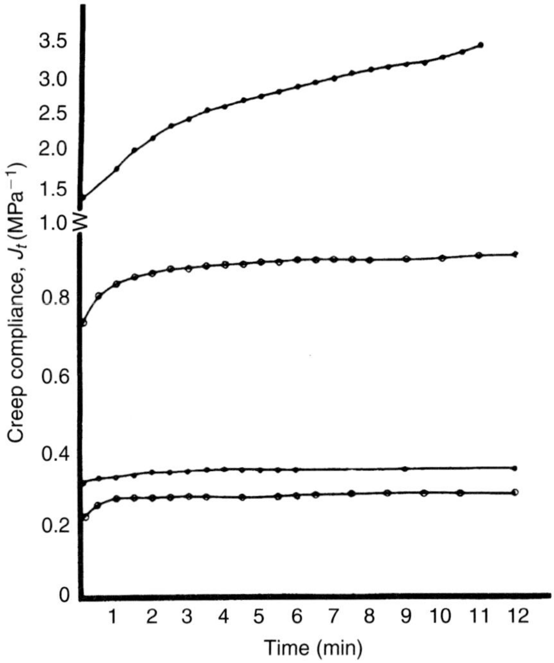

Fig. 12-25 Creep compliance of elastomeric impression materials at the time recommended for removal from the mouth. Curves from *top* to *bottom:* polysulfide, condensation silicone, addition silicone, and polyether.

(From Craig RG: *Mich Dent Assoc J* 59:259, 1977.)

materials are desirable, but compared with the values for hydrocolloid impression materials of 350 to 700 g/cm, they are a major improvement. Although polysulfides have high tear strengths, they also have high permanent deformation that may result in inaccurate impressions.

Creep Compliance Elastomeric impression materials are viscoelastic, and their mechanical properties are time dependent. For example, the higher the rate of deformation, the higher the tear strength; and the longer the impressions are deformed, the higher the permanent deformation. As a result, plots of creep compliance versus time describe the properties of these materials better than stress-strain curves. Creep–compliance time curves for low-consistency polysulfide, condensation silicone, addition silicone, and medium-consistency polyether are shown in Fig. 12-25. The initial creep compliance illustrates polysulfide is the most flexible and polyether is the least flexible. The flatness or parallelism of the curves with respect to the time axis indicates low permanent deformation and excellent recovery from deformation during the removal of an impression material; polysulfides have the poorest elastic recovery, followed by condensation silicone and then addition silicone and polyether.

The recoverable viscoelastic quality of the materials is indicated by differences between the initial creep compliance and the creep compliance value obtained by extrapolation of the linear portion of the curve to zero time. As a result, polysulfides have the greatest viscoelastic quality and require more time to recover the viscoelastic deformation, followed by condensation silicone, polyether, and addition silicone.

Detail Reproduction The requirements of elastomeric impression materials are listed in Table 12-10. Except for the very high–viscosity products, all should reproduce a V-shaped groove and a 0.02-mm wide line in the elastomeric. The impression should be compatible with gypsum products so the 0.02-mm line is transferred to gypsum die materials. Low-, medium-, and high-viscosity elastomeric impression materials have little difficulty meeting this requirement.

WETTABILITY AND HYDROPHILIZATION OF ELASTOMERIC IMPRESSION MATERIALS

Wettability may be assessed by measuring the advancing contact angle of water on the surface of the set impression material or by using a tensiometer to measures forces as the material is immersed and removed (Wilhelmy technique). The advancing contact angles for elastomeric impression materials are listed in Table 12-11. Of all the impression materials discussed in this chapter, only hydrocolloids can be considered truly hydrophilic. All of the elastomeric impression materials possess advancing and receding contact angles greater than 45 degrees. There are, however, differences in wetting among and within types of elastomeric impression materials. Traditional addition silicone is not as wettable as

TABLE 12-11 Wettability of Rubber Impression Materials

Material	Advancing Contact Angle of Water (deg)	Castability of High-Strength Dental Stone (%)
Polysulfide	82	44
Condensation silicone	98	30
Addition silicone		
Hydrophobic	98	30
Hydrophilic	53	72
Polyether	49	70

polyether. When mixes of gypsum products are poured into addition silicone, high contact angles are formed, making the preparation of bubble-free models difficult.

Surfactants have been added to addition silicones by manufacturers to reduce the contact angle, improve wettability, and simplify the pouring of gypsum models. This class with improved wetting characteristics is most accurately called *hydrophilized addition silicone.* Most commonly, nonionic surfactants have gained importance in this area. These molecules consist of an oligoether or polyether substructure as the hydrophilic part and a silicone-compatible hydrophobic part (Fig. 12-26, *A*). The mode of action of these wetting agents is believed to be a diffusion-controlled transfer of surfactant molecules from the polyvinylsiloxane into the aqueous phase, as shown, thereby altering the surface tension of the surrounding liquid. As a result, a reduction in surface tension and therefore greater wettability of the polyvinylsiloxane is observed (Fig. 12-26, *B*). This mechanism differs from polyethers, which possess a high degree of wettability because their molecular structure contains polar oxygen atoms, which have an affinity for water. Because of this affinity, polyether materials flow onto hydrated intraoral surfaces and are therefore cast with gypsum more easily than are addition silicones. This affinity also allows polyether impressions to adhere quite strongly to soft and hard tissues.

By observing water droplets on impression surfaces, it has been shown that hydrophilized addition silicones and polyethers are wetted the best, and condensation silicones and conventional addition silicones the least. Wettability was directly correlated to the ease of pouring high-strength stone models of an extremely critical die, as shown in Table 12-11. Using a tensiometer to record forces of immersed impression specimens (Wilhelmy method), polyether was shown to wet significantly better than hydrophilized addition silicones for both advancing (74° versus 108° C) and receding contact angles (50° versus 81° C).

To evaluate the ability of impression materials to reproduce detail under wet and dry surface conditions, impressions were made of a standard wave pattern used to calibrate surface analyzers. The surfaces of impressions were scanned for average roughness (Ra) after setting to determine their ability to reproduce the detail of the standard, the value of which is shown with a double line in Fig. 12-27. From a clinical standpoint, most impression materials produced acceptable detail under wet and dry conditions. Polyethers produced slightly better detail than did addition silicones, and were generally unaffected by the presence of moisture, whereas detail decreased some for addition silicones under wet conditions, even if hydrophilized.

DISINFECTION OF ELASTOMERIC IMPRESSIONS

All impressions should be disinfected upon removal from the mouth to prevent transmission of organisms to gypsum casts and to laboratory personnel. Several studies confirm that all types of elastomeric impression materials, polysulfide, condensation silicone, addition silicone, and polyether, can be disinfected by immersion in several different disinfectants for up to 18 hours without a loss of surface quality and accuracy.

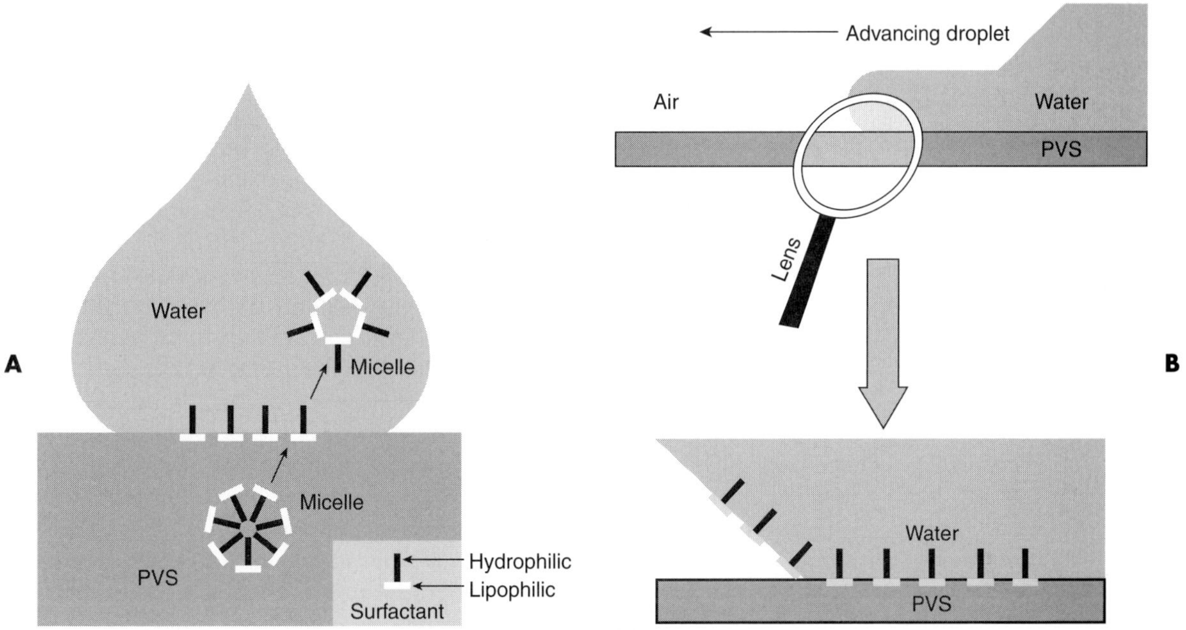

Fig. 12-26 A, The hydrophilization of addition silicones is gained with the incorporation of nonionic surfactants shown as micelles. These molecules consist of a hydrophilic part and a silicone compatible hydrophobic part. The mode of action of these surfactants is thought to be a diffusion-controlled transfer of surfactant molecules from the polyvinylsiloxane into the aqueous phase, as shown. In this manner, the surface tension of the surrounding liquid is altered. **B,** This increased wettability allows the addition silicone to spread more freely along the surface.

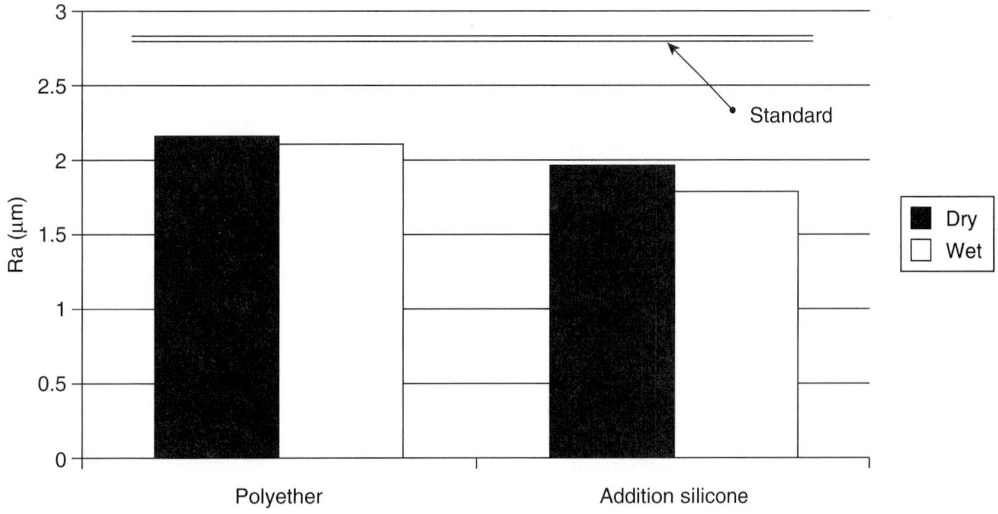

Fig. 12-27 Ability of polyether and hydrophilized addition silicone materials to reproduce detail under dry and wet conditions. The average roughness, *Ra,* of the standard from which impressions were made is shown *(double line).* Polyethers produced the best detail and were unaffected by moisture. The detail captured by addition silicones decreased slightly in the presence of moisture.

(Adapted from Johnson GH, Lepe X, and Berg JC: *J Dent Res* 77 [Spec Iss B]:798, 1998.)

RELATIONSHIP OF PROPERTIES AND CLINICAL APPLICATION

Accuracy, the ability to record detail, ease of handling, and setting characteristics are of prime importance in dental impressions.

Silicones generally have shorter working times than polysulfides but somewhat longer times than polyethers. Single-mix materials have some advantage in that, as a result of shear thinning, they have low viscosities when mixed or syringed but higher viscosities when inserted in a tray. The time of placement of a elastomeric impression material is critical, because viscosity increases rapidly with time as a result of the polymerization reaction. If the material is placed in the mouth after the consistency or viscosity has increased via polymerization, internal stresses induced in the impression are released after the impression is removed from the mouth, resulting in an inaccurate impression.

Thorough mixing is essential; otherwise portions of the mix could contain insufficient accelerator to polymerize thoroughly or may not set at the same rate as other portions of the impression. In this event, removal of the impression would cause high permanent deformation and result in an inaccurate impression. Automixing and mechanical mixing systems produce mixes with fewer bubbles than hand mixing, save time in mixing, and result in a more bubble-free impression.

Polymerization of elastomeric impression materials continues after the material has set, and the mechanical properties improve with time. Removal too early may result in high permanent deformation; however, excessively long times in the mouth are unacceptable to the patient. The manufacturer usually recommends a minimum time for leaving the impression in the mouth, and this minimum is used for testing the materials according to ANSI/ADA Specification No. 19.

Dimensional changes on setting were the highest for condensation silicones and polysulfides. The effect of this shrinkage can be compensated for by use of a double-impression or putty-wash technique. When using a double-impression technique, a preliminary impression is taken in the high- or puttylike-consistency material, providing some space for the final impression in low-consistency material. The preliminary impression is removed, the cavity prepared, and the final impression taken with the low-consistency material, using the preliminary impression as a tray. In this way, the dimensional change in the high consistency or puttylike consistency is negligible, and although the percent dimensional change of the low-consistency material is still large, the thickness is so small that the actual dimensional change is small. The double-impression technique is suitable for use with a stock impression tray, because the preliminary impression serves as a custom tray. With the monophase and simultaneous dual-viscosity technique, a slight improvement in accuracy results when a custom-made tray is used because it provides a uniform thickness of impression material. Several studies have shown, however, that relatively stiff stock plastic or metal trays yield nearly the same accuracy.

Clinical studies have shown that the viscosity of the impression material is the most important factor in producing impressions and dies with minimal bubbles and maximum detail. As a result, the syringe-tray technique produced superior clinical results in the reproduction of fine internal detail of proximal boxes or grooves.

The accuracy of the impression may be affected when the percentage of deformation and the time involved in removing the impression are increased. In both instances, permanent deformation increases, the amount depending on the type of elastomeric impression material.

Because elastomeric impressions recover from deformation for a period after their removal, some increase in accuracy can be expected during this time. This effect is more noticeable with polysulfides than with other impression materials. However, polymerization shrinkage is also occurring, and the overall accuracy is determined by a combination of these two effects. Insignificant recovery from deformation occurs after 20 to 30 minutes; therefore dies should be prepared promptly after that time for greatest accuracy. Addition silicones that release hydrogen are an exception to this guide.

Second pours of gypsum products into elastomeric impressions produce dies that are not quite as accurate as the first, because the impression can be deformed during the removal of the first die; however, they are usually sufficiently accurate to be used as a working die. Materials such as polysulfide are more susceptible to permanent deformation with cast removal than other types.

BITE REGISTRATION MATERIALS

ELASTOMERIC IMPRESSION MATERIALS

Addition silicones and polyethers have been formulated for use as bite registration materials. Most of the products are addition silicones and most are supplied in automix cartridges. Properties of these bite registration materials are listed in Table 12-12. These materials are characterized by short working times and the length of time left in the mouth compared with typical elastomeric impression materials. They are also noted for their high stiffness, indicated by the low percent strain in compression, and for their low flow and dimensional change even after 7 days. The property that distinguishes addition silicones from polyether is their lower dimensional change after removal; however, either is superior to the stability of waxes for taking bite registrations.

ZINC OXIDE–EUGENOL AND IMPRESSION PLASTER

Several materials become rigid when used to record bite relationships and anatomical features. These materials can be used to capture occlusal relationships providing the materials do not flow into undercuts, such as beyond the height of contour of the teeth being recorded. If they do, these brittle materials can distort permanently or fracture upon removal.

Zinc oxide–eugenol, commonly used as a temporary cement or temporary filling material, can also be used to record tooth and arch relationships (Fig. 12-28). In this case, it is often used to reline an area in which the bite was initially recorded, to improve the accuracy of the record. Type I gypsum, also called *impression plaster,* can be used to record relationships of crowns and pontics for soldering and for recording relationships between arches. Detailed descriptions of zinc oxide–eugenol and Type 1 gypsum are given in Chapters 20 and 13, respectively.

WAX REGISTRATIONS

Bite registrations used to articulate upper and lower models have often been taken in wax, as described in Chapter 14. However, the properties of waxes limit their accuracy, because wax registrations (1) can be distorted upon removal, (2) may change dimensions by release of internal stresses, depending on the storage condition, (3) have high flow properties, and (4) undergo large dimensional changes on cooling from mouth to room temperature.

Wax is also used as a corrective impression technique in partial and complete denture prostheses. Impression waxes are available with a variety of softening temperatures, further dis-

TABLE 12-12 Properties of Rubber Impression Materials Used for Taking Bite Registrations

Material	Mixing Type	Working Time (min)	Time in Mouth (min)	Strain in Compression (%)	Flow (%)	Dimensional Change 1 Day (%)	Dimensional Change 7 Days (%)
Addition silicone	Automix	0.5-3.0	1.0-3.0	1.0-2.9	0.0-0.01	0.0 to −0.15	−0.04 to −0.20
Addition silicone	Handmix	1.4	2.5	0.92	0.0	−0.06	−0.08
Polyether	Handmix	2.1	3.0	1.97	0.0	−0.29	−0.32

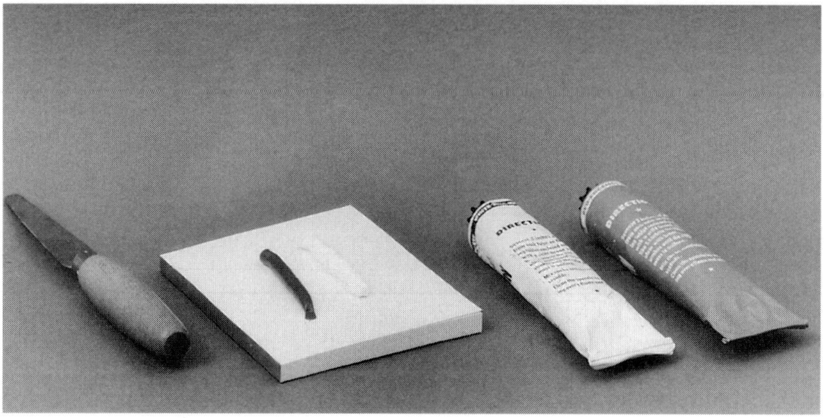

Fig. 12-28 Paper pads and spatula suitable for mixing impression materials of zinc oxide–eugenol type.

cussed in Chapter 14. Waxes with lower softening points are used to register functional impressions. In one case, the posterior palatal seal area is delineated intraorally using a colored pencil. This line is transferred to the final impression. Thereafter, a thin layer of impression wax is placed over the posterior palatal seal area to form a raised area in the final denture, thereby creating a better posterior seal. In other cases, a thin layer of impression wax can be applied to a denture base with occlusal bite rims and left in place in the mouth for a period of time. In this way, the wax flows and adapts itself to the oral tissues under the influence of functional occlusion. Impression waxes with a higher softening point are used in extending the border of the denture base when necessary. The clinical techniques for their use are adequately described in textbooks on prosthetic dentistry.

IMPRESSION COMPOUND

One of the oldest dental impression materials is impression compound. Tray compound has been largely replaced by acrylic and plastic tray materials, but impression compound is still used for border-molding complete denture impressions and is conveniently used to secure rubber dam retainers so they remain stable during clinical procedures. Impression compounds are available in the form of sheets, sticks, cylinders, and cones, some examples of which are shown in Fig. 12-29. Impression compounds are thermoplastic materials and are softened to their working consistency by immersion in hot water or by warming over a flame. Some variation of the temperature at which softening takes place exists among different compounds, and they can be divided into high-fusing (tray) and low-fusing (impression) compounds.

Composition The impression compound shown in Table 12-13 is a mixture of thermoplastic resins and waxes, a filler, and a coloring agent. By varying the proportions of the various ingredients, compounds of differing physical properties can be made. Resins and waxes soften on heating and provide flow and cohesion, and the filler adds body and gives a suitable working consistency. Rouge produces a characteristic reddish brown color and it is the most common pigment.

Thermal Conductivity The thermal conductivity of impression compounds is low. When immersed in hot water or heated over a flame, they rapidly soften on the outside, but time is required before the mass is softened throughout.

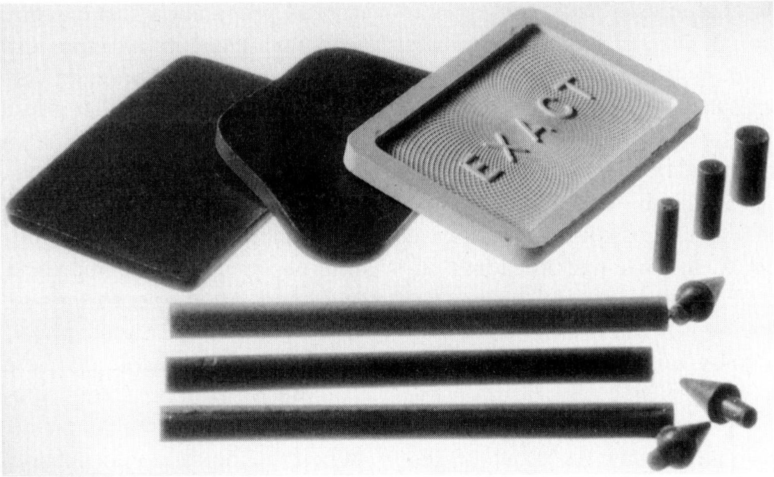

Fig. 12-29 Dental impression compound in the form of sheets, sticks, cylinders, and cones.

TABLE 12-13 Composition of an Impression Compound

Ingredient	Parts
Rosin	30
Copal resin	30
Carnauba wax	10
Stearic acid	5
Talc	75
Coloring agent	Appropriate amount

When heating over a flame, care is needed to prevent the outside from being overheated and the more volatile components from being vaporized or ignited. Prolonged immersion in hot water also leaches out the more soluble components and adversely alters physical properties.

The low thermal conductivity influences the cooling rate of these materials, because the outside of a mass of compound hardens fairly rapidly, whereas the inner regions remain soft. Impressions must be given adequate time to cool completely before they are removed from the mouth.

Softening and Flow Impression compounds should soften at a point just above mouth temperature and exhibit adequate flow to adapt closely to the tissues and register surface detail. They should harden at mouth temperature and exhibit a minimum of flow to reduce the danger of distortion on removal.

ANSI/ADA Specification No. 3 (obsolete) for dental impression compound listed the following criteria for flow qualities of the impression type: the flow at 37° C shall not be more than 6%, and the flow at 45° C shall not be less than 85%.

Sticks or small cones of compound are used for securing rubber dam retainers or for recording occlusal relationships. The sticks or cones should be softened by holding them some distance above a flame to avoid overheating the outside portion and ensure softening the center of the stick. The softened compound may be placed directly around the rubber dam retainer or on the occlusal registration plate, but care must be taken that it is not too hot. For this reason the heated compound should be tempered in air or by a brief immersion in water at a temperature just above the softening point of the compound.

Cooling Impressions formed by placing the softened compound into a suitable copper band for indirect inlay and crown techniques are usually cooled in the mouth with water from a syringe. The water used for cooling should be within the range of 16° to 18° C, because cold water is uncomfortable to the patient and tends to increase the internal stresses in the impression if cooling is too rapid. The exact time required for proper cooling varies with the size of the impression and the particular compound selected.

Effect of Wet Kneading When the compound is softened in a water bath, kneading the material with the fingers is customary to improve the handling qualities. This wet kneading increases the flow of both the softened compound and the hardened impression; this increased flow is believed to be caused by the incorporation of water, which acts as a plasticizer, in the compound.

Wet kneading can modify the flow of the hardened compound to an extent that it exceeds the 6% permissible in the specification (Table 12-14). By kneading for 1 to 3 minutes, the flow of compounds may be more than doubled.

Clinically, excessive wet kneading can increase the flow qualities of the hardened material at mouth temperature to a point at which distortion may occur on removal. Once incorporated, the water remains in the compound for long periods, and subsequent reheating with further kneading has a cumulative effect of increasing flow values.

Accuracy and Dimensional Stability The optimum accuracy and dimensional stability of compound impressions can be ensured by careful preparation and handling of the material and paying attention to the details of the clinical technique in use. Softening the compound by a method that does not adversely affect its physical properties by overheating or prolonged heating is important. Equally important is that adequate flow is developed during softening to allow close adaptation to the tissues and a minimum of internal stresses in the impression. The tray, copper band, or other container used to convey the compound to the mouth must be strong, rigid (inflexible), and stable. In the mouth, adequate cooling of the compound is essential to avoid distortion when the impression is removed. When the impression is obtained, the cast or die should be made as soon as possible to avoid inaccuracies caused by the release of stresses that produce warpage, which may occur on standing. One source of inaccuracy not within the control of the operator is the thermal contraction that the compound exhibits on cooling from mouth to room temperature.

Thermal Contraction The linear contraction of an impression compound on cooling from mouth to room temperature is approximately 0.3%. This quality is inherent in the material and can result in inaccuracy unless it is recognized and adequate compensation is provided.

Tray Compounds The special compounds for making impression trays are similar in composition and working qualities to impression compounds, except that the temperature at which they soften is higher and the property of flow at mouth temperature is minimal. The ANSI/ADA Specification No. 3 requirements for tray compound are listed in Table 12-14. Tray compounds are used primarily to make individual trays for corrective wash impressions. The trays are made when softened tray compound is adapted to a study model and the border of the denture area is trimmed. Compound trays lack strength and dimensional stability; and have been replaced to a large extent by trays made in a similar manner from acrylic resins cured at room temperature.

TABLE 12-14 Permissible Flow Values for Dental Compounds as Defined by ANSI/ADA Specification No. 3*

Material	Flow At 37° C	Flow At 45° C
Type I (impression compound)	Less than 6%	More than 85%
Type II (tray compound)	Less than 2%	70%-85%

*Specification No. 3 is now obsolete.

ANSI/ADA Specification No. 3 for Dental Impression Compound Specification No. 3 has established certain limits for the desirable physical properties of impression compound and tray compound. Impression compounds are required to be homogeneous and to show a smooth, glossy appearance after the surface has been passed through a flame. When trimmed with a sharp knife at room temperature, the cut margins must be firm and smooth. The manufacturer is required to indicate in the package the method of softening, the working temperature, and a curve or data showing the shrinkage of the compound from 40° to 20° C. Two physical tests are required by the specification. One is to test the percent flow at 37° C and at 45° C, and the other is to check the reproduction of the details of a test impression block. The acceptable values of percent flow for impression and tray compounds are shown in Table 12-14.

DIE, CAST, AND MODEL MATERIALS

Dental stones, plaster, electroformed silver and copper, epoxy resin, and casting investment are some of the materials used to make casts or dies from dental impressions. The selection of one of these is determined by the particular impression material in use and by the purpose for which the die or cast is to be used.

Impressions in agar or alginate hydrocolloid can be used only with a gypsum material, such as plaster, stone, or casting investment. Compound impressions, on the other hand, can be used to produce dies of plaster, stone, or electroformed copper. Various rubber impression materials can be used to prepare gypsum, electroformed, or epoxy dies.

DESIRABLE QUALITIES OF A CAST OR DIE MATERIAL

Cast and die materials must reproduce an impression accurately and remain dimensionally stable under normal conditions of use and storage. Setting expansion, contraction, and dimensional variations in response to changes in temperature must be held to a minimum. Not only should the cast be accurate, but it should also satisfactorily reproduce fine detail and have a smooth, hard surface. Such an accurate cast or die must also be strong and durable and withstand the subsequent manipulative procedures without fracture or abrasion of the surface. Qualities of strength, resistance to shearing forces or edge strength, and abrasion resistance are therefore important and are required in varying degrees, according to the purpose for which the cast or die is to be used. For example, because it will not be subjected to much stress in use, a satisfactory study cast might be formed from dental model plaster in which the aforementioned qualities are at a minimum. However, an elastomeric impression used to produce an indirect inlay could be copper- or silver-formed or poured in high-strength stone, thereby producing a die in which these qualities are sufficient to withstand the carving and finishing procedures that are a part of this technique.

The color of a cast or die can facilitate manipulative procedures, such as waxing inlay patterns, by presenting a contrast in color to the inlay wax. The ease with which the material can be adapted to the impression and the time required before the cast or die is ready for use are of considerable practical significance. A contrast in this respect is seen between dental stone, which can be easily vibrated into an impression to produce a cast ready for use within an hour, and a copper die, which requires electroforming and usually won't be ready until the next day.

DENTAL PLASTER AND STONE

The chemistry and physical properties of dental plaster, stone, and high-strength stone are discussed in Chapter 13. These gypsum materials are used extensively to make casts and dies from dental impressions and can be used with any impression material. Stone casts, which are stronger and resist abrasion better than plaster casts, are used whenever a restoration or appliance is to be made on the cast. Plaster may be used for study casts, which are for record purposes only.

Hardening solutions, usually about 30%-silica sols in water, are mixed with stone. The increase in hardness of stone dies poured against impressions varies from 2% for silicones to 110% for polyether, with intermediate increases of 70% for agar and 20% for polysulfide. The dimensional change on setting of stones mixed with hardener is slightly greater than when mixes are made with water, +0.07% versus +0.05%. In most instances the abrasion or scraping resistance of mixes of stone made with hardening solutions is higher than comparable mixes made with water. A range of effects in the abrasion resistance of surface treatments of stone has been reported. Model and die sprays generally increase the resistance to scraping, whereas lubricants can decrease surface hardness and resistance to scraping.

High-strength dental stones make excellent casts or dies, readily reproduce the fine detail of a dental impression, and are ready for use after approximately 1 hour. The resulting cast is dimensionally stable over long periods and withstands most of the manipulative procedures involved in the production of appliances and restorations. However, procedures involving the bending, adapting, or finishing of metals can be accomplished only to a limited extent on high-strength stone dies and are better fulfilled on a metal die.

When wax patterns constructed on high-strength stone dies are to be removed, some separating agent or die lubricant is necessary to prevent the wax from adhering. Oils, liquid soap, detergents, and a number of commercial preparations can be used. Oils are generally to be avoided because some are wax solvents and soften the surface of the wax pattern. In addition, oil on the surface of the wax increases the difficulty of painting the investment on the pattern in subsequent steps of the casting process. The lubricant is applied liberally to the high-strength stone die and allowed to soak in; usually several applications can be made before any excess accumulates on the surface. The excess is blown off with an air blast before proceeding to make the wax pattern.

DIES FORMED BY THE ELECTRODEPOSITION OF METAL

Electroforming Impressions The essential equipment for the electroforming of impressions to form indirect dies for inlay, crown, or bridge restorations is a source of direct electric current and an electrolyte. The electric current may be supplied by storage batteries with a small variable resistance and an ammeter to indicate the energy in the system. Often the alternating current of 110V is converted to direct low-voltage current suitable for plating. In this case, a transformer and rectifier with some fixed resistance are used, with the same variable resistance and ammeter described for storage-battery equipment. A small container for the electrolyte, with inexpensive wire electrodes and a bar of pure copper or silver for the anode, represent the necessary equipment.

A common electrolyte used for plating copper indirect dies is an acidic copper sulfate solution. Silver electrolytes contain silver cyanide in an alkaline solution. Because of the highly poisonous nature of cyanides and shipping restraints on electrolytes, copper plating is more commonly used.

When solution of the copper sulfate occurs in the water, the salt dissociates to give cupric and sulfate ions. During electrolysis, the positive ions are drawn to the negative electrode or cathode by electrostatic attraction. The negative sulfate ($SO^{=}_4$) ions have gained electrons and move toward the positive electrode or anode. Neutral or nondissociated molecules do not move under the influence of an electric field. Hence, if a nondissociated substance such as glucose is present in the electrolyte, it will inhibit only the migration of the copper or sulfate ions, because the molecules are large but are not influenced by the electric current.

The anode is made of pure copper, and during electrolysis copper atoms give up two electrons ($2e$) and become Cu^{++} ions. The metallic copper of the anode therefore regenerates the solution as the plating process occurs with the removal of copper at the cathode. The Cu^{++} ion is attracted to the cathode (the impression), where it gains

$2e$ and is deposited as metallic copper according to the equation $Cu^{++} + 2e \rightarrow Cu^0$. As long as there is free copper at the anode, the solution will maintain a constant composition.

The action at the electrodes is summarized by the following equations:

$$\text{Anode} \quad Cu^0 - 2e \rightarrow Cu^{++}$$
$$\text{Cathode} \quad Cu^{++} + 2e \rightarrow Cu^0$$

Similar reactions occur in the electroforming of silver.

$$\text{Anode} \quad Ag^0 - e \rightarrow Ag^+$$
$$\text{Cathode} \quad Ag^+ + e \rightarrow Ag^0$$

Copper-Formed Dies Metal dies can be made by copper-plating compound or silicone (but usually not polysulfide impressions, where silver-plating is preferred). Such a die is tough and has good strength characteristics, and metal inlays and restorations can be finished and polished satisfactorily on these dies.

A copper-forming apparatus suitable for dental use consists of a transformer and rectifier to reduce the voltage of the domestic supply and convert the alternating current (AC) to direct current (DC), which is needed for electroforming the impression. The low-voltage DC passes through a variable resistor, which is used to regulate the current and modify the rate at which metal is deposited, and a milliammeter, which indicates the current passing through the plating bath. At the anode is attached a copper plate, and at the cathode is the impression to be plated, both of which are immersed in the electrolyte.

The anode is made of electrolytically pure copper and is immersed in the plating solution to the extent that the area of copper immersed is approximately equal to that of the impression to be plated. Copper anodes containing a trace of phosphorus are superior to pure copper.

The plating bath contains an acid solution of copper sulfate, and a number of formulas have been advocated. One acceptable example is given in Table 12-15.

The copper sulfate is the source of the copper, the sulfuric acid increases the conductivity of the solution, and the phenolsulfonic acid assists the penetration of copper ions to the deeper parts of an impression and improves the "throwing power" of the solution. Additives other than phenolsulfonic acid (e.g., dextrose, alcohol, phenol, and molasses) are suggested in some formulas.

TABLE 12-15 Composition of Solution for Copper-Forming Bath

Ingredient	Amount
Copper sulfate (crystals)	200 g
Sulfuric acid (concentrated)	30 ml
Phenolsulfonic acid	2 ml
Water (distilled)	1000 ml

The surface of the impression is coated with a conductor of electricity before it is attached to the cathode lead wire.

When the impression is in compound, a colloidal dispersion of graphite is painted on the surface to be plated and allowed to dry before the impression is placed into the plating bath. When the impression is a silicone rubber, finely divided copper powder is brushed on the surface to be plated before placing the impression into the bath.

About 15 mA is a suitable current to start plating a single-tooth impression. Once a thin layer of copper has covered the entire surface of the impression, the current can be increased to as much as two or three times the initial current. If too high a current setting is used, the copper deposit will be granular and friable in nature, and the die will be unsatisfactory. High current densities also produce a heavier deposit on the areas of the impression nearest the anode, and sometimes rapid plating fails to adequately cover the deeper areas of an impression. Plating is allowed to proceed for 12 to 15 hours; overnight is usually a convenient period.

The quality of the deposit obtained with a freshly made plating solution is often not as good as that achieved when the solution has been in use a short time. Loss of water from evaporation should be replaced to maintain the correct concentration of the electrolyte. The sulfuric acid is slowly decomposed when the solution is in use, and the addition of a few milliliters of acid is required after a few weeks of use to maintain the quality of copper deposit. A sediment or sludge consisting mainly of fine particles of copper may accumulate on the floor of the bath; the solution should then be filtered. When anodes containing a trace of phosphorus are used, the formation of sediment is considerably reduced.

In copper forming, the distance between the anode and the impression to be plated is an important factor in relation to plating the deeper areas of an impression; the greater the distance, the more even is the quantity of copper deposited and the more readily are the deep areas plated. About 15 cm is a suitable distance in practice; if the distance is shorter, there is a tendency for an excess of copper to be deposited on the more superficial areas of the impression, leaving the deeper areas inadequately plated.

The hydrophobic (but not the hydrophilic) addition-silicone impression materials can be satisfactorily copper-formed. The technique followed is as described in the previous paragraph; however, the impression surface is made conductive by the application of finely divided silver powder. The increased cost of silver and the increasing difficulties in obtaining cyanide-silver plating solutions because of transport restrictions have resulted in the return to copper electroformed dies.

Silver-Formed Dies With the advent of the polysulfide impression materials, silver forming was used to make metal dies. Although it is possible to copper-form polysulfide impression materials, consistent results are not always obtained, and the much easier procedure of silver forming lends itself to routine use. The alkaline silver baths used in silver forming soften the surface of impression compound, and silver forming cannot be used. Silicone and polyether impressions can also be silver-formed. A pure silver anode is required, with a silver-cyanide plating solution, an example of which is given in Table 12-16.

TABLE 12-16 Composition of Solution for Silver-Forming Bath

Ingredient	Amount
Silver cyanide	36 g
Potassium cyanide	60 g
Potassium carbonate	45 g
Water (distilled)	1000 ml

This solution is poisonous, and extreme care should be taken that the hands, workbench area, and clothing not become contaminated. This operation should not be used by inexperienced personnel. The addition of acid to the solution produces hydrogen cyanide, an extremely poisonous gas, and for this reason copper-forming solutions should be kept well away, as should any acid. The plating bath should have a cover that can be in place at all times to control evaporation and dissipation of fumes.

The impression is made conductive when the surface is brushed with powdered silver, which adheres well to rubber impressions. Alternatively, dispersions of silver powder in a volatile liquid vehicle are available, and they are painted on and allowed to dry.

A current setting of approximately 5 mA is suitable to start the plating of a single-tooth impression. Once a layer of silver has been deposited over the surface, this current can be doubled or tripled. With larger impressions involving several teeth and the adjacent soft tissue areas, a current of approximately 10 mA/tooth is suitable for initial plating. This can be doubled or tripled once the surface is covered, and usually about 12 to 15 hours of plating produce a suitable thickness of silver.

Distilled water should be added to the electrolyte to replace any loss from evaporation, and the solution should be filtered from time to time. A polysulfide impression that has been silver-formed is shown in Fig. 12-30, *A*. The model made from this silver-formed impression by pouring stone and removing the impression after the stone has set is shown in Fig. 12-30, *B*.

A 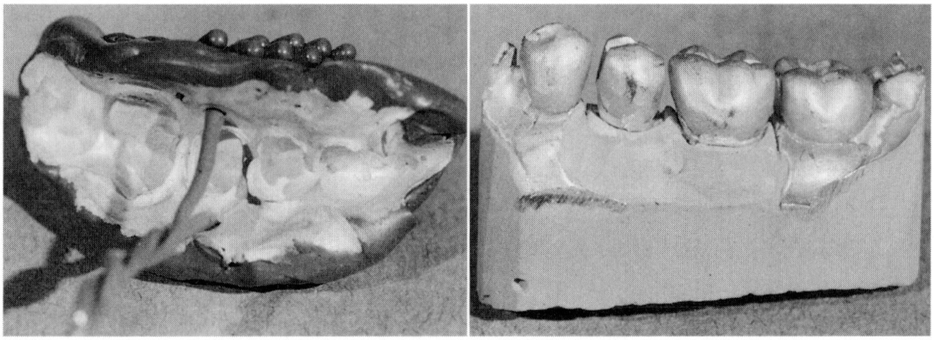 B

Fig. 12-30 A, Polysulfide impression showing connecting wires and layer of silver deposited by electroforming. **B,** Silver-formed model with stone base made from impression in **A.**

Problems in Metal-Forming Among the problems encountered in metal forming are the obvious effects caused by current failure, either in the domestic power line or from some defect in the plating apparatus. However, even if the working apparatus is satisfactory, there are problems related to the procedure itself that are sometimes puzzling.

Faulty Conduction The ammeter may show a current flow, but the impression does not plate or plates irregularly or very slowly. This difficulty is caused by a short circuit through the electrolyte, usually because of exposure of the conducting wire to the solution.

Exhausted Solution Plating is very slow, and the deposit is discolored. The solution should be discarded and replaced with a fresh solution. How long a solution lasts depends on the degree of usage and whether contamination occurs. A well-filtered solution protected from contamination and kept to correct concentration by adding distilled water when required gives the longest life. Cyanide solutions must be disposed of carefully.

Overconcentrated Solution Sometimes the ammeter reading drops rapidly to zero after the impression is placed in the bath. Resetting of the current regulator to establish the correct ammeter setting is followed by another drop of the ammeter reading to zero. This effect is caused by an overconcentrated solution. Adding the required amount of distilled water and rinsing the metal anode in distilled water solves the problem. An overconcentrated solution may also soften the surface of the rubber and discolor any stone areas of the cast.

Metal Anode Too Small An anode that is smaller in area than the impression or impressions to be plated leads to slow and irregular plating.

Friable Metal Deposit If the metal deposit is granular and friable, although of correct color, the current setting is too high.

EPOXY DIE MATERIALS

Until recently, epoxy materials were supplied in the form of a paste to which a liquid activator (amine) was added to initiate hardening. Because the activators are toxic, they should not come into contact with the skin during mixing and manipulation of the unset material. Shrinkage of 0.1% has occurred during hardening, which may take up to 24 hours. The hardened resin is more resistant to abrasion and stronger than a high-strength stone die. The viscous paste is not as readily introduced into the details of a large impression as high-strength dental stone is; a centrifugal casting machine has been developed to assist in the pouring of epoxy resins. Recently, fast-setting epoxy materials have been supplied in automixing systems similar to those described for automixing addition silicones and shown in Fig. 12-31. The epoxy resin is in one cartridge, and the catalyst in the other. Forcing the two pastes through the static mixing tip thoroughly mixes the epoxy material, which can be directly injected into a rubber impression. A small intraoral delivery tip may be attached to the static-mixing tip if desired for injecting into detailed areas of the impression. The fast-setting epoxy hardens rapidly, so dies can be waxed 30 minutes after injecting into the impression. Because water retards the polymerization of resin, epoxy resins cannot be used with water-containing agar and alginate impression materials, and thus are limited to use with rubber impression materials.

COMPARISON OF IMPRESSION AND DIE MATERIALS

High-strength stone dies may be from 0.35% larger to 0.25% smaller than the master, depending on the location of the measurement and the impression material used. In general, occlusogingival (vertical) changes are greater than buccolingual or mesiodistal (horizontal) changes. The shrinkage of the impression material toward the surfaces of the tray in the horizontal direction usually results in dimensions larger than the master. In the vertical direction, shrinkage is away from the free surface of the impression and toward the tray, and dimensions smaller than the master are obtained.

Invariably, metal-formed dies show more vertical change than high-strength stone dies, with the differences being between 0.25% and 0.45%, depending on the impression materials, whereas the horizontal changes are not significantly different for the two die materials. The accuracy of rubber impression materials is in the following order from best to worst, regardless of whether stone or metal dies are used: addition silicone, polyether, polysulfide, and condensation silicone.

Epoxy dies all exhibit some polymerization shrinkage, with values ranging from 0.1% to 0.3%, and as a result the dies are undersized.

Ranking materials by the ability of an impression-die combination to reproduce surface detail produces different results than does ranking by values for dimensional change. If a release agent is not needed on the surface of the impression, epoxy dies are best for reproducing detail (10 μm), followed by metal-formed dies (30 μm), and high-strength stone dies (170 μm). However, polysulfide impressions require the use of a release agent with epoxy dies, and their reproduction of detail is comparable to that obtained with high-strength stone. The silicone-epoxy combination produces the sharpest detail, although not all epoxy die materials are compatible with all silicone impression materials.

Resistance to abrasion and scraping should

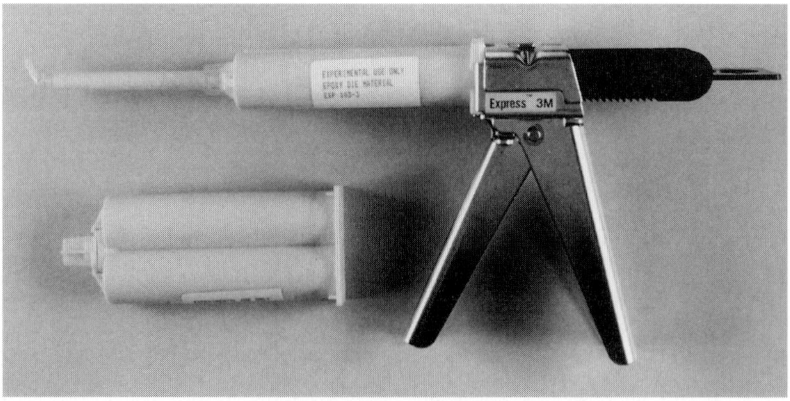

Fig. 12-31 Automix system for fast-setting epoxy die material.

also be considered. Metal-formed dies have superior resistance to abrasion, epoxy dies have good resistance, and high-strength stone dies have the least resistance.

SELECTED PROBLEMS

Problem 1

A mix of alginate was made, and the setting time was shorter than previously experienced with this brand. The material was too stiff at the time of insertion to obtain adequate seating and surface detail. What factors should be considered in the correction of this difficulty?

Solution a

The most common cause for the shorter setting time is too high a temperature of the mix water. The setting reaction is a typical chemical reaction that is accelerated by increases in temperature; a 10° C increase in temperature almost doubles the rate of the reaction. In many operations, a single water faucet is present with a mixing valve to control the temperature of the water. Gradual failure of the mixing valve can inadvertently result in the use of water substantially hotter than the 21° C usually recommended.

Solution b

The setting time can also be shortened by incorrect dispensing resulting in too high a powder/liquid ratio. If the alginate powder is not aerated before each dispensing, the weight of each scoop will be too high, because the apparent density of the powder is higher after standing. The increased amount of powder causes the setting or gelation time to be less than normally experienced.

Solution c

Aging of the alginate powder in a warm, humid atmosphere can affect the setting by reducing the effectiveness of the retarder, resulting in a shorter-than-normal setting time.

Problem 2

A mix of alginate was made, and it appeared thicker than normal. After the impression was taken, its surface seemed grainy and lacking in surface detail. What precautions should be taken to avoid this condition when the impression is retaken?

Solution

A thick consistency can result from lack of aeration of the powder before dispensing, or from an incorrect number of measures of powder or water. However, a thick, grainy mix can occur from inadequate mixing of the correct proportions of powder and water. Inadequate mixing may be caused by casual rather than vigorous spatulation or by not mixing for the full time recommended. Hot water used in combination with the two factors just mentioned accentuates the problem of thick, grainy mixes. If the next mix is carefully dispensed, the temperature of the water checked, and the length of mixing timed, a smooth, creamy consistency should result.

Problem 3

An alginate impression was taken of a patient with a fixed appliance, and tearing of the impression occurred in critical areas as a result of severely undercut areas. What can be done to improve the next impression, because alginate impressions are supposed to be elastic?

Solution

It is true that alginate impressions are flexible, although they are not entirely elastic (they exhibit incomplete recovery) and have rather low resistance to tearing compared with elastomeric impression materials. Several precautions can be taken to improve the chances of an acceptable impression. The severely undercut areas can be blocked out, thus placing less stress on the alginate during removal. Recall that the strength of the alginate improves quite rapidly for 5 to 10 minutes after setting, and the impression can be left in the mouth a few extra minutes before removal. Also, remember that the tear strength is a function of the rate of removal of the impression, and rapid rates enhance the chances of an acceptable impression. Finally, mixes with high powder/liquid ratios have higher tear strengths; however, to obtain a smooth consistency that will record the desired level of surface detail, the ratio must not be increased beyond the limit.

Problem 4

An alginate impression is to be taken of a patient known to have a problem with gagging. What steps can be taken in materials management to reduce the problem and yet obtain a satisfactory impression?

Solution a

The viscosity of mixed alginates remains fairly constant until just before the setting time because the retardation reaction prevents the formation of the calcium alginate gel. When the working and setting times are known accurately, insertion of the impression material into the mouth can be delayed until just before the end of the working time, but allowing enough time to seat the impression. The impression should then be removed at the earliest possible time after it sets but while it still has adequate properties. Thus the impression is in the mouth the shortest possible time.

Solution b

A fast-setting alginate can be selected that not only sets in a shorter time but has better mechanical properties in a shorter time than regular-setting material.

Solution c

Care should be taken during the loading of the maxillary impression tray to avoid excessive amounts of alginate in the posterior portion of the tray. The posterior part of the tray should be seated before the anterior portion, with the patient's head in a position to avoid excess alginate flowing in a posterior direction on the palate.

Problem 5

The set alginate impression separated from the tray during removal from the mouth, resulting in distortion and tearing of the impression. What can be done to avoid this?

Solution

Two choices can be made. A change in the brand of alginate to one that adheres to the metal tray is one option. However, if a non-adhesive alginate is desired, select a tray with perforations that provides mechanical retention. Secondly, use commercial tray adhesives specifically formulated for retention of alginate impressions.

Problem 6

An inaccurate model is obtained despite the use of the correct mixing technique for the alginate and the proper pouring procedure for the gypsum model. What possible factors might have resulted in the inaccurate impression?

Solution a

The tray selected may have been too small, thus providing too little alginate between the tray and the tissues. During the removal of the set alginate, the percent compression may have been too high when the bulge of the tooth compressed the alginate in the undercut areas. This excessive compression results in higher than normal permanent deformation. Correct the problem by selecting a tray that provides about 5 mm of space between the tray and tissues. With the same amount of undercut, the alginate is subjected to lower percent compression, and lower permanent deformation results.

Solution b

A second possible cause of the problem could be the premature removal of the impression. The permanent deformation of the impression on removal decreases with the time after setting. Therefore premature removal of the impression, even though the material is no longer tacky, can be the cause of excessive permanent deformation of the impression in undercut areas.

Solution c

A third possible cause of the inaccurate impression might be a too-slow rate of removal of the set impression material. With everything else being equal, a slow rate of removal rather than a snap removal results in higher than normal amounts of permanent deformation.

Solution d

A fourth reason for the difficulty might be overextension of the alginate to areas not supported by the tray. The weight of these overextended areas can deform the impression; if they are not cut away, deformation and permanent distortion of the impression in these areas can occur.

Solution e

Finally, the alginate impression can be permanently distorted if after removal it is stored in such a manner that the impression is deformed. Two possible conditions could cause this effect: placing the impression down with the weight of the tray on it, and wrapping the impression too tightly in a damp towel.

Problem 7

When an impression was taken using polysulfide impression material, a number of voids appeared on the surface of the impressions of the teeth and abutment preparations. What is the reason for such a failure, and how can it be avoided?

Solution

Some air bubbles are always incorporated into the pastes during the manufacturing process, and these bubbles can be observed when dispensing the pastes onto the paper pad. The mixing of the base and catalyst pastes should be done carefully to avoid incorporating air into the mixture. After the two pastes are initially mixed, the material must be spatulated and spread over the widest area possible and flattened to form a thin layer over the surface of the pad. The spatula must be kept in contact with the mixture so that air bubbles are eliminated. The material is gathered up with the straight edge of the blade and redeposited onto the paper pad, then mixing is continued with a wiping, pressing motion until a homogeneous mix is obtained.

Problem 8

On critical observation of an impression obtained with a polysulfide material, it was found that some areas were incompletely reproduced. What is the cause of these large voids, and how can they be avoided?

Solution

The setting time of polysulfide elastomeric impression materials is affected by humidity. Delay in injecting the low-consistency syringe material results in a higher-viscosity material, reducing the flow, and thus a large area is incompletely produced. Also, the impression does not effectively displace saliva from the surface of the tooth.

This type of failure may be avoided by isolating the field with cotton rolls, drying it carefully with air blasts, and then using a syringe with a low-consistency material (at the correct time after mixing under proper conditions) to cover the teeth and gum surfaces before placing the high-consistency material with the tray.

Problem 9

When a polysulfide impression was withdrawn from the mouth, the impression material was separated from the tray in some areas. What caused this separation, and how accurate are the dies obtained from such an impression?

Solution

The adhesion of an impression material to the custom-made tray is obtained by coating the tray with an adhesive. To get good adhesion to the tray, use enough coats of the adhesive. It is also necessary to wait until the volatile organic solvent evaporates and the adhesive is dry. When the tray is filled with the high-consistency material too soon after applying the adhesive, the retention fails and the impression material separates from the tray. In this instance, a distortion of the impression is always present and results in a distorted model and dies. It is better to remake the impression than to continue with the procedure. When the failure is caused by the adhesive itself, better mechanical retention for the impression material can be obtained by making perforations with a bur in the same type of custom-made tray. These mechanical interlocks retain the impression material in position, and the uniform thickness of impression material in the custom-made tray helps control the polymerization shrinkage of the material.

Problem 10

Preparation of a complete-arch fixed bridge was completed, a wash impression with a condensation silicone was taken, and a single cast was obtained as a master model. The metal frame of the bridge fit perfectly on the cast but did not fit well on all abutments. Is this a problem of the impression material, and how can it be solved? What factors may have produced this problem?

Solution a

Polymerization shrinkage occurs with condensation silicone material. Dimensional change in these silicone materials increases with time up to 24 hours, although about half the change takes place in the first hour. The longer the impression is left on the bench before the cast is poured, the greater the shrinkage of the material. Usually, some castings fit individual abutments, but when such a cast is used as a master model to make the fixed prosthesis, the general accuracy is unsatisfactory.

Solution b

Distortion may be produced as a result of relaxation of stresses in the impression. If the impression is removed from the mouth when polymerization has not progressed sufficiently, stresses may be induced in the mass and a distorted impression is obtained. A distorted impression can result from excessive pressure on the material during setting, which produces residual stresses that can be relieved.

Solution c

Distortion can be produced when the impression is removed with slow movements. Like all elastic impression materials, condensation silicone impressions must be removed from the mouth with a sudden motion. A slow removal induces permanent deformation in the mass, and an inaccurate cast is obtained. If a fixed appliance is made on such a cast, it will not fit on all teeth preparations. Note that less permanent deformation occurs with silicone than with polysulfide impressions.

Solution d

Distortion may result when too much space is provided between the tray and teeth. The amount of silicone impression material between the tray and the abutments should be small. A thin layer is better than a thick mass because less permanent deformation occurs during the removal of the impression and more-accurate dies and models will be obtained.

Problem 11

An impression of a dentulous quadrant was taken with a medium-consistency polyether impression material in a custom-made acrylic tray. The normal relief of 2 mm was provided between the tray and the oral structures. After removal of the impression, tearing was noted at several locations. What adjustments can be made so that the possibility of tearing will be minimized on retaking the impression?

Solution a

Polyethers adhere quite well to hard and soft tissues and the medium consistency is quite stiff when set (low strain in compression). The adhesion and stiffness, combined with moderate tear strength, increases the probability of tearing of the impression. Before removal, first break the seal of the impression to tissues by pulling the impression slightly in the vestibular area. Syringing water into the area can also help break the seal. Finally, increase the relief space between the tray and the tissues to at least 4 mm to allow greater flexibility of impression material, thereby improving the ease of removal.

Solution b

Use the new, softened, medium-consistency polyether impression material in the tray; it is less rigid and possesses reduced Shore A hardness in the set condition. Also, provide additional relief space between the tray and the tissues (at least 4 mm) to increase the effective flexibility of the elastomer.

Problem 12

The manufacturer of an addition-silicone impression specified that high-strength stone dies should not be poured until after 1 hour. An epoxy die was desired, and therefore pouring was delayed for 1 hour. On separation, the die was covered with negative bubbles. What caused the problem, and how can it be avoided?

Solution

Some brands of addition silicones release hydrogen after setting. Waiting 1 hour before pouring the fast-setting, high-strength stone allows the rate of hydrogen release to decrease sufficiently so bubble-free dies can be produced. However, many epoxy die materials set slowly compared with high-strength stone, and sufficient hydrogen is still being released at 1 hour to produce bubbles on the surface of the epoxy die. Even waiting 4 hours may not result in a bubble-free epoxy die. Allowing the impression to stand overnight before pouring the epoxy die solves the problem. Also, note that the accuracy of addition-silicone impressions is excellent at 24 hours, even with the evolution of hydrogen.

Problem 13

An impression, taken in a non-hydrophilized addition silicone, had been mixed by hand spatulation. The resulting high-strength stone die had enough positive and negative bubbles, especially along the internal line angles and finish lines of the preparation, so a retake of the impression was necessary. What could be done to reduce the number of bubbles?

Solution

Changing to an addition silicone supplied in automixing cartridges substantially reduces the number of bubbles in the mix, compared with one prepared by hand spatulation, and minimizes the number of positive bubbles. In addition, changing to hydrophilized, automixing addition silicone decreases the number of negative bubbles in the die because of the better wetting of the impression by the mix of high-strength stone.

BIBLIOGRAPHY

Review Articles—Impression Materials

Allen EP, Bayne SC, Becker IM et al: Annual review of selected dental literature: report of the committee on scientific investigation of the American Academy of Restorative Dentistry, *J Prosthet Dent* 82:50, 1999.

Allen EP, Bayne SC, Donovan TE et al: Annual review of selected dental literature, *J Prosthet Dent* 76:75, 1996.

Craig RG: Review of dental impression materials, *Adv Dent Res* 2:51, 1988.

Jendresen MD, Allen EP, Bayne SC et al: Annual review of selected dental literature: report of the committee on scientific investigation of the American Academy of Restorative Dentistry, *J Prosthet Dent* 80:105, 1998.

Jendresen MD, Allen EP, Bayne SC et al: Annual review of selected dental literature: report of the committee on scientific investigation of the American Academy of Restorative Dentistry, *J Prosthet Dent* 78:77, 1997.

Jendresen MD, Allen EP, Bayne SC et al: Annual review of selected dental literature: report of the committee on scientific investigation of the American Academy of Restorative Dentistry, *J Prosthet Dent* 74:88, 1995.

Lloyd CH, Scrimgeour SN, editors: Dental materials: 1994 literature review, *J Dent* 24:171, 1996.

Lloyd CH, Scrimgeour SN, editors: Dental materials: 1995 literature review, *J Dent* 25:193, 1997.

Whitters CJ, Strang R, Brown D et al: Dental materials: 1997 literature review, *J Dent* 27:421, 1999.

Agar and Alginate Hydrocolloids

Appleby DC, Pameijer CH, Boffa J: The combined reversible hydrocolloid/irreversible hydrocolloid impression system, *J Prosthet Dent* 44:27, 1980.

Bergman B, Bergman M, Olsson S: Alginate impression materials, dimensional stability and surface detail sharpness following treatment with disinfectant solutions, *Swed Dent J* 9:255, 1985.

Brune D, Beltesbrekke H: Levels of airborne particles resulting from handling alginate impression material, *Scand J Dent Res* 86:206, 1978.

Buchan S, Peggie RW: Role of ingredients in alginate impression compounds, *J Dent Res* 45:1120, 1966.

Carlyle LW, III: Compatibility of irreversible hydrocolloid impression materials with dental stones, *J Prosthet Dent* 49:434, 1983.

Craig RG: Mechanical properties of some recent alginates and tensile bond strengths of agar/alginate combinations, *Phillip's J Rest Zahnmed* 6:242, 1989.

Cserna A, Crist R, Adams A et al: Irreversible hydrocolloids: a comparison of antimicrobial efficacy, *J Prosthet Dent* 71:387, 1994.

Durr DP, Novak EV: Dimensional stability of alginate impressions immersed in disinfection solutions, *J Dent Child* 54:45, 1987.

Ellis B, Lamb DJ: The setting characteristics of alginate impression materials, *Br Dent J* 151:343, 1981.

Farah JW, Powers JM, editors: Crown and bridge impression materials, *Dent Advis* 6:1,1989.

Farah JW, Powers JM, editors: Impression materials for fixed prosthodontics, *Dent Advis* 14:4, 1997.

Farah JW, Powers JM, editors: Bite registration materials, *Dent Advis* 15:4, 1998.

Fish SF, Braden M: Characterization of the setting process in alginate impression materials, *J Dent Res* 43:107, 1964.

Ghani F, Hobkirk JA, Wilson M: Evaluation of a new antiseptic-containing alginate impression material, *Br Dent J* 169:83, 1990.

Herrero SP, Merchant VA: Dimensional stability of dental impressions after immersion disinfection, *J Am Dent Assoc* 113:419, 1986.

Hilton T, Schwartz R, Bradley D: Immersion disinfection of irreversible hydrocolloid impressions. Part II: effects on gypsum casts, *Int J Prosthodont* 7:424, 1994.

Hutchings MI, Vanderwalle K, Schwartz R et al: Immersion disinfection of irreversible hydrocolloid impressions in pH-adjusted sodium hypochlorite. Part 2: effect on gypsum casts, *Int J Prosthodont* 9:223, 1996.

Jarvis RG, Earnshaw R: The effects of alginate impressions on the surface of cast gypsum. I. The physical and chemical structure of the cast surface, *Aust Dent J* 25:349, 1980.

Jarvis RG, Earnshaw R: The effect of alginate impressions on the surface of cast gypsum. II. The role of sodium phosphate in incompatibility, *Aust Dent J* 26:12, 1981.

Johnson GH, Chellis KD, Gordon GE et al: Dimensional stability and detail reproduction of alginate and elastomeric impressions disinfected by immersion, *J Prosthet Dent* 79:446, 1998.

Johnson GH, Craig RG: Accuracy and bond strength of combinations of agar/alginate hydrocolloid impression materials, *J Prosthet Dent* 55:1, 1986.

Lewinstein I, Craig RG: The effect of powder/water ratio of irreversible hydrocolloid on the bond strength of irreversible hydrocolloid and agar combinations, *J Prosthet Dent* 62:412, 1989.

MacPherson GW, Craig RG, Peyton FA: Mechanical properties of hydrocolloid and elastomeric impression materials, *J Dent Res* 46:714, 1967.

Matyas J, Dao N, Caputo AS et al: Effects of disinfectants on dimensional accuracy of impression materials, *J Prosthet Dent* 64:25, 1990.

Miller MW: Syneresis in alginate impression materials, *Br Dent J* 139:425, 1975.

Peutzfeldt A, Asmussen E: Effect of disinfecting solutions on accuracy of alginate and elastomeric impressions, *Scand J Dent Res* 97:470, 1989.

Peutzfeldt A, Asmussen E: Effect of disinfecting solutions on surface texture of alginate and elastomeric impressions, *Scand J Dent Res* 98:74, 1990.

Sawyer HF, Sandrik JL, Neiman R: Accuracy of casts produced from alginate and hydrocolloid impression materials, *J Am Dent Assoc* 93:806, 1976.

Schwartz R, Bradley D, Hilton T et al: Immersion disinfection of irreversible hydrocolloid impressions. Part I: microbiology, *Int J Prosthodont* 7:418, 1994.

Vanderwalle K, Charlton D, Schwartz R et al: Immersion disinfection of irreversible hydrocolloid impressions with sodium hypochlorite. Part II: effect on gypsum, *Int J Prosthodont* 7:315, 1994.

Wanis TM, Combe EC, Grant AA: Measurement of the viscosity of irreversible hydrocolloids, *J Oral Rehabil* 20:379, 1993.

Woodward JD, Morris JC, Khan Z: Accuracy of stone casts produced by perforated trays and nonperforated trays, *J Prosthet Dent* 53:347, 1985.

Woody RD, Huget EF, Cutright DE: Characterization of airborne particles from irreversible hydrocolloids, *J Am Dent Assoc* 94:501, 1977.

Duplicating Materials

Craig RG, Gehring PE, Peyton FA: Aging characteristics of elastic duplicating compounds, *J Dent Res* 41:196, 1962.

Craig RG, Peyton FA: Physical properties of elastic duplicating materials, *J Dent Res* 39:391, 1960.

Finger W: Accuracy of dental duplicating materials, *Quint Dent Tech* 10:89, 1986.

Lyon FF, Anderson JN: Some agar duplicating materials: an evaluation of their properties, *Br Dent J* 132:15, 1972.

Peyton FA, Craig RG: Compatibility of duplicating compound and casting investments, *J Prosthet Dent* 12:1111, 1962.

Properties and Use of Elastomeric Impression Materials

Baumann MA: The influence of dental gloves on the setting of impression materials, *Br Dent J* 179:130, 1995.

Bell JW, Davies EH, von Fraunhofer JA: The dimensional changes of elastomeric impression materials under various conditions of humidity, *J Dent* 4:73, 1976.

Boening KW, Walter MH, Schuette U: Clinical significance of surface activation of silicone impression materials, *J Dent* 26:447, 1998.

Braden M: Characterization of the setting process in dental polysulfide rubbers, *J Dent Res* 45:1065, 1966.

Braden M, Causton B, Clarke RL: A polyether impression rubber, *J Dent Res* 51:889, 1972.
Braden M, Inglis AT: Visco-elastic properties of dental elastomeric impression materials, *Biomater* 7:45, 1986.
Bissinger P, Wanek E, Zech J: Polyethercarbosilanes—a new class of wetting agents for impression materials, *J Dent Res* 76 (Spec Issue): 422 (Abstract 3268), 1997.
Bissinger P, Wanek E, Zech J: Disinfection behaviour of hydrophilic polyvinyl siloxane impression materials, *J Dent Res* 77 (Spec Issue B): 946 (Abstract 2517), 1998.
Chai J, Pand IC: A study of the thixotropic property of elastomeric impression materials, *Int J Prosthodont* 7:155, 1994.
Chong YH, Soh G: Effectiveness of intraoral delivery tips in reducing voids in elastomeric impressions, *Quint Int* 22:897, 1991.
Cook WD: Permanent set and stress relaxation in elastomeric impression materials, *J Biomed Mater Res* 15:44, 1981.
Cook WD: Rheological studies of the polymerization of elastomeric impression materials. I. Network structure of the set state, *J Biomed Mater Res* 16:315, 1982.
Cook WD: Rheological studies of the polymerization of elastomeric impression materials. II. Viscosity measurements, *J Biomed Mater Res* 16:331, 1982.
Cook WD: Rheological studies of the polymerization of elastomeric impression materials. III. Dynamic stress relaxation modulus, *J Biomed Mater* Res 16:345, 1982.
Cook WD, Liem F, Russo P et al: Tear and rupture of elastomeric dental impression materials, *Biomater* 5:275, 1984.
Cook WD, Thomasz F: Rubber gloves and addition silicone materials, *Aust Dent J* 31:140, 1986.
Council on Dental Materials and Devices: Status report on polyether impression materials, *J Am Dent Assoc* 95:126, 1977.
Craig RG: Composition, characteristics and clinical and tissue reactions of impression materials. In Smith DC, Williams DF, editors: *Biocompatibility of dental materials,* vol 3, Biocompatibility of dental restorative materials, Boca Raton, Fla, 1982, CRC Press.
Craig RG: Evaluation of an automatic mixing system for an addition silicone impression material, *J Am Dent Assoc* 110:213, 1985.
Craig RG: Properties of 12 addition silicones compared with other rubber impression materials, *Phillip's J Rest Zahnmed* 3:244, 1986.
Craig RG, Sun Z: Trends in elastomeric impression materials, *Oper Dent* 19:138, 1994.
Craig RG, Urquiola NJ, Liu CC: Comparison of commercial elastomeric impression materials, *Oper Dent* 15:94, 1990.
Goldberg AJ: Viscoelastic properties of silicone, polysulfide, and polyether impression materials, *J Dent Res* 53:1033, 1974.
Gordon GE, Johnson GH, Drennon DG: The effect of tray selection on the accuracy of elastomeric impression materials, *J Prosthet Dent* 63:12, 1990.
Herfort TW, Gerberich WW, Macosko CW et al: Viscosity of elastomeric impression materials, *J Prosthet Dent* 38:396, 1977.
Herfort TW, Gerberich WW, Macosko CW et al: Tear strength of elastomeric impression materials, *J Prosthet Dent* 39:59, 1978.
Hondrum S: Tear and energy properties of three impression materials, *Int J Prosthodont* 7:155, 1994.
Idris B, Houston F, Claffey N: Comparison of the dimensional accuracy of one-step techniques with the use of putty/wash addition silicone impression materials, *J Prosthet Dent* 74:535, 1995.
Inoue K, Wilson HJ: Viscoelastic properties of elastomeric impression materials. II. Variation of rheological properties with time, temperature and mixing proportions, *J Oral Rehabil* 5:261, 1978.

Johansson EG, Erhardson S, Wictorin L: Influence of stone mixing agents, impression materials and lubricants on surface hardness and dimensions of a dental stone die material, *Acta Odontol Scand* 33:17, 1975.

Johnson GH, Craig RG: Accuracy of four types of rubber impression materials compared with time of pour and a repeat pour of models, *J Prosthet Dent* 53:484, 1985.

Johnson GH, Craig RG: Accuracy of addition silicones as a function of technique, *J Prosthet Dent* 55:197, 1986.

Johnson GH, Lepe X, Aw TC: Detail reproduction for single versus dual viscosity impression techniques. *J Dent Res* 78 (Spec Issue B):140 (Abstract 273), 1999.

Kim KN, Craig RG, Koran A III: Viscosity of monophase addition silicones as a function of shear rate, *J Prosthet Dent* 67:794, 1992.

Koran A, Powers JM, Craig RG: Apparent viscosity of materials used for making edentulous impressions, *J Am Dent Assoc* 95:75, 1977.

Laufer BZ, Baharav H, Ganor Y et al: The effect of marginal thickness on the distortion of different impression materials, *J Prosthet Dent* 76:466, 1996.

Lee IK, Delong R, Pintado MR et al: Evaluation of factors affecting the accuracy of impressions using quantitative surface analysis, *Oper Dent* 20:246, 1995.

Lepe X, Johnson GH, Berg JC et al: Effect of mixing technique on surface characteristics of impression materials, *J Prosthet Dent* 79:495, 1998.

Lorren RA, Salter DJ, Fairhurst CW: The contact angles of die stone on impression materials, *J Prosthet Dent* 36:176, 1976.

Mansfield MA, Wilson HJ: Elastomeric impression materials: a comparison of methods for determining working and setting times, *Br Dent J* 132:106, 1972.

McCabe JF, Arikawa H: Rheological properties of elastomeric impression materials before and during setting, *J Dent Res* 77:1874, 1998.

McCabe JF, Bowman AJ: The rheological properties of dental impression materials, *Br Dent J* 151:179, 1981.

McCabe JF, Storer R: Elastomeric impression materials. The measurement of some properties relevant to clinical practice, *Br Dent J* 149:73, 1980.

Neissen LC, Strassler H, Levinson PD et al: Effect of latex gloves on setting time of polyvinylsiloxane putty impression material, *J Prosthet Dent* 55:128, 1986.

Norling BK, Reisbick MH: The effect of nonionic surfactants on bubble entrapment in elastomeric impression materials, *J Prosthet Dent* 42:342, 1979.

Ohsawa M, Jorgensen KD: Curing contraction of addition-type silicone impression materials, *Scand J Dent Res* 91:51, 1983.

Pang IC, Chai J. The effect of a shear load on the viscosities of ten vinyl polysiloxane impression materials, *J Prosthet Dent* 71:177, 1994.

Pratten DH, Craig RG: Wettability of a hydrophilic addition silicone impression material, *J Prosthet Dent* 61:197, 1989.

Reusch B, Weber B: In precision impressions—a guide for theory and practice, theoretical section, Seefeld, Germany, 1999, ESPE Dental AG.

Rueda LJ, Sy-Munoz JT, Naylor WP et al: The effect of using custom or stock trays on the accuracy of gypsum casts, *Int J Prosthodont* 9:367, 1996.

Salem NS, Combe EC, Watts DC: Mechanical properties of elastomeric impression materials, *J Oral Rehabil* 15:125, 1988.

Sandrik JL, Vacco JL: Tensile and bond strength of putty-wash elastomeric impression materials, *J Prosthet Dent* 50:358, 1983.

Schelb E, Cavazos E Jr, Troendle KB et al: Surface detail reproduction of Type IV dental stones with selected polyvinyl siloxane impression materials, *Quint Int* 22:51, 1991.

Sneed WD, Miller R, Olean J: Tear strength of ten elastomeric impression materials, *J Prosthet Dent* 49:511, 1983.

Stackhouse JA Jr: The accuracy of stone dies made from rubber impression materials, *J Prosthet Dent* 24:377, 1970.

Stackhouse JA Jr: Relationship of syringe-tip diameter to voids in elastomeric impressions, *J Prosthet Dent* 53:812, 1985.

Tolley LG, Craig RG: Viscoelastic properties of elastomeric impression materials, *J Oral Rehabil* 5:121, 1978.

Vermilyea SG, Huget EF, de Simon LB: Apparent viscosities of setting elastomers, *J Dent Res* 59:1149, 1980.

Williams JR, Craig RG: Physical properties of addition silicones as a function of composition, *J Oral Rehabil* 15:639, 1988.

Disinfection of Elastomeric Impression Materials

Bergman M, Olsson S, Bergman B: Elastomeric impression materials: dimensional stability and surface sharpness following treatment with disinfection solutions, *Swed Dent J* 4:161, 1980.

Drennon DG, Johnson GH: The effect of immersion disinfection of elastomeric impressions on the surface detail reproduction of improved gypsum casts, *J Prosthet Dent* 63:233, 1990.

Drennon DG, Johnson GH, Powell GL: The accuracy and efficacy of disinfection by spray atomization on elastomeric impressions, *J Prosthet Dent* 62:468, 1989.

Johnson GH, Drennon DG, Powell GL: Accuracy of elastomeric impressions disinfected by immersion, *J Am Dent Assoc* 116:525, 1988.

Lepe X, Johnson GH: Accuracy of polyether and addition silicone after long-term immersion disinfection, *J Prosthet Dent* 78:245, 1997.

Lepe X, Johnson GH, Berg JC: Surface characteristics of polyether and addition silicone impression materials after long term disinfection, *J Prosthet Dent* 74: 181, 1995.

Rios MdP, Morgano SM, Stein RS et al: Effects of chemical disinfectant solutions on the stability and accuracy of the dental impression complex, *J Prosthet Dent* 76:356, 1996.

Storer R, McCabe JF: An investigation of methods available for sterilising impressions, *Br Dent J* 151:217, 1981.

Thouati A, Deveraux E, Lost A et al: Dimensional stability of seven elastomeric impression materials immersed in disinfectants, *J Prosthet Dent* 76:8, 1996.

Zinc Oxide–Eugenol Pastes

Brauer GM, White EE, Moshonas MG: Reaction of metal oxides with o-ethoxy benzoic acid and other chelating agents, *J Dent Res* 37:547, 1958.

Copeland HI, Brauer GM, Sweeney WT et al: Setting reaction of zinc oxide and eugenol, *J Res Nat Bur Stand* 55:133, 1955.

Harvey W, Petch NJ: Acceleration of the setting of zinc oxide cements, *Br Dent J* 80:1, 1946; 80:35, 1946.

Kelly EB: Dental impression paste, US Patent No 2,077,418, April 20, 1937.

Myers GE, Peyton FA: Physical properties of the zinc oxide–eugenol impression pastes, *J Dent Res* 40:39, 1961.

Olsson S, Bergman B, Bergman M: Zinc oxide–eugenol impression materials: dimensional stability and surface detail sharpness following treatment with disinfection solutions, *Swed Dent* J 6:177, 1982.

Smith DC: The setting of zinc oxide–eugenol mixtures, *Br Dent J* 105:313, 1958.

Tyas MJ, Wilson HJ: Properties of zinc oxide/eugenol impression pastes, *Br Dent J* 129:461, 1970.

Ullmann's Encyclopedia of Industrial Chemistry, ed 6, (electronic release), ring opening polymerization, 2000.

Vieira DF: Factors affecting the setting of zinc oxide–eugenol impression pastes, *J Prosthet Dent* 9:70, 1959.

Impression Plaster

Jorgensen KD: Study on the setting of plaster of paris, *Odont Tskr* 61:305, 1953.

Sodeau WH, Gibson CS: The use of plaster of paris as an impression material, *Br Dent J* 48:1089, 1927.

Impression Compound

Bevan EM, Smith DC: Properties of impression compound, *Br Dent J* 114:181, 1963.

Braden M: Rheology of dental composition (impression compound), *J Dent Res* 46:620, 1967.

Combe EC, Smith DC: Further studies on impression compounds, *Dent Pract* 15:292, 1965.

Docking AR: Kneading of modelling compounds, *Aust J Dent* 59:225, 1955.

Stanford JW, Paffenbarger GC, Sweeney WT: Revision of ADA Specification No 3 for dental impression compound, *J Am Dent Assoc* 51:56, 1955.

Chapter 13

Gypsum Products and Investments

Gypsum products probably serve the dental profession more adequately than any other materials. Dental plaster, stone, high-strength/high-expansion stone, and casting investment materials constitute this group of closely related products. With slight modification, gypsum products are used for several different purposes. For example, impression plaster is used to make impressions of edentulous mouths or to mount casts, whereas dental stone is used to form a die that duplicates the oral anatomy when poured into any type of impression. Gypsum products are also used as a binder for silica, gold alloy casting investment, soldering investment, and investment for low-melting-point nickel-chromium alloys. These products are also used as a mold material for processing complete dentures. The main reason for such diversified use is that gypsum materials are unique in nature and their properties can be easily modified by physical and chemical means.

The dihydrate form of calcium sulfate, called *gypsum,* is usually white to milky yellowish in color and is found in a compact mass in nature. The mineral gypsum has commercial importance as a source of plaster of paris. The term *plaster of paris* was given this product because it was obtained by burning the gypsum from deposits near Paris, France. Deposits of gypsum, however, are found in most countries.

CHEMICAL AND PHYSICAL NATURE OF GYPSUM PRODUCTS

Most gypsum products are obtained from natural gypsum rock. Because gypsum is the dihydrate form of calcium sulfate ($CaSO_4 \cdot 2H_2O$), on heating, it loses 1.5 g mol of its 2 g mol of H_2O and is converted to calcium sulfate hemihydrate ($CaSO_4 \cdot \frac{1}{2}H_2O$), sometimes written $(CaSO_4)2 \cdot H_2O$. When calcium sulfate hemihydrate is mixed with water, the reverse reaction takes place, and the calcium sulfate hemihydrate is converted back to calcium sulfate dihydrate. Therefore, partial dehydration of gypsum rock and rehydration of calcium sulfate hemihydrate constitute a reversible reaction. Chemically, the reaction is expressed as shown below.

The reaction is exothermic, and whenever 1 g mol of calcium sulfate hemihydrate is reacted with 1.5 g mol of water, 1 g mol of calcium sulfate dihydrate is formed, and 3900 calories of heat are developed. This chemical reaction takes place regardless of whether the gypsum material is used as an impression material, a die material, or a binder in the casting investment.

MANUFACTURE OF DENTAL PLASTER, STONE, AND HIGH-STRENGTH STONE

Three types of base raw materials are derived from partial dehydration of gypsum rock, depending on the nature of the dehydration process. *Plasters* are fluffy, porous, and least dense, whereas the *hydrocal* variety has a higher density and is more crystalline. *Densite* is the most dense of the raw materials. These three types of raw materials are used to formulate the four types of relatively pure gypsum products used in dentistry. They are classified as plasters (model and laboratory), low- to moderate-strength dental stones, high-strength/low-expansion dental stones, and high-strength/high-expansion dental stones, or alternatively as Types 2, 3, 4, and 5 in ANSI/ADA Specification No. 25 (ISO 6873).

Although these types have identical chemical formulas of calcium sulfate hemihydrate, $CaSO_4 \cdot \frac{1}{2}H_2O$, they possess different physical properties, which makes each of them suitable for a different dental purpose. All four forms are derived from natural gypsum deposits, with the main difference being the manner of driving off part of the water of the calcium sulfate dihydrate.

$$\underset{\text{Plaster of paris}}{CaSO_4 \cdot \tfrac{1}{2}H_2O} + \underset{\text{Water}}{1\tfrac{1}{2}H_2O} \rightarrow \underset{\text{Gypsum}}{CaSO_4 \cdot 2H_2O} + 3900 \text{ cal/g mol}$$

Synthetic gypsum can also be used to formulate some products, but is less popular because of higher manufacturing costs.

Mineral gypsum —(dehydration by heat or other means)→ Plasters —(formulation)→ Model plaster, Lab plaster

Hydrocal ——→ Dental stone

Densite ——→ High-strength dental stone

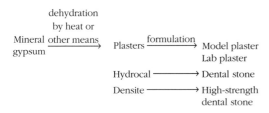

Plasters are produced when the gypsum mineral is heated in an open kettle at a temperature of about 110° to 120° C. The hemihydrate produced is called *β-calcium sulfate hemihydrate.* Such a powder is known to have a somewhat irregular shape and is porous in nature. These plasters are used in formulating model and lab plasters. Crystals of model plaster are shown in Fig. 13-1.

If gypsum is dehydrated under pressure and in the presence of water vapor at about 125° C, the product is called *hydrocal.* The powder particles of this product are more uniform in shape and more dense than the particles of plaster. Crystals of a dental stone are shown in Fig. 13-2. The calcium sulfate hemihydrate produced in this manner is designated as *α-calcium sulfate hemihydrate.* Hydrocal is used in making low- to moderate-strength dental stones.

Types 4 and 5 high-strength dental stones are manufactured with a high-density raw material called *densite.* This variety is made by boiling gypsum rock in a 30% calcium chloride solution, after which the chloride is washed away with hot water (100° C) and the material is ground to the desired fineness. The calcium sulfate hemihydrate in the presence of 100° C water does not react to form calcium sulfate dihydrate because at this temperature their solubilities are the same. The powder obtained by this process is the densest of the types. These materials are generally formulated as high-strength/low-expansion dental stone or high-strength/high-expansion dental stone.

Gypsum products may be formulated with chemicals that modify their handling characteristics and properties. Potassium sulfate, K_2SO_4, and terra alba (set calcium sulfate dihydrate) are

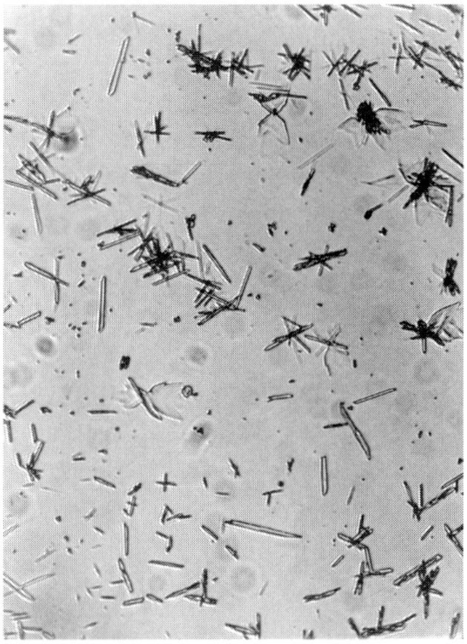

Fig. 13-1 Crystals of model plaster.

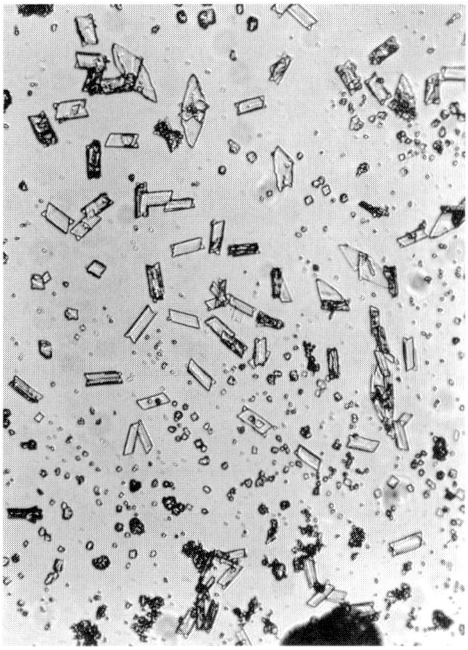

Fig. 13-2 Crystal structure typical of dental stone.

effective accelerators. Sodium chloride in small amounts shortens the setting reaction but increases the setting expansion of the gypsum mass. Sodium citrate is a dependable retarder. Borax, $Na_2B_4O_7$, is both a retarder and accelerator. A mixture of calcium oxide (0.1%) and gum arabic (1%) reduces the amount of water necessary to mix gypsum products, resulting in improved properties. Type 4 gypsum differs from Type 5 in that Type 4 contains extra salts to reduce its setting expansion.

CHEMICAL REACTION

The chemical reaction that takes place during the setting of gypsum products determines the quantity of H_2O needed for the reaction. The reaction of 1 g mol of plaster with 1.5 g mol of water produces 1 g mol of gypsum material. In other words, 145 g of plaster requires 27 g of water to react and form 172 g of gypsum. Therefore 100 g of plaster requires 18.6 g of water to form calcium sulfate dihydrate. As seen in practice, however, model plaster cannot be mixed with such a small amount of water and still develop a mass suitable for manipulation. Table 13-1 shows the recommended mixing water, required water, and excess water for model plaster, dental stone, and high-strength dental stone.

For example, to mix 100 g of model plaster to a usable consistency, use 45 g of water. Note that only 18.6 g of 45 g of water reacts with 100 g of model plaster, and the excess is distributed as free water in the set mass without taking part in the chemical reaction. The excess water is necessary to wet the powder particles during mixing. Naturally, if 100 g of model plaster is mixed with 50 g of water, the resultant mass is thinner and mixes and pours easily into a mold, but the quality of the set gypsum is inferior and weaker than when 45 g of water is used. When model plaster is mixed with a lesser amount of water, the mixed mass is thicker, is more difficult to handle, and traps air bubbles easily when it is poured into a mold, but the set gypsum is usually stronger. Thus, careful control of the proper amount of water in the mix is necessary for proper manipulation and quality of the set mass.

Water/Powder Ratio of Dental Stone and High-Strength Dental Stone The principal difference among model plaster, dental stone, and high-strength dental stone is in the shape and form of the calcium sulfate hemihydrate crystals. Some calcium sulfate hemihydrate crystals are comparatively irregular in shape and porous in nature, as are the crystals in model plaster, whereas the crystals of dental stone and the two high-strength dental stones are dense and more regular in shape, as shown in Figs. 13-1 and 13-2. This difference in the physical shape and nature of the crystals makes it possible to obtain the same consistency with less excess water with dental stone and high-strength dental stones than with model plaster.

In comparison, dental stone requires only about 30 ml of water, and high-strength dental stones require as little as 19 to 24 ml. The difference in their water/powder ratios has a pronounced effect on their compressive strength and resistance to abrasion.

When mixed with water, model plaster, dental stone, or high-strength dental stones set to a hard mass of gypsum. The gypsum products known as

TABLE 13-1 Required and Excess Water for Gypsum Materials*

Gypsum	Mixing Water (ml/100 g of powder)	Required Water (ml/100 g of powder)	Excess Water (ml/100 g of powder)
Model plaster	37-50	18.6	18-31
Dental stone	28-32	18.6	9-13
High-strength dental stones	19-24	18.6	0-5

*Water-powder ratio varies with each product.

high-strength dental stones (Types 4 and 5) are the strongest, the mass produced as model plaster is the weakest, and dental stone produces an intermediate strength material. Note, however, that all gypsum products have the same chemical formula, and that the chemical nature of the masses produced by mixing them with water is also identical; the differences among them are primarily in their physical properties.

Mechanism of Setting The most important and well-recognized theory for the mechanism of the setting is the crystalline theory. It was originated in 1887 by Henry Louis Le Chatelier, a French chemist; in 1907, the theory received the full support of Jacobus Hendricus van't Hoff, a famous Dutch chemist in Berlin at the turn of the century. According to the explanation of van't Hoff, the difference in the solubilities of calcium sulfate dihydrate and hemihydrate causes the setting differences in these materials. Dissolved calcium sulfate precipitates as calcium sulfate dihydrate, because calcium sulfate dihydrate is less soluble than hemihydrate. However, scanning electron microscope and x-ray diffraction studies have shown that not all hemihydrate converts to dihydrate. The residual hemihydrate affects the properties of the set gypsum.

If in a setting mass of plaster two types of centers are distinguished, one for dissolution and the other for precipitation, the dissolution centers are located around the calcium sulfate hemihydrate, and the precipitation centers are around the calcium sulfate dihydrate. The concentration of calcium sulfate is also different in these two centers; it is highest around the dissolution centers and lowest close to the precipitation centers. Calcium and sulfate ions travel in solution by diffusion from the area in which the concentration is greatest to the area in which the concentration is lowest. By understanding the basic concept of the crystalline theory, the effect of different manipulative conditions on some physical properties can be explained.

The effect of manipulative variables and certain chemicals on setting has been studied recently by a kinetic model. An induction time and a reaction constant for crystal growth have been observed. Other theories include the gel theory and the theory of hydration.

Volumetric Contraction Theoretically, calcium sulfate hemihydrate should contract volumetrically during the setting process. However, experiments have determined that all gypsum products expand linearly during setting. As indicated earlier, when 145.15 g of calcium sulfate hemihydrate reacts with 27.02 g of water, the result is the production of 172.17 g of calcium sulfate dihydrate. However, if the volume rather than the weight of calcium sulfate hemihydrate is added to the volume of water, the sum of the volumes will not be equal to the volume of calcium sulfate dihydrate. The volume of the calcium sulfate dihydrate formed is about 7% less than the sum of the volumes of calcium sulfate hemihydrate and water. Instead of 7% contraction, however, in practice about 0.2% to 0.4% linear expansion is obtained. According to the crystalline theory of Le Chatelier and van't Hoff, the expansion results from the thrusting action of gypsum crystals, $CaSO_4 \cdot 2H_2O$, during their growth from a supersaturated solution. The fact that the contraction of gypsum is not visible does not invalidate its existence, and when the volumetric contraction is measured by a dilatometer, it is determined to be about 7%. Because of the linear expansion of the outer dimensions, which is caused by the growth of calcium sulfate dihydrate, with a simultaneous true volumetric contraction of calcium sulfate dihydrate, these materials are porous when set. The gel theory (setting through colloidal state to formation of a gel) may explain the validity of contraction. The theory of hydration interprets expansion through the formation of a hydrate of calcium sulfate.

Effect of Spatulation The mixing process, called spatulation, has a definite effect on the setting time and setting expansion of the material. Within practical limits an increase in the amount of spatulation (either speed of spatulation or time or both) shortens the setting time. Obviously when the powder is placed in water, the chemical reaction starts, and some calcium sulfate dihydrate is formed. During spatulation the newly formed calcium sulfate dihydrate breaks down to smaller crystals and starts new centers of nucleation, around which the calcium sulfate dihydrate can be precipitated. Because an increased amount of spatulation causes more nuclei centers to be formed, the conversion of calcium sulfate hemihydrate to dihydrate requires somewhat less time.

Effect of Temperature The temperature of the water used for mixing, as well as the temperature of the environment, has an effect on the setting reaction of gypsum products. The setting time probably is more affected by a change in temperature than any other physical property. Evidently the temperature has two main effects on the setting reaction of gypsum products.

The first effect of increasing temperature is a change in the relative solubilities of calcium sulfate hemihydrate and calcium sulfate dihydrate, which alters the rate of the reaction. The ratio of the solubilities of calcium sulfate dihydrate and calcium sulfate hemihydrate at 20° C is about 4.5. As the temperature increases, the solubility ratios decrease, until 100° C is reached and the ratio becomes one. As the ratio of the solubilities becomes lower, the reaction is slowed, and the setting time is increased. The solubilities of calcium sulfate hemihydrate and calcium sulfate dihydrate are shown in Table 13-2.

The second effect is the change in ion mobility with temperature. In general, as the temperature increases, the mobility of the calcium and sulfate ions increases, which tends to increase the rate of the reaction and shorten the setting time.

Practically, the effects of these two phenomena are superimposed, and the total effect is observed. Thus, by increasing the temperature from 20° to 30° C, the solubility ratio decreases from 0.90/0.200 = 4.5 to 0.72/0.209 = 3.44, which ordinarily should retard the reaction. At the same time, however, the mobility of the ions increases, which should accelerate the setting reaction. Thus, according to the solubility values, the reaction should be retarded, whereas according to the mobility of the ions, the reaction should be accelerated. Experimentation has shown that increasing the temperature from room temperature of 20° C to body temperature of 37° C increases the rate of the reaction slightly and shortens the setting time. However, as the temperature is raised over 37° C, the rate of the reaction decreases, and the setting time is lengthened. At 100° C the solubilities of dihydrate and hemihydrate are equal, in which case no reaction occurs, and plaster does not set.

Effect of Humidity In the manufacture of plaster it is not practical to convert all the calcium sulfate dihydrate ($CaSO_4 \cdot 2H_2O$) to calcium sulfate hemihydrate ($CaSO_4 \cdot ½H_2O$). During the calcination process most of the gypsum particles are changed to the hemihydrate, although a small portion may remain as the dihydrate, and possibly some particles may further dehydrate completely to form anhydrous soluble calcium sulfate ($CaSO_4$). Soluble calcium sulfate, to a greater degree, and plaster, to a lesser degree, are hygroscopic materials by nature and can easily absorb water vapor from a humid atmosphere to form calcium sulfate dihydrate, which changes the original proportion of each form of calcium sulfate. The presence of small amounts of calcium sulfate dihydrate on the surface of the hemihydrate powder provides additional nuclei for crystallization. Increased contamination by

TABLE 13-2 Solubility of Calcium Sulfate Hemihydrate and Calcium Sulfate Dihydrate at Different Temperatures

Temperature (° C)	$CaSO_4 \cdot ½H_2O$ (g/100 g water)	$CaSO_4 \cdot 2H_2O$ (g/100 g water)
20	0.90	0.200
25	0.80	0.205
30	0.72	0.209
40	0.61	0.210
50	0.50	0.205
100	0.17	0.170

Adapted from Partridge EP, White AH: *J Am Chem Soc* 51: 360, 1929.

moisture produces sufficient dihydrate on the hemihydrate powder to retard the solution of the hemihydrate. Experience has shown that the common overall effect of contamination of gypsum products with moisture from the air during storage is a lengthening of the setting time. For the best results in practice, all gypsum products should be kept in a closed container and well protected from atmospheric humidity. Practically, warmer temperatures and high moisture accelerate the rate of setting of gypsum during mixing.

Effect of Colloidal Systems and pH

Colloidal systems such as agar and alginate retard the setting of gypsum products. If these materials are in contact with $CaSO_4 \cdot \frac{1}{2}H_2O$ during setting, a soft, easily abraded surface is obtained. Accelerators such as potassium sulfate are added to improve the surface quality of the set $CaSO_4 \cdot 2H_2O$ against agar or alginate.

These colloids do not retard the setting by altering the solubility ratio of the hemihydrate and dihydrate forms, but rather by being adsorbed on the $CaSO_4 \cdot \frac{1}{2}H_2O$ or on the $CaSO_4 \cdot 2H_2O$ nucleation sites and thus interfering in the hydration reaction. The adsorption of these materials on the nucleating sites retards the setting reaction more effectively than adsorption on the calcium sulfate hemihydrate.

Liquids with low pH, such as saliva, retard the setting reaction. Liquids with high pH accelerate setting.

PROPERTIES

The important properties of gypsum products include quality, fluidity at pouring time, setting time, linear setting expansion, compressive strength, tensile strength, hardness and abrasion resistance, and reproduction of detail. Some of these property requirements, described by ANSI/ADA Specification No. 25 (ISO 6873), are summarized in Table 13-3.

SETTING TIME

Definition and Importance The time required for the reaction to be completed is called the *final setting time*. If the rate of the reaction is too fast or the material has a short setting time, the mixed mass may harden before the operator can manipulate it properly. On the other hand, if the rate of reaction is too slow, an excessively long time is required to complete the operation. Therefore, a proper setting time is one of the most important properties of gypsum materials.

The chemical reaction is initiated at the mo-

TABLE 13-3 Property Requirements for Gypsum Materials

Type	Setting Time (min)	Setting Expansion Range (%)	Compressive Strength (MPa) min.	Compressive Strength (MPa) max.	Reproduction of Detail (μm)
1 Impression plaster	2.5-5.0	0-0.15	4.0	8.0	75 ± 8
2 Model plaster	± 20%*	0-0.30	9.0	—	75 ± 8
3 Dental stone	± 20%	0-0.20	20.0	—	50 ± 8
4 High-strength/low-expansion dental stone	± 20%	0-0.15	35.0	—	50 ± 8
5 High-strength/high-expansion dental stone	± 20%	0.16-0.30	35.0	—	50 ± 8

*Setting time shall be within 20% of value claimed by manufacturer.

ment the powder is mixed with water, but at the early stage only a small portion of the hemihydrate is converted to gypsum. The freshly mixed mass has a semifluid consistency and can be poured into a mold of any shape. As the reaction proceeds, however, more and more calcium sulfate dihydrate crystals are produced. The viscosity of the mixed mass increases, and the mass can no longer flow easily into the fine details of the mold. This time is called the *working time.*

The final setting time is defined as the time at which the material can be separated from the impression without distortion or fracture. The initial setting time is the time required for gypsum products to reach a certain arbitrary stage of firmness in their setting process. In the normal case, this arbitrary stage is represented by a semihard mass that has passed the working stage but is not yet completely set. Even at final setting, however, the conversion of calcium sulfate hemihydrate to calcium sulfate dihydrate is only partially completed. In high-strength stones, the conversion to dihydrate is never complete. The presence of residual hemihydrate in the set gypsum increases the final strength of the set mass.

Measurement The initial setting time is usually measured arbitrarily by some form of penetration test, although occasionally other types of test methods have been designed. For example, the loss of gloss from the surface of the mixed mass of model plaster or dental stone is an indication of this stage in the chemical reaction and is sometimes used to indicate the initial set of the mass. Similarly, the setting time may be measured by the temperature rise of the mass, because the chemical reaction is exothermic.

The Vicat apparatus shown in Fig. 13-3 is commonly used to measure the initial setting time of gypsum products. It consists of a rod weighing 300 g with a needle of 1 mm diameter. A ring container is filled with the mix, the setting time of which is to be measured. The rod is lowered until it contacts the surface of the material, then the needle is released and allowed to penetrate the mix. When the needle fails to penetrate to the bottom of the container, the material has reached the Vicat or the initial setting time. Other types of instruments, such as Gillmore needles, can be used to obtain the initial and final setting times of gypsum materials.

Control of Setting Time The setting time of gypsum products can be altered rather easily. For example, plaster, which is able to take up water readily, can absorb moisture from the atmosphere and change to gypsum; this absorbance alters the setting time and the other properties of the plaster. The rate of the chemical reaction also can be changed by the addition of suitable chemicals, so it may take from a few minutes to a few hours for the reaction to be completed. According to the crystalline theory discussed earlier, the difference between the solubilities of calcium sulfate hemihydrate and calcium sulfate dihydrate causes the set of the gypsum mass. At a temperature of 20° C, about

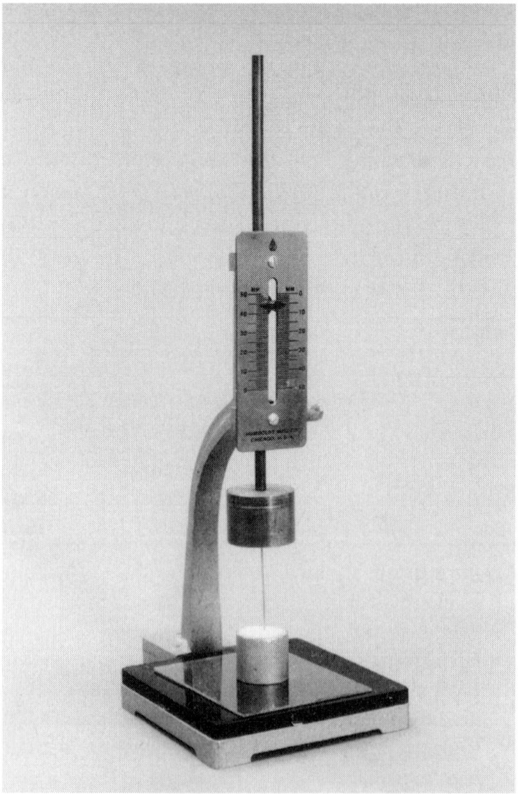

Fig. 13-3 Vicat penetrometer used to determine initial setting time of gypsum products.

4.5 times as much hemihydrate is dissolved in a given amount of water as is dihydrate. If this ratio of 4.5 is increased by the addition of certain salts, the chemical reaction progresses faster and the setting time is shortened. The salt that causes such a change is called an *accelerator*. On the other hand, if by the addition of some salt the ratio of the solubilities of hemihydrate to the dihydrate is decreased, the rate of the reaction is slowed, and the setting time is lengthened. Then the salt is considered a *retarder*.

Although not all accelerators and retarders work on this principle, the change of the solubility ratio may be considered as one way of changing the setting time. In general, setting time can be controlled by manufacturers when they add different chemicals to model plaster or other gypsum products and by operators when they change the manipulative conditions.

Factors Controlled by the Manufacturer

The easiest and most reliable way to change the setting time is to add different chemicals. Potassium sulfate, K_2SO_4, is known as an effective accelerator, and the use of a 2% aqueous solution of this salt rather than water reduces the setting time of model plaster from approximately 10 minutes to about 4 minutes. On the other hand, sodium citrate is a dependable retarder. The use of a 2% aqueous solution of borax to mix with the powder may prolong the setting time of some gypsum products to a few hours.

If a small amount of set calcium sulfate dihydrate is ground and mixed with model plaster, it provides nuclei of crystallization and acts as an accelerator. The set gypsum used as an accelerator is called *terra alba,* and it has a pronounced effect at lower concentrations. The setting time changes significantly if the amount of terra alba present in the mix is changed from 0.5% to 1%. However, terra alba concentrations above 1% have less effect on the setting time. Manufacturers usually take advantage of this fact and add about 1% terra alba to plaster. Thus, the setting time of model plaster is altered less in normal use because of opening and closing the container. When not in use, the model plaster container should be closed tightly to reduce the possibility of moisture contamination, which lengthens the setting time.

Water/Powder Ratio The operator also can change the setting time of model plaster to a certain extent by changing the water/powder (W/P) ratio or the extent of spatulation.

The W/P ratio has a pronounced effect on the setting time. The more water in the mix of model plaster, dental stone, or high-strength dental stone, the longer the setting time, as shown in Table 13-4. The effect of spatulation on setting time of model plaster and dental stone is shown in Table 13-5. Increased spatulation shortens the setting time. Properties of a high-strength dental stone mixed by hand and by a power-driven mixer with vacuum are shown in Table 13-6. The setting time is usually shortened for power mixing compared with hand mixing.

VISCOSITY

The viscosities of several high-strength dental stones and impression plaster are listed in Table 13-7. A range of viscosities from 21,000 to 101,000 centipoises (cp) was observed for five different high-strength stones. More voids were observed in casts made from the stones with the

TABLE 13-4 Effect of Water/Powder Ratio on Setting Time

Material	W/P Ratio (ml/g)	Spatulation Turns	Initial (Vicat) Setting Time (min)
Model plaster	0.45		8
	0.50	100	11
	0.55		14
Dental stone	0.27		4
	0.30	100	7
	0.33		8
High-strength dental stone	0.22		5
	0.24	100	7
	0.26		9

TABLE 13-5 Effect of Spatulation on Setting Time

Material	W/P Ratio (ml/g)	Spatulation Turns	Setting Time (min)
Model plaster	0.50	20	14
	0.50	100	11
	0.50	200	8
Dental stone	0.30	20	10
	0.30	100	8

TABLE 13-6 Properties of a High-Strength Dental Stone Mixed by Hand and by a Power-Driven Mixer with Vacuum

	Hand Mix	Power-Driven Mix with Vacuum
Setting time	8.0	7.3
Compressive strength at 24 hr (MPa)	43.1	45.5
Setting expansion at 2 hr (%)	0.045	0.037
Viscosity, centipoise (cp)	54,000	43,000

From Garber DK, Powers JM, Brandau HE: *Mich Dent Assoc J* 67:133, 1985.

higher viscosities. Impression plaster is used infrequently, but it has a low viscosity, which makes it possible to take impressions with a minimum of force on the soft tissues (mucostatic technique).

COMPRESSIVE STRENGTH

When set, gypsum products show relatively high values of compressive strength. The compressive strength is inversely related to the W/P ratio of the mix. The more water used to make the mix, the lower the compressive strength.

TABLE 13-7 Viscosity of Several High-Strength Dental Stones and Impression Plaster

Material	Viscosity (cp)
High-strength dental stone*	
A	21,000
B	29,000
C	50,000
D	54,000
E	101,000
Impression plaster	23,000

*Adapted from Garber DK,. Powers JM, Brandau HE: *Mich Dent Assoc J* 67:133, 1985. Stones were mixed with 1% sodium citrate solution to retard setting. Viscosity was measured 4 min from the start of mixing.

Model plaster has the greatest quantity of excess water, whereas high-strength dental stone contains the least excess water. The excess water is uniformly distributed in the mix and contributes to the volume but not the strength of the material. The set model plaster is more porous than set dental stone, causing the apparent density of model plaster to be lower. Because high-strength dental stone is the densest, it shows the highest compressive strength, with model plaster being the most porous and thus the weakest.

The 1-hour compressive strength values are approximately 12.5 MPa for model plaster, 31 MPa for dental stone, and 45 MPa for high-strength dental stones. These values are representative for the normal mixes, but they vary as the W/P ratio increases or decreases. The effect of the W/P ratio on the compressive strength of these materials is given in Table 13-8. As shown in Table 13-6, the compressive strength of a high-strength dental stone is improved slightly by vacuum mixing. Evidently, when stone is mixed with the same W/P ratio as model plaster, the compressive strength of dental stone is almost the same as that of model plaster. Similarly, the compressive strength of high-strength dental stone with W/P ratios of 0.3 and 0.5 is similar to the normal compressive strength of dental stone and model plaster.

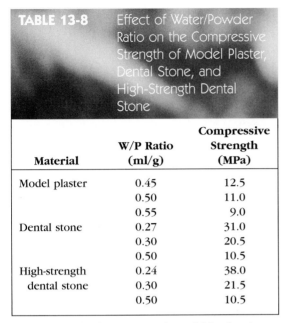

TABLE 13-8 Effect of Water/Powder Ratio on the Compressive Strength of Model Plaster, Dental Stone, and High-Strength Dental Stone

Material	W/P Ratio (ml/g)	Compressive Strength (MPa)
Model plaster	0.45	12.5
	0.50	11.0
	0.55	9.0
Dental stone	0.27	31.0
	0.30	20.5
	0.50	10.5
High-strength dental stone	0.24	38.0
	0.30	21.5
	0.50	10.5

All mixes spatulated 100 turns and tested 1 hr after the start of mixing.

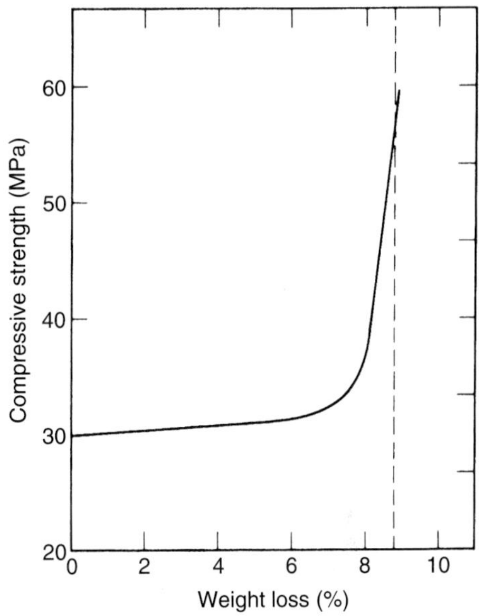

Fig. 13-4 Effect of loss of excess water on compressive strength of dental stone.

At 1 or 2 hours after the final setting time, the hardened gypsum material appears dry and seems to have reached its maximum strength. Actually, this is not the case. The wet strength is the strength of gypsum materials with some or all of the excess water present in the specimen. The dry strength is the strength of the gypsum material with all of its excess water driven out. The dry compressive strength is usually about twice that of the wet strength. Notice that as the hardened mass slowly loses its excess water, the compressive strength of the material does not increase uniformly. The effect of drying on the compressive strength of dental stone is shown in Fig. 13-4. Theoretically, about 8.8% of excess water is in the hardened mass of the stone. As the mass loses up to 7% of the water, no appreciable change develops in the compressive strength of the material. When the mass loses 7.5% of the excess water, however, the strength increases sharply, and when all of the excess (8.8%) is lost, the strength of the material is over 55 MPa.

The drying time for gypsum materials varies according to the size of the gypsum mass and the temperature and humidity of the storage atmosphere. At room temperature and average humidity, about 7 days are necessary for an average denture flask filled with gypsum materials to lose the excess water.

SURFACE HARDNESS AND ABRASION RESISTANCE

The surface hardness of unmodified gypsum materials is related in a general way to their compressive strength. High compressive strengths of the hardened mass correspond to high surface hardnesses. After the final setting occurs, the surface hardness remains practically constant until most excess water is evaporated from the surface, after which its increase is similar to the increase in compressive strength. The surface hardness increases at a faster rate than the compressive strength, because the surface of the hardened mass reaches a dry state earlier than the inner portion of the mass.

Attempts have been made to increase the hardness of gypsum products by impregnating the set gypsum with epoxy or methyl methacrylate monomer that is allowed to polymerize.

Increases in hardness were obtained for model plaster but not for dental stone or high-strength dental stone. Increases in scratch resistance of 15% to 41% were observed for a high-strength dental stone impregnated with epoxy resins or a light-cured dimethacrylate resin. Generally, impregnating set gypsum with resin increases abrasion resistance, but decreases compressive strength and surface hardness.

The idea of drying molds, casts, or dies in an oven to obtain a quick, dry compressive strength and dry surface hardness of a material is not practical, because the gypsum would be dehydrated, which would reduce the strength instead of increasing it. Soaking the gypsum dies or casts in glycerin or different oils does not improve the surface hardness but rather makes the surface smoother, so that a wax carver or other instrument will not cut the stone as it slides over the surface. Mixing high-strength dental stone with a commercial hardening solution containing colloidal silica (about 30%) improves the surface hardness of the set gypsum. The Knoop hardnesses of two commercial high-strength dental stones were 54 and 77 kg/mm^2 when mixed with water. When the hardening solution was used, these values increased to 62 and 79 kg/mm^2, respectively. Increased surface hardness does not necessarily mean improved abrasion resistance, because hardness is only one of many factors that can affect wear resistance. Two-body abrasion studies suggest that the commercial hardening solutions do not improve the abrasion resistance of high-strength dental stones. However, the clinical relevancy of the two-body abrasion test on gypsum has not been established. Further studies of abrasion resistance and methods of measurement are needed. As discussed in the chapter on impression materials, gypsum dies abrade more readily than epoxy dies, even though the gypsum dies are harder.

Although the use of disinfectant chemicals on gypsum dies effectively destroys potentially dangerous organisms, some can damage the surface of a die. Surfaces can be eroded, and the surface hardness can be adversely affected by treatment with some commonly used disinfectants. Other disinfectants, including sodium hypochlorite solutions, have very little effect on the surfaces of gypsum dies.

TENSILE STRENGTH

The tensile strength of model plaster and dental stone is important in structures in which bending tends to occur because of lateral force applications, such as the removal of casts from flexible impressions. Because of the brittle nature of gypsum materials, the teeth on the cast may fracture rather than bend. The diametral compression test for brittle materials is normally used to determine the tensile strength of gypsum products.

Some significant observations have resulted from these studies. First, the 1-hour wet tensile strength of model plaster, 2.3 MPa, is about one half the dry tensile strength, 4.1 MPa, after 40 hours at 45° C. Second, the tensile strength of model plaster in either the wet or dry condition is about one half that of high-strength dental stone in the comparable condition. Third, the tensile strength of model plaster in the wet or dry condition is about one fifth the compressive strength in the same condition (dry, 4.1 MPa in tension; 20 MPa in compression). Fourth, the high-strength dental stone shows an increased

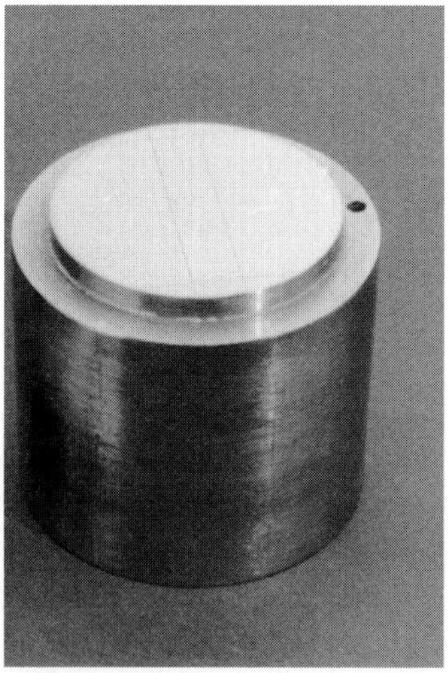

Fig. 13-5 A detail reproduction block.

difference between tensile and compressive values; for example, about 8 MPa in tension and 80 MPa in compression for the dry condition.

REPRODUCTION OF DETAIL

ANSI/ADA Specification No. 25 requires that Types 1 and 2 reproduce a groove 75 μm in width, whereas Types 3, 4, and 5 reproduce a groove 50 μm in width (see Table 13-3). An example of a detail reproduction block is shown in Fig. 13-5. Gypsum dies do not reproduce surface detail as well as electroformed or epoxy dies because the surface of the set gypsum is porous on a microscopic level (Fig. 13-6). Air bubbles are often formed at the interface of the impression and gypsum cast because freshly mixed gypsum does not wet some rubber impression materials (e.g., some silicone types) well. The incorporation of nonionic surfactants in polysulfide and silicone impression materials improves the wetting of the impression by slurry water. The use of vibration during the pouring of a cast reduces the presence of air bubbles. Contamination of the impression in which the gypsum die is poured by saliva or blood can also affect the detail reproduction. Rinsing the impression and blowing away excess water can improve the detail recorded by the gypsum die material.

SETTING EXPANSION

When set, all gypsum products show a measurable linear expansion. The percentage of setting expansion, however, varies from one type of gypsum material to another. Under ordinary conditions, plasters have 0.2% to 0.3% setting expansion, low- to moderate-strength dental stone about 0.15% to 0.25%, and high-strength dental stone only 0.08% to 0.10%. The setting expansion of high-strength/high-expansion dental stone ranges from 0.10% to 0.20%. Typically, over 75% of the expansion observed at 24 hours occurs during the first hour of setting.

The setting expansion may be controlled by different manipulative conditions and by the ad-

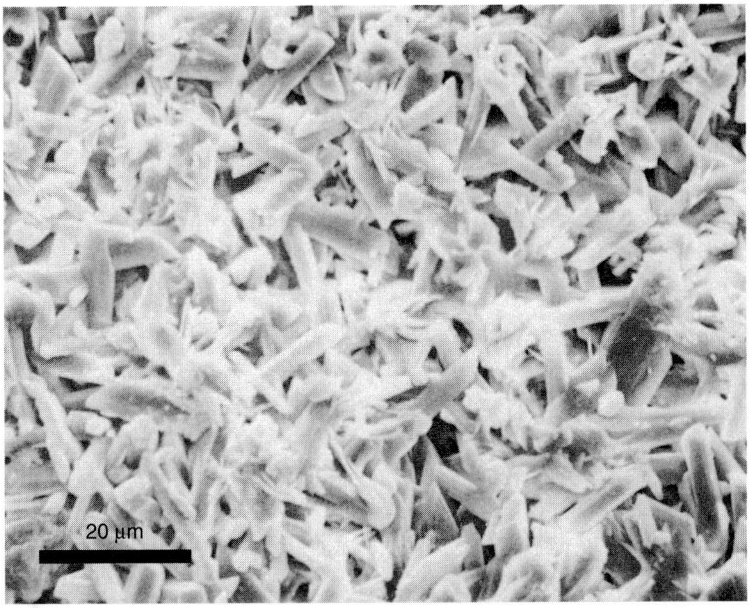

Fig. 13-6 Scanning electron photomicrograph of the surface of a set high-strength stone die. (From Craig RG, Powers JM, Wataha JC: *Dental materials: properties and manipulation*, ed 7, St Louis, 2000, Mosby.)

dition of some chemicals. Mechanical mixing decreases setting expansion. As shown in Table 13-6, a vacuum-mixed high-strength stone expands less at 2 hours than when mixed by hand. Power mixing appears to cause a greater initial volumetric contraction than is observed for hand mixing. The W/P ratio of the mix also has an effect, with an increase in the ratio reducing the setting expansion. The addition of different chemicals affects not only the setting expansion of gypsum products, but may also change other properties. For example, the addition by the manufacturer of sodium chloride (NaCl) in a small concentration increases the setting expansion of the mass and shortens the setting time. The addition of 1% potassium sulfate, on the other hand, decreases the setting time but has no effect on the setting expansion.

If during the setting process, the gypsum materials are immersed in water, the setting expansion increases slightly. This is called *hygroscopic expansion*. A typical, high-strength dental stone has a setting expansion of about 0.08%. If during the setting process the mass is immersed in water, it expands about 0.10%. Increased expansion is observed when dental stone hardens as it comes in contact with a hydrocolloid impression.

MANIPULATION

When any of the gypsum products is mixed with water, it should be spatulated properly to obtain a smooth mix. Water is dispensed into a mixing bowl of an appropriate size and design (Fig. 13-7). The powder is added and allowed to settle into the water for about 30 seconds. This technique minimizes the amount of air incorporated into the mix during initial spatulation by hand. Spatulation can be continued by hand using a metal spatula with a stiff blade (see Fig. 13-7), a hand-mechanical spatulator (Fig. 13-8), or a power-driven mechanical spatulator (Fig. 13-9). A summary of the effect of various manipulative variables on the properties of gypsum products is presented in Table 13-9.

Spatulation by hand involves stirring the mixture vigorously while wiping the inside surfaces of the bowl with the spatula. Spatulation to wet and mix the powder uniformly with the water requires about 1 minute at 2 revolutions per second.

Spatulation with a power-driven mechanical spatulator requires that the powder initially be wet by the water as with hand mixing. The mix is then spatulated for 20 seconds on the low-speed drive of the mixer. Vacuuming during mixing reduces the air entrapped in the mix. Vibration immediately after mixing and during pouring of the gypsum minimizes air bubbles in the set mass.

Pouring an impression with gypsum requires care to avoid trapping air in critical areas. The mixed gypsum should be poured slowly or added to the impression with a small instrument such as a wax spatula. The mass should run into the rinsed impression under vibration in such a manner that it pushes air ahead of itself as it fills the impressions of the teeth. Commonly, the teeth of a cast are poured in dental stone or high-strength dental stone, whereas the base is poured in model plaster for easier trimming.

Once poured, the gypsum material should be allowed to harden for 45 to 60 minutes before the impression and cast are separated and disinfected. Models can be disinfected by immersion in 1:10 dilution of sodium hypochlorite for 30 minutes or with a spray of iodophor following manufacturer's instructions.

CASTING INVESTMENTS

The adoption of the casting practice in dentistry for making gold alloy inlays, crowns, bridges, and other restorations represents one of the major advances in restorative dentistry. In recent years, alloys with higher melting points, the palladium and base metal alloys, have been cast into crowns, bridges, and removable partial denture restorations by using basically the same lost-wax technique used for dental gold alloys. All such

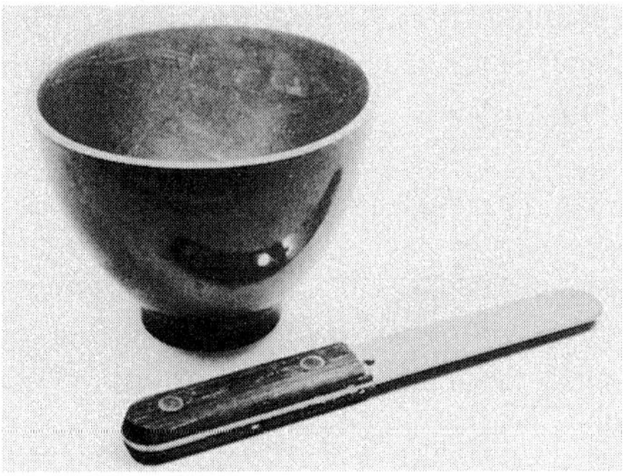

Fig. 13-7 Flexible rubber mixing bowl and metal spatula with a stiff blade.

(From Craig RG, Powers JM, Wataha JC: *Dental materials: properties and manipulation,* ed 7, St Louis, 2000, Mosby.)

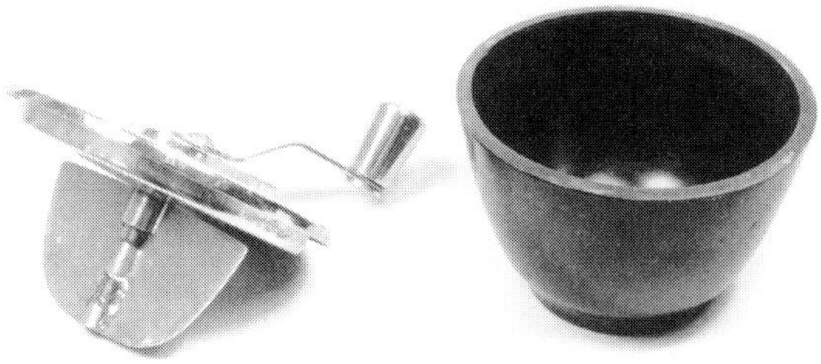

Fig. 13-8 Mechanical spatulator for use with small gypsum mixes.

(From Craig RG, Powers JM, Wataha JC: *Dental materials: properties and manipulation,* ed 7, St Louis, 2000, Mosby.)

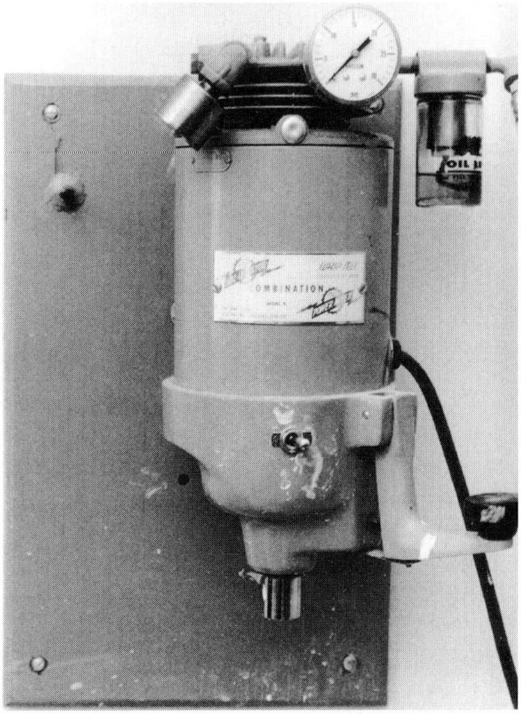

Fig. 13-9 Power-driven mechanical spatulator with a vacuum attachment.

(From Craig RG, Powers JM, Wataha JC: *Dental materials: properties and manipulation,* ed 7, St Louis, 2000, Mosby.)

TABLE 13-9 Summary of Effect of Manipulative Variables on Properties of Gypsum Products

Manipulative Variable	Setting Time	Consistency	Setting Expansion	Compressive Strength
Increase water/powder ratio	Increase	Increase	Decrease	Decrease
Increase rate of spatulation	Decrease	Decrease	Increase	No effect
Increase temperature of mixing water from 23° to 30° C	Decrease	Decrease	Increase	No effect

casting operations involve (1) a wax pattern of the object to be reproduced; (2) a suitable mold material, known as investment, which is placed around the pattern and permitted to harden; (3) suitable furnaces for burning out the wax patterns and heating the investment mold; and (4) proper facilities to melt and cast the alloy. An *investment* can be described as a ceramic material that is suitable for forming a mold into which a metal or alloy is cast. The operation of forming the mold is described as *investing*. Details of the casting technique are described in Chapter 17.

PROPERTIES REQUIRED OF AN INVESTMENT

1. Easily manipulated: Not only should it be possible to mix and manipulate the mass readily and to paint the wax pattern easily, but the investment should also harden within a relatively short time.
2. Sufficient strength at room temperature: To permit ease in handling and provide enough strength at higher temperatures to withstand the impact force of the molten metal. The inner surface of the mold should not break down at a high temperature.
3. Stability at higher temperatures: Investment must not decompose to give off gases that could damage the surface of the alloy.
4. Sufficient expansion: Enough to compensate for shrinkage of the wax pattern and metal that takes place during the casting procedure.
5. Beneficial casting temperatures: Preferably the thermal expansion versus temperature curve should have a plateau of the thermal expansion over a range of casting temperatures.
6. Porosity: Porous enough to permit the air or other gases in the mold cavity to escape easily during the casting procedure.
7. Smooth surface: Fine detail and margins on the casting.
8. Ease of divestment: The investment should break away readily from the surface of the metal and should not have reacted chemically with it.
9. Inexpensive.

These represent the requirements for an ideal investment. No single material is known that completely fulfills all of these requirements. However, by blending different ingredients an investment can be developed that possesses most of the required qualities. These ideal qualities are the basis for considering the behavior and characteristics of casting investments.

COMPOSITION

In general, an investment is a mixture of three distinct types of materials: refractory material, binder material, and other chemicals.

Refractory Material This material is usually a form of silicon dioxide, such as quartz, tridymite, or cristobalite, or a mixture of these. Refractory materials are contained in all dental investments, whether for casting gold or high–melting point alloys.

Binder Material Because the refractory materials alone do not form a coherent solid mass, some kind of binder is needed. The common binder used for dental casting gold alloy is α-calcium sulfate hemihydrate. Phosphate, ethyl silicate, and other similar materials also serve as binders for high-temperature casting investments. These latter investments are described later in conjunction with investment for casting high–melting point alloys.

Other Chemicals Usually a mixture of refractory materials and a binder alone is not enough to produce all the desirable properties required of an investment. Other chemicals, such as sodium chloride, boric acid, potassium sulfate, graphite, copper powder, or magnesium oxide, are often added in small quantities to modify various physical properties. For example, small amounts of chlorides or boric acid enhance the thermal expansion of investments bonded by calcium sulfate.

CALCIUM SULFATE–BONDED INVESTMENTS

The dental literature and patent references describe the quantity and purpose of each of a variety of ingredients in dental casting investments. In general, the investments suitable for casting gold alloys contain 65% to 75% quartz or cristobalite, or a blend of the two, in varying proportions, 25% to 35% of α-calcium sulfate hemihydrate, and about 2% to 3% chemical modifiers. With the proper blending of these basic ingredients, the manufacturer is able to develop an investment with an established group of physical properties that are adequate for dental gold casting practices. A list of specific compositions is of little value, however, because the final product's properties are influenced by both the ingredients present in the investment and the manner in which the mass is manipulated and used in making the mold.

Investments with calcium sulfate hemihydrate as a binder are relatively easy to manipulate, and more information about the effect of different additives, as well as various manipulative conditions, is available for this type than for other types, such as those that use silicates or phosphates as binders. The calcium sulfate–bonded investment is usually limited to gold castings, and is not heated above 700° C. The calcium sulfate portion of the investment decomposes into sulfur dioxide and sulfur trioxide at temperatures over 700° C, tending to embrittle the casting metal. Therefore, the calcium sulfate type of binder is usually not used in investments for making castings of palladium or base metal alloys.

PROPERTIES OF CALCIUM SULFATE–BONDED INVESTMENTS

ANSI/ADA Specification No. 2 (ISO 7490) for gypsum-bonded casting investments applies to two different types of investments suitable for casting dental restorations of gold alloys:

Type 1: For casting inlays and crowns
Type 2: For casting complete and partial denture bases

Both types have calcium sulfate as a binder material. The physical properties included in this specification are appearance of powder, fluidity at working time, setting time, compressive strength, linear setting expansion, and linear thermal expansion. The testing consistency is the W/P ratio recommended by the manufacturer. The values allowed for these properties are summarized in Table 13-10. The test specimens and methods of testing, which also apply to other

TABLE 13-10 Requirements for Dental Gypsum–Bonded Casting Investments

Property	Value
Appearance of powder	Uniform and free from foreign matter and lumps
Fluidity at working time	
Type 1	Diameter of 60 mm
Type 2	Diameter of 40 mm
Setting time	Shall not vary by more than 20% of time claimed by manufacturer
Compressive strength	
Type 1	Minimum 2.3 MPa
Type 2	Minimum 2.6 MPa
Linear setting expansion	Shall not vary by more than 20% of expansion claimed by manufacturer
Linear thermal expansion	Shall not vary by more than 20% of expansion claimed by manufacturer

Modified from ANSI/ADA Specification No. 2 for dental gypsum-bonded casting investments.

types of casting investments, are described in the specification. The manipulation of investments in the inlay casting procedure is discussed in detail in Chapter 17.

EFFECT OF TEMPERATURE ON INVESTMENT

In casting with the lost-wax process, the wax pattern, after being invested, is melted and removed from the investment, leaving a mold cavity into which the molten metal is cast. In this way, regardless of whether the high-heat or hygroscopic casting technique is used, the investment is heated to an elevated temperature. This temperature varies from one technique to another, but in no case is it lower than 550° C or higher than 700° C for calcium sulfate–bonded investments. During the heating process, the refractory material is affected differently by the thermal changes than is the binder.

Effect of Temperature on Silicon Dioxide Refractories Each of the polymorphic forms of silica—quartz, tridymite, and cristobalite—expands when heated, but the percentage of expansion varies from one type to another. Pure cristobalite expands to 1.6% at 250° C, whereas quartz expands about 1.4% at 600° C, and the thermal expansion of tridymite at 600° C is less than 1%. The percentage of expansion of the three types of silica versus temperature is shown in Fig. 3-12. As seen in Fig. 3-12, none of the three forms of silica expands uniformly; instead they all show a break (nonlinearity) in their thermal expansion curves. In the case of cristobalite the expansion is somewhat uniform up to about 200° C. At this temperature its expansion increases sharply from 0.5% to 1.2%, and then above 250° C it again becomes more uniform. At 573° C quartz also shows a break in the expansion curve, and tridymite shows a similar break at a much lower temperature.

The breaks on the expansion versus temperature curves indicate that cristobalite and quartz each exist in two polymorphic forms, one of which is more stable at a higher temperature and the other at a lower temperature. The form that is more stable at room temperature is called the *α-form,* and the more stable form at higher temperatures is designated as the *β-form.* Tridymite has three stable polymorphic forms. Thus the temperatures of 220° C for cristobalite, 573° C for quartz, and 105° and 160° C for tridymite are displacive transition temperatures. A displacive change involves expansion or contraction in the volume of the mass without breaking any bonds. In changing from the α-form (which is the more stable form at room temperature) to the β-form (which is stable at higher temperatures), all three forms of silica expand. The amount of expansion is highest for cristobalite and lowest for tridymite.

The quartz form of silica is found abundantly in nature, and it can be converted to cristobalite and tridymite by being heated through a reconstructive transition during which bonds are broken and a new crystal structure is formed. The α-quartz is converted to β-quartz at a temperature of 573° C. If the β-quartz is heated to 870° C and maintained at that temperature, it is converted to β-tridymite. From β-tridymite, it is possible to obtain either α-tridymite or β-cristobalite. If β-tridymite is cooled rapidly to 120° C and held at that temperature, it is changed to α-tridymite, which is stable at room temperature. On the other hand, if β-tridymite is heated to 1475° C and

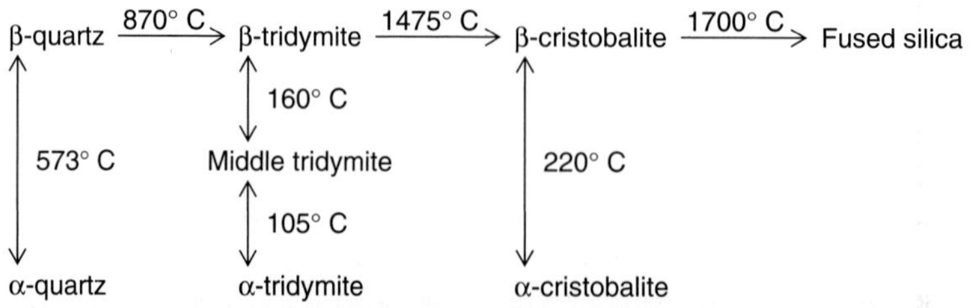

held at that temperature, it is converted to β-cristobalite. Further heating of β-cristobalite produces fused silica, but if it is cooled to 220° C and held at that temperature, α-cristobalite is formed. These transitions are shown in the equation on p. 408.

All forms of silica are in their α-forms in the investment, and during the heating process they are converted completely or in part to their corresponding β-forms. This transition involves an expansion of the mass, which helps to compensate for the casting shrinkages.

Effect of Temperature on Calcium Sulfate Binders The binder used for gold alloy casting investments in dentistry is α-calcium sulfate hemihydrate. During the investing process, some of the water mixed with the investment reacts with the hemihydrate and is converted to calcium sulfate dihydrate, whereas the remainder of the water is uniformly distributed in the mix as excess water. During the early stages of heating, the excess water evaporates. As the temperature rises to about 105° C, calcium sulfate dihydrate starts losing water. The investment mass is then heated still further to the proper temperature for casting the metal. In this way, anhydrous calcium sulfate, silica, and certain chemical additives remain to form the mold into which the gold alloy is cast.

It has been observed experimentally that investment expands when it is first heated from room temperature to about 105° C, then contracts slightly or remains unchanged up to about 200° C, and registers varying degrees of expansion, depending on the silica composition of the investment, between 200 and 700° C. These properties are explained as follows. Up to about 105° C, ordinary thermal expansion occurs. Above 105° C, the calcium sulfate dihydrate is converted to anhydrous calcium sulfate. Dehydration of the dihydrate and a phase change of the calcium sulfate anhydrite cause a contraction. However, the α-form of tridymite (which might be present as an impurity) is expanding and compensates for the contraction of the calcium sulfate sufficiently to prevent the investment from registering a serious degree of contraction. At elevated temperatures, the α-forms of silica present in the investment are converted to the β-forms, which cause some additional expansion.

The thermal expansion curves for a currently available hygroscopic type of investment containing quartz *(A)* and a thermal expansion type of investment containing cristobalite *(B)* are shown in Fig. 13-10, which illustrates the expected degree of expansion at different temperatures. The expansion of the silica content of the investment must not only be sufficiently high to overcome all the contraction, but should also take place at temperatures close to the temperature at which contraction of the hemihydrate occurs.

Cooling of the Investment When the investment is allowed to cool, the refractory and binder contract according to a thermal contraction curve that is different from the thermal expansion curve of the investment (Fig. 13-11). On cooling to room temperature, the investment exhibits an overall contraction compared with its dimensions before heating. On reheating to the temperature previously attained, the investment

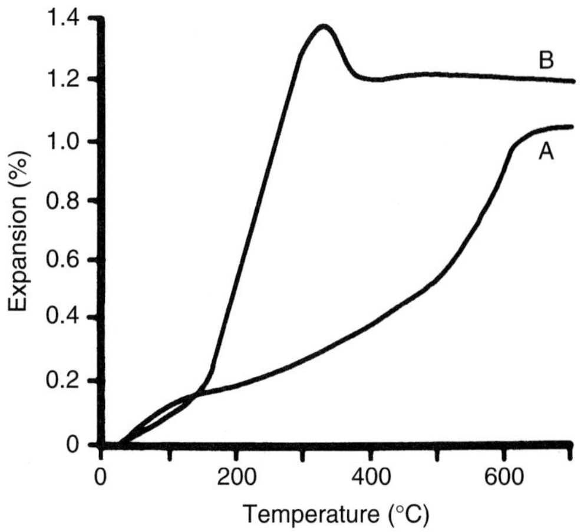

Fig. 13-10 Thermal expansion curves for calcium sulfate–bonded investments. *A*, Hygroscopic type; *B*, thermal expansion type.

(Adapted from Asgar K: Casting restorations. In Clark JW, editor: *Clinical dentistry*, vol 4, New York, 1976, Harper & Row.)

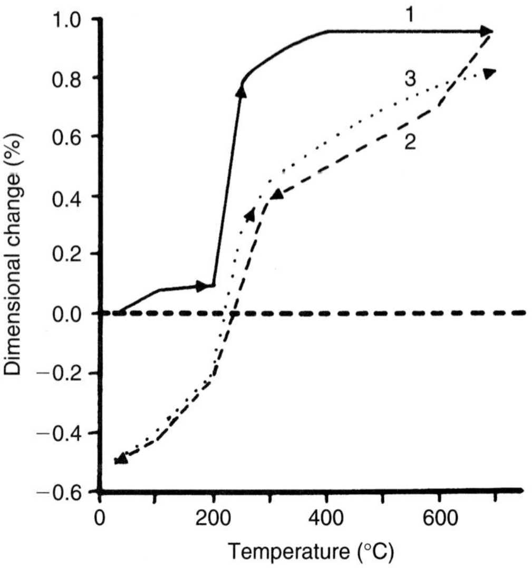

Fig. 13-11 Thermal expansion and contraction curves for calcium sulfate–bonded investment (thermal expansion type). Curve *1* is first heating, curve *2* is cooling, and curve *3* is reheating.

does not expand thermally to the previous level; moreover, the process of cooling and reheating causes internal cracks in the investment that can affect the quality of the casting.

SETTING AND HYGROSCOPIC EXPANSION OF CALCIUM SULFATE–BONDED INVESTMENT

All the calcium sulfate–bonded investments currently available for casting gold alloys have thermal expansion, setting expansion, and hygroscopic expansion. The total dimensional change is a very important property of dental casting investments. The setting expansion of an investment, like that of other gypsum products discussed earlier in this chapter, is the linear expansion that takes place during the normal setting of the investment in air. Hygroscopic expansion, on the other hand, is the linear expansion of the investment that occurs if the investment is in contact with water from any source during the setting process. Such contact with water can be achieved by placing the casting ring, after investing the wax pattern, in a water bath or by using a wet liner inside the casting ring.

Distinguishing between a setting expansion and hygroscopic expansion is difficult, because both take place almost at the same time and end at the same time. In practice, a sum of the hygroscopic and setting expansions of the investment is obtained, which is higher than the setting expansion alone.

The mechanism of hygroscopic expansion has been studied by a number of investigators. According to some of the theories, the addition of water during the setting of an investment increases the surface-film thickness on the inert particles and gypsum crystals, thereby forcing them apart. Some believe that the added water during the setting process permits further hydration of calcium sulfate, thus causing the expansion of the investment, whereas others believe that the added water may force gypsum gel to swell. Another theory states that hygroscopic expansion and setting expansion are the result of the same phenomenon as that occurring with dental stone, which is the outward growth of gypsum crystals. The addition of water or any other liquid provides additional volume into which the gypsum crystals can grow.

Although some question is raised about the exact mechanism of hygroscopic expansion, the effects of many of the manipulative conditions have been studied in detail. The effects of some of these conditions on the setting, hygroscopic, and thermal expansion of calcium sulfate–bonded investment are summarized in Table 13-11. These conditions also have a significant influence on the properties of the casting investment and the quality of the casting.

Water/Powder Ratio As with the setting expansion of gypsum products, the more water in the mix (the thinner the mix or the higher the W/P ratio), the less the setting and hygroscopic expansions. Notice that less thermal expansion is also obtained with a thinner mix.

Spatulation The effect of spatulation on the setting and hygroscopic expansion of the investment is similar to that on the setting expan-

TABLE 13-11 Effects of Manipulative Conditions on the Expansion of Calcium Sulfate–Bonded Investments

Factor	Setting and Hygroscopic Expansion	Thermal Expansion
Water/powder ratio increased	Decreased	Decreased
Time of spatulation increased	Increased	No effect
Rate of spatulation increased	Increased	No effect
Age of investment increased	Decreased	No effect
Delay before immersion increased	Decreased	
Water bath temperature increased	Increased	
Strength of wax for some patterns	More distortion	Less effect
Location of sprue	More critical	Less critical

sion of all gypsum products. As shown in Fig. 13-12, curve *C*, less spatulation produces lower expansion with hygroscopic investment.

Age of Investment Investments that are 2 or 3 years old do not expand as much as freshly prepared investments. Fig. 13-12, curve *D*, shows the effect of aged investment on hygroscopic expansion. For this reason, the containers of investment must be kept closed as much as possible, especially if the investment is stored in a humid atmosphere.

Delay Before Immersion After the wax pattern is invested, the investment mass may be immersed in a water bath to obtain a better fit of the casting. The time between mixing and immersion has an effect on the total amount of expansion. In general, the hygroscopic expansion decreases with increased time between mixing and immersion. However, some investigators claim that if the investment is immersed at about the initial setting time, it expands more than if it is immersed earlier. However, more reproducible results are obtained from one test to another if the immersion is made before the gloss of the investment is lost.

Water-Bath Temperature The temperature of the water bath has a measurable effect on the wax pattern. At higher water-bath temperatures, the wax pattern expands, requiring less

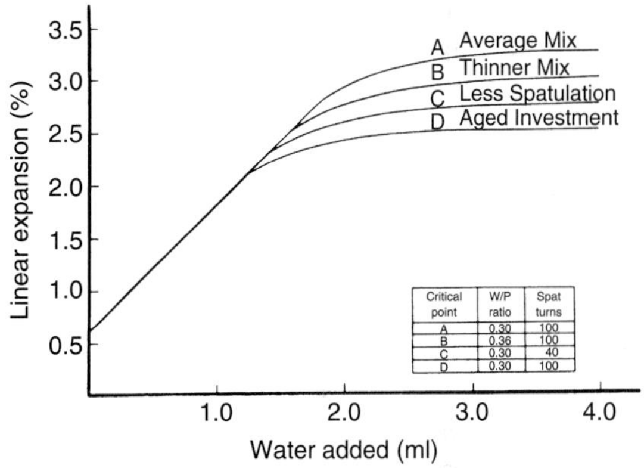

Fig. 13-12 Linear expansion of a hygroscopic investment as a function of the amount of water added and manipulative conditions.

expansion of the investment to compensate for the total casting shrinkage. In addition, higher water-bath temperatures soften the wax. The softened wax then gives less resistance to the expansion of the investment, thus making the setting and hygroscopic expansions more effective. The net effect is higher expansion of the mold with higher water-bath temperatures.

Particle Size of Silica The particle size of calcium sulfate hemihydrate has little effect on hygroscopic expansion, whereas the particle size of silica has a significant effect. Finer silica produces higher setting and hygroscopic expansions.

Silica/Binder Ratio Investments usually contain 65% to 75% silica, 25% to 35% calcium sulfate hemihydrate, and about 2% to 3% of some additive chemicals to control the different physical properties and to color the investments. If the silica/stone ratio is increased, the hygroscopic expansion of the investment also increases, but the strength of the investment decreases.

Role of Water During the setting process, dental casting investments actually absorb water from their surroundings and expand. It also has been observed that, during setting, the more water an investment is permitted to take up from any source, the higher its hygroscopic expansion. The hygroscopic expansion of an investment during setting versus the amount of water added to its surface is shown in Fig. 13-12, curves *A* and *B*. As indicated, the more water added to the surface of the mixed investment, the higher the hygroscopic expansion, up to a point beyond which further additions of water do not create any additional expansion. This degree of expansion and its corresponding quantity of water is called the *critical point*. Note that for an investment to reach its maximum hygroscopic expansion, sufficient water should be available to it. If hygroscopically expanding investments are in contact with less water than they are able to absorb, they will not exhibit their maximum hygroscopic expansion.

HYGROSCOPIC–THERMAL GOLD CASTING INVESTMENT

There is one gold casting investment on the market that was designed for use with either hygroscopic or thermal type of casting techniques. Fig. 13-13 shows the high thermal expansion of this investment in the range between 482° C and 649° C. This expansion is high enough to use the investment with the thermal casting technique, without water immersion. However, when immersed in a water bath, the investment expands hygroscopically (Fig. 13-14). With the hygroscopic technique, the investment needs to be heated to only 482° C to provide the appropriate expansion.

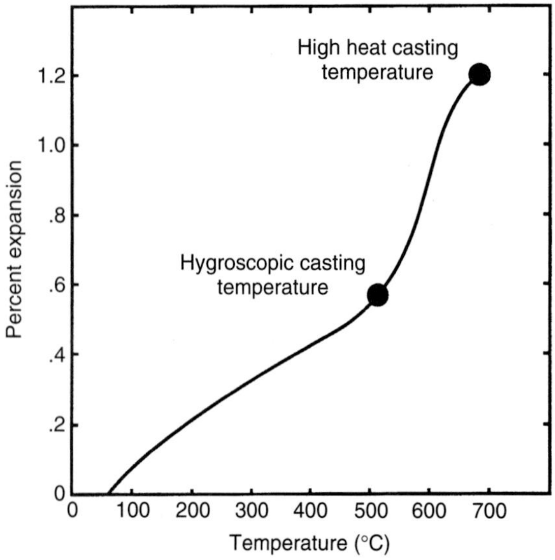

Fig. 13-13 Thermal expansion of mixed hygroscopic–thermal gold casting investment.
(Courtesy Whip Mix Corp., 1992.)

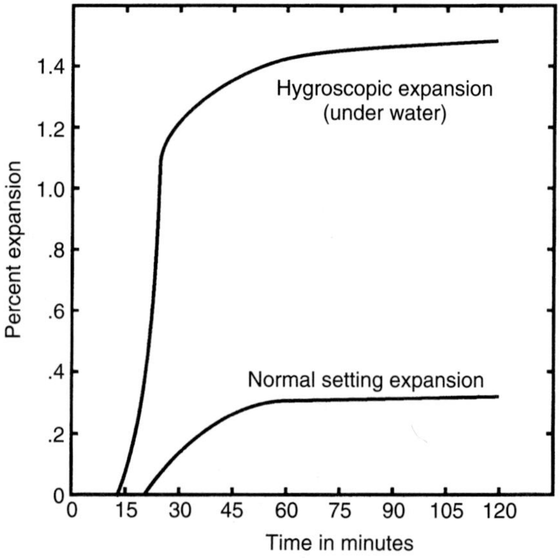

Fig. 13-14 Setting and hygroscopic expansion of mixed hygroscopic–thermal gold casting investment.
(Courtesy Whip Mix Corp., 1992.)

INVESTMENT FOR CASTING HIGH–MELTING POINT ALLOYS

Most palladium and base metal alloys used for partial dentures and porcelain-fused-to-metal restorations have high melting temperatures. They should be cast at a mold temperature greater than 700° C. For this reason, calcium sulfate–bonded investments are usually not used for casting these alloys. Only one base metal alloy for dental applications possesses a low enough melting point to be cast into a mold at 700° C with a calcium sulfate binder. This alloy is an exception, because base metal alloys are usually cast into molds at 850 to 1100° C. To withstand these high temperatures, the molds require different types of binders, such as silicate and phosphate compounds. This type of investment usually has less than 20% binder, and the remainder of the investment is quartz or another form of silica.

Phosphate-Bonded Investment The most common type of investment for casting high–melting point alloys is the phosphate-bonded investment. This type of investment consists of three different components. One component contains a water-soluble phosphate ion. The second component reacts with phosphate ions at room temperature. The third component is a refractory, such as silica. Different materials can be used in each component to develop different physical properties.

The binding system of a typical phosphate-bonded investment undergoes an acid-base reaction between acid monoammonium phosphate ($NH_4H_2PO_4$) and basic magnesia (MgO). The soluble phosphate in water reacts with the sparingly soluble magnesia at its surface, forming a binding media with filler particles embedded in the matrix. The chemical reaction at room temperature can be expressed simply as follows:

$$NH_4H_2PO_4 + MgO + H_2O \rightarrow NH_4MgPO_4 \cdot 6H_2O + H_2O$$

The water produced by this reaction at room temperature lowers the viscosity of the mix as spatulation continues.

As the reaction takes place, colloidal particles are formed with a strong interaction among the particles. During setting and burnout, the sequence of chemical and thermal reactions causes various phase changes, providing room-temperature strength (green strength) and high-temperature strength that enable the investment to withstand the impact of high–melting point alloys. Phases formed at high temperatures include $Mg_2P_2O_7$ and subsequently $Mg_3(PO_4)_2$. To produce higher expansion, a combination of different particle sizes of silica is used.

These investments can be mixed with water or with a special liquid supplied by the manufacturer. The special liquid is a form of silica sol in water. As shown in Fig. 13-15, phosphate-

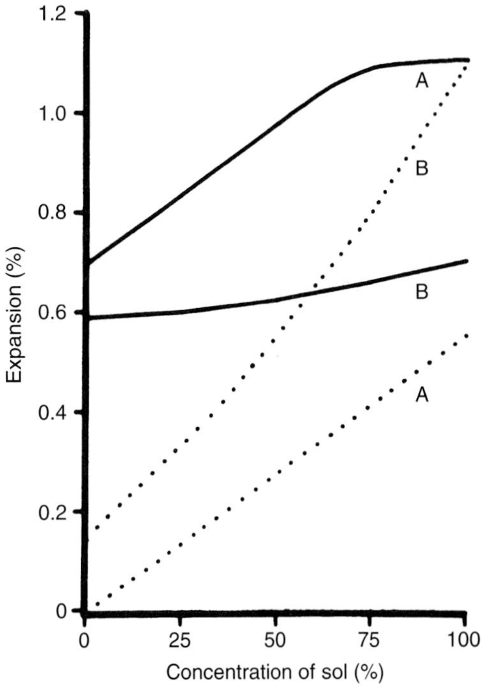

Fig. 13-15 Effect of silica sol concentration on thermal expansion (solid lines) at 800° C and setting expansion (dotted lines) of two phosphate-bonded investments (*A*, thermal expansion type; *B*, hygroscopic expansion type).

(Adapted from Zarb GA, Bergman G, Clayton JA, MacKay HF, editors: *Prosthodontic treatment for partially edentulous patients*, St Louis, 1978, Mosby.)

bonded investments possess higher setting expansion when they are mixed with the silica sol than when mixed with water. With a mix containing silica sol, the investment mass is capable of expanding hygroscopically, whereas if the mix is only water, the hygroscopic expansion of such an investment is negligible. Not all phosphate-bonded investments, however, can expand hygroscopically. Using silica sol instead of water with phosphate-bonded investment also increases its strength considerably. Fig. 13-16 shows thermal expansion curves of two commercial phosphate-bonded investments mixed according to the manufacturers' recommended liquid/powder ratio. Both the setting and thermal expansions must be considered in selecting these investments.

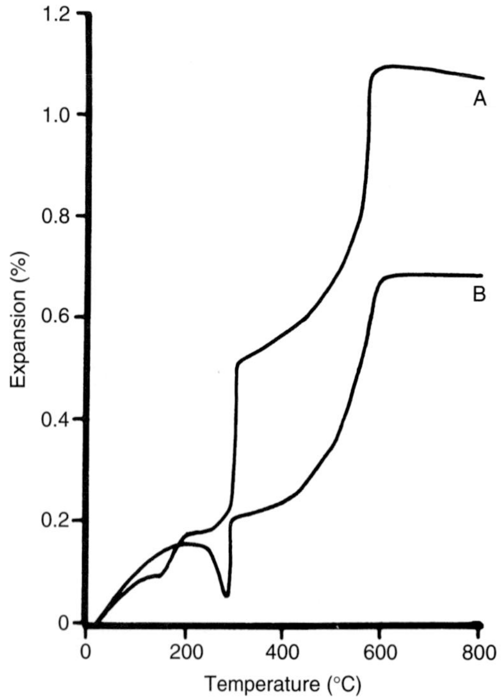

Fig. 13-16 Thermal expansion curves of two phosphate-bonded investments mixed at recommended liquid/powder ratios (*A*, thermal expansion type; *B*, hygroscopic expansion type).

(Adapted from Zarb GA, Bergman B, Clayton JA, MacKay HF, editors: *Prosthodontic treatment for partially edentulous patients,* St Louis, 1978, Mosby.)

ANSI/ADA Specification No. 42 (ISO 9694) for dental phosphate-bonded casting investments specifies two types of investments for alloys having a solidus temperature above 1080° C:

Type 1: For inlays, crowns, and other fixed restorations

Type 2: For partial dentures and other cast, removable restorations

The following properties are specified by the specification: fluidity, initial setting time, compressive strength, and linear thermal expansion. The values allowed for these properties are summarized in Table 13-12.

Silica-Bonded Investment Another type of binding material for investments used with casting high–melting point alloys is a silica-bonding ingredient. This type of investment may derive its silica bond from ethyl silicate, an aqueous dispersion of colloidal silica, or from sodium silicate. One such investment consists of a silica refractory, which is bonded by the hydrolysis of ethyl silicate in the presence of hydrochloric acid. The product of the hydrolysis is a colloidal solution of silicic acid and ethyl alcohol, which can be written as

$$Si(OC_2H_5)_4 + 4H_2O \xrightarrow{HCl} Si(OH)_4 + 4C_2H_5OH$$

In practice, however, the reaction is more complicated, and instead of tetrasilicic acid, which is converted into $SiO_2 \cdot 2H_2O$, a polymerized compound of silicon is formed with the following structure:

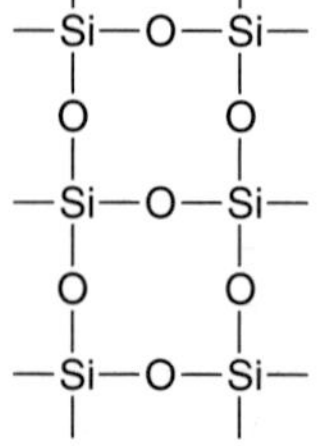

This material has an even higher silica content and better refractory properties than the SiO_2 $2H_2O$.

Ethyl silicate has the disadvantage of giving off flammable components during processing, and the method is expensive; thus other techniques and methods have been developed to reduce the use of this material. Sodium silicate and colloidal silica are more common binders of the silica type.

Today this investment is usually supplied with two bottles of special liquid, instead of water, with which the investment powder should be mixed. In one of the bottles the manufacturer usually supplies a properly diluted water-soluble silicate solution. The other bottle usually contains a properly diluted acid solution, such as a solution of hydrochloric acid. The contents of each bottle can be stored almost indefinitely. Before use, mix an equal volume from each bottle and allow the mixed liquids to stand for a prescribed time, according to the manufacturer's instructions, so hydrolysis can take place and freshly prepared silicic acid forms.

Proposed ANSI/ADA Specification No. 91 (ISO 11246) for ethyl silicate casting investments specifies setting time, compressive strength, and linear thermal expansion. The setting time must not differ by more than 30% from the time stated by the manufacturer. The compressive strength at room temperature shall not be less than 1.5 MPa. The linear thermal expansion must not differ by more than 15% from the time stated by the manufacturer.

BRAZING INVESTMENT

When brazing (soldering) the parts of a restoration, such as clasps on a removable partial denture, the parts must be surrounded with a suitable ceramic or investment material before the heating operation. The assembled parts are temporarily held together with sticky wax until they are surrounded with the appropriate investment material, after which the wax is softened and removed. The portion to be soldered is left exposed and free from investment to permit wax removal and effective heating before it is joined with solder.

ANSI/ADA Specification No. 93 (ISO 11244) for dental brazing investments defines two types of investment:

Type 1: Gypsum-bonded dental brazing investments
Type 2: Phosphate-bonded dental brazing investments

TABLE 13-12 Requirements for Dental Phosphate-Bonded Casting Investments

Property	Value
Appearance of powder	Uniform and free from foreign matter and lumps
Fluidity at working time	
Type 1	Diameter of 90 mm
Type 2	Diameter of 70 mm
Setting time	Shall not vary by more than 30% of time claimed by manufacturer
Compressive strength	
Type 1	Minimum 2.5 MPa
Type 2	Minimum 3.0 MPa
Linear thermal expansion	Shall not vary by more than 15% of expansion claimed by manufacturer

Modified from ANSI/ADA Specification No. 42 for dental phosphate-bonded casting investments.

The specification specifies quality, fluidity, setting time, compressive strength, linear thermal expansion, and linear setting expansion. The values allowed for these properties are summarized in Table 13-13.

The investment for soldering of low-melting-point alloys is similar to casting investments containing quartz and a calcium sulfate hemihydrate binder. For high–melting point alloys, a phosphate-bonded investment is used.

Soldering investments are designed to have lower setting and thermal expansions than casting investments, a feature that is desirable so the assembled parts do not shift in position during the setting and heating of the investment. Soldering investments are often made of ingredients that do not have as fine a particle size as the casting investment, because the smoothness of the mass is less important. Relatively little information is available in the dental literature on the properties of soldering investments.

INVESTMENT FOR ALL-CERAMIC RESTORATIONS

Two types of investment materials have been developed recently for producing all-ceramic restorations. The first type is used for the cast glass technique. This investment is provided by the manufacturer of the glass casting equipment and is composed of phosphate-bonded refractories. The second type of investment for making all-ceramic restorations is the refractory die type of material, which is used for all-ceramic veneers, inlays, and crowns. Refractory dies are made by pouring the investment into impressions. When the investment is set, the die is removed, and is heated to remove gases that may be detrimental to the ceramic (degassing). A refractory die spacer may be added to the surface. Next, porcelain or other ceramic powders are added to the die surface and fired. These materials must accurately reproduce the impression, remain undamaged during the porcelain firing, and have a thermal expansion compatible with that of the ceramic (otherwise the ceramic could crack during cooling). These materials are also phosphate-bonded, and they generally contain fine-grained refractory fillers to allow accurate reproduction of detail. ANSI/ADA Specification No. 92 (ISO 11245) for phosphate-bonded refractory die materials is under development.

TABLE 13-13 Requirements for Dental Brazing Investments

Property	Value
Quality of powder	Uniform and free from foreign matter and lumps
Fluidity	Diameter of 100 mm
Setting time	Shall not vary by more than 30% of time claimed by manufacturer
Compressive strength	Range 2.0-10.0 MPa
Linear setting expansion	Shall not vary by more than 15% of expansion claimed by manufacturer
Linear thermal expansion	Shall not vary by more than 15% of expansion claimed by manufacturer

Modified from ANSI/ADA Specification No. 93 for dental brazing investments.

SELECTED PROBLEMS

Problem 1

High-strength dental stone dies sometimes fracture during separation from rubber impressions. How can this difficulty be minimized?

Solution a

The recommended water/powder ratio should be used. The water/powder ratio can vary from 0.19 to 0.24 for various Type 4 gypsum products. The water and powder should be dispensed accurately. Optimum strength is achieved only at the correct water/powder ratio.

Solution b

Vacuum mixing of high-strength dental stone ensures maximum strength by minimizing porosity.

Solution c

The poured die should be allowed to set for at least 20 minutes or until final set before it is removed from the impression.

Solution d

Increasing the thickness of stiffer impression materials (polyether) increases the ease of removal of the die.

Problem 2

The occlusal surfaces of teeth of a Type 3 gypsum model poured from an alginate impression were chalky and friable. What may have happened, and how can this problem be solved?

Solution

Excess water in the depressions of an alginate impression (or any impression) from rinsing will increase the water/powder ratio of the dental stone. Blood and saliva remaining on the impression retard the setting of the dental stone. Both conditions can cause the dental stone to be chalky and friable. Carefully rinse and remove excess water from an impression before pouring it in dental stone.

Problem 3

The surface of a high-strength dental stone die was abraded during preparation of the wax pattern. Can Type 4 gypsum be treated to create a more abrasion-resistant surface that is less susceptible to damage during construction of the pattern and finishing of the casting?

Solution

Apparently not, because the available hardening solutions and various impregnation techniques have little effect on the abrasion resistance of Type 4 gypsum. Hardening solutions do result in a slightly higher setting expansion of high-strength dental stone dies.

Problem 4

A dental stone master cast for a complete denture was placed in a bowl of water before it was mounted on an articulator. Inadvertently, the cast was left in the water overnight. After the cast was mounted and dried, an unusually rough surface appeared. What happened?

Solution

Dental stone is slightly soluble in water. Leaving the cast in water for an extended time can dissolve some of the surface, roughening the cast. This roughness is transferred to the surface of the denture. If the cast must be stored in water, use a saturated calcium sulfate dihydrate solution (slurry water).

Problem 5

The boxing edge of a dental stone master cast was trimmed on a model trimmer several days after it had been poured. Trimming was much more difficult than when done soon after the dental stone had set. Why was the cast more difficult to trim, and how can this difficulty be corrected?

Solution

As dental stone dries over a period of several days, its compressive strength increases to about twice that when wet. The wet strength may be regained by soaking the cast in slurry water, which is used to minimize dissolution of the surface during soaking.

Problem 6

A gypsum investment was mixed with water in the proportions recommended by the manufacturer, but the working time was too short to invest the wax pattern. What may have happened, and how can this problem be solved?

Solution a

The powder may have been contaminated by water, from high humidity or a wet dispensing spoon. Investment should be stored in an airtight and waterproof container.

Solution b

The temperature of the mixing water may have been higher than 23° C. Water at 20° to 23° C is recommended. Higher temperatures shorten the working time.

Solution c

The spatulation may have been done incorrectly with a mechanical mixer. Overmixing, too long or too rapid, shortens the working time.

Solution d

The mixing bowl or spatula may have been contaminated with particles of set investment containing calcium sulfate dihydrate, accelerating the reaction. Mixing implements should be cleaned before use.

Problem 7

A full crown casting prepared by an immersion hygroscopic technique was too loose. What conditions might have caused this problem, and how can a tighter crown be obtained?

Solution a

The water bath may have been warmer than usual. When warmer water is used, the wax pattern offers less resistance to the expansion of the investment, producing a larger mold. The temperature of the water bath should be monitored regularly.

Solution b

A thicker-than-average mix of investment may have been used, causing an increased setting and hygroscopic expansion. The water/powder ratio recommended by the manufacturer should be used, and the water and powder accurately dispensed.

BIBLIOGRAPHY

Dental Plaster and Stone

Buchanan AS, Worner HK: Changes in the composition and setting characteristics of plaster of paris on exposure to high humidity atmospheres, *J Dent Res* 24:65, 1945.

Chong JA, Chong MP, Docking AR: The surface of gypsum cast in alginate impression, *Dent Pract* 16:107, 1965.

Combe EC, Smith DC: Some properties of gypsum plasters, *Br Dent J* 117:237, 1964.

Docking AR: Gypsum research in Australia: the setting process, *Int Dent J* 15:372, 1965.

Docking AR: Some gypsum precipitates, *Aust Dent J* 10:428, 1965.

Earnshaw R: The consistency of gypsum products, *Aust Dent J* 18:33, 1973.

Earnshaw R, Smith DC: The tensile and compressive strength of plaster and stone, *Aust Dent J* 11:415, 1966.

Fairhurst CW: Compressive properties of dental gypsum, *J Dent Res* 39:812, 1960.

Fan PL, Powers JM, Reid BC: Surface mechanical properties of stone, resin, and metal dies, *J Am Dent Assoc* 103:408, 1981.

Garber DK, Powers JM, Brandau HE: Effect of spatulation on the properties of high-strength dental stones, *Mich Dent Assoc J* 67:133, 1985.

Hollenback GM, Smith DD: A further investigation of the physical properties of hard gypsum, *Calif Dent Assoc J* 43:221, 1967.

Jorgensen KD: Studies on the setting of plaster of paris, *Odont Tskr* 61:305, 1953.

Lindquist JT, Brennan RE, Phillips RW: Influence of mixing techniques on some physical properties of plaster, *J Prosthet Dent* 3:274, 1953.

Mahler DB: Hardness and flow properties of gypsum materials, *J Prosthet Dent* 1:188, 1951.

Mahler DB: Plasters of paris and stone materials, *Int Dent J* 5:241, 1955.

Mahler DB, Asgarzadeh K: The volumetric contraction of dental gypsum material on setting, *J Dent Res* 32:354, 1953.

Neville HA: Adsorption and reaction. I. The setting of plaster of paris, *J Phys Chem* 30:1037, 1926.

Peyton FA, Leibold JP, Ridgley GV: Surface hardness, compressive strength, and abrasion resistance of indirect die stones, *J Prosthet Dent* 2:381, 1952.

Phillips RW, Ito BY: Factors affecting the surface of stone dies poured in hydrocolloid impressions, *J Prosthet Dent* 2:390, 1952.

Sanad MEE, Combe EC, Grant AA: The use of additives to improve the mechanical properties of gypsum products, *J Dent Res* 61:808, 1982.

Sarma AC, Neiman R: A study on the effect of disinfectant chemicals on physical properties of die stone, *Quint Internat* 21:53, 1990.

Stern MA, Johnson GH, Toolson LB: An evaluation of dental stones after repeated exposure to spray disinfectants. Part I: Abrasion and compressive strength, *J Prosthet Dent* 65:713, 1991.

Sweeney WT, Taylor DF: Dimensional changes in dental stone and plaster, *J Dent Res* 29:749, 1950.

Torrance A, Darvell BW: Effect of humidity on calcium sulphate hemihydrate, *Aust Dent J* 35:230, 1990.

von Fraunhofer JA, Spiers RR: Strength testing of dental stone: a comparison of compressive, tensile, transverse, and shear strength tests, *J Biomed Mater Res* 17:293, 1983.

Wiegman-Ho L, Ketelaar JAA: The kinetics of the hydration of calcium sulfate hemihydrate investigated by an electric conductance method, *J Dent Res* 61:36, 1982.

Williams GJ, Bates JF, Wild S: The effect of surface treatment of dental stone with resins, *Quint Dent Technol* 7:41, 1983.

Worner HK: Dental plasters. I. General, manufacture, and characteristics before mixing with water, *Aust J Dent* 46:1, 1942.

Worner HK: Dental plasters. II. The setting phenomenon, properties after mixing with water, methods of testing, *Aust J Dent* 46:35, 1942.

Worner HK: The effect of temperature on the rate of setting of plaster of paris, *J Dent Res* 23:305, 1944.

Casting Investments

Anderson JN: *Applied dental materials,* ed 5, Oxford, 1976, Blackwell Scientific.

Asgar K, Lawrence WN, Peyton FA: Further investigations into the nature of hygroscopic expansion of dental casting investments, *J Prosthet Dent* 8:673, 1958.

Asgarzadeh K, Mahler DB, Peyton FA: The behavior and measurement of hygroscopic expansion of dental casting investment, *J Dent Res* 33:519, 1954.

Chew CL, Land MF, Thomas CC et al: Investment strength as a function of time and temperature, *J Dent* 27:297, 1999.

Delgado VP, Peyton FA: The hygroscopic setting expansion of a dental casting investment, *J Prosthet Dent* 3:423, 1953.

Docking AR: The hygroscopic setting expansion of dental casting investments. I. *Aust J Dent* 52:6, 1948.

Docking AR, Chong MP: The hygroscopic setting expansion of dental casting investments. IV. *Aust J Dent* 53:261, 1949.

Docking AR, Chong MP, Donnison JA: The hygroscopic setting expansion of dental casting investments. II. *Aust J Dent* 52:160, 1948.

Docking AR, Donnison JA, Chong MP: The hygroscopic setting expansion of dental casting investments. III. *Aust J Dent* 52:320, 1948.

Eames WB, Edwards CR, Jr, Buck WH, Jr: Scraping resistance of dental die materials: a comparison of brands, *Oper Dent* 3:66, 1978.

Earnshaw R: The effect of restrictive stress on the thermal expansion of gypsum-bonded investments. I. Inlay casting investments, 'thermal expansion' type, *Aust Dent J* 11:345, 1966.

Earnshaw R: The effects of additives on the thermal behaviour of gypsum-bonded casting investments. I. *Aust Dent J* 20:27, 1975.

Earnshaw R, Morey EF, Edelman DC: The effect of potential investment expansion and hot strength on the fit of full crown castings made with phosphate-bonded investment, *J Oral Rehabil* 24:532, 1997.

Higuchi T: Study of thermal decomposition of gypsum bonded investment. I. Gas analysis, differential thermal analysis, thermobalance analysis, x-ray diffraction, *Kokubyo Gakkai Zasshi* 34:217, 1967.

Jones DW: Thermal analysis and stability of refractory investments, *J Prosthet Dent* 18:234, 1967.

Jones DW, Wilson HJ: Setting and hygroscopic expansion of investments, *Br Dent J* 129:22, 1970.

Lyon HW, Dickson G, Schoonover IC: Effectiveness of vacuum investing in the elimination of surface defects in gold castings, *J Am Dent Assoc* 46:197, 1953.

Lyon HW, Dickson G, Schoonover IC: The mechanism of hygroscopic expansion in dental casting investments, *J Dent Res* 34:44, 1955.

Luk HW-K, Darvell BW: Strength of phosphate-bonded investments at high temperature, *Dent Mater* 7:99, 1991.

Luk HW-K, Darvell BW: Effect of burnout temperature on strength of phosphate-bonded investments, *J Dent* 25:153, 1997.

Luk HW-K, Darvell BW: Effect of burnout temperature on strength of phosphate-bonded investments—part II, *J Dent* 25:423, 1997.

Mahler DB, Ady AB: An explanation for the hygroscopic expansion of dental gypsum products, *J Dent Res* 39:578, 1960.

Mahler DB, Ady AB: The influence of various factors on the effective setting expansion of casting investments, *J Prosthet Dent* 13:365, 1963.

Matsuya S, Yamane M: Thermal analysis of the reaction between II-CaSO4 and quartz in nitrogen flow, *Gypsum Lime* 164:3, 1980.

Miyaji T, Utsumi K, Suzuki E et al: Deterioration of phosphate-bonded investment on exposure to 100% relative humidity atmosphere, *Bull Tokyo Med Dent Univ* 29:53, 1982.

Moore TE: Method of making dental castings and composition employed in said method, US Patent 1,924,874, 1933.

Mori T: Thermal behavior of the gypsum binder in dental casting investments, *J Dent Res* 65:877, 1986.

Neiman R, Sarma AC: Setting and thermal reactions of phosphate investments, *J Dent Res* 59:1478, 1980.

Norling BK, Reisbick MH: Wetting of elastomeric impression materials modified by nonionic surfactant additions, *J Dent Res* 56B (abstr):148, 1977.

O'Brien WJ, Nielsen JP: Decomposition of gypsum investment in the presence of carbon, *J Dent Res* 38:541, 1959.

Phillips RW: Relative merits of vacuum investing of small castings as compared to conventional methods, *J Dent Res* 26:343, 1947.

Ryge G, Fairhurst CW: Hygroscopic expansion, *J Dent Res* 35:499, 1956.

Schilling ER, Miller BH, Woody RD et al: Marginal gap of crowns made with a phosphate-bonded investment and accelerated casting method, *J Prosthet Dent* 81:129, 1999.

Schnell RJ, Mumford G, Phillips RW: An evaluation of phosphate bonded investments used with a high fusing gold alloy, *J Prosthet Dent* 13:324, 1963.

Shell JS, Dootz ER: Permeability of investments at the casting temperature, *J Dent Res* 40:999, 1961.

Shell JS, Hollenback GM: Setting and thermal investment expansion in longitudinal and transverse directions, *J S Calif Dent Assoc* 41:511, 1965.

Tiara M, Okazaki M, Takahashi J et al: Effects of four mixing methods on setting expansion and compressive strength of six commercial phosphate-bonded silica investments, *J Oral Rehabil* 27:306, 2000.

Weinstein LJ: Composition for dental molds, US Patent 1,708,436, 1929.

Chapter 14

Waxes

Few procedures in restorative dentistry can be completed without the use of wax in one of its many forms. Forming an inlay pattern, boxing an impression before it is poured in dental stone, and making an impression for the registration of occlusal bite relationships each requires a specially formulated wax. Some uses for various dental waxes are shown in Fig. 14-1. These examples display how the tasks these waxes perform, and therefore their properties, vary greatly. Accuracy is a requisite for inlay or removable denture patterns, shown in the upper left of Fig. 14-1, whereas for the boxing of an impression, shown in the upper center, the ease and convenient manipulation of the wax are essential. Other applications, such as the denture forms shown in the lower left or the corrective impression wax shown in the upper right of Fig. 14-1, require equally varying qualities in the waxes, as do the applications of wax for the border and palate of the metal tray or for attaching a plaster splint to the model, as shown in the lower right of the figure. Thus the specific use of the dental wax determines the physical properties that are most desirable for a successful application.

WAXES, GUMS, FATS, AND RESINS

Dental waxes may be composed of natural and synthetic waxes, gums, fats, fatty acids, oils, natural and synthetic resins, and pigments of various types. The particular working characteristics of each wax are achieved by blending the appropriate natural and synthetic waxes and resins and other additives, some of which are shown in Table 14-1.

The chemical components of both natural and synthetic waxes impart characteristic physical properties to the wax, which are of primary

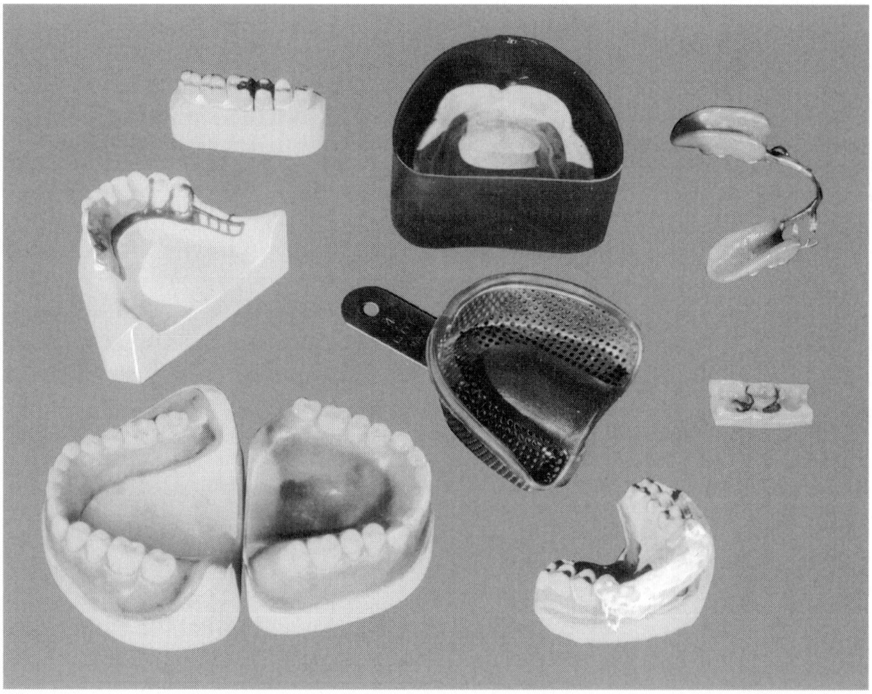

Fig. 14-1 Applications of waxes in dentistry. Inlay pattern, *upper left;* boxing of an impression, *upper center;* baseplate, *lower left;* casting wax, *left center;* utility wax, *center;* sticky wax, *lower right;* corrective impression, *upper right;* and bite, *right center.*

interest because the specific physical properties of a wax or wax blend determine its usefulness for intended applications. Natural waxes are distributed in nature, whereas synthetic waxes are produced by combination of various chemicals in the laboratory or by chemical action on natural waxes. The additives may be natural materials and synthetic products.

NATURAL WAXES

Historically, waxes have been classified according to their origin: (1) mineral, (2) plant, (3) insect, and (4) animal; however, a better classification is based on their chemical composition. The two principal groups of organic compounds contained in waxes are hydrocarbons and esters, although some waxes contain free alcohols and acids as well.

The chief constituents of most mineral waxes are hydrocarbons ranging from 17 to more than 44 carbon atoms, a fact that accounts for odd and even numbers in the chain, as shown in the following formula:

$$CH_3—(CH_2)_{15\text{ to }42}—CH_3$$

The hydrocarbons in plant waxes are saturated alkanes with from 19 to 31 carbon atoms present in odd numbers. Therefore, dental waxes contain molecules having a range of molecular weights that affect the melting and flow properties of the waxes.

Plant and animal waxes contain considerable concentrations of esters, and carnauba (a plant wax) contains 85% alkyl esters of various kinds. The principal ester in beeswax is myricyl palmitate,

$$C_{15}H_{31}—\overset{\overset{\displaystyle O}{\|}}{C}—O—C_{30}H_{61}$$

which is the reaction product of myricyl alcohol and palmitic acid. Plant and animal waxes also contain acids, alcohols, hydrocarbons, and resins; whereas Montan wax (an earth wax) contains large amounts of esters, the main compound being

$$C_{28}H_{57}—\overset{\overset{\displaystyle O}{\|}}{C}—O—C_{24}H_{49}$$

However, there are other esters composed of $C_{20}—C_{29}$ acids and $C_{20}—C_{30}$ alcohols.

This brief description of the composition of natural waxes indicates that they are complex combinations of organic compounds of reasonably high molecular weights. Also, the composition of these waxes varies, depending on the source and the time of collection; therefore, dental manufacturers must blend the particular batches of wax to obtain the properties desired for a particular application. Characteristics of various waxes used in dentistry and described below are summarized in Table 14-2.

Paraffin waxes are obtained principally from the high–boiling point fractions of petroleum. The melting temperatures generally increase

TABLE 14-1 Components of Dental Waxes

Natural Waxes	Synthetic Waxes	Additives
Mineral	Acrawax	Stearic acid
Paraffin	Aerosol OT	Glyceryl tristearate
Microcrystalline	Castorwax	Oils
Barnsdahl	Flexo-wax C	Turpentine
Ozokerite	Epolene N-10	Colorants
Ceresin	Albacer	Natural resins
Montan	Aldo 33	Rosin
Plant	Durawax 1032	Copal
Carnauba		Dammar
Ouricury		Sandarac
Candelilla		Mastic
Japan wax		Shellac
Cocoa butter		Kauri
Insect		Synthetic resins
Beeswax		Elvax
Animal		Polyethylene
Spermaceti		Polystyrene

TABLE 14-2 Characteristics of Various Waxes Used in Dentistry

Wax	Type	Melting Range (° C)	Characteristics in Mixtures with Paraffin Wax
Paraffin	Straight-chain hydrocarbon with 26-30 carbon atoms	40-71	No value
Microcrystalline	Branched-chain hydrocarbon with 41-50 carbon atoms	60-91	Less volumetric change during solidification
Barnsdahl	Microcrystalline wax	70-74	Increases melting range and hardness, reduces flow
Ozokerite	Microcrystalline wax, straight-, branched- and closed-chain hydrocarbons	65	No value
Ceresin	Straight- and branched-chain paraffins	No value	Higher molecular weight, higher hardness, increase melting range
Montan	Long-chain esters with 40-58 carbon atoms, alcohols, acids, resins	72-92	Improves hardness and melting range
Carnauba	Esters, alcohols, acids, hydrocarbons	84-91	Increases melting range and hardness
Ouricury	Esters, alcohols, acids, hydrocarbons	79-84	Increases melting range and hardness
Candelilla	Hydrocarbon with 29-33 carbon atoms, alcohols, acids, esters, lactones	68-75	Increases hardness
Japan wax	Fats—glycerides of palmitic and stearic acids	51	Improves tackiness and emulsifying ability
Cocoa butter	Fats—glycerides of palmitic, stearic, oleic, lauric acids	No value	Improves tackiness and emulsifying ability
Beeswax	Esters—myricyl palmitate, hydrocarbons, organic acids	63-70	Modifies properties of paraffin wax

with increasing molecular weights. The presence of oils in the wax, however, lowers the melting temperature; paraffin waxes used in dentistry are refined waxes and have less than 0.5% oil.

Paraffin waxes produced by current refining procedures can crystallize in the form of plates, needles, or malcrystals, but are usually of the plate type. Many hydrocarbon waxes undergo crystalline changes on cooling, and a transition from needles to plates occurs about 5° to 8° C below their melting temperature. During solidification and cooling, there is a volumetric contraction that varies from 11% to 15%. This contraction is not uniform throughout the temperature range from the melting temperature to room temperature, because the wax is a mixture of hydrocarbons and the wax passes through transition points accompanied by changes in physical properties.

Microcrystalline waxes are similar to paraffin waxes, except they are obtained from the heavier oil fractions in the petroleum industry and, as a result, have higher melting points. These waxes crystallize in small plates and are tougher and more flexible than paraffin waxes. They have an affinity for oil, and their hardness and tackiness may be altered by adding oil. Microcrystalline waxes have less volumetric change during solidification than paraffin waxes.

Barnsdahl is a microcrystalline wax used to increase the melting range and hardness and reduce the flow of paraffin waxes.

Ozokerite is an earth wax found near petroleum deposits in central Europe and the western United States. Ozokerite is similar to microcrystalline wax in that it is composed of straight- and branched-chain hydrocarbons, but it also contains some closed-chain hydrocarbons. It also has great affinity for oil, and in quantities of 5% to 15% greatly improves the physical characteristics of paraffins in the melting range of 54° C.

Ceresin is a term used to describe waxes from wax-bearing distillates from natural-mineral petroleum refining or lignite refining. Like microcrystalline waxes, they are straight- and branched-chain paraffins, but they have higher molecular weights and greater hardness than hydrocarbon waxes distilled from the crude products. These waxes also may be used to increase the melting range of paraffin waxes.

Montan waxes are obtained by extraction from various lignites, and although they are mineral waxes, their composition and properties are similar to those of the plant waxes. Montan waxes are hard, brittle, and lustrous; they blend well with other waxes, and therefore are often substituted for plant waxes to improve the hardness and melting range of paraffin waxes.

Carnauba and *ouricury waxes* are composed of straight-chain esters, alcohols, acids, and hydrocarbons. They are characterized by high hardness, brittleness, and high melting temperatures. Both possess the outstanding quality of increasing the melting range and hardness of paraffin waxes; for example, adding 10% of carnauba wax to paraffin wax with a melting range of 20° C increases the melting range to 46° C. Adding ouricury waxes produces a similar effect, but they are less effective than carnauba wax.

Candelilla waxes consist of 40% to 60% paraffin hydrocarbons containing 29 to 33 carbon atoms, accompanied by free alcohols, acids, esters, and lactones. Like carnauba and ouricury wax, they harden paraffin waxes but are not so effective for increasing the melting range.

Japan wax and *cocoa butter* are not true waxes; they are chiefly fats. Japan wax contains the glycerides of palmitic and stearic acids and higher-molecular-weight acids; cocoa butter is completely fat and composed of glycerides of stearic, palmitic, oleic, lauric, and lower fatty acids. Japan wax is a tough, malleable, and sticky material that melts at about 51° C, whereas cocoa butter is a brittle substance at room temperatures. Japan wax may be mixed with paraffin to improve tackiness and emulsifying ability, and cocoa butter is used to protect against dehydration of soft tissues and to protect glass ionomer products temporarily from moisture during setting or from dehydrating after they are set.

Beeswax is the primary insect wax used in dentistry. It is a complex mixture of esters plus saturated and unsaturated hydrocarbons and high-molecular-weight organic acids. It is a brittle material at room temperature but becomes plastic at body temperature. It is used to modify the properties of paraffin waxes, and is the main component in sticky wax.

Animal waxes such as *spermaceti wax*, obtained from the sperm whale, are not used extensively in dentistry; like beeswax, they are mainly ester waxes. Spermaceti wax has been used as a coating in the manufacture of dental floss.

SYNTHETIC WAXES

In recent years synthetic waxes and resins have become available. Although the use of synthetic waxes and resins is increasing, it is still limited in dental formulations, and the natural waxes continue to be the primary components.

Synthetic waxes are complex organic compounds of varied chemical compositions. Although they differ chemically from natural waxes, they possess certain physical properties, such as melting temperature or hardness, which are akin to those of the natural waxes. They may differ from natural waxes in certain characteristics because of their high degree of refinement, in contrast with the contamination that is common in natural waxes.

Synthetic waxes include (1) polyethylene waxes, (2) polyoxyethylene glycol waxes, (3) halogenated hydrocarbon waxes, (4) hydrogenated waxes, and (5) wax esters from the reaction of fatty alcohols and acids. Polyethylene polymers having molecular weights from 2000 to 4000 are waxes melting at 100° to 105° C. These waxes possess properties similar to high-molecular-weight paraffin waxes obtained from petroleum. Polyoxyethylene waxes are polymers of ethylene glycols and have melting temperatures from 37° to 63° C. They have limited compatibility with other waxes but do function as plasticizers and tend to toughen films of wax. The remaining synthetic waxes are prepared by reactions with natural waxes or wax products, as with chlorine in the preparation of halogenated waxes and hydrogen in the manufacture of hydrogenated waxes. The variability of various batches of synthetic wax is similar to that of natural waxes.

GUMS

Many waxes obtained from plants and animals resemble in appearance a group of substances described as *gums*. Many plants produce a variety of gums that are viscous, amorphous exudates that harden on exposure to air. Most gums are complicated substances. Many are mixtures containing largely carbohydrates; when they are mixed with water, they either dissolve or form sticky, viscous liquids. Gum arabic and tragacanth are two natural gums that do not resemble waxes in either their properties or composition.

FATS

As a class of substances, waxes are harder and have higher melting temperatures than fats, but in some ways they resemble fat. Both are tasteless, odorless, and colorless in the pure form, and they usually feel greasy. Chemically, fats are composed of esters of various fatty acids with glycerol and are known as glycerides, which distinguishes them from waxes. Some examples of fats are glycerides of stearic acid or tristearate, found in tallow, and the mixed glyceride of oleic, palmitic, and butyric acids, found in butter.

Glyceryl tristearate, the chief ingredient of beef tallow, is a fat with a melting temperature of about 43° C. It has a lustrous appearance and is a firm, slightly greasy solid that bears a resemblance to waxes. The fat may be used to increase the melting range and hardness of compounded wax. Oils have a pronounced effect on the properties of waxes, as mentioned earlier in connection with the discussion of paraffin waxes. *Hydrocarbon oils* may be used to soften mixtures of waxes, and small quantities of *silicone oils* may be added to improve the ease of polishing with waxes.

RESINS

In some respects natural resins resemble waxes in appearance and properties, although they form a distinct classification of substances. Many species of trees and other plants produce exudates of natural resins, such as dammar, rosin, or sandarac. Natural resins are relatively insoluble in water, but vary in solubility in certain organic liquids. Generally, resins are complex, amorphous mixtures of organic substances that are characterized by specific physical behavior rather than by any definite chemical composition. Most natural resins are obtained from trees and plants; shellac, however, is produced by insects. Numerous natural resins are blended with waxes to develop waxes for dental applications.

Natural resins such as *dammar* and *kauri* may be mixed with waxes. They are compatible with most natural waxes and produce harder products. Synthetic resins, such as *polyethylene* and *vinyl* resins of various types, may be added to paraffin waxes to improve their toughness, film-forming characteristics, and melting ranges.

Natural and synthetic resins may also be used in organic solvents to produce film-forming materials that may be used as a cavity liner. *Copal* is a natural, brittle resin that has a melting range well above 149° C, but when deposited as a film from an organic solvent, it serves as a liner for prepared cavities. *Polystyrene* is a synthetic resin that may be used in a similar manner.

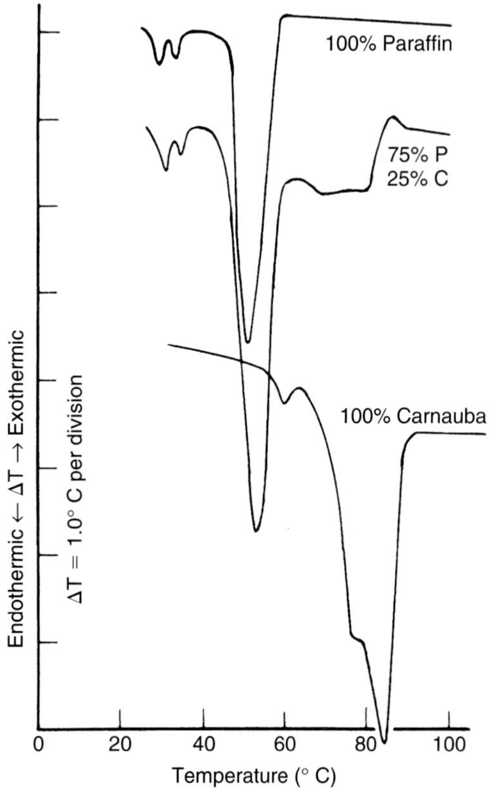

Fig. 14-2 Differential thermograms of paraffin, carnauba, and a 75% paraffin–25% carnauba wax mixture.

CHARACTERISTIC PROPERTIES OF WAXES

Useful and important properties of waxes include melting range, thermal expansion, mechanical properties, flow, residual stress, and ductility.

MELTING RANGE

Because waxes may contain several types of molecules, each having a range of molecular weights, they have *melting ranges* rather than *melting points*. The melting ranges of a paraffin wax, a carnauba wax, and a mixture of these two waxes are illustrated in Fig. 14-2. The curves are differential thermograms obtained in the manner described in the Thermal Properties section of Chapter 3. The melting range for paraffin wax is from 44° to 62° C, and for carnauba wax, from 50° to 90° C. When a mixture of 75% paraffin and 25% carnauba wax was prepared, the paraffin component melted at essentially the same temperatures, but the melting temperature of the carnauba wax was decreased slightly. Note that adding carnauba to paraffin wax dramatically increased the melting range to 44° C, compared with 18° C for paraffin alone.

The effect of the composition of paraffin-carnauba mixtures on the melting range is shown in Fig. 14-3. The presence of 2.5% carnauba wax had little effect on the melting range, but the range increased rapidly as the concentration of carnauba wax was increased to 10%. Al-

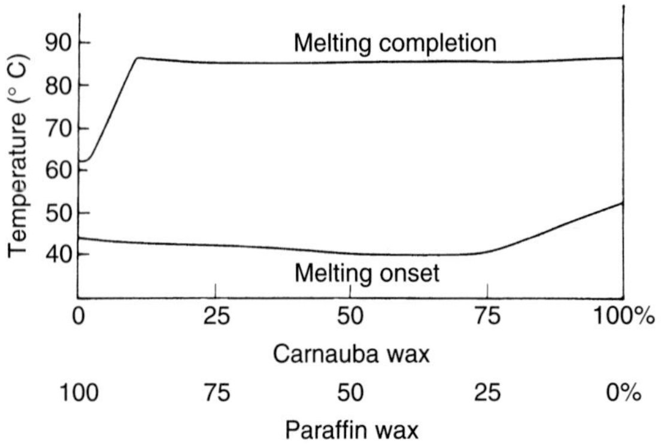

Fig. 14-3 Melting ranges of mixtures of paraffin and carnauba wax.

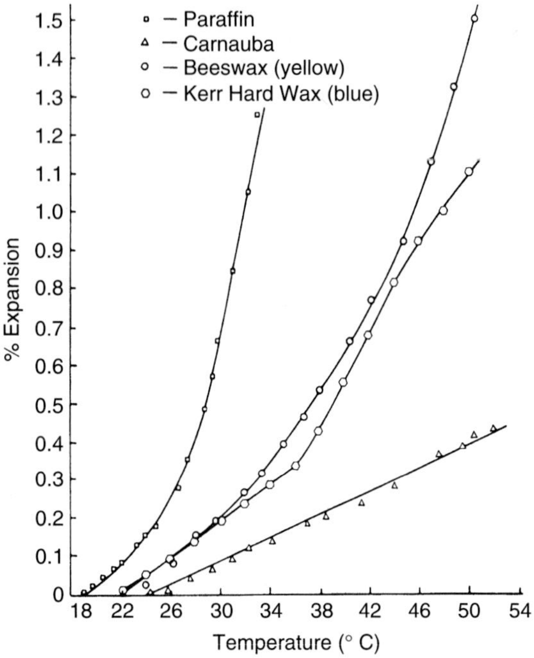

Fig. 14-4 Thermal expansion curves for four waxes.

though concentrations of carnauba wax greater than 10% had no further effect on the melting range, higher amounts are necessary for certain applications to control the flow and mechanical properties. The melting of mixtures of paraffin and higher–melting point waxes can be visualized as the melting of paraffin near its usual temperature, but the entire wax does not appear melted because the matrix of carnauba wax does not melt until a considerably higher temperature is reached.

THERMAL EXPANSION

Like other materials, waxes expand when subjected to a rise in temperature and contract as the temperature is decreased. This fundamental property may be altered slightly when various waxes are blended (Fig. 14-4), but the response to thermal changes cannot be reduced to negligible values. The expansion and contraction of dental waxes with changes in temperature are pronounced, as is illustrated in Table 14-3. In general, dental waxes and their components have the largest coefficient of thermal expansion of any material used in restorative dentistry.

The linear thermal expansion properties of waxes may be explained on the basis of the strength of secondary valence forces and the transition points. Mineral waxes generally have higher coefficients of linear thermal expansion than plant waxes. Mineral waxes expand more because they have weak secondary valence forces, which are easily overcome by the energy absorbed during a rise in temperature. This permits more movement of the wax components, thus allowing a greater amount of thermal expansion.

Plant waxes, on the other hand, have high secondary valence forces because of their high concentrations of esters. Because the secondary valence forces restrict the movement of the wax components, small coefficients of thermal expansion are observed until the melting range of the wax is approached. This phenomenon is illustrated by beeswax; yellow beeswax has much higher coefficients of linear thermal expansion than bleached beeswax.

Many waxes exhibit at least two rates of expansion between 22° and 52° C. These changes in rate of expansion occur at transition points. At these points the internal structural parts become freer to move. For example, during this transition hydrocarbon chains of a mineral wax become free to rotate; consequently, after a wax has been heated through a transition point, it is

TABLE 14-3 Coefficient of Thermal Expansion of Mineral, Plant, Insect, and Inlay Waxes

Wax	Temperature Range (° C)	Coefficient ×10^{-6}/° C
MINERAL		
Paraffin	20.0-27.8	307
	27.8-34.0	1631
Litene	22.0-47.5	205
	47.5-52.0	590
Barnsdahl	22.0-40.4	185
	40.4-52.0	243
Ceresin	22.0-27.4	307
	27.4-34.7	849
	34.7-42.2	471
	42.2-50.0	1434
Montan	22.0-41.5	188
	41.5-52.0	294
PLANT		
Carnauba	22.0-52.0	156
Candelilla	22.0-40.2	182
	40.2-52.0	365
Ouricury	22.0-43.0	186
	43.0-52.0	307
Japan wax	22.0-38.6	304
	38.6-45.0	755
INSECT		
Beeswax (yellow)	22.0-41.2	344
	41.2-50.0	1048
Beeswax (bleached)	22.0-38.6	271
	38.6-50.0	606
INLAY		
Kerr blue inlay wax (hard)	22.0-37.5	323
	37.5-45.0	629
	45.0-50.0	328
Kerr blue inlay wax (regular)	22.0-32.7	263
	32.7-40.9	662
	40.9-46.9	458
	46.9-50.0	1084

freer to expand. Because the ingredient waxes are undergoing transitions that do not coincide with one another, certain inlay waxes exhibit more than two changes in rate of expansion.

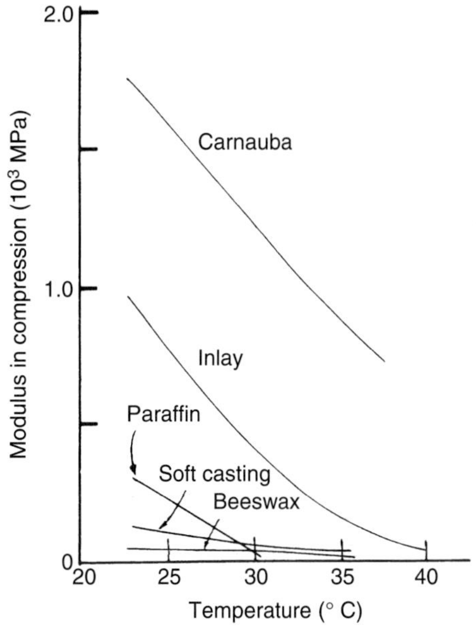

Fig. 14-5 Elastic modulus of various waxes as a function of temperature.

Different waxes may have decidedly different rates and amounts of thermal expansion, as shown in Table 14-3. For example, carnauba and Montan wax have approximately the same melting ranges, but from 22° to 52° C they have dissimilar expansion characteristics.

Some waxes have different rates of expansion in different temperature ranges, as seen by the change of shape of the curves for paraffin, beeswax, and an inlay wax in Fig. 14-4. Because the coefficient of thermal expansion of inlay wax is so great, temperature changes in wax patterns after the critical dimensional relationships are set may be a major contributing factor in inaccuracy of the finished restoration.

MECHANICAL PROPERTIES

The elastic modulus, proportional limit, and compressive strength of waxes are low compared with those of other materials, and these properties depend strongly on the temperature. The elastic moduli of various waxes between 23° and 40° C are shown in Fig. 14-5, with carnauba wax having the highest values and beeswax the lowest. The elastic modulus of carnauba wax decreased from 1790 to 760 MPa from 23° to 37° C. Paraffin wax showed a sharp decrease in modulus from 310 to 28 MPa between 23° and 30° C. The inlay wax, which simulates a mixture of 75% paraffin and 25% carnauba wax, had intermediate changes in modulus of 760 to 48 MPa between 23° and 40° C.

The modulus of the inlay wax is important in the hygroscopic expansion of casting investments, in which the wax pattern is subjected to stresses resulting from the expansion of the investment during setting. Nonuniform deformation of wax patterns, such as crowns, can be minimized by using waxes having different elastic moduli for particular parts of the pattern. For example, in a crown the lateral walls can be prepared with inlay wax, and the occlusal surfaces can be constructed of soft green casting wax (see Fig. 14-5). At the investing temperature, the modulus ratio for the inlay and soft green casting wax is 7:1, which is the approximate ratio needed for many patterns to obtain uniform expansion in the occlusal compared with the marginal areas.

The proportional limits and the compressive strengths of the waxes shown in Fig. 14-5 exhibit the same trends as their elastic moduli. The proportional limit of carnauba wax decreased from 11 to 5.5 MPa over the range of 23° to 37° C. Inlay casting wax experienced a decrease in proportional limit of 4.8 to 0.2 MPa from 23° to 40° C. The compressive strength of inlay wax decreased from 83 to 0.5 MPa over the same temperature range, and the percent compression at rupture varied from 2.7% to 4.3%. Hence the inlay wax would be considered a brittle material, although it possesses flow or viscous properties at stresses below its proportional limit.

FLOW

The property of flow results from the slippage of molecules over each other. A measure of flow in the liquid state of wax would be synonymous with viscosity. Below the melting point of the wax, however, a measure of the flow actually would be a measure of the degree of plastic deformation of the material at a given temperature. Flow is decidedly dependent on the temperature of the wax, the force bringing about the deformation, and the time the force is applied, as shown in Fig. 14-6. Flow greatly increases as the melting point of the wax is approached. Although a high percentage of flow at a given temperature may be required for a specific wax, it may be extremely deleterious at a temperature a few degrees lower. This is especially true for the direct inlay wax. This material must have a relatively high flow a few degrees above mouth temperature so it is workable but not uncomfortably warm when placed in the mouth of the patient. At mouth temperature, an inlay wax to be used for a direct pattern must have essentially no flow to minimize the possibility of distortion of the pattern during removal from the tooth cavity.

The flow of wax at different temperatures is shown in Fig. 14-6. Yellow beeswax does not flow extensively until it reaches 38° C, and at 40° C it flows about 7%. From these data it is easy to understand why beeswax has been used as a major ingredient in dental impression wax. Many mineral waxes have about a 10° C range between 1% and 70% flow, which indicates that these waxes soften gradually over a broad temperature range. Some mineral waxes—paraffin, litene, barnsdahl, and ceresin—flow 50% approximately 20° C below their melting range. This can be explained by the fact that the mineral waxes are straight- or branched-chain hydrocarbons. The secondary valence forces in these waxes are rather weak and are gradually dissipated as the temperature is increased.

Montan wax, another mineral wax, requires a temperature of 71° C, or 8° C below its melting range, to flow 50%. However, this wax is similar to the plant waxes in that it is composed mainly of esters formed in nature by the union of higher alcohols with higher fatty acids. The plant waxes likewise require temperatures close to their melting range to produce 50% flow. As a result of the presence of ester groups in these waxes, the secondary valence forces are rather strong, and a

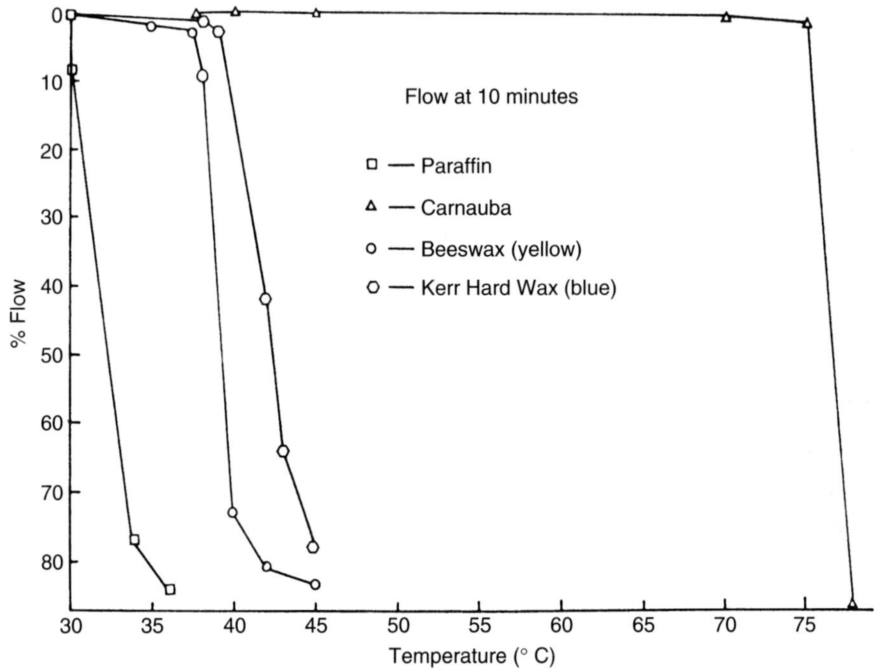

Fig. 14-6 Flow at 10 minutes for four waxes at various temperatures.

high temperature is necessary to overcome these forces. Once the secondary valence forces are overcome, these waxes flow rapidly. Below this point they often appear to fracture in a manner similar to a brittle material.

Yellow beeswax, which is also primarily an ester wax, flows extensively 24° C below its melting range (61° to 63° C) and displays an 8° C temperature difference between 1% and 70% flow. This wax contains a large number of impurities, which interfere with the secondary valence forces. As beeswax goes through the bleaching process and some of these impurities are removed, the secondary valence forces increase. Flow data illustrate this point, because bleached beeswax requires a temperature closer to its melting range to produce a large amount of flow, and the temperature difference between 1% and 70% flow is only 4° C. Note that the flow of various batches of yellow beeswax shows that significant differences may exist between batches. A similar observation is seen with paraffin and carnauba wax.

A plot of percent flow versus time for a hard inlay wax shows that at 40° C the amount of flow in relation to time is linear (Fig. 14-7). The total amount of flow after 10 minutes at this temperature is only 2%. At 42° C, the flow increases enough to cause an increase in the rate of flow. At 43° and 45° C, the rate of flow is very large at the beginning of the test, and the rate decreases rapidly as a result of the increase in diameter of the specimen.

The flow of dental waxes is influenced by the presence of solid-solid and melting transformations that occur in the component waxes. The transformation temperatures can be related to flow indirectly by studying the resistance of the wax to penetration as a function of temperature. In Fig. 14-8, penetration thermograms are compared with a differential thermal analysis curve for an inlay casting wax for annealed, *A*, and unannealed, *U*, specimens tested at two stress levels. At the lower stress level, the high–melting point ester component of the wax influenced penetration. However, at a high stress level the

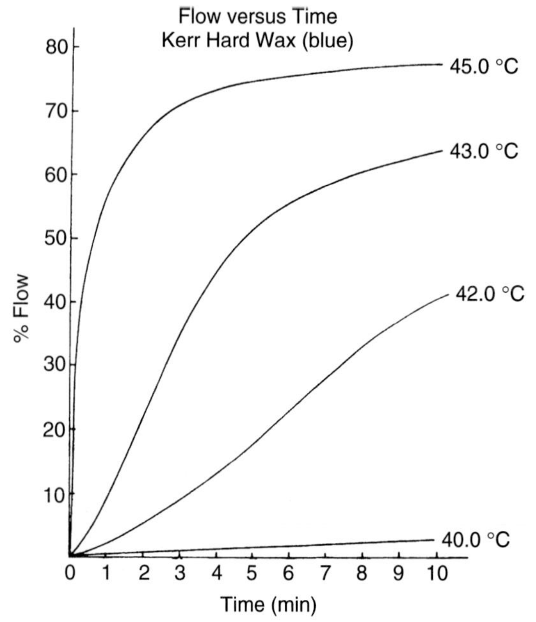

Fig. 14-7 Flow curves at various temperatures for Kerr hard (Type 2) wax.

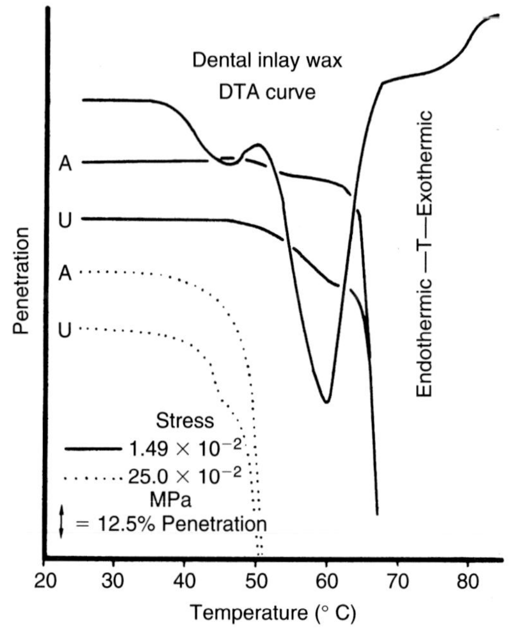

Fig. 14-8 Penetration thermograms for annealed, *A*, and unannealed, *U*, inlay wax compared with a differential thermal analysis (DTA) curve.

temperature of the solid-solid transformation associated with the hydrocarbon component of the wax determined the resistance to penetration. Annealing the wax in an oven at 50° C for 24 hours before testing had the effect of increasing the resistance of the wax to penetration.

RESIDUAL STRESS

Regardless of the method used to prepare a wax pattern, residual stress exists in the completed pattern. The presence of residual stress can be demonstrated by comparing the thermal expansion curves of annealed wax with wax that has been cooled under compression or tension. The thermal expansion of an annealed inlay wax is shown in Fig. 14-9, in which the same curve is obtained on heating or cooling. When the wax specimen is prepared by holding the softened wax under compression during cooling, followed by the determination of the thermal expansion, the thermal expansion is greater than for the annealed specimen. The extent of the deviation from the curve for the annealed wax is a function of the magnitude of the residual internal stress and the time and temperature of storage of the specimen before the thermal expansion curve is determined. Therefore a shaded area is shown rather than a specific curve. When the wax specimen is cooled while being subjected to tensile stress and the thermal expansion is determined, the curve for the wax specimen is lower than that for the annealed specimen. If sufficient residual stress is introduced, a thermal contraction may result on heating; again a shaded area indicates the direction of the effect.

The changes in dimensions resulting from the heating of wax specimens formed under com-

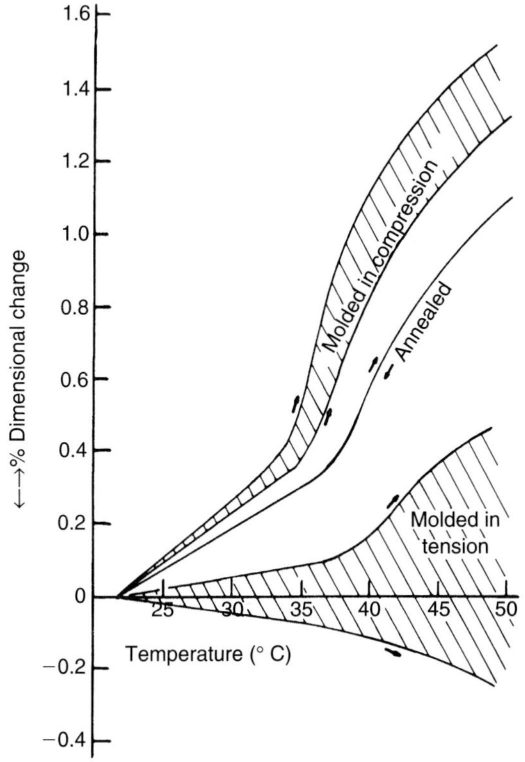

Fig. 14-9 Dimensional change on heating annealed inlay wax patterns, and that of waxes formed under compression and tension.

pression or tension can be explained as follows: When the specimen is held under compression during cooling, the atoms and molecules are forced closer together than when they are under no external stress. After the specimen is cooled to room temperature and the load removed, the motion of the molecules is restricted; this restriction results in residual stress in the specimen. When the specimen is heated, the release of the residual stress is added to the normal thermal expansion, and the total expansion is greater than normal. When the specimen is cooled while under tensile stress and expansion as a result of heating is measured, the release of the residual tensile stress results in a dimensional change that is opposite to the thermal expansion. The sum of these two effects results in a lower thermal expansion curve than for annealed wax. As seen in Fig. 14-9, if a sufficiently large amount of residual stress is introduced, the overall dimensional change on heating results in a contraction of the specimen.

DUCTILITY

Like flow, ductility increases as the temperature of a wax specimen is increased. In general, waxes with lower melting temperatures have a greater ductility at any given temperature than those with higher melting temperatures.

The ductility of a blended wax is greatly influenced by the distribution of the melting temperatures of the component waxes. A blended wax with components that have wide melting ranges generally has greater ductility than blended waxes that have a narrow range. Whenever a wide range of melting temperatures is present, the softening point of the lowest component is approached first. A further temperature rise begins to liquefy this component and approach still closer to the softening points of the higher–softening point components. This tends to plasticize the entire wax mass, thereby enhancing ductility.

Generally, highly refined waxes are quite brittle. The lower–melting point, microcrystalline mineral waxes, which contain appreciable amounts of occluded oil, are moderately soft and exhibit a high degree of plasticity or ductility, even with their comparatively high melting temperatures.

DENTAL WAXES

A variety of natural waxes and resins have been used in dentistry for specific and well-defined applications. In some instances, the most favorable qualities can be obtained from a single wax, such as beeswax, but more often a blend of several waxes is necessary to develop the most desirable qualities.

A classification of dental waxes according to their use and application is given in Table 14-4. Pattern waxes are used to form the general predetermined size and contour of an artificial dental restoration, which is to be constructed of a

TABLE 14-4 A Classification of Dental Waxes

Pattern	Processing	Impression
Inlay	Boxing	Corrective
Casting	Utility	Bite
Sheet	Sticky	
Ready shapes		
Wax-up		
Baseplate		

more durable material such as cast gold alloys, cobalt-chromium-nickel alloys, or acrylic resin. All pattern waxes have two major qualities, thermal change in dimension and tendency to warp or distort on standing, which create serious problems in their use whether an inlay pattern, crown, or complete denture is being constructed.

Processing waxes are used primarily as auxiliary aids in constructing a variety of restorations and appliances, either clinically or in the laboratory. Processing waxes perform numerous tasks that simplify many dental procedures in such operations as denture construction or soldering.

One of the oldest recorded uses of wax in dentistry is for taking impressions within the mouth. Because a wax formulated for use as an impression material exhibits high flow and ductility, it distorts readily when withdrawn from undercut areas. Therefore, the use of wax has been limited to the non-undercut edentulous portions of the mouth. Recently, specially formulated addition-silicone and polyether impression materials have replaced wax as a bite registration material.

INLAY PATTERN WAX

Gold inlays, crowns, and bridge units are formed by a casting process that uses the lost-wax pattern technique. A pattern of wax is first constructed that duplicates the shape and contour of the desired gold casting. The carved wax pattern is then embedded in a gypsum-silica investment material to form a mold with an ingate or sprue leading from the outer surface of the investment mold to the pattern, as described in Chapter 17. The wax is subsequently eliminated by heating and softening, and the mold is further conditioned to receive the molten gold by controlled heating in a furnace.

Composition The principal waxes used to formulate inlay waxes are paraffin, microcrystalline wax, ceresin, carnauba, candelilla, and beeswax. For example, an inlay wax may contain 60% paraffin, 25% carnauba, 10% ceresin, and 5% beeswax. Therefore, hydrocarbon waxes constitute the major portion of this formulation. Some inlay waxes are described as hard, regular (medium), or soft, which is a general indication of their flow. The flow can be reduced by adding more carnauba wax or by selecting a higher–melting point paraffin wax. An interesting example is that a hard inlay wax may contain a lower percentage of carnauba wax than a regular inlay wax, but the flow of the hard inlay wax is less than the regular wax because of the selection of a higher-melting-point paraffin in the formulation of the hard wax. Resins in small amounts, such as 1%, also affect the flow of inlay waxes. Inlay waxes are usually produced in deep blue, green, or purple rods or sticks about 7.5 cm long and 0.64 cm in diameter. Some manufacturers supply the wax in the form of small pellets or cones or in small, metal ointment jars.

Properties The accuracy and ultimate usefulness of the resulting gold casting depend largely on the accuracy and fine detail of the wax pattern. A wax that is able to function well in the gold casting technique must possess certain, very important physical properties.

Revised ANSI/ADA Specification No. 4 (ISO 1561) for dental inlay casting wax has been formulated for waxes used in direct and indirect waxing techniques. A summary of flow requirements of this specification is given in Table 14-5. Because the wax patterns are to be melted and vaporized from the investment mold, it is essential that no excessive residue remain in the mold because of incomplete wax burnout. Excess residue may result in the incomplete casting of inlay

TABLE 14-5 Flow Requirements for Dental Inlay Casting Wax (Flow, in %)

	Wax Temperature					
	30° C	37° C	40° C		45° C	
	Maximum	Maximum	Minimum	Maximum	Minimum	Maximum
Type 1 (soft)	1.0	—	50	—	70	90
Type 2 (hard)	—	1.0	—	20	70	90

Adapted from Dental casting wax ISO 1561:1995(E).

margins. The specification therefore limits the nonvolatile residue of these waxes to a maximum of 0.10% at an ignition temperature of 700° C.

Types 1 (soft) and 2 (hard) dental inlay casting waxes are recognized by Revised ANSI/ADA Specification No. 4. Type 1 wax is a soft wax used as an indirect technique wax. Type 2 wax is a harder wax prescribed for forming direct patterns in the mouth, where lower flow values at 37° C tend to minimize any tendency for distortion of the pattern on its removal from the cavity preparation. Type 1 wax shows greater flow than Type 2 wax at temperatures both below and above mouth temperature. The lower flow of Type 2 wax and the greater ease of carving the softer Type 1 waxes are desirable working characteristics for the techniques associated with each.

The specification also requires the manufacturers to include instructions regarding the method of softening and the working temperature for the wax preparatory to forming a direct pattern. Both types should soften without becoming flaky, and when trimmed to a fine margin during the pattern-carving operation, they should not chip or flake. Thermal expansion data for the Type 2 wax are no longer required by the specification.

Flow When forming a wax pattern directly in the mouth, the wax must be heated to a temperature at which it has sufficient flow under compression to reproduce the prepared cavity walls in great detail. The working temperature, suggested by the manufacturer, which should be satisfactory for making direct wax patterns, must not be so high as to cause damage to the vital tooth structure or be uncomfortable to the patient. Insufficient flow of the wax caused by insufficient heating results in the lack of cavity detail and introduces excess stress within the pattern. An overabundant amount of flow resulting from excessive heating makes compression of the wax difficult because of a lack of "body" in the material.

The values listed in Table 14-5 represent minimum or maximum values of percent flow that occur at various temperatures when Types 1 and 2 wax specimens are subjected to a 19.6 N load for 10 minutes. The temperature that the Type 2 wax must attain to register cavity detail is usually somewhat above 45° C. As seen from these values, the flow of the hard wax is no more than 1% at body temperature. The flow of the Type 1 wax is about 9% at this temperature. Low flow at this temperature tends to minimize distortion of a well-carved pattern as it is withdrawn from an adequately tapered cavity in the tooth.

Thermal Coefficient of Expansion

The curve in Fig. 14-10 shows that the rate of expansion of the Type I inlay wax is greatest from just below mouth temperature to just above 45° C. Knowing the amount of wax expansion or contraction allows one to judge the compensation necessary to produce an accurate casting. Data sufficient to show the thermal contraction of the wax from its working temperature to room temperature may be included in each package of inlay wax. Once the wax pattern is carved, its removal from the tooth cavity and transfer to the laboratory bring about a reduction in tempera-

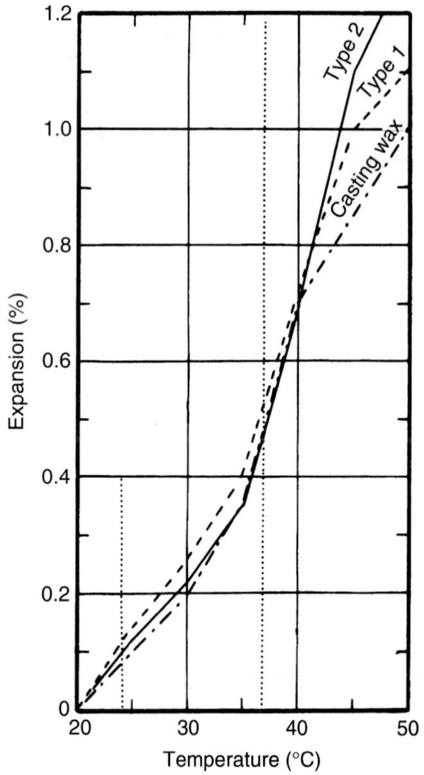

Fig. 14-10 Percent expansion of inlay and casting waxes from 20° to 50° C, showing the percent dimensional change from mouth temperature to average room temperature.

ture and subsequent thermal contraction. A decrease of 12° to 13° C in temperature, from mouth temperature to a room temperature of about 24° C, causes a 0.4% linear contraction of the wax, or about 0.04% change for each degree change in temperature.

Warpage of Wax Patterns Inlay pattern wax has a high coefficient of expansion and tends to warp or distort when allowed to stand unrestrained. The distortion is increased generally as the temperature and time of storage are increased. This quality of wax patterns is related to the release of residual stress developed in the pattern during the process of formation. This characteristic of stress release and warpage is present in all dental waxes, but is particularly troublesome in inlay patterns because of the critical dimensional relations that must be maintained in inlay castings.

Because warpage of the pattern is related to the temperature during pattern formation and storage, the rules related to the pattern temperature must be understood. In general, the higher the temperature of the wax at the time the pattern was adapted and shaped, the less the tendency for distortion in the prepared pattern. This is reasonable, because the residual stress in the pattern causing the distortion is associated with the forces necessary to shape the wax originally. The incorporation of residual stress can be minimized by softening a wax uniformly by heating at 50° C for at least 15 minutes before use, by using warmed carving instruments and a warmed die, and by adding wax to the die in small amounts.

Because the release of internal stress and subsequent warpage are associated with the storage temperature, it follows that greater warpage results at higher storage temperatures. Lower temperature does not completely prevent distortion, but generally the amount is reduced when the storage temperature is kept to a minimum. If inlay wax patterns must be allowed to stand uninvested for a time longer than 30 minutes, they should be kept in a refrigerator. Although some distortion may take place at this temperature, it will be less than at normal room temperature. Such a practice of storage for long periods is not recommended if freedom from warpage is desired. The best way to minimize the warpage of inlay wax patterns is to invest the pattern immediately after it is completely shaped. A refrigerated wax pattern should be allowed to warm to room temperature before it is invested. During spruing, distortion can be reduced by use of a solid wax sprue or a hollow metal sprue filled with sticky wax. If the pattern was stored, the margins should be readapted. Temperature of formation, time and condition of storage, and promptness of investing the pattern are major factors related to all techniques of pattern formation.

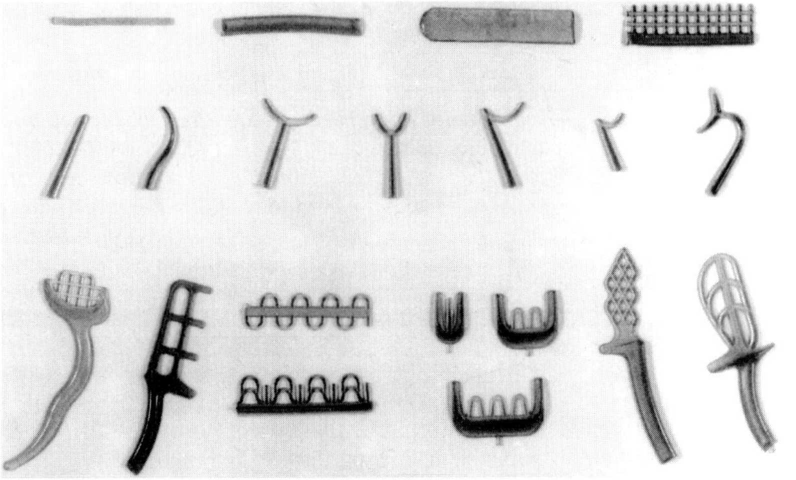

Fig. 14-11 Wax patterns for use in fabrication of metallic framework of removable partial dentures. Preformed bars and mesh, *top;* clasps, *center;* retention forms, *bottom.*

CASTING WAX

The pattern for the metallic framework of removable partial dentures and other similar structures is fabricated from casting waxes. These waxes are available in the form of sheets, usually of 28- and 30-gauge (0.40 and 0.32 mm) thickness, ready-made shapes, and in bulk. As shown in Fig. 14-11, the ready-made shapes are supplied as round, half-round, and half-pear–shaped rods and wires of various gauges in approximately 10-cm lengths. Although casting waxes serve the same basic purpose as inlay waxes in the formation of patterns for metallic castings, their physical properties differ slightly. Little is known of the exact composition of these sheet and shaped waxes, but they include ingredients similar to those found in inlay waxes, with various combinations and proportions of paraffin, ceresin, beeswax, resins, and other waxes being used.

The casting wax sheets are used to establish minimum thickness in certain areas of the partial denture framework, such as the palatal and lingual bar, and to produce the desired contour of the lingual bar. A partial denture framework in the process of being waxed is shown in the left center of Fig. 14-1. The physical nature and form in which the sheet casting wax is supplied resulted in its use for post damming of complete maxillary denture impressions, checking high points of articulation, producing wax bites of cusp tips for the articulation of stone casts, and many other uses.

Physical Characteristics The casting sheets and ready-made shapes of certain types of casting waxes may possess a slight degree of tackiness, which helps to maintain their position on the cast and on each other during assembly of the pattern. This tackiness is not sufficient to prevent changes in position from being made with relative ease, and when the waxes are in final position, they are sealed to the investment cast with a hot spatula.

There is no ANSI/ADA specification for these casting waxes, but a federal specification has been formulated that includes values for softening temperature, amount of flow at various temperatures, general working qualities, and other characteristics. A summary of the properties included in Federal Specification No. U-W-140 is given in Table 14-6. In general, the characteristics most desired include a certain degree of toughness and strength, with a true gauge dimension, combined with a minimum of dimensional

TABLE 14-6 Summary of Requirements of Federal Specifications for Dental Casting Wax

Type of Wax	Flow	Breaking Point	Working Properties
Casting wax Class A—28-gauge, pink Class B—30-gauge, green Class C—ready-made shapes, blue	35° C—maximum, 10% 38° C—minimum, 60%	No fracture at 23° C ± 1°	Pliable and readily adaptable at 40° to 45° C Copies accurately surface against which it is pressed Will not be brittle on cooling Vaporizes at 500° C, leaving no film other than carbon

Adapted from Federal Specification No. U-W-140, March 1948, for casting wax.

change with change in temperature, and the ability to be vaporized completely from the investment mold.

Because the pattern for the removable partial denture framework is constructed on and sealed to an investment cast (from which it is not separated subsequently) at room temperature, there is little need for the casting wax to exhibit low flow at body temperature. The flow characteristics of the casting wax, when measured similarly to the inlay wax, show a maximum of 10% flow at 35° C and a minimum of 60% flow at 38° C. These characteristics are significantly different from the flow values for inlay waxes that comply with the requirements of ANSI/ADA Specification No. 4.

The requirement for ductility of the casting waxes is high. The federal specification requires that the casting wax be bent double on itself without fracture at a temperature of 23° C and that the waxes be pliable and readily adaptable at 40° to 45° C. Heating over a flame and the compression to adapt either the ready-made shapes or the sheet casting wax easily may alter their thickness and contour because of their relatively high ductility and flow.

Because these materials are casting pattern waxes for partial denture cast restorations, as is the inlay wax, they too must vaporize at about 500° C with no residue other than carbon. The mold cavity thus produced will result in more-desirable casting surfaces, because it will be free of foreign materials. Pattern waxes are being replaced to some extent by preformed plastic patterns.

RESIN MODELING MATERIAL

Light-curing resins are available as low- and high-viscosity pastes and as a liquid for the fabrication of patterns for cast metal or ceramic inlays, crowns and bridges, and precision attachments (Fig. 14-12). The modeling pastes are based on diurethane dimethacrylate oligomers with 40% to 55% polyurethane dimethacrylate or poly(methyl methacrylate) fillers. The liquid consistency is mostly urethane dimethacrylate. These resins have a camphorquinone activator. Self-cured acrylic plastics used as inlay patterns are described in Chapter 21.

Modeling resins are characterized by lower heat of polymerization and shrinkage than acrylics, higher strength and resistance to flow than waxes, good dimensional stability, and burnout without residue. Average marginal discrepancies of light-cured resin and self-cured acrylic patterns are similar to those of wax for full-crown patterns but less than those of wax for inlay patterns (Table 14-7). Dimethacrylate resin patterns do not result in cracked investment from heating during burnout, which can occur with acrylic patterns.

Gypsum and resin dies must be treated with a separator and have undercuts blocked out. The modeling resin is applied in layers 3- to 5-mm thick, with each layer cured separately in a

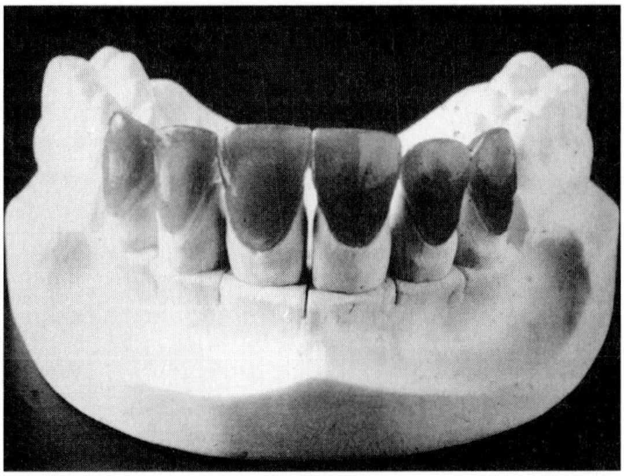

Fig. 14-12 Sculpted anterior crowns made from light-cured resin modeling material.
(Courtesy Heraeus Kulzer, GmbH, Wehrheim, Germany.)

TABLE 14-7 Average Marginal Discrepancies (μm) for Full-Crown and Inlay Patterns Measured 1 Hour and 24 Hours after Forming

Pattern Material	Full Crown	Inlay
Inlay wax (Type II)	11	15
Light-cured resin A	10	8
Light-cured resin B	12	9
Self-cured acrylic	15	7

Adapted from Iglesias A, Powers JM, Pierpont HP: *J Prosthodont* 5:201, 1996.

high-intensity, light-curing chamber for 90 seconds or by using a hand-held, light-curing unit for 20 to 40 seconds per area of irradiation. The liquid material is used first to obtain close adaptation to the die and last to provide a smooth surface. Complete elimination of modeling resins occurs between 670° to 690° C and requires about 45 minutes.

BASEPLATE WAX

Baseplate wax derives its name from its use on the baseplate tray to establish the vertical dimension, plane of occlusion, and initial arch form in the technique for the complete denture restoration. This wax also may be used to form all or a portion of the tray itself. The normally pink color provides some esthetic quality for the initial stage of construction of the denture before processing. Baseplate wax is the material used to produce the desired contour of the denture after teeth are set in position. As a result, the contour wax establishes the pattern for the final plastic denture. Patterns for orthodontic appliances and prostheses other than complete dentures, which are to be constructed of plastics, also are made of baseplate wax. Although these are the primary functions of baseplate wax, it has also been widely used in many phases of dentistry to check the various articulating relations in the mouth and to transfer them to mechanical articulators.

Composition A few formulas are found in the literature for baseplate wax. Baseplate waxes may contain 70% to 80% paraffin-based waxes or commercial ceresin, with small quantities of other waxes, resins, and additives to develop the specific qualities desired in the wax. A typical composition might include 80% ceresin, 12% beeswax, 2.5% carnauba, 3% natural or synthetic resins, and 2.5% microcrystalline or synthetic waxes. Differential thermal analysis and penetration curves of a typical baseplate wax are shown in Fig. 14-13.

Physical Characteristics Baseplate waxes are normally supplied in sheets 7.60 × 15.00 × 0.13 cm in pink or red. The manufacturer usually formulates two types of wax to accommodate the varying climates in which they will be used, because the flow of the wax is influenced greatly by the temperature.

The requirements for dental baseplate wax are listed in Table 14-8, which summarizes ANSI/ADA Specification No. 24 (ISO 12163). Three types of wax are included: Type 1 is a soft wax

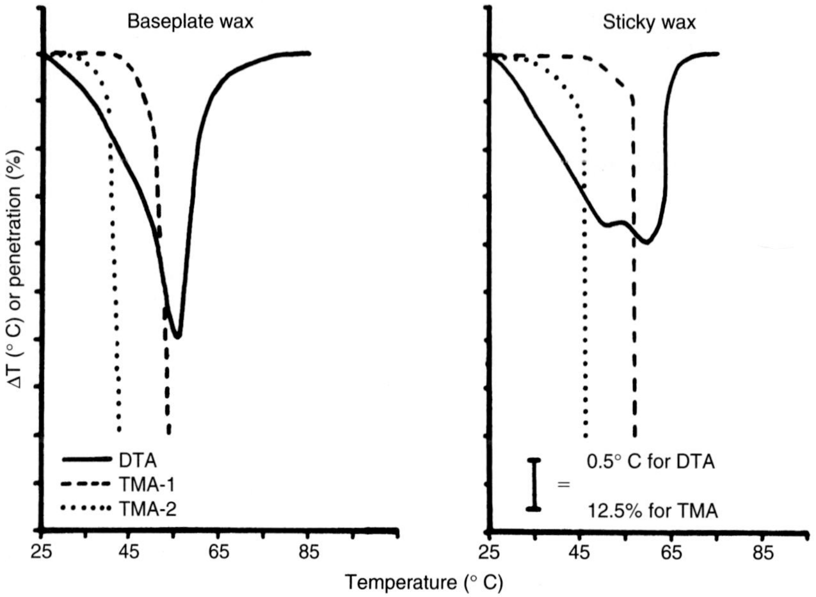

Fig. 14-13 Differential thermal analysis and penetration curves for dental baseplate and sticky waxes. The stresses for TMA-1 and TMA-2 are 0.015 and 0.25 MPa, respectively.

(Adapted from Powers JM, Craig RG: Thermomechanical analysis of dental waxes in the penetration mode. In Porter RS, Johnson JF, editors: *Analytical calorimetry,* vol 3, New York, 1974, Plenum.)

TABLE 14-8 Requirements for Dental Baseplate Wax

	Temperature (° C)	Flow (%)		Practical Requirements
		Minimum	Maximum	
Type 1—Soft, building contours and veneers	23	—	1.0	Softened sheets shall cohere readily without becoming flaky or adhering to fingers
	37	5.0	90.0	
	45	—	—	
Type 2—Hard, patterns in mouth, temperate weather	23	—	0.6	No irritation of oral tissues
	37	—	10.0	Trim easily with a sharp instrument at 23° C
	45	50.0	90.0	
Type 3—Extra-hard, patterns in mouth, hot weather	23	—	0.2	Smooth, glossy surface after gentle flaming
	37	—	1.2	
	45	5.0	50.0	No residue on porcelain or plastic teeth
				Coloring shall not separate or impregnate plaster during processing
				No adhesion to other sheets of wax or separating paper on storage

Adapted from ISO 12163:1999.

for building contours and veneers, Type 2 is a hard wax to be used for patterns to be tried in the mouth in temperate climates, and Type 3 is an extra-hard wax for patterns to be tried in the mouth in tropical weather. The flow values are listed for 23°, 37°, and 45° C when they are applicable. The maximum flow allowed at any given temperature decreases rapidly from Type 1 to Type 3. The flow requirements of Type 3 baseplate wax are comparable to those of the Type 2 (hard) inlay wax, with less flow allowed for the baseplate wax at 45° C.

Because baseplate wax is used both to set denture teeth and to adapt around these teeth to develop proper contour, the dimensional changes that may take place because of variations in temperature are important. Although the need for dimensional stability is not as critical as with the inlay wax, the maintenance of good tooth relationship is important. Although no shrinkage value from a molten state to room temperature is required by the specification, the linear thermal expansion from 26° to 40° C should be less than 0.8%.

A summary of practical requirements is also given in Table 14-8. Baseplate waxes should be easily trimmed with a sharp instrument at 23° C and should yield a smooth surface after gentle flaming. These waxes should not leave any residue on porcelain or plastic teeth, and the coloring agents in the wax should not separate or impregnate the plastic mold during processing.

There is residual stress within the baseplate wax that holds and surrounds the teeth of a wax denture pattern. This stress results from differential cooling, "pooling" the wax with a hot spatula, and physically manipulating the wax below its most desirable working temperature. Remember that both time and temperature affect the relief of these residual stresses; the waxed and properly articulated denture should not be allowed to stand for long periods of time, especially when subjected to elevated temperatures. Such treatment often results in distortion of the wax and movement of the teeth. The waxed denture should be flasked soon after completion to maintain the greatest accuracy of tooth relations.

BOXING WAX

To form a plaster or stone cast from an impression of the edentulous arch, first a wax box must be formed around the impression, into which the freshly mixed plaster or stone is poured and vibrated. This boxing procedure is also necessary for some other types of impressions. The boxing operation usually consists of first adapting a long, narrow stick or strip of wax around the impression below its peripheral height, followed by a wide strip of wax, producing a form around the entire impression, as seen in the upper center of Fig. 14-1.

The dental literature occasionally refers to carding wax for use in the boxing operation. Carding wax was the original material on which porcelain teeth were fixed when received from the manufacturer. The terms *carding wax* and *boxing wax* have been used interchangeably, although boxing wax is more acceptable.

The requirements of Federal Specification No. U-W-138 for boxing wax, which are summarized in Table 14-9, stipulate that this wax should be pliable at 21° C and should retain its shape at 35° C. This broadly defines its lower temperature limit of ductility and flow. Because the impression may be made from a viscoelastic material that is easily distorted, a boxing wax that is readily adaptable to the impression at room temperature is desirable. This property reduces the likelihood of distorting the impression, from the standpoint of both the temperature and stress involved in the boxing procedures. In general, boxing wax should be slightly tacky and have sufficient strength and toughness for convenient manipulation.

UTILITY WAX

An easily workable, adhesive wax is often desired. For example, a standard perforated tray for use with hydrocolloids may easily be brought to a more desirable contour by such a wax, as shown in the center view of Fig. 14-1. This is done to prevent a sag and distortion of the impression material. A soft, pliable, adhesive wax may be used on the lingual portion of a bridge pontic to stabilize it while a labial plaster splint is

TABLE 14-9 Summary of Requirements of Federal Specifications for Dental Boxing, Utility, and Sticky Waxes

Type of Wax	Flow	Color	Working Properties
Boxing	—	Green or black	Smooth, glossy surface on flaming Pliable at 21° C; retains shape at 35° C Seals easily to plaster with hot spatula
Utility	37.5° C—minimum, 65% —maximum, 80%	Orange or dark red	Pliable at 21° to 24° C Tacky at 21° to 24° C; sufficient adhesion to build up
Sticky	30° C—maximum, 5% 43° C—minimum, 90%	Dark or vivid	Sticky when melted Adheres closely Not more than 0.2% residue on burnout Not more than 0.5% shrinkage from 43° to 28° C

Adapted from Federal Specification No. U-W-138, May 1947, for boxing wax; Federal Specification U-W-156, August 1948, for utility wax; Federal Specification U-W-00149a (DSA-DM), September 1966, for sticky wax.

poured. These and many other tasks are performed by the utility wax, justifying its name.

The utility wax is usually supplied in both stick and sheet form in dark red or orange. The ductility and flow of utility waxes, as indicated by the summarized requirements of Federal Specification No. U-W-156 in Table 14-9, are the highest of any of the dental waxes. The utility wax should be pliable at a temperature of 21° to 24° C, which makes it workable and easily adaptable at normal room temperature. The flow of this wax should not be less than 65% nor more than 80% at 37.5° C. Because building one layer on top of another is often desirable, the specification requires a sufficient adhesiveness at 21° to 24° C. Utility wax probably consists of beeswax, petrolatum, and other soft waxes in varying proportions.

STICKY WAX

A suitable sticky wax for prosthetic dentistry is formulated from a mixture of waxes and resins or other additive ingredients. Such a material is sticky when melted and adheres closely to the surfaces on which it is applied. However, at room temperature the wax is firm, free from tackiness, and brittle. Sticky wax should fracture rather than flow if it is deformed during soldering or repair procedures. Although this wax is used to assemble metallic or resin pieces in a fixed temporary position, it is primarily used on dental stones and plasters. The lower right portion of Fig. 14-1 shows an application of sticky wax to seal a plaster splint to a stone model in the process of forming porcelain facings.

According to Federal Specification No. U-W-00149a (DSA-DM), sticky wax should have a dark or vivid color so it is readily distinguishable from the light-colored gypsum materials. The specification, summarized in Table 14-9, also limits the shrinkage of sticky wax to 0.5% at temperatures between 43° and 28° C.

The literature contains several formulas for sticky wax, representing both a high and a low resin content. In addition to rosin and yellow beeswax, which are the usual major constituents, coloring matter and other natural resins such as gum dammar may be present. Differential thermal analysis and penetration curves for a typical dental sticky wax are shown in Fig. 14-13.

CORRECTIVE IMPRESSION WAX

Corrective impression wax is used as a wax veneer over an original impression to contact and register the detail of the soft tissues. It is claimed that this type of impression material records the mucous membrane and underlying tissues in a functional state in which movable tissue is displaced to such a degree that functional contact with the base of the denture is obtained. Corrective waxes are formulated from hydrocarbon waxes such as paraffin, ceresin, and beeswax and may contain metal particles. There are no ANSI/ADA or federal specifications for corrective impression waxes. The flow of several corrective waxes measured by penetration at 37° C is 100%. Differential thermal analysis and penetration curves for a typical corrective impression wax are shown in Fig. 14-14. These waxes are subject to distortion during removal from the mouth.

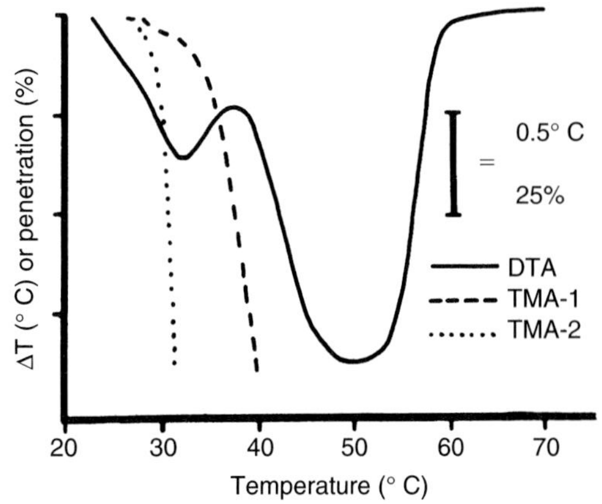

Fig. 14-14 Differential thermal analysis and penetration curves for a dental corrective impression wax. The stresses for TMA-1 and TMA-2 are 0.015 and 0.25 MPa, respectively. Observe that the solid-solid transition temperature occurs below 37° C.

BITE REGISTRATION WAX

Bite registration wax is used to accurately articulate certain models of opposing quadrants. The wax bite registration for the copper-formed die must provide proximal and occlusal relations. Bite registrations are often made from 28-gauge casting wax sheets or from hard baseplate wax, but waxes identified as bite waxes seem to be formulated from beeswax or hydrocarbon waxes such as paraffin or ceresin. Certain bite waxes contain aluminum or copper particles. There are no ADA or federal specifications for bite waxes. The flow of several bite waxes as measured by penetration at 37° C ranges from 2.5% to 22%, indicating that these waxes are susceptible to distortion on removal from the mouth.

SELECTED PROBLEMS

Problem 1

The investing of a wax pattern was delayed for a day, and the gold alloy casting that was produced did not fit. What probably caused this problem and can it be corrected?

Solution a

Residual stresses are always present in wax patterns from manipulation, and they may be released during storage. To minimize distortion, invest the wax pattern promptly.

Solution b

Distortion of the wax pattern may have occurred during spruing or removal of the pattern from the die. A sprued pattern may be replaced on the die to evaluate and readapt the margins.

Problem 2

A wax pattern that had been refrigerated was invested, and the gold alloy casting that was produced did not fit. What probably caused this problem, and how can it be corrected?

Solution

Inlay waxes have high coefficients of thermal expansion. Cooling and heating of a pattern can result in a nonuniform dimensional change. A refrigerated wax pattern should be allowed to warm to room temperature, and its margins should be readapted before proceeding with investing.

Problem 3

The internal surface of a wax pattern prepared on a silver-plated die showed a wrinkled appearance. What caused this problem, and how can it be corrected?

Solution

When molten wax is flowed incrementally onto a cool metal die, the wax next to the die solidifies rapidly. Solidification of adjacent wax occurs more slowly and pulls the previously congealed wax away from the die, resulting in poor surface adaptation. A metal die should be warmed to about 32° C under an electric light or on a heating pad during waxing. An alternative solution is to use a soft wax at the cervical margins.

Problem 4

A wax-up of a complete denture was completed and stored overnight on an articulator. The next day the posterior teeth were no longer in contact. What happened during the storage period, and how can the problem be corrected?

Solution

The esthetic portion of the wax-up is done after the teeth have been articulated. A hot spatula and an alcohol torch are used for shaping the wax, causing it to expand. Subsequent contraction of the wax can occur overnight, thereby moving the teeth out of articulation. This contraction can be minimized by not working in any one area for too long and by not applying too much heat. The waxed denture should be flasked soon after completion of the wax-up to minimize distortion caused by the release of residual stresses in the wax.

Problem 5

The impression wax forming a posterior palatal seal to a maxillary denture impression pulled away from a rubber impression material in several areas when the impression was removed from the mouth. What caused this problem, and how can it be corrected?

Solution

Impression wax adheres poorly to polysulfide and silicone impression materials. The separation can be prevented by applying a very thin layer of sticky wax to the area of the impression material where the impression wax is to be applied. The impression wax will adhere to the sticky wax.

Problem 6

The broken pieces of a denture were joined with baseplate wax, flasked, and processed with heat-cured acrylic. However, the repaired denture did not fit. What may have caused this problem, and how can it be corrected?

Solution

Baseplate wax will flow somewhat if subjected to stress. The denture pieces held together by wax may move relative to each other during the repair process. Pieces to be repaired should be joined with sticky wax. It is brittle and will break rather than distort, thus readily indicating that the pieces have moved.

BIBLIOGRAPHY

Anderson, JN: *Applied dental materials,* ed 5, Oxford, 1976, Blackwell Scientific.

Bennett H: *Industrial waxes,* vols 1 and 2, Brooklyn, NY, 1963, Chemical Publishing.

Coleman RL: Physical properties of dental materials, US Bureau of Standards, Research Paper No 32, *J Res Nat Bur Stand* 1:867, 1928.

Council on Dental Materials, Instruments, and Equipment: Revised ANSI/ADA Specification No 4 for inlay wax, *J Am Dent Assoc* 108:88, 1984.

Craig RG, Eick JD, Peyton FA: Properties of natural waxes used in dentistry, *J Dent Res* 44:1308, 1965.

Craig RG, Eick JD, Peyton FA: Flow of binary and tertiary mixtures of waxes, *J Dent Res* 45:397, 1966.

Craig RG, Eick JD, Peyton FA: Strength properties of waxes at various temperatures and their practical application, *J Dent Res* 46:300, 1967.

Craig RG, Powers JM, Peyton FA: Differential thermal analysis of commercial and dental waxes, *J Dent Res* 46:1090, 1967.

Craig RG, Powers JM, Peyton FA: Thermogravimetric analysis of waxes, *J Dent Res* 50:450, 1971.

Dirksen LC: Composition and properties of a wax for lower impressions, *J Am Dent Assoc* 26:270, 1939.

Farah JW, Powers JM, editors: Bite registration materials, *Dent Advis* 15(4):1, 1998.

Grajower R: A new method for determining the thermal expansion of dental waxes, *J Dent Res* 57:659, 1978.

Grossman LI: Dental formulas and aids to dental practice, Philadelphia, 1952, Lea & Febiger.

Hollenback GM, Rhodes JE: A study of the behavior of pattern wax, *J South Calif State Dent Assoc* 27:419, 1959.

Iglesias A, Powers JM, Pierpont HP: Accuracy of wax, autopolymerized, and light-polymerized resin pattern materials, *J Prosthodont* 5:201, 1996.

Ito M, Yamagishi T, Oshida Y et al: Effect of selected physical properties of waxes on investments and casting shrinkage, *J Prosthet Dent* 75:211, 1999.

Lasater RL: Control of wax distortion by manipulation, *J Am Dent Assoc* 27:518, 1940.

Ludwig FJ Jr: Modern instrumental wax analysis, *Soap & Chem Spec* 42:70, 1966.

Markley MR: The wax pattern, Dental Clinics of North America, Symposium on Dental Materials, Philadelphia, Nov 1958, Saunders.

Maves TW: Recent experiments demonstrating wax distortion on all wax patterns when heat is applied, *J Am Dent Assoc* 19:606, 1932.

McCrorie JW: Dental modelling waxes A new approach to formulation, *Br Dent J* 132:189, 1972.

McCrorie JW: Corrective impression waxes, *Br Dent J* 152:95, 1982.

Morrison JT, Duncanson MG Jr, Shillingburg HT Jr: Wetting effects of surface treatments on inlay wax-investment combinations, *J Dent Res* 60:1858, 1981.

Nelson EA: Practical applications of crowns and inlay casting technics, *J Am Dent Assoc* 27:588, 1940.

Ohashi M, Paffenbarger GC: Melting, flow, and thermal expansion characteristics of some dental and commercial waxes, *J Am Dent Assoc* 72:1141, 1966.

Ohashi M, Paffenbarger GC: Some flow characteristics at 37° C of ternary wax mixtures that may have possible dental uses, *J Nihon Univ Sch Dent* 11:109, 1969.

Phillips RW: *Skinner's science of dental materials,* ed 8, Philadelphia, 1982, Saunders.

Phillips RW, Biggs DH: Distortion of wax patterns as influenced by storage time, storage temperature, and temperature of wax manipulation, *J Am Dent Assoc* 41:28, 1950.

Powers JM, Craig RG: Penetration of commercial and dental waxes, *J Dent Res* 53:402, 1974.

Powers JM, Craig RG: Thermal analysis of dental impression waxes, *J Dent Res* 57:37, 1978.

Powers JM, Craig RG, Peyton FA: Calorimetric analysis of commercial and dental waxes, *J Dent Res* 48:1165, 1969.

Smith DC, Earnshaw R, McCrorie JW: Some properties of modelling and base plate waxes, *Br Dent J* 118:437, 1965.

Taylor NO: Progress report. Research on dental materials: the research program; cooperative work on inlay casting technic, *J Am Dent Assoc* 18:294, 1931.

Taylor NO, Paffenbarger GC: A survey of current inlay casting technics, *J Am Dent Assoc* 17:2058, 1930.

Taylor PB: Inlay casting procedure—its evolution and the effect of manipulatory variables. In Anderson GM, editor: *Proceedings of the Dental Centenary Celebration,* Baltimore, 1940, Maryland State Dental Association.

US General Services Administration, Federal Supply Service, Federal Specification No U-W-135, July 31, 1947, Wax, base plate, dental; No U-W-138, May 12, 1947, Wax, boxing, dental; No U-W-140, March 16, 1953, Wax, casting, dental; No U-W-141a, Dec 6, 1956, Wax, dental (casting inlay); No U-W-00149a (DSA-DM), Sept 9, 1966, Wax, sticky, dental; No U-W-156, Aug 17, 1948, Wax, utility, dental.

Warth AH: *The chemistry and technology of waxes,* ed 2, New York, 1956, Reinhold.

Washburn KC: Inlay wax and its manipulation, *Ill Dent J* 16:409, 1947.

Chapter 15

Noble Dental Alloys and Solders

Noble dental alloys have undergone a tremendous evolution because the U.S. government lifted its support on the price of gold in 1969. Before then, more than 95% of fixed dental prostheses in the United States were made of alloys containing a minimum of 75% gold and other noble metals by weight. However, when the price of gold increased from $35 per ounce to more than $800 per ounce in the early 1980s, the development of alternative alloys increased dramatically to reduce the cost of cast dental restorations. These alternatives included alloys with reduced gold content, but also alloys that contain no gold and alloys that contain no noble metal. Today, the majority of alloys used in the U.S. and a significant portion of those used in other countries are alternative alloys. In 1999, the tremendous increase in the price of palladium, from about $100 to more than $350 per ounce, again encouraged the development of new types of casting alloys.

This chapter will focus on dental casting alloys that have a noble metal content of at least 25% by weight. In addition, wrought noble alloys and solders will be discussed. The limit of 25 wt% is somewhat arbitrary, but represents the limit established by the ADA for alloys that can be classified as noble alloys. Base-metal alloys will be discussed in Chapter 16. The first section of the current chapter will survey the metallic elements classified as noble dental alloys. In subsequent sections, the physical and chemical properties of noble dental alloys, both cast and wrought, will be presented. Finally, the compositions and properties of noble solders will be discussed. Techniques for casting and soldering will be discussed in Chapter 17.

METALLIC ELEMENTS USED IN DENTAL ALLOYS

For dental restorations, it is necessary to combine various elements to produce alloys with adequate properties for dental applications because none of the elements themselves have properties that are suitable. These alloys may be used for dental restorations as cast alloys, or may be manipulated into wire or other wrought forms. The metallic elements that make up dental alloys can be divided into two major groups, the noble metals and the base metals. A general discussion of the principles of alloys and metallurgy that are used in the current chapter can be found in Chapter 6.

NOBLE METALS

Noble metals are elements with a good metallic surface that retain their surface in dry air. They react easily with sulfur to form sulfides, but their resistance to oxidation, tarnish, and corrosion during heating, casting, soldering, and use in the mouth is very good. The noble metals are gold, platinum, palladium, iridium, rhodium, osmium, and ruthenium (Table 15-1, see Fig. 6-1). These metals can be subdivided into two groups. The metals of the first group, consisting of ruthenium, rhodium, and palladium, have atomic weights of approximately 100 and densities of 12 to 13 g/cm^3. The metals of the second group, consisting of osmium, iridium, platinum, and gold, have atomic weights of about 190 and densities of 19 to 23 g/cm^3. The melting points of members of each group decrease with increasing atomic weight. Thus, ruthenium melts at 2310° C, rhodium at 1966° C, and palladium at 1554° C. In the second group the melting points range from 3045° C for osmium to 1064° C for gold. The noble metals, together with silver, are sometimes called *precious metals.* The term *precious* stems from the trading of these metals on the commodities market. Some metallurgists consider silver a noble metal, but it is not considered a noble metal in dentistry because it corrodes considerably in the oral cavity. Thus the terms *noble* and *precious* are not synonymous in dentistry.

Gold (Au) Pure gold is a soft, malleable, ductile metal that has a rich yellow color with a strong metallic luster. Although pure gold is the most ductile and malleable of all metals, it ranks much lower in strength. The density of gold depends somewhat on the condition of the metal, whether it is cast, rolled, or drawn into wire. Small amounts of impurities have a pro-

TABLE 15-1 Properties of Elements in Dental Casting Alloys

Element	Symbol	Atomic Number	Atomic Mass	Density (g/cc)	Melting Temp. (° C)	Color	Comments
NOBLE							
Ruthenium	Ru	44	101.07	12.48	2310.0	White	Grain refiner, hard
Rhodium	Rh	45	102.91	12.41	1966.0	Silver-white	Grain refiner, soft, ductile
Palladium	Pd	46	106.42	12.02	1554.0	White	Hard, malleable, ductile
Osmium	Os	76	190.20	22.61	3045.0	Bluish-white	Not used in dentistry
Iridium	Ir	77	192.22	22.65	2410.0	Silver-white	Grain refiner, very hard
Platinum	Pt	78	195.08	21.45	1772.0	Bluish-white	Tough, ductile, malleable
Gold	Au	79	196.97	19.32	1064.4	Yellow	Ductile, malleable, soft, conductive
BASE							
Nickel	Ni	28	58.69	8.91	1453.0	White	Hard
Copper	Cu	29	63.55	8.92	1083.4	Reddish	Malleable, ductile, conductive
Zinc	Zn	30	65.39	7.14	419.6	Bluish-white	Soft, brittle, oxidizes
Gallium	Ga	31	69.72	5.91	29.8	Grayish-white	Low-melting
Silver	Ag	47	107.87	10.49	961.9		Soft, malleable, ductile, conductive
Tin	Sn	50	118.71	7.29	232.0	White	Soft
Indium	In	49	114.82	7.31	156.6	Gray-white	Soft

nounced effect on the mechanical properties of gold and its alloys. The presence of less than 0.2% lead causes gold to be extremely brittle. Mercury in small quantities also has a harmful effect. Therefore scrap of other dental alloys, such as technique alloy or other base-metal alloys, including amalgam, should not be mixed with gold used for dental restorations. The addition of calcium to pure gold improves the mechanical properties of gold foil restorations (see subsequent discussion).

Air or water at any temperature does not affect or tarnish gold. Gold is not soluble in sulfuric, nitric, or hydrochloric acids. However, it readily dissolves in combinations of nitric and hydrochloric acids (aqua regia, 18 vol% nitric and 82 vol% hydrochloric acids) to form the trichloride of gold ($AuCl_3$). It is also dissolved by a few other chemicals, such as potassium cyanide and solutions of bromine or chlorine.

Because gold is nearly as soft as lead, it must be alloyed with copper, silver, platinum, and other metals to develop the hardness, durability, and elasticity necessary in dental alloys, coins, and jewelry (Table 15-2). Through appropriate refining and purification, gold with an extremely high degree of purity may be produced. Such highly refined ingots of pure gold (99.99% by weight) serve as the starting material for gold foil.

Gold foil is formed by a process known as *gold beating*. High-purity gold is first passed through a series of rollers and then annealed until

TABLE 15-2 Physical and Mechanical Properties of Cast Pure Gold, Gold Alloys, and Condensed Gold Foil

Material	Density (g/cm^3)	Hardness (VHN/BHN) (kg/mm^2)	Tensile Strength (MPa)	Elongation (%)
Cast 24k gold	19.3	28 (VHN)	105	30
Cast 22k gold	—	60 (VHN)	240	22
Coin gold	—	85 (BHN)	395	30
Typical Au-based casting alloy (70 wt% Au)*	15.6	135/195 (VHN)	425/525	30/12
Condensed gold foil†	19.1	60 (VHN)	250	12.8

*Values are for softened/hardened condition.
†Adapted from Rule RW: *J Am Dent Assoc* 24:583, 1937.

the gold is in a ribbon about 0.0025 mm thick, which is comparable to the thickness of tissue paper. The ribbon is cut into small pieces, and each piece is placed between two sheets of paper, which are then placed one over the other to form a packet. The packet, which may contain 200 to 250 pieces of the small gold ribbons, is then beaten by a hammer until the desired thickness of gold is obtained, usually 0.00064 mm. The foil is then carefully weighed and annealed. Purity in the process of manufacturing gold foil is critical to maintaining its cohesive properties.

If uncontaminated, gold foil is cohesive; that is, it can be welded together at room temperature. This cohesive property has been exploited in the use of gold foil as a dental restorative material. If manipulated properly, small pieces of foil can be inserted and condensed into cavity preparations in teeth, providing a restoration with considerable longevity. As Table 15-2 shows, the tensile strength and hardness of condensed gold foil is more than twice that of pure (24 k) cast gold. The reduced elongation of foil compared with cast gold is evidence of the considerable work-hardening that the condensation process has accomplished (see Chapter 6, wrought alloys). It is this improvement of physical properties by work hardening that makes gold acceptable as a restoration in some areas of the mouth; without the improvement, cast gold would lack sufficient strength and hardness. The use of gold foil restorations has declined in recent years because of the time and skill required to properly place these materials and the development of more esthetic (tooth colored) restorative materials for areas where foil restorations were placed.

Platinum (Pt) Platinum is a bluish-white metal, and is tough, ductile, malleable, and can be produced as foil or fine-drawn wire. Platinum has a hardness similar to copper. Pure platinum has numerous applications in dentistry because of its high fusing point and resistance to oral conditions and elevated temperatures. Platinum foil serves as a matrix for the construction of fused porcelain restorations, because it does not oxidize at high temperatures. Platinum foil also has a higher melting point than porcelain and has a coefficient of expansion sufficiently close to that of porcelain to prevent buckling of the metal or fracture of the porcelain during changes in temperature (see Chapter 18). Platinum has been used for pins and posts in crown and bridge restorations, and alloys may be cast or soldered to the posts without damage.

Platinum adds greatly to the hardness and elastic qualities of gold, and some dental casting alloys and wires contain quantities of platinum up to 8% combined with other metals. Platinum is a major component of alloys used for precision attachments in complex crown and bridge restorations because these alloys have excellent wear characteristics and high melting ranges. The high melting range is necessary because other gold alloys must be cast to these attachments without causing distortion of the attachment. Platinum tends to lighten the color of yellow gold–based alloys.

Palladium (Pd) Palladium is a white metal somewhat darker than platinum. Its density is a little more than half that of platinum and gold. Palladium has the quality of absorbing or occluding large quantities of hydrogen gas when heated. This can be an undesirable quality when alloys containing palladium are heated with an improperly adjusted gas-air torch.

Palladium is not used in the pure state in dentistry, but is used extensively in dental alloys. Palladium can be combined with gold, silver, copper, cobalt, tin, indium, or gallium for dental alloys. In the past, palladium was less than half the price of platinum and, because it imparts many of the properties of platinum to dental alloys, was often used as a replacement for platinum. However, in 2000, the price of palladium was greater than platinum because of market shortages, and for economic reasons alone could no longer be substituted for platinum. Alloys are readily formed between gold and palladium, and palladium quantities of as low as 5% by weight have a pronounced effect on whitening yellow gold–based alloys. Palladium-gold alloys with a palladium content of ≥ 10% by weight are white. Alloys of palladium and the other elements previously mentioned are available as substitutes for yellow-gold alloys, and the mechanical properties of the palladium-based alloys may be as good as or better than many traditional gold-based alloys. Although many of the palladium-based alloys are white, some, such as palladium-indium-silver alloys, are yellow.

Iridium (Ir), Ruthenium (Ru), and Rhodium (Rh) Iridium and ruthenium are used in small amounts in dental alloys as grain refiners to keep the grain size small. A small grain size is desirable because it improves the mechanical properties and uniformity of properties within an alloy. As little as 0.005% (50 ppm) of iridium is effective in reducing the grain size. Ruthenium has a similar effect. The grain refining properties of these elements occurs largely because of their extremely high melting points. Iridium melts at 2410° C and ruthenium at 2310° C. Thus these elements do not melt during the casting of the alloy and serve as nucleating centers for the melt as it cools, resulting in a fine-grained alloy.

Rhodium also has a high melting point (1966° C) and has been used in alloys with platinum to form wire for thermocouples. These thermocouples help measure the temperature in porcelain furnaces used to make dental restorations.

Osmium (Os) Because of its tremendous expense and extremely high melting point, osmium is not used in dental casting alloys.

BASE METALS

Several base metals are combined with noble metals to develop alloys with properties suitable for dental restorations. Base metals used in dental alloys include silver, copper, zinc, indium, tin, gallium, and nickel (see Table 15-1, Fig. 6-1).

Silver (Ag) Silver is a malleable, ductile white metal. It is the best known conductor of heat and electricity, and is stronger and harder than gold but softer than copper. At 961.9° C, the melting point of silver is below the melting points of both copper and gold. It is unaltered in clean, dry air at any temperature, but combines with sulfur, chlorine, phosphorus, and vapors containing these elements or their compounds. Foods containing sulfur compounds cause severe tarnish on silver, and for this reason silver is not considered a noble metal in dentistry. Pure silver captures appreciable quantities of oxygen in the molten state, which makes it difficult to cast because the gas is evolved during solidification. As a result, small pits, porosity, and a rough casting surface develop. This tendency is reduced when 5% to 10% by weight of copper is added to the silver, for which reason castings are made of the alloy rather than the pure metal. This combination of elements is also used in silver-based dental solders to prevent pitting during soldering.

Pure silver is not used in dental restorations

because of the black sulfide that forms on the metal in the mouth. Adding small amounts of palladium to silver-containing alloys prevents the rapid corrosion of such alloys in the oral environment. The electroforming of silver of high purity is readily accomplished and represents a popular method of forming metal dies.

Silver forms a series of solid solutions with palladium (see Fig. 15-1, *D*) and gold (see Fig. 15-1, *C*), and is therefore common in gold- and palladium-based dental alloys. In gold-based alloys, silver is effective in neutralizing the reddish color of alloys containing appreciable quantities of copper. Silver also hardens the gold-based alloys via a solid-solution hardening mechanism (see Chapter 6). More recent evidence indicates that a fine lamellar coherent precipitate of an Ag-rich phase at the grain boundaries may contribute to hardening as well. In palladium-based alloys, silver is important in developing the white color of the alloy. Although silver is soluble in palladium, the addition of other elements to these alloys, such as copper or indium, may cause the formation of multiple phases and increased corrosion.

Copper (Cu) Copper is a malleable and ductile metal with high thermal and electrical conductivity and a characteristic red color. Copper forms a series of solid solutions with both gold (Fig. 15-1, *A*) and palladium (Fig. 15-1, *B*), and is therefore an important component of noble dental alloys. When added to gold-based alloys, copper imparts a reddish color to the gold and hardens the alloy via a solid-solution or ordered-solution mechanism. The presence of copper in gold-based alloys in quantities between approximately 40% and 88% by weight causes allows the formation of an ordered phase. Copper is also commonly used in palladium-based alloys, where it can be used to reduce the melting point and strengthen the alloy through solid-solution hardening and formation of ordered phases when Cu is between 15 and 55 wt%. The ratio of silver and copper must be carefully balanced in gold- and palladium-based alloys, because silver and copper are not miscible. Copper is also a common component of most hard dental solders.

Zinc (Zn) Zinc is a blue-white metal with a tendency to tarnish in moist air. In its pure form, it is a soft, brittle metal with low strength. When heated in air, zinc oxidizes readily to form a white oxide of relatively low density. This oxidizing property is exploited in dental alloys. Although zinc may be present in quantities of only 1% to 2% by weight, it acts as a scavenger of oxygen when the alloy is melted. Thus zinc is referred to as a *deoxidizing agent.* Because of its low density, the resulting zinc oxide lags behind the denser molten mass during casting, and is therefore excluded from the casting. If too much zinc is present, it will markedly increase the brittleness of the alloy.

Indium (In) Indium is a soft, gray-white metal with a low melting point of 156.6° C. Indium is not tarnished by air or water. It is used in some gold-based alloys as a replacement for zinc, and is a common minor component of some noble ceramic dental alloys. Recently, indium has been used in greater amounts (up to 30% by weight) to impart a yellow color to palladium-silver alloys.

Tin (Sn) Tin is a lustrous, soft, white metal that is not subject to tarnish in normal air. Some gold-based alloys contain limited quantities of tin, usually less than 5% by weight. Tin is also an ingredient in gold-based dental solders. It combines with platinum and palladium to produce a hardening effect, but also increases brittleness.

Gallium (Ga) Gallium is a grayish metal that is stable in dry air but tarnishes in moist air. It has a very low melting point of 29.8° C and a density of only 5.91 g/cm^3. Gallium is not used in its pure form in dentistry, but is used as a component of some gold- and palladium-based dental alloys, especially ceramic alloys. The oxides of gallium are important to the bonding of the ceramic to the metal.

Nickel (Ni) Nickel has limited application in gold- and palladium-based dental alloys, but is a common component in non-noble dental alloys. Nickel has a melting point of 1453° C and a

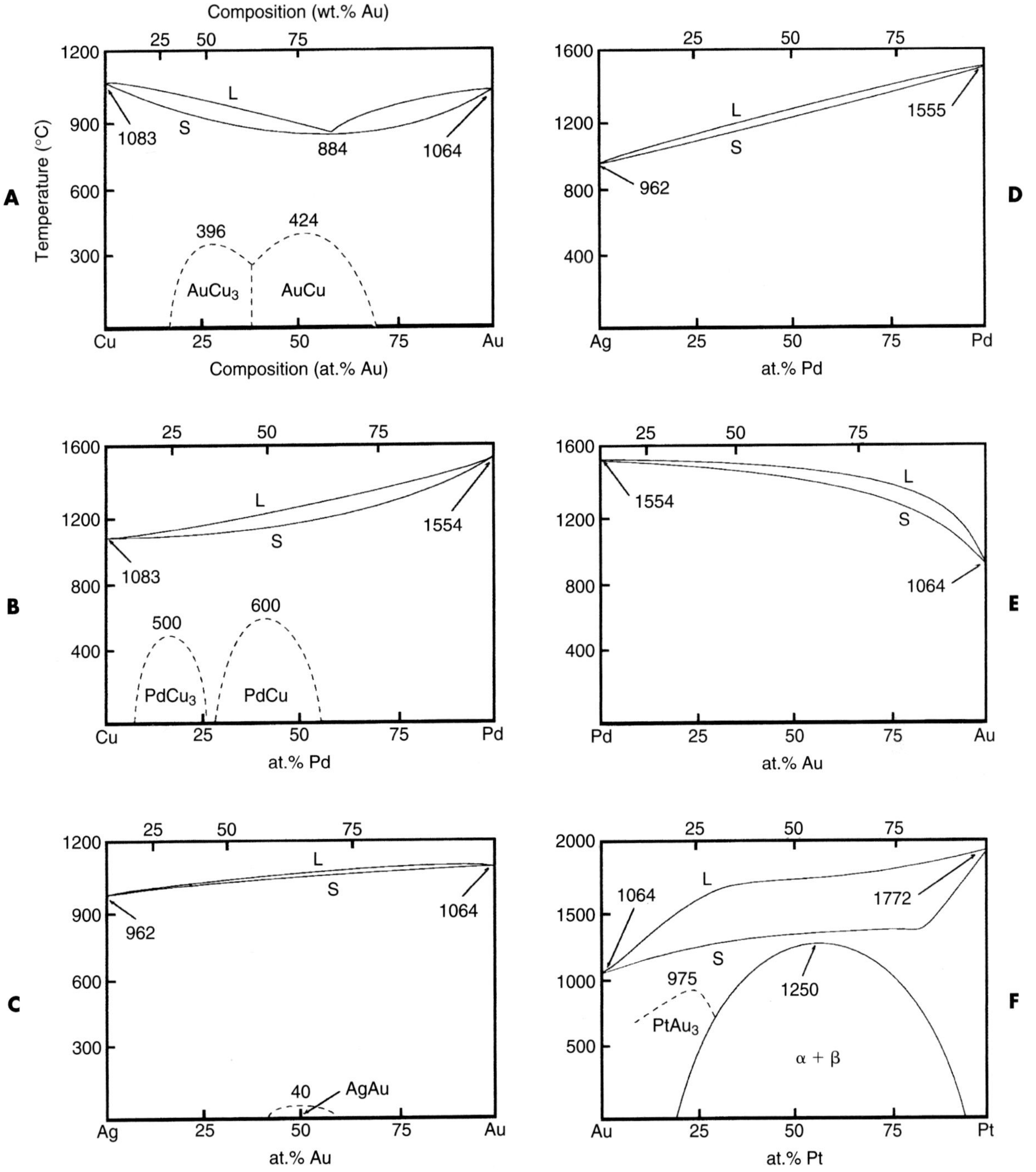

Fig. 15-1 Phase diagrams for binary combinations of **A,** copper and gold; **B,** copper and palladium; **C,** silver and gold; **D,** silver and palladium; **E,** palladium and gold; and **F,** gold and platinum. Atomic percentages are shown along the bottom of each graph; weight percentages are shown along the top. *L,* liquidus; *S,* solidus.

(Adapted from Hansen M; *Constitution of binary alloys,* New York, 1958, McGraw Hill.)

density of 8.91 g/cc. When used in small quantities in gold-based alloys, nickel whitens the alloy and increases its strength and hardness. Ni-based alloys have increased in usage over the past 15 years. A more extensive discussion of these alloys can be found in Chapter 16.

BINARY COMBINATIONS OF METALS

Although most noble casting alloys have three or more elements, the properties of certain binary alloys are important because these binary combinations constitute the majority of the mass of many noble alloys. An understanding of the physical and manipulative properties of these binary alloys is therefore useful in understanding the behavior of the more complex alloys. Among the noble alloys, six binary combinations of elements are important: Au-Cu, Pd-Cu, Au-Ag, Pd-Ag, Au-Pd, and Au-Pt. Phase diagrams for these binary systems are shown in Fig. 15-1. Phase diagrams are powerful tools for understanding the physical and manipulative properties of binary alloys. A review of the theory of phase diagrams can be found in Chapter 6.

Alloy Composition and Temperature

In each phase diagram in Fig. 15-1, the horizontal axis represents the composition of the binary alloy. For example, in Fig. 15-1, *A,* the horizontal axis represents a series of binary alloys of gold and copper ranging in composition from 0% gold (or 100% copper) to 100% gold. The composition can be given in atomic percent (at%) or weight percent (wt%). Weight percent compositions give the relative mass of each element in the alloy, whereas atomic percentages give the relative numbers of atoms in the alloys. It is a simple calculation to convert weight percentages to atomic percentages, or vice versa. Note that for the binary alloys shown in Fig. 15-1, the atomic percent composition is shown along the bottom of the phase diagram whereas the weight percent composition is shown along the top. The atomic and weight percent compositions of the binary alloys can differ considerably. For example, for the Au-Cu system shown in Fig. 15-1, *A,* an alloy that is 50% gold by weight is only 25% gold by atoms. For other systems, like the Au-Pt system in Fig. 15-1, *F,* there is little difference between atomic and weight percentages. The difference between atomic and weight percentages depends on the differences in the atomic masses of the elements involved. The bigger the difference in atomic mass, the bigger the difference between the atomic and weight percentages in the binary phase diagram. Because it more convenient to use masses in the manufacture of alloys, the most common method to report composition is by weight percentages. However, the physical and biological properties of alloys relate best to atomic percentages. It is therefore important to keep the difference between atomic and weight percent in mind when selecting and using noble dental casting alloys. Alloys that appear high in gold by weight percentage may in reality contain far fewer gold atoms than might be thought.

Other aspects of the phase diagrams that deserve attention are the liquidus and solidus lines. The y axes in Fig. 15-1 show temperature. If the temperature is above the liquidus line (marked *L*), the alloy will be completely molten. If the temperature is below the solidus line (marked *S*), the alloy will be solid. If the temperature lies between the liquidus and solidus lines, the alloy will be partially molten. Note that the distance between the liquidus and solidus lines varies among systems in Fig. 15-1. For example, the temperature difference between these lines is small for the Ag-Au system (see Fig. 15-1, *C*), much larger for the Au-Pt system (see Fig. 15-1, *F*) and varies considerably with composition for the Au-Cu system (see Fig. 15-1, *A*). From a manipulative standpoint, it is desirable to have a narrow liquidus-solidus range, because one would like to keep the alloy in the liquid state for as short a time as possible before casting. While in the liquid state, the alloy is susceptible to significant oxidation and contamination. If the liquidus-solidus line is broad, the alloy will remain at least partially molten for a longer period after it is cast. The temperature of the liquidus line is also important, and varies considerably among alloys and with composition. For example the liquidus line of the Au-Ag system ranges from 962° to 1064° C (see Fig. 15-1, *C*) but the liquidus line of the Au-Pd system ranges from 1064° to 1554° C (see Fig. 15-1, *E*). It is often desirable to have an alloy with a liquidus line at lower temperatures; the method of heating is easier, fewer side reactions occur, and shrinkage is generally less of a problem (see Chapter 17, Casting and Soldering Procedures).

Phase Structure of Noble Alloys The area below the solidus lines in Fig. 15-1 is also important to the behavior of the alloy. If this area contains no boundaries, then the binary system is a series of *solid solutions*. This means that the two elements are completely soluble in one another at all temperatures and compositions. The Ag-Pd system (see Fig. 15-1, *D*) and Pd-Au system (see Fig. 15-1, *E*) are examples of solid-solution systems. If the area below the solidus line contains dashed lines, then an ordered solution is present within the dashed lines. An *ordered solution* occurs when the two elements in the alloy assume specific and regular positions in the crystal lattice of the alloy (for a discussion on metallic crystal lattices, see Chapter 6). This situation differs from a solid solution where the positions of the elements in the crystal lattice are random. Examples of systems containing ordered solutions are the Au-Cu system (see Fig. 15-1, *A*) the Pd-Cu system (see Fig. 15-1, *B*) and the Au-Ag system (see Fig. 15-1, *C*). Note that the ordered solutions occur over a limited range of compositions because the ratios between the elements must be correct to support the regular positions in the crystal lattices. If the area below the solidus line contains a solid line, it indicates the existence of a second phase. A *second phase* is an area with a composition distinctly different from the first phase. In the Au-Pt system (see Fig. 15-1, *F*) a second phase forms between 20 and 90 at% platinum. If the temperature is below the phase boundary line within these compositions, two phases exist in the alloy. The presence of a second phase is important because it significantly changes the corrosion properties of an alloy. Fig. 15-2 shows electron micrographs of single- and multiple-phase alloys. The single-phase alloy has little visible microstructure because its composition is more or less homogeneous. In the

A

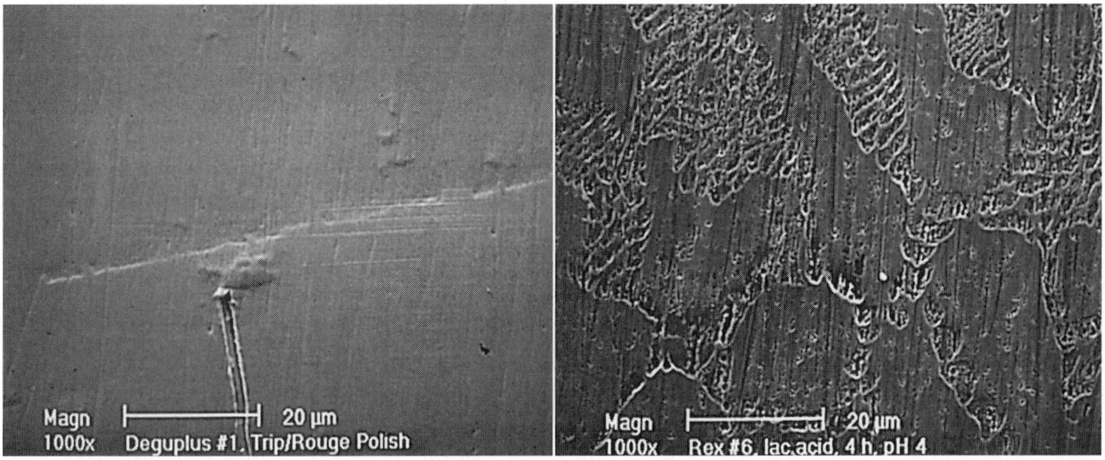

B

Fig. 15-2 Electron micrographs of single-phase **(A)** and multiple-phase **(B)** alloys. **A,** Few distinguishing microstructure characteristics are seen because the alloy is nearly homogeneous. Only a few scratches from polishing and some debris on the surface are visible. **B,** A rich microstructure is evident, reflecting the several phases present. Each phase has a different composition.

multiple-phase alloy, areas that have distinct compositions are clearly visible. These areas correspond to the different phases under the solidus in a phase diagram. Because the different phases may interact electrochemically, the corrosion of multiple-phase alloys may be higher than a single-phase alloy.

Hardening of Noble Alloys The use of pure cast gold is not practical for dental restorations because cast gold lacks sufficient strength and hardness. Solid-solution and ordered-solution hardening are two common ways of strengthening noble dental alloys sufficiently for use in the mouth. By mixing two elements in the crystal lattice randomly (forming a solid solution), the force needed to distort the lattice may be significantly increased. For example, adding just 10% by weight of copper to gold, the tensile strength increases from 105 to 395 MPa and the Brinell hardness increases from 28 to 85 (see Table 15-2). The 90:10 Au-Cu mixture is the composition used in U.S. gold coins. If the positions of the two elements become ordered (forming an ordered solution), the properties of the alloy are improved further (see Table 15-2). For a typical gold-based casting alloy, the formation of an ordered solution may increase yield strength by 50%, tensile strength by 25%, and hardness by at least 10%. It is important to note that the elongation of an alloy is reduced by the formation of the ordered solution. For the typical gold-based alloy, the percentage elongation will decrease from 30% to about 12%.

The formation of ordered solutions has been commonly used to strengthen cast dental restorations, particularly in gold-based alloys. As shown in Fig. 15-1, *A,* the Au-Cu system supports ordered solutions between about 20 and 70 at% gold. However, the manipulation of the alloy during casting will determine if the ordered solution will form. If Au-Cu containing about 50 at% gold is heated to the molten state and then cooled slowly, the mass will solidify at about 880° C as a solid solution. As the mass cools slowly to 424° C, the ordered solution will then form and will remain present at room temperature. However, if the mass is cooled rapidly to room temperature after the initial solidification, the ordered solution will not form because there is insufficient time for the mass to reorganize. Thus the alloy will be trapped in a non-equilibrium state of a solid solution and will be softer, weaker, and have greater elongation. The conversion between the ordered solution and solid solution is reversible in the solid state. By heating an alloy in either condition above 424° C (but below the solidus), the state of the alloy can be selected by picking the cooling rate. Rapid cooling will preserve the solid solution and the soft condition, whereas slow cooling will allow the formation of the ordered solution and the hardened condition. In alloys of gold and copper with other elements, Au-Cu ordered solutions are still possible as long as the ratio of copper to gold is greater than 30:70 (at %). As shown in Fig. 15-2, the formation of ordered solutions is possible in other noble alloy systems, such as Pd-Cu and Au-Pt. The ordered solution of the Ag-Au system exists but cannot be used in practice because the transition temperature is too low (almost body temperature).

The formation of a second phase has also been used to harden dental alloys, but this method is not commonly used for noble dental alloys. The dispersion of the second phase is very important to the effectiveness of the hardening. Recent evidence indicates that some Au-based alloys may contain Ag-rich coherent precipitates that, along with ordered solutions, contribute to alloy hardening. The advantages of the hardening must be balanced against the liabilities of the increased corrosion often seen with multiple-phase systems. It should be noted that, unlike the ordered solutions, the formation of second phases are not usually easily controlled by heat treatments and may not be reversible in the solid state. In fact, heat treatment commonly causes a deterioration of properties with these systems. Further discussion of cast and wrought base-metal alloys can be found in Chapter 17.

Formulation of Noble Alloys The desired qualities of noble dental casting alloys determine the selection of elements that will be used to formulate the alloys. The ideal noble casting alloy should have (1) a low melting range and narrow solidus-liquidus temperature range, (2) adequate strength, hardness, and elongation, (3) a low tendency to corrode in the oral environment, and (4) low cost, among other properties. Traditionally, the noble elements gold and palladium have generally been the foundation to which other elements are added to formulate dental casting alloys. Gold and palladium are preferable to other noble elements because they have relatively low melting points, low corrosion, and form solid solutions with other alloy elements, such as copper or silver (see Fig. 15-1). Solid-solution systems are desirable for the formulation of alloys because they are generally easier to manufacture and manipulate, have a lower tendency to corrode than multiple-phase systems, and provide increased strength through solid-solution or ordered-solution hardening. Furthermore, the systems shown in Fig. 15-1 generally have narrow liquidus-solidus ranges. Thus it is not surprising that combinations of these elements have been extensively used in the formulation of noble dental casting alloys.

The Au-Pt alloys were initially developed out of fear that palladium posed a biological hazard. This fear persisted in spite of a lack of evidence that any hazard existed, other than a low frequency of allergic sensitivity. More recently, palladium-free alloys (Au-Pt and some other systems) have been popular because of the tremendous increase in the cost of palladium. Often, the palladium-free alloys have the disadvantages of high cost and limited compositional flexibility. As shown in Fig. 15-1, *F,* the addition of more than 20 at% platinum to gold forms a multiple-phase alloy. Thus these alloy systems generally have platinum concentrations below 20 at%. Because the Au-Pt systems may not be hard enough for oral applications, the addition of Zn as a dispersed phase–hardener has been used. Thus the corrosion of these alloys may be higher than the Au-Pd compositions they replaced. Furthermore, the cost of platinum is significantly higher than that of gold, and at least as expensive as palladium.

Carat and Fineness of Gold-Based Alloys

For many years the gold content of gold-containing alloys has been described on the basis of the carat, or in terms of fineness, rather than by weight percentage. The term *carat* refers only to the gold content of the alloy; a carat represents a 1/24 part of the whole. Thus 24 carat indicates pure gold. The carat of an alloy is designated by a small letter *k*; for example, 18k or 22k gold.

The use of the term *carat* to designate the gold content of dental alloy is less common now. It is not unusual to find the weight percentage of gold listed or to have the alloy described in terms of fineness. *Fineness* also refers only to the gold content, and represents the number of parts of gold in each 1000 parts of alloy. Thus 24k gold is the same as 100% gold or 1000 fineness (i.e., 1000 fine). The fineness represents a precise measure of the gold content of the alloy and is often the preferred measurement when an exact value is to be listed. An 18k gold would be designated as 750 fine, or, when the decimal system is used, it would be 0.750 fine; this indicates that 750/1000 of the total is gold. A comparison of the carat, fineness, and weight percentage of gold is given in Table 15-3. Both the whole number and the decimal system are in common use, especially for noble dental solders. The fineness system is somewhat less relevant today because of the introduction of alloys that are not gold-based. It is important to emphasize that the terms *carat* and *fineness* refer only to gold content, not noble-metal content.

CASTING ALLOYS

TYPES AND COMPOSITION

The number of dental casting alloys has increased dramatically in recent years. Formerly, the ADA Specification No. 5 classified these alloys as Types I through IV, with the type of alloy depending on its content of gold and platinum group metals. In the old system, the content of

TABLE 15-3 Comparison of Carat, Fineness, and Weight Percentage of Gold in Gold Alloys

Carat	Amount of Gold by Carats	Weight (%) of Gold	Fineness	
			Parts/1000	Decimal
24	24/24	100.0	1000.00	1.000
22	22/24	91.7	916.66	0.916
20	20/24	83.3	833.33	0.833
18	18/24	75.0	750.00	0.750
16	16/24	66.7	666.66	0.666
14	14/24	58.3	583.33	0.583
9	9/24	37.5	374.99	0.375

noble metals (Types I through IV) ranged from 83 to 75 wt%, respectively, and all alloys were gold based. This classification reflected the use of alloys in dentistry at that time. The current ADA specification also classifies alloys by composition, but in a much more inclusive manner, dividing alloys into three groups: (1) *high-noble,* with a noble metal content of ≥60 wt% and a gold content of ≥40%; (2) *noble,* with a noble metal content ≥25% (no stipulation for gold); and (3) *predominately base metal,* with a noble metal content <25%. The newer specification therefore includes non-noble alloys as well as those with no gold but high palladium. Under the current classification, all of the older alloy "types" are considered high-noble alloys. It is important to keep in mind that the percentages used as boundaries in the new specification are somewhat arbitrary.

The current ADA Specification No. 5 (ISO 1562) also uses a Type I through IV classification system in addition to the compositional classification previously described. However, in the current specification, the type of alloy (I through IV) is determined by its yield strength and elongation (Table 15-4). Thus a high-noble alloy might be Type I or Type IV, depending on its mechanical properties. This situation is somewhat confusing, because in the old specification the alloy type was tied to its composition and virtually all alloys were gold-based. In the current system, each type of alloy is recommended for intraoral use based on the amount of stress the restoration is likely to receive. Type I alloys have high elongation and are therefore easily burnished, but can survive only in low-stress environments, such as inlays that experience no occlusal forces. Type IV alloys are to be used in clinical situations where very high stresses are involved, such as long-span, fixed, partial dentures.

Although the number of casting alloys is immense, it is possible to subdivide each ADA compositional group into several classes (Table 15-5). The predominately base-metal alloys are not shown, but will be discussed in Chapter 16. These classes are simply a convenient way of organizing the diverse strategies that have been used to formulate casting alloys. For each class of alloy shown in Table 15-5, there are many variations; the compositions shown are meant only to be representative. Note that both the wt% and at% compositions of the alloys are shown in Table 15-5 (see previous discussion in this chapter). For the sake of simplicity, the following discussion will be in terms of wt% composition.

TABLE 15-4 ANSI/ADA Specification No. 5, Mechanical Properties of Dental Casting Alloys

Alloy Type	Description	Use	Yield Str. (annealed, MPa)	Elong. (annealed, %)
I	Soft	Restorations subjected to low stress: some inlays	<140	18
II	Medium	Restorations subjected to moderate stress: inlays and onlays	140-200	18
III	Hard	Restorations subjected to high stress: crowns, thick-veneer crowns, short-span fixed partial dentures	201-340	12
IV	Extra-hard	Restorations subjected to very high stress: thin-veneer crowns, long-span fixed partial dentures, removable partial dentures	>340	10

TABLE 15-5 Typical Compositions (wt%/at%) of Noble Dental Casting Alloys

Alloy Type	Ag	Au	Cu	Pd	Pt	Zn	Other
HIGH-NOBLE							
Au-Ag-Pt	11.5/19.3	78.1/71.4	—	—	9.9/9.2	—	Ir (trace)
Au-Cu-Ag-Pd-*I*	10.0/13.6	76.0/56.5	10.5/24.2	2.4/3.4	0.1/0.1	1.0/2.0	Ru (trace)
Au-Cu-Ag-Pd-*II*	25.0/30.0	56.0/36.6	11.8/23.9	5.0/6.1	0.4/0.3	1.7/3.4	Ir (trace)
NOBLE							
Au-Cu-Ag-Pd-*III*	47.0/53.3	40.0/24.8	7.5/14.4	4.0/4.7	—	1.5/2.8	Ir (trace)
Au-Ag-Pd-In	38.7/36.1	20.0/10.3	—	21.0/33.3	—	3.8/5.8	In 16.5
Pd-Cu-Ga	—	2.0/1.0	10.0/15.8	77.0/73.1	—	—	Ga 7.0/10.1
Ag-Pd	70.0/69.0	—	—	25.0/25.0	—	2.0/3.3	In 3/2.3

Note: Percentages may not add to exactly 100.0 because of rounding error in calculation of the atomic percentages.

Most of the alloys contain some zinc as a deoxidizer and either Ir or Ru as grain refiners. Some of these compositions are used for both full metal castings and porcelain-metal restorations.

There are three classes of high-noble alloys: the Au-Ag-Pt alloys; the Au-Cu-Ag-Pd alloys with a gold content of >70 wt% (Au-Cu-Ag-Pd-*I* in Table 15-5); and the Au-Cu-Ag-Pd alloys with a gold content of about 50% to 65% (Au-Cu-Ag-Pd-*II*). The Au-Ag-Pt alloys typically consist of 78 wt% gold with roughly equal amounts of silver and platinum. These alloys have been used as casting alloys and porcelain-metal alloys. The Au-Cu-Ag-Pd-*I* alloys are typically 75 wt% gold with approximately 10 wt% each of silver and copper and 2 to 3 wt% palladium. These alloys are identical to the Type III alloys under the old ADA compositional classification. The Au-Cu-Ag-Pd-*II* alloys typically have < 60 wt% gold, with the silver content increased to accommodate the reduced gold content. Occasionally, these alloys will have slightly higher palladium and lower silver percentages.

There are four classes of noble alloys: the Au-Cu-Ag-Pd alloys (Au-Cu-Ag-Pd-*III* in Table 15-5); Au-Ag-Pd-In alloys; Pd-Cu-Ga alloys; and

Ag-Pd alloys. The Au-Cu-Ag-Pd-*III* alloys typically have a gold content of 40 wt%. The reduced gold is compensated primarily with silver, thus the copper and palladium contents are not changed much from the Au-Cu-Ag-Pd-*II* alloys. The Au-Ag-Pd-In alloys have a gold content of only 20 wt%, and have about 40 wt% silver, 20 wt% palladium, and 15 wt% indium. The Pd-Cu-Ga alloys have little or no gold, with about 75 wt% palladium and roughly equal amounts of copper and gallium. Finally, the Ag-Pd alloys have no gold, but have 70 wt% silver and 25 wt% palladium. By the ADA specification, these alloys are considered noble because of their palladium content.

As Table 15-5 shows, the wt% and at% of dental casting alloys can differ considerably. For example, by weight, the Au-Cu-Ag-Pd-*I* alloys have 76% gold. However, only 57% of the atoms in these alloys are gold. Other elements that have less mass than gold increase in atomic percentage. For these same alloys, the copper content by weight is 10%, but by atoms is 24%. For other alloys whose elements have similar mass, the differences between wt% and at% are less pronounced. For example, in the Ag-Pd alloys the weight and atomic percentages are similar. Weight percentages of the alloys are most commonly used by manufacturers in the production and sales of the alloys. However, the physical, chemical, and biological properties are best understood in terms of atomic percentages.

The compositions of casting alloys determine their color. In general, if the palladium content is >10 wt%, the alloy will be white. Thus, the Pd-Cu-Ga and Ag-Pd alloys in Table 15-5 are white, whereas the other alloys are yellow. The Au-Ag-Pd-In alloys are an exception because they have a palladium content of >20% and retain a light yellow color. The color of this alloy results from interactions of the indium with the palladium in the alloy. Among the yellow alloys, the composition will modify the shade of yellow. Generally, copper adds a reddish color and silver lightens either the red or yellow color of the alloys.

GRAIN SIZE

Recent studies have described the influence of minute quantities of various elements on the grain size of dental casting alloys. In the past, many alloys had relatively coarse grain structures. Now, by the addition of small amounts (0.005% or 50 ppm) of elements such as iridium and ruthenium, fine-grained castings are produced (see Fig. 6-12). Adding one of these elements to the alloy is believed to develop centers for nucleating grains throughout the alloy. Most alloy manufacturers use grain refinement in present-day products. The mechanical properties of tensile strength and elongation are improved significantly (30%) by the fine grain structure in castings, which contributes to uniformity of properties from one casting to another. Other properties, however, such as hardness and yield strength, show less effect from the grain refinement.

PROPERTIES

Melting Range Dental casting alloys do not have melting points, but rather melting ranges, because they are combinations of elements rather than pure elements. The magnitude of the solidus-liquidus melting range is important to the manipulation of the alloys (see Fig. 15-1, Table 15-6). The solidus-liquidus range should be narrow to avoid having the alloy in a molten state for extended times during casting. If the alloy spends a long time in the partially molten state during casting, there is increased opportunity for the formation of oxides and contamination. Most of the alloys in Table 15-6 have solidus-liquidus ranges of 70° C or less. The Au-Ag-Pt, Pd-Cu-Ga, and Ag-Pd alloys have wider ranges, which makes them more difficult to cast without problems.

The liquidus temperature of the alloys determines the burnout temperature, type of investment, and type of heat-source that must be used during casting. In general, the burnout temperature must be about 500° C below the liquidus temperature (for details see Chapter 17 on cast-

TABLE 15-6 Physical and Mechanical Properties of Several Types of Noble Dental Casting Alloys

	Property						
Alloy	Solidus (° C)	Liquidus (° C)	Color	Density (g/cm³)	0.2% Yield Strength (Soft/Hard) (MPa)	Elongation (Soft/Hard) (%)	Vickers Hardness (Soft/Hard) (kg/mm²)
HIGH-NOBLE							
Au-Ag-Pt	1045	1140	Yellow	18.4	420/470	15/9	175/195
Au-Cu-Ag-Pd-*I*	910	965	Yellow	15.6	270/400	30/12	135/195
Au-Cu-Ag-Pd-*II*	870	920	Yellow	13.8	350/600	30/10	175/260
NOBLE							
Au-Cu-Ag-Pd-*III*	865	925	Yellow	12.4	325/520	27.5/10	125/215
Au-Ag-Pd-In	875	1035	Light yellow	11.4	300/370	12/8	135/190
Pd-Cu-Ga	1100	1190	White	10.6	1145	8	425
Ag-Pd	1020	1100	White	10.6	260/320	10/8	140/155

ing). For the Au-Cu-Ag-Pd-*I* alloys, therefore, a burnout temperature of about 450° to 475° C should be used. If the burnout temperature approaches 700° C, a gypsum-bonded investment cannot be used because the calcium sulfate will decompose and embrittle the alloys. At temperatures near 700° C or greater, a phosphate-bonded investment is used. As shown in Table 15-6, a gypsum-bonded investment may be used with the Au-Cu-Ag-Pd-*I*, *II*, and *III* and the Au-Ag-Pd-In alloys, but a phosphate-bonded investment is advisable for the other alloys. The gas-air torch will adequately heat alloys with liquidus temperatures below 1100° C. Above this temperature, a gas-oxygen torch or electrical induction method must be used. Again from Table 15-6, a gas-air torch would be acceptable only for the Au-Cu-Ag-Pd-*I*, *II*, and *III* and the Au-Ag-Pd-In alloys.

The composition of the alloys determines the liquidus temperatures. If the alloy contains a significant amount of an element that has a high melting point, it is likely to have a high liquidus. Thus alloys that contain significant amounts of palladium or platinum, both of which have high melting points (see Table 15-1), will have high liquidus temperatures. In Table 15-6, these include the Pd-Cu-Ga, Ag-Pd, and Au-Ag-Pt alloys.

The solidus temperature is important to soldering and formation of ordered phases, because during both of these operations, the shape of the alloys is to be retained. Therefore during soldering or hardening-softening, the alloy may be heated only to the solidus before melting occurs. In practice, it is desirable to limit heating to 50° C below the solidus to avoid local melting or distortion of the casting.

Density Density is important during the acceleration of the molten alloy into the mold during casting. Alloys with high densities will generally accelerate faster and tend to form complete castings more easily. Among the alloys shown in Table 15-6, all have densities sufficient for convenient casting. Lower densities (7 to 8 g/cm³) seen in the predominately base-metal alloys sometimes present problems in this regard. Alloys in Table 15-6 with high densities generally contain higher amounts of denser elements such as gold or platinum. Thus the Au-Ag-

Pt alloys and Au-Cu-Ag-Pd-*I* alloys are among the most dense of the casting alloys.

Strength Strength of alloys can be measured by either the yield strength or tensile strength. Although tensile strength represents the maximum strength of the alloy, the yield strength is more useful in dental applications because it is the stress at which permanent deformation of the alloys occurs (see Chapter 4). Because permanent deformation of dental castings is generally undesirable, the yield strength is a reasonable practical maximum strength for dental applications. The yield strengths for the different classes of alloys are shown in Table 15-6. Where applicable, the hard and soft conditions, resulting from the formation of ordered solutions, are shown. For several alloys, such as Au-Cu-Ag-Pd-*I*, *II*, and *III*, the formation of the ordered phase increases the yield strength significantly. For example, the yield strength of the Au-Cu-Ag-Pd-*II* alloys increases from 350 to 600 MPa with the formation of an ordered phase. For other alloys, such as the Au-Ag-Pt and Ag-Pd alloys, the increase in yield strength is more modest in the hardened condition. The Pd-Cu-Ga alloys do not support the formation of ordered phase because the ratio of palladium and copper are not in the correct range for ordered phase formation (see Table 15-5 and Fig. 15-1, *B*).

The yield strengths of these alloys range from 320 to 1145 MPa (hard condition). The strongest alloy is Pd-Cu-Ga, with a yield strength of 1145 MPa. The other alloys range in strength from 320 to 600 MPa. These latter yield strengths are adequate for dental applications and are generally in the same range as those for the base-metal alloys, which range from 495 to 600. The effect of solid-solution hardening by the addition of copper and silver to the gold or palladium base is significant for these alloys. Pure cast gold has a tensile strength of 105 MPa (see Table 15-2). With the addition of 10 wt% copper (coin gold), solid-solution hardening increases the tensile strength to 395 MPa. With the further addition of 10 wt% silver and 3 wt% palladium (Au-Cu-Ag-Pd-*I*), the tensile strength increases to about 450 MPa and 550 MPa in the hard condition.

Hardness Hardness is a good indicator of the ability of an alloy to resist local permanent deformation under occlusal load. Although the relationships are complex, hardness is related to yield strength and gives some indication of the difficulty in polishing the alloy. Alloys with high hardness will usually have high yield strengths and are more difficult to polish. As Table 15-6 shows, the values for hardness generally parallel those for yield strength. In the hard condition, the hardness of these alloys ranges from 155 kg/mm^2 for the Ag-Pd alloys to 425 kg/mm^2 for the Pd-Cu-Ga alloys. More typically, the hardness of the noble casting alloys is around 200 kg/mm^2. The Ag-Pd alloys are particularly soft because of the high concentration of silver, which is a soft metal. The Pd-Cu-Ga alloys are particularly hard because of the high concentration of Pd, which is a hard metal. The hardness of most noble casting alloys is less than that of enamel (343 kg/mm^2), and typically less than that of base-metal alloys. If the hardness of an alloy is greater than enamel, it may wear the enamel of the teeth opposing the restoration.

Elongation *Elongation* is a measure of the ductility of the alloy. For crown and bridge applications, a low value of elongation for an alloy is generally not a big concern, because permanent deformation of the alloys is generally not desirable. However, the elongation will indicate if the alloy can be burnished. Alloys with high elongation can be burnished without fracture. Elongation is sensitive to the presence or absence of an ordered phase, as shown in Table 15-6. In the hardened condition, the elongation will drop significantly. For example, for the Au-Cu-Ag-Pd-*II* alloys, the elongation is 30% in the soft condition versus only 10% in the hard condition. In the soft condition, the elongation of noble dental casting alloys ranges from 8% to 30%. These alloys are substantially more ductile than the base-metal alloys, which have elongation on the order of 1% to 2% (see Chapter 16).

Biocompatibility The biocompatibility of noble dental alloys is equally important as other physical or chemical properties. A detailed discussion about the principles of biocompatibility can be found in Chapter 5, but a few general principles will be mentioned here. The biocompatibility of noble dental alloys is primarily related to elemental release from these alloys (i.e., their corrosion). Thus any toxic, allergic, or other adverse biological response is primarily influenced by elements released from these alloys into the oral cavity. The biological response is also influenced significantly by exactly which elements are released, their concentrations, and duration of exposure to oral tissues. For example, the short-term (more than 1 to 2 days) release of zinc may not be significant biologically, but longer-term (more than 2 to 3 years) might have more-significant effects. Similarly, equivalent amounts (in moles) of zinc, copper, or silver will have quite different biological effects, because each of the elements is unique in its interactions with tissues.

Unfortunately, there is currently no way of completely assessing the biocompatibility of noble alloys (or any other material), because the effects of elemental release on tissues are not completely understood. However, in general, several principles apply to alloy biocompatibility. The elemental release from noble alloys is not proportional to alloy composition, but rather is influenced by the numbers and types of phases in the alloy microstructure and the composition of the phases. In general, multiple-phase alloys release more mass than single-phase alloys. Some elements, such as copper, zinc, silver, cadmium, and nickel, are inherently more prone to be released from dental alloys than others, such as gold, palladium, platinum, and indium. Alloys with high–noble metal content generally release less mass than alloys with little or no noble-metal content. However, the only reliable way to assess elemental release is by direct measurement, because there are exceptions to each of the generalizations just mentioned. Similarly, it is difficult to predict, even knowing the elemental release from an alloy, what the biological response to the alloy will be. Thus the only reliable way is to measure the biological response directly, either in vitro, in animals, or in humans (see Chapter 5). It is important to also remember that combinations of alloys used in the mouth may alter their corrosion and biocompatibility.

The Identalloy program was developed in an effort to make dentists and patients more aware of the composition of dental alloys that are used. Under this program, each alloy has a certificate (Fig. 15-3) that lists the complete composition of the alloy, its manufacturer, name, and the ADA compositional classification (high-noble, noble, or predominately base metal). When the dental prosthesis is delivered by the laboratory to the dental office, a certificate is placed in the patient's chart. In this manner, all parties know the exact composition of the material used. This information can be invaluable later if there are problems with the restoration;

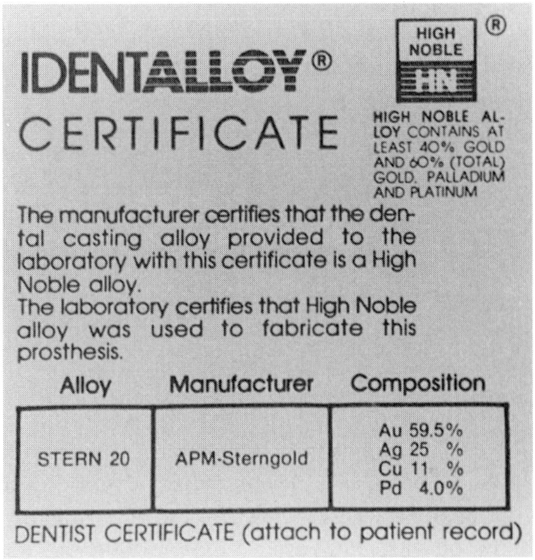
IDENTALLOY®

CERTIFICATE

HIGH NOBLE HN ®

HIGH NOBLE ALLOY CONTAINS AT LEAST 40% GOLD AND 60% (TOTAL) GOLD, PALLADIUM AND PLATINUM

The manufacturer certifies that the dental casting alloy provided to the laboratory with this certificate is a High Noble alloy.
The laboratory certifies that High Noble alloy was used to fabricate this prosthesis.

Alloy	Manufacturer	Composition
STERN 20	APM-Sterngold	Au 59.5% Ag 25 % Cu 11 % Pd 4.0%

DENTIST CERTIFICATE (attach to patient record)

Fig. 15-3 An example of an Identalloy® certificate showing the alloy name, manufacturer, composition, and ADA classification. This section of the certificate is for the dentist's records. A duplicate retained by the laboratory is not shown here. Many dentists will give this information to the patient upon delivery of the crown.

for example, if the patient develops an allergic reaction. This information is also useful when planning additional restorations that may contact the existing restoration, or if some modification (such as occlusal adjustment or contouring) becomes necessary.

GOLD-BASED ALLOYS FOR PORCELAIN-METAL RESTORATIONS

Alloys used for porcelain-to-metal restorations are discussed in detail in Chapter 19. The application of porcelain imposes several additional requirements on alloys to be used for porcelain-metal restorations. However, the principles in the current chapter concerning composition, metallurgy, and physical properties all apply to porcelain-metal alloys. Several sintered (rather than cast) alloy systems have been introduced for porcelain-metal restorations. These systems use gold-based high-noble metals and follow the principles outlined in the current chapter.

WROUGHT ALLOYS

Alloys that are worked and adapted into prefabricated forms for use in dental restorations are described as *wrought alloys.* A wrought form is one that has been worked or shaped and fashioned into a serviceable form for an appliance (Fig. 15-4). The work done to the alloy is usually at a temperature far below the solidus, and is therefore referred to as *cold work.* Wrought forms may include precision attachments, backings for artificial teeth, and wire in various cross-sectional shapes. Wrought alloys are used in two ways in dental prostheses. First, they can be soldered to a previously cast restoration. An example is a wrought wire clasp on a removable partial denture framework. Second, they can be embedded into a cast framework by "casting to" the alloy, as a precision attachment is "cast-to" the retainer of a crown, bridge, or partial denture. The physical properties required of the wrought alloy will depend on the technique used and the composition of the alloy in the existing appliance.

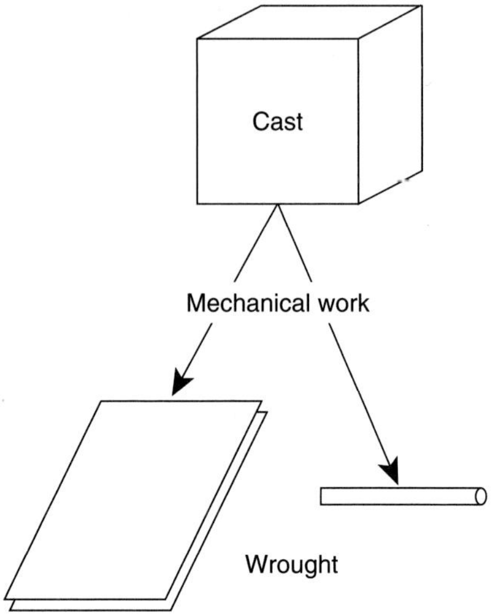

Fig. 15-4 Diagram of the process of mechanical work that transforms cast structures into wrought structures. The microstructure and mechanical properties of cast and wrought forms are fundamentally different (see Chapter 6).

MICROSTRUCTURE

As indicated in Chapter 6, the microstructure of wrought alloys is fibrous. This fibrous structure results from the cold work applied during the operations that shape the alloy into its final form. Wires or other wrought forms normally have a measurable increase in tensile strength and hardness when compared with corresponding cast structures. The increase in these properties results from the entangled, fibrous internal structure created by the cold work.

Wrought forms will recrystallize during heating operations unless caution is exercised (see Figs 6-18, 6-19). During recrystallization, the fibrous microstructure is converted to a grained structure similar to the structure of a cast form. In general, the amount of recrystallization increases as both the heating time and temperature become excessive. For example, in most noble dental wires, a short heating cycle during the soldering operation is not sufficient to appreciably recrystallize the wire, even though the temperature approaches the fusion temperature. However, a prolonged heating period of 30 to

TABLE 15-7 Composition of Typical Wrought Dental Alloys (wt%)

Alloy	Ag	Au	Cu	Pd	Pt	Other
Pt-Au-Pd*	—	27	—	27	45	
Au-Pt-Pd	—	60	—	15	24	Ir 1.0
Au-Pt-Cu-Ag	8.5	60	10	5.5	16	
Au-Pt-Ag-Cu	14	63	9	—	14	
Au-Ag-Cu-Pd	18.5	63	12	5	—	Zn 1.5
Pd-Ag-Cu*	39	—	16	43	1	

*Adapted from Lyman T: *Metals Handbook,* vol 1, *Properties and selection of metals,* ed 8, Metals Park, Ohio, 1961, American Society for Metals.

60 seconds or longer may cause recrystallization, depending on the time, temperature, alloy composition, and manner in which the wire was fabricated. Recrystallization results in a reduction in mechanical properties in proportion to the amount of recrystallization. Severe recrystallization can cause wrought forms to become brittle in the area of recrystallization. Therefore heating operations must be minimized when working with wrought forms.

COMPOSITION

By the current ADA definitions, all alloys used for wrought forms are high-noble alloys except one, which is a noble alloy (Table 15-7). As with the casting alloys, several strategies have been used to formulate alloys with appropriate properties. The compositions in Table 15-7 are not inclusive of all available wrought alloys, but are intended to demonstrate typical alloys. These compositions are designed to provide a range of melting ranges and mechanical properties that are appropriate for wrought alloy applications. The Pt-Au-Pd alloys contain primarily platinum with equal amounts (27 wt%) of palladium and gold. These "PGP" alloys have been commonly used as clasping wires on removable partial dentures. The Au-Pt-Pd alloys are primarily gold with platinum and palladium. The Au-Pt-Cu-Ag, Au-Pt-Ag-Cu, and Au-Ag-Cu-Pd alloys contain approximately 60 wt% gold, but have adopted different strategies for the remaining 40% of the mass. The first two of these alloys contain about 15 wt% platinum with the balance in silver, copper, and palladium, whereas the third of these alloys contains no platinum and higher amounts of silver. The last alloy shown in Table 15-7 contains no appreciable gold or platinum, but consists of palladium and silver in approximately equal amounts with about 16 wt% copper. The Au-Ag-Cu-Pd wrought alloy (see Table 15-7) is similar to the Au-Cu-Ag-Pd-*II* casting alloy (see Table 15-5). These alloys differ only slightly in the gold/silver ratio. Other wrought alloys differ from the casting alloys primarily in their higher platinum contents and absence of iridium or ruthenium grain refiners. Platinum is added to increase the melting temperature of the alloys. The grain refinement is not necessary because these alloys are cold-worked into their final forms.

PROPERTIES

The properties of alloys used for wrought applications are shown in Table 15-8. The solidus of these alloys ranges from 875° C for Au-Ag-Cu-Pd to 1500° C for Pt-Au-Pd. If the wrought form

TABLE 15-8 Properties of Typical Wrought Dental Alloys

	Property				
Alloy	**Solidus (° C)**	**Color**	**0.2% Yield Strength (Soft/Hard) (MPa)**	**Elongation (Soft/Hard) (%)**	**Vickers Hardness (Soft/Hard) (kg/mm²)**
Pt-Au-Pd*	1500	White	750	14	270
Au-Pt-Pd	1400	White	450	20	180
Au-Pt-Cu-Ag	1045	White	400	35	190
Au-Pt-Ag-Cu	935	Light yellow	450/700	30/10	190/285
Au-Ag-Cu-Pd	875	Yellow	400/750	35/8	170/260
Pd-Ag-Cu*	1060	White	515/810	20/12	210/300

*Adapted from Lyman T: *Metals Handbook,* vol 1, *Properties and selection of metals,* ed 8, Metals Park, Ohio, 1961, American Society for Metals.

is to be cast-to or soldered-to, the solidus must be sufficiently high so the form does not melt or lose its fibrous structure during burnout or casting operations. The solidus required will depend on the metals to be joined, the solder, and the burnout and casting temperatures to be used. In general, alloys with high solidus temperatures also have higher recrystallization temperatures. These alloys are mostly white because of the high platinum and palladium contents. Exceptions are the Au-Pt-Ag-Cu and Au-Ag-Cu-Pd alloys, which are light yellow and yellow, respectively. Yield strength, elongation, and hardness are properties relevant to wrought alloys (see Table 15-8). The wrought form must generally have a yield strength low enough to allow for adjustment (of a clasp or attachment), but be high enough that permanent distortion does not occur in service. Furthermore, the elongation must be sufficient to allow for adjustment without fracture. Three of the wrought alloys shown in Table 15-8 can be hardened by formation of ordered phases. The Au-Pt-Ag-Cu and Au-Ag-Cu-Pd alloys are hardened by an Au-Cu ordered phase, whereas the Pd-Ag-Cu alloys are hardened by a Pd-Cu ordered phase. As with the casting alloys, the ordered phase imparts significantly more strength and hardness to the alloy and lower elongation.

SOLDERS AND SOLDERING OPERATIONS

It is often necessary to construct a dental appliance in two or more parts and then join them together by either a soldering or welding process. The terms *soldering, welding,* and *brazing* have specific meanings in industry. The term *welding* is used if two pieces of metal are joined together directly (generally, but not always, without adding a third metal); that is, the metal pieces are heated to a high enough temperature so they attach to each other. The words *soldering* and *brazing* are used if two pieces of metal are joined by adding a third metal. If the temperature used in the process is below 425° C, the operation is soldering; however, if the temperature is above 425° C, the operation is brazing. In dentistry, the parts are joined at temperature above 425° C, so the operation should be called *brazing*. However, because it is most commonly called *soldering,* that is term used in this chapter.

TYPES OF SOLDERS

In general, solders may be divided into two major groups: soft and hard. The soft solders include the lead-tin alloys of eutectic type with a low melting point, sometimes known as "plumber's" solder. The soft solders have several interesting properties, including a low fusion range of about 260° C or less, which permits them to be applied by simple means, such as by a hot soldering iron. Many also possess good working or mechanical properties, making them favorable for use in industry. However, the soft solders lack corrosion resistance, which makes them impractical for dental applications.

Hard solders have a much higher melting temperature than soft solders and possess greater hardness and strength. The high melting range of these solders precludes the use of soldering irons for melting. In industry, special melting methods are used, such as heating with a gas torch, in a furnace, or with other special heating devices.

Two types of hard solders are used in dentistry. Gold-based solders that have good tarnish and corrosion resistance are extensively used in crown and bridge applications. Silver-based solders are commonly used in orthodontic appliances. For dental applications, gold- or silver-based solders are normally melted with a specifically designed dental type of gas blowtorch. Occasionally a method involving an electric furnace or other heating equipment is used, but this is the exception rather than common practice.

Two techniques of dental soldering are used to assemble dental appliances. One is know as *free-hand soldering,* commonly used in assembling orthodontic and other appliances, and the other is *investment soldering,* customarily used in assembling bridges and similar restorations. In freehand soldering, the parts to be assembled are manually held in contact while the heat and solder are applied. As soon as the solder has flowed to position, the heating is discontinued and the appliance is cooled. In investment soldering, the parts to be assembled are mounted in a soldering investment (similar to a casting investment) and held in intimate contact by the hardened investment while the heat and solder are applied. These two techniques are described in detail in appropriate textbooks or manuals on orthodontics, crown and bridge prostheses, and operative dentistry.

Basis of Selecting Solders Certain principles must be observed in selecting solders, regardless of the application. The ideal solder includes qualities such as (1) ease of flow at relatively low temperature, (2) sufficient fluidity to freely flow when melted, (3) strength compatible with that of the structure being soldered, (4) acceptable color to give an inconspicuous joint, (5) resistance to tarnish and corrosion , and (6) resistance to pitting during heating and application. No single, dental, gold-based solder has all of these qualities; therefore manufacturers provide solders that cover a range of fineness and a number of solders that have special qualities. Manufacturers will generally provide detailed information about which solder should be used with each of their alloys. The properties of solders are significantly influenced by the method used during the soldering operation. Thus a recommended procedure must be faithfully followed to obtain the maximum quality from a product.

Composition Gold-based solders for dental use are primarily alloys of gold, silver, and copper, with small quantities of tin, zinc, and sometimes phosphorus included to modify the fusion temperature and flow qualities. The typical composition and resulting fusion temperature values of a variety of gold solders are given in Table 15-9. The compositions of different solders vary considerably from one another. For example, the gold content may vary from 45 to 81 wt%, silver from 8 to 30 wt%, and copper from 7 to 20 wt%, with little variation in the tin or zinc content. Most solders have a copper/gold ratio to support the formation of a Au-Cu ordered phase. The fusion temperature is lower for alloys that have reduced gold content, but the reduction is not as great as sometimes believed. For example, the difference in fusion temperature between solders 1 and 4 is only 69° C when the gold content is reduced by approximately 16%.

In the past, solders were commonly referred to by a carat number. The number did not describe the actual carat of the solder, but rather the carat of the gold alloy on which the solder was to be used. This permitted a wide range of compositions, or actual carat values, to be used for solders described as a specific carat, because the solder was intended for use with an alloy of a definite carat. For example, solders that varied in gold content from 58.5 to 65 wt% might be described as 18k because they were to be used on an casting made of an 18k alloy. The gold content of an 18k alloy should be 75 wt% gold, but the solders contained only 58.5 to 65 wt% gold. This system led to much confusion. In recent years, the degree of fineness has been used to describe the various solders, such as those values designated in Tables 15-9 and 15-10. This

TABLE 15-9 Typical Compositions and Fusion Temperatures of Dental Gold Solders

Solder	Fineness	Composition (% of weight)					Fusion Temperature (° C)
		Au	Ag	Cu	Sn	Zn	
1*	0.809	80.9	8.1	6.8	2.0	2.1	868
2†	0.800	80.0	3-8	8-12	2-3	2-4	746-871
3*	0.729	72.9	12.1	10.0	2.0	2.3	835
4*	0.650	65.0	16.3	13.1	1.7	3.9	799
5†	0.600	60.0	12-32	12-22	2-3	2-4	724-835
6†	0.450	45.0	30-35	15-20	2-3	2-4	691-816

*Adapted from Coleman RL: Res Paper No 32, *J Res Nat Bur Stand* 1:894, 1928.
†Adapted from Lyman T: *Metals handbook,* vol 1, *Properties and selection of metals,* ed 8, Metals Park, Ohio, 1961, American Society for Metals.

TABLE 15-10 Typical Mechanical Properties of Dental Gold Solders

Solder	Fineness	Tensile Strength (Soft/Hard) (MPa)	Proportional Limit (Soft/Hard) (MPa)	Elongation (Soft/Hard) (%)	BHN (Soft/Hard) (kg/mm^2)
1*	0.809	259	142	18	78
3*	0.729	248/483	166/424	7/<1	103/180
4*	0.650	303/634	207/532	9/<1	111/199
	0.730†	221/483	166/405	3/1	112/154
	0.650†	219/436	176/376	3/1	143/192

*Adapted from Coleman RL: Res Paper No 32, *J Res Nat Bur Stand* 1:902, 1928.
†Adapted from Gabel AB, editor: *American textbook of operative dentistry,* ed 9, Philadelphia, 1954, Lea & Febiger, p. 546.

designation is appropriate because it is specific, and when the fineness is changed, the actual carat change is indicated.

Easy-Flowing and Free-Flowing Qualities Dental gold-based solders are frequently described by terms such as *easy-flowing* or *free-flowing*. Although these terms are sometimes interchanged, they refer to two different qualities in the solder alloys. An *easy-flowing* solder is one that has a relatively low fusion temperature; the lower the temperature of fusion, the easier to melt and form the joint. However, the difference in fusion temperatures of high- and low-fineness gold solder is approximately 56° C, so differences in flow caused by a lower fusion temperature are small among these solders (see Table 15-9).

The fusion temperature of the solder must be below that of the alloys being soldered, or the joined pieces will melt during the operation. Previous discussion of casting alloys indicated that the lowest solidus values for the casting alloys are for the Au-Cu-Ag-Pd-*II* and -*III* alloys and the Au-Ag-Pd-In alloys, ranging from 865° to 875° C (see Table 15-6). For wrought alloys, the lowest solidus values ranged from 875° to 935° C, although most of the wrought alloys have substantially higher solidus temperatures (see Table 15-8). As Table 15-9 indicates, most of the solders have fusion temperatures below the solidus temperatures for the casting or wrought alloys. Thus solders are available for even the lowest fusing alloys. In general, the fusion temperature of the solder should be at least 56° C below that of the parts being joined to prevent distortion.

The *free-flowing* quality refers specifically to the ability of the solder to spread and flow freely over the surfaces of the parts begin joined. This quality is closely related to the surface tension of the melted solder. The surface tension (and free-flowing qualities) control the capillary action, which causes the melted solder to penetrate into fine openings between the parts being assembled. In general, lower-fineness solders are more fluid in the molten state than higher-fineness solders because of their lower gold content and the presence of small quantities of alloying metals such as zinc and tin. For this reason, the lower-fineness solders are preferred when joining parts because the solder flows promptly and freely into the available spaces. Solders that spread slowly are often described as being *sticky*, and they resist spreading even when properly heated. As a result, they tend to penetrate or "burn through" the part being soldered if the solder is forced to spread by overheating. Obviously, the easy- and free-flowing qualities work together, because the lower-fineness gold solders have the lowest melting range and greatest freedom of flow.

Mechanical Properties The values in Table 15-10 illustrate typical mechanical properties for dental solders. There are a wide range of strengths and hardness available. As stated previously, it is most desirable to use a solder with a strength similar to that of the parts being joined. All solders in Table 15-10 are subject to hardening by ordered-phase formation except solder 1. Solder 1 does not form an ordered phase because the gold/copper ratio is not appropriate (see Table 15-9). A considerable increase in strength and hardness can be obtained by slow-cooling the solder and allowing the ordered phase to form.

The percentages of elongation in noble solders are notably less than those of many noble casting alloys (see Tables 15-10 and 15-6). Even in the soft condition, the elongation ranges only from 3% to 9% for all of the solders except solder 1. In the hard condition the elongation is most often 1%, which is quite brittle. In general, it is more desirable in most appliances to obtain an improved hardness and proportional limit that accompany the ordered-phase formation than to sacrifice these properties for a small increase in elongation.

Color and Tarnish Resistance The color of dental noble solders varies from deep yellow to light yellow and white in much the same manner as casting alloys. Although the ability to match the color of the appliances is an important quality of a solder, producing an inconspicuous solder joint is not difficult in practice. The location of the solder junction on the restoration and the total amount of solder applied are clearly factors that influence color matching.

Because of their gold content, the solders of high fineness are assumed to be more resistant to tarnish, discoloration, and corrosion in the mouth than the lower-fineness solders. However, there is little evidence or data to support such claims, because no good tests are available for tarnish and discoloration of such structures. High-fineness solders are often recommended to prevent tarnish in service. However, the qualities of increased fluidity and mechanical properties associated with the lower fineness (0.650 or less) may outweigh any increased tendency of those solders to tarnish in service. Actually, the lower-fineness solders are used extensively for the assembly of dental appliances without serious tendencies to discolor.

Biocompatibility Little information exists about the biocompatibility of noble dental solders. However, the same principles govern the biocompatibility of solders as govern alloys (see previous discussion, this chapter). In vitro evidence indicates that the biological properties of solders may be completely different when the solder is tested by itself versus when it is tested in combination with a substrate alloy. Most solders appear to release less mass and have better in vitro biocompatibility when used on an appropriate substrate metal, but a few will be more cytotoxic on the substrate. The character of the substrate alloy also plays a role, as do the surface area of the solder, any pitting present, and other factors. Generally, these results indicate that the biological liabilities of any solder should be assessed with the solder-substrate combination versus the solder by itself.

Pitted Solder Joints Hard solders have a tendency to be pitted after the soldering operation. In general, pitting results from improper heating of the solder, although some compositions of solder may be more susceptible to pitting than others. When solders of typical fineness are used, a pitted solder can often be associated with either excessive heating during the fusion of the solder or with improper fluxing during heating.

If the solder is heated to too high a temperature or for prolonged periods, the lower–melting point tin and zinc in the solder can boil or oxidize and form pits or porosities as the solder solidifies. These pits often become apparent only during finishing and polishing operations. If the solder is underheated and the flux is applied in excess or improperly melted, it may be trapped in the melted solder and form pits that are uncovered during polishing. To avoid pitting from these causes, the solder should be heated promptly to the fusion temperature, and heating should be stopped as soon as the solder has flowed into position.

MICROSTRUCTURE OF SOLDERED JOINTS

Microscopic examination of well-formed soldered joints has shown that the solder does not combine excessively with the parts being soldered. When the solder has fused properly and has not been overheated, a well-defined boundary forms between the solder and the soldered parts. When the joint is heated too high or for too long, diffusion of elements between the solder and the parts occurs in proportion to the time and temperature excess. Studies indicate that diffusion in the soldered joint reduces the strength and quality of the joint.

Fig. 15-5 shows a microscopic view of a soldered joint between a high-noble casting alloy and a section of a Pt-Au-Pd wire used as a clasp on a removable partial denture. The sample has been etched with acid to reveal its microstructure. The wire has a typical fibrous appearance of a wrought form, and the alloy has a typical granular appearance of a cast form. The solder also has a normal granular appearance, and a sharp boundary exists between the solder and wire and the solder and the cast alloy, indicating that time or temperature of the soldering procedure was not excessive.

A less satisfactory soldered joint is shown in Fig. 15-6. The boundary between the wire and the solder is less sharp and wider. This poorer adaptation may have resulted from either im-

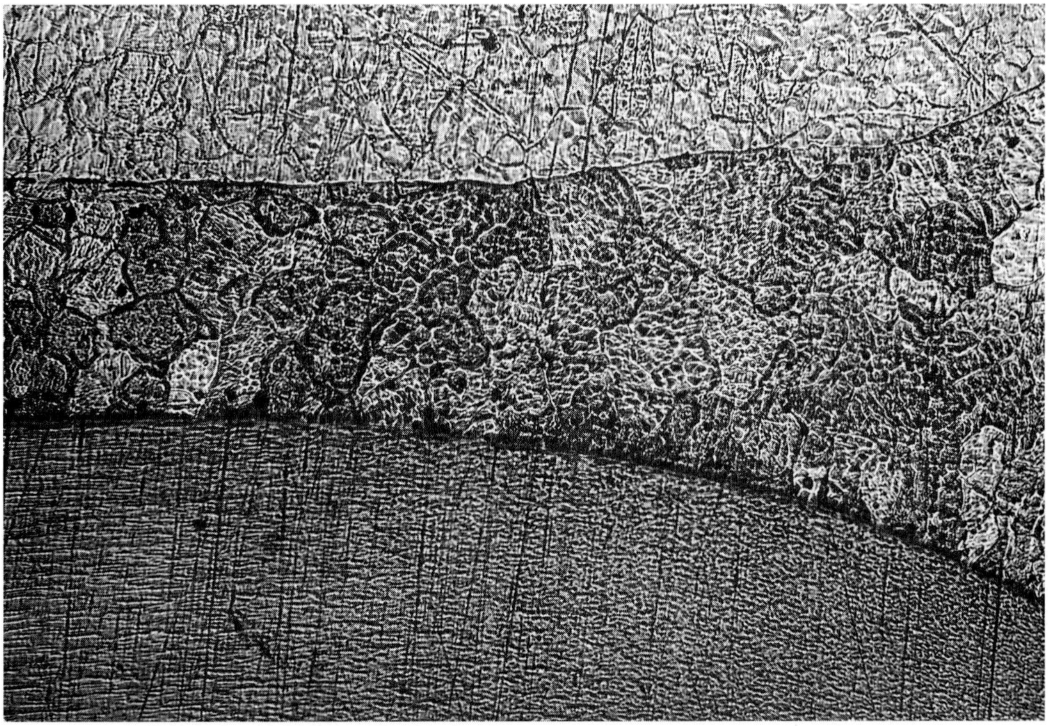

Fig. 15-5 Ideal soldered joint formed between gold-based casting alloy and a gold-based wire. *Top,* Granular microstructure of the cast alloy; *bottom,* fibrous microstructure of the wire. *Middle,* Granular microstructure of the solder.

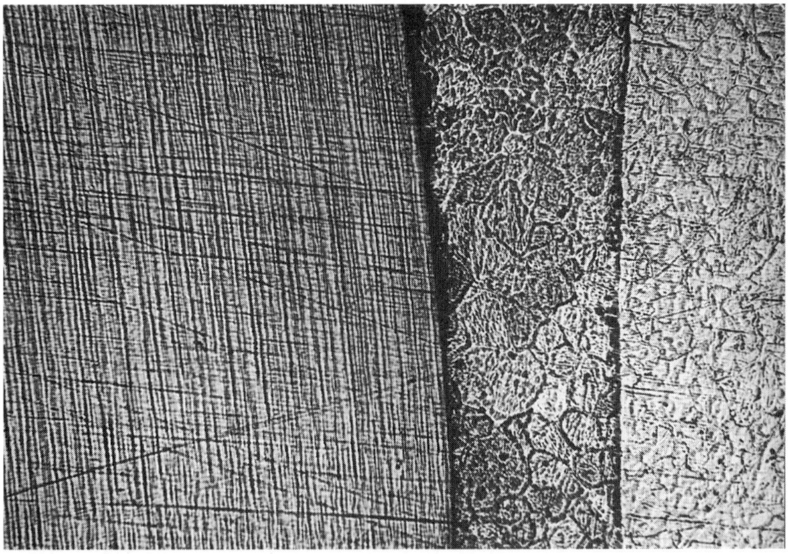

Fig. 15-6 Solder *(middle)* well attached to cast alloy *(right)* but with less satisfactory attachment to the wire *(left).*

proper fluxing or improper heating when the solder was applied. The solder is also not ideally adapted to the cast alloy. However, there is no evidence of recrystallization of the wire and the grain size in the alloy is unchanged, indicating that the time and temperature of heating was not excessive. Overheating would also cause diffusion between the alloys. Recrystallization of the wire, grain growth of the casting alloy, and diffusion are all undesirable because they result in a loss of physical properties necessary for the successful function of the dental appliance.

The microstructure of an overheated wire is shown in Fig. 15-7. Some evidence of the original fibrous wire remains, but recrystallization has taken place throughout most of the wire. The section of wire shown in Fig. 15-7 was 2 mm from the soldered joint. More severe recrystallization occurred close to the solder, and the wire broke in service within the area adjacent to the solder. When cast structures are overheated in the presence of solder, the solder will diffuse into the alloy, resulting in a new alloy that lacks strength and ductility. Overheating can also cause warpage and distortion of the appliance from large dimensional changes.

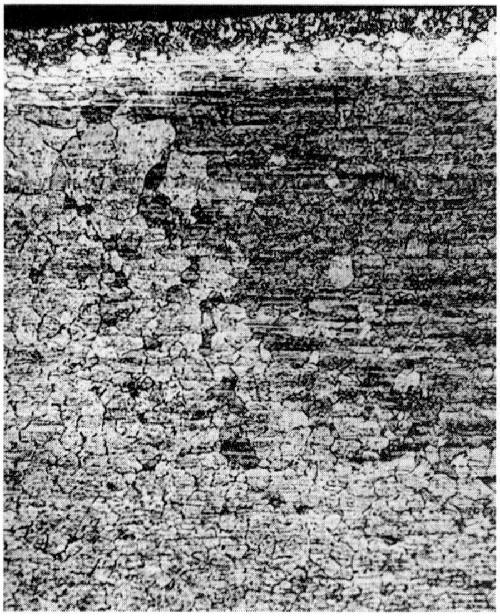

Fig. 15-7 Evidence of recrystallization resulting from excessive heating of gold wire. *Right,* Original fibrous microstructure of the wire; *bottom* and *left,* granular structure resulting from recrystallization. Heat was applied 2 mm from this point on the wire.

Silver Solder Hard solders composed of silver-based alloys are used extensively in some industries, but their application in dentistry has been limited. These solders are also commonly known as *silver solders.* Silver-based solders are used when a low–fusing point solder is needed for soldering onto stainless steel or other base-metal alloys. Orthodontic appliances are commonly soldered using silver-based solders. In general, the resistance of silver solders to tarnish is not as good as gold-based solders, but the strengths of the two types of solders are comparable.

The silver-based solders are composed of silver (10 to 80 wt%), copper (15 to 30%), and zinc (4 to 35%), with some products containing small percentages of cadmium, tin, or phosphorus to further modify the fusion temperature. The formation of the silver-copper eutectic is responsible for the low melting range and higher corrosion rate found in the silver-based solders. The liquidus temperatures for these solders range from 620° to 700° C, which is slightly below those of gold-based solders. This difference is important in the soldering of stainless steel.

SELECTED PROBLEMS

Problem 1

Table 15-2 shows that cast 24k gold has a hardness and strength that are not sufficient for dental restorations, yet gold foil, which is also 24k gold, has three times the hardness and more than twice the tensile strength. Why?

Solution

The manufacturing of gold foil starts with the cast form of the element, then imparts severe cold work until it is very thin. Thus gold foil has a wrought microstructure and exhibits superior mechanical properties because of its fibrous form. Condensation of the foil into the restoration imparts further work hardening to the metal. Note, however, that the elongation of the gold foil is less than half of the original cast 24k gold. Thus by strengthening the gold through work hardening, it has also become more brittle. This trend is typical of wrought metals relative to their cast counterparts.

Problem 2

Inspection of Table 15-5 shows that most noble casting alloys are based either on gold, palladium, or silver, with smaller amounts of copper, platinum, and zinc added. Why do dental manufacturers pick these elements for noble dental casting alloys?

Solution

Gold and palladium are selected as major elements for noble casting alloys because they impart corrosion resistance to the alloys and are miscible (freely soluble) with other the other elements (see Fig. 15-1). In the past, palladium was often used because it was considerably cheaper than gold, and maintained corrosion resistance of the alloy. However, palladium prices have approached and even surpassed those of gold in recent times. Nevertheless, palladium is used to add strength and hardness without sacrificing corrosion resistance. Silver is used as a less expensive alternative to palladium, but cannot provide as much corrosion resistance because it is not a noble metal. Furthermore, silver is not miscible with copper. The other elements in Table 15-5 (copper, zinc, gallium, iridium ruthenium, and indium) are inappropriate as major elements. Copper, zinc, gallium, and indium lack corrosion resistance, and iridium and ruthenium have extremely high melting points and are very expensive. These minor elements are used because they enhance the properties of the major elements. For example, copper provides solid-solution hardening, zinc is a deoxidizer during casting, and iridium is a grain refiner. Platinum, although a noble metal, is not generally used as a major element because of its cost and because it is not miscible with Au or Pd (see Fig. 15-1).

Problem 3

An alloy was listed by a manufacturer as an 11k alloy containing 4.2% Pd, 25% Cu, and 25% Ag (all wt%). What is the atomic percentage of Au in this alloy? Is the carat based on the atomic or weight percent?

Solution

The alloy contains 25.9 atomic percentage of gold. The answer is arrived at in the following manner: an 11-carat alloy contains $11/24 \times 100 = 45.8$ wt% gold. Thus the carat is based on weight percentage. The weight percentage of each element is divided by the respective atomic weight, giving the following results: Au $45.8/197 = 0.232$; Cu $25/63.5 = 0.394$; Ag $25/208 = 0.231$; Pd $4.2/106.5 = 0.039$. The atomic percentage of Au is $0.232 \times 100/(0.232 + 0.394 + 0.231 + 0.039) = 25.9$ atomic percent.

Problem 4

Upon inspection of the elements in Table 15-1, which elements do you think would be candidates as grain refiners and why? (Hint: evaluate the melting range of most alloys in Table 15-6 before answering this question).

Solution

Because Table 15-6 shows that the liquidus of most noble and high-noble casting alloys is below1200° C, any grain refiner would have to have a melting point well above (>500° to 600° C) this value. The elements that are best in this regard are ruthenium, rhodium, osmium, and iridium. All but osmium, which is much too expensive to justify its use over the others, are used in practice.

Problem 5

A dentist tells a laboratory technician that he wants a Type III alloy for a restoration. The laboratory then asks the dentist whether he wants a high-noble or noble alloy. The dentists believes that the laboratory's question is unnecessary, because Type III specifies composition of the alloy. Who is right?

Solution

In this case, the laboratory is correct in asking about the composition of the alloy. Table 15-4 shows that a Type III alloy is a hard alloy suitable for restorations subject to high stress, but Type III gives no indication of composition. Therefore, a number of compositions, noble or high-noble, might meet the requirements for a Type III alloy. Thus the laboratory is correct in asking. Confusion about this issue comes from the past definition of the term *Type III*. In the past, alloy typing for gold-based alloys specified composition and physical properties. However, when the use of alloys other than gold-based varieties became common, the compositions and physical properties were separated. This change still causes confusion among dentists.

Problem 6

In Table 15-5, the atomic percentages of elements in the alloys are sometimes different than their corresponding weight percentages and sometimes quite similar. Why?

Solution

If an alloy contains elements with vastly different atomic weights, then the atomic percentages and weight percentages will be significantly different. The heaviest elements will be lower in atomic percentage than weight percentage and the lightest elements will be higher in atomic percentages than weight percentages. If an alloy contains elements that are comparable in atomic weights, the atomic and weight percentages of the elements will not differ as much. Thus, in Table 15-5, the atomic and weight percentages of the Ag-Pd alloys are similar because the majority of the alloy is composed of silver, palladium, and indium, which are very close to the same atomic weight (Ag = 107.9, Pd = 106.4, and In = 114.8). The other element in this alloy, zinc, does not change much because it is a minor component. If zinc were more prevalent in this alloy, its atomic and weight percentages would be significantly different because its atomic weight (Zn = 65.4) is quite different than that of the other components.

Problem 7

A gold crown made of Au-Cu-Ag-Pd-*I* alloy was inadvertently allowed to slowly cool to room temperature after casting. Because the crown was then in the hardened condition, it was placed into an oven at 400° C for 20 minutes and then quenched in water. However, the casting was still as difficult to finish. Why?

Solution

To convert the hardened alloy to the softened condition, it must be heated above 424° C to affect the conversion (see phase diagram in Fig. 15-1, *A*). Alloys of this composition are often heated to 700° C, which is above the transition temperature of the ordered phase but well below the solidus, to affect the conversion. At this temperature, the alloy converts to the softened condition, then quenching maintains it in the softened condition by cooling it so fast that it does not have enough time to form the ordered phase.

Problem 8

A casting composed of Ag-Pd alloy produced incomplete margins. Why might this have happened?

Solution

Centrifugal casting depends on the density of the molten alloy to create hydrostatic pressure. Low-carat alloys have a lower density, which requires that the casting machine be wound tighter (more turns) for compensation. Alternatively, the fluidity of low-carat alloys is difficult to judge when casting because of a heavier oxide that forms on the surface of the molten mass. If the alloy was not heated sufficiently, then the molten metal cooled before it could reach the fine margin areas of the mold.

Problem 9

Close inspection of Table 15-9 shows that the composition of noble dental solders are quite similar to many noble alloys. Why would this be true?

Solution

Because the solder will be in intimate contact with the alloys, and because corrosion is often enhanced when dissimilar metals are in contact in the mouth, the formulation of solders with compositions similar to noble alloys makes sense. However, the composition of the solders cannot be identical because the solder must have a liquidus below that of the substrate alloy. Also, other elements must be added to ensure good flowability, fluidity, and resistance to pitting.

BIBLIOGRAPHY

Anusavice KJ: *Phillips' science of dental materials,* ed 10, Philadelphia, 1996, W.B. Saunders Company.

Böning K, Walter M: Palladium alloys in prosthodontics: selected aspects, *Int Dent J* 40:289, 1990.

Cartwright CB: Gold foil restorations, *Mich Dent Assoc J* 43:231, 1961.

Corso PP, German RM, Simmons HD: Corrosion evaluation of gold-based dental alloys, *J Dent Res* 64:854, 1985.

Council on Dental Materials, Instruments, and Equipment: Classification system for cast alloys, *J Am Dent Assoc* 109:766, 1984.

Council on Dental Materials, Instruments, and Equipment: Revised ANSI/ADA Specification No. 5 for dental casting alloys, *J Am Dent Assoc* 118:379, 1989.

Craig RG, Powers JM, Wataha JC: *Dental materials: properties and manipulations,* ed 7, St Louis, 2000, Mosby.

Federation Dentaire Internationale: Alternative casting alloys for fixed prosthodontics, *Int Dent J* 40:54, 1990.

German RM, Wright DC, Gallant RF: In vitro tarnish measurement on fixed prosthodontic alloys, *J Prosthet Dent* 47:399, 1982.

Gettleman L: Noble alloys in dentistry, *Current Opinion Dent* 2:218, 1991.

Glantz PO: Intraoral behaviour and biocompatibility of gold versus non precious alloys, *J Biol Buccale* 12:3, 1984.

Hodson JT: Compaction properties of various gold restorative materials, *J Am Acad Gold Foil Op* 12:52, 1969.

Hollenback GM, Collard AW: An evaluation of the physical properties of cohesive gold, *J South Calif Dent Assoc* 29:280,1961.

Johansson BI, Lemons JE, Hao SQ: Corrosion of dental copper, nickel, and gold alloys in artificial saliva and saline solutions, *Dent Mater* 5:324, 1989.

Keller JC, Lautenschlager EP: Metals and alloys. In von Recum AF: *Handbook of biomaterials evaluation,* New York, 1986, Macmillan.

Leinfelder KF: An evaluation of casting alloys used for restorative procedures, *J Am Dent Assoc* 128:37, 1997.

Leinfelder KF, Price WG, Gurley WH: Low-gold alloys: a laboratory and clinical evaluation, *Quint Dent Technol* 5:483, 1981.

Mahan J, Charbeneau GT: A study of certain mechanical properties and the density of condensed specimens made from various forms of pure gold, *J Am Acad Gold Foil Op* 8:6, 1965.

Malhotra ML: Dental gold casting alloys: a review, *Trends Techniques Contemporary Dent Lab* 8:73, 1991.

Malhotra ML: New generation of palladium-indium-silver dental cast alloys: a review, *Trends Techniques Contemporary Dent Lab* 9:65, 1992.

Mezger PR, Stols ALH, Vrijhoef MMA et al: Metallurgical aspects and corrosion behavior of yellow low-gold alloys, *Dent Mater* 5:350, 1989.

Moffa JP: Alternative dental casting alloys, *Dent Clin North Am* 27:733, 1983.

Morris HF, Manz M, Stoffer W et al: Casting alloys: the materials and the 'clinical effects,' *Adv Dent Res* 6:28, 1992.

Nielsen JP, Tuccillo JJ: Grain size in cast gold alloys, *J Dent Res* 45:964, 1966.

O'Brien WJ: *Dental materials and their selection,* ed 2, Carol Stream, IL, 1997, Quintessence.

Richter WA, Cantwell KR: A study of cohesive gold, *J Prosthet Dent* 15:772, 1965.

Richter WA, Mahler DB: Physical properties vs clinical performance of pure gold restorations, *J Prosthet Dent* 29:434, 1973.

Sarkar NK, Fuys RA Jr, Stanford JW: The chloride corrosion of low-gold casting alloys, *J Dent Res* 58:568, 1979.

Shell JS, Hollenback GM: Tensile strength and elongation of pure gold, *J South Calif Dent Assoc* 34:219, 1966.

Stub JR, Eyer CS, Sarkar NK: Heat treatment, microstructure and corrosion of a low-gold casting alloy, *J Oral Rehabil* 13:521, 1986.

Vermilyea SG, Cai Z, Brantley WA et al: Metallurgical structure and microhardness of four new palladium-based alloys, *J Prosthodont* 5:288, 1996.

Wataha JC: Biocompatibility of dental casting alloys, *J Prosthet Dent* 83:223, 2000.

Wendt SL: Nonprecious cast-metal alloys in dentistry, *Current Opinion Dent* 1:222, 1991.

Chapter 16

Cast and Wrought Base-Metal Alloys

Base-metal alloys are used extensively in dentistry for appliances and instruments, as shown in the outline below. Cast cobalt-chromium and nickel-chromium alloys have been used for many years for fabricating partial-denture frameworks and have replaced Type IV gold alloys almost completely for this application. Cast nickel-chromium alloys are used in fabricating crowns and bridges. These alloys were developed as substitutes for Type III gold alloys, and in some cases may be used as a substructure for dental porcelain. Nickel-chromium and cobalt-chromium alloys are used in porcelain-fused-to-metal restorations, and these alloys are discussed in greater detail in Chapter 19. Titanium and titanium alloys are used in cast and wrought forms for crowns, bridges, implants, orthodontic wires, and endodontic files. Stainless steel alloys are used principally for orthodontic wires, in fabricating endodontic instruments, and for preformed crowns.

Dental applications of cast and wrought base-metal alloys are summarized as follows:

1. Cast cobalt-chromium alloys
   a. Partial-denture framework
   b. Porcelain-metal restorations (see Chapter 19)
2. Cast nickel-chromium alloys
   a. Partial-denture framework
   b. Crowns and bridges
   c. Porcelain-metal restorations (see Chapter 19)
3. Cast titanium and titanium alloys
   a. Crowns
   b. Bridges
   c. Partial dentures
   d. Implants
4. Wrought titanium and titanium alloys
   a. Implants
   b. Crowns
   c. Bridges
5. Wrought stainless steel alloys
   a. Endodontic instruments
   b. Orthodontic wires and brackets
   c. Preformed crowns
6. Wrought cobalt-chromium-nickel alloys—orthodontic wires and endodontic files
7. Wrought nickel-titanium alloys—orthodontic wires and endodontic files
8. Wrought beta-titanium alloys—orthodontic wires

GENERAL REQUIREMENTS OF A DENTAL ALLOY

The metals and alloys used as substitutes for gold alloys in dental appliances must possess certain minimal fundamental characteristics:

1. The alloy's chemical nature should not produce harmful toxicologic or allergic effects in the patient or the operator.
2. The chemical properties of the appliance should provide resistance to corrosion and physical changes when in the oral fluids.
3. The physical and mechanical properties, such as thermal conductivity, melting temperature, coefficient of thermal expansion, and strength should all be satisfactory, meeting certain minimum values and being variable for various appliances.
4. The technical expertise needed for fabrication and use should be feasible for the average dentist and skilled technician.
5. The metals, alloys, and companion materials for fabrication should be plentiful, relatively inexpensive, and readily available, even in periods of emergency.

This list of requirements for the ideal substitute for dental gold alloys calls attention to the fact that a combination of chemical, physical, mechanical, and biological qualities is involved in the evaluation of each alloy. Properties depend on material, compositional, and processing factors.

Cast and wrought base-metal alloys, including cobalt-chromium-nickel, nickel-chromium-iron, commercially pure titanium, titanium-aluminum-vanadium, stainless steel, nickel-titanium, and titanium-molybdenum (beta-titanium) alloys are discussed in this chapter. The discussion is based on the synergistic relationship between processing, composition, structure, and properties of the materials.

COBALT-CHROMIUM AND NICKEL-CHROMIUM CASTING ALLOYS

Ever since cobalt-chromium casting alloys became available for cast removable partial-denture restorations, they have continued to increase in popularity. It was estimated as early as 1949 that more than 80% of all partial-denture appliances were cast from cobalt-chromium alloys. By 1969, more than 87% of all partial-denture appliances made in this country were cast from some type of base-metal alloy. Currently, almost all the metal frameworks of partial-denture appliances are made from cobalt-chromium or nickel-chromium alloys.

ANSI/ADA SPECIFICATION NO. 14

According to ANSI/ADA Specification No. 14 (ISO 6871), the weight of chromium should be no less than 20%, and the total weight of chromium, cobalt, and nickel should be no less than 85%. Alloys having other compositions may also be accepted by the ADA, provided the alloys comply satisfactorily with requirements on toxicity, hypersensitivity, and corrosion. Elemental composition to the nearest 0.5% must be marked on the package, along with the presence and percentage of hazardous elements and recommendations for processing the materials. The specification also requires minimum values for elongation (1.5%), yield strength (500 MPa), and elastic modulus (170 GPa).

An important feature of this specification is that it made available a standardized method of testing, which has, in turn, made it possible to compare results from one investigation with those of another.

COMPOSITION

The principal elements present in cast base metals for partial dentures are chromium, cobalt, and nickel, which together account for 82 to 92 wt% of most alloys used for dental restorations. Representative compositions of four commercially available dental casting alloys, including two (on the right) that are used for porcelain-fused-to-metal restorations, are listed in Table 16-1. Chromium, cobalt, and nickel compose about 85% of the total weight of these alloys, yet their effect on the physical properties is rather limited. As discussed in this chapter, the physical properties of these alloys are controlled by the presence of minor alloying elements such as carbon, molybdenum, beryllium, tungsten, and aluminum.

Function of Various Alloying Elements

Chromium is responsible for the tarnish and corrosion resistance of these alloys. When the chromium content of an alloy is higher than 30%, the alloy is more difficult to cast. With this percentage of chromium, the alloy also forms a brittle phase, known as the *sigma* (σ) phase. Therefore cast base-metal dental alloys should not contain more than 28% or 29% chromium. In general, cobalt and nickel, up to a certain percentage, are interchangeable elements. Cobalt increases the elastic modulus, strength, and hardness of the alloy more than does nickel.

The effect of other alloying elements on the properties of these alloys is much more pronounced. One of the most effective ways of increasing the hardness of cobalt-based alloys is by increasing their carbon content. A change in the carbon content of approximately 0.2% changes the properties to such an extent that the alloy would no longer be usable in dentistry. For example, if the carbon content is increased by 0.2% over the desired amount, the alloy becomes too hard and brittle and should not be used for making any dental appliances. Conversely, a reduction of 0.2% in the carbon content would reduce the alloy's yield and ultimate tensile strengths to such low values that, once again, the alloy would not be usable in dentistry. Furthermore, almost all elements in these alloys, such as chromium, silicon, molybdenum, cobalt, and nickel, react with carbon to form carbides, which change the properties of the alloys. Note that, as

TABLE 16-1 Composition of Major Cast Base-Metal Alloys Used in Dentistry

	Alloys (% of Weight)			
Elements	**Vitallium†**	**Ticonium†**	**Beryllium-Containing* Nickel-Chromium Alloy**	**Boron-Containing* Nickel-Chromium Alloy**
Chromium	30.0	17.0	11	20
Cobalt	Balance	–	0.5	0.01
Nickel	–	Balance	Balance	Balance
Molybdenum	5.0	5.0	2	6
Aluminum	–	5.0	2	–
Iron	1.0	0.5	2	0.12
Carbon	0.5	0.1	0.02	0.02
Beryllium	–	1.0	1.6	–
Silicon	0.6	0.5	0.5	4
Manganese	0.5	5.0	0.02	–
Gallium	–	–	–	–
Boron	–	–	–	3

*Alloys for porcelain-fused-to-metal restorations.
†Data from Asgar K: An overall study of partial dentures, USPHS Research Grant DE-02017, NIH; and Baran G: The metallurgy of Ni-Cr alloys for fixed prosthodontics, *J Prosthet Dent* 50:539, 1983.

shown in Table 16-1, the nickel-chromium alloys used with porcelain contain significantly less carbon than the alloys used for partial dentures. The presence of 3% to 6% molybdenum contributes to the strength of the alloys.

Aluminum in nickel-containing alloys forms a compound of nickel and aluminum (Ni_3Al). This compound increases the ultimate tensile and yield strengths of the alloy considerably. The addition of as little as 1% to 2% beryllium to nickel-based alloys lowers the fusion range by about 100° C. However, recent studies suggest that this concentration of beryllium may adversely affect ductility. Corrosion resistance is also compromised, as corrosion occurs preferentially in the Ni-Be eutectic phase, presumably releasing quantities of beryllium greater than the nominal alloy composition of 1% to 2%. Silicon and manganese are added to increase the fluidity and castability of these alloys. Nitrogen, which cannot be controlled unless the castings are made in a controlled atmosphere, such as in a vacuum or under argon, also contributes to the brittle qualities of these cast alloys. When the nitrogen content of the final alloy is more than 0.1%, the castings lose some of their ductility. Numerous other modifications in composition are being proposed to develop more ductile and stronger alloys. There is a remarkable similarity in properties of different alloys having a relatively wide variation in composition. However, as discussed later, it is primarily the minor alloying elements of carbon, nitrogen, and oxygen that influence casting and the properties of a final casting.

MICROSTRUCTURE OF CAST BASE-METAL ALLOYS

The microstructure of any substance is the basic factor that controls properties. In other words, a change in the physical properties of a material is a strong indication that there must have been some alteration in its microstructure. Sometimes this variation in microstructure cannot be distinguished by ordinary means. Neither cobalt-chromium nor nickel-chromium alloys have simple microstructures, and their microstructures change with slight alterations of manipulative conditions.

The microstructure of cobalt-chromium alloys in the cast condition is inhomogeneous, consisting of an austenitic matrix composed of a solid solution of cobalt and chromium in a cored dendritic structure. The dendritic regions are cobalt-rich, whereas the interdendritic regions can be a quaternary mixture consisting of a cobalt-rich γ-phase; a chromium-rich $M_{23}C_6$ phase, where M is Co, Cr, or Mo; an M_7C_3 carbide phase; and a chromium- and molybdenum-rich σ-phase. Interdendritic casting porosity is also associated with this structure.

Many elements present in cast base-metal alloys, such as chromium, cobalt, and molybdenum, are carbide-forming elements. Depending on the composition of a cast base-metal alloy and its manipulative condition, it may form many types of carbide. Furthermore, the arrangement of these carbides may also vary depending on the manipulative condition.

The microstructure of a commercial cobalt-chromium alloy is illustrated in Fig. 16-1. In Fig. 16-1, *A*, the carbides are continuous along the grain boundaries. Such a structure is obtained when the metal is cast as soon as it is completely melted. In this condition, the cast alloy possesses low elongation values with a good and clean surface. Carbides that are spherical and discontinuous, like islands, are shown in Fig. 16-1, *B*. Such a structure can be obtained if the alloy is heated about 100° C above its normal melting temperature; this results in a casting with good elongation values but with a very poor surface because of an increased reaction with the investment. The surface is so poor that the casting cannot be used in dentistry.

Dark eutectoid areas, which are lamellar in nature, are shown in Fig. 16-1, *C*. Such a structure is responsible for very low elongation values but a good and clean casting. From these three examples, it is clear that microstructure can strongly affect physical and mechanical properties. The microstructure of Ni-Cr alloys is strongly dependent on alloy composition. Alloys containing Be form an interdendritic NiBe phase, as shown in Fig 16-1, *D*. In fact, during normal metallographic procedures involving acid etching of alloy specimens, the NiBe phase is dissolved; what is seen in the figure is the void area left behind. The susceptibility of the NiBe phase to acid attack has been taken advantage of in developing resin-bonded retainers. The retainer may be etched in selected areas, where a composite-like luting agent can then mechanically adhere to the retainer after curing.

Alloys not containing Be have complicated, multiphase microstructures such as that shown in Figure 16-1, *E*. The precipitates dispersed within the matrix include complex carbides, and, in alloys where Nb is present, Mo-Nb-Si compounds. All these precipitates are relatively unaffected by the heat treatments the alloys are subjected to during the porcelain firing procedures, although the loss of elements due to oxidation of the alloy surface may be sufficiently great to change the stability of some phases, which then re-dissolve in the alloy matrix.

HEAT TREATMENT OF BASE-METAL ALLOYS

The early base-metal alloys used in partial-denture prostheses were primarily cobalt-chromium and were relatively simple. Heat treating these alloys up to 1 hour at 1000° C did not change their mechanical properties appreciably. Base-metal alloys available today for partial-denture prostheses, however, are more complex. Presently, complex cobalt-chromium alloys, as well as nickel-chromium and iron-chromium alloys, are used for this purpose.

Studies have shown that many heat treatments of cobalt-based alloys reduce both the yield strength and elongation. If for any reason some soldering or welding must be performed on these partial dentures, the lowest possible temperature should be used with the shortest possible time of heating to the elevated temperature.

The coarse grain size and interdendritic carbide and σ-phases present in cast Co-Cr-Mo limit the strength and ductility of the as-cast alloy. Because the interdendritic phases are associated with reduced ductility and reduced corrosion resistance, cast Co-Cr-Mo is typically solution-annealed at approximately 1225° C. If the treatment and chemical composition are well controlled, such a thermal treatment results in the transformation of σ to $M_{23}C_6$ and the partial dissolution of the $M_{23}C_6$ phase, leading to increased yield strength and ductility. In general, yield and fatigue strengths of this alloy are be-

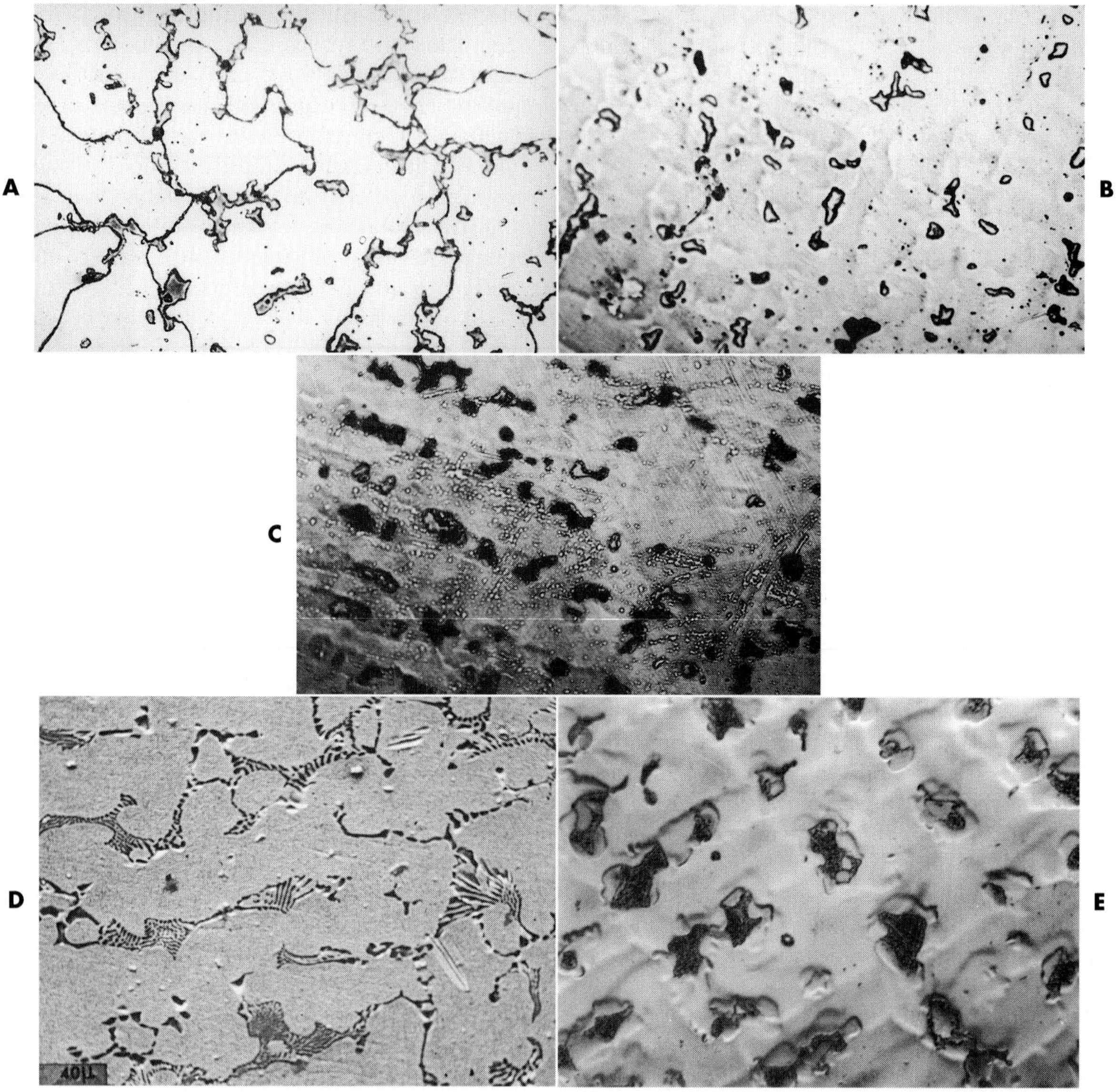

Fig. 16-1 Microstructure of cast cobalt-chromium alloy, **A,** where the carbides are continuous around the grain boundaries. **B,** The islandlike structures are carbides, which are dispersed throughout the entire area. **C,** The dark areas are eutectoid, which are lamellar in nature. **D,** The microstructure of a beryllium-containing nickel-chromium alloy. **E,** The microstructure of a boron- and silicon-containing nickel-chromium alloy.

(**A, B,** and **C,** From Asgar K, Peyton FA: *J Dent Res* 40:68, 1961; **D** and **E,** courtesy G Baran, Temple University.)

lieved to be controlled by the ability of the solute atoms C, Cr, and Mo to inhibit dislocation motion.

Slow cooling to temperatures below those at which incipient melting occurs enhances ductility. A reduction in the carbon content also enhances ductility. However, these increases in ductility are at the expense of yield strength. In general, excess grain-boundary carbide decreases ductility, whereas structures with carbide-free grain boundaries are characterized by markedly reduced yield and tensile strengths.

PHYSICAL PROPERTIES

Melting Temperature The melting temperature of base-metal alloys differs significantly from that of dental gold casting alloys. Most base-metal alloys melt at temperatures of 1400° to 1500° C, as compared with cast gold alloy Types I to IV, which have a melting range of 800° to 1050° C. Only one commonly used nickel-chromium alloy (Ticonium) melts below 1300° C, at a temperature of 1275° C. The addition of 1% to 2% beryllium lowers the melting temperature of Ni-Cr alloys about 100° C. The melting temperature is important in the selection of casting equipment and control of the casting technique.

Density The average density of cast base-metal alloys is between 7 and 8 g/cm^3, which is approximately half the density of most dental gold alloys. Density is of some importance in bulky maxillary appliances, in which the force of gravity causes the relative weight of the casting to place additional forces on the supporting teeth. With certain appliances, therefore, the reduction of weight resulting from the lower density of the cast base-metal alloys can be considered an advantage.

MECHANICAL PROPERTIES

Typical mechanical properties of the partial-denture alloys listed in Table 16-1 have been assembled in Table 16-2, together with a representative range of values for Type IV casting gold alloys subjected to a hardening heat treatment.

Yield Strength The yield strength gives an indication when a permanent deformation of a device or part of a device, such as a clasp, will occur. As such, it is one of the important properties of alloys intended for removable partial-denture restorations. It is believed that dental alloys should have yield strengths of at least 415 MPa to withstand permanent deformation when used as partial-denture clasps. It may be seen from Table 16-2 that base-metal dental alloys have yield strengths greater than 600 MPa.

Tensile Strength The ultimate tensile strength of cast base-metal alloys is less influ-

TABLE 16-2 Mechanical Properties of Alloys Used in Partial Dentures

	Yield Strength, 0.2% Offset (MPa)	Tensile Strength (MPa)	Elongation (%)	Elastic Modulus (GPa)	Vickers Hardness (kg/mm^2)
Cast base-metal alloys*					
Vitallium	644	870	1.5	218	380
Ticonium	710	807	2.4	186	340
Hardened partial-denture gold alloys†	480-510	700-760	5-7	90-100	220-250

*Data from Asgar K, Techow BO, Jacobson JM: *J Prosthet Dent* 23:36,1970; Morris HF, Asgar K: *J Prosthet Dent* 33:36,1975; Moffa JP, Lugassy AA, Guckes AD, Gettleman L: *J Prosthet Dent* 30:424, 1973.
†Data from Oilo G, Gjerdet NR: *Acta Odontal Scand* 41:111, 1983.

enced by variations in specimen preparation and test conditions than are some other properties, such as elongation. Table 16-2 shows that the ultimate tensile strength of cast base-metal dental alloys is greater than 800 MPa. Table 16-2 also demonstrates that hardened partial-denture gold alloys can have ultimate tensile strengths almost equal to those of cast base-metal alloys.

Elongation The percent elongation of an alloy is important as an indication of the relative brittleness or ductility a restoration will exhibit. There are many occasions, therefore, when elongation is an important property for comparison of alloys for removable partial-denture appliances. For example, as described in Chapter 4, the combined effect of elongation and ultimate tensile strength is an indication of toughness of a material. Because of their toughness, partial-denture clasps cast of alloys with a high elongation and tensile strength do not fracture in service as often as do those with low elongation.

The percent elongation is one of the properties critical to accurate testing and to proper control during test preparation. For example, a small amount of microporosity in the test specimen will decrease the elongation considerably, whereas its effect on yield strength, elastic modulus, and tensile strength is rather limited. One can therefore assume that practical castings may exhibit similar variations in elongation from one casting to another. To some degree this is borne out in practice, with some castings from the same product showing a greater tendency toward brittleness than others. This observation indicates that control of the melting and casting variables is of extreme importance if reproducible results are to be obtained.

Although nickel and cobalt are interchangeable in cobalt-nickel-chromium alloys, increasing the nickel content with a corresponding reduction in cobalt generally increases the ductility and elongation. High values of elongation are obtained by casting at the normal melting temperature and by not heating the alloy 100° C above its normal casting temperature. High elongation is achieved without sacrificing strength and is the result of the precise and proper combination of carbon and molybdenum content.

Elastic Modulus The higher the elastic modulus, the more rigid a structure can be expected, provided the dimensions of the casting are the same in both instances. Some dental professionals recommend the use of a well-designed, rigid appliance because it properly distributes forces on the supporting tissues when in service. With a greater elastic modulus, one can design the restoration with slightly reduced dimensions. From Table 16-2, it can be seen that the elastic modulus of base-metal alloys is approximately double the modulus of Type IV cast dental gold alloys.

Hardness Differences in composition of the cast base-metal alloys have some effect on their hardness, as indicated by the values given in Table 16-2. In general, cast base-metal alloys have a hardness about one third greater than gold alloys used for the same purpose.

Hardness is an indication of the ease of finishing the structure and its resistance to scratching in service. The higher hardness of the cast base-metal alloys as compared with gold alloys requires the use of special polishing equipment, which may be considered a disadvantage, but the finishing operation can be completed without difficulty by experienced operators. It is a common practice to use electrolytic polishing for a portion of the finishing operation, which reduces the time and effort necessary for mechanical finishing operations. With an electrolytic polishing procedure, cast base-metal restorations are deplated, and only a very small amount of alloy (a few Ångstroms) is removed from the surface. Electrolytic polishing works on the reverse principle of electroplating, with the restoration serving as the anode. The deplating exposes a new surface, which is smoother than the cast surface because the rough areas are deplated more readily than the smooth ones. The cast base-metal appliances retain their polish well in service. Deplating such a small amount of alloy from the tissue-bearing side of the prosthesis produces a clean, shiny surface, but does not alter the fit. The non–tissue bearing side of the partial denture can be further polished on a high-speed lathe.

Fatigue The fatigue resistance of alloys used for partial denture is important when it is considered that these appliances are placed and removed daily. At these times, the clasps are strained as they slide around the retaining tooth, and the alloy undergoes fatigue. Comparisons among cobalt-chromium, titanium, and gold alloys shows that cobalt-chromium alloys possess superior fatigue resistance, as indicated by a higher number of cycles required to fracture a clasp. Any procedures that result in increasing the porosity or carbide content of the alloy will reduce fatigue resistance. Also, soldered joints, which often contain inclusions or pores, represent weak links in the fatigue resistance of the appliance.

CORROSION

Recent research on dental casting alloys has been dominated by studies on corrosion and potential biological effects of metal ion release. In general, in vitro corrosion tests have evaluated a number of important variables, including effects of electrolytic media and artificial saliva, alloy composition, alloy microstructure, and surface state of the metal. These variables account for 2 to 4 orders of magnitude variation in the amount of species released. The surface state of the metal is an extremely important factor influencing corrosion, because the surface composition is almost always different from that of the bulk alloy. Another important consideration is corrosion coupled with wear. Up to three times the mass of metal ions, such as Ni and Be is released during occlusal rubbing in combination with corrosion than during corrosion alone for Ni-Cr alloys.

CROWN AND BRIDGE CASTING ALLOYS

The nickel-chromium alloys can be divided into those containing or not containing beryllium. Most of the alloys contain 60% to 80% nickel, 10% to 27% chromium, and 2% to 14% molybdenum. As a comparison, cobalt-chromium alloys contain 53% to 67% cobalt, 25% to 32% chromium, and 2% to 6% molybdenum. Those alloys that contain beryllium contain 1.6% to 2.0% of the element. They may also contain small amounts of aluminum, carbon, cobalt, copper, cerium, gallium, iron, manganese, niobium, silicon, tin, titanium, and zirconium. The low atomic weight of about 9 for beryllium, compared with about 59 for nickel and 52 for chromium, results in atomic percentages of beryllium in these alloys of about 11%.

Properties of these alloys are similar to those reported in Table 16-2 for the cobalt-chromium alloys. Crown and bridge casting alloys exhibit a higher hardness and elastic modulus than do noble alloys, but they prove more difficult in casting and soldering. They are also more technique sensitive, and because of their higher solidification shrinkage, producing a restoration with a satisfactory fit is more difficult.

Precautions should be taken to avoid exposure to metallic vapor, dust, or grindings containing beryllium and nickel. The safety standard for beryllium dust is 2 $\mu g/m^3$ of air for a time-weighted, 8-hour day. A higher limit of 25 $\mu g/m^3$ is allowed for a minimum exposure time of less than 30 minutes. Physiological responses may range from contact dermatitis to severe chemical pneumonitis. Therefore efficient local exhaust and filtration systems should be used when casting, finishing, and polishing these beryllium-containing alloys.

The presence of nickel is of greater importance because it is a known allergen. The incidence of allergic sensitivity to nickel has been reported to be from 5 to 10 times higher for females than for males, with 5% to 8% of females showing sensitivity. However, no correlation has been found between the presence of intraoral nickel-based restorations and sensitivity. A cobalt-chromium alloy without nickel or other non–nickel containing alloy should be used on patients with a medical history indicating an allergic response to nickel. The safety standard for nickel is 15 $\mu g/m^3$ of air for a 40-hour week.

To minimize exposure of patients to metallic dust containing nickel or beryllium, intraoral finishing should be done with a high-speed evacuation system.

OTHER APPLICATIONS OF CAST BASE-METAL ALLOYS

Cast cobalt-chromium alloys serve a useful purpose in appliances other than removable partial-denture restorations. In the surgical repair of bone fractures, alloys of this type have been used for bone plates, screws, various fracture appliances, and splints. Metallic obturators and implants for various purposes are formed from cast base-metal alloys. The use of cobalt-chromium alloys for surgical purposes is well established, and these alloys have numerous oral surgical uses. They can be implanted directly into the bone structure for long periods without harmful reactions. This favorable response of the tissue is probably attributable to the low solubility and electrogalvanic action of the alloy; the metal is inert and produces no inflammatory response. The product known as surgical Vitallium is used extensively for this purpose. The primary metal used in oral implantology today is titanium.

TITANIUM AND TITANIUM ALLOYS

Titanium's resistance to electrochemical degradation; benign biological response elicited; relatively light weight; and low density, low modulus, and high strength make titanium-based materials attractive for use in dentistry. Titanium forms a very stable oxide layer with a thickness on the order of angstroms, and it repassivates in a time on the order of nanoseconds (10^{-9} seconds). This oxide formation is the basis for the corrosion resistance and biocompatibility of titanium. Titanium has therefore been called the "material of choice" in dentistry.

Commercially pure titanium (c.p. Ti) is used for dental implants, surface coatings, and, more recently, for crowns, partial and complete dentures, and orthodontic wires. Several titanium alloys are also used. Of these alloys, Ti-6Al-4V is the most widely used. Wrought alloys of titanium and nickel and titanium and molybdenum are used for orthodontic wires. The term *titanium* is often used to include all types of pure and alloyed titanium. However, it should be noted that the processing, composition, structure, and properties of the various titanium alloys are quite different, and also that differences exist between the wrought and cast forms of a given type of titanium.

COMMERCIALLY PURE TITANIUM

Commercially pure Ti is available in four grades, which vary according to the oxygen (0.18 to 0.40 wt%) and iron (0.20 to 0.50 wt%) content. These apparently slight concentration differences have a substantial effect on the physical and mechanical properties.

At room temperature, c.p. Ti has an HCP crystal lattice, which is denoted as the alpha (α) phase. On heating, an allotropic phase transformation occurs. At 883° C, a body-centered cubic (BCC) phase, which is denoted as the beta (β) phase, forms. A component with a predominantly β phase is stronger but more brittle than a component with an α-phase microstructure. As with other metals, the temperature and time of processing and heat treatment dictate the amount, ratio, and distribution of phases, overall composition and microstructure, and resultant properties. As a result, casting temperature and cooling procedure are critical factors in ensuring a successful casting.

The density of c.p. Ti (4.5 g/cm^3) is about half the value of many of the other base metals. The modulus (100 GPa) is also about half the value of the other base metals. The yield and ultimate strengths vary, respectively, from 170 to 480 MPa and 240 to 550 MPa, depending on the grade of titanium.

TITANIUM ALLOYS: GENERAL

Alloying elements are added to stabilize either the α or the β phase, by changing the β transformation temperature. For example, in Ti-6Al-4V, aluminum is an α stabilizer, which expands the α-phase field by increasing the (α + β) to β transformation temperature, whereas vanadium, as well as copper and palladium, are β stabilizers, which expand the β-phase field by decreasing the (α + β) to β transformation temperature.

In general, α-titanium is weldable, but difficult to form or work with at room temperature. Beta-titanium, however, is malleable at room temperature and is thus used in orthodontics. The (α + β) alloys are strong and formable but difficult to weld. Thermal and thermochemical treatments can refine the postcast microstructures and improve properties.

Ti-6Al-4V

At room temperature, Ti-6Al-4V is a two-phase (α + β) alloy. At approximately 975° C, an allotropic phase transformation takes place, transforming the microstructure to a single-phase BCC β alloy. Thermal treatments dictate the relative amounts of the α and β phases and the phase morphologies and yield a variety of microstructures and a range of mechanical properties. Microstructural variations depend on whether working and heat treatments were performed above or below the β-transition temperature and on the cooling rate.

Following forging at temperatures in the range of 700° to 950° C, thermal treatments below the β-transition temperature (typically performed at approximately 700° C) produce recrystallized microstructures having fine equiaxed α grains (Fig. 16-2). Equiaxed microstructures are characterized by small (3 to 10 μm), rounded grains that have aspect ratios near unity. This class of microstructure is recommended for Ti-6Al-4V surgical implants.

The mechanical properties of (α + β) titanium alloys are dictated by the amount, size, shape, and morphology of the α phase and the density of α/β interfaces. The tensile and fatigue properties of Ti-6Al-4V have been studied extensively. Microstructures with a small (<20 μm) α-grain size, a well-dispersed β phase, and a small α/β interface area, such as in equiaxed microstructures, resist fatigue crack initiation best and have the best high-cycle fatigue strength (approximately 500 to 700 MPa). Lamellar microstructures, which have a greater α/β surface area and more oriented colonies, have lower fatigue strengths (approximately 300 to 500 MPa) than do equiaxed microstructures.

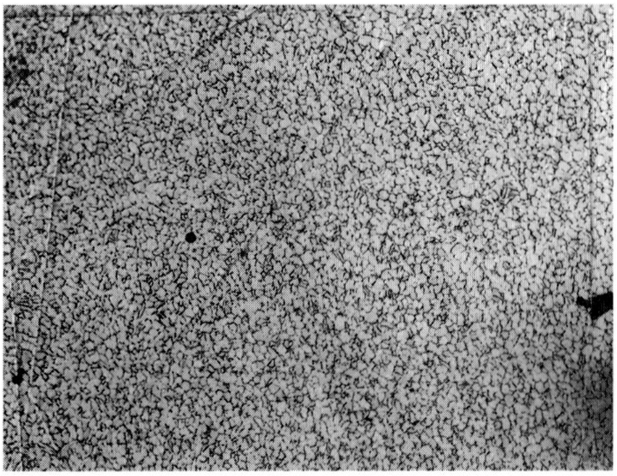

Fig. 16-2 Microstructure of equiaxed Ti-6Al-4V (× 200). Equiaxed microstructures are characterized by small, rounded α-grains, with aspect ratios near unity.

CAST TITANIUM

Based on the attributes, extensive knowledge, and clinical success of wrought titanium implants, interest has developed in cast titanium for dental applications. Although titanium has been cast for more than 50 years, it has only been recently that nearly precision castings have been attainable. For aerospace and medical components, hot isostatic pressing and specific finishing techniques are routinely practiced. However, these techniques are beyond the capabilities and affordability of most dental laboratories.

The two most important factors in casting titanium-based materials are its high melting point (≈ 1700° C for c.p. Ti) and chemical reactivity. Because of the high melting point, special melting procedures, cooling cycles, mold material, and casting equipment to prevent metal contamination are required. Titanium readily reacts with gaseous elements such as hydrogen, oxygen, and nitrogen, particularly at high temperatures (>600° C). As a result, any manipulation of titanium at elevated temperatures must be performed in a well-controlled vacuum. Without a well-controlled vacuum, titanium surfaces will be contaminated with α case, an oxygen-enriched and hardened surface layer, which can be as thick as 100 μm. Surface layers of this thickness reduce strength and ductility and promote cracking because of the embrittling effect of the oxygen. The technology required to overcome these factors is what makes casting titanium so expensive.

Because of the high affinity titanium has for hydrogen, oxygen, and nitrogen, standard crucibles and investment materials cannot be used. Investment materials must have oxides that are more stable than the very stable titanium oxide, and must also be able to withstand a temperature sufficient to melt titanium. If this is not the case, oxygen is likely to diffuse into the molten metal. Investment materials such phosphate-bonded silica and phosphate investment materials with added trace elements achieve this goal. It has been shown that with magnesium oxide–based investments, internal porosity results.

Because of the low density of titanium, it is difficult to cast in conventional, centrifugal-force casting machines. In the last 10 to 15 years, advanced casting techniques, which combine centrifugal, vacuum, pressure, and gravity casting, new investment materials, and advanced melting techniques (e.g., electric arc melting) have been developed. These advances have improved the feasibility of casting titanium-based materials in the dental laboratory.

Pure titanium has been cast into crowns, partial dentures, and complete denture bases. Titanium alloys have a lower melting point than pure titanium. By alloying titanium, the melting temperature can be lowered to the same temperature as that of nickel-chromium and cobalt-chromium alloys. For example, the Ti-Pd and Ti-Cu alloys have melting points of 1350° C. Lower casting temperatures may also reduce the reactivity of titanium with oxygen and other gases. Binary and ternary titanium-based alloys have been cast. Ti-13Cu-4.5Ni has been cast into crowns and partial dentures using vacuum investment-casting technology. Other titanium alloys, such as Ti-6Al-4V, Ti-15V, Ti-20Cu, Ti-30Pd, Ti-Co, and

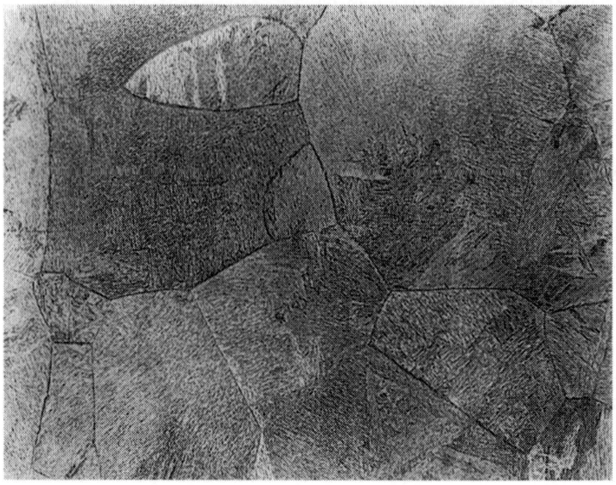

Fig. 16-3 Microstructure of as-cast Ti-6Al-4V.

Ti-Cu are still in the experimental stages and have not yet been implemented in any large clinical studies.

Microstructures of cast titanium materials are similar to those described previously, namely coarse lamellar grains, a result of slow cooling through the β to α or β to (α + β) transformation temperature (Fig. 16-3).

The mechanical properties of cast c.p. Ti are similar to those of Types III and IV gold alloy, whereas cast Ti-6Al-4V and Ti-15V exhibit properties, except for modulus, similar to those of nickel-chromium and cobalt-chromium alloys. Because of the coarse and heterogeneous microstructure, the properties of cast titanium can be nonuniform.

Recently, cast Ti-6Al-4V microstructures have been refined by temporary alloying with hydrogen. The resulting microstructures (Fig. 16-4) can have α-grain sizes less than 1 μm, aspect ratios near unity, and discontinuous grain-boundary α, microstructural attributes that increase tensile and fatigue strength. These changes in microstructural form and structure result in significant increases in yield strength (974 to 1119 MPa), ultimate strength (1025 to 1152 MPa), and fatigue strength (643 to 669 MPa) as compared with respective values for lamellar (902, 994, and 497 MPa) and equiaxed microstructures (914, 1000, and 590 MPa).

Pure titanium has been cast with a pressure-

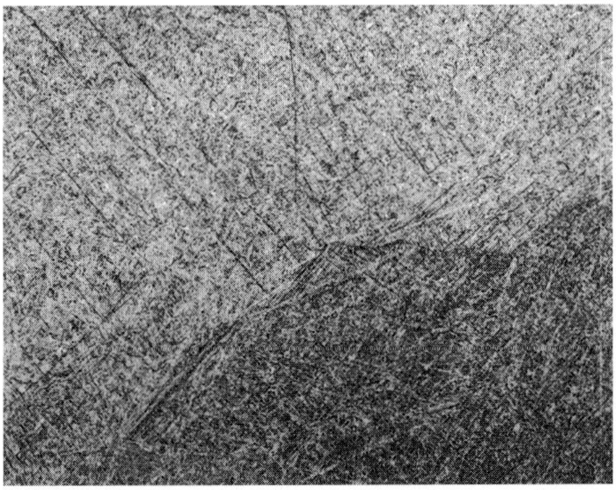

Fig. 16-4 Microstructure of hydrogen-alloy–treated Ti-6Al-4V (× 200).

vacuum casting machine. Other researchers have developed a casting machine that uses an electric arc that melts the titanium in an argon atmosphere. Melting is followed by pressurized casting in a copper crucible and investment in phosphate-bonded silica investment. Such a machine provides a relatively oxygen-free environment and, with the use of a tungsten arc, can reach temperatures of 2000° C. This latter casting regime has been used to cast c.p. Ti crowns and full-denture bases. Crowns cast in this manner have been evaluated clinically, and results revealed that, although fitness was inferior to that of silver-palladium alloy, it was superior to that of nickel-chromium. Occlusal adjustment was no more difficult than with conventional crowns, and discoloration, occlusal wear, and plaque retention were similar to other metals. The clinical results of full-denture bases cast in this manner have not been as good.

Observations of randomly chosen cast crowns have revealed gross surface porosities, to a depth of 75 μm, on both the inside and outside of the surfaces. Mechanical polishing is insufficient to remove this porosity. Internal porosities, sometimes measuring up to 30% of the cross-sectional area, are also readily observed. Surfaces of castings can also be contaminated with α case. The cause of the α case is probably poor vacuum control or mold material contamination. For optimum functionality of the final casting, the surface layer must be removed during finishing. However, even after the α case is removed, internal oxidation can remain and compromise the mechanical properties of the final appliance. Further examination of such castings has also revealed multiple microcracks at the edges of the margins. Some cracks are as long as 100 μm. Cracks of this length are catastrophic to a notch-sensitive material such as titanium.

As outlined, the difficulties with cast titanium for dental purposes include high melting point and high reactivity, low casting efficiency, inadequate expansion of investment, casting porosity, and difficulty in finishing this metal. From a technical standpoint, titanium is difficult to weld, solder, machine, finish, and adjust. Casting titanium requires expensive equipment. As with any new material or technology, specific casting techniques must be developed, which take time, effort, and money.

DENTAL IMPLANTS

The objectives and intended function of dental implants are to restore function to the oral cavity. To fulfill this requirement over an extended period, several other objectives must be met. The implant must be capable of carrying occlusal stresses. In addition, stresses must be transferred to the adjacent bone. Not only must stresses be transferred, they must also be of a "correct" orientation and magnitude so tissue viability is maintained in as near a physiological state as possible. The ability to transmit stress largely depends on attaining interfacial fixation. Thus two further requirements are that (1) the interface stabilize in as short a time as possible postoperatively, and (2) once stable, the interface remain stable for as long a time as possible. Designing an "optimal" implant that meets all of the above objectives requires the integration of material, physical, chemical, mechanical, biological, and economic factors.

In analyzing an implant/tissue system, three aspects are important: (1) the individual constituents, namely the implant materials and tissues; (2) the effect of the implant and its breakdown products on the local and systemic tissues; and (3) the interfacial zone between the implant and tissue. Regarding the ultrastructure of the implant/tissue interface, it is important to understand that, although this zone is relatively thin (on the order of Ångstroms), the constituents of the zone—heterogeneous metallic oxide, proteinaceous layer, and connective tissue—have a substantial effect on the maintenance of interfacial integrity. Furthermore, interfacial integrity depends on material, mechanical, chemical, surface, biological, and local environmental factors, all of which change as functions of time in vivo. Thus implant success is a function of biomaterial and biomechanical factors, as well as of surgical techniques, tissue healing, and a patient's overall medical and dental status.

The physical and material factors affecting implants may be summarized as follows: (1) materials and material processing; (2) mechanisms of implant/tissue attachment; (3) mechanical properties; (4) implant design; (5) loading type; (6) tissue properties; (7) stress distribution; (8) initial stability and mechanisms of enhancing osseointegration; (9) biocompatibility of the implant materials; and (10) surface chemistry, mechanics, and bone-bonding ability of the implant.

Implant Materials and Processing In general, two basic classes of materials—metals and ceramics—are used in implantology, either alone or in hybrid fashion. Metallic implant materials are largely titanium based—either c.p. Ti or Ti-6Al-4V. However, it is essential to note that the synergistic relationships between processing, composition, structure, and properties of the bulk metals and their surface oxides effectively leaves more than two metals. Casting, forging, and machining to form near–net shaped end products can alter the bulk microstructure, surface chemistry, and properties. Similarly, densification of ceramics and deposition of ceramic and metal coatings by hot isostatic pressing or sintering can change bulk and surface composition, structure, and properties. Thus the many material processing sequences necessary to yield the end-stage dental implant have a strong influence on the properties and functionality of the implant, primarily through temperature and pressure effects.

Although cobalt-based alloys have been used experimentally in dentistry, clinically used metallic dental implants are almost exclusively titanium based. The attributes of titanium, namely, corrosion resistance and high strength, have been discussed previously.

The initial rationale for using ceramics in dentistry was based on the relative biological inertness of ceramics as compared with that of metals. Ceramics are fully oxidized materials and therefore chemically stable. Thus ceramics are less likely to elicit an adverse biological response than metals, which oxidize only at their surface. Recently, a greater emphasis has been placed on bioactive and bioresorbable ceramics, materials that not only elicit normal tissue formation, but that may also form an intimate bond with bone tissue and even be replaced by tissue over time.

Mechanisms of Implant/Tissue Attachment Various surface configurations have been proposed as means of improving the cohesiveness of the implant/tissue interface, maximizing load transfer, minimizing relative motion between the implant and tissue, minimizing fibrous integration and loosening, and lengthening the service-life of the construct. The concept of osseointegration around screw-threaded implants represents a situation of bone ongrowth. An alternative method of implant fixation is based on bone tissue ingrowth into roughened or three-dimensional porous surface layers. Such a composite system has been shown to have a higher bone/metal shear strength than have other types of fixation. Increased interfacial shear strength results in a better stress transfer from the implant to the surrounding bone, a more uniform stress distribution between the implant and bone, and lower stresses in the implant. In principle, the result of a stronger interfacial bond is a decreased propensity for implant loosening. A progression of surfaces from the lowest implant/tissue shear strength to the highest is as follows: smooth, textured, screw threaded, plasma sprayed, and porous coated.

Enhancing Osseointegration Because of the necessity of developing a stable interface before loading, effort has been placed on developing materials and methods of accelerating tissue apposition to dental implant surfaces. Materials developments that have been implemented into clinical practice include using surface-roughened implants and ceramic coatings. Other, more-experimental techniques include electrical stimulation, bone grafting, and the use of growth factors.

Important examples of bioactive materials are bioactive glasses and glass ceramics and calcium-phosphate ceramics. Bioactive glasses and glass ceramics include Bioglass, which is a synthesis of several glasses containing mixtures of silica, phosphate, calcia, and soda; Ceravital, which has a different alkali oxide concentration from that of Bioglass; and a glass ceramic–containing crystalline oxyapatite and fluorapatite ($Ca_{10}[PO_4]_6[O,F_2]$) and β-wollastonite (SiO_2-CaO) in a MgO-CaO-SiO_2 glassy matrix (denoted glass-ceramic A-W). Calcium-phosphate ceramics are ceramic materials with varying calcium/phosphate ratios, depending on processing-induced physical and chemical changes. Among them, the apatite ceramics, one of which is hydroxyapatite (HA), have been studied most.

The impetus for using synthetic HA as a biomaterial stems from the perceived advantage of using a material similar to the mineral phase in bone and teeth for replacing these materials. Because of this similarity, better tissue bonding is expected. Additional perceived advantages of bioactive ceramics include low thermal and electrical conductivity, elastic properties similar to those of bone, control of in vivo degradation rates through control of material properties, and the possibility of the ceramic functioning as a barrier to metallic corrosion products when it is coated onto a metal substrate.

However, processing-induced phase transformations provoke a considerable change in the in vitro dissolution behavior, and the different structures and compositions alter the biological reactions. Given the range of chemical compositions available in bioactive ceramics and the resultant fact that pure HA is rarely used, the broader term *calcium-phosphate ceramics* (CPC) has been proposed in lieu of the more specific term *hydroxyapatite*. Each individual CPC is then defined by its own unique set of chemical and physical properties.

Mixtures of HA, tricalcium phosphate, and tetracalcium phosphate may evolve as a result of plasma-spraying deposition processes. Physical properties of importance to the functionality of CPCs include powder particle size, particle shape, pore size, pore shape, pore-size distribution, specific surface area, phases present, crystal structure, crystal size, grain size, density, coating thickness, hardness, and surface roughness.

Results of ex-vivo push-out tests indicate that the ceramic/metal bond fails before the ceramic/tissue bond and is the weak link in the system. Thus the weak ceramic/metal bond and the integrity of that interface over a lengthy service-life of functional loading is reason for concern.

Surface State and Biocompatibility

Implant materials may corrode or wear, leading to the generation of particulate debris, which may in turn elicit both local and systemic biological responses. Metals are more susceptible to electrochemical degradation than are ceramics. Therefore a fundamental criterion for choosing a metallic implant material is that it elicit a minimal biological response. Titanium-based materials are well tolerated by the body because of their passive oxide layers. The main elemental constituents, as well as the minor alloying constituents, can be tolerated by the body in trace amounts. However, larger amounts of metals usually cannot be tolerated. Therefore minimizing mechanical and chemical breakdown of implant materials is a primary objective.

Titanium and other implant metals are in their passive state under typical physiological conditions, and breakdown of passivity should not occur. Both c.p. Ti and Ti-6Al-4V possess excellent corrosion resistance for a full range of oxide states and pH levels. It is the extremely coherent oxide layer and the fact that titanium repassivates almost instantaneously through surface controlled-oxidation kinetics that renders titanium so corrosion resistant. The low dissolution rate and near chemical inertness of titanium dissolution products allow bone to thrive and therefore osseointegrate with titanium. However, even in its passive condition, titanium is not inert. Titanium ion release that does occur is a result of the chemical dissolution of titanium oxide.

Analyses of implant surfaces are necessary to ensure a twofold requirement. First, implant materials cannot adversely affect local tissues, organ systems, or organ functions. Second, the in vivo environment cannot degrade the implant and compromise its long-term function. The interface zone between an implant and the surrounding tissue is therefore the most important entity in defining the biological response to the implant and the response of the implant to the body.

The success of any implant depends on its bulk and surface properties, the site of implantation, tissue trauma during surgery, and motion at the implant/tissue interface. Surface analysis in implantology therefore aids in material characterization, determining structural and composition changes occurring during processing, identifying biologically induced surface reactions, and analyzing environmental effects on the interfaces.

The surface of a material is most always different in chemical composition, form, and structure than is the bulk material. These differences arise from the molecular arrangement, surface reactions, and contamination. In this regard, the interface chemistry is primarily determined by the properties of the metal oxide and not as much by the metal itself. Little or no similarity is found between the properties of the metal and the properties of the oxide, but the adsorption and desorption phenomena can still be influenced by the properties of the underlying metal. Therefore characterization of surface composition, binding state, and form and function are all important in the analysis of implant surfaces and implant/tissue interfaces.

Metallic oxides dictate the type of cellular and protein binding at the implant surface. Surface oxides are continually altered by the inward diffusion of oxygen, and by hydroxide formation and the outward diffusion of metallic ions. Thus a single oxide stoichiometry does not exist.

Summary Although there is no consensus regarding methods of evaluating dental implants and what criteria are most important, clinical evaluations have generally shown that dental implants are successful in about 75% of the cases, 5 years post-implantation. Despite advances in materials' synthesis and processing, surgical technique, and clinical protocols, clinical failures occur at rates of approximately 2% to 5% per year. Causes of failure and current problems with dental implants include: (1) early loosening, stemming from a lack of initial osseointegration; (2) late loosening, or loss of osseointegration; (3) bone resorption; (4) infection; (5) fracture of the implant or abutment; and (6) delamination of the coating from the bulk implant. The most common failure mechanism is alveolar crest resorption, leading to progressive periodontal lesions, decreased areas of supporting tissues, and ultimately implant loosening. Aseptic failures are most often the cumulative result of more than one of the aforementioned factors.

OTHER APPLICATIONS OF WROUGHT TITANIUM

Based on clinical experience with wrought titanium dental implants, wrought titanium crown and bridge applications have been pursued. With the advent of reproducible, high-tolerance machining and processing techniques, such as spark erosion, laser welding and micromachining, and computer-aided design/computer-aided manufacturing, wrought titanium crowns are now possible. Future applications are likely to include partial-denture work, other precision work, implant-supported restorations, and orthodontic components.

WROUGHT STAINLESS STEEL ALLOYS

Steel is an iron-carbon alloy. The term *stainless steel* is applied to alloys of iron and carbon that contain chromium, nickel, manganese, and perhaps other metals to improve properties and give the stainless quality to the steel. These alloys differ in composition from the cobalt-chromium, nickel-chromium, and titanium casting alloys. Usually, stainless steel alloys are not cast, but instead are used in the wrought form in dentistry, which represents the second way that stainless steel differs from the cast base-metal alloys. As a result, the types of appliances formed from these two materials differ. The most common applications of stainless steel for dental purposes at present are in the preparation of orthodontic appliances and fabrication of endodontic instruments, such as files and reamers. Some specialized applications of stainless steel exist for temporary space maintainers, prefabricated crowns, or other appliances placed in the mouth, and for various clinical and laboratory instruments.

COMPOSITION

Several broad classifications of stainless steel are generally recognized. The various groups are referred to as *ferritic, martensitic,* and *austenitic,* and they have different compositions, properties, and applications. The ferritic stainless steels are chromium steels employed in the manufacture of instruments or equipment parts in which some degree of tarnish resistance is desirable. A wide range of compositions is available in this group, in which amounts of chromium, the principal element contributing to stainless qualities, may vary from 15% to 25%. Elements such as carbon, silicon, and molybdenum are included but are all held within narrow limits.

The martensitic steels also are primarily chromium steels with a lower chromium content (about 12% to 18%). These steels can be hardened to some degree by heat treatment, and they have a moderate resistance to tarnish. They are used chiefly in the manufacture of instruments and, to a limited degree, for orthodontic appliances.

The austenitic steels represent the alloys used most extensively for dental appliances. The most common austenitic steel used in dentistry is 18-8 stainless steel, so named because it contains approximately 18% chromium and 8% nickel. The carbon content is between 0.08% and 0.20%, and titanium, manganese, silicon, molybdenum, niobium, and tantalum are present in minor amounts to give important modifications to the properties. The balance ($\approx$ 72%) is, of course, iron.

FUNCTION OF ALLOYING ELEMENTS AND CHEMICAL RESISTANCE

The corrosion resistance of stainless steel is attributed largely to the presence of chromium in the alloy, and no other element added to iron is as effective in producing resistance to corrosion. Iron cannot be used without chromium additions because iron oxide (Fe_2O_3), or rust, is not adherent to the bulk metal. Approximately 11% chromium is needed to produce corrosion resistance in pure iron, and the necessary proportion is increased with the addition of carbon to form steel. Chromium resists corrosion well because of the formation of a strongly adherent coating of oxide on the surface, which prevents further reaction with the metal below the surface. The formation of such an oxide layer is called *passivation*. The surface coating is not visible, even at high magnification, but the film adds to the metallic luster of the metal. The degree of passivity is influenced by a number of factors, such as alloy composition, heat treatment, surface condition, stress in the appliance, and the environment in which the appliance is placed. In dental applications, the stainless characteristics of the alloys can therefore be altered or lost by excessive heating during assembly or adaptation; using abrasives or reactive cleaning agents, which can alter the surface conditions of the appliance; and even by poor oral hygiene practices over prolonged periods.

Of the stainless steel alloys in general use, the austenitic type of 18-8 stainless steel shows the greatest resistance to corrosion and tarnish. In these alloys, chromium and nickel form solid solutions with the iron, which gives corrosion protection. The chromium composition in these alloys must be between 13% and 28% for optimal corrosion resistance. If the chromium content is less than 13%, the adherent chromium oxide layer does not form. If there is more than 28% chromium, chromium carbides form at the grain boundaries, embrittling the steel. The amount of carbon must also be tightly controlled. If not, carbon will react with chromium, forming these grain-boundary chromium-carbides, which lead to depletion of grain-boundary chromium and decrease corrosion resistance in a process known as *sensitization*. Molybdenum increases the resistance to pitting corrosion.

The elements present in small amounts tend to prevent the formation of carbides between the carbon present in the alloy and the iron or chromium and, as a result, often are described as *stabilizing elements*. Some steels, termed *stabilized stainless steels*, contain titanium, niobium, or tantalum, so the carbides that do form are titanium carbides rather than chromium carbides.

The chemical resistance of stainless steel alloys is improved if the surface is clean, smooth, and polished. Irregularities promote electrochemical action on the surface of the alloy. Soldering operations on stainless steel with gold and silver solder may contribute to a reduction in stainless qualities because of electrogalvanic action between dissimilar metals or because of localized, improper composition of the stainless steel wire.

STRESS-RELIEVING TREATMENTS

The 18-8 alloys are not subject to an increase in properties by heat treatment, but they do respond to strain hardening as a result of cold work during adjustment or adaptation of the alloy to form the appliance. Heat treatment above 650° C results in recrystallization of the microstructure, compositional changes, and formation of chromium-carbides, three factors that can reduce mechanical properties and corrosion resistance.

Appliances formed from these alloys may, however, be subjected to a stress-relieving operation to remove the effects of cold working during fabrication, increase ductility, or produce some degree of hardening with some alloys. If heat treatment is to be performed, it should be held to temperatures between 400° and 500° C for 5 to 120 seconds, depending on the temperature, type of appliance, and alloy being heated. A time of 1 minute at 450° C would represent an average treatment to be used on an orthodontic appliance. Keep in mind that temperatures above 650° C will soften or anneal the alloy, and the properties cannot be restored by further treatment. The main advantage of a low-temperature heat-treating operation is that it establishes a uniformity of properties throughout the appliance after adaptation and fabrication, which may reduce the tendency toward breakage in service. Factors affecting an alloy's ability to be heat-treated and stress-relieved include alloy composition, working history (i.e., fabrication procedure), and the duration, temperature, and atmosphere of the heat treatment.

STAINLESS STEEL ORTHODONTIC WIRES

Manipulation Stainless steel wires are processed in the wrought form, through rolling or drawing. *Wrought* means that the near net shape is formed from the material in a solid state. Stainless steel wires can be formed easily into appliances with special orthodontic pliers and instruments. Once an appliance is fabricated, it should be heat-treated for 1 minute at 450° C to relieve stresses created during fabrication.

The soldering of stainless steel appliances requires skill, and the use of suitable materials is essential. Borax fluxes are not satisfactory, and the use of fluoride-containing flux is required for a successful solder joint. Gold and silver solders may be employed to form the union. Silver solders are considered easier to use than are most gold solders, and also provide a stronger solder joint. Silver solders also have the advantage of having slightly lower melting temperatures, 600° to 650° C, than most gold solders, which reduces the hazard of overheating the steel during the soldering operation and thus reducing properties.

The strength of a wire in the vicinity of the soldered joint formed with gold solder is lower than that of one formed with silver solder. Many operators therefore use silver solder with stainless steel or rely entirely on spot welding to assemble the appliance. In one study, which used a standard orthodontic blowtorch as a source of heat with a low-fineness gold solder and a fluoride type of flux, the temperature recorded in the center of a joint was 700° C when the least possible amount of heat was used and 800° C when the maximum amount was applied. The temperature was 650° C at 1 mm from the joint and 635° C at 3 mm, but at 5 mm the temperature in the wire was only 440° C. These observations indicate that higher temperatures are being developed during soldering than were believed to exist, and are no doubt responsible for some of the reduction in strength of stainless steel adjacent to the solder joint.

Cleaning and polishing stainless steel appliances are troublesome operations that become necessary after soldering, heat treating, or periods of service in the mouth. The appliance may be pickled in warmed nitric acid, but a gray satin finish will result that requires buffing or mechanical brushing with a fine abrasive to restore the luster of the original material. An electrolytic polishing bath, also known as an *anodic polisher,* is useful for restoring the surface appearance to stainless steel appliances, the same as for the cast cobalt-chromium structures mentioned previously.

Properties ANSI/ADA Specification No. 32 for orthodontic wires not containing precious metals describes Type I (low-resilience) and Type II (high-resilience) wires. The requirements for flexure yield strength and number of bend cycles are listed in Table 16-3.

Some properties of stainless steel wires when tension, bending, and torsion are applied are listed in Table 16-4 and compared with the properties of nickel-titanium and beta-titanium wires. Of the three types of wires, the stainless steel wire has the highest values of yield strength, elastic modulus, and spring rate and the lowest springback (yield strength/elastic modulus).

Mechanical properties of stainless steel orthodontic wires are listed in Table 16-5 for two sizes of wires in as-received and stress-relieved conditions. The higher values of proportional limit and yield strength of the 0.36-mm diameter wire reflect the increased amount of cold-working used to fabricate this size of wire as compared with that required for 0.56-mm diameter wire. The properties of these wires (except tensile strength) are improved by the stress-relieving heat treatment.

Curves of bending moment versus angular deflection are strongly affected by three factors: (1) the geometry of the wire; (2) the direction of loading, with respect to the wire orientation; and (3) the thermal history of the wire. Curves of bending moment versus angular deflection are

TABLE 16-3 Requirements of ANSI/ADA Specification No. 32 for Orthodontic Wires Not Containing Precious Metals

	Type I–Low Resilience		Type II–High Resilience
Flexure yield strength at 2.9-degree offset, MPa	1700 minimum 2400 maximum		2500 minimum
Number of 90-degree bend cycles (minimum)	0.30-mm diameter	0.30-mm to 0.64-mm diameter	0.64-mm diameter
	15	10	5

TABLE 16-4 Properties of Orthodontic Wires in Tension, Bending, and Torsion

Property	18-8 Stainless Steel	Nickel-Titanium	Beta-Titanium
TENSION			
0.1% yield strength, MPa	1200	343	960
Elastic modulus, GPa	134	28.4	68.6
Springback (YS/E), 10^{-2}	0.89	1.40	1.22
BENDING			
2.9-degree offset yield strength, MPa	1590	490	1080
Elastic modulus, GPa	122	32.3	59.8
Spring rate, mm-N/degree	0.80	0.17	0.37
TORSION			
Spring rate, mm-N/degree	0.078	0.020	0.035

Adapted from Drake SR, Wayne DM, Powers JM, Asgar K: *Am J Orthod* 82:206, 1982. Values are for a 0.43 × 0.64-mm rectangular wire.

TABLE 16-5 Mechanical Properties of 18-8 Stainless Steel Wires

	0.36-mm Diameter		0.56-mm Diameter	
Property	**As Received**	**Stress Relieved***	**As Received**	**Stress Relieved***
Proportional limit,† MPa	1200	1380	1060	912
Yield strength, 0.1% offset,† MPa	1680	1950	1490	1640
Tensile strength, MPa	2240	2180	2040	2160
Hardness (Knoop), kg/mm^2	525	572	536	553
Cold-bending, number of 90-degree bends	37	45	13	21

Adapted from Craig RG, editor: *Dental materials: a problem oriented approach.* St Louis, 1978, Mosby.
*Heated at 482° C for 3 min.
†Properties are measured in tension.

shown in Fig. 16-5 for stainless steel wires having square and rectangular cross-sections. The direction of bending of the rectangular wire has an important effect on the bending moment because the wire is much stiffer in bending in the larger dimension (upper curve versus the middle curve). The curves for the square wire are nearly the same for bending in the direction of the square or the diagonal (bottom curve). The effect of heating on the bending moment–angular deflection curves for round stainless steel wires is shown in Fig. 16-6. Heating the wire even for a short time (15 seconds) causes a decrease in the stiffness in bending and in the angle at which permanent deformation starts as compared with that of the as-received wire. Increased temperature also leads to recrystallization and reduced properties.

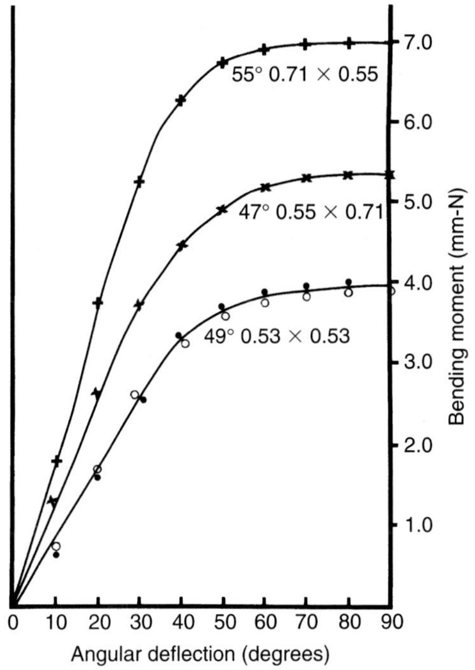

Fig. 16-5 Bending moment–angular deflection curves for square and rectangular 18-8 stainless steel wires. The dimensions of the wires are in mm.

(From Craig RG, editor: *Dental materials: a problem-oriented approach,* St Louis, 1978, Mosby.)

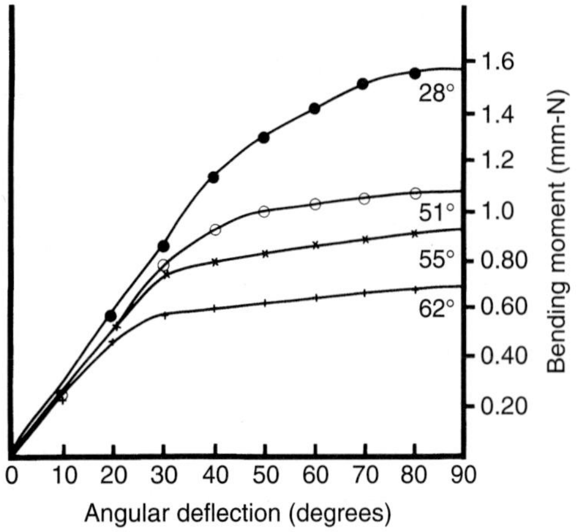

Fig. 16-6 Bending moment–angular deflection curves for 0.46-mm diameter 18-8 stainless steel wire in the as-received condition (●●●) and after 15 seconds (○○○), 60 seconds (xxx), and 120 seconds (+++) at 816° C.

(From Craig RG, editor: *Dental materials: a problem-oriented approach,* St Louis, 1978, Mosby.)

Soldering and spot welding can cause a deterioration in properties if the wire is overheated or underheated. Cross sections of a spot-welded wire are shown in Fig. 16-7. The low setting of the spot welder (underheating) produced an inadequate joint, whereas the high setting (overheating) caused excessive melting and recrystallization of the wrought structure of the wire.

STAINLESS STEEL ENDODONTIC INSTRUMENTS

Numerous endodontic instruments are classified for hand use or as motor-driven instruments. The most common instruments are the K type of root canal files and reamers. These are manufactured by machining a stainless steel wire into a pyramidal blank, either square or triangular in cross section, and then twisting the blank to form a spiral cutting edge. A file with a rhombohedral cross section has also been introduced. Examples of a K file, a K reamer, and a rhombohedral file are shown in Fig. 16-8.

Properties Root canals are rarely straight. Therefore, endodontic files need to be able to follow a curved path. As such, bending and torsional properties of files are important. Similar to orthodontic wires, mechanical properties of endodontic files are dependent upon file geometry, direction of loading and material composition. An example of this is illustrated by the bending moment–angular deflection curves of K and rhombohedral endodontic files (sizes 10 to 35) shown in Fig. 16-9. In bending, the rhombohedral files are less stiff than are the K files, and the increase in stiffness for increasing sizes is smaller and more uniform for the rhombohedral files.

Torsional moment–angular rotation curves of K and rhombohedral endodontic files (sizes 20 and 25) are shown for clockwise and counterclockwise rotation in Fig. 16-10. The rhombo-

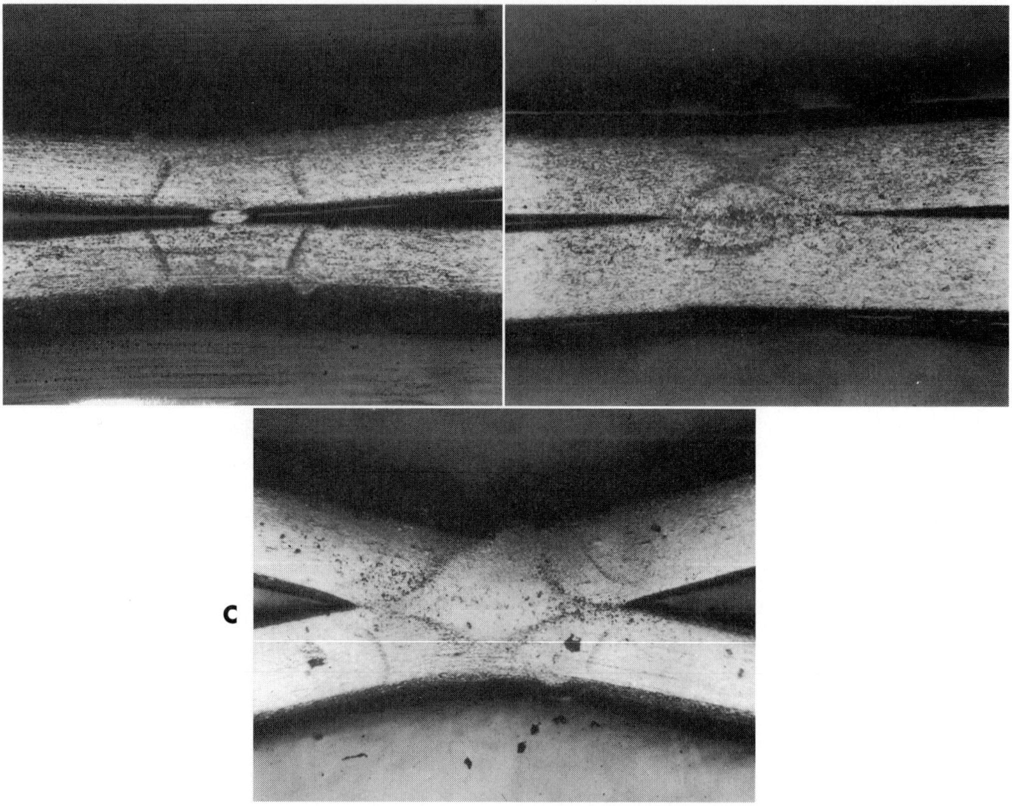

Fig. 16-7 Cross sections of 0.56-mm diameter wires welded at the, **A,** low, **B,** medium, and, **C,** high settings of the spot welder.

(From Craig RG, editor: *Dental materials: a problem-oriented approach,* St Louis, 1978, Mosby.)

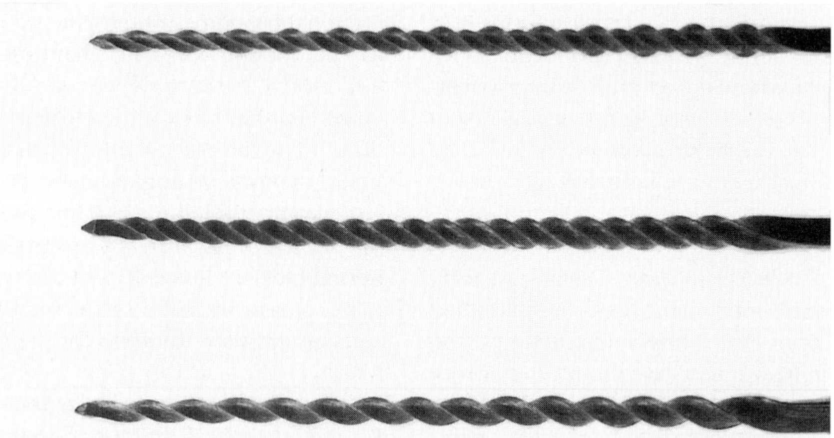

Fig. 16-8 *Top* to *bottom,* Examples of rhombohedral file, K file, and K reamer.

(Courtesy Corcoran JF, Ann Arbor, 1983, University of Michigan School of Dentistry.)

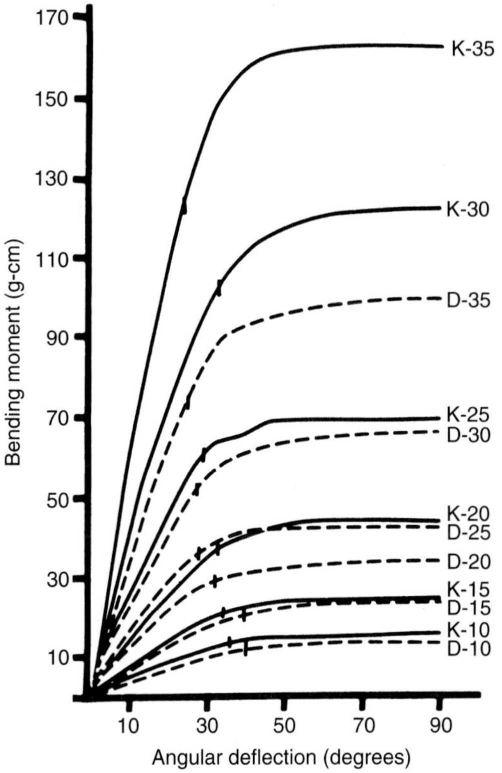

Fig. 16-9 Bending moment–angular deflection curves of endodontic files, sizes 10 to 35. *Vertical marks on curves,* Permanent deformation after 90-degree bending.

(From Dolan DW, Craig RG: *J Endodont* 8:260, 1982.)

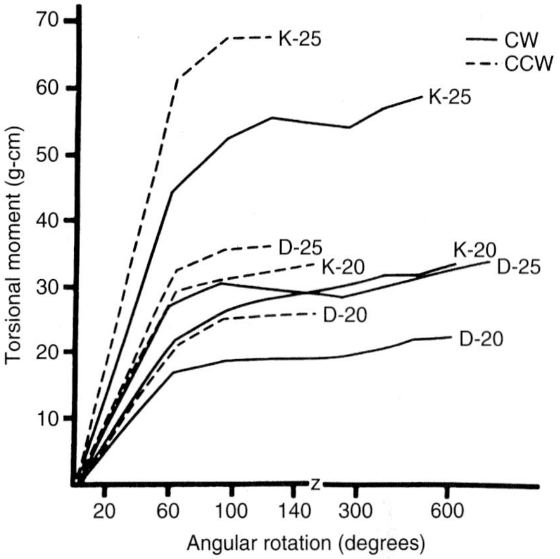

Fig. 16-10 Torsional moment–angular rotation curves of endodontic files, sizes 20 to 25. Clockwise *(CW)* and counterclockwise *(CCW)* rotation.

(From Dolan DW, Craig RG: *J Endodont* 8:260, 1982.)

hedral files are also less stiff than are the K files in torsion, in both directions of rotation. Both types of files fail at lower angular rotation when tested in the counterclockwise direction because counterclockwise rotation increases the tightness of the twist, resulting in brittle fracture, as shown in Fig. 16-11, *A*. Clockwise rotation causes untwisting of the instrument, thereby allowing more rotation before failing in a ductile manner (Fig. 16-11, *B*). Operators are therefore cautioned against twisting a file more than a fourth turn in the counterclockwise direction when a file binds in a canal.

ANSI/ADA Specification No. 28 (ISO 3630-1) for endodontic files and reamers defines geometry, minimum values of torque and angular deflection, and maximum values of stiffness in bending for various sizes of files and reamers. Mechanical tests are made in the clockwise direction. No requirements exist for the counterclockwise direction. Stainless steel instruments are required to be resistant to corrosion when tested according to the specification.

A property not covered in the ANSI/ADA specification, but of importance clinically, is cutting ability. Measurement of cutting ability requires construction of machines that simulate the cutting motion of the instrument. Dentin substrates have been used but produced variation in the data because of biological differences in the hardness of teeth. To overcome this problem, some investigators use acrylic specimens. Cutting ability of individual files varies considerably but is reproducible for the same file with various numbers of strokes. Wear of a file does not appear to affect its cutting ability. Sterilization by dry heat or salt has no effect on the cutting ability of stainless steel files, but autoclave sterilization causes a reduction. Irrigants such as sodium hypochlorite, hydrogen peroxide, and EDTA-urea cause a reduction in cutting ability, whereas a saline irrigant does not cause a reduc-

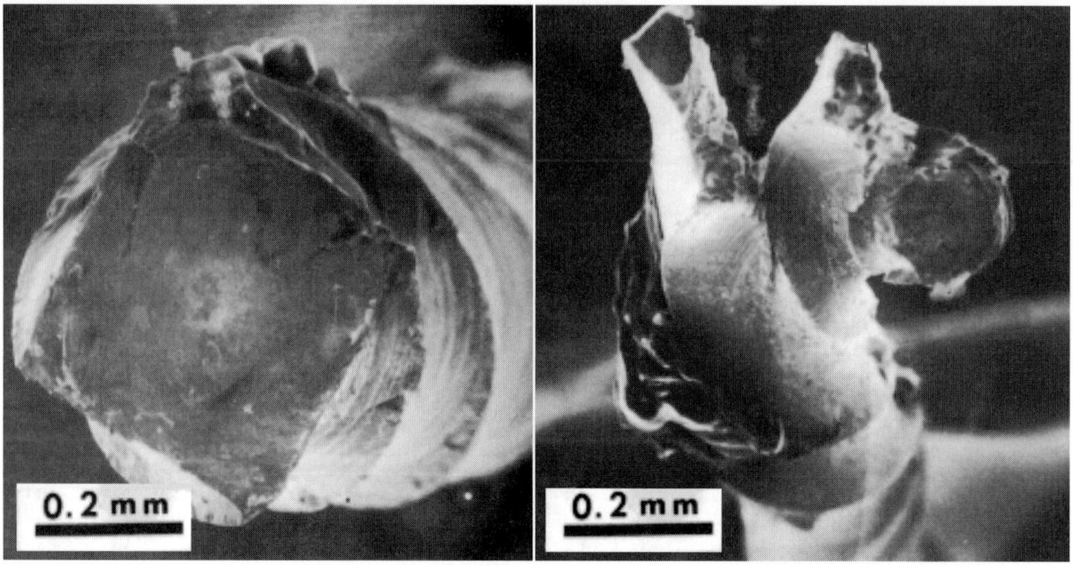

Fig. 16-11 Fracture of K file by counterclockwise torque, **A,** and clockwise torque, **B.** (From Chernick LB, Jacobs JJ, Lautenschlager EP et al: *J Endodont* 2:94, 1976.)

tion. These solutions, excluding saline, also corrode stainless steel at room temperature. Therefore, irrigants should be rinsed from the instruments as soon as possible after use.

NICKEL-TITANIUM ENDODONTIC INSTRUMENTS

The alloys used in nickel-titanium root canal instruments contain about 56% Ni and 44% Ti by weight, which calculate to be 50% of each by atoms. In some instances, <2% of cobalt may be substituted for nickel. Of special interest for this application is that these alloys can change their structure from austenitic (body-centered cubic) to martensitic (close-packed hexagonal) as a function of stress during root canal preparation. When the instrument is used in the canal, the rate of stress levels off due to progressive deformation even if strain is increased due to the transformation to martensite. Note the modulus of Ni-Ti austenite is 120 GPa, and that of martensite is 50 GPa. This effect results in what is termed *super-elasticity.* When the stress decreases, springback occurs without permanent deformation and a return to the austenitic phase.

The super-elasticity of Ni-Ti permits deformations of 8% strain in endodontic files with complete recovery. This value compares to <1% with stainless steel instruments. In addition, the Ni-Ti alloys have higher strengths and lower moduli of elasticity than stainless steel, advantages in preparing curved root canals. Also, it has been shown that Ni-Ti and stainless steel endodontic files do not differ with respect to corrosion resistance.

These improved properties of Ni-Ti root canal instruments have permitted them to be effectively used as engine-driven, rotary instruments. In spite of these improved properties, Ni-Ti instruments can fracture. Studies of cyclic fatigue have shown that the radius of curvature of the file was the most important factor in fatigue resistance, with decreasing radius of curvature (increasing diameter) resulting in decreased fracture time. The fracture was always of a ductile type, suggesting that cyclic fatigue was the major cause of failure.

One drawback of Ni-Ti endodontic instruments is that because of their super-elastic quality they must be manufactured by machining rather than by twisting of tapered wire blanks.

TABLE 16-6 Mechanical Properties of Prefabricated Base Metal Crowns

Types	0.2% Yield Strength (MPa)	Tensile Strength (MPa)	Elongation (%)	Brinell Hardness (kg/mm²)
PERMANENT TYPES				
Stainless Steel 17%-19% Cr, 9%-13% Ni, 0.08%-0.12% C, 0.4%-0.6% Ti	248	593	55	154
Nickel Base 76% Ni, 15.5% Cr, 8% Fe, 0.04% C, 0.35% Mn, 0.2% Si	207	519	42	210
TEMPORARY TYPES				
Tin Base 96% Sn, 4% Ag	24.8	31.7	49	19
Aluminum Base 87% Al, 1.2% Mn, 10% Mg, 0.7% Fe, 0.3% Si, 0.25% Cu	41.4	110	40	28

The instrument design must therefore be ground into the Ni-Ti tapered blanks, thus increasing their cost.

BASE-METAL PREFABRICATED CROWNS

Stainless steel crowns were introduced in 1950 and are recommended for the permanent restoration of primary teeth, particularly in children suffering from rampant caries or in situations where the crowns of the teeth are destroyed. The approximate composition of stainless steel used for crowns and its mechanical properties are listed in Table 16-6. A titanium-stabilized stainless steel may also be used. For purposes of comparison, the properties of a nickel-based alloy used for permanent prefabricated crowns and tin-based and aluminum-based alloys used for temporary prefabricated crowns are also shown. The mechanical properties of stainless steel and nickel-based materials are similar, and the high ductility is important in the clinical adaptation of the crowns. In addition, they have reasonable hardness and strength and, as a result, are classified as permanent restorations. The tin-based and aluminum-based temporary types also have high ductility, but are soft and have lower yield and tensile strengths and thus do not resist clinical wear as do the stainless steel and nickel-based types.

WROUGHT COBALT-CHROMIUM-NICKEL ALLOY

COMPOSITION

A cobalt-chromium-nickel alloy known as Elgiloy is available in wire and band form for various dental appliances. Elgiloy is nominally composed of 40% cobalt, 20% chromium, 15% nickel, 7% molybdenum, 2% manganese, 0.4% beryllium, 0.15% carbon, 15.4% iron, and 0.05% other. Of particular interest is the fact that beryllium serves to decrease the alloy's melting point, facilitating manufacturing. In composition, this alloy resembles the cast base-metal alloys more than it does stainless steel.

PROCESSING AND MANIPULATION

The orthodontic wire is supplied in various tempers (amounts of cold work): soft, ductile, semispring temper, and spring temper. The wires are typically formed in a ductile condition, allowing them to be easily deformed and shaped into appliances and then heat-treated to maximize strength. The standard heat treatment, similar to the treatment used to relieve stress in a stainless steel wire, is 482° C for 7 minutes. Low-temperature heat treatment causes a phase change and stress relief. Excessive heat treatment can cause embrittlement.

The fabrication and soldering techniques used with Elgiloy are similar to those used with stainless steel wires. Elgiloy wires should be soldered with a silver solder in the presence of a fluoride flux or joined by spot welding.

PROPERTIES

The properties of Elgiloy as received are similar to those of stainless steel wires; however, its properties can be modified slightly by the heat treatment (7 minutes at 482° C) used to stress relieve a stainless steel wire. The mechanical properties of spring-temper Elgiloy wire are proportional limit, 1610 MPa; 0.2% yield strength, 1930 MPa; tensile strength, 2540 MPa; and Vickers hardness number, 700 kg/mm^2. The number of 90-degree bends until failure for 0.36-mm and 0.46-mm wires is listed in Table 16-7 for as-received and heat-treated conditions. Note that temper, heat treatment, and wire size all affect this property. Bending moment–angular deflection curves for several Elgiloy wires are shown in Fig. 16-12. The stiffness in bending of the wires is similar; however, the angle at which permanent deformation occurs increases from soft-temper to spring-temper types. The permanent set after a 90-degree bend decreases from soft-temper to spring-temper types. Heat treatment for 7 minutes at 482° C causes an increase in the angle at which permanent deformation occurs but decreases the permanent set.

TABLE 16-7 Cold Bending of Cobalt-Chromium-Nickel (Elgiloy) Wires

	Number of 90-Degree Bends until Fracture		
	0.46-mm Diameter		0.36-mm Diameter
Wire Type	As Received	Heat Treated*	As Received
Soft	15	12	—
Ductile	13	9	—
Semispring temper	12	9	—
Spring temper	5	<1	11

From Craig RG, editor: *Dental materials: a problem oriented approach*, St Louis, 1978, Mosby.
*Heated at 482° C for 7 minutes.

WROUGHT NICKEL-TITANIUM ALLOY

A wrought nickel-titanium alloy known as Nitinol was introduced as a wire for orthodontic appliances in 1972. Nitinol is characterized by its high resiliency, limited formability, and thermal memory.

COMPOSITION AND SHAPE-MEMORY EFFECT

The industrial alloy is 55% nickel and 45% titanium and possesses a temperature transition range (TTR). At temperatures below the TTR, the alloy can be deformed plastically. When the alloy is then heated from below to above the TTR, a temperature-induced crystallographic transformation from a martensitic to an austenitic microstructure occurs and the alloy will return to its original shape. Hence, nickel-titanium is called a *shape-memory alloy*. The orthodontic alloy contains several percent cobalt to lower the TTR. A number of variations of the Ni-Ti alloy have been developed in dentistry. Compositional variations lead to changes in the martensitic and austenitic start and finish temperatures and mechanical properties. Only those wires with austenitic finish temperatures less than 37° C exhibit superelasticity.

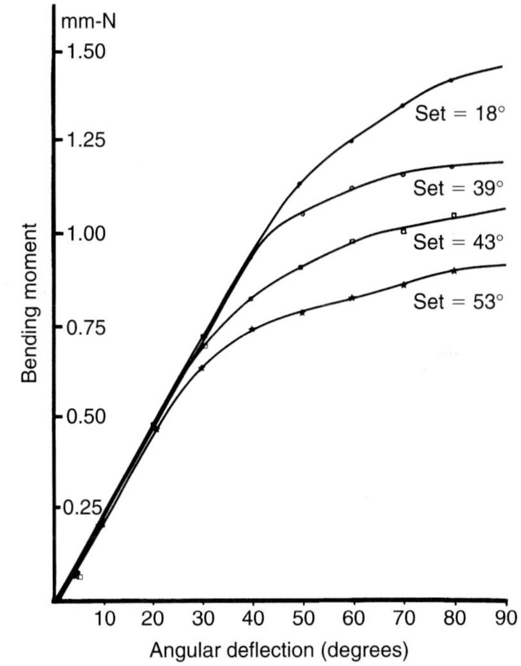

Fig. 16-12 Bending moment–angular deflection curves for 0.46-mm diameter cobalt-chromium-nickel (Elgiloy) wires of the soft (***), ductile (▫▫▫), ductile heat-treated for 7 minutes at 482° C (○○○), and spring temper (●●●) types.

(From Craig RG, editor: *Dental materials: a problem-oriented approach,* St Louis, 1978, Mosby.)

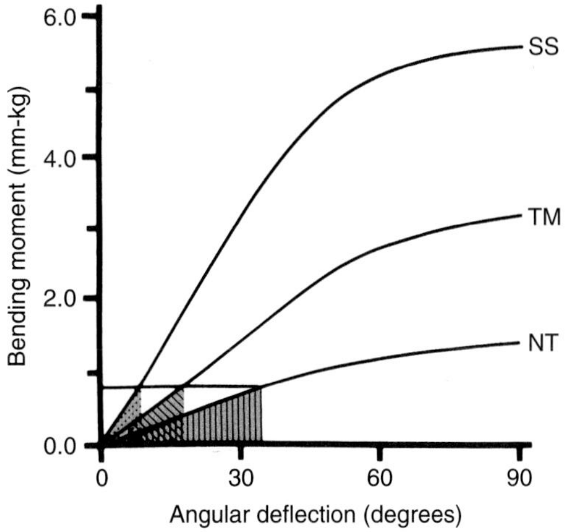

Fig. 16-13 Stored energy at a fixed bending moment below the proportional limit for 0.48-mm by 0.64-mm wires of alloys stainless steel *(SS),* beta titanium *(TM),* and nickel-titanium *(NT).* The stored energy is equal to the shaded areas under the curve for each wire. The spring rate is equal to the slope of each curve.

(From Drake SR, Wayne DM, Powers JM et al: *Am J Orthod* 82:206, 1982.)

PROPERTIES AND MANIPULATION

Mechanical properties of an orthodontic nickel-titanium alloy are compared with those of stainless steel and a beta-titanium alloy in tension, bending, and torsion in Table 16-4. The nickel-titanium alloy has the lowest elastic modulus and yield strength but the highest springback (maximum elastic deflection). As shown in Figs. 16-13 and 16-14, nickel-titanium has the lowest spring rate but the highest resiliency in bending and torsion of the three alloys used for orthodontic wires. Clinically, the low elastic modulus and high resiliency mean that lower and more constant forces can be applied with activations and an increased working range. The high springback is important if large deflections are needed, such as with poorly aligned teeth. Nitinol wire requires special bending techniques and cannot be bent over a sharp edge or into a complete loop; thus the wire is more suited for use with pretorqued, preangulated brackets. The alloy is brittle and therefore cannot be soldered or welded, so wires must be joined mechanically.

WROUGHT BETA-TITANIUM ALLOY

COMPOSITION AND MICROSTRUCTURE

A titanium-molybdenum alloy known as beta-titanium was introduced in 1979 as a wrought orthodontic wire. As discussed previously, c.p. Ti exists in a hexagonal close-packed crystal lattice at temperatures below 883° C and in a body-centered cubic crystal lattice at higher temperatures. These structures are referred to as *alpha-titanium* and *beta-titanium,* respectively. The beta form of Ti can be stabilized at room temperature by alloying with certain elements. Beta-titanium alloy for dental use has the composition 78% titanium, 11.5% molybdenum, 6% zirconium, and 4.5% tin and is supplied as wrought wire.

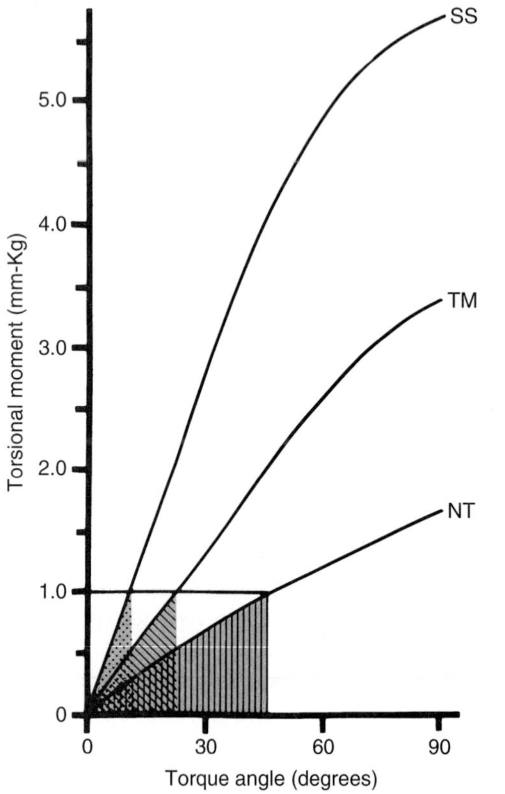

Fig. 16-14 Stored energy at a fixed torsional moment below the proportional limit for 0.48-mm by 0.64-mm wires of alloys stainless steel *(SS)*, beta titanium *(TM)*, and nickel-titanium *(NT)*. The stored energy is equal to the shaded area under the curve for each wire. The spring rate is equal to the slope of each curve.
(From Drake SR, Wayne DM, Powers JM, Asgar K: *Am J Orthod* 82:206, 1982.)

MANIPULATION

Beta-titanium wires can be shaped easily, and the wires can be soldered and welded. Joints can be made by electrical resistance welding. Under proper welding conditions, minimum distortion of the cold-worked microstructure occurs.

PROPERTIES

Compared with stainless steel and Elgiloy wires, beta-titanium wire has lower force magnitudes, a lower elastic modulus, higher springback (maximum elastic deflection), a lower yield strength, and good ductility, weldability, and corrosion resistance. The mechanical properties of beta-titanium alloy in tension, bending, and torsion are compared with stainless steel and nickel-titanium alloys in Table 16-4 and Figs. 16-13 and 16-14. Beta-titanium alloy has values of yield strength, modulus of elasticity, and springback intermediate to those of stainless steel and Nitinol. Its formability and weldability are advantages over Nitinol, and it has a larger working range than do stainless steel or Elgiloy wires.

OTHER ORTHODONTIC WIRES

Recent developments in orthodontic wires include a titanium-based alloy (Ti-15V-3Cr-3Al-3Sn) which is reported to offer a yield strength/modulus ratio slightly greater than that of beta-titanium. Fiber-reinforced thermoplastic wires have also been studied. Candidate fibers include fiberglass and aramid. Candidate resins include polycarbonate and polyethylene terephthalate glycol. For each resin/fiber system, there is a heating or working range where the material can be formed without property degradation. This temperature range is primarily related to the glass transition temperature (T_g) of the resin matrix. A temperature above the T_g is necessary to allow sufficient softening. However higher temperatures will lead to structural changes and reduction in flexural modulus.

SUMMARY OF ORTHODONTIC WIRES

Properties of stainless steel, nickel-titanium, and beta-titanium wires in tension, bending, and torsion are compared in Table 16-4. Of the three types of wires, stainless steel wire has the highest values of yield strength, elastic modulus, and spring rate and the lowest springback (elastic deflection or yield strength/elastic modulus). Elgiloy is easily deformed and shaped.

Nickel-titanium alloy has the lowest elastic modulus and yield strength but the highest springback. Nickel-titanium has the lowest spring rate but highest resiliency in bending and torsion of the three alloys used for orthodontic wires. The disadvantages are that it is hard to bend and cannot be soldered, welded, or heat-treated. Beta-titanium offers an intermediate force delivery system and greater formability and weldability.

SOME OTHER ALLOYS

Certain alloys have considerable value for dental instruments and equipment because of their special properties. For example, Monel metal is an alloy of copper and nickel used for equipment parts because of its good physical properties and resistance to tarnish or corrosion. It has not been popular for constructing appliances placed in the mouth because of difficulties in manipulation. Such an alloy has a composition of approximately 28% copper, 68% nickel, 2% iron, 1.5% manganese, and 0.2% silicon.

Other stainless steels are also used, to lesser extents. A steel with 3% Al may be heat-treated and can be used in wrought condition. Following forming, heat treatment at 900° C for 1 hour leads to an increase in properties. The heat treatment forms coherent precipitate Ni_3Al, which strain-hardens the lattice.

An experimental Co-Cr alloy with addition of 4% to 6% Ti has been developed and reported to have better fatigue resistance than the Co-Cr alloy alone.

Another recently developed alloy is Zr-Pd-Ru with an intermetallic compound structure. This alloy undergoes transformation toughening and has good fracture toughness. The stress-induced microstructural changes are also hypothesized to provide good wear resistance. The 30Ni-30Cu-40Mn alloy is an experimental base-metal casting alloy. The hypothesized advantages of this alloy include a melting point of less than 1000° C and a resultant reduced tendency to absorb oxygen. The secondary alloying elements Al, In, and Sn further reduce the melting point, refine and reduce the dendritic microstructure, and increase hardness and casting accuracy. The secondary alloying elements also segregate to the intermetallic regions, leading to an increase in corrosion resistance.

The possibility of developing satisfactory substitutes for gold in dental appliances is far from being exhausted. Numerous new alloys are being developed for use by the engineering profession, some of which eventually may be found to be satisfactory for dental purposes. Many metals, such as tantalum, molybdenum, columbium, vanadium, and gallium, are becoming available in increasing quantities. These metals and their alloys, along with chromium, nickel, cobalt, titanium, stainless steel, and various copper, aluminum, or magnesium alloys, may be developed to possess physical and chemical qualities that satisfy the requirements of various dental applications.

SELECTED PROBLEMS

Problem 1

The elastic modulus values of nickel-chromium and cobalt-chromium alloys are about twice those of gold alloys, thus the thickness of a restoration in the direction of a bending force can be about halved and still have the same deflection. Is this a justifiable conclusion? (Defend your answer.)

Solution

No. Although a stress-strain curve in tension might lead you to respond affirmatively, it should be remembered that although the deflection of a beam is directly proportional to the modulus, it is inversely proportional to the cube of the thickness. As a result, halving the thickness of the nickel-chromium beam will dramatically increase the deflection as compared with that of the gold beam, even though it has twice the elastic modulus. It can be shown that only small decreases in thickness of the nickel-chromium beam can be made and yet maintain the same stiffness as the gold alloy beam.

Problem 2

During the soldering of a cobalt-chromium partial denture, the temperature of the torch became very high. What might be the expected effect on the properties of the cast framework?

Solution

Excessive heating of the framework will result in a decrease in the yield strength and the percent elongation. This can result from migration of atoms and formation of carbides, resulting in chromium depletion in the grains, which can cause increased corrosion.

Problem 3

Nickel-chromium alloys that can be cast into gypsum-bonded investments contain up to 2% beryllium to reduce the melting temperature. An alloy labeled as containing 77% nickel, 21% chromium, and 2% beryllium will contain 2 at% of Be. Is that statement correct? Defend your response.

Solution

No. The values listed are weight percentages. To obtain the atomic percent, you must first divide the weight percent of each element by the respective atomic number. These quotients are then added, and the atomic percentage calculated by dividing each quotient by the sum times 100. For example, 77 wt% Ni ÷ 59 = 1.305, 21 wt% Cr ÷ 52 = 0.404, and 2 wt% Be ÷ 9 = 0.222. The sum of the quotients is 1.931, and 0.222 ÷ 1.931 × 100 = 11.5 atomic % Be.

Problem 4

An austenitic 18-8 stainless steel orthodontic wire was bent and then heat-treated for 3 minutes, but was inadvertently heated to 816° C rather than the recommended 482° C. What effect would this have on the wire?

Solution

Substantial recrystallization and precipitation of trapped carbon atoms in the iron lattice of the wrought wire would occur, which would result in reduced stiffness and reduced resistance to permanent bending. The recommended heating to 482° C is to relieve stresses introduced during bending of the wire and is sufficiently low so that changes in stiffness and resistance to bending do not occur.

Problem 5

If you wished to select an orthodontic wire with the most constant force without reactivation as the tooth moved, would you select an 18-8 stainless steel, beta titanium, or nickel-titanium wire? Why?

Solution

Based on the bending and torsional moment versus deflection curves, a nickel-titanium wire should be chosen. This wire has the lowest spring rate for a given size but has the highest resiliency and the smallest decrease in force with movement of the tooth. Therefore longer times between activations and a more constant force result.

Problem 6

Endodontic stainless steel K files are used with a 90-degree clockwise rotation and withdrawal. If the tip of a file becomes bound in a root canal, why should care be taken not to rotate it much in the counterclockwise direction?

Solution

The files are twisted during construction so that if the tip is bound in a root canal, continued clockwise rotation will untwist the file, but counterclockwise rotation will twist the file tighter and possibly result in brittle rather than ductile fracture. As a result, these instruments fracture more readily in counterclockwise rotation, frequently in as little as a one-quarter turn.

Problem 7

Why can the carbon content of beryllium- or boron-containing nickel-chromium alloys be such a low value as 0.02% when 0.1% is needed in Ticonium and 0.5% in Vitallium?

Solution

Ticonium and Vitallium are used for partial-denture frameworks and require the high yield strength provided by the carbon content, while the beryllium- and boron-containing nickel-chromium alloys are used for the copings for porcelain-fused-to-metal restorations, where high yield strength is not as critical but some ductility is advantageous.

BIBLIOGRAPHY

Cast Base-Metal Alloys

Asgar K, Allan FC: Microstructure and physical properties of alloy for partial denture castings, *J Dent Res* 47:189, 1968.

Asgar K, Peyton FA: Effect of casting conditions on some mechanical properties of cobalt-base alloys, *J Dent Res* 40:73, 1961.

Asgar K, Peyton FA: Effect of microstructure on the physical properties of cobalt-based alloys, *J Dent Res* 40:63, 1961.

Asgar K, Peyton FA: Flow and fracture of dental alloys determined by a microbend tester, *J Dent Res* 41:142, 1962.

Asgar K, Techow BO, Jacobson JM: A new alloy for partial dentures, *J Prosthet Dent* 23:36, 1970.

Baran GR: The metallurgy of Ni-Cr alloys for fixed prosthodontics. *J Prosthet Dent* 50:639, 1983.

Bates JF: Studies related to the fracture of partial dentures, *Br Dent J* 118:532, 1965.

Bumgardner JD, Lucas LC: Surface analysis of nickel-chromium dental alloys, *Dent Mater* 9:252, 1993.

Ben-Ur Z, Patael H, Cardash HS et al: The fracture of cobalt-chromium alloy removable partial dentures, *Quint Internat* 17:797, 1986.

Bergman M, Bergman B, Soremark R: Tissue accumulation of nickel released due to electrochemical corrosion of non-precious dental casting alloys, *J Oral Rehabil* 7:325, 1980.

Brune D, Beltesbrekke H: Dust in dental laboratories: types and levels in specific operations, *J Prosthet Dent* 43:687, 1980.

Cecconi BT: Removable partial denture research and its clinical significance, *J Prosthet Dent* 39:203, 1978.

Cecconi BT, Asgar K, Dootz ER: Fit of the removable partial denture base and its effect on abutment tooth movement, *J Prosthet Dent* 25:515, 1971.

Cheng TP, Tsai WT, Chern Lin JH: The effect of beryllium on the corrosion resistance of nickel-chromium dental alloys, *J Mater Sci Mater Med,* 1:211, 1990.

Council on Dental Materials, Instruments, and Equipment: Report on base metal alloys for crown and bridge applications: benefits and risks, *J Am Dent Assoc* 111:479, 1985.

Cunningham DM: Comparison of base metal alloys and Type IV gold alloys for removable partial denture frameworks, *Dent Clin North Am* 17:719, 1973.

Frank RP, Brudvik JS, Nicholls JI: A comparison of the flexibility of wrought wire and cast circumferential clasps, *J Prosthet Dent* 49:471, 1983.

Geis-Gerstorfer J, Passler K: Studies of the influence of Be content on corrosion behaviour and mechanical properties of Ni25Cr10Mo alloys, *Dent Mater* 9:177, 1993.

Hinman RW, Lynde TA, Pelleu GB Jr et al: Factors affecting airborne beryllium concentrations in dental space, *J Prosthet Dent* 33:210, 1975.

Lucas LC, Lemons JE: Biodegradation of restorative metal systems, *Adv Dent Res* 65:32, 1992.

Mohammed H, Asgar K: A new dental super alloy system, I, II, III. *J Dent Res* 52:136, 145, 151, 1973.

Morris HF, Asgar K: Physical properties and microstructure of four new commercial partial denture alloys, *J Prosthet Dent* 33:36, 1975.

Morris HF, Asgar K, Rowe AP et al: The influence of heat treatments on several types of base-metal removable partial denture alloys, *J Prosthet Dent* 41:388, 1979.

Rowe AP, Bigelow WC, Asgar K: Effect of tantalum addition to a cobalt-chromium-nickel base alloy, *J Dent Res* 53:325, 1974.

Smith DC: Tissue reaction to noble and base metal alloys. In Smith DC, William DF, editors: *Biocompatibility of dental materials,* vol 4, Boca Raton, FL, 1982, CRC Press.

Strandman E: Influence of different types of acetylene-oxygen flames on the carbon content of dental Co-Cr alloy, *Odontol Revy* 27:223, 1976.

Vallittu PK, Kokkonen M: Deflection fatigue of cobalt-chromium, titanium, and gold alloy cast denture clasps, *J Prosthet Dent* 74:412, 1995.

Wakasa K, Yamaki M: Dental application of the 30Ni-30Cu-40Mn ternary alloy system, *J Mater Sci: Mater Med* 1:44, 1990.

Wakasa K, Yamaki M: Corrosive properties in experimental Ni-Cu-Mn based alloy systems for dental purposes, *J Mater Sci: Mater Med* 1:171, 1990.

Wakasa K, Yamaki M: Tensile behaviour in 30Ni-30Cu-30Mn based alloys for a dental application, *J Mater Sci: Mater Med* 2: 71, 1991.

Wataha JC, Craig RG, Hanks CT: The release of elements of dental casting alloys into cell-culture medium, *J Dent Res* 70:1014, 1991.

Wataha JC, Craig RG, Hanks CT: The effects of cleaning on the kinetics of in vitro metal release from dental casting alloys, *J Dent Res* 71:1417, 1992.

Waterstrat RM: New alloys, *J Am Dent Assoc* 123:33, 1992.

Yong T, De Long B, Goodkind RJ et al: Leaching of Ni, Cr and Be ions from base metal alloys in an artificial oral environment, *J Prosthet Dent* 68:692, 1992.

Wrought Base-Metal Alloys

Andreasen GF, Barrett RD: An evaluation of cobalt-substituted Nitinol wire in orthodontics, *Am J Orthod* 63:462, 1973.

Andreasen GF, Brady PR: A use hypothesis for 55 Nitinol wire for orthodontics, *Angle Orthod* 42:172, 1972.

Andreasen GF, Morrow RE: Laboratory and clinical analyses of Nitinol wire, *Am J Orthod* 73:142, 1978.

Andreasen GF, Bigelow H, Andrews JG: 55 Nitinol wire: force developed as a function of 'elastic memory,' *Aust Dent J* 24:146, 1979.

Braff MH: A comparison between stainless steel crowns and multisurface amalgams in primary molars, *J Dent Child* 46:474, Nov-Dec 1975.

Brantley WA, Augat WS, Myers CL et al: Bending deformation studies of orthodontic wires, *J Dent Res* 57:609, 1978.

Burstone CJ, Goldberg AJ: Beta titanium: a new orthodontic alloy, *Am J Orthod* 77:121, 1980.

Chen R, Zhi YF, Arvy Stas MG: Advanced Chinese NiTi alloy wire and clinical observations, *Angle Orthod* 62:15, 1992.

Council on Dental Materials, Instruments, and Equipment: New American Dental Association Specification No 32 for orthodontic wires not containing precious metals, *J Am Dent Assoc* 95:1169, 1977.

Council on Dental Materials, Instruments, and Equipment: Status report on beta titanium orthodontic wires, *J Am Dent Assoc* 105:684, 1982.

Dolan DW, Craig RG: Bending and torsion of endodontic files with rhombus cross sections, *J Endodont* 8:260, 1982.

Drake SR, Wayne DM, Powers JM et al: Mechanical properties of orthodontic wires in tension, bending, and torsion, *Am J Orthod* 82:206, 1982.

Goldberg J, Burstone CJ: An evaluation of beta titanium alloys for use in orthodontic appliances, *J Dent Res* 58:593, 1979.

Goldberg AJ, Burstone CJ, Hadjinikolaoa I et al: Screening of matrices and fibers for reinforced thermoplastics intended for dental applications, *J Biomed Mater Res* 28:167, 1994.

Haïkel Y, Serfaty R, Bateman G et al: Dynamic and cyclic fatigue of engine-driven rotary nickel-titanium endodontic instruments, *J Endodont* 25:434, 1999.

Kapila S, Sachdeva R: Mechanical properties and clinical applications of orthodontic wires, *Am J Orthod Dentofac Orthop* 96:100, 1989.

Kusy RP: Comparison of nickel-titanium and beta titanium wire sizes to conventional orthodontic arch wire materials, *Am J Orthod* 79:625, 1981.

Neal RG, Craig RG, Powers JM: Cutting ability of K-type endodontic files, *J Endodont* 9:52, 1983.

Neal RG, Craig RG, Powers JM: Effect of sterilization and irrigants on the cutting ability of stainless steel files, *J Endodont* 9:93, 1983.

Newman JG, Brantley WA, Gorstein H: A study of the cutting efficiency of seven brands of endodontic files in linear motion, *J Endodont* 9:316, 1983.

Parmiter OK: Wrought stainless steels. In *ASM metals handbook,* Cleveland, 1948, American Society for Metals.

Patel AP, Goldberg AJ, Burstone CJ: The effect of thermoforming on the properties of fiber-reinfroced composite wires, *J Appl Biomat* 3:177, 1992.

Peterson DS, Jubach TS, Katora M: Scanning electron microscope study of stainless steel crown margins, *ASDC J Dent Child* 45:376, Sept-Oct 1978.

Schwaninger B, Sarkar NK, Foster BE: Effect of long-term immersion corrosion on the flexural properties of Nitinol, *Am J Orthod* 82:45, 1982.

Shastry CV, Goldberg AJ: The influence of drawing parameters on the mechanical properties of two beta-titanium alloys, *J Dent Res* 62:1092, 1983.

Stokes OW, Fiore PM, Barss JT et al: Corrosion in stainless-steel and nickel-titanium files, *J Endodont* 25:17, 1999.

Thompson SA: An overview of nickel-titanium alloys used in dentistry, *Internat Endodont J* 33: 297, 2000.

Waters NE: Superelastic nickel-titanium wires, *Br J Orthod* 19:319, 1992.

Wilkinson JV: Some metallurgical aspects of orthodontic stainless steel, *Am J Orthod* 48:192, 1962.

Wilson DF, Goldberg AJ: Alternative beta-titanium alloys for orthodontic wires, *Dent Mater* 3:337, 1987.

Yoneyama T, Doi H: Superelasticity and thermal behaviour of NiTi orthodontic archwires, *Dent Mater* 11:1, 1992.

Titanium

Ducheyne P, Kohn D, Smith TS: Fatigue properties of cast and heat treated Ti-6Al-4V alloy for anatomic hip prostheses, *Biomater* 8:223, 1987.

Ida K, Togaya T, Tsutsumi S et al: Effect of magnesia investments on the dental casting of pure titanium or titanium alloys, *Dent Mater J* 1:8, 1982.

Ida K, Tani Y, Tsutsumi S et al: Clinical applications of pure titanium crowns, *Dent Mater J* 4:191, 1985.

Kimura H, Izumi O, editors: *Titanium '80 science and technology,* Warrendale, Penn, 1980, The Metallurgical Society of AIME.

Kohn DH, Ducheyne P: A parametric study of the factors affecting the fatigue strength of porous coated Ti-6Al-4V implant alloy, *J Biomed Mater Res* 24:1483, 1990.

Kohn DH, Ducheyne P: Microstructural refinement of beta-sintered and porous coated Ti-6Al-4V by temporary alloying with hydrogen, *J Mater Sci* 26:534, 1991.

Kohn DH, Ducheyne P: Tensile and fatigue strength of hydrogen treated Ti-6Al-4V alloy, *J Mater Sci* 26:328, 1991.

Lutjering G, Gysler A: Critical review-fatigue. In Lutjering G, Zwicker U, Bunk W, editors: *Titanium, science and technology,* Oferursel, West Germany, 1985, Deutsche Gesellschaft Fur Metallkunde.

Margolin H, Williams JC, Chesnutt JC et al: A review of the fracture and fatigue behavior of Ti alloys. In Moser JB, Lin JHC, Taira M et al: Development of dental Pd-Ti alloys, *Dent Mater* 1:37, 1985.

Okabe T, Hero H: The use of titanium in dentistry, *Cells and Mater* 5:211, 1995.

Peters M, Gysler A, Lutjering G: Influence of microstructure on the fatigue behavior of Ti-6Al-4V. In Kimura H, Izumi O, editors: *Titanium '80 science and technology,* Warrendale, Penn, 1980, The Metallurgical Society of AIME.

Szurgot KC, Marker BC, Moser JB et al: The casting of titanium for removable partial dentures, *Dent Mater Sci* QDT Yearbook: 171, 1988.

Taira M, Moser JB, Greener EH: Studies of Ti alloys for dental castings, *Dent Mater* 5:45, 1989.

Voitik AJ: Titanium dental castings, cold worked titanium restorations—yes or no? *Trends and Techniques* 8(10):23, Dec, 1991.

Waterstrat RM: Comments on casting of Ti-13Cu-4.5Ni alloy, Pub No (NIH) 77-1227, DHEW, p 224, 1977.

Yamauchi M, Sakai M, Kawano J: Clinical application of pure titanium for cast plate dentures, *Dent Mater* J 7:39, 1988.

Implants

Adell R, Lekholm U, Rockler B et al: A 15-year study of osseointegrated implants in the treatment of the edentulous jaw, *Int J Oral Surg* 10:387, 1981.

Albrektsson T, Brånemark PI, Hansson HA et al: The interface zone of inorganic implants in vivo: titanium implants in bone, *Ann Biomed Engr* 11:1, 1983.

Brånemark PI, Zarb GA, Albrektsson T: *Tissue-integrated prostheses—osseointegration in clinical dentistry,* Chicago, 1987, Quintessence.

Brånemark PI, Hansson BO, Adell R et al: Osseointegrated implants in the treatment of the edentulous jaw: experience from a 10-year period, *Scand J Plast Reconstr Surg* 11(suppl 16):1-132, 1977.

Brunski JB, Hipp JA: In vivo forces on endosteal implants: a measurement system and biomechanical considerations, *J Prosthet Dent* 51:82, 1984.

Brunski JB, Moccia AF, Pollack SR et al: The influence of functional use of endosseous dental implants on the tissue-implant interface. I. Histological aspects, *J Dent Res* 58:1953, 1979.

Cook SD, Thomas KA, Kay JF et al: Hydroxyapatite-coated porous titanium for use as an orthopedic biologic attachment system, *Clin Orthop* 230:303, 1988.

Deporter DA, Friedland B, Watson PA et al: A clinical and radiographic assessment of a porous-surfaced, titanium alloy dental implant system in dogs, *J Dent Res* 65:1071, 1986.

Ducheyne P: Bioceramics: material characteristics versus in vivo behavior, *J Biomed Mater Res; Appl Biomater* 21(suppl A2):219, Aug 1987.

Ducheyne P, Hench LL, Kagan A et al: The effect of hydroxyapatite impregnation on skeletal bonding of porous coated implants, *J Biomed Mater Res* 14:225, 1980.

Healy KE, Ducheyne P: The mechanisms of passive dissolution of titanium in a model physiological environment, *J Biomed Mater Res* 26:319, 1992.

Hench LL, Ethridge EC: *Biomaterials: an interfacial approach,* New York, 1982, Academic Press.

Hench LL, Splinter RJ, Allen WC et al: Bonding mechanisms at the interface of ceramic prosthetic materials, *J Biomed Mater Res Symp* 2:117, 1972.

Kasemo B: Biocompatibility of titanium implants: surface science aspects, *J Prosthet Dent* 49:832, 1983.

Koeneman J, Lemons J, Ducheyne P et al: Workshop on characterization of calcium phosphate materials, *J Appl Biomater* 1:79, 1990.

Kohn DH: Overview of factors important in implant design, *J Oral Implantol* 18:204, 1992.

Kohn DH: Structure-property relations of biomaterials for hard tissue replacement, in Wise DL, editor, *Encyclopedia of biomaterials and bioengineering,* Matawan, NJ, 83, 1995, Marcel Dekker.

Lemons JE: Dental implant retrieval analyses, *J Dent Ed* 52:748, 1988.

Luthy H, Strub JR, Scharer P: Analysis of plasma flame-sprayed coatings on endosseous oral titanium implants exfoliated in man: preliminary results, *Int J Oral Maxillofac Imp* 2:197, 1987.

Maniatopoulos C, Pilliar RM, Smith DC: Threaded versus porous-surfaced designs for implant stabilization in bone-endodontic implant model, *J Biomed Mater Res* 20:1309, 1986.

National Institutes of Health Consensus Development Conference Statement on Dental Implants, June 13-15, 1988, *J Dent Ed* 52:824, 1988.

Schnitman PA, Schulman LB: Dental implants: benefit and risk. In US Department Health and Human Services, publication no 81-1531, 1980.

Chapter 17

Casting and Soldering Procedures

Casting is the process by which a wax pattern of a restoration is converted to a replicate in a dental alloy. The casting process is used to make dental restorations such as inlays, onlays, crowns, bridges, and removable partial dentures. Because castings must meet stringent dimensional requirements, the casting process is extremely demanding. In dentistry, virtually all casting is done using some form or adaptation of the lost-wax technique. The lost-wax technique has been used for centuries, but its use in dentistry was not common until 1907, when W.H. Taggart introduced his technique with the casting machine.

Soldering is a method of joining two or more cast or wrought pieces using another alloy called a *solder*. Like casting, soldering in dentistry must ensure that the dimensions of soldered pieces are maintained to a high degree of accuracy. Casting and soldering techniques use many of the same laboratory equipment and materials.

This chapter will discuss casting and soldering techniques. These techniques use several materials that are discussed in detail in other chapters. Alloys for casting have been previously discussed in Chapters 15 and 16. Die materials and investments are discussed in Chapter 13, and waxes in Chapter 14. This chapter will focus on techniques used to work with these materials, beginning with an overview of the lost-wax casting process, then reviewing each step in this process: waxing, spruing, investing, burnout, and casting. Finally, some general considerations for dental soldering will be presented. The techniques of casting and soldering are complex and vary considerably for different alloy types, and this chapter is not intended to be a comprehensive discussion of these techniques. For further details, the reader is referred to books on casting and soldering techniques in the dental and metallurgical literature.

CASTING

LOST-WAX TECHNIQUE

The *lost-wax technique* is so named because a wax pattern of a restoration is invested in a ceramic material, then the pattern is burned out ("lost") to create a space into which molten metal is placed or cast. The entire lost-wax casting process is diagrammed in Fig. 17-1. A wax pattern is first formed on a die of the tooth to be restored or, occasionally, directly on the tooth. All aspects of the final restoration are incorporated into the wax pattern, including the occlusion, proximal contacts, and marginal fit. Once the wax pattern is completed, a sprue is attached, which serves as a channel for the molten metal to pass from the crucible into the restoration. Next, the pattern and sprue are invested in a ceramic material, and the invested pattern is heated until all remnants of the wax are burned away. After burnout, molten metal is cast into the void created by the wax pattern and sprue. Once the investment is broken away, the rough casting is pickled to removed oxides. Finally, the sprue is removed and the casting is polished and delivered to the patient. If all steps have been done well, the final restoration will require minimal modification during cementation into the patient's mouth.

Dimensional Changes in the Lost-Wax Technique If materials used during the casting process didn't shrink or expand, the size of the final cast restoration would be the same as the original wax pattern. However, dimensional changes occur in most of the steps in Fig. 17-1 and, in practice, the final restoration may not be exactly the same size as the pattern. The management of these dimensional changes is complex, but can be summarized by the equation:

$$\text{wax shrinkage} + \text{metal shrinkage} = \text{wax expansion} + \text{setting expansion} + \text{hygroscopic expansion} + \text{thermal expansion}$$

This equation balances the shrinkage *(left side of equation)* against the expansion *(right side of equation)* that occurs during the casting process. If the final restoration is to fit the die, the shrinkage and expansion during the casting process must be equal.

Shrinkage forces in the casting process come from two sources: wax and metal. Although the die restricts the wax from shrinking to a large degree while the pattern is on the die, residual

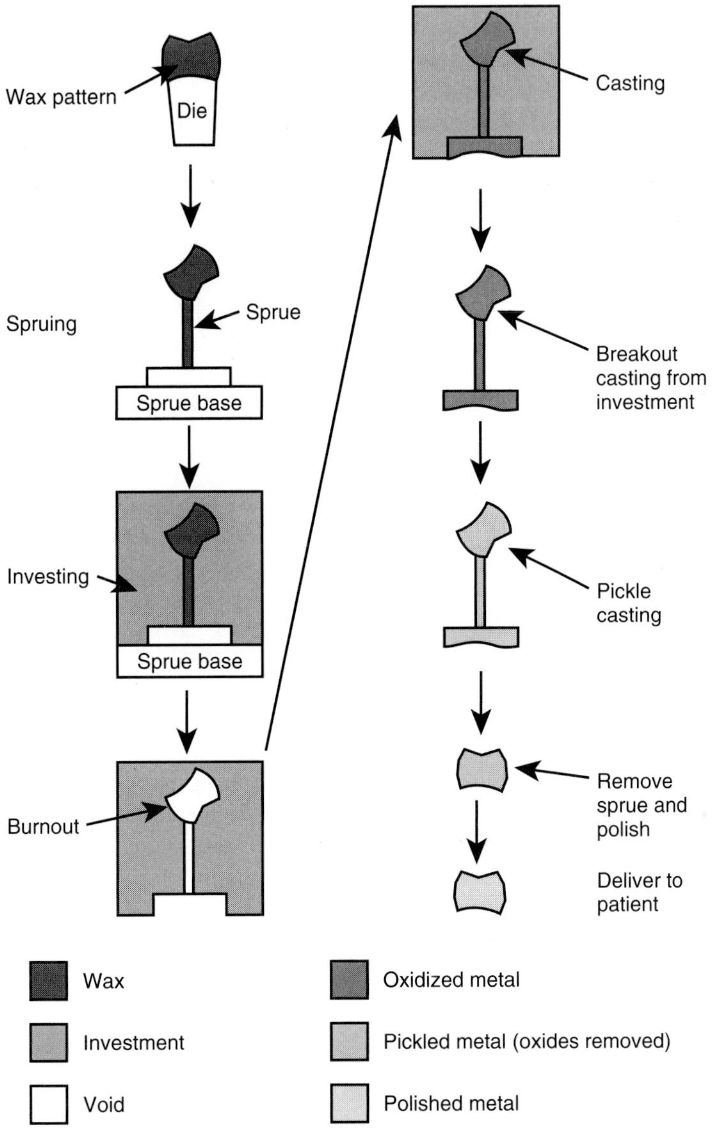

Fig. 17-1 The lost-wax casting process. A wax pattern of the final restoration is made on a die (a replicate of the prepared tooth). A sprue is attached, and the wax pattern is removed from the die and attached to a sprue base and casting ring. The sprue and pattern are invested and the sprue base is removed. The casting ring is placed in an oven to burn out the wax (hence, the term *lost wax*). Metal is melted and cast into the void in the investment created by the wax pattern. After the metal has solidified, the investment is removed and the casting pickled to remove oxides. Finally, the sprue is removed and the casting is polished, cleaned, and delivered to the patient. Note the angles on the sprue base should be rounded.

stresses may be incorporated into the pattern and released during investing, when the pattern is removed from the die. Furthermore, if the investing is done at a temperature lower than that at which the wax pattern was formed, the wax will shrink significantly because of the high coefficient of thermal expansion of waxes (see Chapter 14). Metal shrinkage occurs when the molten metal solidifies, but this shrinkage is normally compensated by introducing more metal as the casting solidifies. However, once the entire casting has reached the solidus temperature of the alloy, shrinkage will occur as the casting cools to room temperature. As for wax, the metallic shrinkage that occurs below the solidus is caused by the coefficient of thermal expansion for the alloy. Cooling shrinkage may reach 2.5% for an alloy that cools from a high solidus temperature (1300° to 1400° C), depending on the coefficient of thermal expansion of the alloy. A typical shrinkage range for most alloys is 1.25% to 2.5%. Furthermore, because the casting is solid at this point, the only possible compensation mechanism is to start with a void space that is 1.25% to 2.5% too large. Thus, shrinkage of wax and metal must be compensated with expansion in the investment if the casting is to have the appropriate dimensions. Fig. 17-2 shows a casting that was too small because of inadequate compensation of the solidification shrinkage of the alloy.

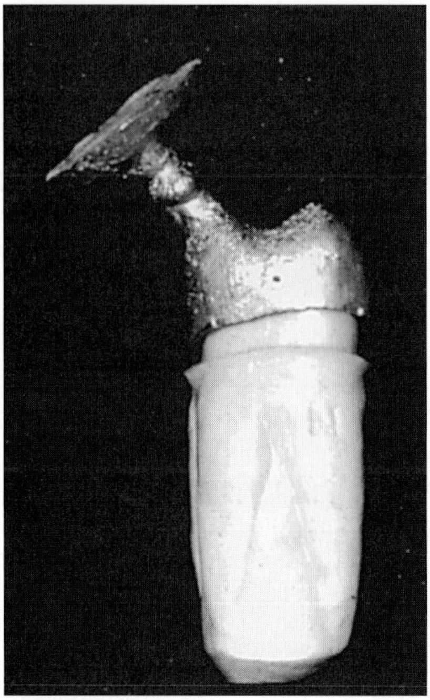

Fig. 17-2 A picture of a casting that is too small and will not seat on the tooth because there was inadequate compensation of solidification shrinkage of the alloy. As the picture shows, the degree of misfit can be substantial.

(Courtesy Dr. Carl W. Fairhurst, Medical College of Georgia School of Dentistry.)

Sources for expansion of the investment are listed in the equation previously presented and come from two sources: expansion of the wax pattern or expansion of the investment itself. Investment expansion may be setting, hygroscopic, or thermal; these phenomena are discussed in detail in Chapter 13. The relative contributions of these three expansions are not important as long as the total expansion is sufficient to balance the shrinkage of metal previously discussed. Expansion of the wax pattern before investing is theoretically possible, but impractical because of the release of residual stresses that distort the pattern (see Chapter 14). Thus, in the shrinkage-expansion equation, the primary shrinkage comes from cooling of the solidified casting, and this shrinkage must be compensated by an appropriate total expansion of the investment.

Accuracy of the Lost-Wax Technique

A casting should be as accurate as possible, although a tolerance of ±0.05% for an inlay casting is acceptable. If the linear dimension of an average dental inlay casting is assumed to be 4 mm, ±0.05% of this value is equal to only ±2 μm, which suggests that if two castings made for the same tooth have a variation of 4 μm, the difference may not be noticeable. To visualize this dimension, recall that the thickness of an average human hair is about 40 μm. Therefore the tolerance limits of a dental casting are approximately one-tenth the thickness of a human hair. To obtain castings with such small tolerance limits, rigid requirements must be placed not only on the investment material but also on the impression materials, waxes, and die materials. Naturally, technical procedures and the proper handling of these materials are equally important. The values for the setting, hygroscopic, and thermal expansions of investment materials may vary from one product to another, and slightly different techniques may be used with different investments. In each case, the values obtained for any one property should be reproducible from one batch to another and from one casting to another.

FORMATION OF THE WAX PATTERN

The fabrication of a restoration in wax is convenient because it involves few materials and is inexpensive, fast, reversible, and customizable. However, the properties of wax, such as its high coefficient of thermal expansion and tendency to flow and harbor residual stresses, must be kept in mind. These properties are reviewed in detail in Chapter 14. Failure to accommodate for these properties will result in inaccurate castings. There are two fundamental ways to prepare a wax pattern for a dental restoration. In the direct method, the pattern is prepared on the tooth in the mouth. This method can only be used for small inlay restorations. In the indirect method, a model (die) of the tooth is first made, and the pattern is made on the die. The indirect method is used for all types of restorations. Each of these techniques will be discussed at length.

Direct Wax Patterns As mentioned in Chapter 14, the wax for a direct wax pattern must be heated sufficiently to have adequate flow and plasticity under compression to reproduce all details of the cavity walls. Adequate compression of the wax is required in forming direct wax patterns. Also, overheating of the wax should be avoided because of possible tissue damage and discomfort to the patient, as well as the difficulty encountered in compression of very fluid wax when it is overheated.

When wax is heated to the proper working temperature of approximately 50° to 52° C for a short period, the previously induced stress from manufacturing and handling tends to be dissipated. A stress-free piece of wax at the proper consistency should be obtained so that the pattern, when formed under pressure, remains relatively stress free. Thus minimal distortion results when the pattern is subsequently removed from the tooth. This heating and annealing of the wax before insertion into the cavity preparation is accomplished most easily and effectively in a small dry-heat oven. A nonuniform consistency and possible volatilization of some of the wax mass tends to result form excessively heating the wax over a Bunsen burner flame. Although wax may be annealed in water that is at a proper temperature, it should not be stored for long periods under these conditions. Prolonged heating of the wax in water, especially at high temperatures, may result in a crumbly mass.

Because wax has a rather low thermal conductivity, cooling from the working temperature to mouth temperature occurs slowly, and ample time for cooling should be allowed. The decrease in temperature of the wax to mouth temperature results in a contraction. This contraction is offset to some degree when the pattern is held under pressure until mouth temperature is reached, because the compression stresses tend to be released, to some degree, when the wax is removed from the prepared tooth. However, the degree and distribution of these stresses vary from one pattern to another. Although these induced stresses are undesirable, their presence is unavoidable.

Because carving a wax pattern directly in the mouth demands a high degree of dexterity, any property that makes manipulation easier is desirable. Therefore ANSI/ADA Specification No. 4 (ISO 1561) for inlay wax states that the wax color should contrast with the hard and soft tissues of the mouth; the wax should soften without becoming flaky; and the wax should not show appreciable chipping or flaking when trimmed to a fine margin. Carving instruments that have been sufficiently warmed are desirable to soften, but not melt, the wax as the marginal adaptation and contour are developed. The warm instrument brings the portion of the wax that is being manipulated to its proper working temperature, so that less stress is induced in these areas. A cool carving instrument burnishing over or cutting through the wax introduces tensile and compressive stresses into the pattern, which are detrimental to the ultimate fit of the casting.

Indirect Wax Patterns When a wax pattern is formed by the indirect method, a metal or stone die is used, which is the positive replica of the prepared tooth and at least some of its surrounding structure. This tooth replica permits the pattern to be formed outside the mouth. Forming the wax pattern on a die permits a change in the type of wax and certain manipulative procedures that are necessary for the direct technique. The convenience provided by the indirect method makes the property of wax flow less critical, because the pattern may be removed from the die at a lower temperature and with greater ease.

Some laboratories will coat the die with a die spacer on stone dies to allow space for the cement in the final restoration. The spacer is brushed onto the die as a viscous liquid, then allowed to dry before applying wax lubricant and wax. The thickness of the spacer, which can be difficult to control, ranges from 10 to 30 μm and is a function of the manipulative technique. Die spacers should not be used to compensate for improper manipulation of the other materials in the casting process, nor should they be used on the margins of the restoration.

When adapting wax to stone or some metal dies, some form of lubricant must be used to release the wax pattern from the die. In the mouth no such lubricant is required because a thin film of saliva or dentinal fluid serves as a lubricant. A variety of fluids is currently available to prevent the attachment of the wax to the die. These fluids produce a separator film of minimum thickness. An excess of separator is to be avoided because it leads to inaccuracies in the wax pattern and a poor surface of the cast alloy.

The wax may be adapted to the die either by flowing small melted increments from a spatula to build up the desired contour or by the compression method, as is suggested in the direct technique. By either method the temperature of a stone die is of little concern in wax adaptation because the stone is a poor thermal conductor. Likewise, the temperature of a metal die is not critical when compression of the wax is used to form the pattern. However, this temperature is critical when molten increments are used to build up the pattern because the manner of solidification of the wax depends on the temperature of the metal die.

When molten wax flows onto a cool metal die, the wax immediately adjacent to the die solidifies rapidly because the heat from the molten wax is rapidly dissipated. The wax adjacent to the air stays molten for a period; as it solidifies and contracts, it pulls the previously congealed wax away from the metal, as shown in Fig. 17-3, *A*. Conversely, if the metal die is warmed throughout to near body temperature, the wax solidifies more evenly throughout its mass, resulting in better adaptation, as shown in 17-3, *B*. The die can be warmed by placing it under an electric lamp or with the carving instruments on an elec-

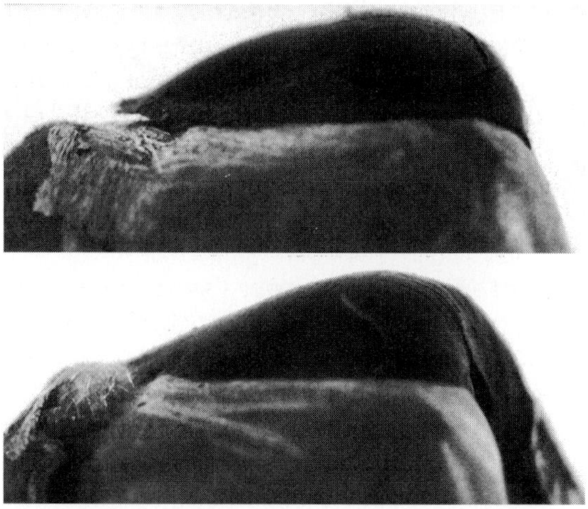

A

B

Fig. 17-3 Improper manipulation of the wax pattern can cause the pattern to distort significantly. **A,** The wax was cooled too quickly and residual stresses have been released, causing the pattern to pull away from the die. **B,** A proper cooling rate and manipulation results in a pattern that remains adapted to the die.

tric heating pad at a suitable temperature. The indirect wax pattern is carved with a warm instrument, as is the direct pattern, again to minimize the formation of stresses in the wax.

Because of the basic physical nature of wax, distortion of the pattern is a continual hazard. Not only does wax have one of the highest coefficients of thermal expansion of any dental material, it also possesses a relatively low softening temperature, which may cause stress release or flow to occur. Stresses are easily induced in forming any pattern; in fact, the formation of a completely stress-free wax pattern would appear improbable. However, with knowledge of the physical characteristics of the wax, an operator can minimize the stresses in the pattern by applying the appropriate manipulative procedures.

SPRUING THE WAX PATTERN

The purpose of the sprue is to provide a conduit for the molten metal to reach the void formed by the wax pattern after burnout. Proper spruing technique and sprue design is critical to the successful casting of the restoration. Before spruing, the wax pattern is generally briefly removed from the die. After the die is cleaned and relubricated, the pattern is replaced on the die and the margins of the restoration are finalized. The type, number, location of attachment, diameter, length, and direction of the sprues are all important to the success of the casting.

Several types of materials are used for sprues, depending on the type of restoration being cast. For small inlays, a hollow-metal sprue may be used. The metal is stronger than a comparably sized wax sprue. The core of the hollow pin should be filled with sticky wax to preclude sucking of the pattern wax into the sprue when attaching the sprue to the pattern. Of course, the metallic sprue cannot be burned out, but must be carefully removed after investing of the pattern. Round wax is a commonly used sprue material for many restorations of all sizes. Wax has the advantages of being inexpensive, easy to manipulate, easy to burn out, and available in a variety of diameters. Wax sprues can also be easily designed for complex castings that require multiple sprues and vents. Plastic sprues have also been used for casting. Plastic has the rigidity of metal, an advantage, but can still be burned out, although longer burnout times may be required than with wax.

For most common crowns and inlays, a single sprue is sufficient. However, bridges and removable partial dentures may require multiple sprues in a complex configuration (Fig. 17-4). Sprues of small diameter may also be attached to the pattern to act as vents to enhance the displacement of gases from the mold during the entry of the molten metal. Two sprues in the configuration of a "Y" may also be used on some relatively small restorations to prevent warpage of the wax pattern susceptible to distortion. The Y-sprue design is often used on MOD inlay restorations.

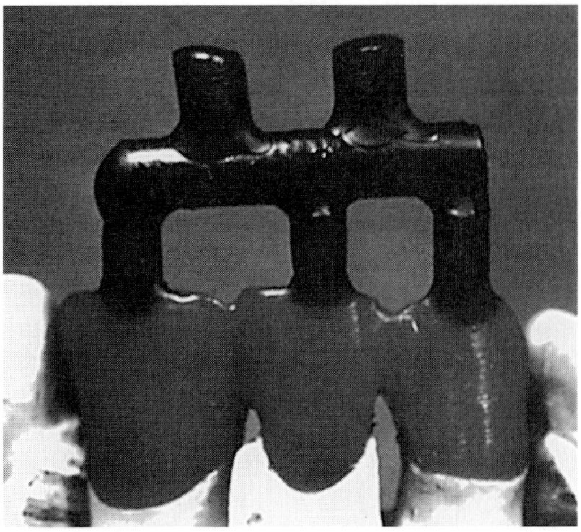

Fig. 17-4 Picture of a complex sprue design for a 3-unit fixed partial denture. The restoration is on the bottom (lighter colored wax). Each unit has a sprue feeding to it from a horizontal feeder bar. Two large-diameter sprues feed into the feeder bar; to encourage turbulence of the molten metal, they are purposely not aligned with the unit sprues. The use of complex arrangements such as this ensures that the molten metal will cause the sprue bar area to become hotter and freeze last. Note that the attachments of the sprues to the individual units are broad and flared. (Courtesy Carl W. Fairhurst, Medical College of Georgia School of Dentistry.)

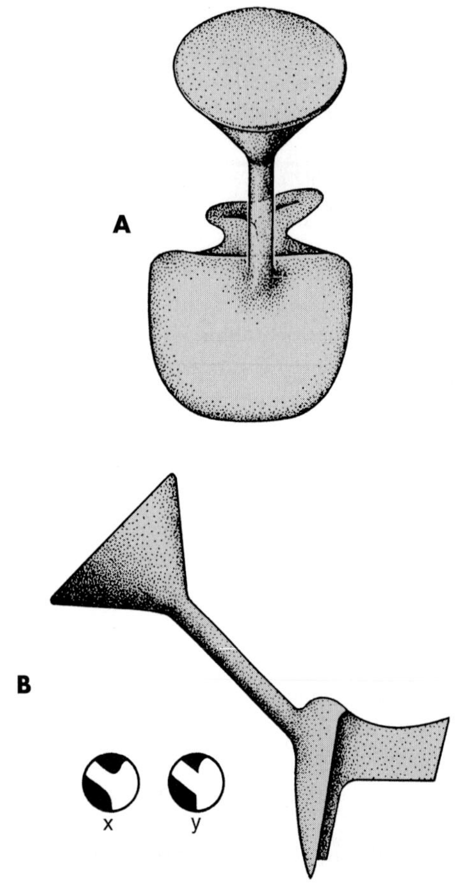

Fig. 17-5 Diagram showing the position and area of attachment of a single sprue to a small inlay restoration pattern. The location **(A),** diameter, length, and angle of the sprue **(B)** are critical to preserving the proper freezing order during casting. Furthermore, the attachment of the sprue to the restoration is critical. In *x*, the sprue is attached with rounded corners to avoid turbulence and the risk of investment fracture. In *y*, the sharp corners of attachment are not desirable.

The location of the sprue attachment to the wax pattern is paramount for proper casting. In general, the sprue should be attached to the bulkiest portion of the wax pattern, as shown in Fig. 17-5. Placing the sprue away from the fine margins minimizes distortion of this delicate area of the pattern. When attaching the sprue, the point of contact should be flared, as shown in insert *x* of Fig. 17-5, *B*. This allows more-even flow of the metal into the mold and less porosity in the casting at the point of contact. In addition, not flaring the sprue connections, as shown in insert *y*, results in the formation of sharp projections of investment that can break off and incorporate into the metal during casting. The direction of the sprue is another factor to consider. In general, the sprue should be directed toward the margins such that it minimizes the turbulence of the flow of the molten metal and favors the fine margins of the wax pattern. Finally, the point of attachment of the sprue should be selected, keeping in mind that the contour of the restoration will be altered by the sprue's presence. Although the contour can be restored once the casting is complete, such recontouring is often much more difficult in metal.

The diameter of the sprue, in conjunction with the pressure of the casting machine and density of the molten metal, controls the rate of flow of the molten metal into the mold cavity. The larger the diameter of the sprue and the higher the density of the molten metal, the faster the molten metal should enter the mold cavity. However, the mold cavity is filled with various gases before the entry of the molten metal, and the mold cavity cannot be filled completely unless all gases are driven out through the pores of the investment. As mentioned in Chapter 13, a requirement of dental investments is that they be sufficiently porous to allow gases to escape. Thus not only do the sprue diameter and pressure of the casting machine have an effect on the rate of filling the mold cavity, but the rate of elimination of gases from the mold cavity also has an effect. Incomplete castings may result from using a sprue with a diameter that is too small. In this case, the molten metal may solidify in the sprue area before completely filling the mold cavity. The proper sprue diameter for dental castings, depending on the size of the wax pattern, may vary between 6 and 12 gauge (4.1 and 2.0 mm, respectively). Theoretically, the diameter of the sprue should be larger than the thickest part of the wax pattern; however, practically it could be slightly smaller.

The length of the sprue is also important to ensure a good casting. The wax pattern should be positioned approximately 6 mm from the end

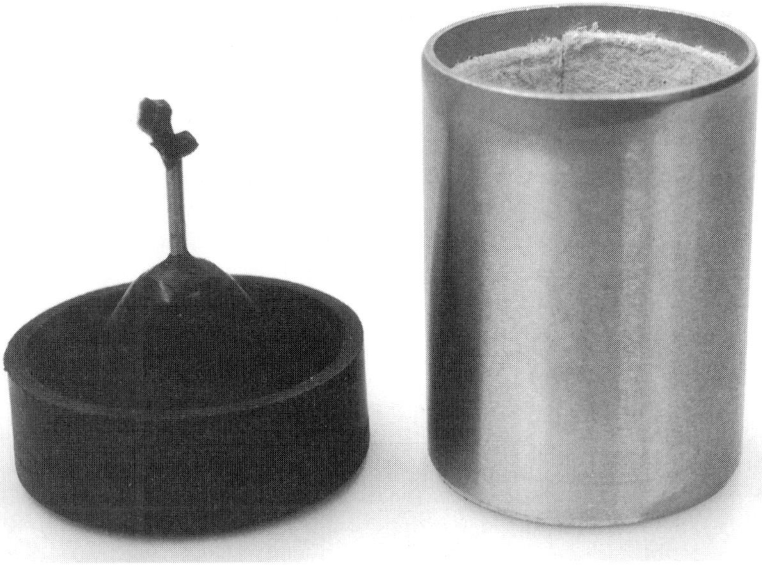

Fig. 17-6 Picture of an inlay restoration on a single sprue pin *(left)*. The single sprue pin is attached to the sprue base. Next, the casting ring lined with a ceramic paper *(right)* will be placed onto the sprue base and the pattern will be invested. Once the investment has set, the metallic sprue pin will be removed before burnout of the pattern.

of the casting ring (Fig. 17-6). This position provides sufficient thickness of investment to contain the molten metal and reduces the amount of investment through which gases must escape. Positioning the pattern close to the surface also ensures that the casting cools more rapidly than the more centrally located sprue. When this is done, the metal in the sprue remains liquid and flows to the casting until the casting is completely solidified.

Once the sprue is attached to the restoration, the other end of the sprue is attached to a sprue base usually made of hard rubber (see Fig. 17-6). As with the attachment of the sprue to the restoration, the base-sprue attachment should avoid sharp corners to ensure smooth, nonturbulent flow of the metal into the pattern during casting. Sharp corners may also encourage fracture of pieces of the investment during casting, sending these pieces of investment into the mold and possibly the restoration. Once the pattern has been completely sprued on the base, it is ready for investing.

INVESTING THE WAX PATTERN

Investing is the process by which the sprued wax pattern is embedded in a material called an *investment*. The investment must be able to withstand the heat and forces of casting, yet must conform to the pattern in a way such that the size and surface detail are exactly reproduced. In dentistry, gypsum- and phosphate-bonded investment materials are the two types of materials used for this purpose; details about the composition, setting reaction, and expansion properties of these materials are covered in Chapter 13. After spruing, the pattern appears as shown in Fig. 17-6 *(left)*. A casting ring is added to contain the investment while the investment material is poured carefully around the pattern.

For the setting and hygroscopic expansion of an investment to take place more uniformly, some allowance must be made for the lateral expansion of the investment. Solid rings do not permit the investment to expand laterally during the setting and hygroscopic expansions of the mold. To overcome this lateral restriction, a ceramic paper liner is placed inside the ring. A drawing of the sprue base, wax patter, inlay ring, and liner in position is shown in Fig. 17-7. The ceramic paper liner is cut to fit the inside of the metal ring and is held in place with the finger. The ring containing the liner is then dipped into water until the liner is completely wet and water is dripping from it. The ring is shaken gently to remove the excess water. After the liner has been soaked, it should not be touched or adapted further with a finger because this reduces its cushioning effect, which is needed for the lateral expansion of the investment. A liner that is about 3 mm short at each end of the ring is preferred. When the liner is equally short at each end of the ring, the investment is locked into the ring, and uniform expansion of the cavity form occurs.

During investing, the water-based gypsum material must flow around the pattern and capture every surface detail. However, the wax surfaces generally are not easily wetted by water. The surface of a wax pattern that is not completely wetted with investment results in surface irregularities in the casting that destroy its accuracy. These irregularities can be minimized by applying a surface-active wetting agent on the wax. The function of the wetting agent is to reduce the contact angle of a liquid with the wax surface. Wetting agents also remove any oily film that is left on the wax pattern from the separating medium. The spreading of water is illustrated by the comparison in Fig. 17-8, which show silhouettes of advancing water droplets on a polished inlay wax surface, *A,* and on the same surface treated with the surface-active agent before the water droplet was applied, *B.* In *B,* the agent was applied and blotted dry with lens paper. The contact angles are 98° for the plain wax surface and 61° for the treated wax surface. The lower contact angle indicates that the treated wax surface has an affinity for water, which results in the investment being able to spread more easily over the wax. Because the surface-active agents are quite soluble, rinsing the wax pattern with water after the application defeats the purpose of their

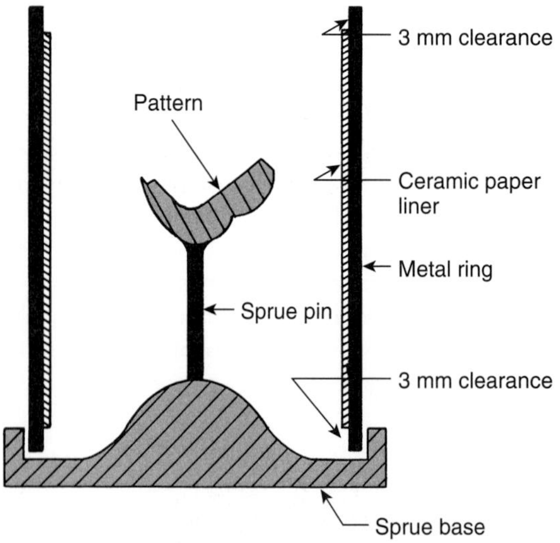

Fig. 17-7 Cross-sectional diagram of the assembled sprue-based and metal casting ring shown in Fig. 17-6. A single sprue connects the sprue base to the inlay pattern. After investing but before burnout, this metallic sprue pin will be removed. If the sprue is made of wax, its removal is not necessary. The ceramic liner is 3 mm short of the top and bottom of the ring to lock in the investment during burnout and casting.

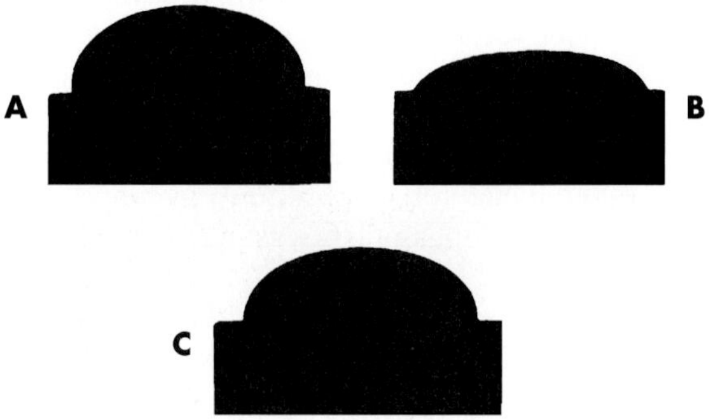

Fig. 17-8 Diagram illustrating the contact angle of a liquid like water on the wax pattern. In **A,** the water has a high contact angle and does not wet the wax well. In **B,** a wetting agent was applied, which decreases the contact angle and improves the wetting. In **C,** the contact angle is increased again because the wetting agent was rinsed off. For successful investing, the water-based investment must wet the wax pattern well.

use, as shown in Fig. 17-8, *C*. The same wax as was used in Fig. 17-8, *B*, was rinsed with tap water and blotted dry. The contact angle in this case was 91°, closely approaching that of the original untreated wax surface.

The distortion of the wax pattern after its removal from the die is a function of the temperature and time interval before investing. The nearer the room temperature approaches the softening point of the wax, the more readily internal stresses are released. Also, the longer a pattern is allowed to stand before investing, the greater the deformation that may occur, even at room temperature. A pattern should therefore be invested as soon as possible after it is removed from the die, and it should not be subjected to a warm environment during this interval. In any case, a pattern should not stand for more than 20 to 30 minutes before being invested. Once it is properly invested and the investment has set, there is no danger of further pattern distortion, even if it remains for some hours before the final stages of wax elimination (burnout) and casting.

Investment Techniques During investing of the pattern, the correct water/powder ratio of the investment mix, a required number of spatulation turns, and a proper investing technique are essential to obtain acceptable casting results. There are two methods of investing the wax pattern: hand investing and vacuum investing. In both cases, the proper amount of investment powder and water should be used, following the manufacturer's instructions exactly. The water is added first, followed by the slow addition of the powder to encourage the removal of air from the powder. The powder and liquid are mixed briefly with a plaster spatula until all the powder is wetted.

In hand investing, the cover of the bowl containing the investment mix is placed over the bowl (Fig. 17-9). The cover contains a mechanical mixer, and the mixing is done by hand, usually for 100 turns of the spatulator. The setting rate of an investment depends on the number of spatulation turns, which also affects the hygroscopic expansion. The investment, after being spatulated, is placed on the vibrator to eliminate some of the air bubbles from the mix and to collect all of the mix from the sides of the rubber bowl into the center. The sprue base, which holds the sprue and wax pattern, is held with one hand, and the investment is painted over the wax pattern with a camel-hair brush. In painting the pattern, the investment should be teased ahead of the brush to prevent incorporation of air ad-

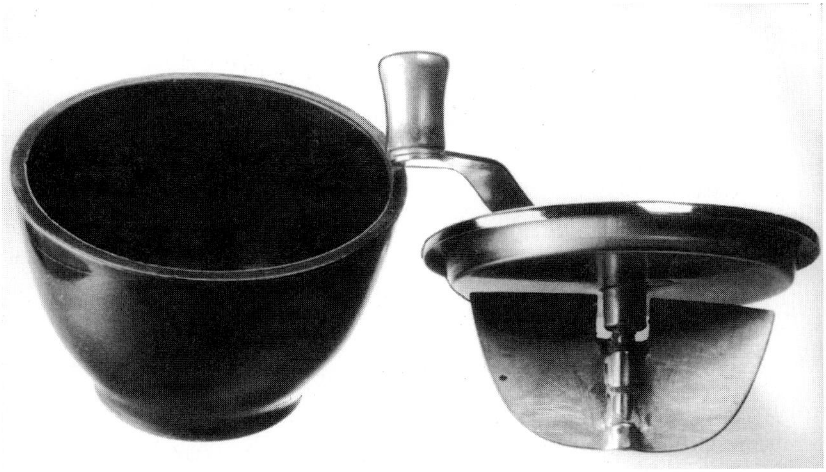

Fig. 17-9 Picture of a device for hand mixing investment. The hand mechanical spatula is placed over the bowl and the investment is then mixed before pouring it into the casting ring.

jacent to the pattern. Furthermore, to avoid distorting the pattern, the brush itself should not touch the pattern. After the painting is completed, the pattern is vibrated very gently with the sprue base held firmly with the fingers and the underside of the hand resting on the vibrator. This method relieves any minor air bubbles that might have been trapped around the wax pattern.

After the pattern has been painted with investment, the mixed investment is poured into the ring, which is held at a slight angle so the investment flows slowly down its side to fill from the bottom to the top. In this manner, the possibility of trapping air in the ring or around the pattern is reduced to a minimum. It is often helpful to hold the assembled ring and the sprue base in one hand, which rests gently on a vibrator, while the investment is being poured into the ring. When the ring is completely filled, it is leveled with the top by the edge of a plaster spatula. The filled ring is then set aside for the investment to set completely, which usually requires 45 to 60 minutes. When a phosphate-bonded investment is used, the ring is slightly overfilled, the top of the ring is not leveled off, and the investment is allowed to set. After the investment has set, the excess investment is ground off using a model trimmer. This procedure is necessary because a nonporous, glassy surface results, which must be ground off to improve the permeability of the investment and allow for gases to readily escape from the mold during casting.

In vacuum investing, special equipment is used to facilitate the investing operation. A popular vacuum machine used in dentistry is shown in Fig. 17-10. With this equipment, the powder and water (or special liquid) are mixed under vacuum and the mixed investment is permitted to flow into the ring and around the wax pattern with the vacuum present. Although vacuum investing does not remove all the air from the investment and the ring, the amount of air is usually reduced enough to obtain a smooth adaptation of the investment to the pattern. Vacuum investing often yields castings with improved surfaces when compared with castings produced from hand-invested patterns. The degree of difference between the two procedures depends largely on the care used in hand investing. Whether hand- or vacuum-investing procedures are used in filling the casting ring, the investment should be allowed to harden in air before burnout of the wax.

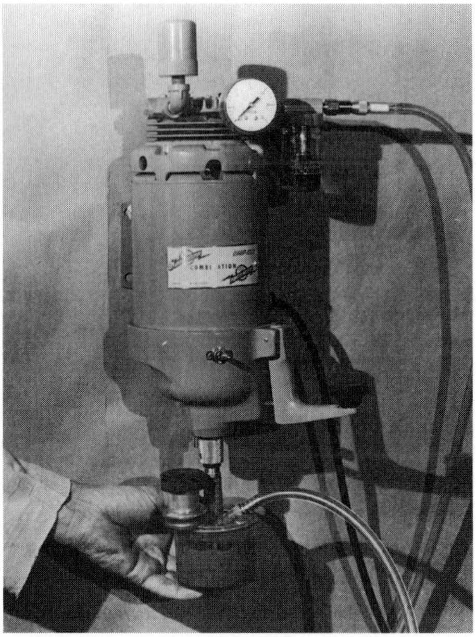

Fig. 17-10 Picture of a powered vacuum unit for investing. The investment powder and liquid are added to the mixing bowl and mixed with a spatula to ensure wetting of the powder. A vacuum line is then attached to the mixing bowl and the top of the power unit. The casting ring is inverted and attached to the mixing container. The power is switched on, and the mixing bowl is attached to the bottom of the mixer, causing the mixing blades to rotate in the bowl. After mixing 10 to 15 seconds, the mixing bowl is inverted such that the investment slowly enters the casting ring. Vibration is applied by the lever protruding from the right side of the mixer. Alternatively, the mixer may be removed from the mixing bowl after mixing and the investment poured by hand into the ring.

BURNOUT OF THE WAX PATTERN

After the wax pattern has been invested, it should be set aside until the investment has hardened, usually 45 to 60 minutes. The metallic ring is

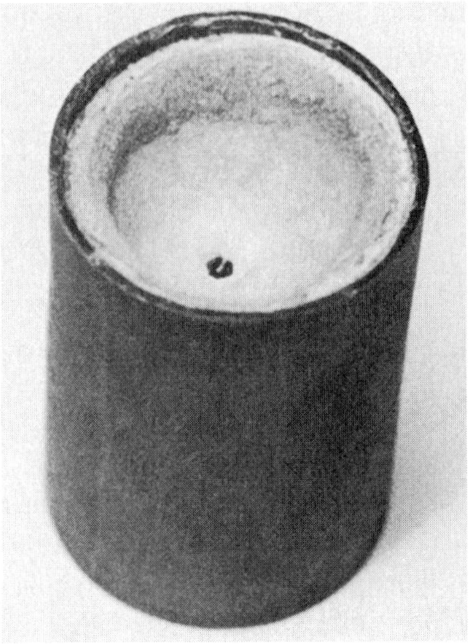

Fig. 17-11 Picture of a casting ring that has been filled with investment, but before burnout. The wax sprue is visible as a small dark dot in the middle of the investment. The casting ring is inverted and the sprue base has been removed. This ring is ready for burnout.

placed directly into the burnout oven to begin eliminating wax from the mold. As discussed previously, investment must withstand the impact force exerted by the molten metal when it enters the hot mold during casting. These forces can be considerable. The metallic ring will support the investment as the molten metal enters the mold (Fig. 17-11). In spite of the support given by the ring, it is imperative that the investment be mixed properly and allowed to set completely so it will obtain a sufficient strength.

During burnout, the mold is placed in an oven to completely eliminate the wax, thereby forming a cavity into which the molten metal is cast. During wax elimination, the investment expands thermally, which is necessary to compensate for the casting shrinkage. Although wax melts at a comparatively low temperature, its complete elimination requires much higher temperatures. Usually, if elimination is not complete, small bits of the wax residue are retained in the fine margins of the mold and prevent the formation of a complete casting. When the molten metal enters the sprue hole, the resulting force causes the air in the mold cavity to be driven out through the pores of the investment, thus the mold cavity is filled completely. This process takes less than a second. The presence of any foreign material in the mold cavity slows or possibly prevents the air or other gases from being driven out of the mold before the molten metal solidifies. As a result, the castings may be incomplete or the margins irregular, in which case the casting should be repeated, starting with a new wax pattern.

Because waxes are organic materials, they are composed of carbon, hydrogen, oxygen, and nitrogen. When heated to higher temperatures, any organic material decomposes and forms carbon dioxide (CO_2), water (H_2O), or nitrogen oxide (NO_2), all of which are gases and can be easily eliminated. However, formation of these gases depends on the presence of a sufficient supply of oxygen, the relatively high temperature of the oven, and adequate heating time of the ring. If insufficient oxygen is available to the wax in the mold cavity, the temperature of the oven is not high enough, or the wax pattern is heated for only a short time, incomplete reaction between the wax and oxygen may result. The internal walls of mold cavities placed in a room-temperature oven, set at 500° C, and left for different times are shown in Fig. 17-12. The longer the ring remained in the oven, the better the elimination of carbon residue from the mold cavity. Castings made under these four conditions showed that for conditions seen in Fig. 17-12, *A* and *B,* the castings were not complete and part of the pattern did not cast. For the condition seen in Fig. 17-12, *C,* depending on the total amount of wax used, the number of investment rings in the oven at the same time, and other such variables, the castings were either incomplete (as shown in *A* and *B*) or appeared complete but had short and rounded margins. These results indicated that elimination of gases from mold cavities was rather slow because of the presence of carbon deposits, and the molten alloy solidified before all the gases around the marginal area could escape. For all three condi-

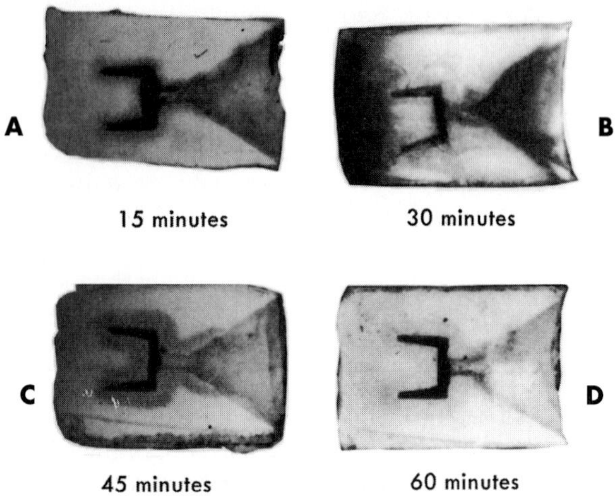

Fig. 17-12 Effect of burnout time of wax in investment molds on the presence of carbon residue. Each mold was placed in a room-temperature furnace that was then set at 500° C, heated for the times indicated (**A** to **D**), and sectioned to examine the internal appearance. Notice the dark gray area of carbon residue around the mold cavity in **C** even after 45 minutes of heating.

tions, the surfaces of the castings were black and could not be cleaned by normal pickling (deoxidization) action. This black color indicated that the surfaces were covered with fine particles of carbon residue, because the acid in pickling solutions is not effective in dissolving or removing carbon particles. Castings made under the condition shown in Fig. 17-12, *D,* were complete, with sharp margins, and on pickling the casting surfaces had a typical yellow color. These experiments demonstrate the importance of adequate burnout time.

A satisfactory way of eliminating the wax pattern is to set the mold in the furnace with the sprue hole placed downward at first, so most of the wax drains out and is eliminated as a liquid. The ring is then inverted with the sprue hole placed upward. In this position the oxygen in the oven atmosphere can circulate more readily into the cavity, react with the wax, and form gases rather than the fine carbon that interferes with the venting of the mold cavity. The lower the mold temperature and larger the wax pattern, the longer the mold should be left in the oven. For a 500° C oven temperature and larger wax patterns, the mold should remain in the oven for approximately 1 hour, with the sprue hole placed downward during half of this time and upward during the other half. If more than one ring is placed in an oven, a longer period is required for wax elimination. The general rule is to add 5 minutes to the burnout time for every extra ring placed in the oven at 500° C. With an oven temperature of 600° to 700° C, a shorter time may be sufficient to completely eliminate the wax.

Investment materials are poor heat conductors, which results in a temperature difference between the inner core and the outside portion of the mold. Although this difference is relatively great at the beginning of the burnout, it diminishes as time progresses and is zero at the time of casting. The difference in temperature between the inner and outer portions of the mold are even greater if the mold is placed in a hot oven or if the heating rate of the oven is too rapid. The outside of the mold, being exposed to a higher temperature, expands somewhat more than does the inner part. This expansion may cause the mold to crack during heating. Because of the high thermal expansion of investments containing cristobalite, these temperature differences may be especially important. For best results, this type of investment should always be placed into a room-temperature oven and the oven temperature increased slowly. These temperature differences do not affect quartz-containing investments, probably because their rate of thermal expansion is slower than that of cristobalite investments.

When the wax pattern is completely eliminated and the mold has reached the casting temperature, the gold alloy is melted by an appropriate method and cast into the mold cavity immediately upon removal of the mold from the burnout oven. However, the investment should never be allowed to cool before casting because the expansion of the investment during burnout is essentially irreversible (see Chapter 13). If the mold cools before it is cast, the only recourse is to discard the mold and start over by making a new wax pattern.

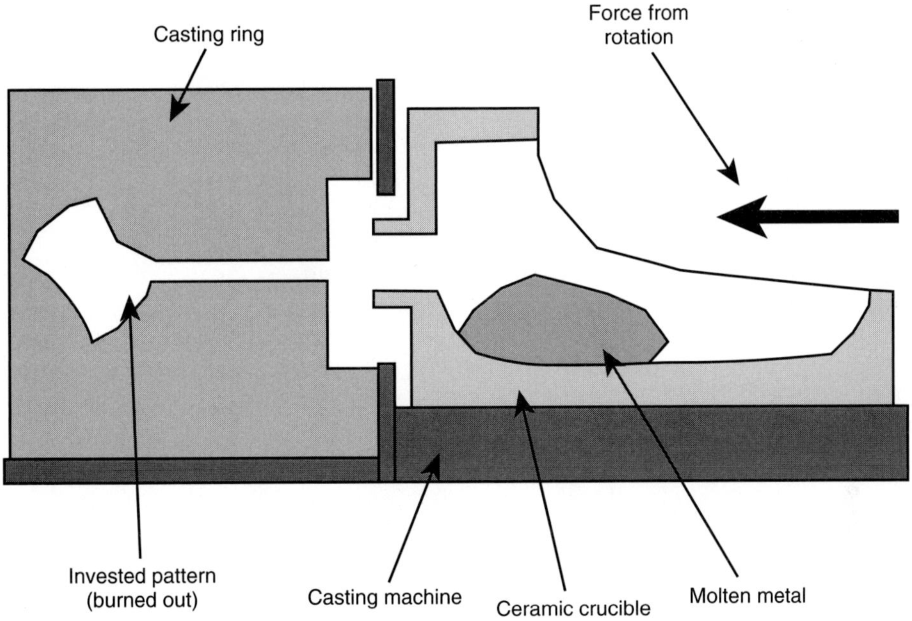

Fig. 17-13 Diagram showing the relationship between the ceramic crucible used to melt the alloy and the casting ring in a centrifugal casting machine. Both the crucible and the ring are placed on the casting machine. Once molten, the metal is rapidly driven centrifugally out of the crucible and into the mold in the casting ring. The traverse of the molten metal takes less than one second. The oxidized elements and flux, which are less dense, lag behind the molten metal as slag.

CASTING

Casting Machines Several types and designs of casting machines are used to make dental castings. All casting machines accelerate the molten metal into the mold either by centrifugal force or air pressure. Numerous modifications and variations of these methods are used in different machines. The selection of the casting and melting techniques is heavily influenced by the type of alloy and restoration to be cast.

A variety of centrifugal machines are available. Some spin the mold in a plane parallel to the table top on which the machine is mounted, whereas others rotate in a plane vertical to the table top. Some are spring-driven, and others are operated by electric power. An electric heating unit is attached to some machines to melt the alloys before spinning the mold to throw in the metal. Others have a refractory crucible in which the alloy is melted by a torch before the casting operation is completed. Each of these machines depends on the centrifugal force applied to the molten metal to cause it to completely fill the mold with properly melted metal (Fig. 17-13). Concerning the quality of the casting, a preference for either machine is not known. The main advantage of the centrifugal machines is the simplicity of design and operation, with the opportunity to cast both large and small castings on the same machine. Typical examples of centrifugal machines are shown in Fig. 17-14.

With the air pressure type of machine, either compressed room air or some other gas, such as carbon dioxide or nitrogen, can be used to force the molten metal into the mold. The air pressure is applied to the molten metal through a suitable

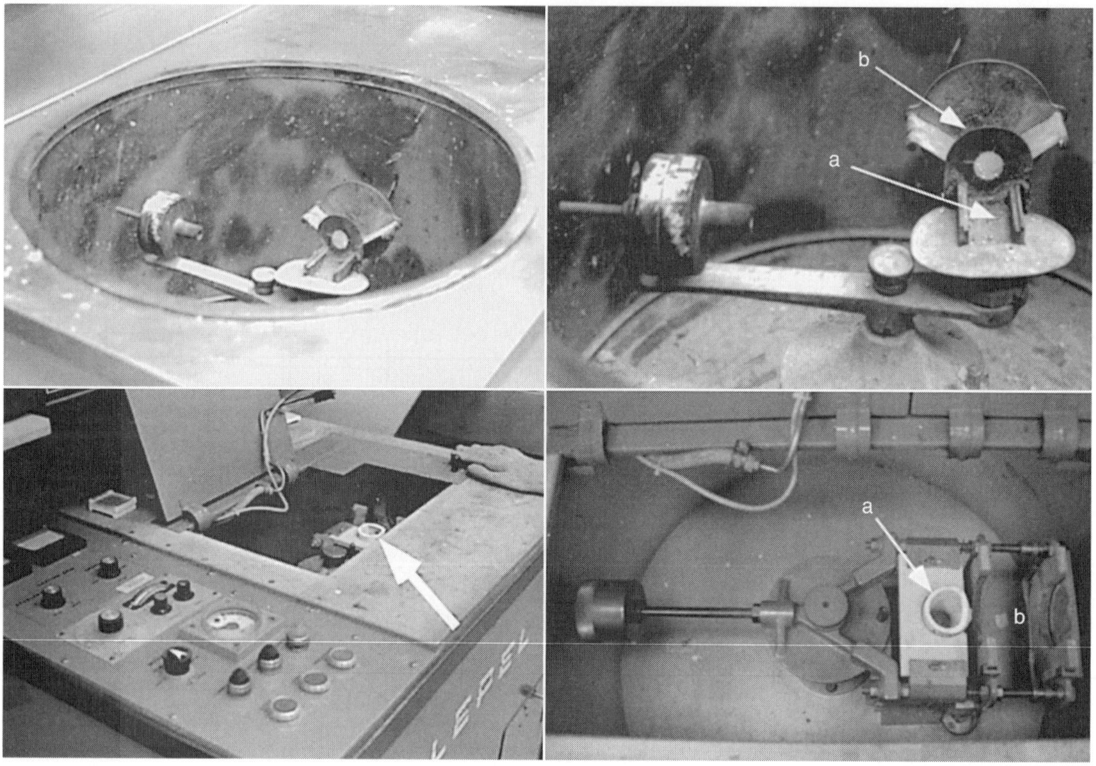

Fig. 17-14 Pictures of centrifugal casting machines. In **A,** the centrifugal force is created with a spinning motion powered by a spring and the alloy is heated with a torch. The casting device is in a well to protect the operator from any debris that might fly out during casting. **B,** A close-up view of the casting machine in **A.** The crucible *(not shown)* is placed into the cradle at *a,* and the casting ring onto the sling at *b* (see Fig. 17-13). The counterweight of the casting arm is visible at the left, which balances the device as it spins rapidly to centrifugally drive the metal from the crucible into the ring. **C,** Induction casting machine. In this machine, the metal is melted by an electrical current, so no casting torch is necessary. The crucible is visible in the casting well *(arrow).* **D,** A close-up view of the casting apparatus in **C.** The crucible is visible at *a,* and the ring *(not shown)* is placed into the space at *b.* The spinning motion is motor driven, not spring-driven as in **A.** The counterweight is visible at the left.

valve mechanism. This type of machine is satisfactory only for making small castings.

Casting machines, both the centrifugal and gas pressure, are available with an attached vacuum system designed to assist the molten metal in filling the mold. In some castings, the added vacuum may be advantageous, but in general, this addition shows little evidence of producing superior quality castings.

Melting the Alloy To cast a metal restoration, a suitable torch or other heating equipment to melt the alloy is necessary. Various devices are available for each of these operations. The most common method of heating dental alloys for full cast-metal restorations is by using a gas-air torch. A properly adjusted torch develops an adequate temperature for melting dental alloys whose melting ranges are between 870° and 1000° C. Completing the melting operation promptly also depends on the proper adjustment of the torch flame. Poorly adjusted flames can waste time during melting and considerably damage the alloy through excessive oxidation or gas inclusion. Small and irregularly shaped flames should not be used to melt moderate or large quantities of alloy for casting purposes. A well-defined torch flame is the hottest and most effective for such melting operations.

The literature contains many descriptions of the proper flame for heating metals and alloys. One practical method of checking and interpreting the flame condition is to apply the flame to a small piece of copper, approximately the size of a coin, placed on a soldering block. The torch is adjusted as it would be for making a casting and is then directed on the copper. If the copper turns bright and clean as it is heated, the flame and the torch manipulation are correct. If the copper turns to a dark, dull red color, oxidation is occurring and the heating is ineffective. The operator should make the necessary adjustments to eliminate these conditions.

The properly adjusted flame contains well-defined component parts described as inner and out cones or portions having differing color intensities. For example, the inner, well-defined, light blue central cone is usually accepted as the most effective for heating because it is the least oxidizing portion of the flame. Although an improper flame is the most common cause of oxidation of the base metals in alloys, even a properly adjusted flame causes oxidation if it is held too close to the metal being heated, too far from it, to one side or another, or if it is moved over the surface or away from the alloy. The dramatic oxidation and ineffective heating that can be seen on the copper are not as evident with noble and high-noble alloys, yet may be observed by the experienced operator who is aware of such conditions.

Modified torches may be used that combine natural gas and oxygen or certain "tank" gases, such as acetylene and oxygen. The natural gas and oxygen combination is mainly used for melting alloys designed for construction of porcelain-metal restorations. The combination of acetylene and oxygen has been used mostly to melt cobalt-chromium and nickel-chromium alloys, which have higher fusion temperatures and are used for removable partial dentures.

Electric melting units of various designs are used in some laboratories to melt the alloys during casting. The advantage of using these units is that slightly less skill is required than is necessary for controlling the torch. However, many of these electric heating units have no limiting controls, and the operator must therefore exercise judgment regarding the proper condition of the alloy to be cast. The electric units are heated either by induction or by resistance heating systems. Those units heated by induction melt alloy much faster than do those heated by torch; if the procedure is not watched closely, the alloy can easily be overheated. An electronic monitor is useful for indicating proper temperature. Melting units with resistance heating take longer to complete the heating and casting operation than do torch-heated units. The slightly longer heating time does not appreciably increase the temperature of the molten alloy, nor does it cause any significant problems.

Regardless of the method of melting the alloy or the type of casting machine used, the following objectives should be kept in mind when casting: (1) the alloy should be heated as quickly as possible to a completely molten condition (above the liquidus temperature); (2) oxidation of the alloy should be prevented by heating the metal with a well-adjusted torch (or other method) and a small amount of flux on the metal surface; and (3) adequate force should be applied to force the well-melted metal into the mold. Finally, after the molten metal is forced into the mold cavity, the casting machine should be allowed to continue to provide pressure on the metal while the metal is solidifying. This pressure encourages complete casting of the margins. Although each of these operations demands care and attention, they are not difficult to master.

SPECIAL CASTING SITUATIONS

Casting Porcelain-Fused-To-Metal Alloys

Because of the characteristically high melting temperature of the alloys used in porcelain-fused-to-metal restorations, special investments and casting facilities are necessary. Calcium sulfate–bonded investment materials and conventional melting facilities are inadequate for most available alloys because the melting range of the alloys is too high. Generally, phosphate-bonded investments and gas-oxygen torch are used in casting this type of alloy. Phosphate investments are stronger and denser than are gypsum-bonded investments (see Chapter 13). Although the technique for using these special alloys and investments is not complicated or elaborate, the technique recommended by the manufacturers should be followed faithfully to achieve satisfactory surface character and fit of the casting.

Because the phosphate-bonded investment used for porcelain-fused-to-metal castings is dense, special attention should be given to the manner of spruing of the wax pattern. Proper spruing should facilitate the escape of gases from the mold cavity before the molten metal solidifies completely. The bar type of spruing used for casting these alloys is shown in Fig. 17-4. With this type of spruing, the sprue bar is placed inside the mold as a reservoir to help keep the alloy in the molten stage for a longer time so a more complete casting can be attained. For single units, the bar is shortened or a ball is used. Note that with a normal spruing method, the pattern is sprued in such a manner as to reduce turbulence in the flow of molten alloy. However, with the bar-spruing method, an attempt is made to increase the turbulence so the investment close to the sprue maintains a higher temperature, which keeps the alloy molten for a longer time. The main disadvantage of the bar type of sprue is the increased amount of alloy required to make castings; for this reason the bar type is not used to make castings of alloys with low melting ranges and gypsum-bonded investments.

If a bar type of sprue is used with a centrifugal casting machine, the casting ring should be placed in the casting machine so the bar sprue is vertical. The leader from the sprue button to the bar should be attached 1 to 2 mm below the top of the bar. In this manner, when the alloy at the tip of the bar sprue freezes, the alloy 1 to 2 mm below the tip remains molten, and feeding from the sprue button to the bar is still possible. The leader from the bar to the wax pattern should be attached to the highest part of the wax pattern. Centrifugal casting machines tend to feed molten alloy straight (as a result of the centrifugal force) and down (from gravity). If the leaders from the sprue button to the bar or from the bar to a one-piece cast bridge are placed in the middle of the bar or bridge, there is a high probability of a miscast. In such a sprue arrangement, the molten alloy must fill the lower portion of the bar and the mold cavity before being forced upward against gravity to fill the upper portion of the bar and the bridge. Proper attachment of the leaders to the bar and to three copings are shown in Fig. 17-4.

Other steps in the investing and casting procedure of porcelain-fused-to-metal alloys normally include vacuum investing, careful wax elimination, a gas-oxygen torch or other high-temperature melting facility, and centrifugal casting with adequate casting pressure. Special solders may be required with these alloys for certain techniques; with some alloys and solders, the operation requires skilled management only obtained with extensive practical experience.

Casting Co-Cr and Ni-Cr Alloys and Partial Denture Frameworks Posterior crowns are often cast in base-metal alloys but, because of their high melting temperatures, phosphate investments are almost always used. Also, as a result of their high freezing temperatures, more shrinkage of the alloy must be compensated for than in gold-based alloys to obtain accurately fitting castings. The extra compensation can be obtained by (1) painting a die spacer (varnish) on the die, but short of the margins, before preparing the wax pattern; and/or (2) using two layers of ceramic paper liner in the investing ring to make the setting expansion of the investment more effective.

The methods of casting relatively large partial-denture frameworks in base metals differ from the casting of simple restorations such as crowns, although the two operations are similar in principle. In cast partial-denture construction, a suitable cast of refractory material serves as the structure on which the wax pattern is formed. This is done because the wax pattern is too large to be freestanding and must be supported during investing and casting. This refractory cast is prepared by duplicating the master stone model, usually by using the agar duplicating materials described in Chapter 12. Fig. 17-15, *A*, shows a duplicating flask containing the master model before pouring the duplicating material. Fig. 17-15, *B*, shows the duplicate impression in agar and the separated refractory cast that was prepared in the agar mold.

Once the refractory cast is prepared, the wax pattern for the partial framework is prepared on the cast and invested, in place, on this cast. Fig. 17-16, *A*, shows a wax pattern on a refractory cast. Note that the pattern is sprued through the base of the cast. After the wax pattern is formed, the refractory cast with the wax pattern is invested in a casting ring as shown in Fig. 17-16, *B*, where the sprue button–former has been removed. A gypsum-bonded investment is used when a low–fusing point (<1300° C liquidus) alloy is used, but a phosphate- or silica-bonded investment is used when high–fusing point alloys (>1300° C solidus) are to be cast. The invested pattern is burned out and the investment is heated to the casting temperature, causing thermal expansion. As for any casting, the sum of the setting and thermal expansions compensates for the casting shrinkage of the base metals. A cast restoration is shown in Fig. 17-17.

Because the minor alloying elements of carbon, nitrogen, and oxygen influence the properties of a base metal, it is generally recognized that a pronounced variation in properties can result from the use of variable casting conditions (see Chapter 16). Variables such as mold temperature, temperature of the molten alloy, and the sprue size and arrangement affect the properties of the finished casting as much as does the composition. Therefore, Co-Cr and Ni-Cr alloys are generally considered technique-sensitive. Another reason for this sensitivity is that almost all elements in these alloys, such as chromium, silicon, molybdenum, cobalt, and nickel, react with carbon to form carbides, even though only a relatively small amount of carbon is present in the alloys. Depending on the mold and alloy casting temperature, cooling rate, and other technical variables, carbides of any one of these elements may form, which changes the properties of the alloy. Careful control of manipulative variables in the casting operations is therefore essential.

The alloy melting temperature is an important factor in the selection and control of the melting and casting equipment and in the choice of technique and mold equipment used for the casting of base-metal alloys. Only a base-metal alloy that melts below 1300° C can be cast into a calcium sulfate–bonded investment. It is also possible to cast a low–melting point nickel-chromium alloy against wrought platinum-gold-palladium wire when a flexible partial–denture clasp is required. Because of their higher melting points, other cast base-metal alloys cannot be melted with the conventional blowtorch used for gold-based alloys. It has therefore been necessary to develop special electric or induction melting facilities or, less commonly, to melt the alloy with an oxygen-acetylene torch. Either method is acceptable in the hands of a skillful operator.

Regardless of the method employed to melt the alloy, it is possible to cause severe damage to the properties of a base-metal casting if proper melting practices are not observed. Two sprue buttons from base-metal alloy casting, one sound and free from defects and the other with some porosity and surface irregularities, are shown in Fig. 17-18. More-severe damage from excessive overheating and resulting porosities and surface reaction with the mold materials is not uncommon. Castings with poor surface appearance usually also possess inferior physical properties. It is probable that the proper control of the factors related to the casting operation is more important in controlling the properties of the finished structure than are the variations in composition or the choice of different products.

When casting any of the base metals into molds designed to accommodate the higher melting temperatures of these alloys, certain problems may be encountered that are less common when casting alloys of lower melting temperatures. One problem is that of trapping gases in the mold during the casting process. To have sufficient strength and resistance to thermal

A

B

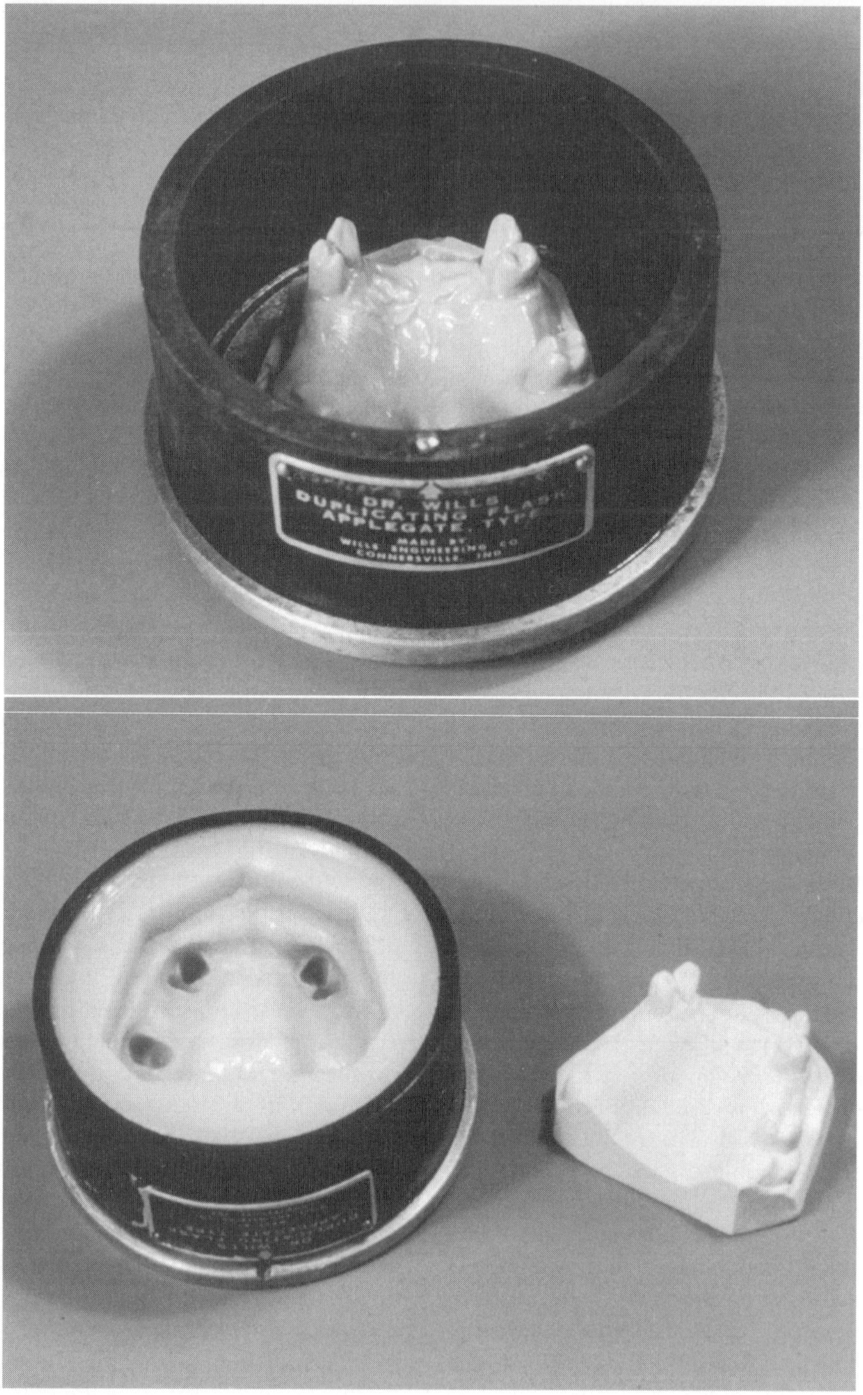

Fig. 17-15 A duplicating flask used to make a refractory cast onto which a partial denture framework will be waxed and cast. In **A,** the flask contains the gypsum master cast and is ready to be invested with the agar duplicating material. In **B,** the agar has set and the original gypsum cast has been removed. The refractory material will then be poured into the mold to create the refractory cast.

(Courtesy Dootz ER, Ann Arbor, 1995, University of Michigan School of Dentistry.)

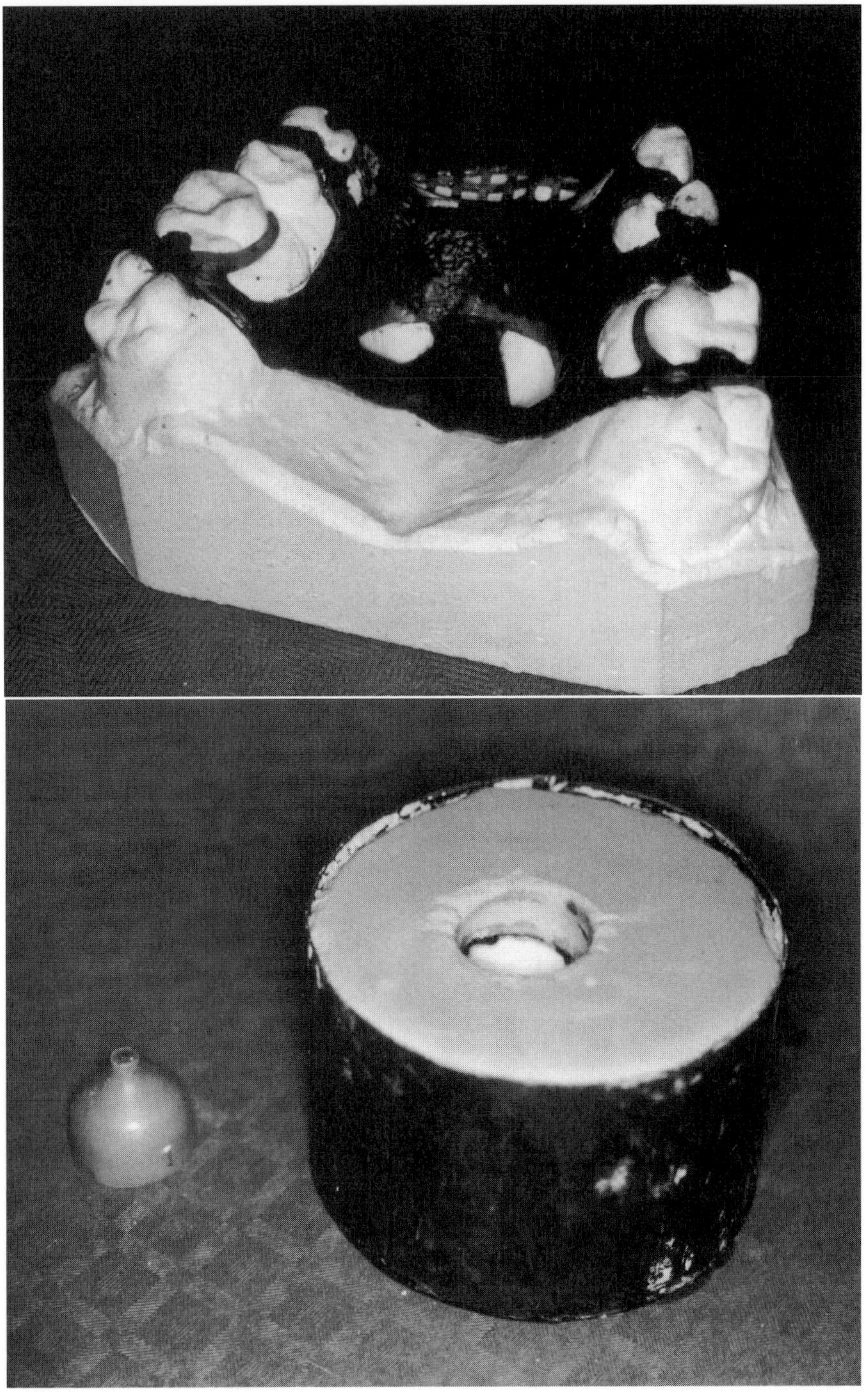

A

B

Fig. 17-16 In **A,** the wax pattern for a partial denture framework has been waxed onto a refractory cast. The sprue for this pattern is through a hole in the base of the cast. In **B,** the wax pattern and refractory cast have been invested and the sprue button–former has been removed. The pattern is now ready for burnout and casting.

(Courtesy Dootz ER, Ann Arbor, 1995, University of Michigan School of Dentistry.)

A

B

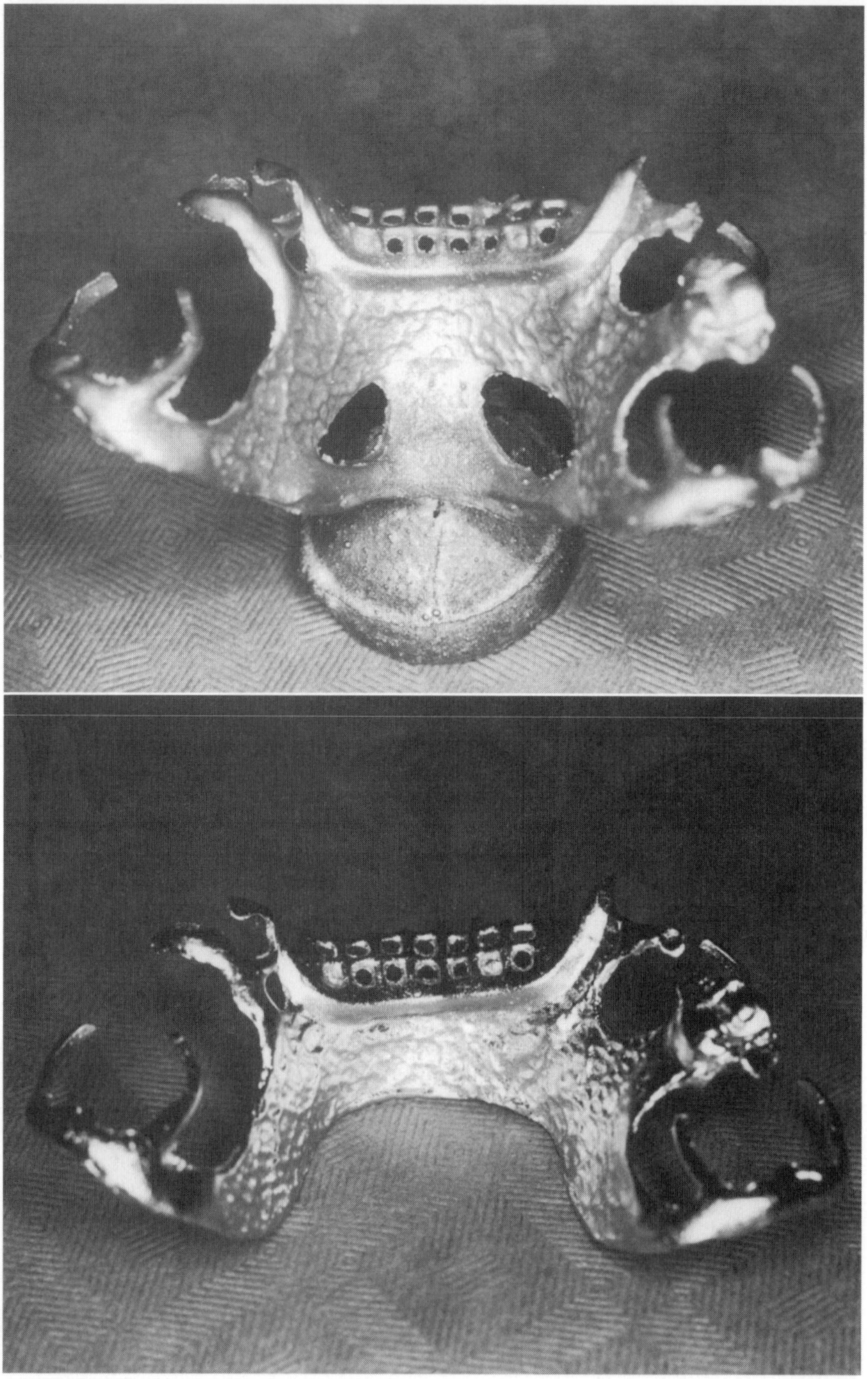

Fig. 17-17 A, A partial-denture framework has been cast and divested from the investment and refractory cast. The casting button is visible at the bottom of the picture. **B,** The framework has been polished and the button removed. The framework is now ready to be tried in the mouth.

(Courtesy Dootz ER, Ann Arbor, 1995, University of Michigan School of Dentistry.)

shock, some investments for cast base-metal alloys lack sufficient porosity for the rapid escape of gases from the mold cavity when the hot metal enters. Gases may therefore be trapped in the mold cavity and produce voids and casting defects. The effect of such trapped gases on one casting of a cobalt-chromium alloy is clearly shown in Fig. 17-19. The general view of the casting in *A* shows the location of the defect in a critical area of the appliance. The magnified view of the defective area in *B* reveals that a large gas bubble became trapped in the molten metal at the time the mold was filled. Before it could be dissipated, the metal solidified. A higher temperature of the casting alloy would have assisted in overcoming this difficulty. Numerous other

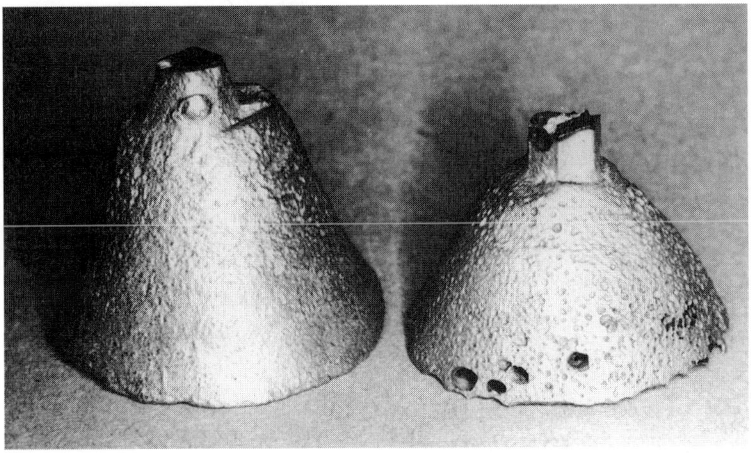

Fig. 17-18 Sprue buttons from base-metal alloy showing an alloy that was properly heated *(left),* and one that was slightly overheated *(right).* Overheating caused the inclusion of several porosities in the alloy.

A

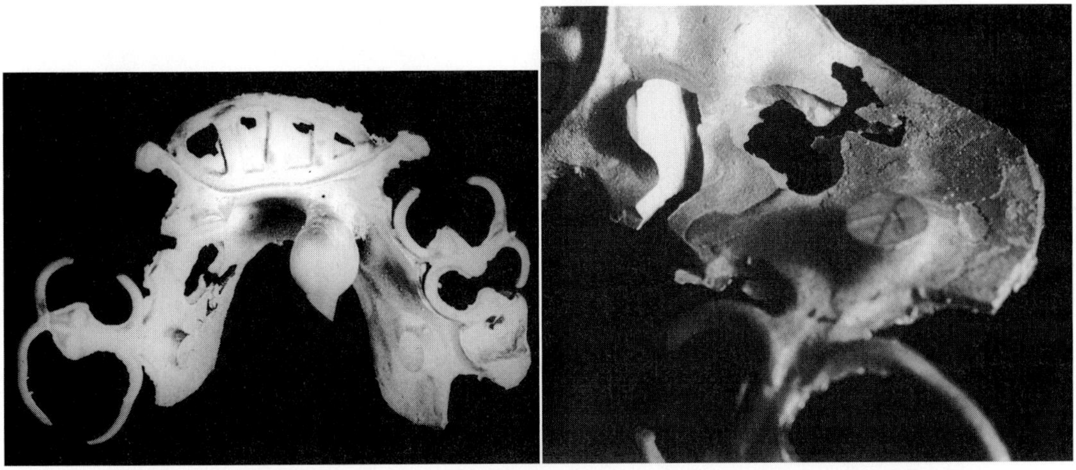

B

Fig. 17-19 Pictures of removable partial-denture frameworks with flaws from poor casting techniques. **A,** The framework has a void in the major connector *(left center area).* **B,** A magnified view of the defect in **A** showing that the defect was caused by metal that was too cold and by gas inclusion in the mold.

methods have been proposed to overcome such defects, such as venting to the surface of the mold to permit rapid elimination of gases. Such a method is used in the preparation of cast test bars for specification testing purposes. The skillful spruing and venting of the mold, combined with complete elimination of the wax residue and adequate heating of the metal, tend to reduce this type of defective casting.

When properly designed and cast, the cast base-metal alloys give acceptable removable partial-denture restorations. A typical appliance of this type, with an acrylic denture base material and artificial teeth attached in the proper relationship is shown in Fig. 17-20. Much clinical study has been given to the choice of clasp material and the proper design of the appliance to give stability and support to the appliance and to the remaining teeth. The mechanics of the design of such restorations are an important aspect of clinical procedures, and rely on the appropriate physical properties of properly cast alloys.

Casting Titanium Titanium has many desirable properties for use in dentistry, but it is difficult to cast in comparison with the common dental casting alloys because it requires relatively complex and expensive equipment. Two problems in casting titanium are its high melting point and the tendency for the molten metal to become contaminated. The melting point of commercially pure titanium is 1671° C, whereas other dental casting alloys have liquidus temperatures below 1500° C. Titanium readily absorbs several gases when in the molten state. If hydrogen, oxygen, and nitrogen are absorbed, the mechanical properties are adversely effected. To prevent absorption of gases, titanium is cast under the protective atmosphere of argon or in a vacuum. To achieve the high melting temperatures, arc melting in either graphite or water-cooled copper crucibles is used. The casting systems force the metal into the mold using either pressure or centrifugal casting techniques.

The casting design for titanium casting is similar to that of other more common dental alloys. A wax pattern is prepared and sprued, as before, but here only the more temperature resistant investments can be used. Both phosphate-bonded and silica and magnesia investments produce good castings and give casting dimensions

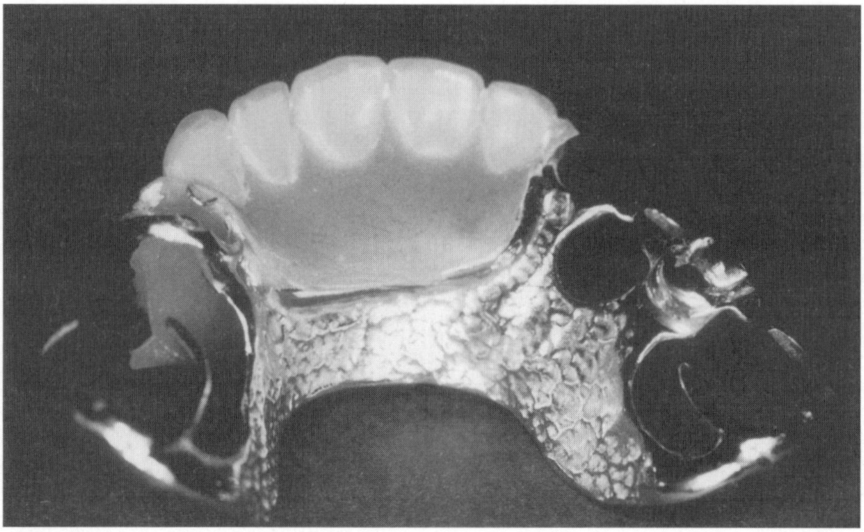

Fig. 17-20 Partial denture framework with artificial teeth attached by acrylic denture base material.

(Courtesy Dootz ER, Ann Arbor, 1995, University of Michigan School of Dentistry.)

that are within the accepted range for base-metal partial-denture and crown castings.

CASTING PROBLEMS

Unless every step in the casting operation is handled properly, the cast restoration may not fit the prepared tooth with the desired accuracy. Naturally, a proper cavity design, an accurate impression of the prepared cavity, a good and accurate die, and proper waxing and investing are all important steps in achieving an acceptable cast restoration. Some common casting problems are described in the following paragraphs and Fig. 17-21. The complete description of casting problems is beyond the scope of this chapter; detailed information is available in books on casting and metallurgy.

Improper solidification of metal causes many casting problems. As discussed earlier in this chapter, the shrinkage of wax and alloy is compensated for by various types of expansion of the investment. However, the shrinkage of alloys takes place in two stages as a result of (1) the transformation of the alloy from liquid to solid and (2) the coefficient of expansion of the solid alloy. While the molten alloy is cooling, the temperature eventually reaches the solidification range, causing the alloy to change from a liquid to a solid. This change of state is accompanied by a large shrinkage, which is compensated for only by adhering to a proper casting technique because the expansion of the investment cannot offset such a large shrinkage. The result of not having this expansion is shown in Fig. 17-22. Ideally, molten alloy located farthest from the sprue button should freeze first and molten alloy in the sprue and the sprue button should feed the rest of the pattern, thus compensating for the shrinkage as a result of the change of state.

As long as the remaining alloy is in the liquid state and the casting machine is rotating, molten alloy will feed the solidified portion of the casting, thereby compensating for the shrinkage. The next layer then solidifies, and this process continues until all the shrinkage resulting from the change of state is compensated for by the available molten alloy in the casting, sprue, and sprue button. If solidification does not occur in this systematic manner and a portion of the alloy in the sprue freezes before the alloy in the casting, what is known as *suckback porosity* occurs, as shown in 17-21, *A,* and Fig. 17-22, *B.* Expansion of the investment material cannot compensate for this type of porosity.

Improper sprue design can also cause suckback porosity. As seen in Fig. 17-22, molten alloy may enter the mold cavity through a single sprue. Investment at the pulpal floor of a full crown pattern therefore heats up because of the higher temperature of the molten alloy, and it keeps the alloy in this area molten somewhat longer than other areas. Thus if alloy in the sprue solidifies before the alloy in the pulpal floor area, the molten alloy in this area would feed the solidifying alloy in the sprue area. When molten alloy in the pulpal floor area solidifies and shrinks because of the change of state, it cannot be fed. As a result, a large suckback porosity under the sprue occurs. Because the cause of the suckback porosity is the improper sequence in the solidification of the alloy, the precautions in the following paragraphs may help to prevent it.

A Y-shaped sprue can be used instead of a single sprue. In this instance, only half of the molten alloy enters the mold cavity through each leg of the Y-sprue, so the temperature of the investment under the sprue does not rise as high. However, the arms of the Y must be widely separated to prevent the investment between the arms from overheating, which could also cause suckback porosity. If a Y-sprue has already been employed, the diameter of each leg of the Y can be increased or an extra 1 to 2 g of gold alloy can be used, which will keep the alloy in the sprue and the sprue button in the molten state somewhat longer and will better feed the solidifying alloy.

Another possible solution to prevent suckback is to increase the mold temperature from 500° C, which is used with many investments and techniques, to 650° or 700° C. With a higher mold temperature, the difference in temperature between the investment located around the sprue and the investment in the area of the pulpal floor of the full crown is decreased. This decrease

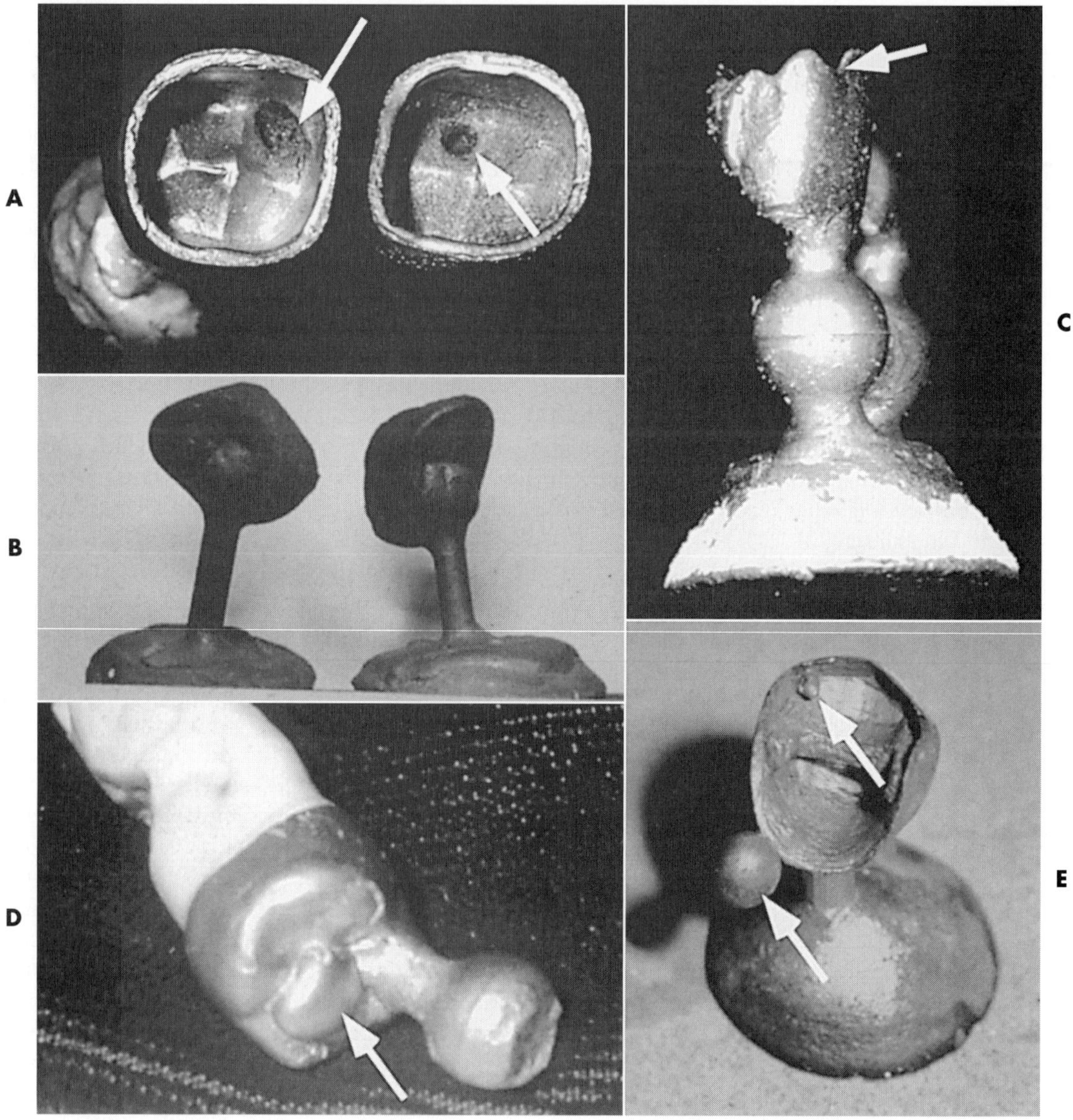

Fig. 17-21 Pictures of various common casting problems. **A,** Suckback porosity visible at arrows. **B,** Dark castings resulting from incomplete burnout of the wax. The black coating is from carbon particles on the alloy and cannot be removed by pickling. **C,** Incomplete casting of the margins *(arrow)* and rounded margins. This defect can be caused by inadequate heating of the metal, lack of sufficient porosity in the investment, or inadequate casting pressure (force). **D,** Positive bubble *(arrow)* on the external part of the casting was caused by air entrapment during investing. **E,** Positives on the margins and internal portions of the casting *(arrows)* caused by air entrapment during investing. Marginal and internal positives are difficult to manage and may require recasting the restoration.

(Courtesy Dr. Carl W. Fairhurst, Medical College of Georgia School of Dentistry.)

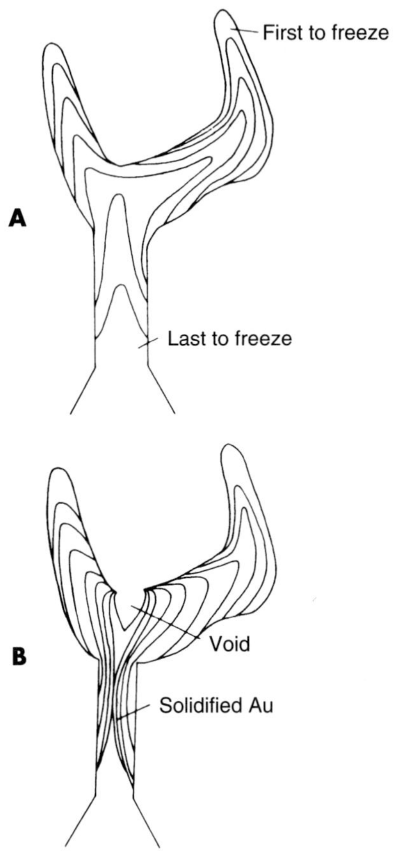

Fig. 17-22 A, Correct sequence of solidification of an alloy in the investment mold of a full cast crown. The margins of the casting should freeze first and the button should freeze last. This order allows the molten metal to compensate for the shrinkage realized when each increment of metal goes from the liquid to solid state. **B,** Incorrect solidification sequence that results in a suckback porosity. The sprue area froze before the cusp area of the crown and the metal in the crown had to feed the shrinking alloy, causing a void in the crown.

helps the molten alloy at the pulpal floor to solidify before the alloy at the sprue. Studies have shown that when a gold alloy with a solidification temperature of 940° C was heated to 1040° C and cast into a mold with a temperature of 500° C, the temperature of the investment 1 mm away from the sprue reached only 585° C, whereas the temperature of the investment 1 mm away from the area of the pulpal floor was as high as 900° C. Thus the difference between the solidification temperature of the alloy and the temperature of the investment at the pulpal floor was only 40° C, whereas the difference near the sprue was 355° C. Therefore the molten alloy decreased in temperature faster around the sprue than at the pulpal floor, and the sprue solidified sooner. When the temperature of the mold was increased from 500° to 700 ° C, the temperature of the investment 1 mm away from the pulpal floor increased from 900° C to 906° to 910° C, whereas the temperature of the investment around the sprue area increase from 585° to 800° C. Thus the difference between the solidification temperature of the alloy and the temperature of the investment in the area of the pulpal floor was 30° to 35° C, whereas around the sprue it was 140° C. In other words, by increasing the mold temperature before casting, the variation of the mold temperature in different areas after casting is reduced.

Increasing the temperature of the molten alloy or using an extra turn on a centrifugal casting machine in an attempt to drive the alloy more completely into the mold does not help eliminate suckback porosity. In fact, this strategy may increase suckback porosity by increasing the temperature of the investment in local areas as the alloy is driven across the investment at a higher rate. The higher forces of alloy entry also increase the chances of cracking the investment, either from thermal shock or from mechanical failure. Miscasts can be caused by a host of other factors, including incomplete wax elimination, overheating of alloys, insufficient casting pressure, insufficient escape of mold gases, and incorrect spruing. These topics have been discussed in other parts of this chapter.

Other Casting Problems With calcium sulfate–bonded investments, when the color of a casting is black after removal from the investment, the cause is probably one of the following: (1) the wax was not completely eliminated, (2) the mold remained in the oven too long, (3) the oxidizing flame was used in melting the alloy, or (4) the investment did not contain any deoxidizing agents. As mentioned earlier, when wax is not completely eliminated, very fine particles of carbon cover the investment pores through which the gas in the mold cavity is supposed to escape. Depending on the amount of carbon remaining on the walls of the mold cavity when the molten metal enters, the casting may be complete but black in color (see Fig. 17-21, *B*), or it may be incomplete (see Fig. 17-21, *C*). The black color in this instance cannot be cleaned by routine pickling action, which is described later in this chapter, because most pickling solutions are acidic and most acids are not effective in removing carbon from the surface of noble and high-noble alloys.

However, if the black color of the gold casting is removed by the normal pickling procedure, it was caused mainly by copper oxides formed during casting. Most casting investments contain some reducing agents to provide a reducing atmosphere when the molten alloys are entering the mold cavity. If the investment mold is left too long in an oven, all the deoxidizers will be decomposed and eliminated. Thus when the molten alloy enters the mold cavity, the oxidation of the copper is not prevented, and the casting will be black. Some investments routinely produce blackened castings because the manufactures do not add any deoxidizing agents. Also, if an oxidizing flame is used in melting the alloy, the casting will be black. Castings that are black because of oxidation of some of the elements in the alloy can easily be cleaned, and the original alloy color can be restored by normal pickling procedures.

Insufficient casting pressure or underheating of alloys usually results in castings with rounded margins (see Fig. 17-21, *C*). The rounded margins are caused by freezing of the alloy before the gases are forced from the mold cavity. As mentioned previously, the slow escape of mold gases can be caused by the investment being too thick over the end of the ring or by a phosphate-bonded investment that has a glassy surface coating that has not been removed. However, rounded margins can also be caused when the alloy cannot exert enough force while entering the mold cavity. This situation can be caused by an underheated alloy that is too viscous or does not stay in the liquid state long enough to force the gases out and reach the marginal areas of the mold. Alternatively, the rounded margins can be caused when the casting machine is underwound and the force on the molten alloy is insufficient to drive the alloy into the mold before the alloy freezes.

Finally, investment errors can result in miscasts that are apparent only after the casting process is complete. Perhaps the most common problem is the trapping of air in the investment during the investing process (see Fig. 17-21, *D*, *E*). These air bubbles may occur on the outside or inside of the casting. If they occur on the outside (see Fig. 17-21, *D*), they are theoretically removable, but often at great expense of time and money (lost metal). However, the fit of the casting is not effected. If the voids occur on the margins or inside of the casting (see Fig. 17-21, *E*), successful removal is extremely difficult and often the restoration will have to be recast.

CLEANING AND PICKLING ALLOYS

The surface oxidation or other contamination of dental alloys is a troublesome occurrence. The oxidation of base metals in most alloys can be kept to a minimum or avoided by using a properly adjusted method of heating the alloy and a suitable amount of flux when melting the alloy (see discussion on fluxes later in this chapter). Despite these precautions, as the hot metal enters the mold, certain alloys tend to become contaminated on the surface by combining with the hot mold gases, reacting with investment ingredients, or physically including mold particles in the metal surface. The surface of most cast, soldered, or otherwise heated metal dental appliances is cleaned by warming the structure in suitable solutions, mechanical polishing, or other treatment of the alloy to restore the normal surface condition.

Surface tarnish or oxidation can be removed by the process of *pickling*. Castings of noble or high-noble metal may be cleaned in this manner by warming them in a 50% sulfuric acid and water solution (Fig. 17-23). Today, most commercially available pickling solutions are not made of

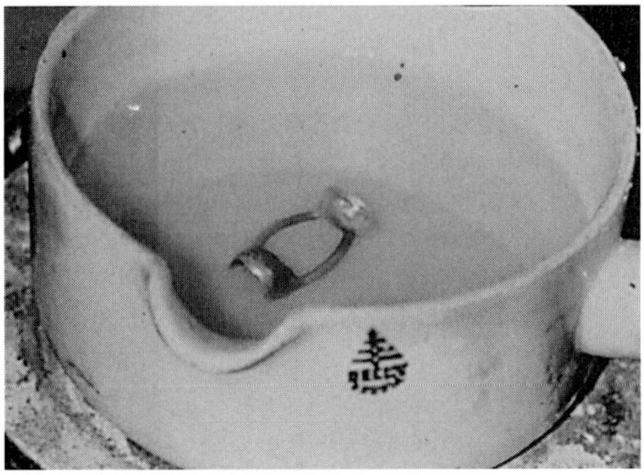

Fig. 17-23 Pickling an alloy. After casting, the alloy (with sprue attached) is placed into the warmed pickling solution for a few seconds. The pickling solution will reduce oxides that have formed during casting. However, pickling will not eliminate a dark color caused by carbon deposition (see Fig. 17-21, *B*). The effect of the solution can be seen by comparing the submerged surfaces to those that have still not contacted the solution.

(Courtesy Dr. Carl W. Fairhurst, Medical College of Georgia School of Dentistry.)

the ordinary inorganic acid solutions and do not release poisonous gases on boiling (as sulfuric acid does). In either case, the casting to be cleaned is placed in a suitable porcelain beaker with the pickling solution and warmed gently, but short of the boiling point. After a few moments of heating, the alloy surface normally becomes bright as the oxides are reduced. When the heating is completed, the acid may be poured from the beaker into the original storage container and the casting is thoroughly rinsed with water. Periodically, the pickling solution should be replaced with fresh solution to avoid excessive contamination.

There are several important notes about pickling. With the diversity of compositions of casting alloys available today, it is prudent to follow the manufacturer's instructions for pickling precisely, as all pickling solutions may not be compatible with all alloys. Furthermore, the practice of dropping a red-hot casting into the pickling solution should be avoided. This practice may alter the phase structure of the alloy or warp thin castings, and splashing acid may be dangerous to the operator. Finally, steel or stainless steel tweezers should not be used to remove castings from the pickling solutions. The pickling solution may dissolve the tweezers and plate the component metals onto the casting. Rubber-coated or Teflon tweezers are recommended for this purpose.

SOLDERING TECHNIQUES

GENERAL SUGGESTIONS FOR SOLDERING

The details for dental soldering are adequately described in textbooks related to other fields of dentistry. Certain principles of the freehand and investment techniques are emphasized here. For successful soldering, both the technique and the selection of solder are important. Many of the materials and techniques used in casting are also useful in soldering.

Dental solders are supplied in a variety of shapes, such as strips, rods, wires, or cubes, each of which is convenient for certain operations. Thin strips are the conventional form for general applications, and small cubes, approximately 1-mm square, are convenient for soldering a contact area on an inlay or crown. Rods are often notched along two sides, which permits them to hold flux better than a smooth form. Also, when melted, the notched forms do not roll back into a ball as easily as smooth forms. Choosing a particular shape depends on the operation to be performed; each shape is available in a range of fineness.

Proper application of fluxes provides a protective coating that prevents oxidation of the solder and parts being soldered. The *flux* dissolves surface oxides and allows the melted solder to wet and flow onto the adjoining alloy surfaces. The fluxes used for soldering gold alloys are combinations of borax and boric acid, with potassium fluoride added to some. Too much flux is as undesirable as not enough flux. See the discussion on fluxes at the end of this chapter.

The careful and skillful use of the soldering torch flame is important to a high quality soldered joint. A well-defined, not-too-large, pointed flame is advisable for the final heating of solder in a localized area, but a larger, less well-defined flame of the "brush" type may be used for the initial heating. The flame should not be applied directly to the parts to be joined until the flux has melted and formed a uniform layer over the surface. Applying a hot flame to the flux too quickly causes the flux to form droplets rather than a film. Once the flame has been applied to the spot to be soldered, it should not be withdrawn until soldering is completed. A protective envelope should be created around the spot to be soldered with the reducing portion of the flame. The operation should be completed in the shortest time possible to avoid oxidation of the base metal ingredients of the alloys involved and to prevent damage to the microstructures of the alloys.

Overheating during the soldering operation will cause (1) pits in the solder, (2) penetration or burning through thin sections, and (3) a loss of strength because of diffusion of the solder into the other metals or loss of fibrous microstructure. Underheating will cause pitting from the retention of unmelted flux and failure of the solder to flow and adhere to all surfaces. Good wetting of the surfaces by the solder is imperative for satisfactory joining of the parts. Solder that is not well heated tends to "ball" and fails to spread properly. Both overheating and underheating will result in a weaker solder joint. For this reason, the proper and careful heating and fluxing of the solder are essential.

Sometimes the flow of the solder should be restricted from parts of the restoration, such as the margins or the occlusal grooves. Flow into these areas can be prevented with an *antiflux* material, which should be applied to the surface before the flux or solder is applied. Solder does not flow into an area contaminated with graphite; a soft lead pencil is therefore an effective antiflux. Other materials, such as rouge (iron oxide) or whiting (calcium carbonate) in an alcohol and water suspension, are effective antifluxes for prolonged heating or high-temperature heating, which can burn off the graphite.

The distance between the parts to be joined can influence the accuracy of the final appliance. If the parts are in intimate contact, they tend to expand and push apart on heating, whereas if the distance is too great, the parts tend to draw together as the solder solidifies. A clearance of a few hundredths of a millimeter (0.13 mm) between the parts to be joined is optimal when using the investment-soldering technique. This thickness can be practically estimated by the thickness of a typical business card. When attempting free hand soldering of wires for orthodontic or other appliances, a closer adaptation of the parts is possible. The shape of the joint and the purpose of the appliance will ultimately determine the appropriate distance between the soldered parts.

Despite certain well-established principles, soldering is an art. The timing and type of heating, selection of the type and shape of the solder, contour of parts to be joined, and application of flux cannot always be dictated by specific rules. Ultimately, the experience of the operator plays a significant role in any successful soldering operation.

INFRARED SOLDERING

Instead of using a torch to provide heat, an infrared heating unit is available specifically for dental soldering. The unit uses the light from a 1000-watt, tungsten-filament, quartz-iodine bulb, which is mounted at the primary focal point of a gold-plated, elliptical reflector. The material to be soldered is placed at the reflector's secondary focal point, at which the reflected infrared energy of the tungsten light source is focused. This equipment, shown in Fig. 17-24, can be used for the high-temperature soldering of alloys for porcelain-fused-to-metal bridges at 1150° C. The main problem in the use of this unit is locating the focal center of the light on the spot to be soldered. The infrared energy must be focused on the crowns and not on the solder itself. Failure to focus on the right spot on the crown can result in cold joints that are porous.

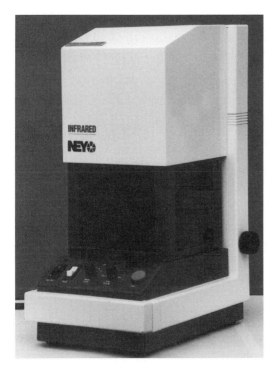

Fig. 17-24 An infrared soldering unit that uses a focused light beam for melting the solder. The appliance is placed into the lower half of the unit and the infrared beam is focused on the area to be soldered.

CASTING AND SOLDERING FLUXES

A *flux* is a substance applied to the surface of molten metal primarily to prevent oxygen from contacting the hot metal and thereby causing oxidation. In addition, flux dissolves oxides that may form while the metal is heated; the resulting solution of oxides or other extraneous matter in the flux constitutes a slag. A flux also facilitates the free flow of solder; it helps solder to wet and spread over the metal surface. For a flux to be effective, it must have a fusion temperature below that of the alloy being heated, but should not burn or volatilize readily.

NOBLE AND HIGH-NOBLE ALLOYS

Borax, or sodium tetraborate ($(Na_2B_4)_7 \cdot 10H_2O$), can dissolve the metal oxides (mainly copper oxides) that occur on noble and high-noble alloys, and therefore is commonly used as a flux in dentistry. Dehydrated sodium tetraborate is known as *borax glass* and can be used in the dry powder form. When melted, borax glass is a clear, viscous liquid that does not volatilize readily when heated. It can be made more fluid by adding boric acid or other salts, which aid in spreading of the flux on the hot metal surface. Boric acid is not used alone for fluxing purposes, as is sometimes done with borax. Dehydrated borax glass is preferred to the ordinary hydrated borax, which liberates water vapor on being heated and, as a result, effervesces and bubbles up over the surface of the hot meal without forming an effective surface covering.

Fluxes are available in a variety of forms, which are usually designated for specific applications in soldering or casting operations. Liquid flux is principally a solution of borax and boric acid in water, and is applied in soldering operations of orthodontic appliances and bridge structures in which a minimum of flux is desired. A saturated solution, or lower concentration, of the ingredients may be used, and smaller quantities of other salts, such as potassium carbonate or ammonium chloride, may be added to some liquid fluxes. Also available are paste fluxes formed from mixtures of about one-third borax added to a mineral grease, such as petroleum jelly, with other chemicals added as desired. Pastes are convenient for soldering operations in which a large quantity of flux is desired and its application is directed to a specific area. Powder fluxes, which are normally used for metals during the melting for a casting operation, are sprinkled lightly on the metal. Powder fluxes may contain finely divided charcoal or other ingredients mixed with borax and boric acid; this combination gives added protection by producing what is described as a *reducing flux*. The charcoal not only helps prevent the formation of oxides on the metal surface, but also reduces oxides that have already formed to free metal. Fluxes in the powder form also may contain a very small percentage (1% to 2%) of finely divided silica flour, which holds the molten flux in position on the surface of the hot metal.

CHROMIUM-CONTAINING ALLOYS

When soldering stainless-steel or cast cobalt-based alloys that contain chromium, a special flux is required because borax and boric acid alone do not dissolve chromium oxides. Normally the fluxes for these soldering operations should contain about 50% to 60% potassium fluoride, or another fluoride, mixed with 25% to 35% boric acid (H_3BO_4), 6% to 8% borax glass, and 8% to 10% potassium or sodium carbonate. An equal mixture of boric acid and the fluoride salt may be formed into a paste for soldering when they are ground together with a few drops of water, which is considered effective in such soldering operations. Other similar compositions have been recommended. Pastes should not be formulated with petroleum grease for these applications because the carbon formed in heating alters the properties of the alloy being soldered or cast.

Choosing the proper flux (borax or fluoride) for the soldering operation is important. The choice of flux is dictated by the type of alloy to be soldered or cast, not by the type of solder used. If the alloy contains chromium, such as stainless steel wires for orthodontics or cobalt-chromium alloys for partial dentures, the proper choice is fluoride flux, regardless of whether gold- or silver-based solder is used. If noble or high-noble alloys are to be soldered, the proper choice is borax flux, regardless of the solder employed.

A principle governing the use of fluxes for any purpose is that neither too much nor too little should be applied to the metal during the heating operation. When too little flux is applied, it tends to burn off and be ineffective; when too much flux is applied, it may become entangled in the molten metal to produce a defect by inclusion.

SELECTED PROBLEMS

Problem 1

An invested casting ring was removed from the oven in preparation for melting and casting the alloy; however, there was a delay of several minutes before the alloy was cast. The casting did not fit. What was the probable cause of this problem, and how can it be corrected?

Solution

When the casting ring is removed from the oven and placed into the casting machine, the investment rapidly cools and contracts. A delay of more than a minute generally results in sufficient shrinkage to produce an undersized casting. The recommended procedure is to premelt the gold alloy in the crucible of the casting machine before removing the casting ring from the oven and to cast promptly. Reheating the ring is not recommended because the contraction of most investments is not fully reversible. Allowing the investment to cool too much also risks its fracture during the rapid contraction.

Problem 2

A casting that did not seat well had external and internal surface irregularities. How were these surface irregularities produced, and how might they be avoided?

Solution a

Air bubbles become attached to the wax pattern during investing, thereby producing nodules on the casting. Their removal can alter the fit of the casting. To avoid air bubbles, a wetting agent should be applied to the wax pattern, and the investment should be mixed and the pattern invested under vacuum.

Solution b

When too much water is used in mixing the investment, a rougher surface of the casting can result. The powder and liquid of the investment should be dispensed accurately.

Solution c

The position and direction of the sprue affect the turbulence of the molten alloy as it is introduced into the mold cavity. Localized roughness can result from abrasion of the mold. Attach the sprue to the bulkiest portion of the wax pattern. The point of contact should be flared, and the sprue should be directed toward the margins.

Solution d

Prolonged heating of a gypsum-bonded investment at a temperature above 650° C caused a breakdown of the investment, resulting in a rough surface on the casting. Casting should be completed promptly when wax burnout has been achieved.

Solution e

Phosphate-bonded investments produce water droplets as a byproduct of the reaction. These droplets can attach to the pattern and result in a positive defect in the casting. This problem can be prevented by accurately measuring the investment and liquid solution and following the mixing times and procedures exactly.

Problem 3

A full-crown casting was made by reheating an invested casting ring; the ring had been heated to the burnout temperature the day before, then cooled when the procedure could not be completed. The resulting crown did not fit. What caused this problem, and how can it be corrected?

Solution

Irreversible chemical and physical changes in the binder and refractory of the investment occur when the investment is heated and then cooled. On reheating, the dimensional changes of the mold will be less than normal. Therefore, the casting was likely too small. If a casting procedure cannot be completed promptly with a heated investment, a new wax pattern should be invested and cast.

Problem 4

A soldered joint showed a large amount of porosity. What caused the porosity, and how can it be avoided?

Solution

Porosity in the soldered joint is usually associated with excessive heat applied during the fusion of the solder or with improper fluxing. Scrupulously clean and properly flux the surfaces to be soldered. The reducing part of the flame should be used, and the solder should be heated only as much as necessary to ensure adequate flow.

Problem 5

During a soldering operation, the fine margins of a casting were fused. What factor produced this problem, and how can it be avoided?

Solution a

If the layer of soldering investment protecting the margins of a casting is too thin or is porous, the refractory material will not be able to act effectively as a thermal barrier. The margins of a casting should be protected with a thick layer of investment carefully painted onto the occlusal areas and along the proximal walls.

Solution b

If the soldering investment is mixed with a high water/powder ratio, the strength of the investment will be low. Portions of the investment may fracture during heating, thereby exposing margins to the soldering operation. The powder and liquid of the soldering investment should be dispensed accurately.

Solution c

Overheating the investment assembly for a long period can transfer heat to the protected margins, thus causing them to melt. Adequate temperature should be reached in the furnace, after which the reducing flame of the torch should be applied properly. The solder should be fused promptly.

Problem 6

During a soldering operation, the flow of the solder appears good, but the soldered crown no longer fits the die or the tooth after soldering. What could have happened?

Solution a

If the solder flowed onto the margins of the crown or into the interior of the crown, it will prevent the crown from seating properly on the die or tooth. This can be prevented by using antiflux appropriately to prevent the flow of solder into undesirable areas. The judicious use of soldering investment can also protect the margins somewhat.

Solution b

If the crown was heated to too high a temperature, then sag or other distortion of the crown can occur, which then prevents the crown from fitting. For this reason, a solder should be selected that has a liquidus at least 50° C less than that of the crown. Furthermore, the solder and crown should be heated only to the extent necessary to melt the solder.

Problem 7

A full-crown wax pattern was sprued to the bulkiest portion with a single sprue. After casting, porosity was observed on the pulpal floor of the gold crown. What could have caused the problem, and how can the problem be avoided on the next casting?

Solution

The porosity, commonly known as *suckback porosity,* resulted from improper freezing of the alloy so that molten alloy could not compensate for shrinkage of the solidifying alloy. Several conditions could have caused the problem: (1) The diameter of the sprue may have been too small or the length of the sprue too long, resulting in the alloy's freezing in the sprue before freezing in the crown. A shorter, larger-diameter sprue should be used. (2) The single sprue directed the molten alloy to an area of the pulpal floor, and the investment in this area became much hotter than the surrounding investment. This condition, coupled with the poor thermal conductivity of the investment, may have caused the alloy in this area to stay molten after it had frozen in the sprue. The direction of the sprue should be toward the margins of the restoration, and a Y-shaped sprue should be used to distribute the flow of the alloy more uniformly. Increasing the temperature of the high-heat investment before casting reduces the differences in the temperature of the investment from the impingement of the molten alloy. (3) The amount of alloy forming the sprue button may have been too small in relationship to the size of the pattern; again, the sprue and button froze before the alloy in the crown, causing the porosity.

Problem 8

A removable, cobalt-chromium partial-denture alloy was melted with an oxygen-acetylene flame. There were problems adjusting the torch, however, and the alloy was heated three times longer than normal. What, if any, problems might be expected with the cast framework?

Solution

Extended heating of the alloy with such a flame will probably increase the carbon content of the cast alloy. The alloy contains several elements that form carbides under such conditions, and their precipitation increases the brittleness and decreases the elongation of the alloy. The clasps of the cast partial denture will therefore be susceptible to fracture during minor adjustments.

Problem 9

A low–fusing point (Be-containing) nickel-chromium alloy was to be cast to embedded platinum-gold-palladium (PGP) wire in the preparation of a partial-denture framework. A gypsum-bonded investment was used, but after the investment had been heated to the casting temperature, casting of the alloy was delayed for four hours. Later, when the PGP wire was bent to form a clasp, it was brittle and broke. What caused this embrittlement and could it have been prevented?

Solution

Low–fusing point nickel-chromium alloys melt at substantially higher temperatures than gold-based alloys, just under 1300° C (compared to 900° to 1100° C). Therefore special gypsum-bonded investments are often used that contain oxalic acid, oxalates, carbonates, and carbon, which release CO_2 at various temperatures during heating and keep the mold cavity flushed with CO_2 to remove any sulfur oxides from the calcium-sulfate binder. On extended heating these CO_2 sources are used up and the sulfur oxides react with the PGP wire, causing embrittlement. Embrittlement will also occur if a gypsum-bonded casting investment (designed for gold alloys) that does not contain these protective chemicals is used, even if there is no delay in the casting procedure. Thus casting of the nickel-chromium alloy to the embedded PGP wire should be done promptly after the investment has reached proper temperature.

Problem 10

Why is it necessary to prepare a duplicate investment cast from the master stone model when preparing a wax pattern for partial-denture framework?

Solution

The large wax pattern is too fragile to be handled and sprued as a free-standing wax pattern as is done for crowns and bridges. Waxing must therefore be done on a cast that becomes part of the investment mold. If the stone model (master cast) were used, it would not survive the temperatures necessary during casting and burnout, and its decomposition during heating would embrittle the alloy. Furthermore, the model would be destroyed in the process of casting and there would then be no model on which to add the acrylic portions of the partial denture. Thus a duplicate model, called the *refractory cast,* is made and the wax pattern is constructed on this model and invested in place. After casting, the framework (now in metal) is transferred to the master cast for subsequent steps in the fabrication process.

BIBLIOGRAPHY

Anusavice KJ, editor: *Phillips' science of dental materials,* Philadelphia, 1996, WB Saunders.

Asgar K: Casting restorations. In Clark, JW, editor: *Clinical dentistry,* vol 4, New York, 1976, Harper and Row.

Craig RG, Powers JM, Wataha JC: *Dental materials: properties and manipulation,* ed 7, St Louis, 2000, Mosby.

Dootz ER: Technology of casting and soldering alloys for metal-ceramic applications, *Ceramic Eng Sci Proc* 6:84, 1985.

Mackert JR: An expert system for analysis of casting failures, *Int J Prosthodont* 1:268, 1988.

O'Brien WJ, editor: *Dental materials and their selection,* ed 2, Carol Stream, IL, 1997, Quintessence.

Tuccillo JJ, Nielsen JP: Sprue design for cast gold alloys, *Dent lab Rev* 39:14 (June), 14 (July), 1964.

Wagner AW: Causes and cures for porosities in dental casting, *Quint Dent Technol* 3:57, 1979.

Chapter 18

Ceramics

The term *ceramic* is defined as any product made essentially from a nonmetallic material by firing at a high temperature to achieve desirable properties. The term *porcelain* refers to a family of ceramic materials composed essentially of kaolin, quartz, and feldspar, also fired at high temperature. Dental ceramics for *ceramic-metal* restorations belong to this family and are commonly referred to as *dental porcelains.*

The art of processing dental ceramics has remained, to a great extent, with those persons who have learned the art directly from others. The laboratory portion of a ceramic restoration is usually made in a commercial dental laboratory by a skilled technician working with specialized equipment to the shape and shade specifications provided by the dentist. Skilled technicians and artisans are also employed by the manufacturers of artificial denture teeth to produce the many forms, types, and shades necessary in this application of porcelain.

HISTORICAL BACKGROUND

Dental ceramics were first used in dentistry in the late 1700s. Porcelain jacket crowns were developed in the early 1900s. They consisted of feldspathic or aluminous porcelain baked on a thin platinum foil and can be considered the ancestors of all-ceramic crowns. Because their low strength, however, porcelain jacket crowns were limited to anterior teeth. In the 1960s, the poor match in thermal expansion (and contraction) between framework alloys and veneering ceramics, which often led to failures and fractures upon cooling, stimulated the development of leucite-containing feldspathic porcelains. The problem was solved by mixing controlled amounts of high-expansion leucite with feldspar glass at the manufacturing stage. This allowed the adjustment of the coefficient of thermal expansion of feldspathic porcelains to very narrow specifications. This invention led to considerable improvement in the reliability of ceramic-metals and allowed ceramic materials to be bonded to a metal framework. During cooling, the thermal contraction of the metal framework is slightly higher than that of the veneering ceramic, thus placing the internal surface of the ceramic in compression. Because ceramics are stronger in compression than in tension, this property is used to advantage to provide increased resistance to shattering.

The end of the twentieth century saw the introduction of several innovative systems for fabricating all-ceramic dental restorations. The first was a castable glass-ceramic system in which the restoration was cast using the lost-wax technique and later heat-treated to promote its transformation into a glass-ceramic. This castable system was later abandoned due to processing difficulties and the high incidence of fractures. Ceramics for slip-casting, heat-pressing, and machining were developed concurrently within the past fifteen years. New materials for all-ceramic restorations are introduced every year and attest to the increasing popularity of ceramics in dentistry.

CLASSIFICATION OF DENTAL CERAMICS

Dental ceramics can be classified according to their fusion temperature, application, fabrication technique, or crystalline phase (Table 18-1).

FUSION TEMPERATURE

The high-fusing ceramics have a fusing range from 1315° to 1370° C; the medium-fusing ceramics, from 1090° to 1260° C; and the low-fusing ceramics, from 870° to 1065° C. This classification dates back to the early 1940s. It was employed more intensively with the earlier dental ceramic compositions, which belong to the triaxial porcelain compositions. The term *triaxial* means the composition has three major ingredients: quartz (or flint), feldspar, and clay (or kaolin). The fusion temperature is dictated by the relative amounts of these three ingredients. It is interesting to note that these temperature ranges vary from textbook to textbook and are not continuous. This is related to the fact that the processing of ceramic materials was initially monitored us-

TABLE 18-1 Classification of Dental Ceramic Materials

	Fabrication	Crystalline Phase
ALL-CERAMIC	Machined	Alumina (Al_2O_3) Feldspar ($KAlSi_3O_8$) Mica ($KMg_{2.5}Si_4O_{10}F_2$)
	Slip-cast	Alumina (Al_2O_3) Spinel ($MgAl_2O_4$)
	Heat-pressed	Leucite ($KAlSi_2O_6$) Lithium disilicate ($Li_2Si_2O_5$)
	Sintered	Alumina (Al_2O_3) Leucite ($KAlSi_2O_6$)
CERAMIC-METAL	Sintered	Leucite ($KAlSi_2O_6$)
DENTURE TEETH	Manufactured	Feldspar

ing pyrometric ceramic cones of specific composition. These cones are placed in the furnace and bend under their own weight when the temperature is reached. The medium- and high-fusing ceramics are used for denture teeth. Dental ceramics for ceramic-metal or all-ceramic fixed restorations belong to the low- or medium-fusing categories. Ultra-low-fusing dental ceramics with firing temperatures below 870° C have been recently introduced.

The medium- and low-fusing porcelains powders are usually modified by the manufacturer with chemicals or fluxes (boron oxide or alkali carbonates) of low melting temperature. They are melted together (prefused) and reduced to powder form. The addition of fluxing agents results in narrower fusing ranges and increases the tendency for the porcelain to slump during repair or when making additions, staining, or glazing. Prefusing and regrinding, however, increase the homogeneity of the powder, which may be an advantage in the handling and fusing operations. Low firing temperatures are a definite asset in the fusion of porcelain to metal, because the differences in the coefficients of expansion of the porcelain and metal can be tolerated better at lower temperature ranges.

High-fusing porcelains are considered superior in strength, insolubility, translucency, and maintenance of accuracy in form during repeated firings. Recent tests of low-fusing products, however, indicate that they are essentially as strong as the high-fusing types, and their solubility and translucency are adequate. The principal practical advantage of high-fusing porcelain is therefore its ability to be repaired, added to, stained, or glazed without distortion.

APPLICATIONS

Ceramics have three major applications in dentistry: (1) ceramics for metal crowns and fixed partial dentures, (2) all-ceramic crowns, inlays, onlays, and veneers, when esthetics is a priority, and (3) ceramic denture teeth.

FABRICATION TECHNIQUE

This classification is summarized in Table 18-1. One of the most common fabrication techniques for dental ceramics is called *sintering*. Sintering is the process of heating the ceramic to ensure densification. This occurs by viscous flow when the firing temperature is reached. Ceramics fired

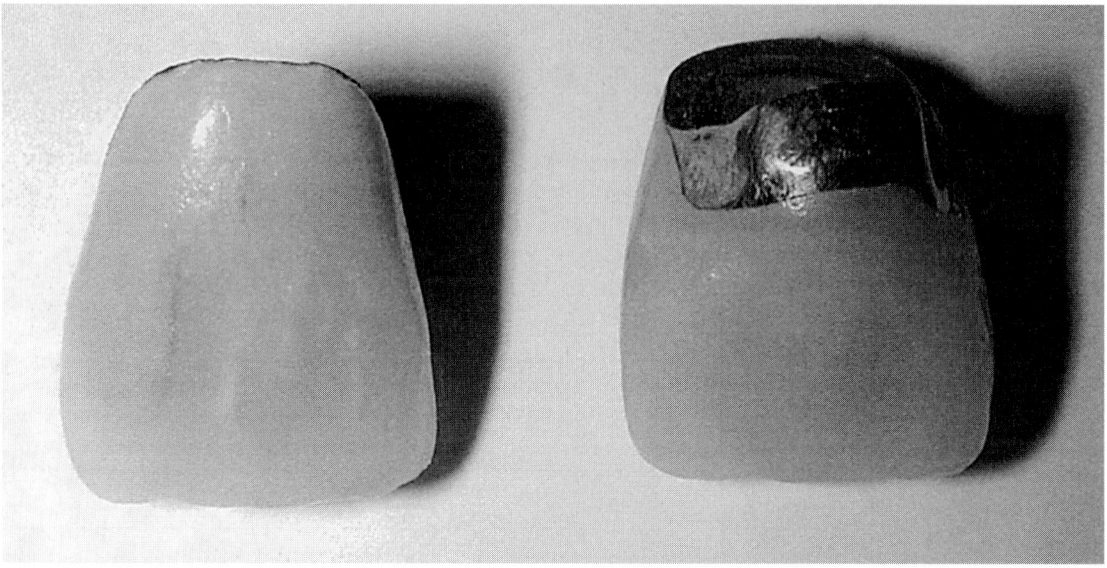

Fig. 18-1 Lingual and labial view of a ceramic-metal restoration.

to metals are processed by sintering, whereas all-ceramic materials encompass a wider range of processing techniques, including heat-pressing, machining, and slip-casting.

CRYSTALLINE PHASE

Regardless of their applications or fabrication technique, after firing, dental ceramics are composed of two phases: a glassy (or vitreous) phase surrounding a crystalline phase. Depending on the nature and the amount of crystalline phase present, the mechanical and optical properties of dental ceramics vary widely. Increasing the amount of glassy phase lowers the resistance to crack propagation but increases translucency. Materials for all-ceramic restorations have increased amounts of crystalline phase (between 35% and 90%) for better mechanical properties. Table 18-1 lists the various crystalline phases found in dental ceramics.

CERAMIC-METAL RESTORATIONS

Ceramic-metal restorations consist of a cast metallic framework (or core) on which at least two layers of ceramic are baked. The first layer applied is the opaque layer, consisting of ceramic, rich in opacifying oxides. Its role is to mask the darkness of the oxidized metal framework to achieve adequate esthetics. As the first layer, it also provides ceramic-metal bond. The next step is the buildup of dentin and enamel (most translucent) ceramics to obtain an esthetic appearance similar to that of a natural tooth. Opaque, dentin and enamel ceramics are available in various shades. After building up or modelling the porcelain powders, the ceramic-metal crown is sintered in a porcelain furnace.

Fig. 18-1 illustrates a ceramic-metal restoration, and Fig. 18-2 shows a three-unit ceramic-metal fixed partial denture. When fabricated by skilled technicians, these restorations can provide excellent esthetics, along with good strength because of the alloy framework. The alloys used for casting the substructure are usually gold-based containing tin and indium. Gold-palladium, silver-palladium, and nickel-chromium alloys were initially developed as lower-cost alternatives. However, the recent steep increase in the price of palladium have changed the palladium-containing alloys into a higher-cost alternative.

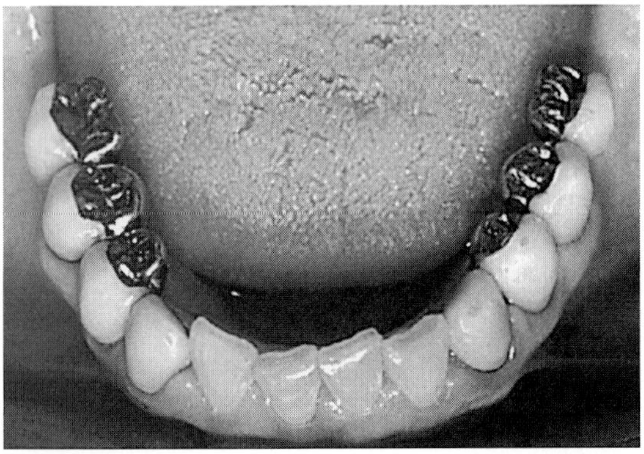

Fig. 18-2 View of ceramic-metal fixed partial denture.
(Courtesy Dr. Julie A. Holloway.)

It is essential that the coefficient of thermal expansion of the veneering ceramic be slightly lower than that of the alloy to ensure that the ceramic is in slight compression after cooling. This will establish a better resistance to crack propagation of the ceramic-metal restoration. The ceramic-metal systems are described in detail in Chapter 19.

COMPOSITION AND MANUFACTURE

COMPOSITION

The quality of any ceramic depends on the choice of ingredients, correct proportioning of each ingredient, and control of the firing procedure. Only the purest ingredients are used in the manufacture of dental porcelains because of the stringent requirements of color, toughness without brittleness, insolubility, and translucency, as well as the desirable characteristics of strength and thermal expansion. In many instances, the manufacturer must formulate a product that is a compromise.

In its mineral state, feldspar, the main raw ingredient of dental porcelains, is crystalline and opaque with an indefinite color between gray and pink. Chemically it is designated as potassium aluminum silicate, with a composition of $K_2O \cdot Al_2O_3 \cdot 6SiO_2$. The fusion temperature of feldspar varies between 1125° and 1170° C, depending on its purity.

Iron and mica are commonly found as impurities in feldspar. It is particularly important to remove the iron, because metallic oxides act as strong coloring agents in porcelain. To remove iron, each piece of feldspar is broken with a steel hammer, and only the uniformly light-colored pieces are selected for use in the porcelain. These pieces are ground in mills to a fine powder. The final particle size is carefully controlled by screening to remove the coarser particles, and flotation processes are used to remove the excessively fine particles. The dry powder is then slowly vibrated down inclined planes equipped with a series of narrow ledges formed by induction magnets. In this way the remaining iron contaminants are separated and removed, and the feldspar is made ready for use.

Pure quartz (SiO_2) crystals are used in dental porcelain and ground to the finest grain size possible. Silica is added, and contributes stability to the mass during heating by providing a glassy framework for the other ingredients.

MANUFACTURE

Feldspathic dental porcelains in recent years are made mainly with potash feldspar ($K_2O \cdot Al_2O_3 \cdot 6SiO_2$) and small additions of quartz (SiO_2). During the manufacturing process, the ground ingredients are carefully mixed together. Alkali metal carbonates are added as fluxes and the mix is heated to about 1200° C in large crucibles. At high temperature, the feldspar decomposes to form a glassy phase with an amorphous structure, as illustrated in Fig. 18-3, and a crystalline (mineral) phase consisting of leucite ($KAlSi_2O_6$ or $K_2O \cdot Al_2O_3 \cdot 4SiO_2$). The crystalline structure of tetragonal leucite is illustrated in Fig. 18-4.

The mix of leucite and glassy phase is then cooled very rapidly (quenched) in water which causes the mass to shatter in small fragments. The product obtained, called a *frit,* is ball-milled to

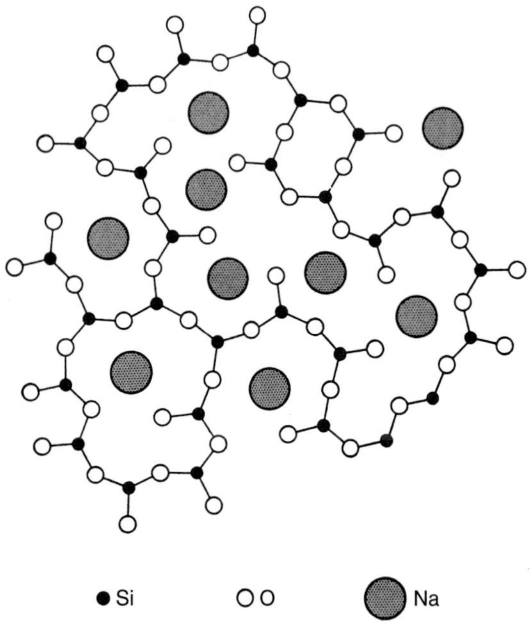

Fig. 18-3 Two-dimensional structure of sodium silicate glass.
(Modified from Warren BE, Biscoe J: *J Am Ceram Soc* 21:259, 1938.)

achieve proper particle size distribution. Coloring pigments in small quantities are added at this stage, to obtain the delicate shades necessary to mimic natural teeth. The metallic pigments include titanium oxide for yellow-brown shades, manganese oxide for lavender, iron oxide for brown, cobalt oxide for blue, copper or chromium oxides for green, and nickel oxide for brown. In the past, uranium oxide was used to provide fluorescence; however, because of the small amount of radioactivity, lanthanide oxides (such as cerium oxide) are being substituted for this purpose. Tin, titanium, and zirconium oxides are used as opacifiers.

After the manufacturing process is completed, feldspathic dental porcelain consists of two phases. One is the vitreous (or glass) phase, and the other is the crystalline (or mineral) phase. The glass phase formed during the manufacturing process has properties typical of glass, such as brittleness, nondirectional fracture pattern, translucency, and high surface tension in the fluid state. The crystalline phase is leucite, a potassium alumino-silicate with high thermal expansion (>20 × 10^{-6}/° C). The amount present (10% to 20%) controls the thermal expansion coefficient of the porcelain. Leucite also contributes strength to the porcelain; high-leucite porcelains are approximately twice as strong as those containing low concentrations. The microstructure of conventional feldspathic porcelain is shown in Fig. 18-5; the glassy phase has been lightly acid-etched to reveal the leucite crystals.

Typical compositions for opaque and dentin porcelain powders are given in Table 18-2.

PROCESSING

The production of a satisfactory porcelain restoration requires careful attention to the principles and details of the operation.

Porcelain Application and Condensation After the tooth has been prepared, an elastomeric impression is made, and a working model or die is formed of a suitable die material. A wax framework is fabricated and the wax is cut back by 1 mm in the esthetic areas to ensure enough space for porcelain application. The framework is cast by the lost wax technique. It is extremely important that all sharp angles be rounded to avoid stress concentrations and wedge effects in the fired porcelain. After careful cleaning of the metal framework, a thin layer of opaque porcelain is applied and baked. Dentin porcelain powder, in the shade selected for the body or dentin portion, is mixed with modeling liquid (mainly distilled water) to a creamy consistency and is applied on the opaque layer, with allowances made for shrinkage. To produce minimum shrinkage and a dense, strong porcelain, it is important to achieve a thorough condensation of the particles at this stage. Various means of condensation may be employed. The vibration method is particularly efficient in driving the excess water towards the surface. The wet porcelain mix is applied with a spatula and vibrated gently until the particles settle together. The excess water is then removed with a clean tissue or an absorbent medium. A cross section of

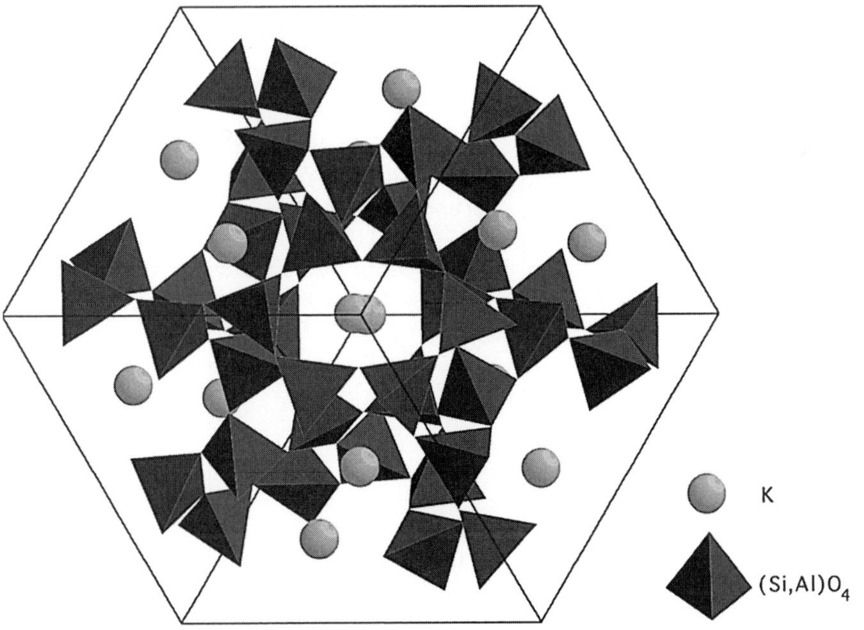

Fig. 18-4 Three-dimensional structure of leucite ($KAlSi_2O_6$).

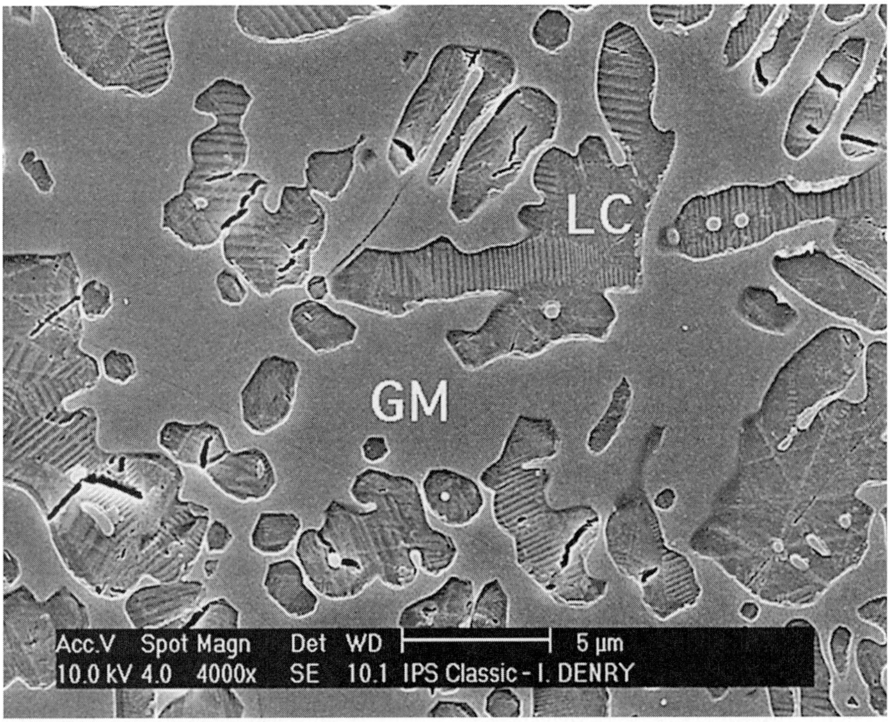

Fig. 18-5 Scanning electron micrograph showing the microstructure of feldspathic porcelain for ceramic-metal restorations. *GM*, Glassy matrix; *LC*, leucite crystal.

TABLE 18-2 Composition of Dental Ceramics for Fusing to High-Temperature Alloys

Compound	Biodent Opaque BG 2 (%)	Ceramco Opaque 60 (%)	V.M.K. Opaque 131 (%)	Biodent Dentin BD 27 (%)	Ceramco Dentin T 69 (%)
SiO_2	52.0	55.0	52.4	56.9	62.2
Al_2O_3	13.55	11.65	15.15	11.80	13.40
CaO	—	—	—	0.61	0.98
K_2O	11.05	9.6	9.9	10.0	11.3
Na_2O	5.28	4.75	6.58	5.42	5.37
TiO_2	3.01	—	2.59	0.61	—
ZrO_2	3.22	0.16	5.16	1.46	0.34
SnO_2	6.4	15.0	4.9	—	0.5
Rb_2O	0.09	0.04	0.08	0.10	0.06
BaO	1.09	—	—	3.52	—
ZnO	—	0.26	—	—	—
UO_3	—	—	—	—	—
B_2O_3, CO_2, and H_2O	4.31	3.54	3.24	9.58	5.85

From Nally JN, Meyer, JM: *Schweiz Monatsschr Zahnheilkd* 80:250, 1970.

a ceramic-metal crown is shown in Fig. 18-6, *right.*

Other methods of condensation include the spatulation and brush techniques. The spatulation method consists of smoothing the wet porcelain with a suitable spatula until the excess water is brought to the surface, where it is absorbed with a tissue. The brush or capillary attraction method depends on the action of dry porcelain powder to remove the excess water by capillary attraction. The dry powder is applied with a brush to a small area of the wet porcelain mass, and as the water is withdrawn toward the dry area, the wet particles are pulled closely together. This process is repeated as dry powder is placed on the opposite side of each new addition of the wet mix.

Drying After the porcelain mix has been applied and condensed, the restoration is placed in front of an open preheated porcelain furnace to be dried. This drying stage, which lasts between 5 and 8 minutes, is a very important step; it ensures that any remaining excess water is removed from the porcelain mix. During the drying stage, the water diffuses towards the surface and then evaporates. If the piece is dried too quickly, the water evaporation rate becomes greater than the diffusion rate and the unfired porcelain can undergo spontaneous breakage. After the mass is placed in the furnace, remaining free and combined water is removed in various stages of heating until a temperature of 480° C is reached.

Firing/Sintering Porcelain restorations may be fired either by temperature control alone or by controlled temperature and a specified time. In the first method the furnace temperature is raised at a constant rate until a specified temperature is reached. In the second method the temperature is raised at a given rate until certain levels are reached, after which the temperature is maintained for a measured period until the desired reactions are completed.

Either method gives satisfactory results, but the time and temperature method is generally preferred because it is more likely to produce a

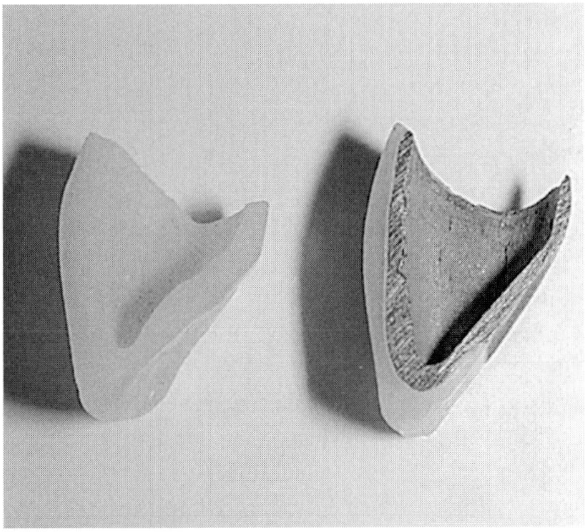

Fig. 18-6 Cross sectional micrograph of a ceramic-metal crown *(right)*. Cross sectional view of an all-ceramic crown *(left)*.

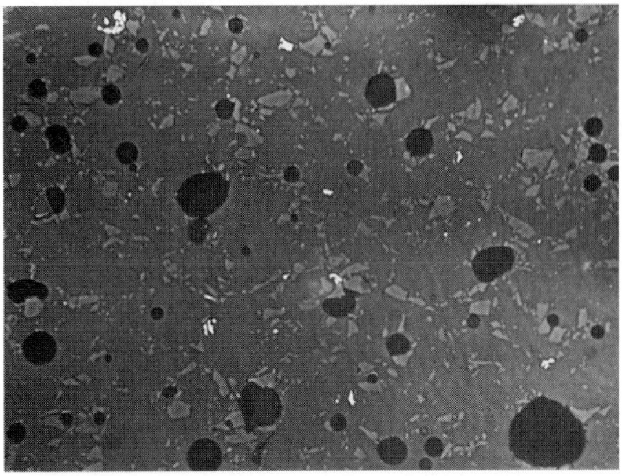

Fig. 18-7 Microscopic view of air-fired porcelain, showing porosity.

(Courtesy Semmelman JO, York, Pa, 1959, Dentsply International.)

uniform product. Porcelain is a poor thermal conductor, and thus too rapid heating may overfuse the outer layers before the inner portion is properly sintered.

As the temperature is raised, the particles of porcelain fuse by sintering. Sintering is the process responsible for the fusion of the porcelain particles to form a continuous mass. During this densification, the volume change, ΔV, in the early stages is related to the surface tension of the porcelain, γ, viscosity, η, the particle radius, r, and sintering time, t, as shown in the following equation:

$$\frac{\Delta V}{V_0} = \frac{9\gamma}{4\eta r}t$$

As this equation indicates, the lower the viscosity and the finer the particle size, the greater the rate of densification. A minimum number of three firing operations are needed in the fabrication of a ceramic-metal restoration: one for the opaque portion, one for the dentin and enamel portion, and another for the stain and glaze. However, due to the shrinkage associated with the sintering process, it is necessary to oversize the porcelain buildup. For this reason, only experienced operators can complete a porcelain restoration in only three firings.

During the second firing, the dentin and enamel portion, which is formed approximately 13% oversize, is heated to the biscuit (or bisque) bake. This temperature is 56° C below the fusing temperature of the porcelain. Virtually all the shrinkage takes place during this firing.

The presence of gas bubbles (pores) has always been a problem in the production of dental porcelain. The extent to which pores may exist in air-fired porcelain is shown in Fig. 18-7. The specimen shown was ground and polished, and the round black spots are the cross-sectioned pores. It has been calculated that air-fired porcelain contains as much as 6.3% voids. This not only results in undesirable roughness and pits when a porcelain crown must be ground, but also exerts an even more undesirable effect on the strength and optical properties of the porcelain.

Pores are caused by air trapped during the sintering process. Air spaces become spherical under the influence of surface tension and expand with increased temperature. Porcelains for ceramic-metal restorations are fired under vacuum. As the porcelain furnace door closes, the pressure is lowered to 0.1 atmosphere. The temperature is raised until the firing temperature is reached; the vacuum is then released and the furnace pressure returns to 1 atmosphere. The increase in pressure from 0.1 to 1 atmosphere helps compress and close the residual pores. This occurs by viscous flow at the firing temperature. The result is a dense, relatively pore-free porcelain, as illustrated in Fig. 18-8. Studies have shown that sintering under vacuum reduces the amount of porosity to 0.56% (from 5.6%) in air-fired dental porcelains. Vacuum-firing improves the translucency and decreases the surface roughness of feldspathic porcelains, and increases impact strength approximately 50%.

An alternate method uses the principle of diffusion to secure improved density in fused porcelain. A diffusible gas such as helium may be introduced to the furnace at low pressure during the sintering (densification) stage. The helium gas (instead of air) is therefore entrapped in the interstitial spaces, and because its molecular diameter is smaller than the porcelain lattice, it diffuses outward under the pressure of the shrinking porcelain.

Before the development of these improved firing methods, fine texture and translucency were not possible at the same time. Maximum translucency was obtained only by use of coarse powders that trapped only a few relatively large pores, but which also produced an undesirable granular appearance. Fine-grained powders developed a better texture but increased the opacity because of the large number of small pores. Vacuum-firing achieved both fine texture and translucency in ceramic-metal restorations; however, another property was still missing. Human enamel exhibits a specific optical property called *opalescence:* a scattering effect that makes it appears bluish when viewed in reflected light and orange when viewed in transmitted light. Studies of pigment particle size and dispersion have made it possible to produce partially opalescent restorations that compare favorably with natural teeth.

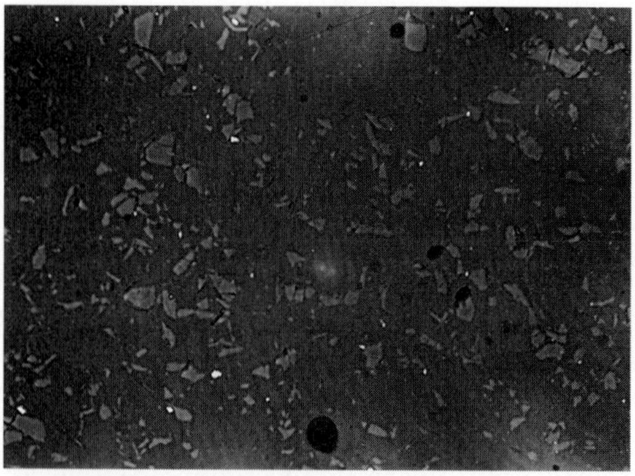

Fig. 18-8 Microscopic view of vacuum-fired porcelain showing minimal porosity.
(Courtesy Semmelman JO, York, Pa, 1959, Dentsply International.)

Glazing After the porcelain is cleaned and any necessary stains are applied, it is returned to the furnace for the final glaze firing. Usually, the glazing step is very short; when the glazing temperature is reached, a thin glassy film (glaze) is formed by viscous flow on the porcelain surface. Overglazing is to be avoided, because it gives the restoration an unnatural shiny appearance and causes loss of contour and shade modification. Glazing temperatures and times vary with the type and brand of porcelain employed.

Cooling It is commonly accepted that the cooling stage is a critical one in the fabrication of ceramic-metal restorations and that extreme (too fast or too slow) cooling rates should be avoided. Too-rapid cooling of the outer layers may result in surface crazing or cracking; this is also called *thermal shock.* Very slow cooling (e.g., in a furnace) as well as multiple firings, might induce the formation of additional leucite and increase the overall coefficient of thermal expansion of the ceramic, and may also result in surface cracking and crazing. Slow cooling is preferred, and is accomplished by removing the fired restoration from the furnace as soon as the firing is finished and placing it under a glass cover to protect it from air currents and possible contamination by dirt.

ALL-CERAMIC RESTORATIONS

Materials for all-ceramic restorations use a wide variety of crystalline phases as reinforcing agents and contain up to 90% by volume of crystalline phase. The nature, amount, and particle size distribution of the crystalline phase directly influence the mechanical and optical properties of the material. The match between the refractive indexes of the crystalline phase and glassy matrix is an important factor for controlling the translucency of the porcelain.

As mentioned earlier, several processing techniques are available for fabricating all-ceramic crowns: sintering, heat-pressing, slip-casting, and machining. Fig. 18-6, *left,* illustrates the cross section of an all-ceramic crown.

SINTERED ALL-CERAMIC MATERIALS

Two main types of all-ceramic materials are available for the sintering technique: alumina-based ceramic and leucite-reinforced ceramic.

Alumina-Based Ceramic Aluminous core ceramic is a typical example of strengthening by dispersion of a crystalline phase. Alumina has a high modulus of elasticity (350 GPa) and high fracture toughness (3.5 to 4 MPa · $m^{0.5}$). Its dispersion in a glassy matrix of similar thermal expansion coefficient leads to a significant strengthening of the core. It has been proposed that the excellent bond between the alumina and the glass phase is responsible for this increase in strength compared with leucite-containing ceramics. The first aluminous core porcelains contained 40% to 50% alumina by weight. The core was baked on a platinum foil and later veneered with matched-expansion porcelain. Aluminous core ceramic is now baked directly on a refractory die. Aluminous core porcelains have flexural strengths of about 138 MPa and shear strengths of 145 MPa.

Leucite-Reinforced Feldspathic Porcelain A feldspathic porcelain containing up to 45% by volume tetragonal leucite is available for the fabricating all-ceramic sintered restorations. Leucite acts as a reinforcing phase; the greater leucite content (compared with conventional feldspathic porcelain for ceramic-metal applications) leads to higher flexural strength (104 MPa) and compressive strength. The large amount of leucite in the material also contributes to a high thermal contraction coefficient. In addition, the large thermal contraction mismatch between leucite (22 to 25 × 10^{-6}/° C) and the glassy matrix (8 × 10^{-6}/° C) results in the development of tangential compressive stresses in the glass around the leucite crystals upon cooling. These stresses can act as crack deflectors and contribute to increased resistance of the weaker glassy phase to crack propagation.

Magnesia-Based Core Porcelain A high-expansion magnesia core material has been developed that is compatible with the same dentin porcelains used for ceramic-metal restorations. The flexural strength of unglazed magnesia core ceramic is twice as high (131 MPa) as that of conventional feldspathic porcelain (70 MPa), with an average coefficient of expansion of 14.5 × 10^{-6}/° C. The main advantage of this core material is that it allows a laboratory to veneer it with the more widely available porcelains for ceramic-metal restorations. The magnesia core material can be significantly strengthened by glazing, thereby placing the surface under residual compressive stresses that have to be overcome before fracture can occur.

Sintered all-ceramic restorations are slowly being replaced by heat-pressed all-ceramic restorations that simplify the processing steps.

Heat-Pressed All-Ceramic Materials

Heat-pressing relies on the application of external pressure to sinter and shape the ceramic at high temperature. Heat-pressing is also called *high-temperature injection molding.* It is used in dentistry to produce all-ceramic crowns, inlays, onlays, veneers, and more recently, fixed partial dentures. Heat-pressing classically helps avoid large pores and promotes a good dispersion of the crystalline phase within the glassy matrix. The mechanical properties of many ceramic sys-

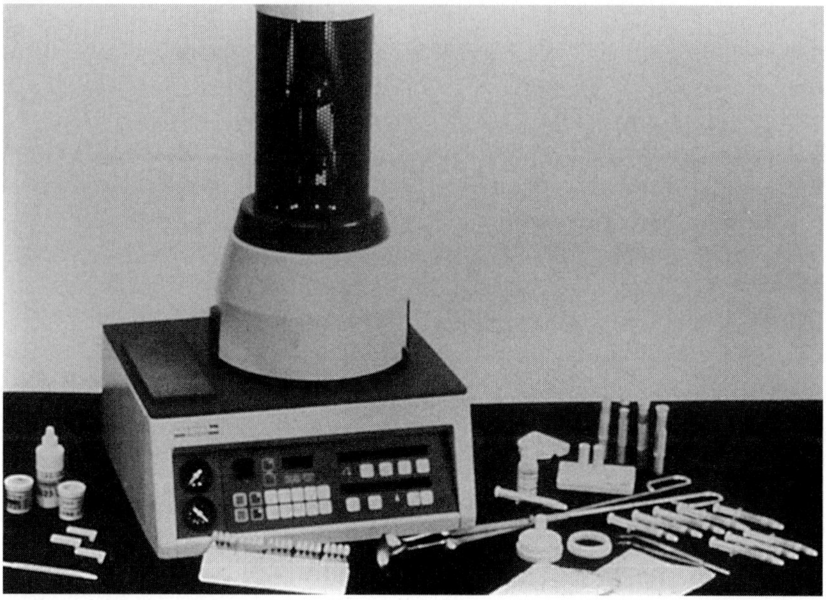

Fig. 18-9 The Empress high-temperature injection molding systems for all ceramic restorations. (Courtesy Ivoclar Inc., Amherst, NY, 1995.)

tems are maximized with high density and small crystal size.

Leucite-Based Leucite-based ceramics are available for heat-pressing. Leucite ($KAlSi_2O_6$ or $K_2O \cdot Al_2O_3 \cdot 4SiO_2$) is used as a reinforcing phase in amounts varying from 35% to 55%. Ceramic ingots are pressed between 1150° and 1180° C (under a pressure of 0.3 to 0.4 MPa) into the refractory mold made by the lost-wax technique (Fig. 18-9). This temperature is held for about 20 minutes in a specially designed automatic press furnace. The ceramic ingots are available in different shades. The final microstructure of these heat-pressed ceramics consists of leucite crystals, 1 to 5 micrometers in size and dispersed in a glassy matrix (Fig. 18-10, *A*). Two techniques are available: a staining technique or a layering technique involving the application of veneering porcelain. The two techniques lead to comparable mean flexural strength values for the resulting porcelain composite. To ensure compatibility with the thermal expansion coefficient of the veneering porcelain, the thermal expansion coefficient of the material for the veneering technique ($14.9 \times 10^{-6}/°$ C) is lower than that of the material for the staining technique ($18 \times 10^{-6}/°$ C). The flexure strength of these ceramics (120 MPa) is about double that of conventional feldspathic porcelains. The main disadvantages are the initial cost of the equipment and relatively low strength compared with other all-ceramic systems.

Lithium Disilicate–Based In recent years, new all-ceramic materials for heat-pressing have become available. These materials contain lithium disilicate ($Li_2Si_2O_5$) as a major crystalline phase. They are heat-pressed in the 890° to 920° C temperature range, using the same equipment as for the leucite-based ceramics. The heat-pressed restoration is later layered with glasses of matching thermal expansion. The final microstructure consists of about 60% elongated lithium-disilicate crystals (0.5 to 5 micrometers long) dispersed in a glassy matrix (Fig. 18-10, *B*). The main advantage of the lithium disilicate–containing ceramics is their superior flexural strength

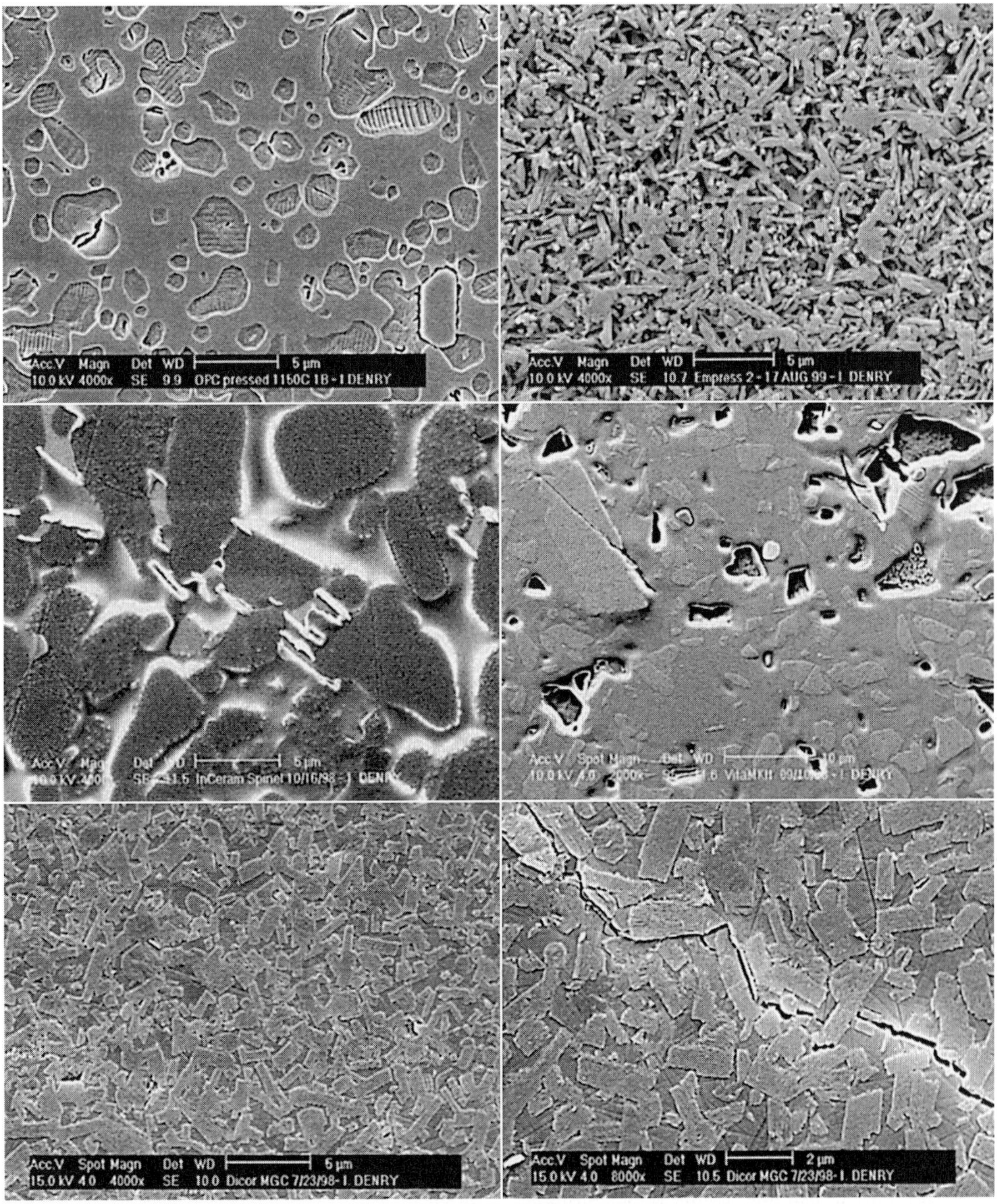

A B C D E F

Fig. 18-10 Scanning electron micrographs showing the microstructure of selected all-ceramic materials (polished and etched surfaces). **A,** Leucite-reinforced pressable ceramic; **B,** lithium-disilicate pressable ceramic; **C,** slip-cast alumina-spinel ceramic; **D,** feldspar-based machinable ceramic; **E,** mica-based machinable ceramic; **F,** crystal/crack interaction in mica-based machinable glass-ceramic.

(350 MPa) and fracture toughness (3.2 MPa · $m^{0.5}$), which extend their range of applications. The fabrication of fixed partial dentures is theoretically possible with these materials. However, no long-term clinical data is presently available.

The advantages of heat-pressed ceramics include good esthetics for the leucite-reinforced materials, high strength (but higher opacity) for the lithium disilicate–based materials and ability to use the well known lost-wax technique. Processing times are short and margin accuracy is within an acceptable range.

SLIP-CAST ALL-CERAMIC MATERIALS

Slip-casting involves the condensation of an aqueous porcelain slip on a refractory die. The porosity of the refractory die helps condensation by absorbing the water from the slip by capillary action. The piece is then fired at high temperature on the refractory die. Usually the refractory shrinks more than the condensed slip so that the piece can be separated easily after firing. The fired porous core is later glass-infiltrated, a unique process in which molten glass is drawn into the pores by capillary action at high temperature. Materials processed by slip-casting tend to exhibit reduced porosity, fewer defects from processing, and higher toughness than conventional feldspathic porcelains.

Alumina-Based An alumina-based slip is applied to a gypsum refractory die designed to shrink during firing. The alumina content of the slip is more than 90%, with a particle size between 0.5 and 3.5 μm. After firing for 4 hours at 1100° C, the porous alumina coping is shaped and infiltrated with a lanthanum-containing glass during a second firing at 1150° C for 4 hours. After removal of the excess glass, the restoration is veneered using matched-expansion veneer porcelain. This processing technique is unique in dentistry and leads to a high-strength material due to the presence of densely packed alumina particles and the reduction of porosity. The microstructure of this material is shown in Fig. 18-10, *C*. The flexural strength of this slip-cast alumina material is around 450 MPa. Because of the high strength of the core, short span anterior fixed partial dentures can be made using this process.

Spinel- and Zirconia-Based Two modified ceramic compositions for this technique have been recently introduced. One contains a magnesium spinel ($MgAl_2O_4$) as the major crystalline phase with traces of alpha-alumina, which improves the translucency of the final restoration. The second material contains tetragonal zirconia and alumina. The spinel-based material has a lower modulus of rupture than the alumina-based material, whereas the zirconia-based material has a reported flexural strength neighboring 600 MPa.

The main advantage of slip-cast ceramics is their high strength; disadvantages include high opacity (with the exception of the spinel-based materials) and long processing times.

MACHINABLE ALL-CERAMIC MATERIALS

Machinable ceramics can be milled to form inlays, onlays, and veneers using special equipment. One system uses CAD/CAM (computer assisted design/computer assisted machining) technology to produce restorations in one office visit. After the tooth is prepared, the preparation is optically scanned and the image is computerized. The restoration is designed with the aid of a computer, as shown in Fig. 18-11. The restoration is then machined from ceramic blocks by a computer-controlled milling machine. The milling process takes only a few minutes. Although convenient, the CAD/CAM system is very expensive and its marginal accuracy is poor, with values of 100 to 150 μm. Bonding of the restorations with resin cements may help compensate for some of the problems of poor marginal fit.

Another system for machining ceramics is to form inlays, onlays, and veneers using copy milling. In this system, a hard resin pattern is made on a traditional stone die. This handmade pattern is then copied and machined from a ceramic

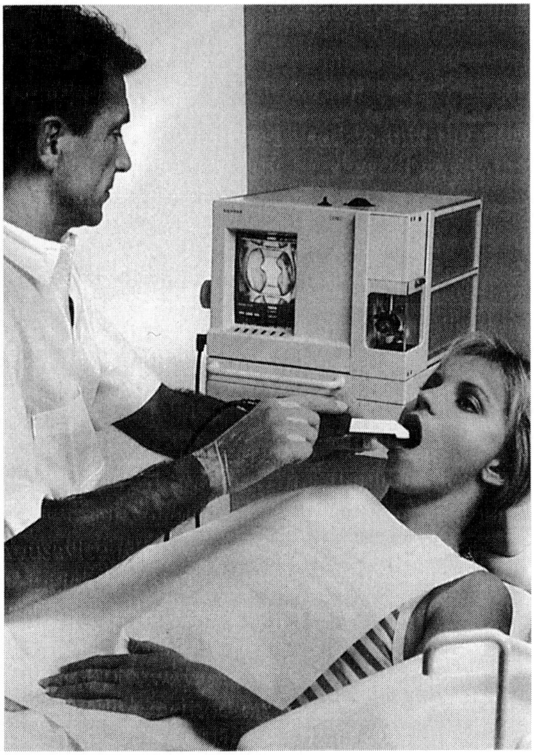

Fig. 18-11 The Cerec chairside CAD/CAM system for porcelain inlay fabrication.
(Courtesy Siemens Corp., Bad Soligman, Germany, 1995.)

block using a pantographic device similar in principle to those used for duplicating house keys. Again, marginal accuracy is a concern and there are high equipment costs.

Several machinable ceramics are presently available for use with these systems. One contains a potassium feldspar as a major crystalline phase dispersed in a glassy matrix (Fig. 18-10, *D*) It is available in several shades. Its flexural strength can be ranked as moderate (105 MPa).

Mica-based glass-ceramics are also available with this system. Their microstructure consists of mica crystals (50% to 70% by volume) dispersed in a glassy matrix. The mica crystals are elongated and randomly oriented (Fig. 18-10, *E*). Because of the crystalline structure of the mica crystals, cracks are deflected along the crystals, as shown in Fig. 18-10, *F*. This microstructure and the cleavage properties of mica crystals gives this type of glass-ceramic its good machinability and a flexural strength around 230 MPa.

Pre-sintered slip-cast alumina blocks can be machined using the copy-milling system to generate copings for crowns and fixed partial dentures. The alumina copings are further infiltrated with glass, resulting in a final marginal accuracy within 50 μm.

A more recent system involves an industrial CAD/CAM process to produce crowns. The die is mechanically scanned by the technician and the data is sent to a workstation where an enlarged die is milled using a computer-controlled milling machine. This enlargement is necessary to compensate for the sintering shrinkage. Aluminum oxide powder is then compacted onto the die and the coping is milled before sintering at very high temperature (>1550° C). The coping is further veneered with an aluminous ceramic with matched expansion.

As mentioned earlier, the main advantage of the machining process in making dental ceramic restorations is the ability to accomplish the restoration in one office visit. This is not true for the last system reviewed in which the restoration is fabricated in a laboratory. High equipment costs, poor marginal accuracy (compared to gold restorations) of the machining process, and the high opacity of the ceramic materials available constitute the main disadvantages of this process. Except for the alumina-based systems, strength remains a concern.

GENERAL APPLICATIONS OF CERAMICS IN RESTORATIVE DENTISTRY

Ceramics are probably the best material available for matching the esthetics of a complex human tooth. They are used for ceramic-metal crowns, fixed partial dentures, all-ceramic restorations, and to fabricate denture teeth. However, ceramics are brittle and fragile in tension, and the quality of the final product is very technique-sensitive, in terms of strength and esthetics.

CERAMIC-METAL CROWNS AND FIXED PARTIAL DENTURES

Ceramic is widely used as the veneering material in ceramic-metal crowns and fixed partial dentures. This development was the result of successfully matching the coefficients of thermal expansion of porcelain with alloys and achieving a proper bond. The glazed surface produces a restoration that is color-stable, tissue-friendly, biocompatible, chemically durable and has low thermal diffusivity. Ceramic-metal restorations are still widely used; their failure rate at 10 years is considerably lower than most all-ceramic crown systems. It should be noted, however, that no survival data are available for some of the newest all-ceramic systems.

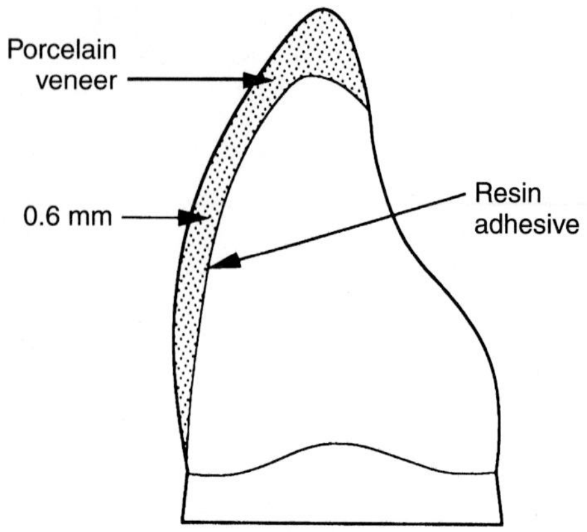

Fig. 18-12 Diagram of porcelain veneer bonded to facial surface of tooth.

(From Craig RG, Powers JM, Wataha JC: *Dental materials: properties and manipulation*, ed. 7, St Louis, 2000, Mosby.)

ALL-CERAMIC CROWNS, INLAYS, ONLAYS, AND VENEERS

Ceramics have been used to fabricate jacket crowns since the early 1900s. At that time feldspathic porcelain was used in the fabrication. Alumina-reinforced ceramics were later introduced to improve the mechanical properties. In the past 20 years, novel materials and techniques for the fabricating all-ceramic restorations have been introduced. They include slip-cast, machined, and heat-pressed all-ceramic materials. These new materials and techniques have widened the range of applications of all-ceramic materials, and in some cases made their processing easier.

Ceramic inlays and onlays are becoming increasingly popular as an alternative to posterior composite resins. They have better abrasion resistance than posterior composite resins and therefore are more durable. However, occlusal adjustments are more difficult and can lead to subsequent wear of the opposing tooth if not properly polished. The marginal gap is greater than with gold inlays or onlays. These restorations are not indicated when high occlusal loads are expected.

A porcelain esthetic veneer (laminate veneer) is a layer of porcelain bonded to the facial surface of a prepared tooth to cover an unsightly area (Fig. 18-12). Porcelain veneers are custom made and are fabricated in a dental laboratory. Initially, porcelain veneers were made of feldspathic porcelain and sintered. Currently, most porcelain veneers are fabricated by heat-pressing, using either a leucite-reinforced or lithium-disilicate ceramic. To obtain sufficient adhesion, the tooth enamel is etched with phosphoric acid and the bonding surface of the porcelain is etched with diluted hydrofluoric acid and treated with a silane coupling agent. Resin composites specifically formulated for bonding to ceramic are used as the adhesive.

MECHANICAL AND THERMAL PROPERTIES OF DENTAL CERAMICS

The properties of dental ceramics depend on their composition, microstructure, and flaw population. The nature and amount of reinforcing crystalline phase present dictate the material's strength and resistance to crack propagation and its optical properties.

Ceramics are brittle and contain at least two populations of flaws: fabrication defects and surface cracks.

Fabrication defects are created during processing and consist of inclusions at the condensation stage or voids generated during sintering.

TABLE 18-3 Flexural Strength of Selected Dental Ceramics

Processing Technique	Crystalline Phase	Flexural Strength (MPa)
Sintered ceramic-metal	Leucite	70
Sintered all-ceramic	Leucite	104
Sintered all-ceramic	Alumina	139
Heat-pressed all-ceramic	Leucite	121
Heat-pressed all-ceramic	Lithium disilicate	350
Slip-cast all-ceramic	Alumina	446
Slip-cast all-ceramic	Spinel-alumina	378
Slip-cast all-ceramic	Zirconia-alumina	604
Machinable all-ceramic	Fluormica	229
Machinable all-ceramic	Feldspar	122

From Seghi R, Sorensen J: *Int J Prosthodont* 8(3):239-246, 1995; Seghi RR, Daher T, Caputo A: *Dent Mater* 6(3):181-184, 1990.

Inclusions are often linked to improper cleaning of the metal framework or use of unclean instruments. Porosity on the internal side of clinically failed glass-ceramic restorations has been identified as the fracture initiation site. Microcracks also develop upon cooling in feldspathic porcelains and can be due to thermal contraction mismatch between the leucite crystals and the glassy matrix, or to thermal shock if the porcelain is cooled too rapidly.

Surface cracks are induced by machining or grinding. The average natural flaw size varies from 20 to 50 μm. Usually, failure of the ceramic originates from the most severe flaw.

Dental ceramics are subjected to repeated (cyclic) loading in a humid environment (chewing), conditions that are ideal for the extension of the preexisting defects or cracks. This phenomenon, called *slow crack growth,* can contribute to a severe reduction of the survival probability of ceramic restorations.

TEST METHODS

Numerous test methods are available to evaluate the mechanical properties of ceramics. Studies of the influence of test method on the failure stress of brittle dental materials have shown that important test parameters are the specimen thickness, contact zone at loading, homogeneity and porosity of the material, and loading rate. For this reason, discrepancies exist amongst the published values of mechanical properties for a given material.

Sometimes, researchers use devices that try to simulate dental morphology. However, the experimental variables can become extremely complex and difficult to reproduce in this type of testing. Finite element analysis (FEA) constitutes another approach to the simulation of clinical conditions. Failure predictions of ceramic inlays by the FEA technique have successfully matched fractographic analyses of clinically failed restorations.

Fractography is well established as a failure-analysis technique for glasses and ceramics. It has been recognized as a powerful analytical tool in dentistry. The in vivo failure stress of clinically failed all-ceramic crowns can be determined using fractography.

COMPARATIVE DATA

The flexural strengths of dental ceramics are summarized in Table 18-3. Feldspathic porcelains for ceramic-metal restorations have a mean flexural strength of about 70 MPa. This value is lower than those listed for all-ceramic materials;

however, because ceramic-metal restorations are supported by a metallic framework, their probability of survival is usually higher.

Among the currently available all-ceramic materials, slip-cast ceramics exhibit the highest values (378 to 604 MPa), followed by lithium-disilicate heat-pressed ceramics (350 MPa). The flexural strength of leucite-reinforced heat-pressed ceramics is around 100 MPa. Among the machinable ceramic materials, mica-based material has the highest flexural strength value (229 MPa). As mentioned previously, the nature and amount of the crystalline phase present in the ceramic material strongly influences the mechanical properties of the final product.

The flexural strength of feldspathic porcelain is between 62 and 90 MPa, the shear strength is 110 MPa, and the diametral tensile strength is lower at 34 MPa. The compressive strength is about 172 MPa, and the Knoop hardness is 460 kg/mm^2.

Fracture toughness is also an important property of ceramics; it is a measure of the energy absorbed by the material as it fails. The fracture toughness of conventional feldspathic porcelains is very similar to that of soda lime glass (0.78 $MPa \cdot m^{0.5}$). Leucite-reinforced and mica-based ceramics have a fracture toughness about double that of soda-lime glass and four times that of glass for lithium-disilicate ceramics.

The elastic constants of dental ceramics are of interest as they are needed in the calculations of both flexural strength and fracture toughness values. Poisson's ratio lies between 0.21 and 0.26 for dental ceramics. The modulus of elasticity is 69 GPa for feldspathic porcelain, varies from 62 to 72 GPa for machinable ceramics, and reaches 110 GPa for lithium-disilicate heat-pressed ceramics.

The amount of shrinkage in ceramic bodies depends on the average pore size, which is directly related to the particle size distribution. The smaller pores obtained from a broader particle size distribution generate higher capillary pressure, leading to more shrinkage. The linear firing shrinkage of feldspathic porcelains has been reported to be approximately 14% for low-fusing porcelain (ceramic-metals) and 11.5% for high-fusing porcelain (denture teeth). Overglazed porcelain has a greater percentage of shrinkage for both the low- and high-fusing types, and the volumetric shrinkage shows even greater differences of approximately 8%. Several studies have shown the low-fusing type to have a volumetric shrinkage of from 32% to 37% and the high-fusing porcelain to shrink as much as 28% to 34%. The medium-fusing porcelain has shrinkage values between the high- and low-fusing types. As pointed out earlier in this chapter, precise control of the condensation and firing technique is required to compensate for such shrinkage values during the construction of the porcelain restoration. The greatest dimensional change will occur where porcelain is thickest.

Shrinkage remains an issue for all ceramic materials with the exception of machined ceramics from fully sintered ceramic blocks and heat-pressed ceramics. Shrinkage of the veneering ceramics applied on all-ceramic cores has to be carefully compensated for during porcelain buildup.

The density of fully sintered feldspathic porcelain is around 2.45 g/cm^3 and will vary with the porosity of the material. The density of all-ceramic materials, which depends on the amount of crystalline phase present, is between 2.4 and 2.5 g/cm^3.

The thermal properties of feldspathic porcelain include a conductivity of 0.0030 $cal/sec/cm^2$ (° C/cm), a diffusivity of 0.64 mm^2/sec, and a linear thermal coefficient of expansion of $12.0 \times 10^{-6}/°$ C between 25 and 500° C. This coefficient is about $10 \times 10^{-6}/°$ C for aluminous ceramics and lithium-disilicate ceramics, and 14 to $18 \times 10^{-6}/°$ C for leucite-reinforced ceramics.

OPTICAL PROPERTIES OF DENTAL CERAMICS

Color matching is a critical problem in replacing portions of natural teeth. Porcelain, being partially amorphous in structure, does not resemble crystalline enamel completely. As a result, various kinds of light are reflected and absorbed in different manners by the tooth tissue and porcelain, and restorations viewed from an angle may not appear the same as they do when viewed from the front. The cementing medium is an important factor in the final appearance of an all-ceramic restoration. Because of its opacity, an aluminous all-ceramic restoration may be cemented with a wide range of luting agents, but not with resin-modified glass ionomer cements (associated with fracture). However, a more translucent all-ceramic restoration such as a leucite-reinforced heat-pressed crown or veneer, or a machined inlay or veneer, usually requires the use of translucent resin luting agents that are available in different shades.

The colors of commercial premixed dental porcelain powders are in the yellow to yellow-red range. Because the range of colors of natural teeth is much greater than the range available in a kit of premixed porcelains, modifier porcelains are also supplied for adjustments. These modifiers are strongly pigmented porcelains usually supplied in blue, yellow, pink, orange, brown, and gray. The dental technician may add the modifier porcelain to the opaque and body porcelains during the building of the crown. Extrinsic surface staining, another way of changing the color of a dental porcelain crown, involves the application of highly pigmented glazes. The main disadvantages of surface staining are a lowered durability (a result of solubility) and the reduction of translucency.

Translucency is another critical property of dental porcelains. The translucency of opaque, dentin (body), and enamel (incisal) porcelains differs considerably. Opaque porcelains have very low translucency, allowing them to mask metal substructure surfaces. Dentin porcelain translucency values range between 18% and 38%, as seen in Table 18-4. Enamel porcelains have the highest values of translucency, ranging between 45% and 50%. The translucency of materials for all-ceramic restorations varies with the nature of the reinforcing crystalline phase. Alumina-based systems are opaque, whereas leucite-reinforced systems are more translucent. The translucency of spinel-based systems is comparable with that of lithium disilicate–based systems and intermediate between alumina-based and leucite-reinforced systems.

Because dental enamel is fluorescent under ultraviolet light, uranium oxide had been added to produce fluorescence with porcelain. However, because of the low but detectable radioactivity of uranium, newer formulations contain rare earth oxides (such as cerium oxide) to produce fluorescence.

Because the outer layers of a porcelain crown are translucent, the apparent color is affected by reflectance from the inner opaque or core porcelain. Color mixing results from combining the light reflected from the inner, opaque porcelain surface and the light transmitted through the body porcelain. The thickness of the body porcelain layer determines the color obtained with a given opaque porcelain. This thickness effect may be minimized if the body porcelain and the opaque porcelain are the same color as that of some commercial systems.

TABLE 18-4 Percent Light Transmission of 1-mm Thick Dentin Porcelains

Shade	Ceramco	Vita	Neydium	Will-Ceram	Steeles
59	29.97	22.66	31.93	26.06	27.23
62	27.85	—	—	27.88	—
65	23.31	20.39	35.39	33.50	22.10
67	26.32	18.04	23.58	19.03	23.42
91	31.81	—	38.41	—	—

Adapted from Brodbelt RHW, O'Brien WJ, Fan PL: *J Dent Res* 59:70, 1980.

PROPERTIES OF PORCELAIN DENTURE TEETH

Porcelain denture teeth are commercially manufactured and their composition and properties set them apart from ceramics for fixed restorations. Individual or complete sets of teeth of excellent quality are available in a wide range of shapes and shades from a number of manufacturers. They have been used for complete dentures. The anterior teeth have one or two gold-covered pins to provide retention to the denture base. The posterior teeth have diatoric holes located centrally in the underside of the teeth for retention to the denture base. A typical set of porcelain teeth is shown in Fig. 18-13.

The ceramic composition of porcelain denture teeth belongs to the triaxial porcelain compositions (quartz, clay, kaolin). The teeth are made in split molds, fired under vacuum and slowly cooled to prevent crazing.

The main advantages of porcelain denture teeth are their superior esthetics, resistance to abrasion, and excellent shade stability. One disadvantage is the difficulty of polishing the surface after occlusal adjustment, resulting in significant wear of the opposing teeth.

The physical properties of tooth porcelain are perhaps best shown when compared with the properties of plastic teeth and, when possible, with those of natural teeth. These properties, however, are often so radically different that they cannot be measured with the same equipment or compared quantitatively. The hardness values of porcelain compared with plastic and natural tooth structures are shown in Table 4-16.

It is evident from these values that the two standard tooth-replacement materials are quite different in hardness. Porcelain is harder than enamel, whereas the best plastic teeth are softer than dentin.

In regard to abrasion resistance, dental porcelain has been clinically evaluated as being equal to or slightly more wear resistant than natural tooth structure. At present, clinical data represent the only measure of abrasion believed to be of real significance. On this basis, porcelain has

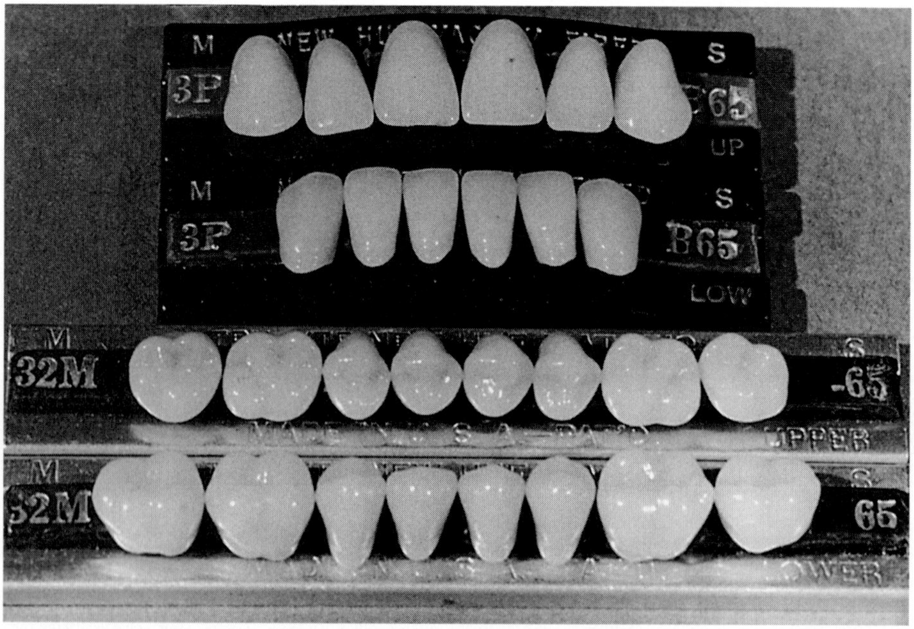

Fig. 18-13 A complete set of porcelain teeth as supplied by the manufacturer.

been estimated to have from 10 to 20 times the abrasion resistance of plastic teeth.

Porcelain is resistant to the action of solvents, with only hydrofluoric acid known to have any significant effect on it. The cross-linked plastics are relatively craze resistant and are immune to reasonable amounts of ordinary solvents. They may, however, be softened to some extent by a number of organic solvents.

Water bleaching and sunlight have no effect on porcelain, but repeated cycles of drying and water immersion may cause whitening and loss of color in plastic teeth. Continued exposure to ultraviolet light may cause a slight yellowing. When plastic is softened by solvents, organic dyes may penetrate the outer layer and cause discoloration.

The flexural strength of dental plastics is unquestionably superior to that of the dental porcelains. The pin anchorage and the strength of the porcelain that surrounds it are the determining factors in the basic strength of a porcelain tooth. Retention is adequate for most service conditions.

The high impact strength of plastic gives it a definite advantage. Vacuum-firing has improved the fracture resistance of dental porcelain by about 50%, but this does not preclude the possibility of fracture from sudden shock.

In dimensional stability or permanence of form, plastic is less acceptable than porcelain. The superior strength of plastic is indicated by its ability to cushion the impact blow of mastication and avoid fracture caused by brittleness. Unfortunately, plastic does not return to its original form each time it yields, and there is cumulative loss of dimension; this loss is described as *flow*. Porcelain, like tooth enamel, is incapable of cold flow.

It is often necessary to "spot" grind porcelain denture teeth or to heat them in a flame momentarily during the waxing of a denture. Overheating during these procedures may cause a small area to expand and become too large to be compatible with the remainder of the tooth. This may result in immediate breakage, or perhaps only in cracking the tooth, so that failure occurs in service. It is therefore advisable to keep a porcelain tooth wet during all grinding operations and to avoid rapid heating or cooling.

Both porcelain and plastic withstand heating well enough for the usual dental procedures. Plastic teeth will withstand temperatures of approximately 200° C, and porcelain is unaffected by temperatures in excess of 1100° C if the heat is applied slowly.

A direct and more complete comparison of the characteristic properties of porcelain and plastic teeth is discussed under "Properties of Dental Plastics" in Chapter 21.

SELECTED PROBLEMS

Problem 1

A porcelain that normally glazes at 982° C was found to require 1010° C for glazing. Explain.

Solution a

The pyrometer of the porcelain furnace requires periodic calibration, usually with silver disks that are supplied by the furnace manufacturer.

Solution b

If the particle size is changed, the sintering and glazing temperatures change also. It is important to shake the porcelain before using it to counteract any settling of particles.

Problem 2

A porcelain crown fractured as a result of excessive porosity. What can be done to avoid porosity?

Solution a

The mix of porcelain should not be stirred too much because bubbles may be entrapped.

Solution b

Porcelain should be heated gradually when first fired to evaporate the water holding the particles together without creating steam. Rapid heating results in steam, which can create porosity.

Solution c

The vacuum level in the porcelain furnace was improperly set. Air-firing does not allow proper elimination of pores during sintering.

Problem 3

A patient showed considerable wear of enamel on the teeth in occlusion with porcelain crowns. Explain.

Solution

Dental porcelain is harder than tooth enamel and can wear it away. Porcelain fused to metal with metal lingual surfaces on anterior crowns results in less wear. However, because the porcelain crowns are already cemented, the use of a bite splint in the case of bruxism may be indicated.

Problem 4

A heat-pressed leucite-reinforced crown fractured after firing of the veneering ceramic. Explain.

Solution a

Improper core material was used. Heat-pressed ceramic ingots are available either for the staining technique or for the veneering technique. These ingots have different coefficients of thermal expansion. If the veneering ceramic was fired on a core material for the staining technique, the thermal expansion mismatch between the materials can lead to fracture or cracking upon cooling.

Solution b

Improper veneering ceramic was used; for example, an aluminous veneering ceramic with unmatched coefficient of thermal expansion.

Problem 5

A heat-pressed, all-ceramic crown pressed incompletely. Explain the possible causes of incomplete pressing.

Solution a

The pressing temperature was not reached because of an erroneous temperature calibration. Heat-pressing furnaces should be calibrated regularly. If the pressing temperature was not reached, the viscosity of the ceramic ingot was too high to allow complete pressing of the crown.

Solution b

The air-pressure in the heat-pressing furnace was too low. Ideal pressure should be at least 65 psi for proper pressing.

Solution c

Only one ceramic ingot was used when two were needed. Wax-patterns should be weighed before pressing to ensure that enough material is available for pressing.

Problem 6

The porcelain on a ceramic-metal crown fractured at the drying stage. Explain.

Solution a

The recommended drying time was improperly set or the heating rate was too high.

Solution b

The ceramic slurry was insufficiently condensed.

Problem 7

The surface of a ceramic-metal crown exhibits several dark inclusions. What are the possible causes of these defects?

Solution a

The inclusions are metallic inclusions created during framework grinding; They were not eliminated because of inadequate cleaning after grinding.

Solution b

Dirty instruments were used to mix the porcelain powder or dirty brushes to apply the ceramic.

Solution c

Metallic instruments were used at any time during porcelain preparation or application.

BIBLIOGRAPHY

Anusavice KJ, Gray A, Shen C: Influence of initial flaw size on crack growth in air-tempered porcelain, *J Dent Res* 70:131, 1991.

Asaoka K, Nuwayama N, Tesk JA: Influence of tempering method on residual stress in dental porcelain, *J Dent Res* 71:1623, 1992.

Baran GR, O'Brien WJ, Tien TY: Colored emission of rare earth ions in a potassium feldspar glass, *J Dent Res* 56:1323, 1977.

Barreiro MM, Riesgo O, Vicente EE: Phase identification in dental porcelains for ceramo-metallic restorations, *Dent Mater* 5:51, 1989

Brodbelt RHW, O'Brien WJ, Fan PL: Translucency of dental porcelain, *J Dent Res* 59:70, 1980.

Denry IL, Rosenstiel SF, Holloway JA et al: Enhanced chemical strengthening of feldspathic dental porcelain, *J Dent Res* 72:1429, 1993.

Dong JK, Luthy H, Wohlwend A et al: Heat-pressed ceramics: technology and strength, *Int J Prosthodont* 5:9, 1992.

Gray HS: The porcelain jacket crown, *NZ Dent J* 59:283, 1963.

Hodson JT: Some physical properties of three dental porcelains, *J Prosthet Dent* 9:235, 1959.

Johnston WM, O'Brien WJ: Color analysis of dental modifying porcelains, *J Dent Res* 60 (Spec Issue A):441, 1981.

Jones DW, Wilson HJ: Some properties of dental ceramics, *J Oral Rehabil* 2:379, 1975.

Kelly JR, Giordano R, Pober R et al: Fracture surface analysis of dental ceramics: clinically failed restorations, *Int J Prosthodont* 3:430, 1990.

Kelly JR, Nishimura I, Campbell SD: Ceramics in dentistry: historical roots and current perspectives, *J Prosthet Dent* 75:18, 1996.

Kelly JR, Tesk JA, Sorensen JA: Failure of all-ceramic fixed partial dentures in vitro and in vivo: Analysis and modeling, *J Dent Res* 74:1253, 1995.

Kingery WD, Bowen HK, Uhlmann DR: *Introduction to ceramics,* (ed 2) New York, 1976, John Wiley & Sons.

Kulp PR, Lee PW, Fox JE: Impact test for dental porcelain, *J Dent Res* 40:1136, 1961.

Kurzeja R, O'Brien WJ: The fluorescence of porcelain containing cerium, *J Dent Res* 60 (Spec Issue A):435, 1981.

Leone EF, Fairhurst CW: Bond strength and mechanical properties of dental porcelain enamel, *J Prosthet Dent* 18:155, 1967.

Mackert JRJ, Rueggeberg FA, Lockwood PE et al: Isothermal anneal effect on microcrack density around leucite particles in dental porcelains, *J Dent Res* 73:1221, 1994.

Mackert JR Jr, Twiggs SW, Evans-Williams AL: Isothermal anneal effect on leucite content in dental porcelains, *J Dent Res* 74:1259, 1995.

McLaren EA, Sorensen JA: High-strength alumina crowns and fixed partial dentures generated by copy-milling technology, *Quint Dent Technol* 18:31, 1995.

McLean JW: A higher strength porcelain for crown and bridge work, *Br Dent J* 119:268, 1965.

McLean JW: The alumina reinforced porcelain jacket crown, *J Am Dent Assoc* 75:621, 1967.

McLean JW, Hughes TH: The reinforcement of dental porcelain with ceramic oxides, *Br Dent J* 119:251, 1965.

Meyer JM, O'Brien WJ, Yu R: Sintering of dental porcelain enamels, *J Dent Res* 55:696, 1976.

Milleding P, Örtengren V, Karlsson S: Ceramic inlay systems: some clinical aspects, *J Oral Rehabil* 22:571, 1995.

Mora GP, O'Brien WJ: Thermal shock resistance of core reinforced all-ceramic crown systems, *J Biomed Mater Res* 28:189, 1994.

Morena R, Lockwood PE, Fairhurst CW: Fracture toughness of commercial dental porcelains, *Dent Mater* 2:58-62, 1986.

O'Brien WJ: Ceramics, *Dent Clin North Am* 29:851, 1985.

O'Brien WJ: Recent developments in materials and processes for ceramic crowns, *J Am Dent Assoc* 110:547, 1985.

O'Brien WJ, Craig RG, editors: *Proceedings of conference on recent developments in dental ceramics,* Ceramic Eng and Sci Proc, Columbus, Ohio, 1985, American Ceramic Society.

O'Brien WJ, Johnston WJ, Fanian F: Filtering effects of body porcelain on opaque color modifiers, *J Dent Res,* IADR Abstracts 61:330, 1982.

O'Brien WJ, Nelson D, Lorey RE: The assessment of chroma sensitivity to porcelain pigments, *J Prosthet Dent* 49:63, 1983.

Piché PW, O'Brien WJ, Groh CL et al: Leucite content of selected dental porcelains, *J Biomed Mater Res* 28:603, 1994.

Preston JD, Bergen SF: *Color science and dental art,* St Louis, 1980, Mosby.

Pröbster L, Diehl J: Slip-casting alumina ceramics for crown and bridge restorations, *Quint Int* 23:25, 1992.

Rekow ED: A review of the developments in dental CAD/CAM systems, *Curr Opin Dent* 2:25, 1992.

Seghi R, Sorensen J: Relative flexural strength of six new ceramic materials. *Int J Prosthodont* 8(3):239-246, 1995.

Sherrill CA, Jr, O'Brien WJ: The transverse strength of aluminous and feldspathic porcelains, *J Dent Res* 53:683, 1974.

Smith BB: Esthetic restoration of anterior teeth, with emphasis on rapid fabrication of fired porcelain units, *J Am Acad Gold Foil Oper* 6:6, 1963.

Smith BB: Porcelain inlays for the general practitioner, *Dent Clin North Am* 191, Mar. 1967.

Thompson JY, Anusavice KJ, Naman A et al: Fracture surface characterization of clinically failed all-ceramic crowns, *J Dent Res* 73(12):1824-1832, 1994.

Thompson JY, Anusavice KJ: Effect of surface etching on the flexure strength and fracture toughness of Dicor disks containing controlled flaws, *J Dent Res* 73:505, 1994.

Vaidyanathan TK, Vaidyanathan J, Prasad A: Properties of a new dental porcelain. *Scanning Microscopy* 3:1023-1033, 1989.

Vines RF, Semmelman JO: Densification of dental porcelain, *J Dent Res* 36:950, 1957.

Wagner WC, O'Brien WJ, Mora GP: Fracture surface analysis of a glaze-strengthened magnesia core material, *Int J Prosthodont* 5:475-478, 1992.

Weinstein M, Katz S, Weinstein AB: Fused porcelain-to-metal teeth. US Patent No. 3,052,982, September 11, 1962.

Wozniak WT, Moore BK, Smith E: Fluorescence spectra of dental porcelain, *J Dent Res* 55(Spec Issue B):B186, 1976.

Yamada HN: *Dental porcelain, the state of the art—1977,* Los Angeles, 1977, University of Southern California.

Chapter 19

Ceramic-Metal Systems

All-ceramic anterior restorations can appear very natural. Unfortunately, the ceramics used in these restorations are brittle and subject to fracture from high tensile stresses. Conversely, all-metal restorations are strong and tough but, from an esthetic viewpoint, acceptable only for posterior restorations. Fortunately the esthetic qualities of ceramic materials can be combined with the strength and toughness of metals to produce restorations that have both a natural toothlike appearance and very good mechanical properties. As a result they are more successful as posterior restorations than all-ceramic crowns. A cross section of a ceramic-metal anterior crown is shown in Fig. 19-1. The cast metal coping provides a substrate on which a ceramic coating is fused. The ceramics used for these restorations are porcelains, hence the common name, porcelain-fused-to-metal restorations. These ceramic-metal restorations are highly popular and are used for most of the crown and bridge restorations made today.

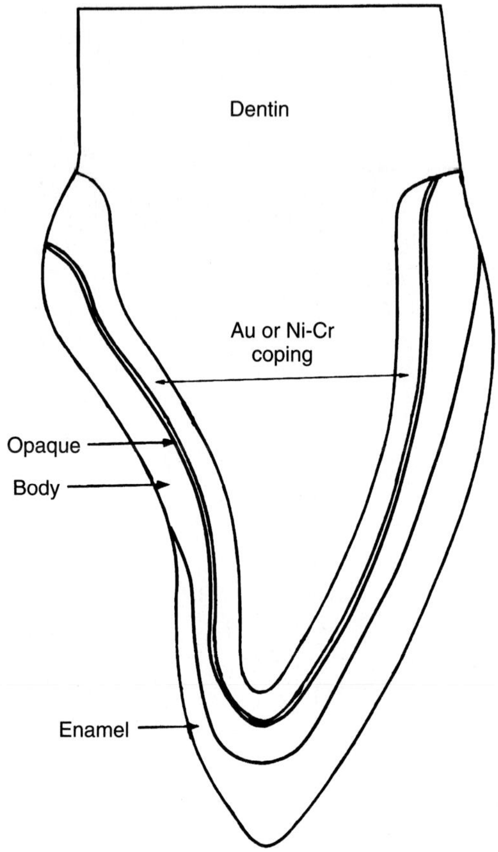

Fig. 19-1 Cross section of a ceramic-metal crown showing a gold alloy or base metal coping, the opaque body (dentin), and enamel ceramic layers.

REQUIREMENTS FOR A CERAMIC-METAL SYSTEM

1. High fusing temperature of the alloy. The fusing temperature must be substantially higher (>100° C) than the firing temperature of the ceramic and solders used to join segments of a bridge.
2. Low fusing temperature of the ceramic. The fusing temperature must be lower than ceramic used for all-ceramic restorations so no distortion of the coping takes place during fabrication.
3. The ceramic must wet the alloy readily when applied as a slurry in order to prevent voids forming at the interface. In general, the contact angle should be 60 degrees or less.
4. A good bond between the ceramic and metal is essential and is achieved by the interactions of the ceramic with metal oxides on the surface of metal (Fig. 19-2) and by the roughness of the metal coping.
5. Compatible coefficients of thermal expansion of the ceramic and metal so the ceramic does not crack during fabrication. The system is designed so the value for the metal is slightly higher than for the ceramic, thus putting the ceramic in compression (where it is stronger) during cooling (Fig. 19-3).
6. Adequate stiffness and strength of the alloy core. This requirement is especially important for fixed bridges and posterior crowns. High stiffness in the alloy reduces stresses in the ceramic by reducing deflection and strain. High strength is essential in the interproximal regions in fixed bridges.
7. High sag resistance is essential. The alloy copings are relatively thin; no distortion should occur during firing of the ceramic

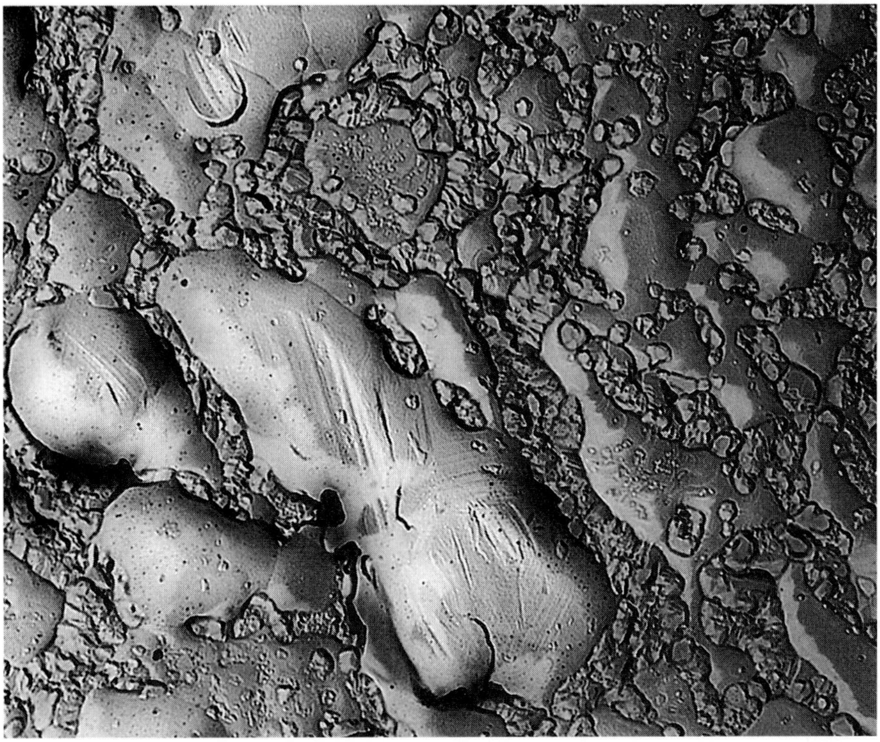

Fig. 19-2 Electron micrograph of replicated oxidized surface of a Au-Pt-Pd alloy (×8000). (From Kelly M, Asgar K, O'Brien WJ: *J Biomed Mater Res* 3:403, 1969.)

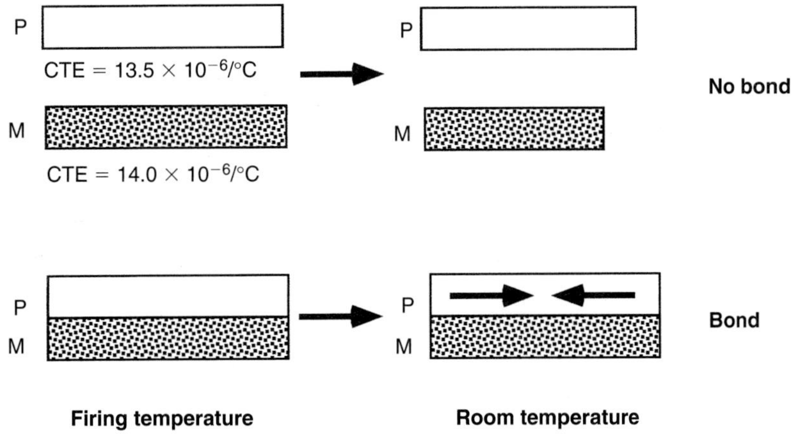

Fig. 19-3 Diagram of the ceramic-metal bond at the firing temperature and at room temperature when the thermal coefficient of expansion of the metal is $0.5 \times 10^{-6}/°$ C greater than the ceramic, thus placing the ceramic in compression at room temperature.

(From Craig RG, Powers JM, Wataha JC: *Dental materials: properties and manipulation,* ed. 7, St. Louis, 2000 Mosby.)

or the fit of the restoration will be compromised.
8. An accurate casting of the metal coping is required even with the higher fusing temperature of the alloy.
9. Adequate design of the restoration is critical. The preparation should provide for adequate thickness of alloy (see 5 on p. 576) and also provide enough space for an adequate thickness of ceramic to yield an esthetic restoration. In some instances, a ceramic-metal restoration has an advantage over an all-ceramic restoration because less tooth structure needs to be removed to provide adequate bulk for the all-ceramic restoration. However, in cases of small, lower, anterior teeth, an all-ceramic restoration has an advantage with respect to esthetics, because with a ceramic-metal restoration it is difficult to remove enough tooth structure to provide space for the coping and the esthetic ceramic layer. The geometry of the shoulder should be flat with a rounded angle or a chamfer to allow enough bulk of ceramic and avoid fracture in this area. If full ceramic coverage is not used (e.g., a metal occlusal) the position of the ceramic-metal joint should be located as far as possible from areas of contact with opposing teeth.

CERAMIC-METAL BONDING

The bond strength between the ceramic and metal is perhaps the most important requirement and thus will be given special attention. In general, the bond is a result of chemisorption by diffusion between the surface oxides on the alloy and in the ceramic. These oxides are formed during wetting of the alloy by the ceramic and firing of the ceramic. The most common mechanical failure of these restorations is ceramic debonding from the metal. Many factors control metal-ceramic adhesion: the formation of strong chemical bonding, mechanical interlocking between the two materials, and residual stresses. In addition, as noted earlier the ceramic must wet and fuse to the surface to form a uniform interface with no voids. These factors are also important for ceramic coatings on metallic implants.

An interface between a metal and a ceramic with many strong chemical bonds between them, with the bonds acting as tags that hold the two materials together, would obviously lead to strong bonding. However, methods producing a ceramic-metal interface with strong chemical bonding have not been developed. But the formation of oxides on the surface of the metal have been proven to contribute to the formation of strong bonding. Noble metals, which are resistant to oxidizing, must have other, more easily oxidized elements added, such as indium and tin, to form surface oxides. When these more easily oxidized elements are added, bonding is improved. The common practice of "degassing" or preoxidizing the metal coping before ceramic application creates surface oxides that improve bonding.

Base-metal alloys contain elements, such as nickel, chromium, and beryllium, which form oxides easily during degassing, and care must be taken to avoid too thick an oxide layer. Manufacturers' specify conditions to form the optimal oxide and often indicate the color of the oxide. Oxides rich in NiO tend to be dark gray, whereas those rich in Cr_2O_3 are greenish. These oxides dissolve in the ceramic during fixing and may discolor it or be visible through thin layers of ceramic near the gingival edge of the restoration.

The oxides are not completely dissolved during the fusion of the ceramic and thus the oxide-alloy interface can be the site of mechanical failure. This situation is especially true with some alloys that form layers rich in Cr_2O_3, which does not adhere well to the alloy. These alloys typically require the application of a bonding agent to the alloy surface to modify the type of oxide formed.

Alloys containing Be normally form well-adhering oxides. BeO is a slow-growing oxide that does not delaminate from the surface of the alloy. Rare earth elements such as yttrium can be added to the alloy to improve adherence by forming oxides, tying the alloy to the oxide layer.

From both theoretical and practical standpoints, the roughness, or more generally the topography, of a ceramic-metal interface plays a large part in adhesion. The ceramic penetrating into a rough metal surface can mechanically interlock with the metal, like Velcro, improving adhesion. The increased area associated with a rougher interface also provides more room for chemical bonds to form. However, rough surfaces can reduce adhesion if the ceramic does not penetrate into the surface and voids are present at the interface; this may happen with improperly fired porcelain or metals that are poorly wetted by the porcelain. Sandblasting is often used to remove excess oxide and to roughen the surface of the metal coping to improve the bonding of the ceramic.

High residual stresses between the metal and ceramic can lead to failure. If the metal and ceramic have different thermal expansion coefficients, the two materials will contract at different rates during cooling and strong residual stresses will form across the interface. If these stresses are strong enough the ceramic on the restoration will crack or separate from the metal. Even if the stresses are less strong and do not cause immediate failure, they can still weaken the bond. To avoid these problems the ceramics and alloys are formulated to have closely matched thermal expansion coefficients. Most porcelains have coefficients of thermal expansion between 13.0 and 14.0 $\times$ $10^{-6}/°$ C, and metals between 13.5 and 14.5 $\times$ $10^{-6}/°$ C. The difference of 0.5 $\times$ $10^{-6}/°$ C in thermal expansion between the metal and ceramic causes the metal to contract slightly more than does the ceramic during cooling after firing. This condition puts the ceramic under slight residual compression, which makes it less sensitive to applied tensile forces.

Wetting is important to the formation of good ceramic-metal bonding. During firing, the ceramic must wet and flow over the metal surface. The contact angle between the ceramic and metal is a measure of the wetting and, to some extent, the quality of the bond that forms. The wetting of the alloy surface by the fused ceramic indicates an interaction between surface atoms in the metal with the ceramic. Low contact angles indicate good wetting. The contact angle of ceramic on a gold type of ceramic alloy is about 60 degrees. The surface of the noble alloys containing tin and indium after heating have these oxides present, and they diffuse into and interact with the ceramic, forming an adhesive bond. The oxide surface of an Au-Pt-Pd 98% noble alloy is shown at high magnification in Fig. 19-2.

EVALUATION OF CERAMIC-METAL BONDING

Many tests have been used to determine the bond strength between ceramics and metals; however, the ideal test currently does not exist. In addition, data obtained from different tests are often not comparable. One of the established bond-strength tests is the planar shear test. Other commonly used tests are the flexural tests. The flexural tests require layers of ceramic to be bonded to a strip or plate of metal. The coated metal plate is flexed in a controlled manner until the ceramic fractures off. In the 3-point flexure bend test, ceramic is fired to one side of a rectangular strip of metal. The metal-ceramic strip is supported by two knife edges, and the specimen is loaded in the center with the ceramic surface down until failure of the ceramic occurs.

An adequate bond occurs when the fracture stress is >25 MPa; however, with many metal-ceramic systems values of 40 to 60 MPa are common. In a variant of this test, opaque and body ceramics are applied and fired to a thickness of approximately 1 mm on a 20-mm $\times$ 5-mm $\times$ 0.5-mm alloy sheets. The specimen is then bent over a 1-cm-diameter rod (with the ceramic on the outside) and then straightened. The surface is viewed under low magnification and the percent of the surface with retained ceramic is reported. Tests based on tensile and torsional loading schemes have also been used.

A ceramic-metal bond may fail in any of three possible locations (Fig. 19-4). Knowing the location of the fracture provides considerable information. The highest strength metal-ceramic specimens will fracture in the ceramic when tested (see Fig. 19-4, *C*); this is observed with some alloys that were properly prepared and had

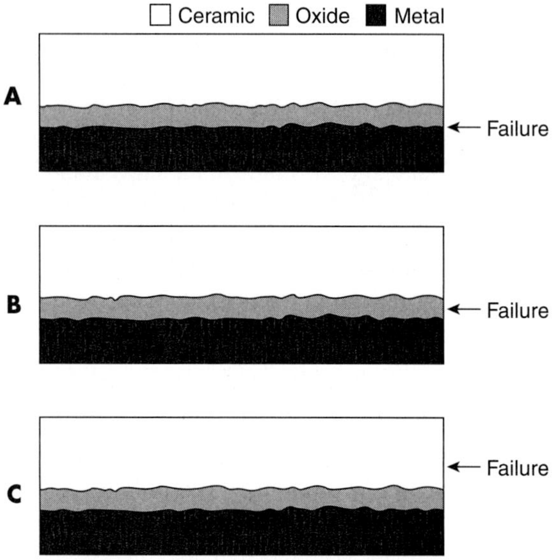

Fig. 19-4 Diagram showing three observed types of bond failure in ceramic-metal systems: **A,** metal–metal oxide; **B,** metal oxide–metal oxide; and **C,** ceramic-ceramic. *Note:* The dimensions of the layers are not to scale.

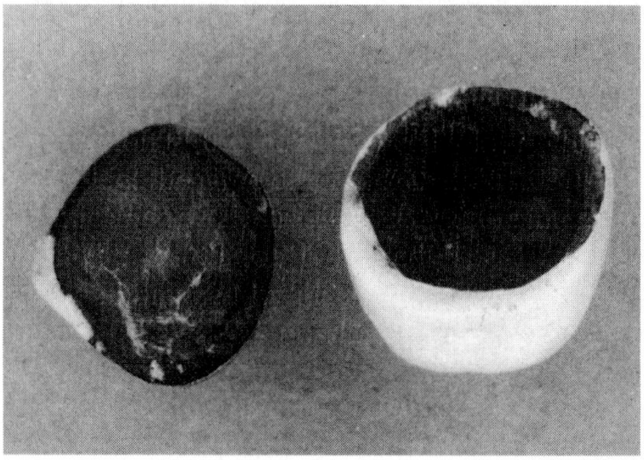

Fig. 19-5 Bond failure through the metal oxide layer of a nickel-based ceramic-metal crown.
(From O'Brien WJ, in Yamada H, editor: *Dental porcelain: the state of the art–1977,* Los Angeles, 1977, University of Southern California.)

ceramic applied and fused. Testing these high-strength specimens using the push-through shear test shows the maximum strengths are approximately the same as the shear strength of the ceramic. Fractures through the oxide (see Fig. 19-4, *B*) and metal–metal oxide fracture (see Fig. 19-4, *A*) are commonly observed with poor bonding. Base-metal alloys commonly fracture through the oxide (Fig. 19-5) if an excessively thick oxide layer is present. Interfacial fracture is observed with metals that are resistant to forming surface oxides, such as pure gold or platinum.

CERAMICS FOR CERAMIC-METAL RESTORATIONS

The ceramics used for porcelain-fused-to-metal restorations must fulfill five requirements: (1) they must simulate the appearance of natural teeth, (2) they must fuse at relatively low temperatures, (3) they must have thermal expansion coefficients compatible with the metals used for ceramic-metal bonding, (4) they must withstand the oral environment, and (5) they must not unduly abrade opposing teeth. The ceramic is carefully formulated to achieve these requirements. These ceramics are composed of crystalline phases in an amorphous and glassy (vitreous) matrix. They comprise primarily SiO_2, Al_2O_3, Na_2O, and K_2O (Table 19-1). Opacifiers (TiO_2, ZrO_2, SnO_2) and various heat-stable pigments are also added to the ceramic. Because of their composition, they can be considered a type of glass. To match the appearance of tooth structures, small amounts of fluorescing pigments such as rare earth oxides (CeO_2) are added. The nature of ceramics, with their glassy matrix and crystalline phases, produces a translucency much like that of teeth, whereas pigments and opacifiers control the color and translucency of the restoration. The ceramic is supplied as a fine powder.

In developing ceramics for ceramic-metal bonding, a major breakthrough was formulating products that had sufficiently high thermal expansion coefficients to match those of dental alloys. This higher expansion was made possible

TABLE 19-1 Composition Ranges of the Main Constituents in Ceramics for Ceramic-Metal Restorations

Component	Opaque Powder (%)	Dentin (Body) Powder (%)
SiO_2	50-59	57-62
Al_2O_3	9-15	11-16
Na_2O	5-7	4-9
K_2O	9-11	10-14
TiO_2	0-3	0-0.6
ZnO_2	0-5	0.1-1.5
SnO_2	5-15	0-0.5
Rb_2O	0-0.1	0-0.1
CeO_2	—	0-3
Pigments	—	Trace

by the addition of potassium oxide and the formation of a high-expansion phase called *leucite* ($KAlSi_2O_6$). This phase increased the thermal expansion of the porcelain so it could match that of dental alloys.

These materials have other qualities that make them well suited for ceramic-metal restorations. They fuse at lower temperatures than do many other ceramic materials, lessening the potential of distorting the metal coping. Sodium and potassium oxides in the glassy matrix are responsible for lowering the fusing temperatures to the range 930° to 980° C; low-fusing ceramics have hydroxyl groups and more Na_2O to lower fusing temperatures to as low as 660° C. These ceramics do not corrode, and are also resistant to the fluids present in the oral environment. They can, however, be abrasive to opposing teeth because of their hardness; this becomes a significant problem if the porcelain surface is rough due to improper processing or becomes rough in the oral environment. Newer products have been shown to be less abrasive to natural teeth. These new ceramics are also strong in compression, which permits their use on the occlusal surfaces of the restorations. The ceramics used to bond to metals have tensile strengths of 35 MPa, compressive strengths of 860 MPa, shear strengths of 120 MPa, and flexural strengths of 60 MPa.

ALLOYS FOR CERAMIC-METAL RESTORATIONS

Chronologically the alloys developed for ceramic-metal restorations were Au-Pt-Pd, Ni-Ci, Co-Cr, Au-Pd-Ag, Pd-Ag, Au-Pd, Pd-Cu, and Ti.

COMPOSITION AND PROPERTIES OF NOBLE METAL ALLOYS

The composition ranges and color of five types of noble alloys for ceramic-metal restorations are listed in Table 19-2. The properties of these alloys are given in Table 19-3.

Au-Pt-Pd Types These alloys contain a very high noble metal content, mainly gold with platinum and palladium to increase the melting range. The high-noble content provides good corrosion resistance. Indium, tin, and iron are present and form oxides to produce a ceramic-metal bond. Rhenium is added as a grain refiner. Hardening of Au-Pt-Pd type alloys results from solid solution hardening and the formation of an $FePt_3$ precipitate. Optimum heat treatment for hardening is 30 minutes at 550° C, but practically the hardening occurs during firing of the ceramic. During the casting of these alloys some of these base elements are lost; it is therefore recommended that 50% new alloy be used with a sprue button if it is used to make a second casting. The new alloy will provide enough of the base elements so adequate oxides and hardening result.

From Table 19-3 it is seen that these alloys have high stiffness (elastic modulus), strength, and hardness and reasonable elongation; however, they have somewhat low sag resistance. The alloys are very costly because of their high noble-metal content and high density; they are sold on a weight basis but used on a volume basis. The casting temperature is reasonably high, and although reasonably easy to solder, care must be taken because the soldering temperature is only about 50 ° C below the melting

TABLE 19-2 Composition Ranges and Color of Types of Noble Alloys for Ceramic-Metal Restorations (wt%)

Type	Au (%)	Pt (%)	Pd (%)	Ag (%)	Cu (%)	Other (%)	Total Noble Metal Content (%)	Color
Au-Pt-Pd	84-86	4-10	5-7	0-2	—	Fe, In, Re, Sn 2-5	96-98	Yellow
Au-Pd	45-52	—	38-45	0	—	Ru, Re, In 8.5, Ga 1.5	89-90	White
Au-Pd-Ag	51-52	—	26-31	14-16	—	Ru, Re, In 1.5, Sn 3-7	78-83	White
Pd-Ag	—	—	53-88	30-37	—	Ru, In 1-5, Sn 4-8	49-62	White
Pd-Cu	0-2	—	74-79	—	10-15	In, Ga 9	76-81	White

TABLE 19-3 Properties and Casting Temperatures of Noble Alloys Used in Ceramic-Metal Restorations

Type	Ultimate Tensile Strength (MPa)	0.2% Yield Strength (MPa)	Elastic Modulus (GPa)	Elongation (%)	Hardness (DPH, kg/mm^2)	Density (g/cm^3)	Casting Temperature (° C)
Au-Pt-Pd	480-500	400-420	81-96	3-10	175-180	17.4-18.6	1150
Au-Pd	700-730	550-575	100-117	8-16	210-230	13.5-13.7	1320-1330
Au-Pd-Ag	650-680	475-525	100-113	8-18	210-230	13.6-13.8	1320-1350
Pd-Ag	550-730	400-525	95-117	10-14	185-235	10.7-11.1	1310-1350
Pd-Cu	690-1300	550-1100	94-97	8-15	350-400	10.6-10.7	1170-1190

temperature of the alloys. Finally, although considerable Pt and Pd are present, these alloys are still yellow, which makes producing pleasing esthetics with the ceramic easier than with white alloys.

Au-Pd Types This high-noble type with good corrosion resistance has decreased gold but increased palladium content. These alloys contain no platinum or iron and thus are solution- rather than precipitation-hardened. They contain In for bonding, gallium to decrease the fusion temperature, rhenium for grain refining, and ruthenium for castability. Because of their high palladium content, the alloys are white (some call it gray) rather than yellow, even though they contain about 50% gold. This color causes increased difficulty in producing esthetic restorations.

These alloys are stronger, stiffer, and harder than the Au-Pt-Pd type and have higher elongation (more ductile) and casting temperatures (easier to solder). They have lower densities, and when they were introduced were less costly than the Au-Pt-Pd type, because Pd was cheaper than Au. With Pd being more costly than Au, there is no longer a cost advantage. The decrease in density indicates more care should be taken during casting because of the decrease in the force with which the alloy enters the casting ring. However, these alloys are easy to cast, and soldering is easy because of the higher casting temperature.

Au-Pd-Ag Types These alloys contain less palladium than the Au-Pd type; the decrease is made up by adding silver. However, they still have good corrosion resistance. Again, In and Sn are added for bonding with the ceramics, ruthenium (Ru) for castability, and rhenium (Re) for grain refining. Hardening results from solution hardening. As seen in Table 19-3, the properties of the Au-Pd-Ag type are similar to those of the Au-Pd type.

Pd-Ag Types These alloys, which contain no gold and have a moderately high silver content, have the lowest noble-metal content of the five noble alloys. They contain In and Sn for bonding and Ru for castability. Their properties are similar to the Au-Pd-Ag type, except they are less dense (~11 g/cm^3 vs. 14 g/cm^3). They were developed at a time when the cost of Au was about \$800/oz and the cost of Pd was low; those conditions no longer exist. Some ceramics used with these high-Ag alloys resulted in what was called "greening," really a color shift toward yellow. Contamination and technique was blamed to some extent for this problem.

Pd-Cu Types These alloys contain very high Pd content with 10% to15% Cu. They contain In for bonding and Ga for controlling casting temperature. These alloys have high strength and hardness, moderate stiffness and elongation, and low density. However, they have low sag resistance and form dark oxides. They are white alloys, like all the other types except the yellow Au-Pt-Pd type.

COMPOSITION AND PROPERTIES OF BASE-METAL ALLOYS

The range of compositions of base metal alloys for ceramic-metal restorations are given for Ni-Cr, Co-Cr, and Ti type in Table 19-4, and typical properties of these alloys are listed in Table 19-5. Considerable variation in composition and properties are shown in these tables.

Ni-Cr Types Chromium provides tarnish and corrosion resistance, whereas alloys containing Al and Ti are strengthened by the formation of coherent precipitates of Ni_3Al or Ti_3Al. Mo is added to decrease the thermal coefficient of expansion, and Be to improve castability (by reducing the melting point) and hardening. Note because of the wide differences in atomic weight of Be, Ni, and Cr, 2 wt% is roughly equal to 6 at%. The use of Be may cause some toxicity problems and surface oxidation at high temperatures.

These alloys are harder than noble alloys but usually have lower yield strengths. They also have higher elastic moduli, and it was hoped thinner copings and frameworks could result. They have much lower densities (7 to 8 g/cm^3)

TABLE 19-4 Composition Ranges of Base Metals for Ceramic-Metal Restorations (wt%)

Type	Ni	Cr	Co	Ti	Mo	Al	V	Fe	Be	Ga	Mn	Nb	W	B	Ru
Ni-Cr	69-77	13-16	—	—	4-14	0-4	—	0-1	0-2	0-2	0-1	—	—	—	—
Co-Cr	—	15-25	55-58	—	0-4	0-2	—	0-1	—	0-7	—	0-3	0-5	0-1	0-6
Ti	—	—	—	90-100	—	0-6	0-4	0-0.3	—	—	—	—	—	—	—

TABLE 19-5 Properties of Base-Metal Alloys for Ceramic-Metal Restoration

Type	Ultimate Tensile Strength (MPa)	0.2% Yield Strength (MPa)	Elastic Modulus (GPa)	Elongation (%)	Hardness (DPH, kg/mm^2)	Density (g/cm^3)	Casting Temperature (° C)
Ni-Cr	400-1000	255-730	150-210	8-20	210-380	7.5-7.7	1300-1450
Co-Cr	520-820	460-640	145-220	6-15	330-465	7.5-7.6	1350-1450
Ti	240-890	170-830	103-114	10-20	125-350	4.4-4.5	1760-1860

and generally higher casting temperatures. Adequate casting compensation is at times a problem, as is the fit of the coping.

Co-Cr Types Again, Cr provides tarnish and corrosion resistance. Unlike Co-Cr partial-denture alloys, the alloys for ceramic-metal restorations are strengthened by solution hardening rather than carbide formation. Mo helps lower the coefficient of expansion and Ru improves castability. They are stronger and harder than noble and Ni-Cr alloys and have roughly the same densities and casting temperature as Ni-Cr alloys. Casting and soldering of these alloys is more difficult than noble alloys, as is obtaining a high degree of accuracy in the castings.

Ti Types Pure Ti and Ti-6Al-4V may become important for ceramic-metal restorations, but they present processing difficulties, as indicated by casting temperatures of 1760° to 1860° C and their ease of oxidation. However, newer techniques, such as machine duplication and spark erosion to fabricate copings, may increase the use of these metals.

In summary, the noble alloys have good corrosion resistance, but only the Au-Pt-Pd alloys have a desirable yellow color. The other types are white (gray), which is more difficult to mask with the ceramic. The Au-Pd, Au-Pd-Ag, and Pd-Ag types have excellent mechanical properties coupled with high fusion temperatures and ease of casting and soldering. However, the Pd-Ag type has caused some problems with discoloration of the ceramic. The Pd-Cu types are characterized by the formation of dark oxides, which may cause problems with masking by the ceramic. The Ni-Cr and Co-Cr types are noted for high hardness and elastic modulus, although some Ni-Cr alloys have lower yield strengths. They are also noted for high casting temperatures. In general the Ti types have lower mechanical properties than the other base metal alloys but notably lower density and higher casting temperatures. Good bonding of ceramic and alloy can be achieved with all alloys, but bonding with some base metal alloys is more technique sensitive.

PREPARATION OF CERAMIC-METAL RESTORATIONS

The processing of the metal coping for ceramic-metal restorations is much like that of all-metal crowns and bridges. One significant difference relates to the reuse of metal. As mentioned earlier, when the metal is melted and cast, certain alloying elements can be lost, especially the elements that readily form oxides. These elements are important for bonding with noble metal alloys. To conserve metal, portions of the casting are commonly remelted. Each time the metal is remelted, some of these easily oxidized elements are lost. Therefore a certain portion of new alloy (usually half) should be added each time the metal is reused to replenish the lost alloying elements.

Surface treatment of the metal coping before ceramic application is important for good bonding. These treatments are used to roughen the coping surface and form surface oxides. The surface may be roughened by blasting with a fine abrasive (25 to 50 μm alumina); in some cases this results in a large increase in bond strength. In most cases the metal coping is heat-treated either in air or under partial vacuum to produce a surface oxide to improve bonding. In some palladium alloys, the heat treatment forms not only surface oxides but also internal oxides that penetrate the metal from the surface and effectively roughen the surface, thereby improving bonding. Some base-metal alloys tend to form excessively thick interfacial oxides, which weaken the metal-ceramic bond (see Fig. 19-5). With these alloys, the coping is heat-treated and then blasted to remove enough oxide to achieve higher bonding. If this process is not used, failure through the oxide may occur.

Ceramic application is similar to that described in Chapter 18. However, there are several important considerations. The first layer of ceramic is especially important with ceramic-metal restorations because it must hide the metal; special opaque ceramic must be used (see Table 19-1). After the opaque layer has been applied and fired the dentin (or body) ceramic, which contains less of the opaque oxides (such as SnO_2 and ZnO_2), pigments, and fluorescing oxides, is applied and fired. Finally, once the correct contour has been established an essentially transparent glaze layer is applied and fired. The ceramic-alloy compatibility is another important consideration. As pointed out earlier, the thermal expansions must be matched and the porcelain firing temperatures must be low enough that the alloy will not sag; the manufacturer usually supplies compatibility information. Titanium alloys require special ceramics, otherwise processing of the ceramic is similar to that of the other alloys.

EFFECT OF DESIGN ON CERAMIC-METAL RESTORATIONS

Because ceramics are weak in tension and can withstand very little strain before fracturing, the alloy copings must be rigid to minimize deformation of the ceramic. However, you would like the coping to be as thin as possible to allow space for the ceramic to hide the color of the alloy without overcontouring the ceramic. This consideration is especially true for alloys that are white (gray). This might lead to the conclusion that Ni-Cr or Co-Cr alloys would be superior to the noble alloys because their moduli (stiffness) are 1.5 to 2 times greater and the thickness of the coping could be halved. However, loading the restoration places it in bending, and the bending equation shows that deformation is a function of only the first power of the modulus, whereas it is a function of the cube of the thickness. It can be shown that for a typical dental ceramic-metal restoration, the thickness of a base-metal coping can be reduced only about 7% because of the higher elastic modulus. Thus, the advantage of the higher modulus for the base-metal alloys is minimal.

When full ceramic coverage of the coping is done, the shoulder of the crown should be flat with a rounded angle. This design provides for bulk of ceramic and minimizes fracture compared with a knife-edge shoulder geometry. A somewhat easier preparation is a chamfer, which provides for adequate bulk of ceramic and resists fracture essentially as well as the flat-shoulder geometry. In any case, sharp angles in the ceramic are to be avoided.

When using partial coverage by ceramics, such as when a metal occlusal surface is desired, the position of the ceramic-metal joint is critical. Because of the large difference in modulus of the ceramic and metal, stresses occur at the interface when the restoration is loaded. These stresses can be minimized by placing the ceramic-metal joint as far away as possible from contact with opposing teeth.

In the design of a ceramic-metal bridge, the geometry of the interproximal area between the crown and pontic is critical. The occlusal-gingival length of the joint should be as long as clinically feasible; because deflection is decreased as the cube of the length, greater length will minimize deflection of the ceramic. It should be remembered that the bridge is not a uniform beam; maximum deflection on loading will occur at the thinnest cross section, the interproximal area.

SELECTED PROBLEMS

Problem 1

The ceramic of a metal-ceramic crown placed in the mouth fractured from the metallic substructure. What factors might have produced such a failure, and how can it be avoided?

Solution a

Surface contamination of the alloy before placing the ceramic may be a causative factor. Impurities on the metal surface, such as organic powder from the grinding stones or grease and oils from fingers, may prevent a good wetting of the ceramic, and air bubbles will be present at the ceramic-metal interface. To avoid this problem, you should use vitrified grinding stones, protect the metal surface from polishing debris, and not touch the metal with the fingers.

Solution b

Underfired opaquer may be a factor. When the opaque ceramic has not been brought up to its fusing point, a complete fusion into the surface of the metal has not been achieved. Proper firing technique with the opaque material will eliminate this trouble.

Solution c

Another cause for the fracture may be improper metallic thickness. A uniform metal thickness is very important to prevent failures in the metal-ceramic bond. A minimum thickness of 0.4 mm is allowable. Thinner metal substructure will not protect the ceramic from fracture.

Solution d

The reuse of alloys may cause a fracture in the substructure. When sprue buttons are used to cast a new substructure, tin, or indium may be decreased or eliminated, and a very weak bonding with the porcelain is the result. The use of fresh alloys for casting the substructure is ideal, but a combination of a 50% (75% is better) fresh alloy and 25% to 50% used alloy may be used without detrimental effects on the metal-ceramic bond.

Problem 2

When a ceramic-metal restoration was removed from the oven, cracks in the ceramic were observed. What factors may have caused this failure, and how can it be avoided?

Solution a

Improper selection of ceramic and alloy will cause such cracks. Manufacturers often produce ceramic with special characteristics to match the thermal properties of a particular alloy. When another metal is tried with the same ceramic, a mismatch in the thermal expansion may be sufficient to cause cracking. Only the alloy and the ceramic suggested by the manufacturer should be used.

Solution b

Another causative factor may be overglazed or overfired ceramic. An overglazed or overfired ceramic no longer matches the alloy properly. Irregularities on ceramic surfaces should be finished before glazing to avoid overglazing.

Solution c

When the ceramic-metal restoration is allowed to cool in the furnace after the ceramic has been baked, cracks in the ceramic material will be produced. The ceramic should never be cooled in the furnace because slow cooling may change some physical properties of the ceramic, creating a mismatch with the alloy.

Solution d

When hot ceramic is touched with a cold instrument, a thermal shock can produce cracks.

Problem 3

When a metal-ceramic fixed appliance was completed, the shades appeared too gray. What could be the cause of such a dark ceramic, and how can it be avoided?

Solution a

When the coating of opaque ceramic is too thin or incomplete, the transparency of the body ceramic will allow the gray coping to show through. The opaque bake should be examined for gray areas and reopaqued if any are present. Two thin coats of opaque ceramic with separate firings are often recommended.

Solution b

When opaque ceramic has been fired to maturity at the opaque bake, by the time a third or fourth bake is made, the ceramic may have become too glazed and lost some of its opacifying qualities, thereby allowing the metal to reflect through the opaque layer, creating a gray shade. The manufacturer's suggested technique to bake the opaque should be carefully followed.

Solution c

When a crucible contaminated by an alloy containing base metals is used, a dark shade may be obtained. To avoid this problem, do not use a crucible that has been used to cast any other alloy. Only clean crucibles without ceramic liners or fluxes should be employed to cast the alloys for metal-ceramic restorations.

Solution d

Nonprecious alloys may contaminate the oven. Another source of oven contamination is the formation of volatilized impurities when the ceramic furnace has been used often for degassing and soldering operations. When the contamination accumulates in the oven, ceramic fired there will be dark. To avoid this problem you should purge the ceramic oven frequently.

Problem 4

A metal-ceramic restoration was cemented in the mouth. After insertion, flaking or chipping of the ceramic was observed. What may have been the cause of this failure?

Solution

The main problem with ceramic is it does not withstand much bending without fracture. When fired on a thin or flexible substructure, deformation of the metal under stress may deform the ceramic beyond its limit, and flakes or chips in the ceramic material are produced. The alloy selected to prepare ceramic-metal restorations or appliances should be built with enough bulk and have a high enough rigidity to withstand masticatory stresses without excessive deformation.

Problem 5

A crown preparation was made on a small lower anterior tooth that allowed little space for a metal coping. A Ni-Cr alloy was selected for the coping because its stiffness was reported to be twice that of the noble alloys. Because of the higher stiffness, the thickness of the coping was halved. In service the ceramic fractured. Why?

Solution

It is a mistake to halve the thickness in response to a higher modulus. In the deflection of the coping, the thickness of the coping is much more important than the modulus. If inadequate space is available for the coping and the desired color of a normally thick coping cannot be achieved without overcontouring the ceramic, an all-ceramic crown should be considered.

BIBLIOGRAPHY

Anthony DH, Burnett AP, Smith DL et al: Shear test for measuring bonding in cast gold alloy-porcelain composites, *J Dent Res* 49:27, 1970.

Anusavice KJ, Dehoff PH, Fairhurst CW: Comparative evaluation of ceramic-metal bond tests using finite element stress analysis, *J Dent Res* 59:608, 1980.

Anusavice KJ, Ringle RD, Fairhurst CW: Bonding mechanism evidence in a ceramic nonprecious alloy system, *J Biomed Mater Res* 11:701, 1977.

Anusavice KJ, Ringle RD, Fairhurst CW: Identification of fracture zones in porcelain-veneered-to-metal bond test specimens by ESCA analysis, *J Prosthet Dent* 42:417, 1979.

Anusavice KJ, Ringle RD, Morse PK et al: A thermal shock test for porcelain metal systems, *J Dent Res* 60:1686, 1981.

Baran GR: Phase changes in base metal alloys along metal-porcelain interfaces, *J Dent Res* 58:2095, 1979.

Baran GR: Oxide compounds on Ni-Cr alloys, *J Dent Res* 63:1332, 1984.

Baran GR, Meraner M, Farrell P: Transient oxidation of multiphase Ni-Cr base alloys, *Oxides of Metals* 29:409, 1988.

Baran GR, Woodland EC: Forming of cast precious metal alloys, *J Dent Res* 60:1767, 1981.

Bartolotti RL, Moffa JP: Creep rate of porcelain-bonding alloys as a function of temperature, *J Dent Res* 59:2062, 1980.

Council on Dental Materials and Devices: How to avoid problems with porcelain-fused-to-metal restorations, *J Am Dent Assoc* 95:818, 1977.

Dent RJ, Preston JD, Moffa JP et al: Effect of oxidation on ceramometal bond strength, *J Prosthet Dent* 47:59, 1982.

Donachie MJ Jr, editor: *Titanium, a technical guide,* Metals Park, OH, 1988, ASM International.

Dorsch P, Ingersoll C: A review of proposed standards for metal-ceramic restorations, Ivoclar-Vivadent Report, Ivoclar AG, Schoen, Liechtenstein, Feb 4, 1988.

Duncan JD: Casting accuracy of nickel-chromium alloys: marginal discrepancies, *J Dent Res* 59:1164, 1980.

Duncan JD: The casting accuracy of nickel-chromium alloys for fixed prostheses, *J Prosthet Dent* 47:63, 1982.

Duncanson MG Jr: Nonprecious metal alloys for fixed restorative dentistry, *Dent Clin North Am* 20:422, 1976.

Eden GT, Franklin OM, Powell JM et al: Fit of porcelain fused-to-metal crown and bridge casting, *J Dent Res* 58:2360, 1979.

Fairhurst CW, Anusavice KJ, Hashinger DT et al: Thermal expansion of dental alloys and porcelains, *J Biomed Mater Res* 14:435, 1980.

Farah JW, Craig RG: Distribution of stresses in porcelain-fused-to-metal and porcelain jacket crowns, *J Dent Res* 54:255, 1975.

Faucher RR, Nicholls JI: Distortion related to margin design in porcelain-fused-to-metal restorations, *J Prosthet Dent* 43:149, 1980.

German RM: Hardening reactions in a high-gold content ceramo-metal alloy, *J Dent Res* 59:1960, 1980.

Huget EF, Dvivedi N, Cosner HE Jr: Characterization of gold-palladium-silver and palladium-silver for ceramic-metal restoration, *J Prosthet Dent* 36:58, 1976.

Huget EF, Dvivedi N, Cosner HE Jr: Properties of two nickel-chromium crown and bridge alloys for porcelain veneering, *J Am Dent Assoc* 94:87, 1977.

Jones DW: Coatings of ceramics on metals. In Ducheyne P, Lemons JE, editors: *Bioceramics: materials characteristics versus in vivo behavior,* vol 523, New York, 1988, New York Academy of Science.

Könönen M, Kivilahti J: Bonding of low-fusing dental porcelain to commercially pure titanium, *J Biomed Mater Res* 28:1027, 1994.

Lautenschlager EP, Greener EH, Elkington WE: Microprobe analysis of gold-porcelain bonding, *J Dent Res* 48:1206, 1969.

Lenz J, Schwarz S, Schwickerath H et al: Bond strength of metal-ceramics systems in three-point flexure bond test, *J Appl Biomater* 6:55, 1955.

Lubovich RP, Goodkind RJ: Bond strength studies of precious, semiprecious, and non-precious ceramic-metal alloys with two porcelains, *J Prosthet Dent* 37:288, 1977.

Mackert JR Jr, Twiggs SW, Evans-Williams AL: Isothermal anneal effect on leucite content in dental porcelains, *J Dent Res* 74:1259, 1995.

Malhotra ML, Maickel LB: Shear bond strength of porcelain-fused-to-alloys of varying noble metal contents, *J Prosthet Dent* 44:405, 1980.

Meyer JM, Payan J, Nally JM: Evaluation of alternative alloys to precious ceramic alloys, *J Oral Rehabil* 6:291, 1979.

O'Brien WJ: Ceramics, *Dent Clin North Am* 29: 851, 1985.

Ohno H, Kanzawa I, Kawashima I et al: Structure of high-temperature oxidation zones of gold alloys for metal-porcelain bonding containing small amounts of In and Sn, *J Dent Res* 62:774, 1983.
Ringle RD, Fairhurst CW, Anusavice KJ: Microstructures in non-precious alloys near the porcelain-metal interaction zone, *J Dent Res* 58:1987, 1979.
Saxton PL: Post soldering of non-precious alloys, *J Prosthet Dent* 43:592, 1980.
Shell JS, Nielsen JP: Study of the bond between gold alloys and porcelain, *J Dent Res* 41:1424, 1962.
Smith DL, Burnett AP, Brooks MS, Anthony DH: Iron-platinum hardening in casting golds for use with porcelain, *J Dent Res* 49:283, 1970.
Valega TM, editor: Alternatives to gold alloys in dentistry, proceedings of a conference held at NIH, January 1977, Bethesda, MD, DHEW Publication No (NIH) 77-1227.
Vermilyea SG, Huget EF, Vilca JM: Observations on gold-palladium-silver and gold-palladium alloys, *J Prosthet Dent* 44:294, 1980.

Chapter 20

Cements

A variety of cements have been used in dentistry through the years for two primary purposes: as restorative filling materials, either alone or with other materials, and to retain restorations or appliances in a fixed position within the mouth. In addition, certain cements are used for specialized purposes in the restorative, endodontic, orthodontic, periodontic, and surgical fields of dentistry.

When the properties of dental cements are compared with those of other restorative materials, such as amalgams, resin composites, gold, or ceramics, cements exhibit less favorable strength, solubility, and resistance to oral conditions. As a result, the general use of cements for restorations exposed to the oral environment is quite limited.

Zinc phosphate, glass ionomer, and zinc oxide–eugenol (ZOE) cements can be applied as a base in deep cavities to insulate the pulp from possible chemical and thermal trauma. A metallic, ceramic, or composite filling material may then be placed over the cement base in sufficient bulk and in proper adaptation to the cavity walls to form the final restoration. The sedative effect of ZOE mixtures has made them valuable for a variety of applications. The ability of the glass and hybrid ionomer and compomer cements to release fluoride and to bond chemically to tooth structure has resulted in their uses as bases and for cementation. Resin cements are used for retention of orthodontic brackets, all-ceramic veneers, crowns and inlays, and resin-bonded bridges because of their strength and ability to bond to acid-etched enamel and dentin treated with a dentin bonding agent.

The following is a classification of dental cements, based on their chief chemical ingredients and application:

GLASS AND HYBRID IONOMERS

Class 5 restorations (see Chapter 8)
Retention of alloy restorations
Retention of orthodontic bands
High-strength bases
Provisional restorations

ZINC POLYACRYLATE

Retention of alloy restorations
Retention of orthodontic bands
High-strength bases

ZINC PHOSPHATE

Retention of alloy restorations
Retention of orthodontic bands
High-strength bases
Provisional restorations

ZINC OXIDE–EUGENOL

Low- and high-strength bases
Provisional restorations
Temporary and permanent retention of restorations

NON-EUGENOL–ZINC OXIDE

Temporary retention of restorations
Root canal sealers
Gingival tissue packs
Surgical dressings

CALCIUM HYDROXIDE

Low-strength bases

COMPOMERS

Bonded conventional crowns and bridges
Retention of orthodontic brackets
High-strength bases

COMPOSITES AND ADHESIVE RESINS

Bonded conventional crowns and bridges
Bonded ceramic veneers, inlays, and onlays*
Bonded laboratory composites*
Bonded posts and cores*
Bonded Maryland bridges*
Retention of provisional restorations

*Used with bonding agents

Retention of orthodontic brackets
High-strength bases

Ten types of cements are currently available. Although members of the profession are not in unanimous agreement regarding the purposes of each cement or the necessity for all the types, they are available to the dental profession and have been employed principally in the ways listed.

ZINC PHOSPHATE CEMENT

Zinc phosphate cement is a traditional crown and bridge cement used for alloy restorations. It is supplied as a powder and a liquid, both of which are carefully compounded to react with one another during mixing to develop a mass of cement possessing desirable physical characteristics.

TABLE 20-1 Typical Composition of Zinc Phosphate Cement Powder and Liquid

Composition	Weight (%)
Powder	
ZnO	90.2
MgO	8.2
SiO_2	1.4
Bi_2O_3	0.1
Misc. BaO, Ba_2SO_4, CaO	0.1
Liquid	
H_3PO_4 (free acid)	38.2
H_3PO_4 (combined with Al and Zn)	16.2
Al	2.5
Zn	7.1
H_2O	36.0

Adapted from Paffenbarger GC, Sweeney WT, Issacs A: *J Am Dent Assoc* 20:1960, 1933.

COMPOSITION

Powder The principal ingredient of the zinc phosphate cement powder is zinc oxide. Magnesium oxide, silicon dioxide, bismuth trioxide, and other minor ingredients are used in some products to alter the working characteristics and final properties of the mixed cement. A typical formulation of a zinc phosphate cement powder and liquid is shown in Table 20-1. The magnesium oxide, usually in quantities of about 10%, is added to the zinc oxide to reduce the temperature of the calcination process. The silicon dioxide is an inactive filler in the powder and during manufacture aids in the calcination process. Although the bismuth trioxide is believed to impart a smoothness to the freshly mixed cement mass, in large amounts it may also lengthen the setting time. Tannin fluoride may be added to provide a source of fluoride ions in some products.

The ingredients of the powder are heated together at temperatures ranging from 1000° to 1300° C for 4 to 8 hours or longer, depending on the temperature. Calcination results in a fused or sintered mass. The mass is then ground and pulverized to a fine powder, which is sieved to recover selected particle sizes. The degree of calcination, fineness of particle size, and composition determine the reactivity of the powder with the liquid.

Liquid Zinc phosphate cement liquids are produced by adding aluminum and sometimes zinc, or their compounds, to a solution of orthophosphoric acid. Although the original acid solution contains about 85% phosphoric acid and is a syrupy fluid, the resulting cement liquid usually contains about one-third water, as shown in Table 20-1. The partial neutralization of the phosphoric acid by the aluminum and zinc tempers the reactivity of the liquid and is described as *buffering*. This reduced rate of reaction helps establish a smooth, nongranular, workable cement mass during the mixing procedure. The zinc phosphate cement liquid is adjusted by both partial neutralizing or buffering and dilution so it reacts with its powder to produce a cement mass with proper setting time and mechanical qualities.

SETTING REACTION

When an excess of zinc phosphate cement powder is brought into contact with the liquid to begin the cement mix, wetting occurs and a chemical reaction is initiated. The surface of the alkaline powder is dissolved by the acid liquid, resulting in an exothermic reaction.

The set zinc phosphate cement is essentially a hydrated amorphous network of zinc phosphate that surrounds incompletely dissolved particles of zinc oxide. This amorphous phase is extremely porous. There is no evidence that the magnesium oxide present in the powder reacts with the phosphoric acid. Although no crystalline phosphate is involved in the setting process of the cement, there can be subsequent growth of crystalline hopeite, $Zn_3(PO_4)_2 \cdot 4H_2O$, in the presence of excess moisture during setting.

MANIPULATION

The manner in which the reaction between the zinc phosphate cement powder and liquid is permitted to occur determines to a large extent the working characteristics and properties of the cement mass. Incorporate the proper amount of powder into the liquid slowly on a cool slab (about 21° C) to attain the desired consistency of cement. Certain requirements must be met to carry out this type of manipulation.

Mixing Slab A properly cooled, thick glass slab will dissipate the heat of the reaction. Should a rapid reaction occur, ample working time would not be available for proper manipulation of the cement before hardening or setting occurs. The mixing slab temperature should be low enough to effectively cool the cement mass but must not be below the dew point unless the frozen slab technique is used; this method is described subsequently. A temperature of 18° to 24° C is indicated when room humidity permits. The moisture condensation on a slab cooled below the dew point contaminates the mix, diluting the liquid and shortening the setting time. The ability of the mixing slab to be cooled and yet be free of moisture greatly influences proper control of the reaction rate of the zinc phosphate cement.

Powder/Liquid Ratio The amount of powder that can be incorporated into a given quantity of liquid greatly determines the properties of the mixed mass of cement. Because an increase in the ratio of powder to liquid generally provides more desirable properties, incorporate as much powder as possible to obtain a particular consistency.

Care of the Liquid When zinc phosphate cement liquid is exposed to a humid atmosphere, it will absorb water, whereas exposure to dry air tends to result in a loss of water. The addition of water causes a more rapid reaction with the powder, resulting in a shorter setting time. A loss of water from the liquid results in a lengthened setting time. Therefore keep the bottle tightly closed when not dispensing the material. Polyethylene squeeze bottles do not require removal of a dropper and therefore eliminate the tendency for gain or loss of water from the liquid.

Mixing Procedure By initially incorporating small portions of powder into the liquid, minimal heat is liberated and easily dissipated. The heat of the reaction is most effectively dissipated when the cement is mixed over a large area of the cooled slab. Use a relatively long, narrow-bladed stainless steel spatula to spread the cement across this large area to control the temperature of the mass and its setting time.

During the neutralization of the liquid by the powder, the temperature of the mixing site is inversely proportional to the time consumed in mixing. Thus if a large volume of powder is carried to the liquid all at once rather than spatulated over a large area of the slab for a sufficient time, the temperature at the site of the reaction becomes higher. This temperature rise speeds the reaction and hinders control over the consistency. In this case the consistency of the mass is achieved by the rapid approach of the initial setting rather than by the establishment of a higher powder/liquid ratio under more ideal mixing conditions.

During the middle of the mixing period, larger amounts of powder may be incorporated to further saturate the liquid with the newly forming complex zinc phosphates. The quantity of unreacted acid is less at this time because of the prior neutralization gained from initially adding small increments of powder. The amount of heat liberated will likewise be less, and it can be dissipated adequately by the cooled slab.

Finally, smaller increments of powder are again incorporated, so the desired ultimate consistency of the cement is not exceeded. Thus the mixing procedure begins and ends with small increments, first to achieve slow neutralization of the liquid with the attendant control of the reaction and last to gain a critical consistency.

Depending on the product, 60 to 90 seconds of mixing appears adequate to accomplish a proper zinc phosphate cementing mass. When the mixing time is unduly long, the cementing mass may be ultimately weakened by the breaking down of the matrix because it tends to form and bind the undissolved powder particles together.

Frozen Slab Method The mixes used in the normal mixing procedure have adequate working and setting times for the cementation of inlays and crowns. However, in the cementation of orthodontic bands, the short working time of normal mixes allows the cementation of only a few bands with one mix, and the setting times are too long for clinical convenience. The frozen slab method has been developed to overcome these difficulties.

In this method, a glass slab is cooled in a refrigerator at 6° C or a freezer at –10° C. No attempt is made to prevent moisture from condensing on the slab when it is brought to room conditions. A mix of cement is made on the cold slab by adding the powder until the correct consistency is reached. The amount of powder incorporated with the frozen slab method is 50% to 75% more than with the normal procedures. The compressive and tensile strengths of cements prepared by the frozen slab method are not significantly different from those prepared from normal mixes, however, because incorporation of condensed moisture into the mix in the frozen slab method counteracts the higher powder/liquid ratio. No difference exists in the solubility of frozen slab and normal mixes.

The advantages of the frozen slab method are a substantial increase in the working time (4 to 11 minutes) of the mix on the slab and a shorter setting time (20% to 40% less) of the mix after placement into the mouth. This method has also been advocated for cementation of bridges with multiple pins.

CHARACTERISTIC PROPERTIES

Zinc phosphate cements exhibit certain properties during setting and when hardened. The more important of the properties are included in ANSI/ADA Specification No. 96 (ISO 9917) for dental water-based cements. A summary of these requirements is given in Table 20-2.

Selected properties of a typical zinc phosphate cement and of other luting materials are listed in Tables 20-3 and 20-4.

Consistency and Film Thickness The desired consistency of the zinc phosphate cement mix depends on the particular purpose of the material and the working convenience needed, as expressed by the setting time. Two arbitrary consistencies, termed *inlay seating,* or luting, and *cement base,* or filling, are in general use. A third consistency of zinc phosphate cement, which lies midway between the inlay seating and the cement base, is used for the retention of orthodontic bands and has been termed a *band-seating consistency.*

The inlay-seating consistency of zinc phosphate cement is used to retain alloy restorations. Although the unhardened zinc phosphate cement is somewhat tenacious, the retaining action in its hardened state is one of mechanical interlocking between the surface irregularities of the tooth and the restoration. This interlocking is illustrated in the photomicrograph of the inter-

TABLE 20-2 Specification Requirements for Dental Water-Based Cements

Cement	Film Thickness, Maximum (μm)	Net Setting Time (min)	Compressive Strength (MPa)	Acid Erosion, Maximum (mm/hour)	Opacity, $C_{0.70}$	Acid-Soluble Arsenic Content (mg/kg)	Acid-Soluble Lead Content (mg/kg)
Glass ionomer (luting)	25	2.5-8.0	70	0.05	—	2	100
Zinc phosphate (luting)	25	2.5-8.0	70	0.1	—	2	100
Zinc polycarboxylate (luting)	25	2.5-8.0	70	2.0	—	2	100
Glass ionomer (base/liner)	—	2.5-6.0	70	0.05	—	2	100
Zinc phosphate (base/liner)	—	2.5-6.0	70	0.1	—	2	100
Zinc polycarboxylate (base/liner)	—	2.5-6.0	70	2.0	—	2	100
Glass ionomer (restorative)	—	2.5-6.0	130	0.05	0.35-0.90	2	100

Modified from ANSI/ADA Specification No. 96 for dental water-based cements.

TABLE 20-3 Mechanical Properties of Luting Cements*

	Compressive Strength (MPa)	Tensile Strengih (MPa)	Elastic Modulus (GPa)	Bond Strength to Dentin (MPa)
CEMENTS FOR FINAL CEMENTATION				
Adhesive resin	52-224	37-41	1.2-10.7	11-24 with bonding agent
Compomer	100	—	3.6	18-24 with bonding agent
Composite	180-265	34-37	4.4-6.5	18-30 with bonding agent
Glass ionomer	93-226	4.2-5.3	3.5-6.4	3-5
Hybrid ionomer	85-126	13-24	2.5-7.8	10-12 without bonding agent, 14-20 with bonding agent
Zinc oxide-eugenol (Type II)				
EBA-alumina	64	6.9	5.4	0
Polymer-modified	37	3.8	2.7	0
Zinc phosphate	96-133	3.1-4.5	9.3-13.4	0
Zinc polyacrylate	57-99	3.6-6.3	4.0-4.7	2.1
CEMENTS FOR TEMPORARY CEMENTATION				
Non-eugenol–zinc oxide	2.7-4.8	0.39-0.94	—	0
Composite resin	25-70	—	—	0
Zinc oxide–eugenol unmodified (Type I)	2.0-14	0.32-2.1	0.22	0

*Properties measured at 24 hours.

TABLE 20-4 Physical Properties of Luting Cements

Cements	Solubility in H_2O (% in 24 hr)	Setting Time at 37° C (100% Humidity) (min)	Film Thickness (μm)
Compomer	Low	3	—
Composite	0.13	4-5	13-20
Glass ionomer	0.4-1.5	6-8	22-24
Hybrid ionomer	0.07-0.40	5.5-6.0	10-22
Zinc oxide–eugenol			
Polymer-modified	0.08	9	25
EBA-alumina	0.02-0.04	7-9	25-35
Zinc polyacrylate	<0.05	7-9	25-48
Zinc phosphate	0.2 maximum	5-9	25 maximum

face of a gold alloy casting and the opposing dentin and enamel wall shown in Fig. 20-1. The gold alloy casting and the dentin are separated slightly and mechanically locked by cement.

The film thickness of the zinc phosphate cement greatly determines the adaptation of the casting to the tooth. The strength of the retention bond may also be influenced by the film thickness. ANSI/ADA Specification No. 96 has requirements for cements designed for the seating of precision appliances. The maximum film thickness is 25 μm. The heavier the consistency, the

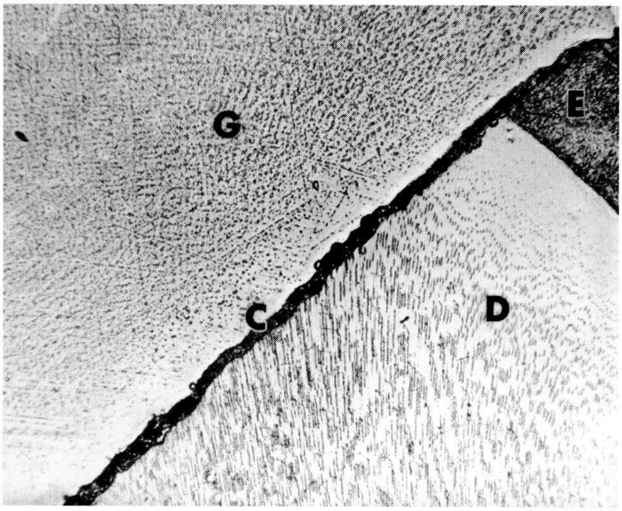

Fig. 20-1 Cement film between gold inlay and tooth. *G,* Gold inlay; *C,* cement; *D,* dentin; *E,* enamel.

greater the film thickness (as shown in Fig. 20-2) and the less complete the seating of the restoration. The ultimate film thickness that a well-mixed, nongranular cement attains depends first on the particle size of the powder and second on the concentration of the powder in the liquid, or the consistency of the cement. The film thickness also varies with the amount of force and the manner in which this force is applied to a casting during the cementation. The type of restoration being cemented influences the ease of the cement escaping from around the margins of the restoration. A full-crown casting presents the greatest problem in obtaining maximum displacement of the cement.

Obviously, the consistency of the zinc phosphate cement to be used in the cementation of a casting is critical. An increased amount of powder incorporated into the liquid will increase the consistency of the cement mass. Heavier-than-normal inlay-seating consistencies of cement are more difficult to express from under a casting, and incomplete seating of the inlay or crown may result from their use. The operator must frequently test each mass as the end of the mixing time is approached. The final consistency will be fluid, yet the cement will string up from the slab

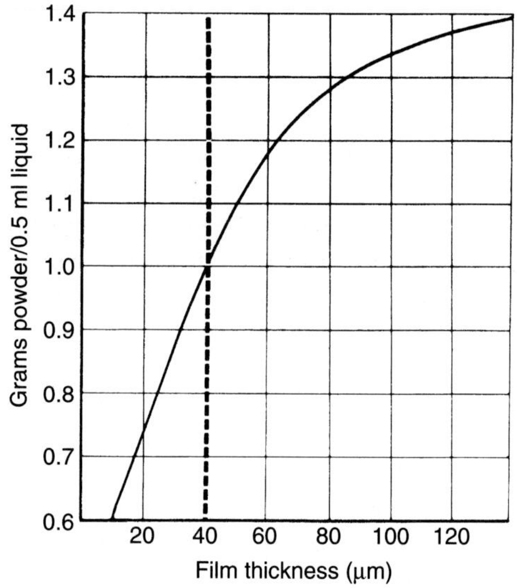

Fig. 20-2 Relation of powder/liquid ratio to film thickness.

on the spatula about 2 to 3 cm as the spatula is lifted away from the mass.

A heavy, puttylike consistency of zinc phosphate cement is used as a thermal and chemical insulating barrier over thin dentin and as a high-strength base. This same consistency may also

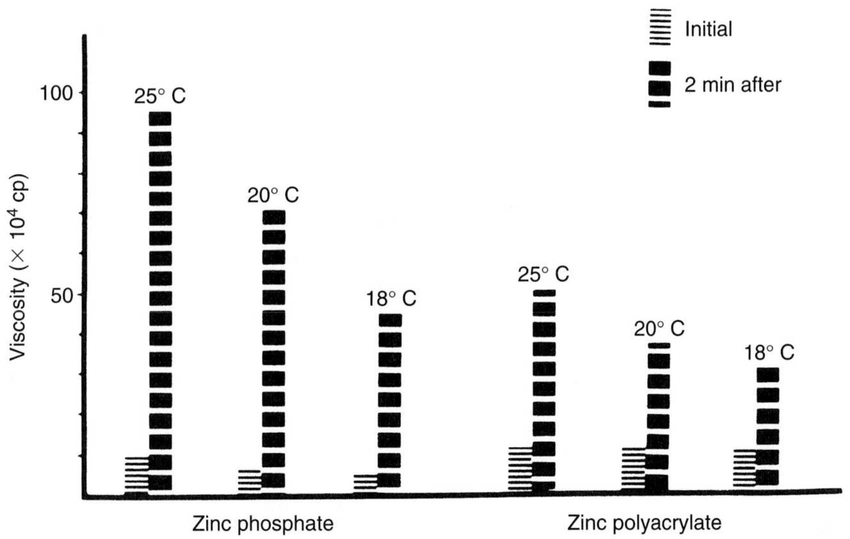

Fig. 20-3 Viscosity of zinc phosphate and zinc polyacrylate cements as a function of temperature and time.
(Modified from Vermilyea SG, Powers JM, Craig RG: *J Dent Res* 56:762, 1977.)

serve as a fairly durable provisional filling material. As such, the cement is exposed to dissolution in saliva, abrasion of mastication, and other oral conditions for an extended period of time. The cement base or filling consistency is achieved when using a powder/liquid ratio higher than that used for the inlay-seating or band-seating consistency.

Viscosity The consistency of cements can be quantified by measuring viscosity. The initial viscosity of mixes of zinc phosphate cements of inlay consistency is shown in Fig. 20-3 for mixes made at 18°, 20°, and 25° C. A small but significant increase in viscosity is seen at the higher temperatures. The viscosities of the mixes 2 minutes after completion of mixing are also shown. In all instances, pronounced increases in viscosity occurred during this time interval, with greater increases at the higher temperatures. Values for mixes of zinc polyacrylate cements are also listed. The rapid increase in viscosity demonstrates that restorations should be cemented promptly after completion of the mixing to take advantage of the lower viscosity of the cement. Delays in cementation can result in considerably larger values of film thickness and insufficient seating of the restoration.

Setting Time Of equal importance to the consistency of the cement is its setting time. A sufficient period of time must be available after the mixing to seat and finally adapt the margins of a casting, to seat and adjust a series of orthodontic bands, or to properly contour a base or provisional restoration. Adequate working time is expressed by proper net setting time, which, as determined by ANSI/ADA Specification No. 96 and based on an inlay-setting consistency, is between 2.5 and 8 minutes at a body temperature of 37° C. The first 60 to 90 seconds are consumed by mixing the powder and liquid, so the net setting time is the time elapsed between the end of mixing and the time of setting, as measured by resistance to a standard indentor. The setting time at mouth temperature of one brand of zinc phosphate cement, as the powder/liquid ratio is increased, is shown in Fig. 20-4.

The setting time for the band-seating or cement-base consistency is only slightly shorter because of the greater quantity of powder used to establish the heavier consistency.

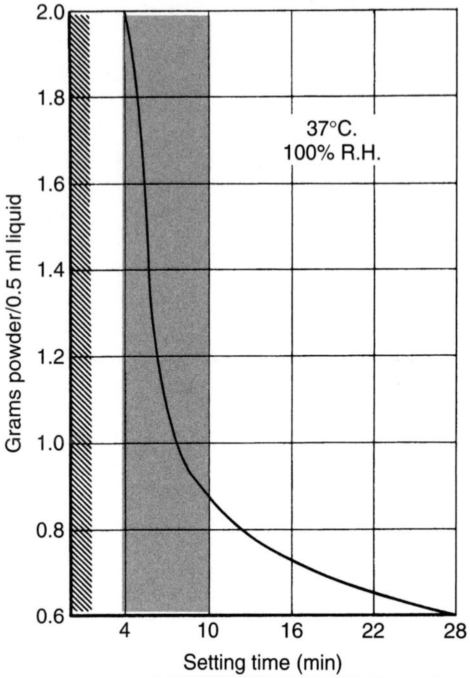

Fig. 20-4 Effect of powder/liquid ratio on setting time.

Several factors influence the rate of set of zinc phosphate cement. Those factors under the control of the manufacturer and the operator are listed in Tables 20-5 and 20-6. Although the manufacturer initially adjusts the setting time, improper handling of the powder and liquid can greatly modify the setting time. Anything that tends to speed the rate of reaction will shorten the setting time.

Strength The strength of zinc phosphate cement is influenced by the initial powder and liquid composition, the powder/liquid ratio and manner of mixing, and the handling of the cement during its placement.

ANSI/ADA Specification No. 96 (ISO 9917) stipulates that a standard inlay-seating consistency must exhibit a minimum 24-hour compressive strength of 70 MPa. The compressive strength of the zinc phosphate cement develops rapidly, with the inlay-seating consistency reaching at least two thirds of its final strength within 1 hour.

TABLE 20-5 Factors Governing the Rate of Set of Zinc Phosphate Cement

Controlled by Manufacturer	Controlled by Operator
Powder composition	Powder/liquid ratio
Degree of powder calcination	Rate of powder incorporation
Particle size of powder	Mixing temperature
Buffering of liquid	Manner of spatulation
Water content of liquid	Water contamination or loss from liquid

A proper mixing technique ensures a higher powder/liquid ratio for the consistency of cement desired, increasing the compressive strength of the cement mass. A cement base consistency, when properly achieved, offers greater strength than the inlay-seating consistency does. The maximum powder/liquid ratio is reached, however, when further amounts of powder do not increase the strength but may in fact decrease it because of the presence of excess unattached powder. For this reason a mass of mixed cement should evenly incorporate the powder throughout the mix.

Solubility and Disintegration The premature contact of the incompletely set cement with water results in the dissolution and leaching of that surface. Prolonged contact, even of the well-hardened cement, with moisture demonstrates that some erosion and extraction of soluble material does occur from the cement. ANSI/ADA Specification No. 96 allows a maximum rate of erosion of 0.1 mm/hr when the cement is subjected to lactic acid erosion by an impinging jet technique. Even the filling cement mixes show considerable loss of material in the mouth over a period of time, indicating that zinc phosphate cement can be regarded as only a temporary filling material. Wear, abrasion, and attack of food decomposition products accelerate the dis-

TABLE 20-6 Effects of Manipulative Variables on Selected Properties of Zinc Phosphate Cement

	Property				
Manipulative Variables	**Compressive Strength**	**Film Thickness**	**Solubility**	**Acidity**	**Setting Time**
Decreased powder/liquid ratio	Decrease	Decrease	Increase	Increase	Lengthen
Increased rate of powder incorporation	Decrease	Increase	Increase	Increase	Shorten
Increased mixing temperature	Decrease	Increase	Increase	Increase	Shorten
Water contamination	Decrease	Increase	Increase	Increase	Shorten

From Craig RG, Powers JM, Wataha JC: *Dental materials: properties and manipulation,* ed 7, St Louis, 2000, Mosby.
*Water contamination should not be confused with water incorporated in the frozen slab method.

integration of zinc phosphate cements within the oral cavity. Greater resistance to solution and disintegration is obtained by increasing the powder/liquid ratio. A thicker mix of cement therefore exhibits less solubility and disintegration than a thinner mix.

The difference between the resistance to abrasive and chemical attack intraorally and the passive resistance to solution and disintegration in distilled water causes a different clinical observation between zinc phosphate and other cements. This lack of correlation has been demonstrated in a clinical study in which the order of solubility of cements tested in the mouth was, from least to most soluble, glass ionomer, zinc phosphate, ZOE reinforced with ethoxybenzoic acid, and polyacrylate cements. Laboratory tests in distilled water indicate that glass ionomer cements are the most soluble and that polyacrylate, ZOE, and zinc phosphate cements are the least soluble.

ANSI/ADA Specification No. 96 specifies the maximum acid-soluble arsenic and lead contents as 2 and 100 mg/kg, respectively.

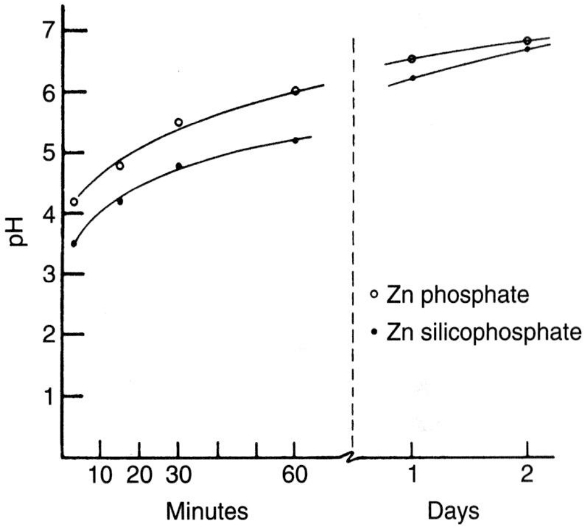

Fig. 20-5 Direct pH values determined on external surface of cements stored in humidor. *Note:* Zinc silicophosphate cements are no longer used.
(Adapted from Norman RD, Swartz ML, Phillips RW: *J Dent Res* 45:136, 1966.)

Dimensional Stability Zinc phosphate cement exhibits shrinkage on hardening. The normal dimensional change when properly mixed cement is brought into contact with water after it has set is that of slight initial expansion, apparently from water absorption. This expansion is then followed by a slight shrinkage on the order of 0.04% to 0.06% in 7 days.

Acidity During the formation of zinc phosphate cement, the union of the zinc oxide powder with the phosphoric acid liquid is accompanied by a change in pH, as shown in Fig. 20-5. In the early manipulative stage this increase in pH is relatively rapid, with a standard mix reaching a pH of 4.2 within 3 minutes after mixing is started. At the end of 1 hour this value increases to about 6 and is nearly neutral at 48 hours.

Investigation has shown that the initial acidity of zinc phosphate cement at the time of placement into a tooth may excite a pulpal response, especially where only a thin layer of dentin exists between the cement and the pulp. In a normal, healthy tooth this response may be entirely reversible, whereas in a tooth whose pulp has already been put under stress from other trauma the response may be irreversible, with pulp death ensuing. When zinc phosphate cement is to be used, exercise precaution in a deep cavity to protect the nearby pulp tissue from further trauma by the initial acidity of the cement. Such precautions include the use of resinous, film-forming, cavity varnishes; calcium hydroxide and zinc oxide suspensions; ZOE or calcium hydroxide bases; and, more recently, dentin bonding agents.

Gross decalcifications occasionally observed after the removal of orthodontic bands that have been retained in place with zinc phosphate cement are most probably attributable to the loss of the luting material between the band and the tooth, resulting in a favorable environment for bacterial action.

Thermal and Electrical Conductivity

One of the primary uses of zinc phosphate cement is as an insulating base beneath metallic restorations. Recent studies have shown that as a base material this cement is an effective thermal insulator, although not more effective than dentin itself. Although the presence of moisture does not have a significant effect on the thermal conductivity of the cement, the moisture present under clinical conditions greatly reduces the potentially good electrical insulating properties of the material.

APPLICATIONS

Zinc phosphate cement is used most commonly for luting permanent metal restorations and as a base. Other applications include cementation of orthodontic bands and the use of the cement as a provisional restoration.

Cementation of Orthodontic Bands

Zinc phosphate cement has been used for the cementation of orthodontic bands to the teeth for many years. The orthodontic consistency lies somewhere between the luting and base consistencies. Apparently the most important requirement is working time. Longer working times have been achieved by using the frozen slab method.

ZINC OXIDE–EUGENOL AND NON-EUGENOL CEMENTS

When certain types of zinc oxide are mixed with eugenol, the mix sets to a hard cement that is compatible with both the hard and soft tissues of the mouth. Cements of this type have been used extensively since the 1890s. Simple mixtures of these two materials do not have great strength when compared with zinc phosphate cements, and their use has been limited to situations in which strength is not important. Quite early it was found that they had a sedative effect on exposed dentin. For many years, ZOE cements have been used as provisional restorations, soft tissue packs in oral surgery and periodontics, and root canal sealers. Because eugenol acts as an inhibitor for free-radical polymerized materials, select other materials for provisional restorations when bonding of the permanent restoration is anticipated.

Non-eugenol–zinc oxide cements are also available for temporary cementation. These cements are suitable for patients sensitive to eugenol.

COMPOSITION

A typical formula for a ZOE cement compounded as a provisional filling material is shown in Table 20-7. The powder is mainly zinc oxide, with added white rosin to reduce the brittleness of the set cement, zinc stearate as a plasticizer, and zinc acetate to improve the strength of the cement. The liquid is eugenol with olive oil as a plasticizer. Two compositional changes have been used to increase the strength of the cement for luting purposes. In one, methyl methacrylate polymer is added to the powder, and in the other, alumina (Al_2O_3) is added to the powder and ethoxybenzoic acid (EBA) to the liquid.

A typical polymer-reinforced cement has 80% zinc oxide and 20% poly(methyl methacrylate) in the powder and eugenol in the liquid. These cements are sufficiently strong for final cementation of fixed prostheses and are used also as cement bases and provisional restorations. A typical EBA-alumina–reinforced ZOE cement contains 70% zinc oxide and 30% alumina by weight in the powder. In some cases, rosin and copolymers may be added to reduce the brittleness and film thickness and improve the mixing qualities. The liquid of the EBA-alumina–reinforced cements contains 62.5% ortho-EBA by weight and 37.5% eugenol by weight. The compressive strength of a typical EBA cement is shown in Table 20-3.

The non-eugenol–zinc oxide cements typically contain an aromatic oil and zinc oxide. Other ingredients may include olive oil, petroleum jelly, oleic acid, and beeswax.

TABLE 20-7 Formula for a Typical Zinc Oxide-Eugenol Temporary Filling Cement

Ingredients	Weight (%)
Powder	
Zinc oxide	69.0
White rosin	29.3
Zinc stearate	1.0
Zinc acetate	0.7
Liquid	
Eugenol	85.0
Olive oil	15.0

Adapted from Wallace DA, Hansen HL: *J Am Dent Assoc* 26: 1536, 1933.

SETTING REACTION

The setting of ZOE cements is a chelation reaction in which an amorphous, zinc eugenolate is formed. The setting reaction is shown below, where two molecules of eugenol react with ZnO in the presence of water to form the chelate, zinc eugenolate. Excess zinc oxide is always used, so the set material consists of a matrix of amorphous zinc eugenolate that binds the unreacted zinc oxide particles together. The setting reaction is accelerated by increases in temperature or humidity. EBA also forms a chelate with zinc oxide, and its presence allows some crystalline zinc eugenolate to form, which provides additional strength. The reaction is not measurably exothermic, and the presence of moisture is essential for setting to occur.

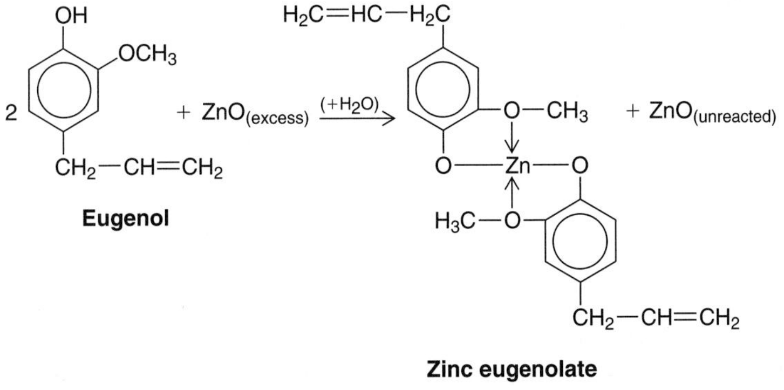

MANIPULATION

Dispensing The unmodified ZOE and non-eugenol–zinc oxide cements are typically two-paste systems. Equal lengths of each paste are dispensed and mixed to a uniform color.

For some cements used for temporary cementation or for provisional restorations, powder is often incorporated into a dispensed amount of liquid until a suitable consistency is achieved for the operation at hand. The dentist makes this determination from experience. A considerable amount of powder can be incorporated into the liquid by heavy spatulation with a stiff spatula. In general, the more powder incorporated, the stronger the cement and the more viscous the mixed cement.

Cements intended for final cementation of restorations carry manufacturers' directions and measuring devices that are important to use. Because of the deceptive flow qualities of these cements, adding powder until the operator feels the mix is of suitable consistency for cementing a restoration will lead to a cement deficient in powder and a lowered strength in the set cement. To those accustomed to the handling qualities of zinc phosphate cement as a luting medium, a correctly proportioned and mixed ZOE luting cement appears far too viscous.

Mixing Procedures Because the setting reaction is not significantly exothermic, a cooled mixing slab is not required. Usually a paper mixing pad with disposable sheets is used, which facilitates the cleanup procedures after cementation. A glass slab is recommended for mixing the EBA-alumina–modified cements. There is no need to incorporate the powder in small increments; usually the bulk of the powder is incorporated in the initial step, the mix is thoroughly spatulated, and a series of smaller amounts is then added until the mix is complete. The mix is thoroughly kneaded with the spatula (a stiff-bladed steel spatula is the most effective type). The EBA-alumina–modified cement is dispensed according to the instructions, kneaded for 30 seconds, and then stropped for 60 seconds to develop a creamy consistency. Oil of orange can be used to clean eugenol cements from instruments.

CHARACTERISTIC PROPERTIES

The variety of compositions of the ZOE cements and the many uses to which they are applied make it difficult to write a specification for these cements. ANSI/ADA Specification No. 30 (ISO 3107) for dental zinc oxide–eugenol cements and zinc oxide non-eugenol cements gives standards for temporary cements, permanent cements, filling materials and bases, and cavity liners. It sets requirements for the general characteristics of the powders, liquids, and pastes used in these cements and for the important physical properties of setting time, compressive strength, disintegration, film thickness, and acid-soluble arsenic content, where these are applicable. The limiting values established for these properties for each type of cement are shown in Table 20-8.

Film Thickness Film thickness is an important factor in the complete seating of restorations at the time of cementation. The film thickness should be not more than 25 μm for cements used for permanent cementation and not more than 40 μm for cements used for temporary cementation, as determined by the specification test. This requirement is not applied to cements used for purposes other than cementation.

Setting Time For all except two of the cements, a range of setting times from 4 to 10 minutes is required. For cements intended for filling materials and bases, the preference of some operators for a faster setting cement is recognized in the specification by extending the lower end of the range to 2 minutes.

Compressive Strength A maximum value of 35 MPa is required for cements intended for temporary cementation. A minimum of 35 MPa is required for cements intended for permanent cementation and 25 MPa for filling materials and bases. Lining materials are required to have a minimum compressive strength of 5 MPa. Clinical studies have shown that for temporary cementing of restorations a variety of cements with compressive strengths varying from 1.4 to 21 MPa is desirable. The strength of a cement for temporary cementation is selected in

TABLE 20-8 Specification Requirements for Zinc Oxide–Eugenol and Zinc Oxide–Non-Eugenol Cements

Cement	Setting Time at 37° C (min)	Compressive Strength (24 hr) (MPa)	Maximum Disintegration (24 hr) (%)	Maximum Film Thickness (µm)	Maximum Acid-Soluble Arsenic Content (mg/kg)
Type I. Temporary Cement					
Class 1. Powder-liquid	4-10	35 maximum	2.5	40	2
Class 2a. Paste-paste (eugenol)	4-10	35 maximum	2.5	40	2
Class 2b. Paste-paste (non-eugenol)	4-10	35 maximum	2.5	40	2
Class 3. Paste-paste (nonsetting)	—	—	—	40	2
Type II. Permanent cement					
Class 1. Powder-liquid	4-10	35 minimum	1.5	25	2
Type III. Filling materials and bases					
Class 1. Powder-liquid	2-10	25 minimum	1.5	—	2
Class 2. Paste-paste	2-10	25 minimum	1.5	—	2
Type IV. Cavity liners					
Class 1. Powder-liquid	4-10	5 minimum	1.5	—	2
Class 2. Paste-paste	4-10	5 minimum	1.5	—	2

Modified from ANSI/ADA Specification No. 30 for dental zinc oxide–eugenol cements and zinc oxide–non-eugenol cements, 2000.

relation to the retentive characteristics of the restoration and the expected problems of removing the restoration when the time arrives.

For permanent cementation the strongest cement possible is preferable. Most ZOE cements for permanent cementation have compressive strength values considerably higher than the 35 MPa required by the specification. The strength of the non-eugenol–zinc oxide cements is similar to that of the unmodified ZOE cements intended for temporary cementation. A comparison of the compressive strengths of several types of cements is given in Table 20-3.

Disintegration The disintegration of cement is generally regarded as less critical for cements used as provisional restorations or for temporary cementation. This is reflected in the maximum specification values for disintegration in 24 hours. A maximum value of 2.5% is acceptable for provisional cementing materials, but a value of 1.5% is required for the other cements. The test used is the amount of disintegration, measured by weight loss, which occurs in a disk of the cement immersed in distilled water for 24 hours. There is no close correlation between this test and the clinical behavior of these cements, and the test serves only to compare cements of known clinical acceptability with other products. It is a useful monitoring method for evaluating new products and ensuring quality control of manufacturing processes.

APPLICATIONS

A range of ZOE and modified ZOE cements are suitable for many uses in restorative dentistry, and the practitioner should become familiar with each type and its application.

Base Materials having a compressive strength of 5.5 to 39 MPa are used as a cement base, and the strength reaches a maximum in about 12 to 15 minutes. They are normally used under zinc phosphate cement, which acquires about three times the strength in the same time. The ZOE cements have the advantage that the thermal insulating properties of the cements are excellent and are approximately the same as those for human dentin. Bases are discussed later in this chapter.

Temporary Cementation Unmodified ZOE cements are also used as luting materials for provisional crowns and temporary cementation of metal restorations in crown and bridge prosthodontics. Laboratory studies have shown that the retention of metal restorations with unmodified cements is proportional to the compressive strength of the cements. Unmodified ZOE cements are available in compressive strengths varying from 1.4 MPa to 21 MPa. A clinical study of the use of various unmodified cements for luting provisional crowns indicated that a cement with a compressive strength of 15 to 24 MPa was the most appropriate cement, based on: (1) retention, (2) taste, (3) ease of removal, and (4) ease of cleaning. Another clinical study indicated that an unmodified ZOE cement with a compressive strength of 6.9 MPa was the most commonly used material for the temporary cementation of complete crown and bridge restorations, although a range of cements with compressive strengths from 1.4 to 21 MPa was found to be desirable.

The non-eugenol–zinc oxide cements do not adhere as well to preformed metal crowns as the eugenol-containing cements, and they are slower setting. The non-eugenol cements, however, do not soften provisional acrylic crowns.

Provisional Restorations The EBA-alumina–modified cements have been tried as provisional restorations based on their physical properties. Clinical studies showed these cements were handled easily and had improved carvability, which prevented chipping during trimming, and that symptomatic teeth without pulp exposure showed no symptoms. The EBA-alumina–modified cements, despite their low solubility in water, disintegrated and wore excessively in the mouth. A thick mix, 2.6 g/0.4 ml of polymer-modified ZOE, was more serviceable than the EBA-alumina–modified type, and although some chipping was observed at the margins, all provisional restorations of ZOE were serviceable for 2 to 10 months of observation.

Permanent Cementation The use of EBA-alumina–modified ZOE cements has been clinically successful for the permanent cementation of crowns and bridges. The film thickness of these cements is therefore important, and, as indicated in Table 20-4, a film thickness of 25 to 35 μm is readily obtained. Other properties are shown in Tables 20-3 and 20-4.

Endodontic Sealers Endondontic ZOE preparations have been used as a root canal sealer alone and with gutta-percha. There are two major groups of products based on ZOE cements—conventional and therapeutic sealers.

Composition and Setting Conventional sealers are generally based on the formulas of Grossman or Rickert, as summarized in Table 20-9. The setting reaction occurs between zinc oxide and eugenol. Resins improve the mixing characteristics and retard setting. Radiopacity is improved by adding barium or bismuth salts or silver powder. The conventional sealers are used with gutta-percha points.

Therapeutic sealers are usually used without a core material and are formulated with ingredients such as iodoform, paraformaldehyde, or trioxymethylene, which may have therapeutic value. The use of these sealers is controversial.

ANSI/ADA Specification No. 57 (ISO 6876) covers materials used in endodontics within the tooth to seal the root canal space. The physical properties specified include working time, flow, film thickness, setting time, dimensional change following setting, solubility, and radiopacity. A summary of these requirements is given in Table 20-10.

Viscosity The ability of a sealer to penetrate into irregularities and accessory canals has been termed *flow,* though *viscosity* is a more correct term. Viscosity has been shown by several different tests to decrease during the mixing procedure (an example of shear thinning). Values of viscosity range from 8 to 680,000 cp (centipoise).

Setting Time The setting time of cements is measured by a penetration test and ranges from 15 minutes to 12 hours at mouth temperature. Sealers set much more rapidly at mouth temperature than at room temperature.

Film Thickness Film thickness, measured as directed by ANSI/ADA Specification No. 57, is influenced by viscosity, setting time, and the size

TABLE 20-9 Composition of Typical Zinc Oxide–Eugenol Endodontic Sealers

Rickert's Formula		Grossman's Formula		Therapeutic Formula
POWDER	**%**	**POWDER**	**%**	**POWDER**
Zinc oxide	41*	Zinc oxide	42	Zinc oxide
Silver	30	Staybelite resin	27	Bismuth subnitrate
White rosin	17	Bismuth subcarbonate	15	Iodoform
Thymol iodide	12	Barium sulfate	15	Rosin
		Sodium borate anhydrate	1	
LIQUID		**LIQUID**		**LIQUID**
Oil of cloves	78	Eugenol	100	Eugenol
Canada balsam	22			Creosote
				Thymol

*Percent by weight.

TABLE 20-10 Specification Requirements for Types II and III Endodontic Filling Materials

Working Time	Minimum Flow (mm)	Maximum Film Thickness (μm)	Setting Time	Maximum Linear Dimensional Change at 30 Days (%)	Maximum Solubility (%)	Minimum Radiopacity (mm of Aluminum)
±10% of manufacturer's claimed value	20	50	±10% of manufacturer's claimed value	1.0 shrinkage 0.1 expansion	3.0	3.0

Adapted from ANSI/ADA Specification No. 57 for endodontic sealing materials, 1993.

of filler particles in the cement. Lower values of film thickness are considered desirable for condensation of gutta-percha. Values range from 80 to 500 μm, depending on the testing load.

Compressive Strength The strength of a sealer is an indication of its ability to support tooth structure weakened by the cleaning of the canal and its durability. Values range from 8 to 50 MPa.

Solubility Solubility is an undesirable characteristic in a root canal sealer, because the process of dissolution can cause the sealer to release components that may be biologically incompatible. Solubility has been measured in water, and typically values range from 0.1% to 3.5%.

Radiopacity Radiopacity is desirable, and a minimum value has been established at the equivalent of 3 mm of aluminum. Values of radiolucency range from 0.10 to 0.98 among various sealers and 0.78 for gutta percha. These are relative values with lower numbers for more radiopaque materials.

Dimensional Change Most root canal sealers shrink as a result of setting. This shrinkage affects the integrity of the bond between the sealer and the tooth or core material. Values of volume loss after 90 days in a capillary tube range from −0.7% to −5.0%.

Biological Properties These properties have been studied by in vivo and in vitro tests of HeLa cells, human skin fibroblasts, and bovine pulp tissue; endodontic fillings in dogs, monkeys, and rats; and implants in tibias and in subcutaneous connective tissues of animals. Conventional ZOE sealers generally elicit mild to moderate reactions, whereas several of the therapeutic sealers elicit severe reactions.

Tissue Management Another variation of the ZOE cements has been necessitated by the special requirements imposed in the management of gingival tissues. This group of cements is used in two ways: (1) to mechanically displace soft tissue, and (2) to dress soft tissues after surgery. When these cements are used as a mechanical tissue pack, a thin consistency is incorporated into cotton fibers that are placed into the gingival sulcus. As a surgical dressing, this preparation affords greater comfort to the patient during eating, obtunds the surgerized tissue, promotes epithelial growth, and helps prevent the overgrowth of granulation tissue.

The setting times of these ZOE surgical cements must be quite long to facilitate the mixing of rather large quantities and to permit the proper placement and contouring of the dressing. Usually no accelerator is added to these materials. On placement of the packs in the mouth, the moisture and increased temperature tend to hasten the setting reaction. When mixed to a proper consistency, the cement must be soft enough to permit placement and contouring with gentle pressures, and yet firm enough to maintain the desired form.

These formulations generally have greater quantities of mineral, peanut, or almond oil present to increase plasticity over that of filling cements. Cotton fibers are often added to increase the strength and durability. In addition to the normal ingredients (zinc oxide, rosin, and eugenol), tannic acid is often added as a hemostatic agent and to decelerate the setting reaction. Aromatic oils and coloring agents may be incorporated to improve the taste and color of the dressing. Chlorhexidine has also been added as an antibacterial agent.

ZINC POLYACRYLATE CEMENT

COMPOSITION

Zinc polyacrylate cements (or zinc polycarboxylate) are supplied as a powder and a liquid or as a powder that is mixed with water. The liquid is a water solution of polyacrylic acid, the formula being:

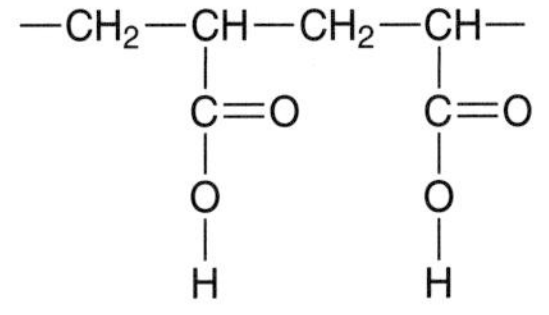

Most commercial liquids are supplied as a 32% to 42% solution of polyacrylic acid, having a molecular weight of 25,000 to 50,000. The manufacturer controls the viscosity of the cement liquid by varying the molecular weight of the polymer or by adjusting the pH by adding sodium hydroxide. Itaconic and tartaric acids may be present to stabilize the liquid, which can gel on extended storage.

The cement powder is essentially zinc oxide and magnesium oxide that have been sintered and ground to reduce the reactivity of the zinc oxide. The cement powder that is mixed with water contains 15% to 18% polyacrylic acid coated on the oxide particles.

SETTING REACTION

The set cement is a zinc polyacrylate ionic gel matrix that unites unreacted zinc oxide particles. The gel is bound to the polyanion chains by electrostatic interactions rather than by stronger specific ion binding. The matrix appears to be amorphous. The setting reaction can be retarded by a cool environment or accelerated by a warm environment.

MANIPULATION

The cements supplied with the polyacrylic acid in the liquid are usually mixed at a powder/liquid ratio of 1:1 to 2:1. One cement mixed with water has a powder/liquid ratio of 5:1 for cementation consistency. The consistency of the mixes is creamy compared with that of zinc phosphate cements. The mixed cement is *pseudoplastic;* that is, the viscosity decreases as the shear rate increases, or, in other terms, the flow increases as spatulation increases or as force is placed on the material. The correct consistency is found in a mix that is viscous but that will flow back under its own weight when drawn up with a spatula.

Dispense the liquid immediately before mixing to prevent evaporation of water and subsequent thickening. A nonabsorptive surface, such as a glass slab or treated paper, will keep all the liquid available for the reaction and facilitate spatulation. Mix polyacrylate cements within 30 to 60 seconds, with half to all of the powder incorporated at once to provide the maximum length of working time (typically 2.5 to 6 minutes). Extend the working time to 10 to 15 minutes by mixing on a glass slab chilled to 4° C. The strength of the mixed cement is not compromised by this technique. Some manufacturers supply the cement as a capsulated powder-liquid system for mixing in a mechanical mixer.

Polyacrylate cements have been used to cement metal inlays and crowns and to make bases. Apply the cement to clean cavity walls that are well isolated in a dry field. Use the mixed cement only as long as it appears glossy on the surface. Once the surface becomes dull, the cement develops stringiness and the film thickness becomes too great to seat a casting completely.

PROPERTIES

ANSI/ADA Specification No. 96 This specification establishes maximum values of setting time, film thickness, acid erosion, and arsenic and lead content, and a minimum value of compressive strength for zinc polyacrylate cement. A summary of these requirements is given in Table 20-2.

Viscosity The effect of temperature on the initial viscosity of zinc polyacrylate cement and the viscosity 2 minutes after mixing is shown in Fig. 20-3. The initial viscosity was essentially unaffected by the temperature increase from 18° to 25° C, although the viscosity was higher than the initial viscosity for comparable mixes of zinc phosphate cement. The viscosity of zinc polyacrylate cement 2 minutes after mixing increased modestly at all three temperatures; however, the increases in viscosity were substantially less than those for comparable zinc phosphate cement mixes. Thus the initial viscosity of zinc polyacrylate cements is higher than zinc phosphate cements, and a delay of 2 minutes in cementation reverses the situation.

Setting Time The setting-time test measures the time at which the cement is sufficiently hard to resist indentation by a standard indenter. The net setting time should occur within 2.5 to 8 minutes so final finishing procedures associated with the restoration can occur. As shown in Table 20-4, setting of the zinc polyacrylate cements usually occurs within 7 to 9 minutes from the start of mixing.

Film Thickness The film thickness test excludes materials that might have excessively large powder particles or a short working time, because complete seating of a casting with zinc polyacrylate cement might not occur. The film thickness of the polyacrylate cements is slightly higher than that of zinc phosphate cements but is well within clinical limits, as shown in Table 20-4.

Strength The compressive strength test excludes materials that have a compressive strength of less than 70 MPa. Clinical studies have shown that cements of this strength or greater will satisfactorily retain castings with a good fit.

The 24-hour compressive strength of polyacrylate cements for luting is lower than that of zinc phosphate cements, 98 to 133 MPa compared with 57 to 99 MPa; however, the tensile strength of polyacrylate cements is about 40% higher than that of zinc phosphate cements. The higher tensile strength may be influenced by the test method. In the diametral compression test, zinc polyacrylate cement specimens deform somewhat before breaking. The deformation results in a higher load before fracture is recorded than would occur if brittle fracture occurred. The modulus of elasticity of the zinc polyacrylate cements is about one third that of the zinc phosphate cements mixed to a luting consistency.

Bond Strength An interesting feature of polyacrylate cement is its bonding to enamel and dentin, which is attributed to the ability of the carboxylate groups in the polymer molecule to chelate to calcium. The bond strength to enamel has been reported to be from 3.4 to 13 MPa, and the bond strength to dentin has been found to be 2.1 MPa. Optimum bonding, however, requires cleaned tooth surfaces. The bonding of the polyacrylate cements to gold casting alloy is likewise highly dependent on surface preparation. Sandblasting or electrolytic etching of the gold alloy surface is necessary to achieve optimum bonding. Clinical studies have not demonstrated improved retention of crowns and bridges as a result of cementation with polyacrylate cements, however.

Because of the adhesion of polyacrylate cements to enamel, the cements were used at one time for direct bonding of orthodontic brackets to teeth. Presently, direct bonding is accomplished with composite cements.

Solubility and Disintegration The solubility and disintegration test excludes materials that are excessively soluble in distilled water. Solubility in distilled water does not always correlate with solubility in vivo. Solubility in water at 1 day varies from 0.12% to 0.25% for typical zinc polyacrylate cements. One cement tested increased in solubility from 0.25% at 1 day to 0.60% at 1 month in water. Other cements were not affected by longer-term storage. ANSI/ADA Specification No. 96 specifies the maximum rate of acid erosion of zinc polyacrylate cements as 2.0 mm/hr.

Dimensional Stability The zinc polyacrylate cements show a linear contraction when setting at 37° C. The amount of contraction varies from 1% for a wet specimen at 1 day to 6% for a dry specimen at 14 days. These contractions are more pronounced than those observed for zinc phosphate cements and start earlier.

Acidity Zinc polyacrylate cements are slightly more acidic than zinc phosphate cements when first mixed, but the acid is only weakly dissociated, and penetration of the high–molecular weight polymer molecules toward pulpal tissue is minimal. Histological reactions to polyacrylate cements appear similar to those of ZOE cements, although the production of reparative dentin under the polyacrylate cements is more evident.

APPLICATIONS

Zinc polyacrylate cements are used primarily for luting permanent alloy restorations and as bases. These cements have also been used in orthodontics for cementation of bands.

GLASS IONOMER CEMENT

COMPOSITION

Glass ionomer cements are supplied as a powder and a liquid or as a powder that is mixed with water. Several products are encapsulated. The liquid typically is a 47.5% solution of 2:1 polyacrylic acid/itaconic acid copolymer (average molecular weight 10,000) in water. The itaconic acid reduces the viscosity of the liquid and inhibits gelation caused by intermolecular hydrogen bonding; D(+) tartaric acid (5%, the optically active isomer) in the liquid serves as an accelerator by facilitating the extraction of ions from the glass powder.

The powder of glass ionomer cement is a calcium fluoroaluminosilicate glass with a formula of

$$SiO_2—Al_2O_3—CaF_2—Na_3AlF_6—AlPO_4$$

The nominal composition of the glass is listed in Table 20-11. The maximum grain size of the powder appears to be between 13 and 19 μm. The powder is described as an ion-leachable glass that is susceptible to acid attack when the Si/Al atomic ratio is less than 2:1. Barium glass or zinc oxide may be added to some powders to provide radiopacity.

In some products the polyacrylic acid is coated on the powder. The liquids of these products may be water or a dilute solution of tartaric acid in water.

TABLE 20-11 Nominal Composition of Calcium Fluoroaluminosilicate Glass Used in Powder of Glass Ionomer Cement

Chemical	Percent by Weight
SiO_2	29.0
Al_2O_3	16.6
CaF_2	34.3
Na_3AlF_6	5.0
AlF_3	5.3
$AlPO_4$	9.8

Adapted from Prosser HJ, Richards CP, Wilson AD: *J Biomed Mater Res* 16:431, 1982.

SETTING REACTION

The setting reaction is an acid-base reaction between the acidic polyelectrolyte and the aluminosilicate glass, as diagrammed below.

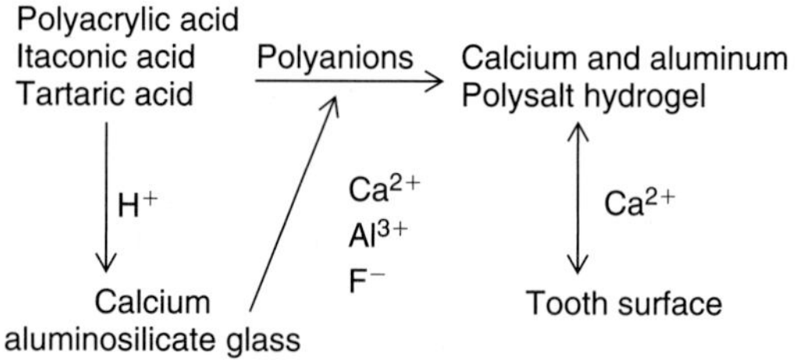

The polyacid attacks the glass to release cations and fluoride ions. These ions, probably metal fluoride complexes, react with the polyanions to form a salt gel matrix. The Al^{3+} ions appear to be site bound, resulting in a matrix resistant to flow, unlike the zinc polyacrylate matrix. During the initial setting reaction in the first 3 hours, calcium ions react with the polycarboxylate chains. Subsequently, the trivalent aluminum ions react for at least 48 hours. Between 20% and 30% of the glass is decomposed by the proton attack. The fluoride and phosphate ions form insoluble salts and complexes. The sodium ions form a silica gel. The structure of the fully set cement is a composite of glass particles surrounded by silica gel in a matrix of polyanions cross-linked by ionic bridges. Within the matrix are small particles of silica gel containing fluorite crystallites.

Glass ionomer cements bond chemically to enamel and dentin during the setting process. The mechanism of bonding appears to involve an ionic interaction with calcium and/or phosphate ions from the surface of the enamel or dentin. Bonding is more effective with a cleaned surface provided the cleansing process does not remove an excessive amount of calcium ions. Treating dentin with an acidic conditioner followed by a dilute solution of ferric chloride improves the bonding. The cleansing agent removes the smear layer of dentin while the Fe^{3+} ions are deposited and increase the ionic interaction between the cement and dentin.

MANIPULATION

Glass ionomer cements mixed with the more viscous carboxylic acid liquids have a powder/liquid ratio of 1.3:1 to 1.35:1, whereas those mixed with water or a liquid with a consistency like that of water have a powder/liquid ratio of 3.3:1 to 3.4:1. The powder and liquid are dispensed onto a paper or glass slab. The powder is divided into two equal portions. The first portion is incorporated into the liquid with a stiff spatula before the second portion is added. The mixing time is 30 to 60 seconds. Encapsulated products are typically mixed for 10 seconds in a mechanical mixer and dispensed directly onto the tooth and restoration. The cement must be used immediately because the working time after mixing is about 2 minutes at room temperature (23° C). An extension of the working time to 9 minutes can be achieved by mixing on a cold slab (3° C), but because a reduction in compressive strength and in the modulus of elasticity is observed, this technique is not recommended. Do not use the cement once a "skin" forms on the surface or when the viscosity increases noticeably.

Glass ionomer cements are very sensitive to contact with water during setting. The field must be isolated completely. Once the cement has achieved its initial set (about 7 minutes), coat the cement margins with the coating agent supplied with the cement.

PROPERTIES

ANSI/ADA Specification No. 96 (ISO 9917) Requirements of this specification for glass ionomer cements used as cements, bases, and restorative materials are given in Table 20-2.

Film Thickness The film thickness of glass ionomer cements is similar to or less than that of zinc phosphate cement (see Table 20-4) and is suitable for cementation.

Setting Time Glass ionomer cements set within 6 to 8 minutes from the start of mixing. The setting can be slowed when the cement is mixed on a cold slab, but this technique has an adverse effect on the strength.

Strength The 24-hour compressive strength of glass ionomer cements ranges from 90 to 230 MPa and is greater than that of zinc phosphate cement. Values of tensile strength are similar to those of zinc phosphate cement. Unlike zinc polyacrylate cements, glass ionomer cements demonstrate brittle failure in the diametral compression test. The elastic modulus of glass ionomer cements is less than that of zinc phosphate cement, but more than that of zinc polyacrylate cement. The rigidity of glass ionomer cement is improved by the glass particles and the ionic nature of the bonding between polymer chains.

The compressive strength of glass ionomer cements increases between 24 hours and 1 year, unlike that of zinc polyacrylate cement. A glass ionomer cement formulated as a filling material showed an increase from 160 to 280 MPa over this period. The strength of glass ionomer cements improves more rapidly when the cement is isolated from moisture during its early life.

Bond Strength Glass ionomer cements bond to dentin with values of tensile bond strength reported between 1 and 3 MPa. The bond strength of glass ionomer cements to dentin is somewhat lower than that of zinc polyacrylate cements, perhaps because of the sensitivity of glass ionomer cements to moisture during setting. The bond strength has been improved by treating the dentin with an acidic conditioner followed by an application of a dilute aqueous solution of $FeCl_3$. Glass ionomer cements bond well to enamel, stainless steel, tin oxide–plated platinum, and gold alloy.

Solubility Values of solubility of glass ionomer cements as measured in water are substantially higher than those measured for other cements (see Table 20-4). However, when these cements are tested in acid (0.001 N lactic acid), the values are quite low compared with values for zinc phosphate and zinc polyacrylate cements. The rankings determined by solubility tests in acid correlate well with clinical evaluations.

ANSI/ADA Specification No. 96 specifies the maximum acid erosion rate as 0.05 mm/hr. This specification also sets limits on the acid-soluble arsenic content and lead content (see Table 20-2).

Biological Properties Biological evaluations of glass ionomer cements have been done by tissue culture and animal tests. The culture cells showed a weaker reaction to glass ionomer cement than to ZOE or zinc polyacrylate cements. Pulp tissue reactions of monkeys tested in vivo showed no difference between glass ionomer and ZOE cements. These reactions have been described as mild.

Glass ionomer luting cements may cause prolonged hypersensitivity, varying from mild to severe. Microleakage has been suggested as an explanation, but a recent study showed no increase in bacterial counts 56 days after cementation of crowns with a glass ionomer cement. These cements may be bacteriostatic or bactericidal, however, because of fluoride release. Good isolation appears essential when glass ionomer cements are used. The use of the proper powder/liquid ratio and the application of a calcium hydroxide base in areas closest to the pulp are recommended.

APPLICATIONS

Glass ionomer cements are used primarily for permanent cement, as a base, and as a Class 5 filling material (see Chapter 8). The cement has been evaluated as a pit and fissure sealant and as an endodontic sealer. The sensitivity of the cement to moisture and desiccation may minimize its use in these latter applications. Glass ionomer cements are being used clinically for cementation of orthodontic bands because of their ability to minimize decalcification of enamel by means of fluoride release during orthodontic treatment.

HYBRID IONOMER CEMENT

Self-cured and light-cured hybrid ionomers (or resin-modified glass ionomers) are available for cementation. Hybrid ionomer restorative materials are described in Chapter 8.

COMPOSITION

One self-cured hybrid ionomer cement powder contains a radiopaque, fluoroaluminosilicate glass and a micro-encapsulated potassium persulfate and ascorbic acid catalyst system. The liquid is an aqueous solution of polycarboxylic acid modified with pendant methacrylate groups. It also contains 2-hydroxyethylmethacrylate (HEMA) and tartaric acid. Another self-cured cement contains a mixture of fluoroaluminosilicate and borosilicate glasses in the powder. Its liquid is a complex monomer containing carboxylic acid groups that can undergo an acid-base reaction with glass and vinyl groups that can polymerize when chemically activated. A light-cured hybrid ionomer cement contains fluoroaluminosilicate glass in the powder and a copolymer of acrylic and maleic acids, HEMA, water, camphorquinone, and an activator in the liquid.

SETTING REACTION

Setting of hybrid ionomer cements generally results from an acid-base glass ionomer reaction and self-cured or light-cured polymerization of the pendant methacrylate groups. Some cements, however, are light-cured only.

MANIPULATION

The powder is fluffed before dispensing. The liquid is dispensed by keeping the vial vertical to the mixing pad. For one product, the powder/liquid ratio is 1.6 g of powder to 1.0 g of liquid, and the powder is incorporated into the liquid within 30 seconds to give a mousse-like consistency. The working time is 2.5 minutes. The cement is applied to a clean, dry tooth that is not desiccated. Some products recommend the use of a conditioner for enhanced bonding to dentin. No coating agent is needed. HEMA is a known contact allergen; therefore use of protective gloves and a no-touch technique are recommended.

PROPERTIES

Requirements for light-activated cements, which are water-based and set by multiple reactions, including an acid-base reaction and polymerization (Type I), and by cements that set only after light-activation (Type II), are described by ANSI/ADA Specification No. 96 (ISO 9917, Part 2). Properties for liners and bases and restoratives are given in Table 20-12.

The compressive and tensile strengths of hybrid ionomer cements are similar to those of glass ionomer cements (see Table 20-3). The fracture toughness is higher than that of other water-based cements but lower than composite cements. The bond strength to moist dentin ranges from 10 to 14 MPa and is much higher than that of most water-based cements. Hybrid ionomer cements have very low solubility when tested by lactic acid erosion. Water sorption is higher than

TABLE 20-12 Specification Requirements for Light-activated Dental Water-based Cements*

Property	Bases and Liners	Restoratives
Sensitivity to ambient light	No change with 30-second exposure	
Setting time w/o activating radiation (Type 1 materials)	Less than 60 minutes	
Initial hardening time (Type 1 materials)	Not less than value stated by manufacturer	
Depth of cure	Not less than 1 mm; within 0.5 mm of value claimed by manufacturer	
Flexural strength	≥10 MPa	≥20 MPa
Radiopacity	At least the same as equivalent thickness of Al, if radiopacity claimed by manufacturer, and not more than 0.5 mm below value claimed	
Opacity	Not applicable	0.35-0.90
Shade	Not applicable	Matches shade guide
Color stability	Not applicable	No more than slight color change after 7 days

*Modified from ANSI/ADA Specification No. 96 for dental water-based cements—Part 2: Light-activated cements. Type 1 cements are light cured but also set in absence of activating light; Type 2 cements require light activation.

for resin cements. Delayed fracture of ceramic restorations cemented with hybrid ionomer cements has been reported. Recently, some hybrid ionomer cements have been modified to have less water sorption. Fluoride release and rechargeability are similar to glass ionomer cements. The early pH is about 3.5 and gradually rises. Clinical experience indicates minimal postoperative sensitivity.

APPLICATIONS

Self-cured hybrid ionomer cements are indicated for permanent cementation of porcelain-fused-to-metal crowns; bridges; metal inlays, onlays, and crowns; post cementation; and luting of orthodontic appliances. Additional uses include adhesive liners for amalgam, bases, provisional restorations, and cementation of specific ceramic restorations. Light-cured hybrid ionomer cements are used primarily for liners and bases. Restorative applications of light-cured hybrid ionomer cements are discussed in Chapter 8. One light-cured product is recommended for direct bonding of orthodontic brackets and bands.

COMPOMERS

Compomer cement is the newest resin-based cement indicated for cementation of cast alloy crowns and bridges, porcelain-fused-to-metal crowns and bridges, and gold cast inlays and onlays. Cementation of all-ceramic crowns, inlays, onlays, and veneers, with some exceptions, is contraindicated. The cement should not be used as a core or filling material. Compomers are also known as *poly acid–modified composites.* A compomer cement was recently introduced for orthodontic bonding.

COMPOSITION

The cement powder contains strontium aluminum fluorosilicate glass, sodium fluoride, and self- and light-cured initiators. The liquid contains polymerizable methacrylate/carboxylic acid monomer, multifunctional acrylate/phosphate monomer, diacrylate monomer, and water.

SETTING REACTION

Setting is the result of self- and light-cured polymerization. Once the cement comes into contact with oral fluids, an acid-base reaction may occur. The carboxylic acid groups contribute to the adhesive capability of the cement.

MANIPULATION

Dry the tooth to be cemented but do not desiccate. The powder/liquid ratio is 2 scoops to 2 drops. Tumble the powder before dispensing. Mix the powder and liquid rapidly for 30 seconds. Place the mixed cement in the crown only and then seat the crown. A gel state is reached after 1 minute, at which time the excess cement is removed with floss and a scaler. Light-cure the exposed margins to stabilize the restoration. Setting occurs 3 minutes after start of mix. Once set, compomer cement is very hard.

PROPERTIES

Compomer cement has high values of retention, bond strength, compressive strength, flexural strength, and fracture toughness (see Table 20-3). The cement has low solubility and sustained fluoride release.

COMPOSITES AND ADHESIVE RESINS

Cements based on resin composites have been used for cementation of crowns, conventional bridges, and resin-bonded bridges; for bonding of esthetic ceramic and laboratory-processed composite restorations to teeth; and for direct bonding of orthodontic brackets to acid-etched enamel. Recently, composite cements have been developed for cementation of provisional restorations.

ISO 4049 for polymer-based filling, restorative, and luting materials (ANSI/ADA No.

27) describes the following three classes of composite cements:

Class 1—self-cured materials

Class 2—light-cured materials

Class 3—dual-cured materials

Property requirements based on ISO 4049 can be summarized as follows:

Class 1, 2, 3: film thickness, max.—50 μm

Class 1, 3: working time, min.—60 seconds

Class 1, 3: setting time, max.—10 minutes

Class 2: depth of cure, min.—0.5 mm (opaque), 1.5 mm (others)

Class 1, 2, 3: water sorption, max.—40 $\mu g/mm^3$

Class 1, 2, 3: solubility, max.—7.5 $\mu g/mm^3$

CEMENTATION OF ALLOY CROWNS AND BRIDGES, RESIN-BONDED BRIDGES, AND PROVISIONAL RESTORATIONS

Synthetic resin cements based on methyl methacrylate have been available since 1952 for use in cementation of inlays, crowns, and appliances. In the early 1970s, a resin composite was introduced as a crown and bridge cement.

Composition and Setting Reaction

Self-cured, composite cements are typically two-paste systems. One major component is a diacrylate oligomer diluted with lower–molecular weight dimethacrylate monomers. The other major component is silanated silica or glass. The initiator-accelerator system is peroxide-amine.

One adhesive resin cement is a self-cured, powder-liquid system formulated with methacryloxyethylphenyl phosphate or 4-methacryloxyethyl-trimellitic anhydride (4-META). The 4-META cement is formulated with methyl methacrylate monomer and acrylic resin filler and is catalyzed by tri-butyl-borane. Another adhesive resin cement is a phosphonate cement supplied as a two-paste system, containing Bis-GMA resin and silanated quartz filler. The phosphonate molecule is very sensitive to oxygen, so a gel is provided to coat the margins of a restoration until setting has occurred. The phosphate end of the phosphonate reacts with calcium of the tooth or with a metal oxide. The double-bonded ends of both 4-META and phosphonate cements react with other double bonds when available. Setting of resin cements results from self- or light-cured polymerization of carbon-carbon double bonds.

Properties Some properties of composite and adhesive resin cements are listed in Tables 20-3 and 20-4. A comparison of bond strengths of adhesive and conventional resin-bonded bridge cements is given in Table 20-13. Adhesive resin cements have superior bonding to sandblasted Ni-Cr-Be and Type IV gold alloys. Composite cements used for cementation of provisional restorations (25 to 70 MPa) have a substantially

TABLE 20-13 Bond Strengths of Adhesive and Conventional Resin-Bonded Bridge Cements to Various Substrates

	Bond Strength (MPa)	
Substrate	**Adhesive Resin Cement**	**Conventional Resin Cement**
Dentin (unetched)	4.1	0.0
Enamel (etched)	15.0	10.0
Ni-Cr-Be alloy		
Sandblasted	24.0	14.1
Electrolytically etched	27.4	25.2
Type IV gold alloy		
Sandblasted	22.0	9.4
Tin-plated	25.5	12.8

From Powers JM, Watanabe F, Lorey RE: *In vitro* evaluation of prosthodontic adhesives. In Gettleman L, Vrijhoef MMA, Uchiyama Y: *Adhesive prosthodontics—adhesive cements and techniques,* Nijmegen, 1986, Academy of Dental Materials; and Watanabe F, Powers JM, Lorey RE: *J Dent Res* 67:479, 1988.

lower compressive strength than composite cements used for permanent cementation (180 to 265 MPa).

Applications Adhesive resin cements and composite cements in conjunction with bonding agents are being used as cements for posts and cores. Bond strengths of 14 MPa have been reported for silica-treated posts cemented with 4-META resin cement in extracted teeth. The use of resin-bonded bridges declined dramatically in the late 1980s.

BONDING OF ESTHETIC RESTORATIONS

The bonding of all-ceramic, tooth-colored crowns, veneers, inlays, and onlays became popular in the late 1980s. Dual-cured composite resin cements are ideal for bonding cast or CAD/CAM-prepared ceramic restorations or laboratory-processed composite inlays. Light-cured composite cements are useful for bonding thin ceramic veneers where achieving adequate depth of cure is not a problem.

Composition Composite cements are microfilled or hybrid composites formulated primarily from Bis-GMA or urethane dimethacrylate resins and fumed silica or glass fillers (20% to 75% by weight) or both. Dual-cured cements come in a base-catalyst form and must be mixed before use. Light-cured composites are photoinitiated in the presence of a camphoroquinone-amine system. They provide a wide selection of shades, tints, and opaquers.

Manipulation A bonding agent is necessary to bond the resin cement to tooth structure, whereas various surface preparations (sandblasting) and treatments (silanation or chemical softening) are used to prepare the ceramic or laboratory-fabricated composite restorations for bonding. Based on in vitro studies, composite cements bond well to post-cured composite inlays.

Properties Compressive strengths of dual- and light-cured resin composite cements have been reported from 180 to 265 MPa (see Table 20-3). Viscosity has been measured subjectively to range from low to high. Film thicknesses on vented crowns range from 13 to 20 μm. The cements are radiopaque for use in the posterior portion of the mouth.

RESIN-METAL BONDING

Bonding composite to the metal framework of a bridge and denture acrylic to a partial denture framework can be improved by the use of silica coatings. Presently there are three processes for applying silica to either noble or base-metal alloys. One method applies pyrogenic silica using a propane flame. Other methods use heat in an oven or ceramic blasting to coat the restoration or appliance. Bond strengths of composites to silica-coated Au-Pd or Ni-Cr-Be alloys range from 16 to 22 MPa. Silica coating of noble alloys eliminates the need for tin plating these alloys to improve adhesion of composites. The bond strength of denture acrylics to Ni-Cr-Be alloys range from 7 to 23 MPa when the alloy is treated with a silica coating or primed with adhesive resin cement. Liquid primers based on thiosulfates have recently become available for treatment of alloys. Recently, metal primers based on thiophosphate chemistry have been introduced as a treatment for resin-metal bonding.

BONDING OF ORTHODONTIC BRACKETS

Resin cements were evaluated for direct bonding of orthodontic brackets (without bands) in the late 1960s. Advances in acid etching of enamel substantially increased the popularity of the technique in the mid-1970s. Now resin composite cements have completely replaced acrylic resin cements for orthodontic bonding. Composite cements are used with metal, plastic, or ceramic orthodontic brackets.

Composition and Setting Composite cements are formulated from various diacrylate oligomers diluted with lower–molecular weight dimethacrylate monomers and fillers of silica, glass, or colloidal silica. The highly filled cements typically contain silanated inorganic particles (more than 60% by weight). The slightly filled cements contain 28% colloidal silica. The initiator-accelerator systems of these composite cements depend on the mode of initiating the polymerization. Amine-cured systems include conventional two-paste products and one-step products. Light-cured systems are polymerized by visible light.

Manipulation The success of composite cements used for direct and indirect bonding is highly dependent on proper isolation and acid etching of the enamel. The acid-etching technique involves etching the tooth for 15 to 60 seconds with a solution of phosphoric acid, followed by rinsing and drying. If the enamel is contaminated, re-etching of the tooth is necessary. Acid etching of enamel is discussed in greater detail in Chapter 10. A commercial self-etching primer is available as an alternative to phosphoric acid etching for orthodontic bonding to enamel.

Two-paste composite cements require mixing for 20 to 30 seconds before they are applied to the enamel and bracket base. A primer such as methyl methacrylate monomer in a solvent usually must be applied to a plastic bracket base. Sometimes a sealant formulated from an unfilled diacrylate is applied initially to the acid-etched enamel. The two-paste cements set several minutes after mixing.

The one-step (no-mix) cements require no mixing. A priming liquid is applied to the etched enamel, and the paste is applied to the bracket base. A plastic bracket may require a bracket primer. Polymerization is initiated when the bracket is placed on the primed tooth. The effect of film thickness on the polymerization of these cements has been investigated. Generally, there is a decrease in tensile bond strength as the thickness of one-step cements increases. Failures are characterized by incomplete polymerization of the resin. Bond strength of one-step cements decreases if the primer is exposed to a simulated oral environment for a minute or more, so bases should be placed promptly after the primer is applied to the teeth.

Light-cured composite cements are single-paste systems that require no mixing. The resin is applied to the tooth and bracket base, and polymerization is activated by the light source. A sealant may be used for bonding to the teeth, and a primer may be required for bonding to a plastic bracket. Recently, high-intensity, visible lights and argon lasers have been used in orthodontics to save time.

Properties Two important properties of composite cements for orthodontic bonding are esthetics and bond strength to tooth structure and the bracket base.

Changes in color of composite cements can result from staining or from the formation of colored reaction products. After accelerated aging or exposure to a tea stain, the cements were darker and more chromatic. Exposure to the tea stain caused a greater change in color than the aging test.

The bond strength of composite cements to tooth structure appears clinically adequate if proper isolation and manipulative techniques are followed. Bonding to tooth structure results from the resin matrix penetrating into the etched areas of enamel.

Bonding to orthodontic bracket bases depends on the type of bracket base (metal, plastic, or ceramic) and the type of cement (hybrid ionomer, highly filled composite, or slightly filled composite), as shown in Table 20-14. Failures typically occur at the cement-base interface or, less often, within the cement or base. Bonding to plastic bases appears to be chemical, whereas bonding to metal and ceramic bases is mechanical. Failures at the cement-metal base interface are initiated at areas of stress concentration in the metal base, such as weld spots or damaged mesh (Fig. 20-6). Plastic brackets tend to fail at the wings rather than debonding in laboratory testing. Failure at the interface of the cement-ceramic bracket is influenced by the amount of penetration of resin into the retention areas of the base.

Improved metal bases, including photographically etched and grooved types, have been tested with surface treatments such as silanation, etching, and activation. Etching of the grooved

TABLE 20-14 Effect of Types of Cement and Bracket Base on Bond Strength of Direct-Bonding Cements

Type of Cement	Bond Strength (MPa) Type of Bracket		
	Base Metal	**Ceramic**	**Plastic**
Hybrid ionomer	2.9-4.2	5.8-7.4	1.4-4.5
Slightly filled composite	8.8	4.6	8.3*
Highly filled composite	13.0	5.1	8.1

Adapted from Buzzitta VAJ, Hallgren SE, Powers JM: *Am J Orthod* 81:87, 1982; de Pulido LG, Powers JM: *Am J Orthod* 83:124, 1983; and Blalock KA, Powers JM: *Am J Orthod Dentofac Orthop* 107:596, 1995.
*With bracket primer.

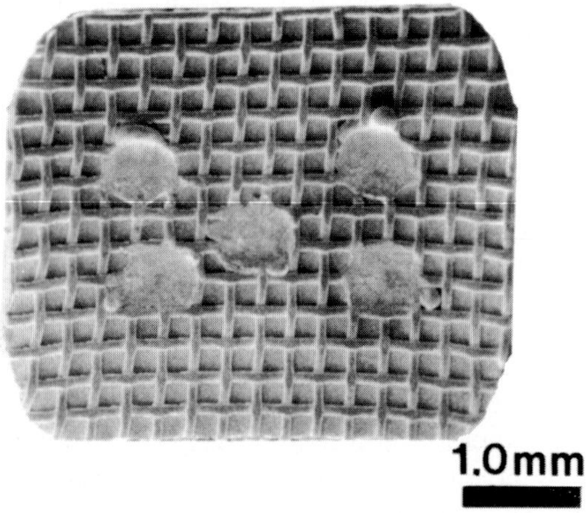

Fig. 20-6 Scanning electron photomicrograph of direct-bonding metal mesh base damaged by spot welds.
(From Dickinson PT, Powers JM: *Am J Orthod* 78:630, 1980.)

base was most effective in improving the bond strength. Studies of the new alumina and glass-ceramic brackets indicate that high bond strengths can be attained. Most clinical failures are attributed to breakage of the wings of the ceramic brackets.

Reconditioning of metal bases by thermal treatment, chemical treatment, and grinding with a green stone have been evaluated. Reconditioning caused a 20% to 56% decrease in bond strength of several composite cements to a mesh metal base.

CAVITY VARNISHES

A cavity varnish is used to provide a barrier against the passage of irritants from cements or other restorative materials and to reduce the penetration of oral fluids at the restoration-tooth interface into the underlying dentin. Varnishes help reduce postoperative sensitivity when applied to dentinal surfaces under newly placed restorations. Cavity varnishes are rapidly being replaced by bonding agents.

COMPOSITION

A cavity varnish is a solution of one or more resins from natural gums, synthetic resins, or rosin. Copal and nitrated cellulose are typical examples of a natural gum and synthetic resin, respectively. The solvents that may be used to dissolve these materials are chloroform, alcohol, acetone, benzene, toluene, ethyl acetate, and amyl acetate. Medicinal agents such as chlorobutanol, thymol, and eugenol also have been added. The volatile solvents evaporate quickly when the varnish is applied to the prepared tooth surface, thus leaving a thin resin film. The addition of fluoride to cavity varnish has not been established as effective.

MANIPULATION

Varnish solutions are usually applied by means of a small cotton pledget at the end of a wire or root canal reamer. Apply thin layers of the varnish with a partially saturated pledget. Use a gentle stream of air for drying, but take care to avoid forming ridges. Add a new layer only to a previously dried one. Two thin layers have been found more protective than one heavy layer. To prevent contamination of the cavity varnish, use a new cotton pledget for each application. Tightly cap varnish solutions immediately after use to minimize loss of solvent. Most varnishes are supplied with a separate bottle of pure solvent. This solvent may be used to keep the varnish from becoming too thick. Replace the loss from evaporation by adding solvent to keep the bottle at least half full by diluting the contents with the solvent. Eventually the solvent will be exhausted and a new supply should be purchased. The solvent is also useful for removing varnish from external tooth surfaces.

PROPERTIES

Cavity varnishes reduce but do not prevent the passage of constituents of the phosphoric acid cements into underlying dentin. Variations in results and the mere reduction rather than the prevention of the passage of acid appear to be a result of pinpoint holes in the varnish film formed during volatilization of the organic solvent. Greater continuity of the dried varnish film is possible by the use of successive layers of thin varnish; this technique is more effective than using just one layer of thicker varnish.

Thin films of resinous cavity varnishes significantly reduce leakage around the margins and walls of metallic restorations. Although the effect of the cavity varnishes is not completely known, it can be hypothesized that this reduction of fluid penetration around cavity margins would minimize postoperative sensitivity. These varnishes are applied to prepared cavity walls, including the margins. The integrity of the resin film is destroyed when composite restorative materials are placed in contact with them. The monomer contained in these resin materials dissolves the film.

Varnishes neither possess mechanical strength nor provide thermal insulation because of inadequate film thickness. Values of film thickness have been measured at between 1 and 40 μm for different commercial varnishes. Contact angles of varnishes on dentin range from 53 to 106 degrees. Improved integrity of a varnish film might be achieved by improvement in the spreading of the varnish on the tooth surface.

APPLICATIONS

Cavity varnishes are indicated for use (1) on dentinal surfaces to minimize the penetration of acid from zinc phosphate cements, and (2) on enamel and dentinal walls to reduce the penetration of oral fluids around metallic restorations. Cavity varnishes appear also to retard the penetration of discolored corrosion products from dental amalgam into dentin. Varnishes are not used under composite restorations, because bonding agents effectively seal the dentin tubules. A cavity varnish is applied to the dentinal walls of those tubules in direct contact with the pulp when a base of zinc phosphate cement is used. When therapeutic action is expected from a low-strength base or liner or when the cement base material itself is bland in its action on the pulp, a cavity varnish is not used on the underlying dentin. The varnish may be applied over the cement base in these situations.

CAVITY LINERS

A cavity liner is used like a cavity varnish to provide a barrier against the passage of irritants from cements or other restorative materials and to reduce the sensitivity of freshly cut dentin. Unlike a varnish, a liner may provide some therapeutic benefits to the tooth. Liners, however, do not set as the calcium hydroxide pulp-capping agents do.

COMPOSITION

Cavity liners are suspensions of calcium hydroxide in an organic liquid such as methyl ethyl ketone or ethyl alcohol or in an aqueous solution of methyl cellulose. The methyl cellulose functions as a thickening agent. Liners also may contain acrylic polymer beads or barium sulfate. Fluoride compounds such as calcium monofluorophosphate have been added to some liners. On evaporation of the volatile solvent, the liner forms a thin film on the prepared tooth surface.

MANIPULATION

Cavity liners are fluid in consistency and are easily flowed or painted over dentinal surfaces. The solvents evaporate to leave a thin film residue that protects the underlying pulp. Certain products are claimed to have better integrity and pulpal protection when used with composite restorative materials.

PROPERTIES

Like varnishes, cavity liners neither possess mechanical strength nor provide any significant thermal insulation. The calcium hydroxide liners are soluble and should not be applied at the margins of restorations.

Fluoride compounds have been added to some cavity liners to reduce the possibility of secondary caries around permanent restorations or to reduce sensitivity. Effectiveness of the fluoride for either purpose would depend on its availability to enamel and dentin through its solubility. Although in vitro studies with one material have shown reduced solubility of tooth tissue, clinical studies have not yet demonstrated its efficacy. However, such an investigation has shown an absence of bacteria at the resin composite–tooth tissue interface when a cavity liner containing calcium monofluorophosphate is used.

LOW-STRENGTH BASES

Low-strength (low-rigidity) bases are two-paste calcium hydroxide or ZOE cements that set to a hard mass when mixed. These cements are commonly referred to as *liners, intermediary bases,* or *pulp-capping agents* (calcium hydroxide products only). Glass ionomer, hybrid ionomer, and compomer bases are discussed in the section on high-strength bases.

COMPOSITION AND CHEMISTRY OF SETTING

Calcium Hydroxide Bases The base paste of a typical product contains calcium tungstate, tribasic calcium phosphate, and zinc oxide in glycol salicylate. The catalyst paste contains calcium hydroxide, zinc oxide, and zinc stearate in ethylene toluene sulfonamide. The ingredients responsible for setting are calcium hydroxide and a salicylate, which react to form an amorphous calcium disalicylate. Fillers such as calcium tungstate or barium sulfate provide radiopacity.

A light-cured calcium hydroxide base consists of calcium hydroxide and barium sulfate dispersed in a urethane dimethacrylate resin.

Zinc Oxide–Eugenol Bases These bases are non-modified (Type IV) ZOE cements as described in ANSI/ADA Specification No. 30 (ISO 3107). They are typically two-paste systems in which the zinc oxide and eugenol are formulated with inert oils and fillers. The cement sets to a hard mass when mixed. The setting reaction is accelerated by moisture and an increase in temperature.

MANIPULATION

Calcium hydroxide bases and ZOE low-strength bases are supplied as two-paste systems. Equal lengths of the different-colored pastes are dispensed on a paper pad and then mixed to a uniform color.

PROPERTIES

Calcium hydroxide cements are used for lining deep cavities or for direct pulp capping. The antibacterial action of calcium hydroxide makes these cements useful in indirect pulp-capping procedures involving carious dentin. ZOE cements are used in deep cavities to retard penetration of acids and reduce possible discomfort to the pulp. Both calcium hydroxide and ZOE low-strength bases are often used with a high-strength base in restoring a tooth. Root canal sealers containing calcium hydroxide have been developed.

Calcium Hydroxide Bases The important properties of these bases are mechanical and thermal properties, solubility, and pH. Calcium hydroxide (self-cured) bases have low values of tensile strength and compressive strength, or elastic modulus, compared with high-strength bases (Table 20-15). Although setting times vary between 2.5 and 5.5 minutes, compressive strengths of these cements continue to increase over a 24-hour period. For a group of five commercial products, compressive strengths ranged from 6.5 to 14.3 MPa at 10 minutes to from 9.8 to 26.8 MPa at 24 hours. The low elastic modulus of calcium hydroxide bases restricts their usage to areas not critical to the support of restorations. Mechanical support should be provided by sound dentin or by a high-strength base. Calcium hydroxide bases are, however, considered strong enough to support the forces of condensation of amalgam.

Calcium hydroxide bases may provide some thermal insulation to the pulp if used in sufficiently thick layers. A thickness greater than 0.5 mm is not suggested. Practically, thermal protection should be provided by the overlying high-strength base.

The solubility of calcium hydroxide bases has been measured in several solvents for various periods of immersion. For a group of five commercial products, values ranged from 0.4% to 7.8% in distilled water at 37° C for 24 hours, from 0.1% to 6.2% in 35% phosphoric acid for 60 seconds, and from 0.3% to 1% in ether for 10 seconds. One product that was resistant to dissolution in water and in acid disintegrated when exposed to ether. Some solubility of the calcium hydroxide is necessary to achieve its therapeutic properties, although an optimum value is not known. Clearly the use of acid-etching procedures and varnish in the presence of calcium hydroxide bases must be done with care. Over a long term, some calcium hydroxide products seem to "disappear" from the cavity. The cause of this dissolution is unclear, but some products have been reformulated in an attempt to minimize the problem.

The pH of commercial products has been

TABLE 20-15 Mechanical Properties of Low- and High-Strength Cement Bases

	Compressive Strength (MPa)	Tensile Strength (MPa)	Elastic Modulus (GPa)
LOW-STRENGTH (LOW-RIGIDITY) BASES			
Calcium hydroxide (light-cured)	96	38	—
Calcium hydroxide (self-cured)	12-26	1	0.4
Glass ionomer (light-cured)	90-110	11-14	3.0-4.0
Glass ionomer (self-cured)	40-175	—	1.8-2.8
Zinc oxide–eugenol (Type III)	5.5	0.41	0.3
HIGH-STRENGTH (HIGH-RIGIDITY) BASES			
Glass ionomer	70-210	3.9-8.3	3.7-9.0
Hybrid ionomer	150-200	20-40	8-20
Polymer-reinforced zinc oxide–eugenol (Type IV)	38	3.4	2.1
Zinc phosphate	130-160	8	22
Zinc polyacrylate	80	16	5.0

measured at between 9.2 and 11.7. Free calcium hydroxide in excess of that necessary to form the calcium disalicylate stimulates secondary dentin in proximity to the pulp and shows antibacterial activity.

One light-cured calcium hydroxide base is reported to have a surface pH of 11.9, low dissolution in acid (<0.5%), low 24-hour solubility in water (<1.0%), and high compressive strength (80 MPa). Whereas two-paste calcium hydroxide bases show antibacterial activity, a light-cured type did not.

ZINC OXIDE–EUGENOL BASES

ANSI/ADA Specification No. 30 (ISO 3107) requirements for zinc oxide–eugenol liners are listed in Table 20-8. The mechanical properties of these cements are compared with those of calcium hydroxide bases and high-strength bases (see Table 20-15). ZOE products tend to be weaker and less rigid than calcium hydroxide pastes that set. Because the base is used in thin layers, it provides little thermal insulation. The eugenol has a sedative (obtundent) effect on the pulp. The base should not be used when a composite is to be placed, because eugenol can inhibit polymerization of the bonding agent and composite.

HIGH-STRENGTH BASES

High-strength bases are used to provide thermal protection for the pulp and mechanical support for a restoration. Bases are usually prepared from a base or secondary consistency (higher powder/liquid ratio) of zinc phosphate, zinc polyacrylate, glass ionomer, hybrid ionomer, or compomer cements. A polymer-reinforced ZOE base is also available.

Recently, self-cured and light-cured glass ionomer and hybrid ionomer cements have become available as low- and high-strength bases. The low-strength bases (liners) typically flow more readily than the high-strength bases and are less rigid, as shown in Table 20-15. Light-cured glass ionomers are water-based cements but have a unique chemistry of setting that involves both an acid-base reaction between carboxylate ions and the glass particles and a light-accelerated polymerization of dimethacrylate oligomers. Most of the light-cured liners are premixed pastes or powder-liquid systems mixed by hand, but one recent light-cured liner is encapsulated. The composition and setting reaction of the hybrid ionomers used as bases are identical to those of the luting cements discussed earlier in this chapter.

PROPERTIES

The tensile strength, compressive strength, and elastic modulus of five types of high-strength bases are compared in Table 20-15. The secondary consistencies of these cements result in higher values of strength and elastic modulus than values obtained from mixes of a primary (luting) consistency (see Table 20-3). Zinc phosphate cements are the most rigid of the five types, whereas the polymer-modified ZOE cements (Type III) have the lowest properties. ANSI/ADA Specification No. 96 specifies the net setting time, minimum compressive strength, and maximum values of acid erosion and acid-soluble arsenic and lead content for zinc phosphate, zinc polyacrylate and glass ionomer bases, as listed in Table 20-2.

The ability of a cement base to support a restoration during function has been studied by stress analysis techniques, as described in Chapter 4. The thickness and elastic modulus of the base affect the deflection of the base and restoration. Mismatches in the moduli of the base and restorative material can cause tensile stresses at the cement-restoration interface that can lead to failure of either material. Studies have recommended that a zinc phosphate base be used to support an amalgam restoration, whereas zinc phosphate, glass ionomer, or zinc polyacrylate may be used to support a Class 1 resin composite restoration.

The glass ionomer lining cements and bases are unique in their ability to bond to dentin. Bond strengths measured in tension vary from 2.0 to 4.9 MPa. These cements also can be etched to provide additional retention to a composite restoration (so-called *sandwich technique*). Glass ionomer lining cements and bases release fluoride ions and are radiopaque.

The thermal conductivity and diffusivity of dental cements (see Tables 3-4 and 3-6) are similar to those of enamel and dentin. Thus cement bases provide thermal protection to the pulp if used in a sufficiently thick layer (>0.5 mm).

SELECTED PROBLEMS

Problem 1

A provisional acrylic crown was difficult to remove, and upon removal was found to be soft. What caused these problems, and how can they be resolved?

Solution

The use of reinforced ZOE cement makes the removal of a provisional acrylic crown difficult, and the eugenol softens the acrylic. Therefore a low-strength, non-eugenol–zinc oxide or provisional resin cement is recommended for use with acrylic crowns.

Problem 2

A low-gold alloy bridge with normal retention is to be temporarily cemented. Which cement is recommended for this application?

Solution

Low-strength ZOE cement is suggested to allow for easy removal and cleanup of the bridge for final cementation.

Problem 3

A low–gold content MOD inlay with normal retention is to be cemented permanently. Which cements are recommended for this application? Which are not?

Solution a

Glass ionomer, hybrid ionomer, zinc phosphate, and zinc polyacrylate cements are sufficiently strong and insoluble in oral fluids for this application.

Solution b

EBA ZOE cements are weaker and more soluble in oral fluids than are other cements and are generally not recommended for final cementation.

Problem 4

A gold alloy casting seated properly before cementation but failed to seat when cemented with zinc phosphate cement. What factors might have caused this difficulty, and how can it be corrected?

Solution

An excessive film thickness of zinc phosphate cement may result from (1) too high a mixing temperature, (2) too high a powder/liquid ratio, (3) water contamination during mixing, (4) a glass slab temperature below the dew point, (5) too long a time between completion of mixing and cementation, or (6) cement being placed on the tooth before being placed on the casting.

Problem 5

A clinician experienced difficulties in reproducing the consistency of mixes of a zinc polyacrylate cement. The mixes were too thick. What were the probable causes of this problem, and how can they be corrected?

Solution a

The liquid of a zinc polyacrylate cement (excluding the anhydrous type) is very viscous and difficult to dispense accurately. The dropper bottle should be held perpendicular to the mixing pad when the liquid is dispensed. Try to dispense drops of uniform size.

Solution b

The loss of water by evaporation will increase the powder/liquid ratio. The liquid should be dispensed just before mixing, and a water-resistant mixing pad should be used.

Solution c

A mixing temperature higher than 23° C or overmixing will result in a mix that is too thick. Use a cool slab for mixing, and carefully follow the recommended mixing time for more consistent mixes.

Problem 6

During the insertion of a zinc phosphate cement base into an extensive cavity preparation, the mix became dry and friable and did not adhere well to the cavity walls. What factors might be related to such a change in consistency, and how can the consistency be improved?

Solution a

The heat of reaction accelerates the setting reaction of zinc phosphate cement, thereby causing the working time to decrease. Mixing the cement with incremental additions of powder and over a large area of a cool slab will reduce the temperature rise and allow a longer working time.

Solution b

Too much powder incorporated into a mix as it approaches secondary consistency decreases the working time and causes the cement base to be weak and friable because of insufficient matrix to bind the powder together. The base should be slightly tacky after it is rolled in powder at the completion of mixing.

Problem 7

A properly mixed zinc phosphate cement base became contaminated with saliva during placement. Should there be any deleterious effect expected from the contamination?

Solution

Yes, a soft, friable surface results from the dilution of acid and leaching of the matrix of a setting cement base by saliva.

Problem 8

A calcium hydroxide base appeared to disintegrate when acid came into contact with it during an acid-etching procedure. Are there bases that can be used in conjunction with acid-etching procedures for a composite?

Solution a

Yes, acid-resistant calcium hydroxide bases containing disalicylates are available.

Solution b

Glass ionomer bases can be etched to enhance the bond between the base and the composite.

Solution c

Use hybrid ionomer cement. Its bond to composite is not affected by etching.

Problem 9

When an amalgam is placed over a ZOE base, the cement sometimes crumbles and becomes incorporated into the amalgam mass. Should a thicker layer of ZOE cement or a different cement base be placed to provide better support?

Solution a

The ZOE base is a material with a low rigidity. Increasing its thickness will result in less rather than more support. Maintain the thickness of a low-strength base at less than 0.5 mm.

Solution b

A more rigid cement base, such as zinc phosphate cement, should be placed over the ZOE base to provide additional support for condensation and for the amalgam from occlusal forces.

Problem 10

A paste-primer (one-step) composite orthodontic cement failed shortly after the appliance was activated. Composite remained on the tooth and the metal bracket. What factors might explain these observations, and how can the problem be corrected?

Solution a

The bond strength of a one-step composite cement can be very low if too thick a layer of the paste is placed on the bracket. The primer cannot diffuse through the thick layer of paste, causing insufficient polymerization of the cement. Keep the thickness of the cement paste to less than 0.25 mm.

Solution b

The enamel primer of a one-step cement remaining in the warm, humid environment of the mouth too long before the bracket is placed will cause a decrease in the cohesive strength of the cement. Apply the brackets to the teeth within 1 minute after applying the primer.

BIBLIOGRAPHY

General

American Dental Association Council on Scientific Affairs: Products of excellence, *J Am Dent Assoc* (suppl) 129:1, 1998.

Barakat MM, Powers JM: In vitro bond strength of cements to treated teeth, *Aust Dent J* 31: 415, 1986.

Craig RG, Peyton FA: Thermal conductivity of tooth structure, dental cements, and amalgam, *J Dent Res* 40:411, 1961.

Craig RG, Peyton FA, Johnson DW: Compressive properties of enamel, dental cements, and gold, *J Dent Res* 40:936, 1961.

Dennison JB, Powers JM: A review of dental cements used for permanent retention of restorations. I. Composition and manipulation, *Mich Dent Assoc J* 56:116, 1974.

McCabe JF, Wilson HJ: The use of differential scanning calorimetry for the evaluation of dental materials. I. Cements, cavity lining materials and anterior restorative materials, *J Oral Rehabil* 7:103, 1980.

Mesu FP: Degradation of luting cements measured in vitro, *J Dent Res* 61:655, 1982.

Mitchem JC, Gronas DG: Clinical evaluation of cement solubility, *J Prosthet Dent* 40:453, 1978.

Myers ML, Staffanou RS, Hembree JH Jr et al: Marginal leakage of contemporary cementing agents, *J Prosthet Dent* 50:513, 1983.

Norman RD, Swartz ML, Phillips RW: Studies on film thickness, solubility, and marginal leakage of dental cements, *J Dent Res* 42:950, 1963.

Norman RD, Swartz ML, Phillips RW: Direct pH determinations of setting cements. I. A test method and the effects of storage time and media, *J Dent Res* 45:136, 1966.

Norman RD, Swartz ML, Phillips RW: Direct pH determinations of setting cements. II. The effects of prolonged storage time, powder/liquid ratio, temperature, and dentin, *J Dent Res* 45:1214, 1966.

Oilo G, Espevik S: Stress/strain behavior of some dental luting cements, *Acta Odontol Scand* 36:45, 1978.

Osborne JW, Swartz ML, Goodacre CJ et al: A method for assessing the clinical solubility and disintegration of luting cements, *J Prosthet Dent* 40:413, 1978.

Paddon JM, Wilson AD: Stress relaxation studies on dental materials. I. Dental cements, *J Dent* 4:183, 1976.

Phillips LJ, Schnell RJ, Phillips RW: Measurement of electric conductivity of dental cement. III. Effect of increased contact area and thickness; values for resin, calcium hydroxide, zinc oxide–eugenol, *J Dent Res* 34:597, 1955.

Powers JM, Craig RG: A review of the composition and properties of endodontic filling materials, *Mich Dent Assoc J* 61:523, 1979.

Powers JM, Farah JW, Craig RG: Modulus of elasticity and strength properties of dental cements, *J Am Dent Assoc* 92:588, 1976.

Richter WA, Ueno H: Clinical evaluation of dental cement durability, *J Prosthet Dent* 33:294, 1975.

Tanizaki K, Inoue K: Effect of tannin-fluoride preparation on the reduction of secondary caries, *J Osaka Univ Dent Sch* 19:129, 1979.

Vermilyea S, Powers JM, Craig RG: Rotational viscometry of a zinc phosphate and a zinc polyacrylate cement, *J Dent Res* 56:762, 1977.

Walls AW, McCabe JF, Murray JJ: An erosion test for dental cements, *J Dent Res* 64:1100, 1985.

Watts DC, Smith R: Thermal diffusion in some polyelectrolyte dental cements: the effects of powder/liquid ratio, *J Oral Rehabil* 11:285, 1984.

Wilson AD: The chemistry of dental cements, *Chem Soc Rev* 7:265, 1978.

Zinc Phosphate Cements

Crisp S, Jennings MA, Wilson AD: A study of temperature changes occurring in the setting dental cements, *J Oral Rehabil* 5:139, 1978.

Kendziar GM, Leinfelder KF, Hershey HG: The effect of cold temperature mixing on the properties of zinc phosphate cement, *Angle Orthod* 46:345, 1976.

Mitchem JC, Gronas DG: Clinical evaluation of cement solubility, *J Prosthet Dent* 40:453, 1978.

Muhler JC (Indiana Univ Foundation, Bloomington, Ind): Dental cement. Canadian Patent 912,026 (Cl 6-36), Oct 17, 1972; Appl July 20, 1970, 23 pp.

Servais GE, Cartz L: Structure of zinc phosphate dental cement, *J Dent Res* 50:613, 1971.

Wilson AD: Specification test for the solubility and disintegration of dental cements: a critical evaluation, *J Dent Res* 55:721, 1976.

Zinc Oxide–Eugenol Cements

Brauer GM: A review of zinc oxide–eugenol type filling materials and cements, *Rev Belg Med Dent* 20:323, 1965.

Brauer GM, McLaughlin R, Huget EF: Aluminum oxide as a reinforcing agent for zinc oxide-eugenol-o-ethoxy-benzoic acid cements, *J Dent Res* 47:622, 1968.

Civjan S, Brauer GM: Physical properties of cements, based on zinc oxide, hydrogenated rosin, o-ethoxybenzoic acid, and eugenol, *J Dent Res* 43:281, 1964.

Civjan S, Brauer GM: Clinical behavior of o-ethoxy-benzoic acid-eugenol-oxide cements, *J Dent Res* 44:80, 1965.

Civjan S, Huget EF, Wolfhard G et al: Characterization of zinc oxide–eugenol cements reinforced with acrylic resin, *J Dent Res* 51:107, 1972.

El-Tahawi HM, Craig RG: Thermal analysis of zinc oxide–eugenol cements during setting, *J Dent Res* 50:430, 1971.

Farah JW, Powers JM, editors: Temporary cements, *Dent Advis* 15(9):1, 1998.

Gilson TD, Myers GE: Clinical studies of dental cements. I. Five zinc oxide–eugenol cements, *J Dent Res* 47:737, 1968.

Gilson TD, Myers GE: Clinical studies of dental cements. II. Further investigation of two zinc oxide–eugenol cements for temporary restorations, *J Dent Res* 48:366, 1969.

Gilson TD, Myers GE: Clinical studies of dental cements. III. Seven zinc oxide–eugenol cements used for temporarily cementing completed restorations, *J Dent Res* 49:14, 1970.

Gilson TD, Myers GE: Clinical studies of dental cements. IV. A preliminary study of a zinc oxide–eugenol cement for final cementation, *J Dent Res* 49:75, 1970.

Grossman LI: Physical properties of root canal cements, *J Endodont* 2:166, 1976.

Harvey W, Petch NJ: Acceleration of the setting of zinc oxide cements, *Br Dent J* 80:1, 1946.

Higginbotham TL: A comparative study of the physical properties of five commonly used root canal sealers, *Oral Surg Oral Med Oral Pathol* 24:89, 1967.

McComb D, Smith DC: Comparison of physical properties of polycarboxylate-based and conventional root canal sealers, *J Endodont* 2:228, 1976.

Molnar EJ, Skinner EW: Study of zinc oxide-rosin cements. I. Some variables which affect the hardening time, *J Am Dent Assoc* 29:744, 1942.

Nielsen TH: Sealing ability of chelate root filling cements. Part I. Device for measuring linear changes of setting chelate cements, *J Endodont* 6:731, 1980.

Powers JM, Craig RG: A review of the composition and properties of endodontic filling materials, *Mich Dent Assoc J* 61:523, 1979.

Silvey RG, Myers GE: Clinical studies of dental cements. V. Recall evaluation of restorations cemented with a zinc oxide–eugenol cement and a zinc phosphate cement, *J Dent Res* 55:289, 1976.

Silvey RG, Myers GE: Clinical studies of dental cements. VI. A study of zinc phosphate, EBA reinforced zinc oxide–eugenol and polyacrylic acid cements as luting agents in fixed prostheses, *J Dent Res* 56:1215, 1977.

Silvey RG, Myers GE: Clinical studies of dental cements. VII. A study of bridge retainers luted with three different dental cements, *J Dent Res* 57:703, 1978.

Vermilyea SG, Huget EF, DeSimon LB: Extrusion rheometry of fluid materials, *J Dent Res* 58:1691, 1979.

Wilson AD, Mesley RJ: Chemical nature of cementing matrixes of cements formed from zinc oxide and 2-ethoxy benzoic acid-eugenol liquids, *J Dent Res* 53:146, 1974.

Zinc Polyacrylate Cements

Ady AB, Fairhurst CW: Bond strength of two types of cements to gold casting alloy, *J Prosthet Dent* 29:217, 1973.

Bertenshaw BW, Combe EC: Studies on polycarboxylate and related cements. I. Analysis of cement liquids, *J Dent* 1:13, 1972.

Bertenshaw BW, Combe EC: Studies on polycarboxylate and related cements. II. Analysis of cement powders, *J Dent* 1:65, 1972.

Brannstrom M, Nyborg H: Pulpal reaction to polycarboxylate and zinc phosphate cements used with inlays in deep cavity preparations, *J Am Dent Assoc* 94:308, 1977.

Chamberlain BB, Powers JM: Physical and mechanical properties of three zinc polyacrylate dental cements, *Mich Dent Assoc J* 58:494, 1976.

Crisp S, Lewis BG, Wilson AD: Zinc polycarboxylate cements: a chemical study of erosion and its relationship to molecular structure, *J Dent Res* 55:299, 1976.

Crisp S, Prosser HJ, Wilson AD: An infra-red spectroscopic study of cement formation between metal oxides and aqueous solutions of poly(acrylic acid), *J Mater Sci* 11:36, 1976.

Jendresen MD, Trowbridge HO: Biological and physical properties of a zinc polycarboxylate cement, *J Prosthet Dent* 28:264, 1972.

Jurecic A (Pennwalt Corporation): Acrylic acid copolymers in dental cements, Canadian Pat 909,414, Sept 5, 1972.

McLean JW: Polycarboxylate cements—five years' experience in general practice, *Br Dent J* 132:9, 1972.

Mizrahi E, Smith DC: The bond strength of a zinc polycarboxylate cement, *Br Dent J* 127:410, 1969.

Oilo G: Linear dimensional changes during setting of two polycarboxylate cements, *J Oral Rehabil* 3:161, 1976.

Plant CB: The effect of polycarboxylate cement on the dental pulp—a study, *Br Dent J* 129:424, 1970.

Powers JM, Johnson ZG, Craig RG: Physical and mechanical properties of zinc polyacrylate dental cements, *J Am Dent Assoc* 88:380, 1974.

Smith DC: A new dental cement, *Br Dent J* 125:381, 1968.

Truelove EL, Mitchell DG, Phillips RW: Biologic evaluation of a carboxylate cement, *J Dent Res* 50:166, 1971.

Glass Ionomer and Hybrid Ionomer Cements

Barry TI, Clinton DJ, Wilson AD: The structure of a glass-ionomer cement and its relationship to the setting process, *J Dent Res* 58:1072, 1979.

Berry EA III: The clinical uses of glass ionomer cements (vol. 4, Chap. 20A). In Hardin JF, *Clark's clinical dentistry,* Philadelphia, 1993, J.B. Lippincott.

Berry EA III, Powers JM: Bond strength of glass ionomers to coronal and radicular dentin, *Oper Dent* 19:122, 1994.

Council on Dental Materials, Instruments, and Equipment: Biocompatibility and postoperative sensitivity, *J Am Dent Assoc* 116:767, 1988.

Crisp S, Kent BE, Lewis BG et al: Glass ionomer cement formulations. II. The synthesis of novel polycarboxylic acids, *J Dent Res* 59:1055, 1980.

Crisp S, Lewis BG, Wilson AD: Characterization of glass-ionomer cements. I. Long term hardness and compressive strength, *J Dent* 4:162, 1976.

Crisp S, Lewis BG, Wilson AD: Characterization of glass-ionomer cements. 5. The effect of the tartaric acid concentration in the liquid component, *J Dent* 7:304, 1979.

Crisp S, Lewis BG, Wilson AD: Characterization of glass-ionomer cements. 6. A study of erosion and water absorption in both neutral and acidic media, *J Dent* 8:68, 1980.

Crisp S, Pringuer MA, Wardleworth D et al: Reactions in glass ionomer cements. II. An infrared spectroscopic study, *J Dent Res* 53:1414, 1974.

Crisp S, Wilson AD: Reactions in glass ionomer cements. I. Decomposition of the powder, *J Dent Res* 53:1408, 1974.

Crisp S, Wilson AD: Reactions in glass ionomer cements. III. The precipitation reaction, *J Dent Res* 53:1420, 1974.

Finger W: Evaluation of glass ionomer luting cements, *Scand J Dent Res* 91:143, 1983.

Fitzgerald M, Heys RJ, Heys DR et al: An evaluation of a glass ionomer luting agent: bacterial leakage, *J Am Dent Assoc* 114:783, 1987.

Forss H: Release of fluoride and other elements from light-cured glass ionomers in neutral and acidic conditions, *J Dent Res* 72:1257, 1993.

Forsten L: Fluoride release from a glass ionomer cement, *Scand J Dent Res* 85:503, 1977.

Friedl K-H, Powers JM, Hiller K-A: Influence of different factors on bond strength of hybrid ionomers, *Oper Dent* 20:74, 1995.

Hunt PR, editor: The Next Generation; Proceedings of the 2nd International Symposium on Glass Ionomers. Philadelphia, PA, 1994.

Johnson GH, Herbert AH, Powers JM: Changes in properties of glass-ionomer luting cements with time, *Oper Dent* 13:191, 1988.

Kawahara H, Imanishi Y, Oshima H: Biological evaluation on glass ionomer cement, *J Dent Res* 58:1080, 1979.

Maldonado A, Swartz ML, Phillips RW: An in vitro study of certain properties of a glass ionomer cement, *J Am Dent Assoc* 96:785, 1978.

Mitra SB, Li MY, Culler SR: Setting reaction of Vitrebond light cure glass-ionomer liner/base, 130. In Watts DC, Setcos JC: Proceedings of the Conference on Setting Mechanisms of Dental Materials, *Trans Academy Dent Mater* 5(2):175, 1992.

Negm MM, Beech DR, Grant AA: An evaluation of mechanical and adhesive properties of polycarboxylate and glass ionomer cements, *J Oral Rehabil* 9:161, 1982.

Nicholson JW: The setting of glass-polyalkenoate ("glass-ionomer") cements, 113. In Watts DC, Setcos JC: Proceedings of the Conference on Setting Mechanisms of Dental Materials, *Trans Acad Dent Mater* 5(2), 1992.

Oilo G: Bond strength of new ionomer cements to dentin, *Scand J Dent Res* 89:344, 1981.

Prosser HJ, Richards CP, Wilson AD: NMR spectroscopy of dental materials. II. The role of tartaric acid in glass-ionomer cements, *Biomed Mater Res J* 16:431, 1982.

Ryan MD, Powers JM, Johnson GH: Properties of glass ionomer luting cements, *Mich Dent Assoc J* 67:17, 1985.

Shalabi HS, Asmussen E, Jorgensen KD: Increased bonding of a glass-ionomer cement to dentin by means of $FeCl_3$, *Scand J Dent Res* 89:348, 1981.

Wilson AD: Resin-modified glass-ionomer cements, *Int J Prosthodont* 3:425, 1990.

Wilson AD, Crisp S, McLean JW: Experimental luting agents based on the glass ionomer cements, *Br Dent J* 142:117, 1977.

Wilson AD, Crisp S, Prosser HJ et al: Aluminosilicate glasses for polyelectrolyte cements, *I&EC Prod Res & Develop* 19:263, 1980.

Resin Cements

Balderamos LP, O'Keefe KL, Powers JM: Color accuracy of resin cements and try-in paste, *Int J Prosthodont* 10:111, 1997.

Blackman R, Barghi N, Duke E: Influence of ceramic thickness on the polymerization of light-cured resin cement, *J Prosthet Dent* 63:295, 1990.

Blalock KA, Powers JM: Retention capacity of the bracket bases of new esthetic orthodontic brackets, *Am J Orthod Dentofac Orthop* 107:596, 1995.

Buzzitta VAM, Hallgren SE, Powers JM: Bond strength of orthodontic direct-bonding cement-bracket systems as studied in vitro, *Am J Orthod* 81:87, 1982.

Chan KC, Boyer DB: Curing light-activated composite cement through porcelain, *J Dent Res* 68:476, 1989.

Cochran D, O'Keefe KL, Turner DT et al: Bond strength of orthodontic composite cement to treated porcelain, *Am J Orthod Dentofac Orthop* 111:297, 1997.

DeSchepper EJ, Tate WH, Powers JM: Bond strength of resin cements to microfilled composites, *Am J Dent* 6:235, 1993.

Dickinson PT, Powers JM: Evaluation of fourteen direct-bonding orthodontic bases, *Am J Orthod* 78:630, 1980.

Evans LB, Powers JM: Factors affecting in vitro bond strength of no-mix orthodontic cements, *Am J Orthod* 87:508, 1985.

Farah JW, Powers JM, editors: Esthetic resin cements, *Dent Advis* 17(3):1, 2000.

Faust JB, Grego GN, Fan PL et al: Penetration coefficient, tensile strength, and bond strength of thirteen direct bonding orthodontic cements, *Am J Orthod* 73:512, 1978.

Jordan RE, Suzuki M, Sills PS et al: Temporary fixed partial dentures fabricated by means of the acid-etch resin technique: a report of 86 cases followed for up to three years, *J Am Dent Assoc* 96:994, 1978.

Livaditis GJ, Thompson VP: Etched castings: an improved retentive mechanism for resin-bonded retainers, *J Prosthet Dent* 47:52, 1982.

Mennemeyer VA, Neuman P, Powers JM: Bonding of hybrid ionomers and resin cements to modified orthodontic band materials, *Am J Orthod Dentofac Orthop* 115:143, 1999.

Miller BH, Nakajima H, Powers JM et al: Bond strength between cements and metals used for endodontic posts, *Dent Mater* 14:312, 1998.

Noie F, O'Keefe KL, Powers JM: Color stability of resin cements after accelerated aging, *Int J Prosthodont* 8:51, 1995.

O'Keefe KL, Miller BH, Powers JM: In vitro tensile bond strength of adhesive cements to new post materials, *Int J Prosthodont* 13:47, 2000.

O'Keefe K, Powers JM: Light-cured resin cements for cementation of esthetic restorations, *J Esthet Dent* 2:129, 1990.

O'Keefe K, Powers JM, McGuckin RS et al: In vitro bond strength of silica-coated metal posts in roots of teeth, *Int J Prosthodont* 5:373, 1992.

Powers JM: Adhesive Resin Cements, *Shigaku* 79:1140, 1991.

Powers JM, Kim H-B, Turner DS: Orthodontic adhesives and bond strength testing, *Semin Orthod* 3:147, 1997.

de Pulido LG, Powers JM: Bond strength of orthodontic direct-bonding cement-plastic bracket systems in vitro, *Am J Orthod* 83:124, 1983.

Rabchinsky DS, Powers JM: Color stability and stain resistance of direct-bonding orthodontic cements, *Am J Orthod* 76:170, 1979.

Rochette AL: Attachment of a splint to enamel of lower anterior teeth, *J Prosthet Dent* 30:418, 1973.

Siomka LV, Powers JM: In vitro bond strength of treated direct-bonding metal bases, *Am J Orthod* 88:133, 1985.

Tate WH, DeSchepper EJ, Powers JM: Bond strength of resin cements to a hybrid composite, *Am J Dent* 6:195, 1993.

Wright WL, Powers JM: In vitro tensile bond strength of reconditioned brackets, *Am J Orthod* 87:247, 1985.

Cavity Varnishes, Liners and Bases

Bryant RW, Wing G: A simulated clinical appraisal of base materials for amalgam restorations, *Aust Dent J* 21:322, 1976.

Chong WF, Swartz ML, Phillips RW: Displacement of cement bases by amalgam condensation, *J Am Dent Assoc* 74:97, 1967.

Costa CAS, Mesas AN, Hebling J: Pulp response to direct capping with an adhesive system, *Am J Dent* 13:81, 2000.

Farah JW, Hood JAA, Craig RG: Effects of cement bases on the stresses in amalgam restorations, *J Dent Res* 54:10, 1975.

Farah JW, Powers JM, Dennison JB et al: Effects of cement bases on the stresses and deflections in composite restorations, *J Dent Res* 55:115, 1976.

Fisher FJ: The effect of three proprietary lining materials on micro-organisms in carious dentin, *Br Dent J* 143:231, 1977.

Gordon SM: Gum copal solution for cavity lining and varnish, *J Am Dent Assoc* 23:2374, 1936.

Gourley JM, Rose DE: Comparison of three cavity base materials under amalgam restorations, *J Can Dent Assoc* 38:406, 1972.

Hilton TJ: Cavity sealers, liners, and bases: Current philosophies and indications for use, *Oper Dent* 21:134, 1996.

Leinfelder KF: Changing restorative traditions: The use of bases and liners, *J Am Dent Assoc* 125:65, 1994.

McComb D: Comparison of physical properties of commercial calcium hydroxide lining cements, *J Am Dent Assoc* 107:610, 1983.

Plant GC, Wilson HJ: Early strengths of lining materials, *Br Dent J* 129:269, 1970.

Soremark R, Hedin M, Rojmyr R: Studies on incorporation of fluoride in a cavity liner (varnish), *Odontol Rev* 20:189, 1969.

Swartz ML, Phillips RW, Norman RD et al: Role of cavity varnishes and bases in the penetration of cement constituents through tooth structure, *J Prosthet Dent* 16:963, 1966.

Chapter 21

Prosthetic Applications of Polymers

Poly(methyl methacrylate) polymers were introduced as denture base materials in 1937. Previously, materials such as vulcanite, nitrocellulose, phenol formaldehyde, vinyl plastics, and porcelain were used for denture bases. The acrylic resins were so well received by the dental profession that by 1946, 98% of all denture bases were constructed from methyl methacrylate polymers or copolymers. Other polymers developed since that time include vinyl acrylic, polystyrene, epoxy, nylon, vinyl styrene, polycarbonate, polysulfone-unsaturated polyester, polyurethane, polyvinylacetate-ethylene, hydrophilic polyacrylate, silicones, light-activated urethane dimethacrylate, rubber-reinforced acrylics, and butadiene-reinforced acrylic.

Acrylic polymers have a wide variety of applications in prosthetic dentistry as artificial teeth, denture repair materials, facings in crown and bridge restorations, impression trays, record bases, temporary crowns, and obturators for cleft palates.

PROPERTIES OF DENTURE BASE MATERIALS

The following list indicates the requirements for a clinically acceptable denture base material.

1. Strength and durability
2. Satisfactory thermal properties
3. Processing accuracy and dimensional stability
4. Chemical stability (unprocessed as well as processed material)
5. Insolubility in and low sorption of oral fluids
6. Absence of taste and odor
7. Biocompatible
8. Natural appearance
9. Color stability
10. Adhesion to plastics, metals, and porcelain
11. Ease of fabrication and repair
12. Moderate cost

There are many commercially available materials that meet these requirements. The vast majority of dentures made today are fabricated from heat-cured poly(methyl methacrylate) and rubber reinforced poly(methyl methacrylate). Fractures of dentures still occur, but are usually associated with carelessness or unreasonable use by the patient. Considering functional stresses, the oral environment, and expected service life, denture base materials perform remarkably well.

TABLE 21-1 Principal Ingredients of Acrylic Denture Base Powder and Liquid

Powder	Liquid
Acrylic polymer (or copolymer) beads	Monomer
Initiator	Inhibitor
Pigments	Accelerator
Dyes	Plasticizer
Opacifiers	Cross-linking agent
Plasticizer	
Dyed organic fibers	
Inorganic particles	

PHYSICAL FORM AND COMPOSITION

Denture base plastics are commonly supplied in a powder-liquid or a gel form. The powder-liquid type may contain the materials listed in Table 21-1.

Powder Most commercial materials contain poly(methyl methacrylate), modified with small amounts of ethyl, butyl, or other alkyl methacrylates to produce a polymer somewhat more resistant to fracture by impact. The powder also contains an initiator such as benzoyl peroxide (see formula below) or diisobutylazonitrile to initiate the polymerization of the monomer liquid after being added to the powder.

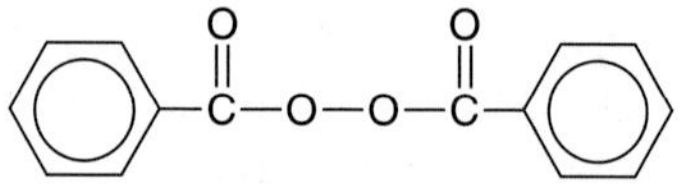

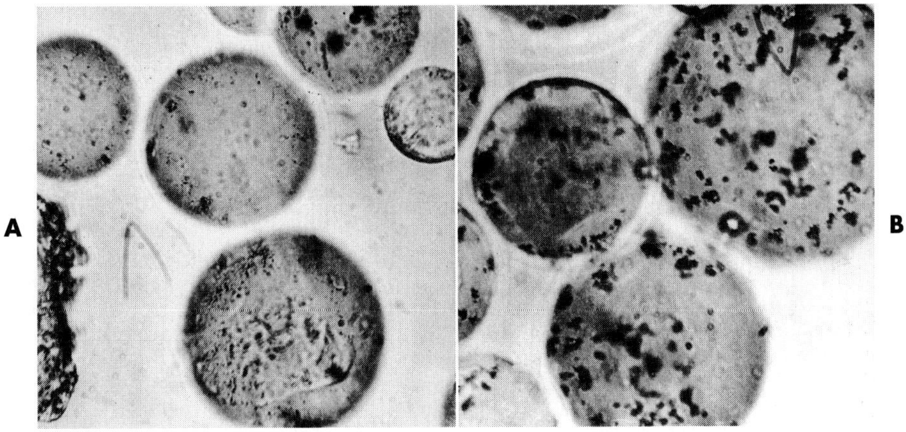

Fig. 21-1 Polymer beads with the pigment locked into the polymer, **A,** and mechanically mixed with the polymer, **B.** (× 450.)
(Courtesy The LD Caulk Co, Milford, Del, 1959.)

The peroxide initiator may be added to the polymer or be present as a residual from the polymerization reaction and is present in amounts from 0.5% to 1.5%.

Pure polymers, such as poly(methyl methacrylate), are clear and are adaptable to a wide range of pigmentation. The pigments used to obtain the various tissuelike shades are compounds such as mercuric sulfide, cadmium sulfide, cadmium selenide, ferric oxide, or carbon black, although the use of cadmium salts is suspect because of demonstrated toxicity. These pigments may be locked into the polymer beads by addition during the commercial polymerization, or mechanically mixed with the polymer beads after polymerization, as shown in Fig. 21-1. Generally, the latter method is used, and the uneven distribution of the pigment in the final denture provides a mottled, natural appearance. Dyes are occasionally used, but generally are not as satisfactory because they tend to be leached out of the plastic by oral fluids, thereby gradually lightening the shade. In addition to coloring agents, zinc or titanium oxides are used as opacifiers, with titanium dioxide being most effective. Dyed synthetic fibers made from nylon or acrylic are usually added to simulate the minute blood vessels of oral mucosa.

Plasticizers such as dibutyl phthalate may be incorporated in the powder or the monomer. Inorganic particles such as glass fibers and beads or zirconium silicate have been added to plastics. The particles are usually treated with a coupling agent such as an unsaturated triethoxysilane to improve the wetting and bonding of the inorganic particles and the plastic. Studies have reported on the addition of whiskers of alumina, silicon carbide, boron nitride, and carbon fibers to dental plastics. Adding glass fibers and alumina (sapphire) whiskers increases the stiffness, decreases the thermal coefficient of expansion, and increases thermal diffusivity. Polyethylene-woven yarn and polyaramid fabric have also been used to reinforce acrylic polymers.

Most denture bases are transparent on x-ray examination. Pieces of fractured dentures or temporary acrylic crowns have been aspirated by patients during traumatic injury and are difficult if not impossible to locate. A few denture base materials contain heavy metal compounds of elements such as barium or radiopaque glass fillers added to improve the radiopacity. It is necessary to add up to 20% by weight of these compounds to give sufficient radiopacity, and this results in a reduction in the strength of the material and a change in the appearance of the denture. A 3-year clinical study of a commercial radiopaque polymer, however, showed the dentures performed well and remained radiopaque. Other additives that provide radiopacity include bismuth or uranyl salts at concentrations of 10% to 15% and zirconyl dimethacrylate at 35%. Recently a new radiopaque terpolymer has been synthesized containing [2′3′5′-triodobenzyoyl]-ethyl methacrylate, methyl methacrylate and 2-hydroxyethyl methacrylate. This methacrylate terpolymer may find use as a radiopaque denture base material. It has been shown that esthetically pleasing radiopaque plastics can be made that do not demonstrate cytotoxicity or mutagenicity and have reasonable properties for prosthetic applications. In the future, efforts must be made to improve the handling properties, transverse deflection, and water sorption of radiopaque denture base materials.

Liquid The liquid component of the powder-liquid type acrylic resin is methyl methacrylate, but it may be modified by the addition of other monomers. Because these monomers may be polymerized by heat, light, or traces of oxygen, inhibitors are added to give the liquid adequate shelf life. The inhibitor most commonly used to prevent premature polymerization is hydroquinone, shown below, which may be present in concentrations of 0.003% to 0.1%.

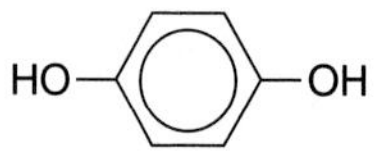

When a chemical accelerator rather than heat is used to speed up the peroxide decomposition and enable the polymerization of the monomer at room temperature, an accelerator is included in the liquid. These accelerators are tertiary amines, sulfinic acids, or the more stable salts of sulfinic acid. Commonly used amines are *N,N*-dimethyl-para-toluidine, and *N,N*-dihydroxyethyl-para-toluidine.

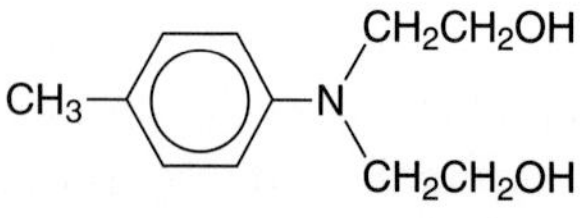

These are referred to as *self-curing, cold-curing,* or *autopolymerizing resins.* The pour type of denture resin is included in this category.

Plasticizers are sometimes added to produce a softer, more resilient polymer. They are generally relatively low–molecular weight esters, such as dibutyl phthalate.

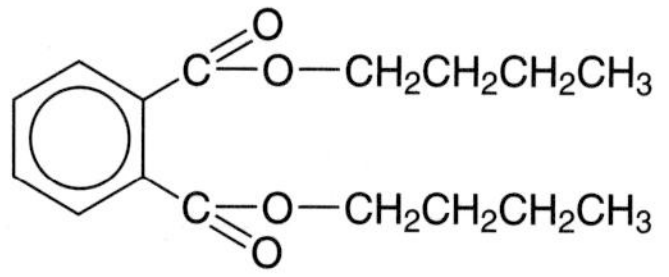

Plasticizer molecules do not enter the polymerization reaction but do interfere with the interaction between polymer molecules. This makes the plasticized polymer softer than the pure polymer. One disadvantage in using plasticizers is that they gradually leach out of the plastic into oral fluids, resulting in hardening of the denture base. A polymer also may be plasticized by the addition of some higher ester such as butyl or octyl methacrylate to methyl methacrylate. The esters polymerize and form a more flexible plastic. This type of internal plasticizing does not leach out in the oral fluids, and the material remains flexible.

If a cross-linked polymer is desired, organic compounds such as glycol dimethacrylate are added to the monomer.

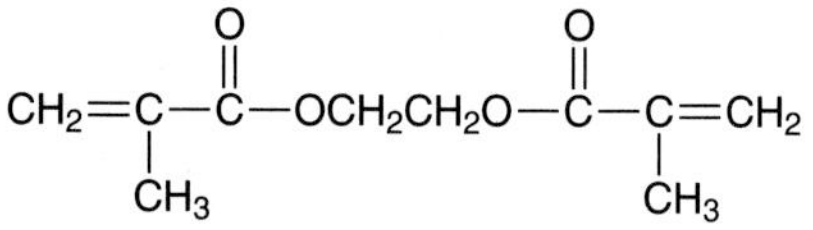

Cross-linking compounds are characterized by reactive –CR=CH– groups at opposite ends of the molecules and serve to link long polymer molecules together. Using cross-linking agents provides greater resistance to minute surface cracking, termed *crazing,* and may decrease solubility and water sorption. Cross-linking materials may be present in amounts of 2% to 14%, but have little effect on the tensile strength, transverse properties, or hardness of acrylic plastics, although recovery from an indentation by a metal ball such as a Rockwell Superficial Hardness indenter is somewhat improved.

Gel Types It also is possible to supply denture base plastics such as vinyl acrylics in a gel form. These gels have, in general, the same components as the powder-liquid type, except the liquid and powder have been mixed to form a gel and shaped into a thick sheet. Chemical accelerators cannot be used in a gel, because the initiator, accelerator, and monomer would be in intimate contact. The storage temperature of a gel and the amount of inhibitor present have a pronounced effect on the shelf life of the material. When stored in a refrigerator, the shelf life is about 2 years.

OTHER DENTURE MATERIALS

Several modified poly(methyl methacrylate) materials have been used for denture base applications. These include pour type denture resins, hydrophilic polyacrylates, high-impact strength resins, rapid heat-polymerized acrylics, and light-activated materials.

Pour Type Denture Resin The chemical composition of the pour type denture resins is similar to poly(methyl methacrylate) materials that are polymerized at room temperature. The principal difference is in the size of the polymer powder or beads. The pour type denture resins, commonly referred to as *fluid resins,* have much smaller powder particles; when mixed with monomer, the resulting slurry is very fluid. The mix is quickly poured into an agar-hydrocolloid or modified plaster mold and allowed to polymerize under pressure at 0.14 MPa. Centrifugal casting and injection molding are techniques used to inject the slurry into the mold.

High-Impact Strength Materials Denture base materials that have greater impact strength have been introduced. These polymers are reinforced with butadiene-styrene rubber. The rubber particles are grafted to methyl methacrylate to bond to the acrylic matrix. These materials are supplied in a powder-liquid form and are processed in the same way as other heat-accelerated methyl methacrylate materials.

Rapid Heat-Polymerized Resins Dentists and technicians are always looking for ways to do things quicker and better. The rapid heat-polymerized materials were introduced with that in mind. These are hybrid acrylics that are polymerized in boiling water immediately after being packed into a denture flask. The initiator is formulated from both chemical- and heat-activated initiators to allow rapid polymerization without the porosity one might expect. After placing the denture in boiling water, the water is brought back to a full boil for 20 minutes. After bench cooling to room temperature, the denture is deflasked, trimmed, and polished in the conventional manner.

Light-Activated Denture Base Resins This denture base material consists of a urethane dimethacrylate matrix with an acrylic copolymer, microfine silica fillers, and a photoinitiator system. It is supplied in premixed sheets having a claylike consistency. The denture base material is adapted to the cast while it is still pliable. The denture base can be polymerized in a light chamber without teeth and used as a record base. The teeth are processed to the base with additional material and the anatomy is sculptured while the material is still plastic. The acrylic is polymerized in a light chamber with blue light of 400 to 500 nm. The denture rotates in the chamber to provide uniform exposure to the light source. Various formulations of light activated acrylic are used for many prosthetic applications.

ANSI/ADA SPECIFICATION NO. 12 (ISO 1567) FOR DENTURE BASE RESINS

The scope, requirements, and procedures for evaluating denture base plastics are listed in ANSI/ADA Specification No. 12. The specification includes acrylic, vinyl, and styrene polymers, or mixtures of any of these polymers, as well as copolymers. Denture base resins may be heat-curing or self-curing.

The specification lists a number of general requirements for the non-processed materials. The liquid should be as clear as water and free of extraneous material, and the powder, plastic

TABLE 21-2 Properties of Various Types of Denture Acrylics According to ANSI/ADA Specification No. 12

Property	Conventional	Rubber Reinforced	Vinyl	Light-activated Acrylic*	Pour Type	Rapid Heat Cure
Transverse deflection (mm)						
at 3500 g	2.0	2.4	1.8	1.9	2.2	1.7
at 5000 g	4.1	5.0	3.8	3.6	Fractured	3.5
Water sorption (mg/cm^2)	0.60	0.55	0.50	0.64	0.50	0.64
Water solubility (mg/cm^2)	0.02	0.02	0.02	0.01	0.01	0.02
Color change	None	Slight	Slight	Slight	Slight-Moderate	Slight

*Data supplied by Densply International, York, Pa.

cake, or precured blank should be free of impurities such as dirt and lint. The specification further states that (1) a satisfactory denture shall result when the manufacturer's instructions are followed; (2) the denture base should be nonporous and free from surface defects; (3) the cured plastic should take a high gloss when polished; (4) the processed denture should not be toxic to a normal, healthy person; (5) the color should be as specified; (6) the plastic should be translucent; and (7) the cured plastic should not show any bubbles or voids.

The specific requirements are that (1) within 5 minutes after reaching the proper consistency, indicated by clean separation from the walls of a glass mixing jar, the material shall have adequate flow properties so it will intrude to a depth of at least 0.5 mm into a 0.75-mm diameter hole when a load of 5000 g is placed on a plate 5 mm thick and 50 mm^2 in area (this test is modified for pour type of plastics); (2) the water sorption shall not be more than 0.8 mg/cm^2 after immersion for 7 days at 37° C; (3) the solubility shall not be more than 0.04 mg/cm^2 after the water sorption specimen is dried to constant weight; (4) the plastic shall show no more than a slight color change when exposed 24 hours to a specified ultraviolet lamp test; and (5) the transverse deflection shall be within the limits listed in the discussion on transverse deflection.

Properties for various types of plastics are shown in Table 21-2. Although the values are typical for each group, they can vary considerably for different commercial products.

PROPERTIES OF DENTAL PLASTICS

STRENGTH PROPERTIES

Conventional heat-accelerated acrylic resins are still the predominant denture base materials in use. These materials are typically low in strength, soft and fairly flexible, brittle on impact, and fairly resistant to fatigue failure. The properties of poly(methyl methacrylate) and polyvinyl acrylic are shown in Table 21-3. Several properties of newer denture base materials are seen in Table 21-4.

TABLE 21-3 Strength Characteristics of Denture Base Plastics

Property	Poly(methyl methacrylates)	Polyvinyl Acrylics
Tensile strength (MPa)	48.3-62.1	51.7
Compressive strength (MPa)	75.9	70.0-75.9
Elongation (%)	1-2	7-10
Elastic modulus (GPa)	3.8	2.8
Proportional limit (MPa)	26.2	29.0
Impact strength, Izod (kg m/cm notch)	0.011	0.023
Transverse deflection (mm)		
At 3500 g	2.0	1.9
At 5000 g	4.0	3.9
Fatigue strength (cycles at 17.2 MPa)	1.5×10^6	1×10^6
Recovery after indentation (%)		
Dry	89	86
Wet	88	84
KHN (kg/mm^2)		
Dry	17	16
Wet	15	15

Tensile and Compressive Strength Table 21-3 reveals small differences between poly(methyl methacrylate) and polyvinyl acrylic. The two plastics have adequate tensile and compressive strength for complete or partial denture applications. Fractures in these materials are usually caused by accidental dropping of a denture or by faulty fabrication. Fractures may also be caused by flexure fatigue from cyclic stresses of low magnitude in service.

Elongation Elongation, in combination with the ultimate strength, is an indication of the toughness of the plastic. The larger the area under the stress-strain curve, the tougher the material is. Materials having a combination of reasonable tensile strength and elongation will be tough materials, and those with low elongation will be brittle. Examples of tough materials are polyvinylchloride or polyethylene, whereas poly(methyl methacrylate) is more brittle.

Values for percent elongation of polyvinyl acrylics are considerably higher than for poly(methyl methacrylate) and, as expected, the polyvinyl acrylics are tougher and permit larger deformation before fracture.

Elastic Modulus The higher strain or elastic deformation for a given stress for polyvinyl acrylic is reflected in the lower value for elastic modulus of 2.8 GPa. This value may be compared with that of 3.8 GPa for poly(methyl methacrylates). A denture constructed of polyvinyl acrylic will deform elastically to a greater extent under the forces of mastication than a comparable poly(methyl methacrylate) denture. The modulus of elasticity for several newer denture base materials is seen in Table 21-4. When compared with metals used as denture bases, the elastic moduli of all plastics are quite low.

Proportional Limit There is some question as to whether dental plastics possess a true proportional limit, because they may be permanently deformed at low stresses, and, as a result, the proportional limit obtained is a function of

TABLE 21-4 Mechanical Properties of New Denture Resins

Material	Processing Condition	Knoop Hardness (kg/mm^2)	Rockwell Indentation (μm)	Rockwell Recovery (%)	Flexural Strength (MPa)	Flexural Modulus (GPa)	Izod Impact Strength (J/m)
20 min cure PMMA	100° C, 20 min	15-17	70-74	74-78	79-86	1.3-1.6	12-15
Light-cured resins	10 min in light chamber	18	73	72	80	2.1	13
Rubber reinforced PMMA	74° C, 9 hr	14	79	73	78	1.1	31
Autopolymerizing PMMA	45° C, 0.14 MPa	16	73	76	84	1.6	15
Microwave-cured PMMA	3 min, 500 W	17	74	75	92	1.7	14

Adapted with permission from Smith LT, Powers JM, Ladd D: *Int J Prosthodont* 5:315, 1992.

the rate of stress application. Despite this characteristic, the proportional limit determined under standard conditions is important. A plastic with a low proportional limit will begin to deform permanently at a low stress. If the percent elongation is relatively high, it may deform permanently to a considerable extent before rupture. If the proportional limit is high, considerable stress is required before permanent deformation will occur. A denture material should have a proportional limit sufficiently high that permanent deformation does not result from the stress applied during mastication. Permanent deformation may result in loss of retention or loosening of the teeth embedded in the denture base. The values reported in Table 21-3 for the proportional limit of poly(methyl methacrylates) and polyvinyl acrylics are approximately the same and the dimensional stability of dentures made of these materials would be expected to be similar.

Impact Strength Impact strength is a measure of the energy absorbed by a material when it is broken by a sudden blow.

The impact strength for polyvinyl acrylics is about twice that of poly(methyl methacrylates) (see Table 21-3), which indicates that polyvinyl acrylic absorbs more energy on impact and is more resistant to fracture.

Although the addition of plasticizers may increase the impact strength of plastics, the increases are accompanied by decreases in hardness, proportional limit, elastic modulus, and compressive strength. Ideally, a denture base plastic should have a sufficiently high impact strength to prevent breakage on accidental dropping, but not at the expense of the other properties.

The impact strength of several denture base materials is listed in Tables 21-4 and 21-5. There are differences in relative impact strength with all tests. However, the impact strength of rubber-reinforced acrylic plastic is considerably higher in all instances. When surface defects are present, this improved impact resistance is significantly reduced.

TABLE 21-5 Impact Strength of Denture Base Plastics

Material	Charpy Impact* Strength (Joules)	Hounsfield Impact† Test (Nm × 10^{-4})
Conventional heat-cured acrylic	0.26	455
Vinyl acrylic	0.20	578
Rubber-reinforced acrylic	0.58	1063
Hydrophilic acrylic	0.18	NA

*Adapted from Soni PM, Powers JM, Ctaig RG: *J Mich Dent Assoc* 59:418, 1977.
†Adapted from Stafford GD, Bates JF, Hugget R, Handley RW: *J Dent* 8:292, 1980.
NA, Not applicable.

Transverse Strength and Deflection In the evaluation of denture plastics, transverse strength measurements are used to a greater extent than either tensile or compressive strength, because this test more closely represents the type of loading in vivo. Transverse strength is determined by applying an increasing load until fracture at the center of a test specimen, as shown in Fig. 21-2. The deflection in millimeters at the middle of the plastic specimen is recorded at a load of 3500 and 5000 g. Transverse strength is therefore a combination of tensile and compressive strength and includes some of the elements of proportional limit and elastic modulus. The values listed in Table 21-4 show that the transverse strength varies from 78 to 92 MPa for various denture base materials.

A transverse deflection test has been used to evaluate denture base resins. The requirements are that the deflection in the center of the specimen shall be no more than 2.5 mm for a load of 1500 to 3500 g, and between 2.0 and 5.5 mm for a load of 1500 to 5000 g. All specimens are tested in water at 37° C after storage in water for 2 days at 37° C.

A comparison of the transverse deflection of several types of materials is seen in Table 21-2.

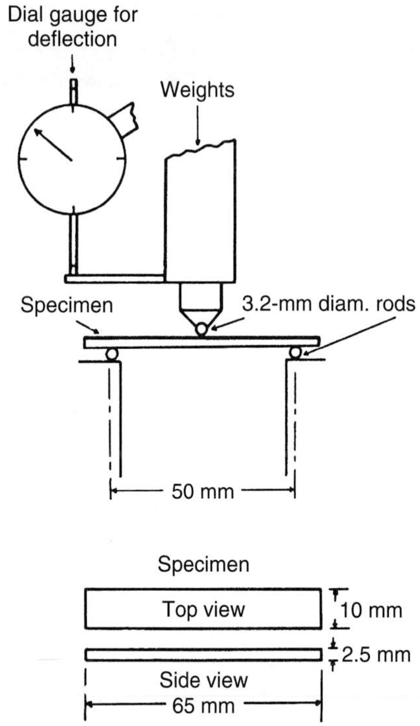

Fig. 21-2 Simplified sketch of equipment for determining transverse deflection and strength.

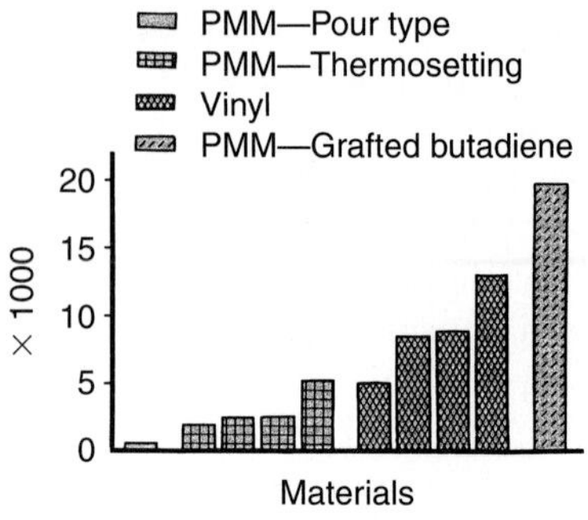

Fig. 21-3 Flexural fatigue of various types of denture base materials.

(Adapted from Johnson EP: *J Prosthet Dent* 46:478, 1981.)

Note that the pour-type resin fractured in this test and the rapid heat-cured acrylic was slightly less flexible than the other materials.

Fatigue Strength Dentures are subjected to a large number of smaller cyclic stresses during mastication. For this reason, the fatigue properties of denture plastics are important. Fatigue strength represents the number of cycles before failure at a certain stress. Values of the fatigue strength at a stress of 17.2 MPa for poly(methyl methacrylates) and polyvinyl acrylic plastics are 1.5×10^6 and 1×10^6, respectively. Because the current denture base plastics hold up well in service, a value of 1×10^6 cycles at 17.2 MPa is apparently an adequate fatigue strength value.

There are many flexural fatigue tests reported in the literature for denture base resins. Results from one of these tests are shown in Fig. 21-3. The samples were repeatedly flexed under a load of 3650 g at 342 flexures per minute in a fatigue-testing machine. The flexural fatigue strength of the rubber-reinforced acrylic plastic was superior to the other materials, and the pour type of acrylic plastic had the lowest value.

Fracture Toughness Because the geometry of denture bases is complex and stresses can be concentrated in flaws on the surface or in frenum notches, cracks can occur in the denture base. Several tests are available for determining fracture toughness. One method for testing fracture toughness is to bend a notched specimen and record the force required for crack propagation (Fig. 21-4). Several denture base materials are compared in Table 21-6. The fracture toughness of the high-impact resin appears to be no better than that of vinyl or conventional acrylic resin. The rapid heat-cured resin had the highest fracture toughness, and the pour type of resin the lowest toughness. The fracture toughness of acrylic is greater when samples are saturated with water rather than dry.

Compressive Creep When denture base resins are placed under a load they will deform (creep) with time. The lowest compressive creep rates are found for heat-polymerized materials. Chemically accelerated acrylics, both dough and pour type, have higher values for compressive creep. At low stress levels, the type and quantity of cross-linking agents have no major affect on creep. However, at higher stress levels, creep values decrease with increasing quantities of cross-linking agents. For heat-polymerized mate-

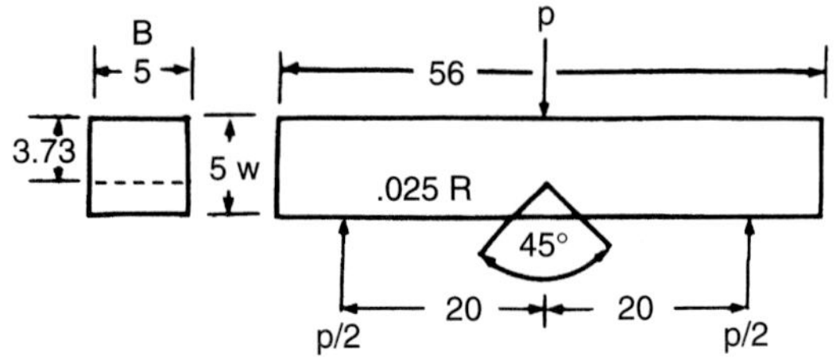

Fig. 21-4 Sketch of specimens for measuring fracture toughness. *p*, Load; *R*, radius; *W*, thickness; *B*, width. Dimensions in millimeters.

(Adapted from Stafford GD, Bates JF, Huggett R, Handley RW: *J Dent* 8:292, 1980.)

TABLE 21-6 Fracture Toughness of Denture Base Plastics

Material	$MN/m^{-3/2}$
High impact resin	2.0
Rapid heat cure	3.0
Conventional acrylic	2.3
Pour type of acrylic	1.5

Adapted from Stafford GD, Bates JF, Hugget R, Handley RW: *J Dent* 8:292, 1980.

rials, when the temperature is increased from 37° to 50° C the mode of failure changes from brittle to ductile. For autopolymerizing acrylics, the materials fail in a ductile manner at both temperatures.

Recovery After Indentation Indentation recovery of plastics in equilibrium with water is generally lower than when dry. The recovery from indentation of a 1.27-cm diameter steel ball loaded for 10 minutes at 30 kg is given in Table 21-3. The time allowed for recovery was 10 minutes. Recovery was 86% to 89% for dry specimens and 84% to 88% for wet specimens. The results for several new products are seen in Table 21-4.

A modified Wallace hardness tester has been used to measure the hardness, creep, and recovery of denture base polymers and the effects of cyclic loading. Results demonstrate the viscoelastic nature of denture base polymers. A torsional pendulum also may be used to evaluate the viscoelastic properties of denture base resins. These tests are useful in evaluating the effect of free monomer, plasticizers, and degree of cross-linking.

TABLE 21-7 Abrasion Resistance of Denture Base Plastics

Material	Material Loss ($mm \times 10^{-3}$)
Conventional acrylic	595
Rubber-reinforced acrylic	588
Vinyl acrylic	499
Rapid heat-curcd acrylic	530
Pour type of acrylic	611

Hardness The low Knoop hardness number of the denture base plastics (see Tables 21-3 and 21-4) indicates these materials may be scratched easily and abraded. Cross-linked poly(methyl methacrylate) is only slightly harder than regular poly(methyl methacrylate) (about 1 kg/mm^2). The incorporation of fillers in plastics may alter the resistance to abrasion, but the hardness of the plastic matrix remains unchanged. Polishing, shell blasting, and cleaning denture bases by brushing should be carried out with this in mind.

Abrasion Resistance Abrasion resistance of denture base resins has been evaluated by abrading specimens against 600-grit silicon carbide paper for 1 hour under a stress of 0.26 MPa in water at 37° C and measuring loss of material (Table 21-7). All materials had similar wear characteristics. However, the vinyl acrylic had the best and the pour type of acrylic had the least wear resistance.

THERMAL CHARACTERISTICS

The thermal properties of plastics are important because plastic materials are usually processed at 74° C and in service are in contact with

TABLE 21-8 Thermal Characteristics of Denture Base Plastics

Property	Poly(methyl methacrylates)	Polyvinyl Acrylics
Thermal conductivity (cal/sec/cm^2) (° C/cm)	5.7×10^{-4}	2.2×10^{-4}
Specific heat (cal/° C/g)	0.35	0.2-0.28
Thermal coefficient of expansion (/° C)	81×10^{-6}	71×10^{-6}
Heat distortion temperature (° C)	71-91	54-77

hot and cold foods and beverages. If a chemical accelerator is used rather than heat, the material is still subjected to exothermic heat resulting from the polymerization reaction.

Thermal Conductivity Dental plastics are poor thermal and electrical conductors. Compared with gold, cobalt alloys, or even human dentin, which have thermal conductivities of 0.7, 0.16, and 1.3×10^{-3} cal/sec/cm^2 (° C/cm), respectively, the values for the various types of plastics listed in Table 21-8 are low. Low thermal conductivity allows plastic denture bases to serve as an insulator between the oral tissues and hot or cold materials placed in the mouth. It has been shown that the inclusion of sapphire whiskers in poly(methyl methacrylate) increases heat conductivity.

Specific Heat Specific heat, or the heat required to raise the temperature of a gram of plastic 1° C, is a thermal property closely related to thermal conductivity. Although it is not obvious, it may be shown that the ratio of thermal conductivity to the product of specific heat and density is a constant for a particular material and represents the velocity of temperature disturbance in a plastic. The higher this ratio, termed *diffusivity*, the greater the velocity of heat transfer through a material. The specific heats for poly(methyl methacrylates) and polyvinyl acrylics are similar, and the respective thermal conductivities are not greatly different; therefore the diffusivity of plastics will be roughly equivalent, 0.123 mm^2/sec.

Thermal Coefficient of Expansion

The temperature change from processing temperature to room temperature or mouth temperature indicates the importance of the thermal coefficient of expansion. Plastics have relatively high thermal coefficients of expansion (71 to 81×10^{-6} /° C) compared with other dental materials. Gold, amalgam, and tooth structure have values of 14.4×10^{-6}/° C, 22 to 28×10^{-6} /° C, and 11.4×10^{-6} /° C, respectively. The addition of fillers such as glass reduces the thermal coefficient of expansion, although the reduction is not a linear function of the amount of the filler present. Thermal expansion is important in the fit of denture bases. It is apparent that a denture that fits a cast accurately at room temperature will not fit exactly the same at mouth temperature.

Heat Distortion Temperature Heat distortion temperature is a measure of the ability of a plastic to resist dimensional distortion by heat. This is the temperature at which a specimen loaded in a transverse manner at 1.8 MPa stress deflects a distance of 0.25 mm. These temperatures are sufficiently high that they are of little concern except in the repair of dentures. The heat distortion temperature for polyvinyl acrylic is 54° to 77° C and for poly(methyl methacrylates) 71° to 91° C. These values suggest the need for keeping repair temperatures low by using chemically or light-polymerized materials for this purpose.

Plastics or polymers, when heated, are transformed from a glassy or brittle condition to a

TABLE 21-9 Miscellaneous Properties of Denture Base Plastics

Property	Poly(methyl methacrylates)	Polyvinyl Acrylics
Density (g/cm^3) Polymerization shrinkage (% by volume)	1.16-1.18 6*	1.21-1.36 6*
Dimensional stability Water sorption (mg/cm^2; ADA Test)	Good 0.69	Good 0.26
Water solubility (mg/cm^2) Resistance to weak acids	0.02 Good	0.01 Excellent
Resistance to weak bases Effect of organic solvents	Good Soluble in ketones, esters, and aromatic and chlorinated hydrocarbons	Excellent Soluble in ketones and esters and swells in aromatic hydrocarbons
Processing ease Adhesion to metal and porcelain	Good Poor	Good Poor
Adhesion to acrylics Colorability	Good Good	Good Good
Color stability Taste or odor	Yellows very slightly None	Yellows slightly None
Tissue compatibility Shelf life	Good Powder and liquid, good; gel, fair	Good Gel, fair

*Monomer shrinkage in mixes with polymer/monomer ratios of approximately 3:1.

rubbery condition. The temperature of this transition is called the glass transition, *Tg*. Molecular motions are allowed above this temperature that are not permitted at lower temperatures, thus plastics are easier to deform above *Tg*.

OTHER PROPERTIES OF DENTURE PLASTICS

Density The density, or the weight in grams of a cubic centimeter (g/cm^3) of material, varies in plastics because of variations in molecular weight. Denture base plastics have densities ranging from 1.16 to 1.36 g/cm^3 (Table 21-9), or slightly greater than the density of water.

Polymerization Shrinkage The density of methyl methacrylate monomer is only 0.945 g/cm^3 at 20° C, compared with 1.16 to 1.18 g/cm^3 for poly(methyl methacrylate). This increase in density is mainly accounted for by an approximate 21% decrease in volume of monomer during polymerization. Because the ratio of polymer to monomer used in the preparation of dental poly(methyl methacrylates) and polyvinyl acrylics is usually 3:1, the free volumetric shrinkage amounts to approximately 6%. The light-activated denture base material has low polymerization shrinkage of 3% because higher molecular weight oligomers are used.

TABLE 21-10 Polymerization Shrinkage of Posterior of Maxillary Denture Bases

Material	Shrinkage (%)
Conventional acrylic	0.43
High impact acrylic	0.12
Vinyl acrylic	0.33
Rapid heat-cured acrylic	0.97
Pour type of acrylic	0.48

Adapted from Stafford GD, Bates JF, Huggett R, Handley RW: *J Dent* 8:292, 1980.

It should be pointed out that the linear shrinkage values reported in the literature are generally much less than would be expected (Table 21-10) on the basis of the free volumetric shrinkage, because a portion of the polymerization takes place after the plastic has attained a solid condition, resulting in residual stresses in the plastic rather than additional shrinkage. An ideal plastic would be one that had no polymerization shrinkage, but thermal dimensional change would still result from cooling the plastic from molding temperature to room temperature.

Dimensional Stability and Accuracy

The dimensional stability of the denture during processing and in service is important in the fit of the denture and the satisfaction of the patient. In general, if the denture is properly processed, the original fit and the dimensional stability of the various denture base plastics are good. However, excess heat generated during finishing of the denture can easily distort a denture base by releasing residual stresses.

It has been shown that chemically activated denture bases processed by dough molding with a dimensional accuracy of –0.1% were more accurate than heat-activated denture bases at –0.4%. The most accurate dentures were produced using either a chemically activated pour resin processed under pressure at 45° C or a microwave-activated resin. A visible light–activated resin was more accurate than a conventional heat-activated resin. In the past, injection-molded dentures were less accurate than compression-molded materials. Recent studies demonstrate that dentures processed by new injection molding methods are more accurate than standard compression molding. The increase in vertical dimension of occlusion was very small for the injection-molded acrylic when compared with the conventional compression-molded acrylic.

In another report, six different denture base materials were processed by heat, light, or microwave energy. The denture bases were removed from the casts, finished, and polished. After storage in distilled water for 42 days to allow for water sorption, the dentures were placed back on the stone casts on which they were made and ranked for accuracy of fit by five evaluators. Denture bases processed by microwave energy, low heat at 45° C (autopolymerizing resins), or visible light fit better than resins processed at either 74° C (conventional resins) or 100° C (rapid heat-cured resins).

When evaluated in two dimensions, the dimensional stability of denture bases is usually reported at <1%. In one study the accuracy of maxillary dentures was measured at six locations from anterior to posterior. For all materials studied, the accuracy was better from the anterior of the denture to the middle of the palate (generally <100 μm) and became worse toward the posterior of the denture. In a recent study of three-dimensional stability of several products, changes ranged from 0.2% to 8.1% in the frontal dimension, and 0.2% to 9% in the lateral dimension. Changes were greatest in the cross-arch dimension.

There are numerous articles in the literature that report conflicting results for accuracy of denture base resins. However, it is encouraging that emphasis is being placed on dimensional accuracy and some of the newer materials appear superior to older products.

Water Sorption and Solubility The sorption of water also alters the dimensions of acrylic dentures. This change in dimension is, for the most part, reversible and the plastic may go through numerous expansions and contractions when alternately soaked in water and dried. However, repeated wetting and drying of dentures should be avoided by the patient, because irreversible warpage of the denture bases may result. Denture plastics of the same type may vary considerably in water sorption because of the presence of additives. Poly(methyl methacrylates) have relatively high water sorption values of 0.69 mg/cm^2. Polyvinyl acrylics have lower values of 0.26 mg/cm^2. The thickness of the plastic specimen and the type of polymer influence whether equilibrium water sorption will be attained in 24 hours.

Temperature also affects the rate at which water is absorbed, because the diffusion coefficient is increased by a factor of two between room and oral temperature and the equilibrium absorption value does not change.

Denture plastics can be tested for water sorption where a dried plastic disk 50 mm in diameter and 0.5 mm thick is stored in distilled water at 37° C for 7 days, after which the increase in water is determined and the sorption recorded in milligrams per square centimeter. In addition, the solubility of the plastic is measured on the same specimen by re-drying to constant weight in a desiccator and re-weighing to determine the loss in weight in milligrams per square centimeter. A denture plastic should have a water sorption value of not more than 0.8 mg/cm^2 and a solubility not greater than 0.04 mg/cm^2 (see Table 21-2).

Resistance to Acids, Bases, and Organic Solvents The resistance of denture plastics to water solutions containing weak acids or bases is good to excellent. Denture plastics are quite resistant to organic solvents, with poly(methyl methacrylate) being more resistant than polyvinyl acrylic. Both are soluble in aromatic hydrocarbons, ketones, and esters. Alcohol will cause crazing in certain denture plastics. Ethanol also functions as a plasticizer and can reduce the glass transition temperature. Therefore solutions containing alcohol should not be used for cleaning or storing dentures. Incorporating ethylene glycol dimethacrylate as a cross-linking agent in denture base resins has little effect on water sorption, but significantly improves solvent resistance.

Processing Ease A comparison of the processing ease of the various types of denture plastics is difficult. In general, with the proper equipment and facilities all of the denture plastics have satisfactory processing properties.

Adhesion Properties The adhesion of denture plastics to untreated porcelain or metals is generally poor. As a result, porcelain teeth or combined metal and plastic bases should be designed so that the porcelain or metal is held by mechanical retention. It has been shown that the lack of adhesion between a plastic base and porcelain teeth provides an area in which microorganisms present in the oral fluids may incubate, and this makes maintenance of a clean denture more difficult. This problem can be avoided by the use of plastic teeth, which form a bond with denture base materials or by organosilane treatment of porcelain teeth (although this treatment is not routinely used). The silane coupling agent, γ-methacryloxypropyltrimethoxysilane, provides a bond between the porcelain and the plastic surface. Many studies have demonstrated the effectiveness of bonding denture base resins to partial denture alloys or titanium using the following ingredients alone or in combination: silica blasting, metal etching, silane coupling agents, 4-META adhesive resin, other organic primers such as 10-methacryloxydecyl dihydrogen phosphate.

Esthetics The esthetic qualities of denture base plastics include such properties as colorability, color stability, taste, and odor. The ability of the plastics to be colored and their compatibility with dyed synthetic fibers for characterization are both good. Color-measuring systems have been used to compare the actual color of denture base resins with the color of gingival tissues. Results indicate that few commercial products actually match the color of the tissue they are replacing. A color stability test requires that a specimen exposed for 24 hours to an ultraviolet light source shall not show more than a slight change in color when compared with an original specimen. One study questioned the stain resistance of the light-activated denture acrylic. Current denture products have no taste or odor when properly processed.

Tissue Compatibility The tissue compatibility or allergic sensitization of the skin to the components of denture plastics or to processed plastics has been a subject of considerable contention. It may be concluded that completely polymerized poly(methyl methacrylate) or polyvinyl acrylics rarely cause allergic reactions but that methyl methacrylate monomer or other trace components in the monomer may produce an allergic reaction. Dentures prepared by polymerization of methyl methacrylate with a chemical accelerator may have sufficient residual methyl methacrylate monomer present in the finished denture to cause an allergic reaction in patients who are sensitive to methyl methacrylate monomer. This reaction diminishes as residual monomer leaches out of the plastic. Allergic reactions to heat-processed denture base plastics also occur but less often than with chemically accelerated plastics. Again, residual monomer is considered the allergen, and strict adherence to processing instructions recommended by the manufacturer can keep the residual monomer to a minimum. When patients are known to have suffered from an allergic reaction, processing the denture for extended periods (such as 24 versus 8 hours) may be helpful. Residual monomer levels can also be reduced dramatically by processing heat-polymerized poly(methyl methacrylate) in a water bath for 7 hours at 70° C, followed by boiling for 1 hour. Boiling has only a slight effect on the dimensional accuracy of the processed dentures. Vinyl acrylic or light-activated denture base materials are an alternative for those patients who are sensitive to methyl methacrylate monomer.

In one study, 53 patients wearing dentures and suffering from "burning-mouth syndrome" were evaluated for allergies related to various components of denture base plastics. Epicutaneous patch tests were used. Approximately 15 patients demonstrated a positive skin test to one or more of the following: *N,N*-dimethyl-para-toluidine, hydroquinone, formaldehyde, methyl methacrylate, and p-phenylenediamine, as well as several metallic compounds. Pigments also may be toxic. There is one case reported of a patient who had an extensive systemic reaction to dentures. Patch testing was used and the patient had a positive reaction to the pure dye supplied by the manufacturer. She had no reaction to the unpigmented acrylic.

Plasticizers are used to lower the glass transition temperature of poly(methyl methacrylate), which in turn produces a tougher, less brittle material. In addition, the use of plasticizers decreases water sorption because they are hydrophobic. There is evidence that plasticizers fill microvoids within acrylic. This "microvoid concept" is also related to water sorption where water may replace the plasticizer in the microvoids over time. Plasticizers are commonly used in fairly high concentrations in soft denture liners. Unfortunately, some plasticizers, particularly phthalates, are known toxins; products that contain these materials should be evaluated for biocompatibility. With the demand for safety from health-related products, greater attention will be focused on the tissue compatibility of denture base materials.

The growth of *Candida albicans* on the surface of dentures is a concern for many denture patients. This organism is associated with denture stomatitis. An in vitro study has demonstrated the effectiveness of chlorhexidine gluconate in eliminating this organism. The chlorhexidine apparently can bind to acrylic surfaces for at least 2 weeks. Treating acrylic with Nystatin, followed by drying, produces similar results. The use of phenolic disinfectants can cause surface damage to denture base resins and is not recommended.

In addition to *Candida albicans,* many other microorganisms can adhere to denture base acrylics, such as *Streptococcus oralis, Bacteroides gingivalis, B. intermedius,* and *S. sanguis.* It is not surprising that many organisms adhere more to rougher surfaces than to those that are highly polished.

Shelf Life The shelf life, or useful storage time at room temperature, for denture base plastics varies considerably. Acrylic plastics packaged in the powder-liquid form have excellent shelf life, because the powder is almost indefinitely stable and the liquid usually is adequately protected from polymerization during storage by a hydroquinone inhibitor. Vinyl acrylic plastics, packaged as a gel in which the monomer is in contact with the polymer, must be stored at refrigerator temperature (about 2° C) to have a reasonable storage life of 1 to 2 years. The shelf life of light-activated denture base materials has not been reported.

Summary It is fortunate that many types of denture base materials are available that will produce satisfactory dentures. The requirements may vary for different patients, and the processing facilities can dictate which material to use. There are also significant differences between products in each category, and it is wise to choose materials that have passed ANSI/ADA Specification No. 12.

MANIPULATION AND PROCESSING OF DENTURE BASE PLASTICS

As mentioned previously, denture base plastics are supplied in several forms. The techniques used to process these materials into a finished complete or partial denture are briefly described subsequently, as are the justifications for the various procedures are presented.

Texts on prosthetic dentistry describe impression techniques, pouring master stone casts, setting denture teeth, preparing the waxed denture, investing in a denture flask, removing the wax, and coating the stone mold to prevent adhesion of the plastic. A set of waxed dentures on stone casts with the teeth in position is shown in Fig. 21-5, and a flask that contains maxillary porcelain teeth ready for packing the plastic dough is shown in Fig. 21-6.

HEAT-ACCELERATED ACRYLIC DENTURE PLASTICS

The general method for processing a heat-accelerated acrylic denture base material consists of proportioning and mixing the polymer powder and the liquid monomer and allowing the monomer to react physically with the polymer in a sealed jar until a doughy consistency is

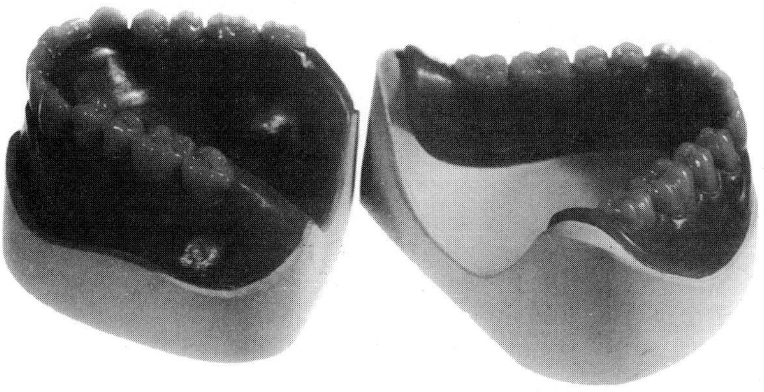

Fig. 21-5 Waxed maxillary and mandibular dentures on the stone casts.

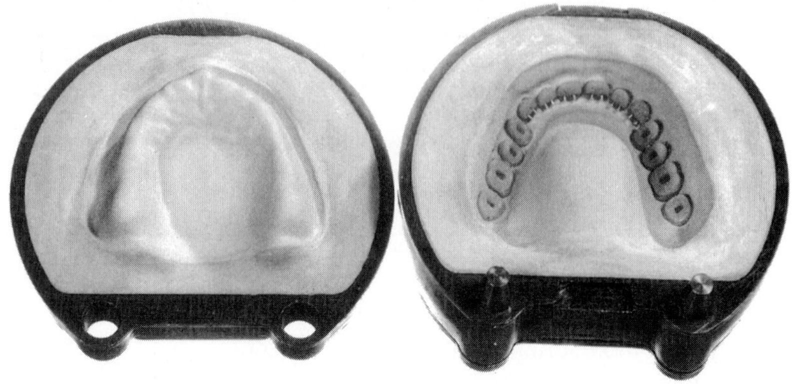

Fig. 21-6 Flask containing maxillary porcelain teeth, ready for packing the plastic dough.

$$\underbrace{\text{Polymer} + \text{Peroxide initiator}}_{\text{Powder}} + \underbrace{\text{Monomer} + \text{Inhibitor}}_{\text{Liquid}} + \underset{\text{(external)}}{\text{Heat}} \longrightarrow \text{Polymer} + \underset{\text{(reaction)}}{\text{Heat}}$$

reached. Before packing, all stone surfaces of the mold are coated with an alginate separator and allowed to dry. The dough is then packed into the treated denture mold containing the artificial teeth and "trial packed" by repeated application of slow pressure with a flask press until no excess flash remains and the material has a glossy surface. Polymerization is accomplished by applying heat and pressure, which are maintained until polymerization is complete. The flask is then bench cooled to room temperature, and the denture is deflasked, finished, and polished.

The reaction involved in the heat-accelerated powder-liquid type of acrylic is outlined in a simplified equation above. The powder, consisting of the polymer plus the initiator, and the liquid monomer, containing the inhibitor, are proportioned in the ratio of approximately 3:1 by volume.

Proportioning There must be sufficient liquid to completely wet the polymer powder. The powder and liquid are mixed with a stainless steel spatula and then kept in the sealed jar during the initial stages of reaction to avoid loss of monomer by evaporation. Incompletely wetted portions can result in a streaked or blanched appearance in the denture because of incomplete polymerization of the plastic during processing. Care should be taken to avoid breathing the monomer vapor. Animal studies have shown that the monomer can affect respiration, cardiac function, and blood pressure.

The polymer-monomer mixture, on standing, goes through several distinct consistencies, which may be qualitatively described as (1) sandy, (2) stringy or sticky, (3) doughy or puttylike, (4) rubbery or elastic, and (5) stiff. When the mixture is doughy it has desirable qualities for packing into a denture flask. Different products vary considerably in the time required to reach the doughy condition and the length of time they remain at the packing consistency. These stages or consistencies are represented by a model of the viscosity of the polymer/monomer mix (Fig. 21-7). *Nf* represents the final viscosity and *nf/2* is one half of this value. The powder-liquid mixture of a denture base plastic should be at the packing consistency when the mixture separates cleanly from the walls of the glass mixing jar and that this consistency be attained in less than 40 minutes from the start of mixing. The consistency, determined 5 minutes after the packing consistency is reached, should

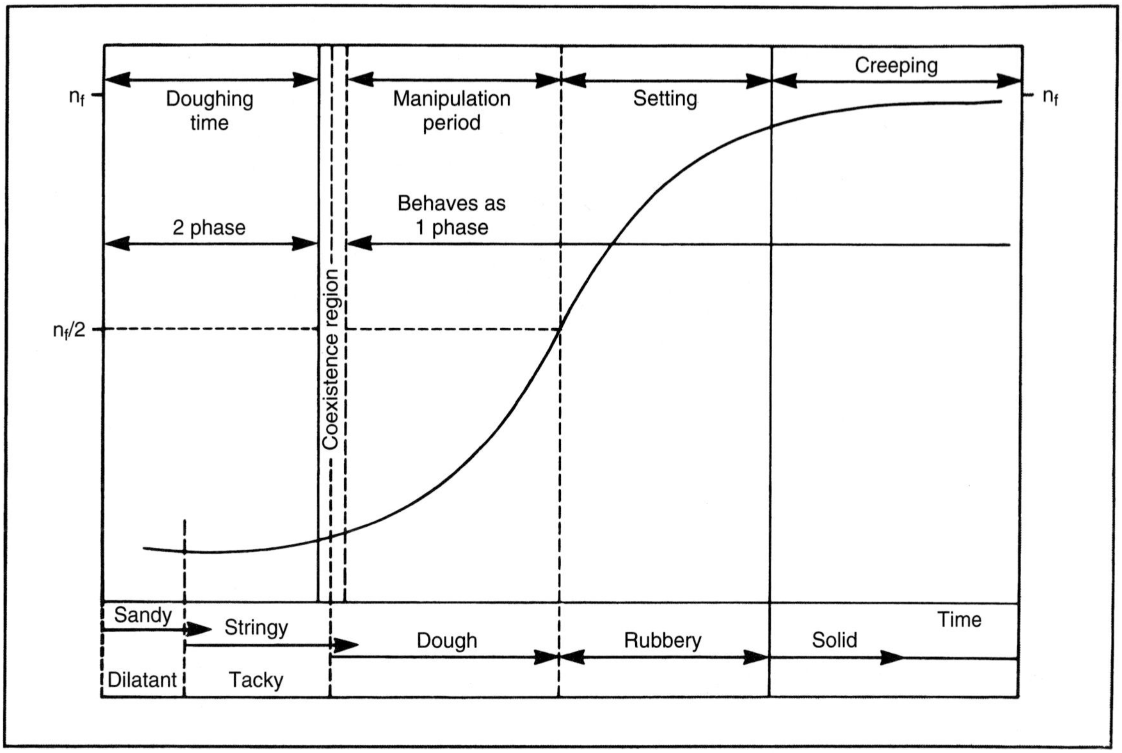

Fig. 21-7 Rheology stages of pre-polymerized denture acrylic after mixing of powder and liquid. *Nf* is the final viscosity and *nf/2* is half of the final value.
(From Mutlu G, Huggett R, Harrison P, Goodwin JW, Hughes RW: *Dent Mater* 6:288, 1990.)

be such that when 6 to 10 g of the material are placed over 0.75-mm diameter holes in a brass plate and loaded with a 5000 g weight, the dough intrudes into the holes to a depth of not less than 0.5 mm. If the material passes this test, adequate time should be available for trial packing of the denture mold and for final closure. During the various consistency stages, little polymerization is taking place and the reaction occurring is physical in nature. This reaction includes some solution of the polymer in the monomer and some absorption of the monomer by the polymer, as well as wetting of the polymer particles. For conventional acrylic plastics, no substantial polymerization occurs until the denture flask is heated to above 70° C. If too much monomer is used in the mixture, polymerization shrinkage will be greater, additional time will be required to reach the packing consistency, and there will be a tendency for porosity to occur in the denture. If too little monomer is used, the polymer will be insufficiently wetted, the dough will be difficult to manage, and the quality of the final denture will be compromised.

Packing The powder-liquid mixture should be packed into the flask at the doughy stage (Fig. 21-8, *A*) for several reasons. If it is packed at the sandy or stringy stages, too much monomer will be present between the polymer particles, the material will be of too low a viscosity to pack well, and it will flow out of the flask too easily. Packing too early may also result in porosity in the final denture base. If packed at the rubbery-to-stiff stage, the material will be too viscous to flow well under the pressure of the flask press, and metal-to-metal contact of the flask halves will not be obtained. Delayed packing will result in

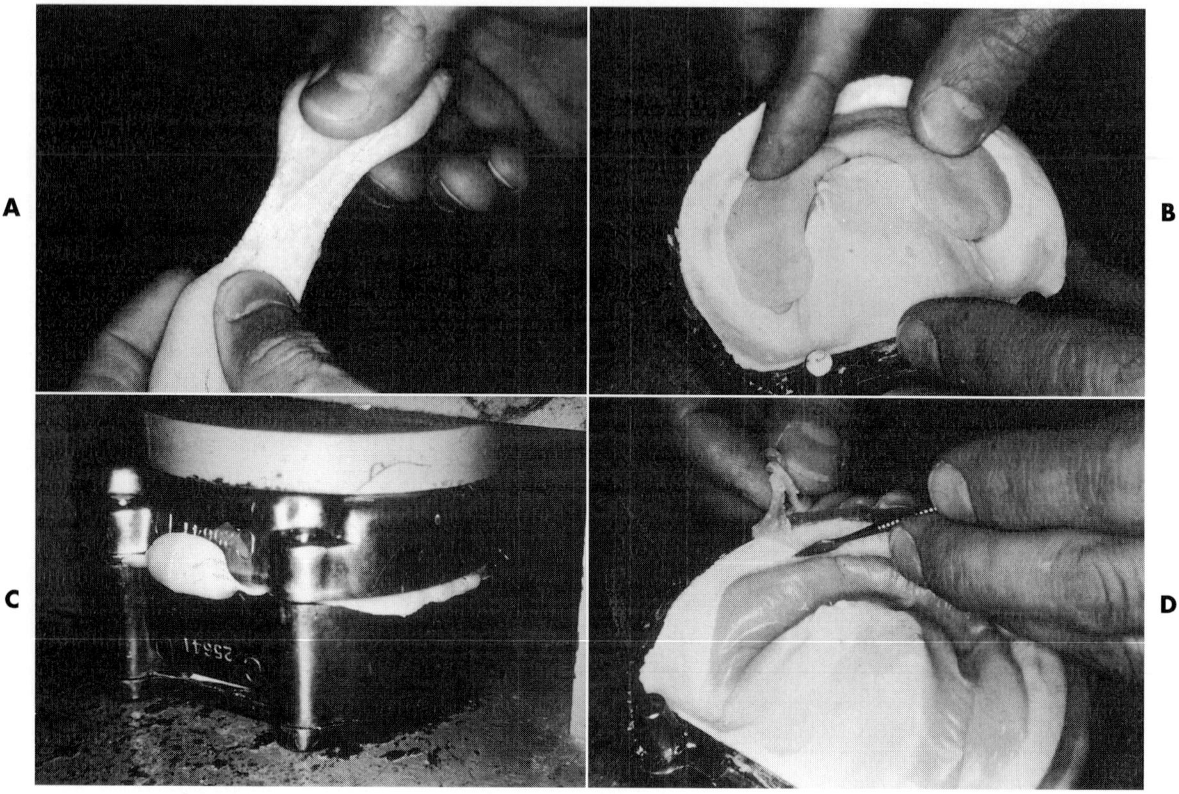

Fig. 21-8 A, Powder-liquid acrylic denture base material in the dough consistency. **B,** An excess being placed in the mold. **C,** The excess being forced out between the two portions of the flask. **D,** The flash being trimmed away.

(Adapted from Craig RG, Powers JM, Wataha JC: *Dental materials: properties and manipulation*, ed 7, St Louis, 2000, Mosby.)

loss of detail in the denture, movement or fracture of the teeth, and an increase in the contact vertical dimension of the denture. Some plastics now have increased working time and remain in the doughy stage for periods approaching 1 hour. This permits the packing of several dentures at the same time. Other products, particularly the rubber-reinforced materials, have shorter working times, and in some instances only one or two dentures should be packed with one mix. The plastic dough should not be manipulated excessively with bare hands. The monomer is a good solvent for body oils and may pick up dirt from the hands, resulting in a nonesthetic denture. Monomer may also enter the bloodstream through the skin.

The acrylic dough is packed into the flask in slight excess by use of a hydraulic, pneumatic, or mechanical press (Fig. 21-8, *B*), and this excess is removed by trial packing procedures, with a damp cellophane or polyethylene film used as a separator for the upper half of the flask. The film separator allows easy separation of the flask halves during trial packing procedures. The closing force of the press is applied slowly during the trial packing to allow the excess or flash to flow out between the halves of the flask (Fig. 21-8, *C*). The flask is opened at intervals and the flash trimmed away (Fig. 21-8, *D*). Before final closure, the separating film is removed and discarded. During final closure of the flask, metal-to-metal contact of the flask halves is completed in the

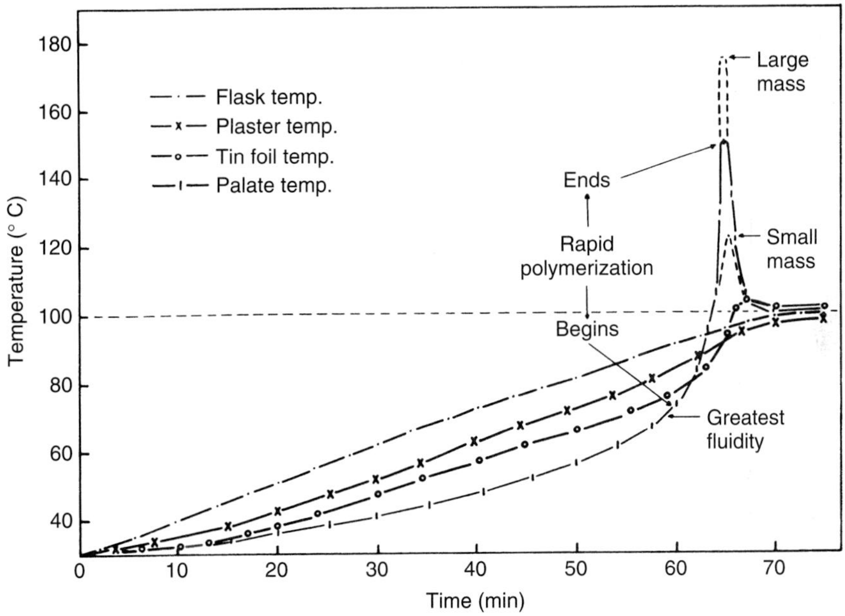

Fig. 21-9 Temperature observed at various positions in a denture flask during processing. (Adapted from Tylman SD: *J Am Dent Assoc* 29:1845, 1942.)

press, the flasks are placed in a flask press that maintains pressure, and the denture is processed.

Processing For heat-polymerized plastics the curing temperature must be maintained close to 74° C, because the polymerization reaction is strongly exothermic. The heat of reaction will be added to the heat used to raise the material to the polymerization temperature. The temperature rise at various positions in a denture flask during a curing cycle is illustrated in Fig. 21-9. The initial temperature increases are in the following order—flask, plaster or stone, tinfoil, and plastic—because the outside of the flask is in contact with the water bath. The temperatures in the different areas increase at approximately the same rate until the temperature of the plastic dough reaches about 70° C. At this point the material becomes quite fluid, and the decomposition rate of the benzoyl peroxide initiator is rapid enough for a substantial amount of polymerization to take place. As the polymerization reaction proceeds, the exothermic heat of reaction increases the temperature of the plastic to values considerably above the surrounding materials and above the boiling point of the methyl methacrylate monomer. This occurs because both the plastic and stone are poor thermal conductors and the heat of reaction is dissipated slowly. Also the larger the mass or bulk of material, the higher the peak temperature attained in the plastic. In thick sections of a denture the temperature rise will be greater than in thin sections. It has been demonstrated that the strength of thin sections of a denture may be less than that of the thick sections because of a lower degree of polymerization. Because of the excessive temperature rise, porosity will more likely occur in thick sections of the denture.

The porosity that developed in two plastics cured at 74°, 82°, and 100° C is shown in Fig. 21-10. Product *A* showed no porosity at 74° C, a negligible amount at 82° C, and moderate porosity at 100° C. Product *B*, however, evidenced no porosity at 74° C, a moderate amount at 82° C, and severe porosity at 100° C. On the basis of a large number of studies, a satisfactory processing temperature for most products is between 71° and 77° C, although, as indicated in Fig. 21-10, some products can be processed at higher temperatures without serious difficulty. A satisfactory processing procedure is to cure the plastic in a constant temperature water bath at 74° C for 8 hours or longer. Longer curing times, such as overnight, will not result in any degradation of properties. Another satisfactory processing method, which permits curing in a shorter time, is to heat at 74° C for 1.5 hours and then increase the temperature of the water bath to boiling for an additional hour.

The porosity shown in the specimens in Fig. 21-10 is in the center. The absence of porosity in the periphery of the specimens results from lower temperatures in these areas because the heat can be dissipated to the surrounding dental stone. The center of the specimens experience higher temperatures because poor thermal conductivity of the plastic prevents the dissipation of heat. Porosity in thick sections of dentures therefore may exist below the surface of the plastic, and in pigmented materials it may not be noticed until grinding or polishing exposes the deeper layers.

Porosity also results when insufficient pressure is maintained on the flask during processing, but the distribution of the porosity is different from that shown in Fig. 21-10. Porosity resulting from insufficient pressure is distributed uniformly throughout the material, rather than concentrated in the center.

Other problems associated with rapid initial heating of the acrylic dough above 74° C are production of internal stresses, warpage of the denture after deflasking, and checking or crazing around the necks of the artificial teeth. High internal stresses resulting from rapid heating combined with the heat of polymerization may be released later and cause distortion and misfit of the denture base.

A variety of other methods of supplying the necessary heat to accelerate the polymerization reaction have been used. They include steam, dry heat supplied by electric platens, dry-air oven, infrared heating, induction or dielectric heating, and microwave radiation. The results of various processing studies have shown that equally satisfactory clinical results may be obtained with any of these methods compared with

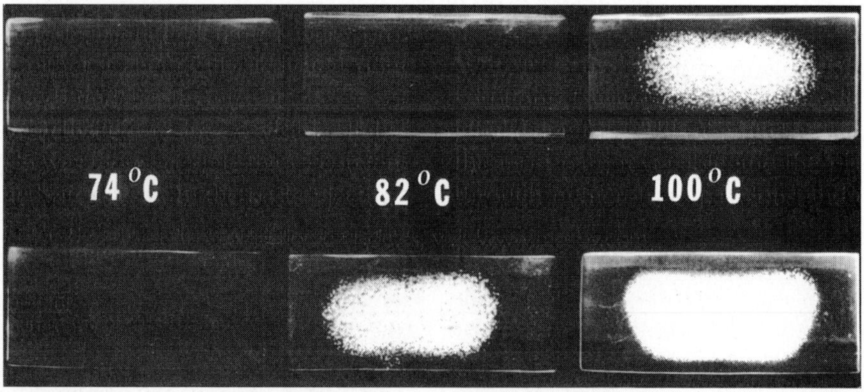

Fig. 21-10 Effect of the processing temperature on the porosity of two acrylic dental plastics. (From Peyton FA: *J Am Dent Assoc* 40:525, 1950.)

the water bath method if adequate temperature control and pressure are maintained.

Deflasking and Finishing After polymerization, the flask is removed from the water bath and allowed to cool to room temperature. If the flask is opened prematurely while the plastic is still warm, warpage is likely to occur. Rapid cooling also tends to increase stresses in the denture, which may be released at a later time. During the cooling process, thermal shrinkage occurs. The thermal shrinkage takes place as a result of the relatively high thermal coefficient of expansion of the plastic. The magnitude of this thermal shrinkage will depend on the difference between the temperature at which the plastic hardens and room or mouth temperature, whichever is the final reference point. It is apparent that as long as the plastic is soft, it will shrink with the stone cast, which has a different thermal coefficient. When the plastic hardens, stresses are induced as cooling continues, because the plastic is forced to follow the shape of the cast despite the differences in thermal coefficients. Deflasking of the denture after cooling, however, allows some of the stresses in the denture to be released, and warpage occurs. Numerous studies dealing with the linear shrinkage of denture bases, measured across the posterior region, have shown that for normal processing conditions, the linear shrinkage is 0.3% to 0.5%. Usually more shrinkage is observed in mandibular than in maxillary dentures because of their shape.

A change in the contact vertical dimension of a denture during processing, as measured on an articulator, is also important. These changes are caused by variations in flask pressure, flask temperature, consistency of the dough, and strength of the stone mold. The pressure developed during closure of the flask is possibly the most important factor. If proper precautions are taken, the vertical opening may be held to 0.5 mm rather than reported variations of 2 to 5 mm.

After cooling, the denture is ejected from the flask and the stone is removed. Stone adhering to the plastic may be removed by shell blasting, a process where ground walnut shells are used to abrade the stone with little or no effect on the plastic. After deflasking, the denture is trimmed with an arbor band and acrylic burs and polished. A wet polishing wheel and a slurry of pumice and water should be used to avoid heating the acrylic, which can cause measurable warpage. Tin oxide has been used to produce the final polish. However, tin oxide has been identified as a biological hazard and should be used with caution. After finishing, the denture should be stored in water.

Residual Monomer During the polymerization process the amount of residual monomer decreases rapidly at first, then more slowly. The amount of residual monomer in a denture plastic processed at 70° C and at 100° C is shown as a function of the time and processing in Fig. 21-11. At zero time the monomer content was 26.2%. After 1 hour at 70° C it decreased to 6.6%, and at 100° C to 0.31%. After 4 hours the residual monomer was 4.0% and 0.29%, respectively. It required 168 hours at 70° C for the residual monomer to approximate the value obtained after 1 hour at 100° C. These data support the use of a

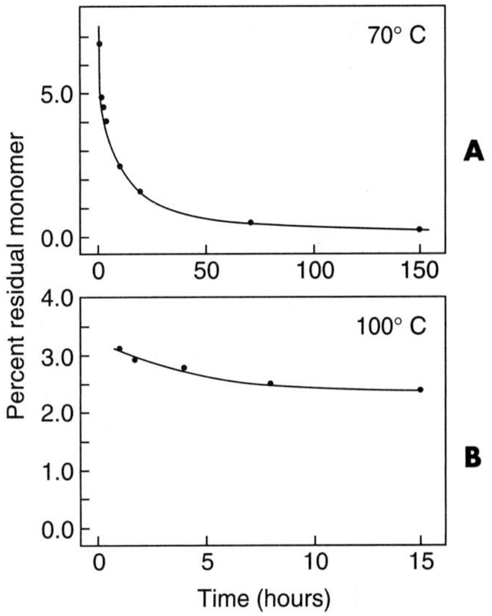

Fig. 21-11 Residual monomer concentration in the polymerization of methyl methacrylate in dental plastics at 70° C, **A,** and 100° C, **B,** as a function of the time of processing.

(Adapted from Smith DC: *Br Dent J* 105:86, 1958.)

1-hour terminal boil for processing dentures, as described earlier. However, the processing temperature should not be raised to boiling until most of the polymerization is completed, or porosity may result.

The highest residual monomer level is observed with chemically accelerated denture base plastics at 1% to 4% shortly after processing. Storing the denture for several days at elevated temperatures (up to 50° C) and excluding oxygen can significantly reduce the monomer level. However, this may be impractical. The rapid heat-cured denture base materials have significant residual monomer levels from 1% to 3% when they are processed in less than 1 hour in boiling water. If they are processed for 7 hours at 70° C and then boiled for 3 hours, the residual monomer content may be less than 0.4%.

If heat-processed materials are to be used for patients sensitive to residual monomer, processing for longer times in boiling water should reduce the monomer to an acceptable level. Because there is evidence that poly(methyl methacrylate) monomer has poor biocompatibility, every effort should be made to eliminate residual monomer or reduce it to very low levels.

Dimensional Changes Dimensional changes take place when dentures are stored in water or are in contact with oral fluids. A considerable number of studies have reported on dimensional changes occurring during processing and storage of dentures. The area described with the most uniform results has been the posterior region. In general, heat-cured dentures stored in water show a linear expansion in this region of 0.1% to 0.2%, which partially but not completely compensates for the processing shrinkage of 0.3% to 0.5%. The net linear change can vary from a shrinkage of 0.1% to 0.4%. The major portion of the expansion in water takes place during the first month, and changes are insignificant after 2 months.

In a study comparing the fit of maxillary dentures made from five different commercial products, denture bases were placed on their respective casts after being stored in water at 37° C for 42 days to ensure equilibrium. The materials were ranked from best fit to worst fit by a panel of trained observers. The relative fit was determined by the space between the base and the cast in the palatal region. One rubber-modified acrylic had the worst fit, whereas another had a fit that was similar to the conventional acrylic. The best fit was observed with the vinyl-modified and the hydroxyethyl acrylics. There was no correlation with water sorption values, and therefore the fit of the denture bases may be related more to the glass transition temperature (glassy to brittle transition) than to water sorption for these materials.

There is always concern regarding what a net shrinkage of 0.1% to 0.4% represents clinically. A number of other steps in the preparation of a complete denture may cause dimensional inaccuracies, such as making the impression, pouring the stone cast, and preparing and investing the waxed denture. The oral tissues apparently accommodate small dimensional changes in dentures.

Injection Molding Denture Base Resins

Several manufacturers have re-introduced injection molding materials and equipment and the process is gaining in popularity. The flasking and boiling out of the waxed denture is similar to that used for compression molding. For injection molding, a hollow sprue connects the mold cavity created by wax boilout to an external opening on the flask and a high-pressure injection cylinder is connected to the opening. The denture base resin is mixed and placed in the cylinder. When the material reaches the proper consistency it is injected into the mold cavity under high pressure. The pressure is maintained during the polymerization cycle, and as polymerization shrinkage occurs additional material enters the flask. There are several studies noting increased dimensional accuracy with this technique. Injection molding is also used for microwavable and pour type resins.

$$\underbrace{\text{Polymer} + \text{Peroxide initiator}}_{\text{Powder}} + \underbrace{\text{Monomer} + \text{Inhibitor} + \text{Amine accelerator}}_{\text{Liquid}} \longrightarrow \text{Polymer} + \underset{\text{(reaction)}}{\text{Heat}}$$

CHEMICALLY ACCELERATED ACRYLIC DENTURE PLASTICS—COMPRESSION MOLDING

Chemically accelerated dental plastics, often called *chemically curing resins, self-curing resins, cold-curing resins,* or *autopolymerizing resins,* are similar to heat-accelerated dental plastics. The principal difference is that the polymerization reaction is accelerated by a chemical, such as *N,N*-dihydroxyethyl-para-toluidine, rather than by heat, as indicated by the simplified equation above (compare with the equation given in the earlier section on heat-accelerated acrylic denture plastics).

The amine accelerator reacts with the peroxide initiator at room temperature and sufficient free radicals are produced to initiate the polymerization reaction. Except for initiation, the remainder of the polymerization reaction is the same as for the heat-accelerated type. The reaction is exothermic and polymerization still results in volumetric shrinkage, but the plastic does not reach as high a peak temperature.

Manipulation and Processing The general procedure for compression molding a chemically accelerated plastic is much the same as for the heat-accelerated type, except after final flask closure the dough is allowed to polymerize at room temperature or in a warm water bath in a pressure vessel.

The denture mold is packed when the polymer-monomer mixture reaches the doughy stage. Several trial closures are made and the flash removed. Care must be taken to make both the trial and final closure before the dough becomes so stiff that final closure is not possible. The chemically accelerated materials start to polymerize soon after the powder and liquid are mixed and proceed more rapidly through the various consistency stages than the heat-accelerated types. The average time needed to reach packing consistency is only 5 minutes for the chemically accelerated type, compared with 15 minutes for the heat-polymerized acrylic. It is more difficult to pack a number of denture flasks from one mix and still obtain complete flask closure. Additional working time may be obtained when the ingredients and the mixing jar are cooled in a refrigerator.

Properties After the flask is packed it should remain closed and under clamp pressure for a minimum of 2.5 hours to ensure polymerization. Compared with heat-cured plastics, chemically cured types do not reach the same degree of polymerization. The higher residual monomer acts as a plasticizer, which results in higher transverse deflection values and lower transverse strengths. After 15 days in water, however, chemically cured acrylics are nearly as hard as heat-cured. If, after 2.5 hours of curing at room temperature, the flask is boiled for 0.5 to 1 hour, properties comparable to the heat-cured type are obtained, and the residual monomer content is considerably reduced.

Peak temperatures observed at various positions in a denture cured by chemical acceleration are not as high as for heat-polymerized types. The linear shrinkage across the posterior region of a chemically cured maxillary denture after deflasking is about 0.3% compared with 0.5% for a heat-cured maxillary denture. As in the case of heat-cured dentures, mandibular dentures prepared with chemically accelerated denture plastics show more dimensional change than corresponding maxillary dentures. The lower dimensional change of the chemically cured type results because less residual stress is produced in the denture during the processing cycle. This is substantiated by the fact that the chemically accelerated denture plastics produce less shrinkage when processed at 20° to 25° C rather than at 37° C. When chemically cured dentures are placed in water, an increase in the molar-to-molar distance is observed. After 1 month this expansion amounts to about 0.3%, which approximately compensates for the processing shrinkage of 0.3%. Additional storage up to 9 months results in a total expansion of 0.4%, and the net dimensional change at this time is +0.1%, compared with the master model. It should be noted that water sorption of the chemically cured acrylics is between 0.5 and 0.7 mg/cm^2, or about the same as the heat-cured type. However, the solubility is 0.05 mg/cm^2 for the chemically cured type compared with 0.02 mg/cm^2 for the heat-cured type. This larger value for solubility is caused by the loss of residual monomer from the chemically cured acrylic.

On the basis of these observations, it can be concluded that chemically cured acrylic dentures are generally about 0.1% oversize after several months of service and heat-cured acrylic dentures are 0.3% to 0.4% undersize.

In addition to strength, water sorption, solubility, and dimensional changes, the color stability of chemically cured denture base should be considered. The presence of some amine accelerators may cause problems in color stability. These amines produce colored products on oxidation, and therefore the color stability of chemically cured acrylics may not be as good as that of heat-cured acrylics, although definite improvements have been made since their introduction. Several products are now available that comply with the ANSI/ADA Specification No. 12 color stability test. Activators such as organic sulfinic acids can be used to improve color stability, but these compounds have certain disadvantages, such as chemical instability.

FLUID RESIN ACRYLIC DENTURE PLASTICS

The fluid resin technique takes advantage of the flow properties of polymer-monomer mixtures in the early consistency stage and the smaller size of the polymer powder particles. A very fluid mix also results from a much higher monomer-polymer ratio of about 1:2.5. The polymer and monomer are mixed and then poured into the mold in the denture flask, and no trial packing is required. This procedure is advantageous in the preparation of the saddles for partial dentures, in which trial packing is difficult and flow of plastic around the metal framework is required. It also requires less expensive equipment than the heat-accelerated acrylic. Manufacturers claim that a denture can be produced in much less time using this procedure. This was not substantiated in a laboratory survey.

This technique involves the use of agar or alginate hydrocolloid or, less commonly, a soft stone or silicone mold. The presence of water in the hydrocolloid does not interfere with the polymerization of the slurry of polymer and monomer. The technique involves preparation of a hydrocolloid gel mold of the waxed-up denture, as shown in Fig. 21-12, *A*. After the gel is formed, the model, including the waxed denture, is removed. The wax is removed from the model and teeth, and the teeth are reinserted into the mold (Fig. 21-12, *B*). The model is repositioned in the mold after an alginate separator has been applied and allowed to dry. The denture flask is constructed so that two or three circular holes can be cut from the side of the flask through the gel to the posterior portion of the model. A slurry of chemically activated acrylic is poured through one of these holes into the mold space provided by the loss of the wax (Fig. 21-12, *C*). The remaining hole or holes provide vents for the excess acrylic slurry, thus ensuring adequate filling of the mold space. After pouring the acrylic the flask is placed in a pressure vessel containing warm water, and air pressure of 0.1 to 0.2 MPa is applied. Only 30 to 45 minutes are necessary for polymerization. After processing, the gel is easily broken away from the denture and the denture looks as clean as the one shown in Fig. 21-12, *D*. Because of higher polymerization shrinkage, dentures fabricated by this technique are slightly less accurate than heat-activated dentures processed in a stone mold. When compared with heat-cured resins, pour-type acrylics are characterized by lower impact and fatigue strengths,

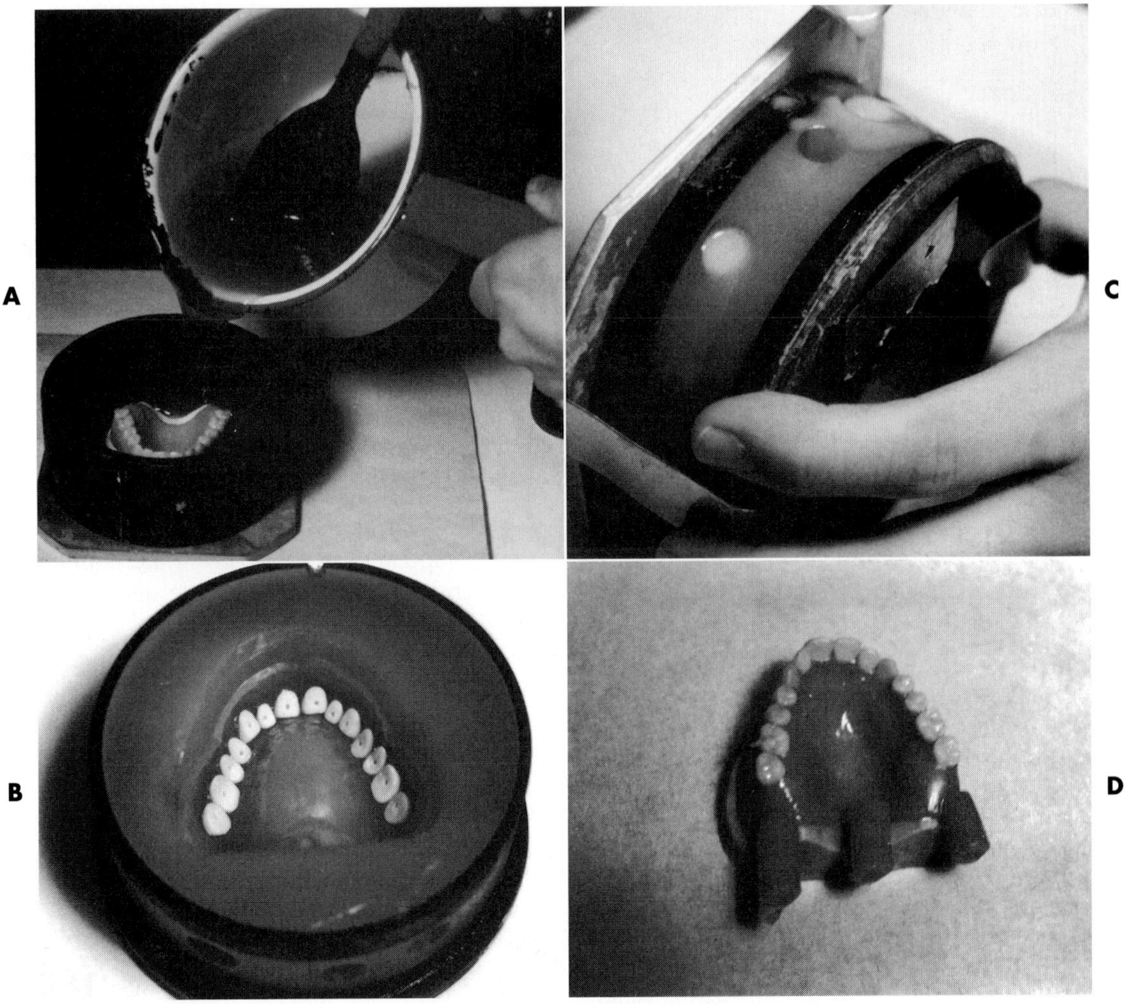

Fig. 21-12 Slurry casting of chemically accelerated acrylic denture base material. **A,** Pouring of agar mold. **B,** Agar mold with denture teeth in position. **C,** Pouring of powder-liquid slurry into the agar mold. **D,** Appearance of denture after processing.

higher creep values, lower transverse bend strength, lower water sorption values, and higher solubility. The technique is interesting, because the hydrocolloid mold is easy to prepare, processing time is shortened considerably, the agar hydrocolloid may be reused, problems of broken teeth are eliminated, and deflasking is simplified.

Commercial fluid resins may vary considerably in apparent viscosity. Fig. 21-13 demonstrates the dramatic increase in apparent viscosity of six different fluid resins as a function of time and at a constant shear rate (rotational speed). It illustrates the importance of pouring the fluid resins into the mold soon after the powder and liquid phases are mixed if lower viscosities are to be obtained. The apparent viscosity of fluid resins appears to be an important factor when fluid resin denture materials are evaluated.

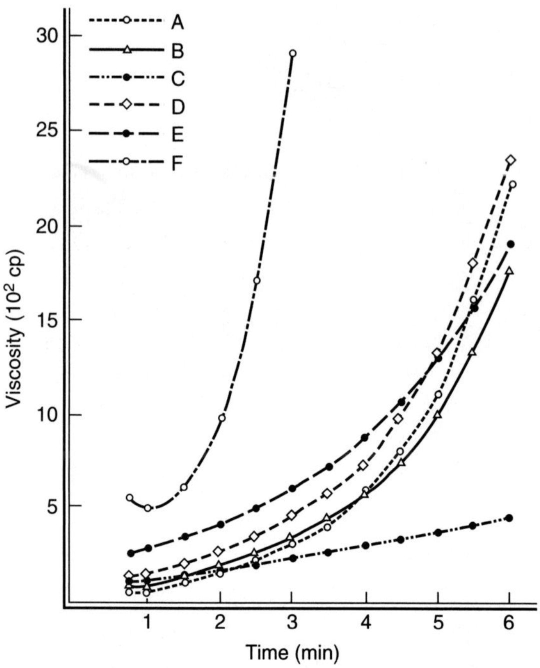

Fig. 21-13 Viscosity of six fluid resins as a function of time at 10 rpm.
(From Vermilyea SG, Powers JM, Koran A: *J Dent Res* 57:227, 1978.)

LIGHT-CURED DENTURE PLASTIC

Light curing of a denture is a novel method compared with other processing methods. After the try-in of the waxed-up trial denture is completed, a roll of light-activated acrylic is placed over the occlusal surfaces of the teeth to form a template having three reference areas on the master cast (Fig. 21-14, *A*). The template is cured in the light chamber for 10 minutes, then the teeth are removed from the trial denture. Removal is simple because the wax softens under the heat of the high-intensity light bulbs. The teeth, the attached template, and the cast are placed in boiling water to remove all traces of wax (Fig. 21-14, *B*).

After coating the master cast with a release agent, a sheet of the light-activated denture base material is adapted to the cast and trimmed to the boxing edge (Fig. 21-14, *C*). The base is then polymerized in the light chamber.

A strip of the light-activated acrylic is placed on the underside of the teeth after they have been coated with a bonding agent. The teeth are then repositioned in the original position on the denture base using the template (Fig. 21-14, *D*). The teeth are held in position by polymerization in the light chamber.

The anatomical portion of the denture is completed using more of the base material to sculpt the surface and develop the final shape of the denture (Fig. 21-14, *E*). After contouring, final polymerization is accomplished in the light chamber and the denture is removed from the cast and finished in a conventional manner.

FACTORS INVOLVED IN DENTURE RETENTION

Accuracy of fit has been cited as an important factor in the retention of dentures. Other factors are (1) capillary forces involving the liquid film between the oral tissues and the denture base; (2) surface forces controlling the wetting of the plastic denture base by the saliva; (3) the thickness of the saliva film between the denture and the oral tissues; (4) the surface tension of the saliva; (5) the viscosity of the saliva; and (6) atmospheric pressure. High surface tension, area, and wetting increase retention, as does a thin film of saliva (see Chapter 2). A technical discussion of all factors involved in the retention of dentures is not within the scope of this text.

EFFECT OF AUXILIARY MATERIALS ON DENTURE PLASTICS

A number of materials are used in making a denture. These materials may affect the final properties and function of the denture. Examples of such materials are (1) dental plaster and stone, (2) impression materials, (3) wax, (4) mold separators, (5) artificial teeth, (6) characterization materials, (7) metal inserts, (8) repair and reline materials, and (9) denture cleansers.

Plaster and Stone The strength of the plaster or stone used to invest the wax denture is of concern, because a weak investment resulting from a thin mix or incomplete mixing will not adequately support the artificial teeth during packing of the denture mold. As a result of teeth

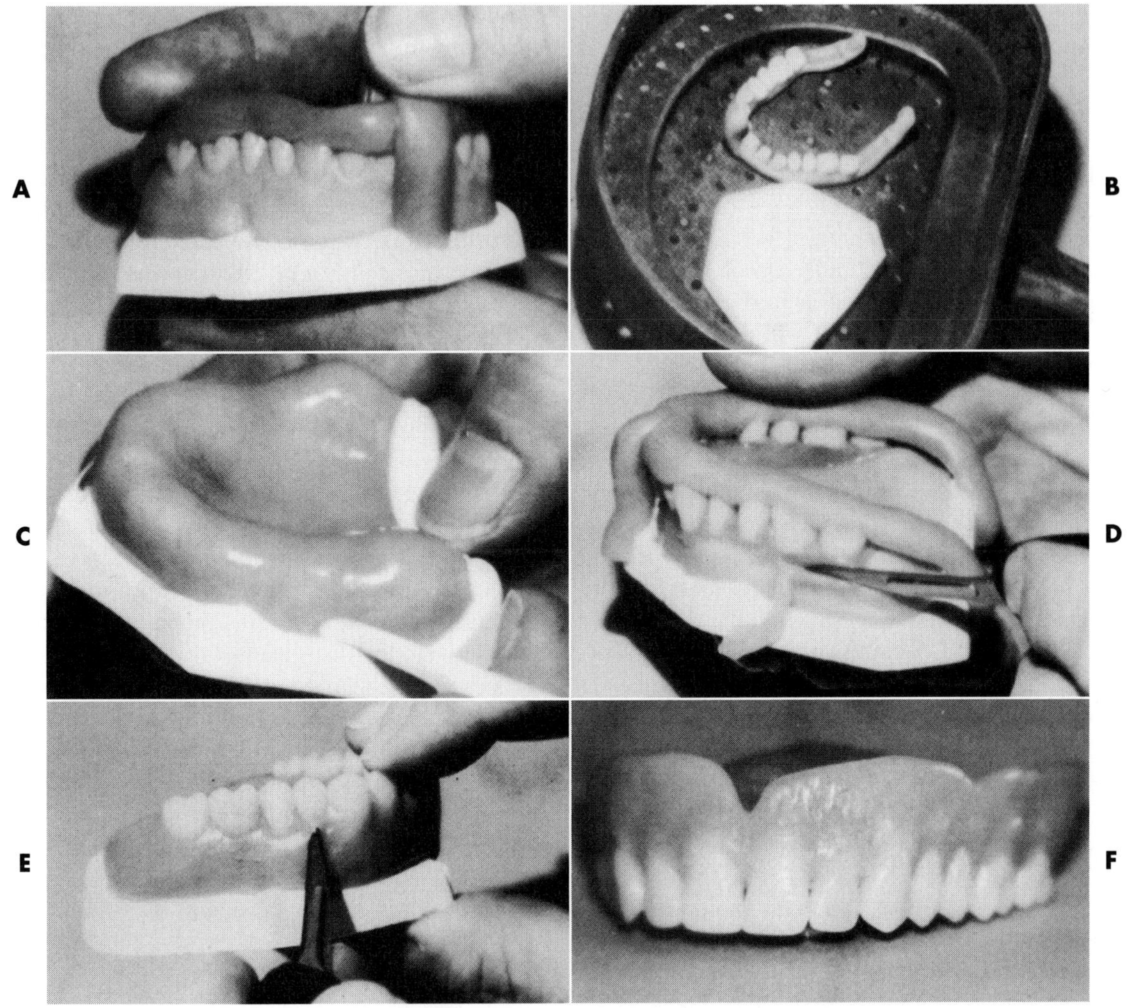

Fig. 21-14 Processing of a light-activated denture base. **A,** Pick-up of the denture teeth from the waxed trial denture using a rope of the light-activated acrylic. **B,** Removal of all traces of wax from the teeth and master cast. **C,** Adaptation of light-activated denture base material to the master cast. **D,** Reseating the teeth on the master cast and beginning the shaping of the anatomical portion of the denture. **E,** Final adaptation of the anatomical portion of the denture, just before polymerization in the light chamber. **F,** Completed light-activated acrylic denture. (Courtesy Dentsply International, York, Pa, 1987.)

shifting, the finished dentures may have faulty occlusion. Another problem involved in the use of a stone mold is that the thermal coefficient of expansion, or contraction, is different from the thermal coefficients of the teeth and the plastic used to form the denture. After the polymerization reaction, the plastic and investment cool to room temperature and attempt to contract according to their individual thermal coefficients. The stone cast with a different thermal coefficient creates residual stresses in the acrylic as it cools. These stresses may be released after the processed denture is deflasked and deformation or crazing may result. One study suggests that using a high expansion dental stone in the final impression will compensate for the polymerization shrinkage of the denture base resin and provide greater accuracy in the denture base.

Impression Materials When alginate materials are used to make an impression, it is important that the cast be poured as soon as possible. If dimensional changes occur in the impression, these inaccuracies will be reflected in the final fit of the denture base. When zinc oxide–eugenol impression materials are used, residual eugenol in the cast will function as an inhibitor in the polymerization of the plastic.

Waxes Baseplate wax that is not removed from the crown portion of the teeth before the denture is flasked will cause problems. During the removal of the wax in boiling water, the wax on the coronal area of the teeth is also removed and will result in shifting of the teeth, poor articulation, or broken teeth when the denture is packed. A more common problem is the presence of a residual wax film on the gingival portions of the artificial teeth after the boilout of the wax, which prevents the adherence of the denture base to the teeth. This may be avoided by the addition of detergent to the water used in the boilout procedure, followed by rinsing with clear boiling water.

Mold Separators For many years tinfoil was the most acceptable separating medium. Tinfoil, however, is difficult to apply and as a result a number of tinfoil substitutes have been developed. Materials such as aqueous solutions of sodium silicate, calcium oleate, or sodium or ammonium alginate have been used. The common alginate separators contain about 2% sodium alginate in water with small amounts of glycerin, alcohol, sodium phosphate, and preservatives. Care must be exercised to avoid coating plastic teeth with these release agents because this will interfere with the bond between the denture base and the teeth.

Characterization Materials A variety of materials are used for the characterization of dentures. Included in this group of materials are dyed synthetic fibers, pigments, dyes, and clear plastic powder. These materials have the effect of improving the esthetics of the dentures and have no substantial effects on the strength or other properties of dental plastics. For example, the addition of dyed acrylic fibers to simulate the blood vessels of the oral mucosa does not alter the water sorption or strength of the dental plastic significantly. There is a justified concern over the toxicity of some of the pigments used to color denture base materials.

Denture Cleansers Denture cleansers and cleaning methods may scratch and wear dentures. Denture acrylic has been tested for wear using various commercially available denture cleaning pastes, an experimental paste, soap and water, and water against a reciprocating soft toothbrush. The results shown in Fig. 21-15 are dramatic. The use of water, or soap and water, produced little or no wear compared with the commercial denture cleansers and toothpaste. Daily brushing with a very soft brush (similar to the toothbrushes used in periodontal therapy) is very effective in keeping dentures clean and will not abrade the denture or teeth appreciably if abrasive cleansers are not used. Most immersion

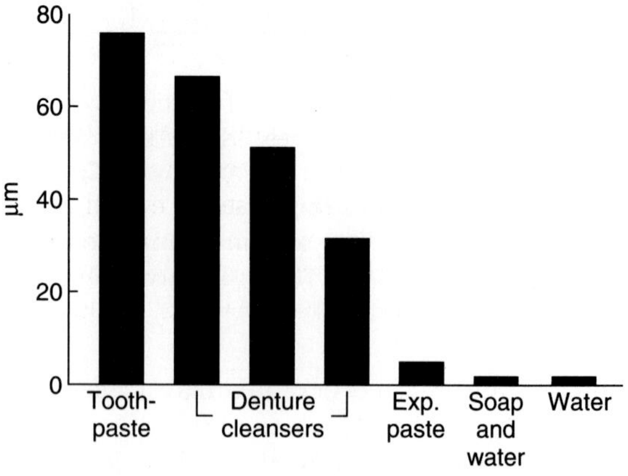

Fig. 21-15 Wear of denture base acrylic in various media, as illustrated by a histogram showing loss of thickness after 60,000 stokes.

(Adapted from Heath JR, Davenport JC, Jones PA: *J Oral Rehabil* 10:159, 1983.)

denture cleansers are effective in the removal of mucin, stains, and loosely attached food debris. Some immersion cleaners have been demonstrated to be effective sanitizing agents. A water solution containing a hypochlorite and a glassy phosphate (Calgon) is an effective denture cleanser that does not cause discoloration of the dental plastic or the metal retainer pins in porcelain artificial teeth when used occasionally. A solution consisting of 1 tsp of a hypochlorite, such as Clorox, and 2 tsp of Calgon in half a glass of water has been recommended for occasional overnight immersion of plastic dentures. This cleanser is not recommended for use on prostheses containing cobalt-chromium or nickel-chromium alloys because chlorine solutions tend to darken these metals.

REPAIR MATERIALS

An important application of plastics in prosthetic dentistry is in the repair of broken dentures. Repair materials are usually acrylic plastics of the powder-liquid type, similar to those used for denture bases, and are usually either heat-accelerated or chemically accelerated. Light-activated acrylic has also been shown to be a fast and effective repair material. The material of choice will depend on the following factors: (1) length of time required for making the repair, (2) transverse strength obtainable with the repair material, and (3) degree to which dimensional accuracy is maintained during repair.

One technique for making a repair requires holding, or luting, the broken pieces together with sticky wax, pouring a stone model on the inside of the denture, and investing the model and denture in a flask. Then the wax is removed, the fracture line is opened with a bur to allow for a reasonable amount of repair plastic, and the ground surfaces are painted with monomer or a 4:1 mixture of monomer and polymer. Acrylic dough is packed into the area being repaired, and the material is cured, cooled, deflasked, and finished.

If a heat-accelerated acrylic is used, the denture should be completely flasked, and curing of the repair material preferably should be carried out at temperatures no greater than 74° to 77° C for 8 hours or longer. This procedure minimizes the dimensional change of the denture base.

In a similar manner, the repair may be done without flasking, by use of a chemically accelerated acrylic. After a cast is poured, the fracture line is opened and the acrylic is painted into the defect. The denture is then placed in a pressure vessel under air pressure until polymerization is complete. Repairs using light-activated acrylic are done in a similar manner. After the acrylic dough is packed into the defect, curing is done in the light chamber. A bonding agent is used to increase the strength of the repair.

The use of chemically accelerated and light-activated acrylic resins for repairs does not require flasking. The procedure is rapid and may be done while the patient waits. The dimensional accuracy is maintained because not enough heat is present during polymerization to cause warpage from the release of stresses. The chemically accelerated acrylic resins, however, have the disadvantage of lower transverse strength in the repaired area than a heat-cured acrylic. In general, the transverse strength of a heat-cured repair is about 80% of that of the original plastic, and the transverse strength of a chemically cured repair is approximately 60% of the original material. Light-activated acrylic is affected by water storage, resulting in lower transverse strength than the self-cured repair resin. Regardless of the type of plastic used for repair, the shape of the edges in the repair area should be tapered and all corners rounded to avoid areas of high stress concentration. These ground edges are painted with monomer to soften the plastic to obtain a chemical bond between the repair material and the denture.

The use of chemically accelerated repair material without flasking at room temperature and pressure may result in a repair area containing porosity. Polymerization in the center of the repair proceeds rapidly, but polymerization at the surface is slowed by the inhibiting effect of the oxygen. When the repair is done in water, under air pressure of 0.2 MPa and a temperature of 30° C, the porosity is greatly reduced. The residual monomer content of specimens processed either in air or under pressure is approximately 3%.

The reported net dimensional change across the molar region of a maxillary denture for a heat-cured repair conducted at 73.5° C is –0.3%, whereas for a chemically cured repair it is +0.2%. It also has been reported that a denture repaired with chemically accelerated plastic will fit the model better. This may be the result of less warpage or because the denture is slightly oversized. Studies have been done on the contour of denture bases before they were broken and after repair. The results indicate that better reproduction of dimensions results when chemically accelerated repair materials are used to repair dentures originally prepared from heat-cured or self-cured acrylic plastics. Superior results also are obtained when a heat-curing acrylic repair material is used to repair a denture prepared from a chemically accelerated acrylic plastic. Less satisfactory reproduction of dimensions is obtained when a heat-curing repair material is used to repair a heat-cured denture. If the cause of breakage is not corrected, such as faulty occlusion, fit, or both, repairs usually will fail regardless of which repair material is used.

ANSI/ADA Specification No. 13 for Denture Self-Curing Repair Resins The requirements of the chemically accelerated repair plastics or the self-curing repair resins are listed in ANSI/ADA Specification No. 13. The specification includes self-curing powder-liquid plastics, which may be either pink or clear. These materials must satisfy the requirements for denture base plastics, with two exceptions. First, the plasticity test shall be conducted as in the denture base specification, except the test should be started 3 minutes rather than 5 minutes after the proper plasticity is reached. This change allows for the faster setting of the repair materials.

Second, the transverse deflection between a 1500- and 2500-g load shall be not more than 1.5 mm, and the deflection between a 1500- and 4000-g load shall be not less than 1 mm and not more than 4.5 mm. This transverse deflection requirement is difficult to compare with the test for chemically accelerated denture base plastics, because the loads used are different and therefore the deflection limits are not the same. It does appear, however, that the deflection limits for the repair materials are somewhat more lenient.

In general, the color stability test is difficult for chemically accelerated repair materials to pass.

RELINING AND REBASING DENTURES

The fit of a denture may be satisfactory when it is first delivered to the patient. However, because of changes in the contour of the soft tissues and resorption of underlying bone, the denture may gradually lose retention. If the occlusion and vertical dimension of the dentures have not been greatly altered, the retention may be regained by either relining or rebasing.

Relining *Relining* is a process in which a film of plastic is added to the inside of the denture to obtain an improved fit with the denture-bearing mucosa. This is accomplished by (1) making an impression of the denture-bearing mucosa using the denture as a tray, reflasking the denture, removing the impression material, and packing and curing the new liner; or (2) making a chairside reline where the reline material is used to make the impression.

Two different types of reline materials may be used—one permanent, the other temporary. The former may be either a heat-accelerated, chemically accelerated, or light-activated acrylic. The relining process is carried out either by a flasking procedure or curing in a light chamber, depending on the type of material. Permanent reline materials may be identical to those from which permanent denture bases are made.

The problems involved in relining a denture are much the same as those encountered in repairing a denture: (1) a good chemical bond is desired between the reline plastic and the denture plastic; (2) satisfactory strength of the relined denture is necessary; (3) no warpage or dimensional change should result in the denture because of the relining procedure; and (4) relining should take as short a time as possible for patient convenience. For heat-polymerized reline materials the area to be relined is softened by monomer and the acrylic is packed soon after reaching the doughy consistency to achieve a chemical bond between the two materials. The polymerization should occur at temperatures between 74° to 77° C to prevent warpage. Chemically accelerated reline materials have an advantage because lower peak temperatures during polymerization may minimize warpage.

The light-activated material is used directly in the denture to record the tissue surface. A bonding agent is used before placing the material in the denture. Polymerization is achieved in a light chamber. The light-activated acrylic allows the entire reline procedure to be completed in 30 to 45 minutes.

Temporary relining plastics are used directly in the mouth, and a chemically accelerated curing system is used. These materials are considered temporary because they are porous and stain easily or foul with microorganisms. In addition, most of these products are not color stable. Temporary reline materials polymerize at mouth temperature and the reaction is exothermic, with peak polymerization temperatures of 59° to 79° C and peak temperature times of 6 to 11 minutes. The lower temperatures generally correspond to longer times. Peak temperatures of 79° C can cause tissue injury. To avoid burning of the tissues, the denture is usually taken from the mouth after a few minutes, chilled in cool water, and returned to the mouth. In addition to the exothermic heat, direct contact of monomer on the oral tissues may elicit a burning sensation. Temporary reline plastics, however, do not cause any clinically significant warpage of the denture.

ANSI/ADA Specification No. 17 for Denture Base Temporary Relining Resin

ANSI/ADA Specification No. 17 for temporary relining resin is for hard-setting, self-curing plastics of the powder-liquid type. This specification contains requirements for the consistency, temperature rise, hardening time, ease of polishing, translucency, porosity, hardness, water sorption and solubility, and color stability. The peak temperature reached during processing should not be more than 75° C, and the time of hardening should be between 6 and 15 minutes. The processed plastic should have a smooth glossy surface when polished by usual methods and should be translucent and free of large numbers or sizes of bubbles. The Knoop hardness shall be not less than 10 kg/mm^2. The water solubility and sorption shall be less than 0.07 and 0.7 mg/cm^2, respectively, when stored for 24 hours at 37° C. The requirements for hardness and solubility in water therefore are less demanding for temporary relining materials than for denture base plastics. Temporary relining plastics, however, must pass the color stability test for denture plastics, which requires that the specimen show no more than a slight color change after an exposure of 24 hours. This requirement may be difficult to satisfy, because many products show noticeable color changes when exposed to ultraviolet light.

Rebasing *Rebasing* refers to a technique in which the dimensional relations of the teeth are maintained and the entire denture base is replaced. A cast is prepared from an impression made in the denture. After flasking, all of the old plastic is removed except around the teeth. The denture is then processed according to standard procedures with new acrylic. The end result is a new denture base retaining the original teeth in the same position as in the original denture.

Tissue Conditioners Tissue conditioners are soft elastomers used to treat an irritated mucosa supporting a denture. They are mixed at chairside, placed in the denture, and seated in the patient's mouth. These materials will conform to the anatomy of the residual ridge, gel in that position, and continue to flow slowly after application. They are used only for short-term applications and should be replaced every 3 days. Inhibition of the growth of oral bacterial flora is associated with some materials, and this should promote healing of inflamed tissues.

Tissue conditioners are composed of a powder containing poly(ethyl methacrylate) and a liquid containing an aromatic ester-ethyl alcohol (up to 30%) mixture. Tissue conditioners are very soft elastomers with a hardness of from 13 to 49 Shore A hardness units 24 hours after mixing. They will show a weight loss of from 4.9% to

9.3% after 24 hours as a result of the loss of alcohol. These materials deform easily, and with a stress of 200 g/cm^2 applied 15 minutes after the set of the material, the compression will range from 60% to 83% of the original length. When the stress is removed, there will be a recovery of from 22% to 48%. When unstrained samples are left in a humidifier for 24 hours, they will tend to "slump" or shorten under their own weight. Within a few days, tissue conditioners become stiffer as a result of the loss of alcohol.

Tissue conditioners are formulated to have specific viscoelastic properties. The viscosities of a number of tissue conditioners are listed in Table 21-11. The values were obtained 2 hours after mixing and under prolonged static loads. Under cyclic loading, which parallels cyclic masticatory forces, the materials demonstrate elastic behavior, particularly when the frequency is more than 1 Hz.

The properties that make tissue conditioners effective are (1) viscous behavior, which allows adaptation to the irritated denture-bearing mucosa over a period of several days; and (2) viscoelastic and elastic behavior, which cushions the cyclic forces of mastication and bruxism. The viscoelastic properties are influenced by the molecular weight of the polymer powders and the power/liquid ratio.

It has been suggested that the initial flow depends on the time of loading, volume of the material, and load applied when seating the denture. A rheologic study has shown that different products must be seated in the mouth at different times from the start of mixing because they may differ both in viscosity or gelation time. The gelation time is related to the molecular weight and particle size of the polymer powder, the ethanol content, and the plasticizer used.

An evaluation of the viscoelastic properties of tissue conditioners consisting of poly(ethyl methacrylate) powders and butyl phthalate/butyl glycolate–ethanol liquids demonstrates that the elastic modulus, relaxation time, and instantaneous modulus increase as a function of time. The rate of increase in the coefficient of viscosity is greater than the elastic modulus in all cases. This confirms that compliance measurements and the Maxwell model are the most useful when describing the viscoelastic properties of tissue conditioners.

Viscoelastic finite element analysis has been used to evaluate the stress concentrations caused by simulated dentures with soft liners during function. The results indicate that the viscous flow of soft liners and tissue are affected by the load and the duration of the load placed on the denture. This affects the stress distribution in the supporting tissues.

TABLE 21-11 Viscosity of Tissue Conditioners 2 Hours after Mixing

Material	Liquid/ Powder Ratio	Viscosity (10^6 poise) (20° C)	(37.4° C)
A	1.03	2.00	1.20
B	0.98	7.40	4.90
C	0.97	2.73	1.30
D	0.98	5.75	1.87
E	0.89	6.75	3.78
F	1.03	2.70	1.23
	0.8	5.80	2.455
G	1.04	0.187	0.029
	0.77	3.98	—
H	1.15	0.78	—
I	1.01	1.16	2.66
J	0.92	1.47	—

Adapted from Braden M: *J Dent Res* 49:496, 1970.

Soft or Resilient Denture Liners Soft or plasticized acrylic, vinyl polymers, and copolymers, as well as natural and silicone rubber products, have been used as denture liners. As mentioned previously, these soft liners are suggested for use in patients with irritation of the denture-bearing mucosa, areas of severe undercuts, or congenital or acquired defects of the palate. Some products reportedly have an inhibitory effect on the growth of *Candida albicans* whereas others appear to support the growth of microorganisms. Desirable properties are

(1) high bond strength to the denture base, (2) dimensional stability of the liner during and after processing, (3) permanent softness or resilience, (4) low water sorption, (5) color stability, (6) ease of processing, and (7) biocompatibility. Soft liners may be mouth cured or processed in the laboratory.

Mouth-Cured Soft Liners Conventional mouth-cured soft liners are used for periods to improve the comfort and fit of an old denture until it can be remade or permanently relined. After several weeks they may begin to foul and debond from the denture. They are mixed chairside, placed in the denture, and seated in the patient's mouth until polymerized, which generally takes a few minutes. Three types of materials are generally used:

1. Powder—poly(ethyl methacrylate) and peroxide initiator; liquid—aromatic esters, ethanol, and tertiary amines
2. Powder—poly(ethyl methacrylate), plasticizers such as ethyl glycolate, and a peroxide initiator; liquid—methyl methacrylate and tertiary amines
3. Addition silicone elastomers

Biocompatibility of these materials is of interest because it has been demonstrated both in vitro and in vivo that both tissue conditioners and chairside soft liners leach out significant amounts of alcohol and phthalate esters.

Processed Soft Liners Processed soft liners are used with denture patients who experience chronic soreness with their dentures because of heavy bruxism or poor health. The cushioning effect of soft liners has been evaluated using an impact test with an accelerometer. Of four soft liners tested, all were found to reduce impact forces compared with denture base resin. Although these materials fulfill a need, they will generally not last long in use. A year is considered good service. These materials tend to pull away from the denture base or become porous and foul smelling. They are processed in the laboratory in a manner similar to processing of a denture base. Several addition-silicone elastomers can be processed either intraorally or in the laboratory. Finishing of soft denture liners is often difficult because the materials are soft. Several types of processed soft liners are available, including plasticized acrylics, plasticized vinyl acrylics, heat- and room temperature–cured silicones, hydrophilic acrylates, and polyphosphazine. The compositions of various commercial products of plasticized acrylic and silicones are shown in Tables 21-12 and 21-13.

TABLE 21-12 Composition of Plasticized Acrylic Soft Lining Materials

Material	Polymer	Monomer	Plasticizer	Percentage of Plasticizer
A	Poly(ethyl methacrylate)	Methyl methacrylate	Butyl phthalyl butyl glycollate	31.2
B	Poly(ethyl methacrylate)	*n*-Butyl methacrylate	Butyl phthalyl butyl glycollate	24.9
C	Poly(methyl methacrylate)	Methyl methacrylate	Butyl phthalyl butyl glycollate	58.8
D	Poly(ethyl methacrylate)	Methyl methacrylate + Ethyl acetate	Di-*n*-butyl phthalate	36.2
E	Poly(ethyl methacrylate)	Ethyl methacrylate	2-Ethylhexyl diphenyl phosphate	39.0

Adapted from Wright RS: *J Dent* 9:210, 1981.

TABLE 21-13 Composition of Silicone Soft Lining Materials

Material	Polymer	Cross-Linking Agent	Catalyst	Percentage of Filler	Adhesive
A	α-ω-dihydroxy end-blocked poly(dimethyl siloxane)	Triethoxy silanol	Dibutyltin dilaurate	34.5	Silicone polymer in solvent
B	α-ω-dihydroxy end-blocked poly(dimethyl siloxane)	Ethyl polysilicate	Dibutyltin dilaurate	16.5	Silicone polymer in solvent
C	α-ω-dihydroxy end-blocked poly(dimethyl siloxane)	Tetraethoxy silane	Stannous octoate	42.6	Silicone polymer in solvent
D	α-ω-dihydroxy end-blocked poly(dimethyl siloxane)	Methyltriacetoxy silane	Moisture	11.35	Silicone polymer in solvent
E	α-ω-dihydroxy end-blocked poly(dimethyl siloxane)	Acryloxyalkyl silane	Heat + Benzoyl peroxide	21.5	γ-Methacryloxypropyl trimethoxysilane

Adapted from Wright RS: *J Dent* 9:210, 1981.

Several physical properties of four categories of laboratory processed soft liners, determined 24 hours after processing, are presented in Table 21-14. The properties of these materials show a wide range of values. This variability is difficult to interpret because there is no ANSI/ADA specification for laboratory processed soft liners. For example, a plasticized acrylic may have very high tear resistance *and* a high Shore A hardness value. Because softer materials are generally considered kinder to the tissues, the gain in tear resistance is offset by hardness. Conversely, a silicone soft liner may have a low Shore A hardness value and low tear resistance. Many of these materials tend to increase in hardness with time, and their physical and mechanical properties are also affected by prolonged storage in water or in the oral environment.

The water solubility and sorption of soft liners is complex. When placed in water, plasticizers and other components may leach out over extended periods while water is absorbed until equilibrium is reached. Absorbed water can have a detrimental effect on the adhesion of soft liners to acrylic denture bases, particularly if the rate of diffusion is rapid. At 1 week, water sorption will be from 0.2 to 5.6 mg/cm^2 and solubility from 0.03 to 0.40 mg/cm^2 for various commercial products. An ideal processed soft liner would have no soluble components and low water sorption.

Processed soft liners are intended to be used for extended periods. In some patients it has been observed that a yeast, *Candida albicans,* and other microorganisms may grow on and within the liner, resulting in a rough and hardened surface. Antimicrobial agents have been proposed to eliminate this problem. Color changes have also been demonstrated for some liners subjected to accelerated aging.

The bond strengths for the materials listed in Table 21-14 are seen in Table 21-15. The materials were tested in a two-phase tensile test. Two test conditions were used; the soft liners were processed against both polymerized and unpolymerized acrylic resin. Again the results were variable. For both test conditions the polyphosphazine material demonstrated higher bond strength. It also was surprising that for three of

TABLE 21-14 Properties of Laboratory-Processed Soft Liners

Materials	Tensile Strength (MPa)	Percent Elongation	Hardness Shore A	Tear Resistance (N/cm)
Plasticized poly(methyl methacrylate)	0.8-8.3	150-300	30-95	29-260
Plasticized vinyl acrylics	2.0-3.6	250-280	35-55	49-110
Silicones	2.4-4.3	325-340	25-45	49-69
Polyphosphazine	3.6	240	50	88

Adapted from Dootz ER, Koran A, Craig RG: *J Prosthet Dent* 67:707, 1992.

TABLE 21-15 Bond Strength of Laboratory-Processed Soft Denture Liners

Materials	Processed to Unpolymerized PMMA (MPa)	Processed to Polymerized PMMA (MPa)
Plasticized poly(methyl methacrylate)	0.5-1.3	1.1-1.7
Plasticized vinyl acrylics	2.6	1.1
Silicones	0.8-1.4	1.0-1.8
Polyphosphazine	2.0	2.5

Adapted from Kawano F, Dootz ER, Koran A, Craig RG: *J Prosthet Dent* 68:367, 1992.

the four groups, the bond strength was higher to polymerized acrylic than to unpolymerized acrylic. Most manufacturers recommend processing the soft liner and the denture base acrylic at the same time to improve the bond strength. Only the plasticized vinyl acrylic had a higher bond strength when processed against unpolymerized acrylic. Recently, bonding agents have been introduced that significantly increase the bond strength of several addition-silicone elastomers to denture base resin.

Dynamic viscoelastic measurements are effective for evaluating the elastic behavior of elastomers over time. In one study evaluating a plasticized acrylic, a fluoroelastomer, a heat-cured silicone, and a self-curing addition silicone, the acrylic and fluoroelastomer demonstrated viscoelastic behavior whereas the silicones exhibited elastic behavior. The silicones were more stable over time than the other materials.

Growth of *Candida albicans* and other microorganisms continues to challenge the use of short- and long-term soft denture liners. Unfortunately, researchers and manufacturers have yet to develop materials that will not support the growth of microorganisms. At this time, only excellent oral and denture hygiene and the use of antimicrobial agents are effective in minimizing this problem.

Unfortunately, many of the short- and long-term resilient denture liners contain significant amounts of plasticizers, many of which have questionable biocompatibility. Phthalate esters have caused epithelial changes when polymer disks containing these esters have been implanted in the hamster cheek pouch. The potentially premalignant changes are a cause for concern because the amount of this plasticizer leached from a typical soft liner may be between 10 and 40 times greater than environmental and food uptake. Although even this amount of plasticizer is low, demonstrated biocompatibility of soft denture liners should be considered.

Soft liners have an important place in denture prosthetics, but require improved strength, improved adhesion to the denture base, and the ability to inhibit the growth of microorganisms before they will be considered permanent.

DENTURE TEETH

Plastic teeth are prepared from acrylic and modified acrylic materials similar to denture plastics. Different pigments are used to produce the various tooth shades, and usually a cross-linking agent is used to improve strength and prevent crazing. Plastic teeth are prepared in layers of different colors so the shade is gradually lightened toward the incisal and occlusal portions to give these areas a translucent appearance. The gingival or body portion may not be as highly cross-linked as the incisal or occlusal portion. This is done to improve the chemical bond between the teeth and the denture base. Fillers may be added to increase resistance to wear. Recently, the use of composite materials as denture tooth materials has received some interest and new, modified tooth materials that appear to have increased wear resistance have been introduced.

As indicated in the discussion on the physical properties of dental plastics, poly(methyl methacrylate) has satisfactory chemical properties for use as plastic teeth. It is nontoxic and insoluble in oral fluids but is soluble to some extent in ketones and aromatic hydrocarbons. The mechanical properties of compressive strength (76 MPa), abrasion resistance, elastic modulus (2700 MPa), elastic limit (55 MPa), and hardness (18 to 20 kg/mm^2) are low when compared with other restorative materials or with human enamel and dentin.

Of necessity, a discussion of the merits of plastic teeth includes a general comparison of the properties of plastic and porcelain teeth, a number of which are listed in Table 21-16. Certain properties may be listed as a disadvantage or an advantage depending on the particular purpose and point of view involved. For example, the softness and low abrasion resistance of plastic teeth may be cited as a disadvantage, because the teeth are more easily abraded and the occlusion and vertical dimension of the denture may be altered. On the other hand, low wear resistance also has been cited as an advantage, because plastic teeth are easy to grind and polish and tend to be self-adjusting in service. The hardness of porcelain teeth compared with plastic teeth is an advantage, whereas the resulting brittleness of

TABLE 21-16 Comparison of Properties of Plastic and Porcelain Teeth

Plastic Teeth	Porcelain Teeth
High resilience	Very brittle
Tough	Friable
Soft—low abrasion resistance	Hard—high abrasion resistance
Insoluble in mouth fluids—some dimensional change	Inert in mouth fluids—no dimensional change
Low heat-distortion temperature, cold flow under pressure	High heat-distortion temperature; no permanent deformation under forces of mastication
Bond to denture base plastic	Poor bond-to-denture base plastic*; mechanical retention provided in tooth design
Natural appearance	Natural appearance
Natural feel—silent	Possible clicking sound in use
Easy to grind and polish	Grinding removes surface glaze
Crazing and blanching—if non-cross linked	Occasional cracking

*Does not apply if silane-treated.

porcelain compared with the toughness of plastic teeth is a disadvantage.

The main difference between porcelain and plastic teeth is that plastic teeth are softer but tougher than porcelain teeth. Other differences are the low elastic modulus, low resistance to cold flow, low abrasion resistance, and high impact strength of plastic teeth. Both plastic and porcelain teeth are insoluble in oral fluids. Porcelain teeth are resistant to organic solvents such as ketones and aromatic hydrocarbons, which will react with non–cross linked plastic teeth. Plastic teeth composed of poly(methyl methacrylate) show small dimensional changes when placed in water. As expected, vinyl acrylic teeth do not show as much dimensional change as the totally acrylic teeth. Porcelain teeth show no dimensional change when stored in water and exhibit no permanent deformation from forces exerted on them in the mouth.

For denture teeth, the coefficient of friction of acrylic against acrylic in the presence of water or saliva is lower than the coefficient for porcelain against porcelain. The lowest coefficients of friction, however, are obtained when porcelain and acrylic specimens oppose each other.

In Fig. 21-16, the frictional behavior of acrylic denture teeth is shown for central incisors from two manufacturers. The tangential force on a diamond slider being drawn across the teeth was measured under various loads in distilled water. The width of the wear track was also measured. In general, low values of track width occurred with low tangential force values, and higher track widths and more severe surface failure were associated with higher values of tangential force. The "enamel" surfaces, which were the labial surfaces of the teeth, were more resistant to penetration and surface damage than the "dentin" surfaces, which were prepared by removing

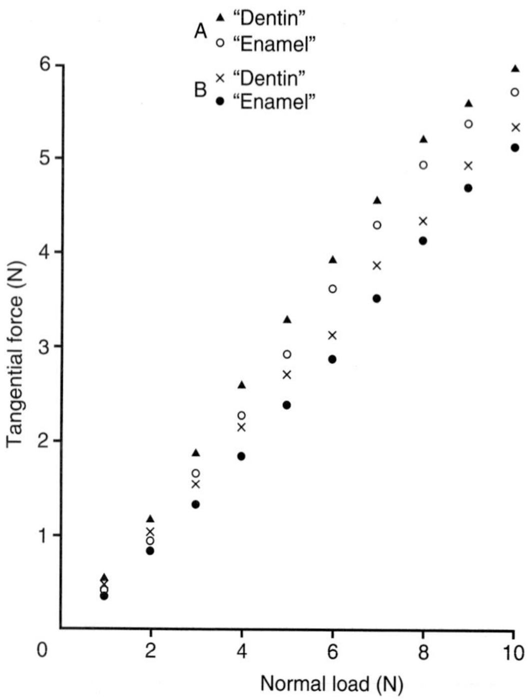

Fig. 21-16 Tangential force versus normal load for a diamond slider on "enamel" and "dentin" surfaces of two manufacturers' acrylic teeth (*A* and *B*) in water. (Adapted from Raptis CM, Powers JM, Fan PL: *J Dent Res* 60:908, 1981.)

1 mm of acrylic from the ridge lap area of the tooth.

Plastic teeth possess low heat-distortion temperatures, although the use of cross-linked plastics has improved this property considerably. Care should be taken not to flame plastic teeth during the preparation of a waxed denture. Porcelain teeth have high heat-distortion temperatures; however, sudden temperature changes may cause cracking or fracture. As indicated previously, plastic teeth exhibit cold flow, or permanent deformation, under stresses below their elastic limit, and their dimensions may be altered slightly during use. Plastic teeth are of a similar material to the denture base and may be chemically bonded to the base. The bond strength between chemically accelerated acrylics and plastic teeth is lower, and the use of mechanical retention on the underside of the teeth may prove useful. Highly cross-linked acrylic denture teeth may be treated with 4-methacryloxyethyl trimellitic anhydride to improve the bond strength to denture base resins. An adhesive containing this compound is also available for bonding acrylic to nickel-chromium and cobalt-chromium denture bases or partial dentures. This allows acrylic posterior palatal seals to be added to metal bases and metal base dentures to be relined, when necessary.

Porcelain teeth are usually fabricated with mechanical retention for bonding to the denture base. It has been shown that treating porcelain teeth with a silane coupling agent, such as γ-methacryloxypropyl-trimethoxy silane, provides a surface treatment that allows the teeth to be chemically bonded to the denture base material. When the bond was tested in tension, the porcelain ruptured rather than the bond. Because the use of cross-linked acrylic teeth has made the chemical bonding to the denture base more difficult, mechanical retention is often provided for plastic teeth. The chemical bond produced between plastic and porcelain teeth and the denture base has the distinct advantage of preventing capillary spaces around the teeth, which are difficult to clean and in which microorganisms may grow.

Both types of artificial teeth have a realistic appearance, but the noise or clicking of porcelain teeth against each other is about three times greater than plastic against porcelain or plastic against plastic. The processing of a single tooth replacement and the characterization of plastic teeth are considerably easier than for porcelain teeth. In addition, plastic teeth may be ground and polished with ease, whereas grinding of porcelain teeth removes the surface glaze, making repolishing more difficult. Porcelain teeth should not be used opposing natural teeth or gold restorations because excessive wear will occur.

The choice between plastic and porcelain teeth depends to a great extent on the preferences of the dentist and the patient. In the last few decades acrylic teeth have become much more popular than porcelain. Plastic teeth are used opposite natural teeth or gold restorations and in patients with poor ridge conditions or limited space. Porcelain teeth may be used for patients with good ridge support, adequate space, and those with both maxillary and mandibular dentures. There is no ANSI/ADA specification available for porcelain teeth, although one is available for plastic teeth.

ANSI/ADA SPECIFICATION NO. 15 (ISO 3336) FOR SYNTHETIC POLYMER TEETH

ANSI/ADA Specification No. 15 presents the desired properties for plastic teeth. Only an abstract of this specification is included here, because a large number of requirements are listed.

1. Dimensions of teeth: The dimensions shall be within 5% of those stated by the manufacturer.
2. Color and blend: Sets of anterior and posterior teeth, representing each shade from the same manufacturer, shall exhibit no perceptible color differences between each other and the manufacturer's shade guide.
3. Freedom from biologic hazard: Refer to ISO 10993-1, Biological Evaluation of Medical Devices.
4. Surface finish: No stain will occur in service.
5. Retention of finish: After processing and reprocessing, the teeth shall be capable of being polished to restore the original finish.
6. Repolishing: The teeth shall be capable of being ground and repolished to a finish equivalent to their original appearance.
7. Quality of bonding to denture-base polymers: The teeth shall be capable of being bonded to heat-polymerized denture-base materials.
8. Color stability: There shall be no perceptible color change in the exposed teeth.
9. Resistance to blanching, distortion and crazing: When tested as outlined, no tooth shall exhibit blanching or distortion.
10. Dimensional stability: When tested as outlined, the dimensional change of a tooth shall be within ±2% of its original mesial-distal dimension.

MAXILLOFACIAL MATERIALS

Maxillofacial materials are used to correct facial defects resulting from cancer surgery, accidents, or even congenital deformities. Noses, ears, eyes and orbits, or any other part of the head and neck may be replaced by these prostheses (Fig. 21-17).

Maxillofacial prostheses are difficult to fabricate and have a relatively short life of 6 months to several years in service. They fail as a result of inherent problems with static and dynamic properties over varying periods and because of color degradation. The prostheses are expensive to fabricate, and many patients cannot afford frequent replacement.

The several types of materials for maxillofacial prostheses vary considerably in ease of preparation and physical properties.

POLY(METHYL METHACRYLATE)

Poly(methyl methacrylate) was once commonly used for maxillofacial prostheses, and is still used occasionally to make artificial facial parts. When properly pigmented, these prostheses can look quite realistic. The main disadvantages are that the acrylic is hard and heavy, does not flex when the face moves, and does not have the feel of skin. Stone molds are generally used with poly(methyl methacrylate), and these are sacrificed when the prosthesis is deflasked after processing.

PLASTICIZED POLYVINYLCHLORIDE

Polyvinylchloride has been used widely for maxillofacial applications, but it has been replaced by newer materials with superior properties. Polyvinylchloride is a rigid plastic with a glass transition temperature higher than room temperature. For maxillofacial applications, plasticizers are added to produce an elastomer at room

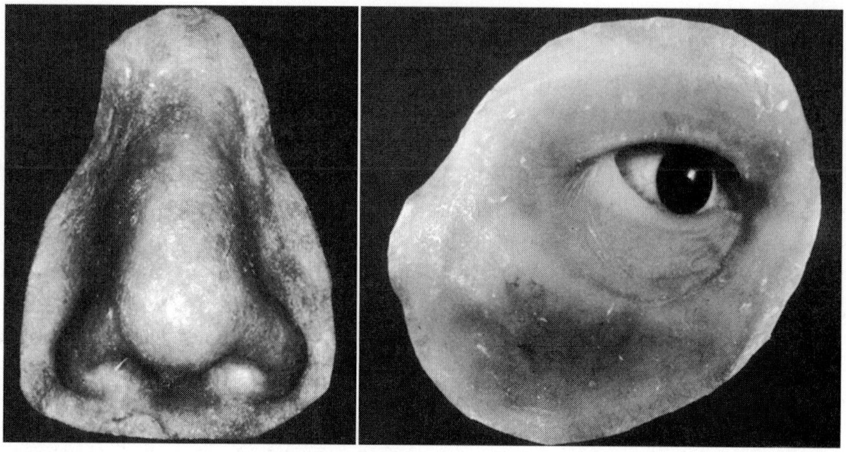

Fig. 21-17 Maxillofacial appliances. **A,** Nose. **B,** Eye and orbit.
(From Craig RG, editor: *Dental materials: a problem-oriented approach,* St Louis, 1978, Mosby.)

$$O=C=N-R-N=C=O \ + \ OH\text{\textasciitilde\textasciitilde\textasciitilde}OH \ \xrightarrow{\text{Initiator}}$$

Diisocyanate **Polyol**

$$O=C=N-R-\overset{\overset{\displaystyle H}{|}}{N}-\overset{\overset{\displaystyle O}{\|}}{C}-O\text{\textasciitilde\textasciitilde\textasciitilde}O-\overset{\overset{\displaystyle O}{\|}}{C}-\overset{\overset{\displaystyle H}{|}}{N}-R-\overset{\overset{\displaystyle H}{|}}{N}-\overset{\overset{\displaystyle O}{\|}}{C}-O-$$

Polyurethane

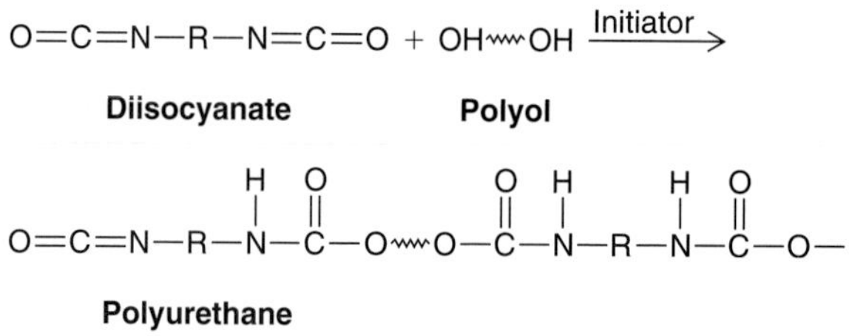

temperature. Other ingredients added to polyvinylchloride include cross-linking agents for added strength and ultraviolet stabilizers for color stability. There is no chemical reaction involved when the material is processed. The product is supplied as finely divided polyvinylchloride particles suspended in a solvent. When the fluid is heated above a critical temperature, the polyvinylchloride will dissolve in the solvent. When the mix is cooled, an elastic solid is formed. Plasticized polyvinylchloride is processed at 150° C, and metal molds are generally used.

POLYURETHANE

Polyurethanes are used as maxillofacial materials. The formation of polyurethane is the result of the direct addition of diisocyanate to a polyol in the presence of an initiator, as shown in the

equation above. Isophorone polyurethane has also been used as a maxillofacial material.

The reaction must be carried out in a dry atmosphere, or carbon dioxide will be produced and a porous elastomer will result. The diisocyanates are very toxic and must be handled with extreme care. The processing temperature of 100° C is reasonable, and stone molds can be used.

HEAT-VULCANIZED SILICONE

Heat-vulcanized silicones are used occasionally for maxillofacial prostheses. The vulcanization mechanism is achieved by an addition reaction. The components of heat-vulcanized silicones are a polydimethylvinyl siloxane copolymer with approximately 0.5% vinyl side chains, 2,4-dichlorobenzoyl peroxide as an initiator, and a silica filler obtained from burning methyl silanes (see below). Vulcanization results from thermal decomposition of the initiator to form free radicals that cross-link the copolymer into a three-dimensional structure. The processing temperature is 220° C, and metal molds are used. The copolymer is supplied as a rubbery solid with a high viscosity. The pigments are incorporated into the polymer with roller mills. Although this material is more difficult to pigment and process, excellent results can be obtained.

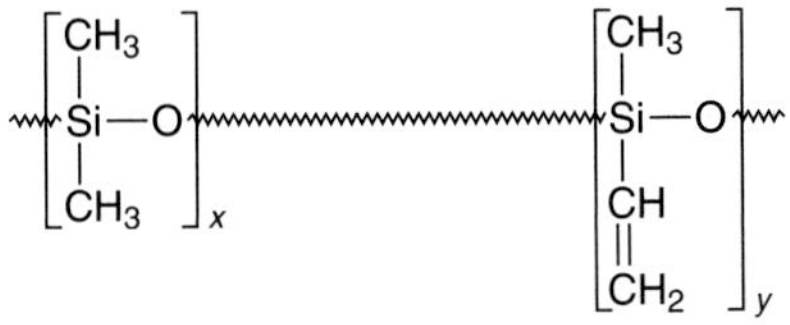

Polydimethylvinyl siloxane

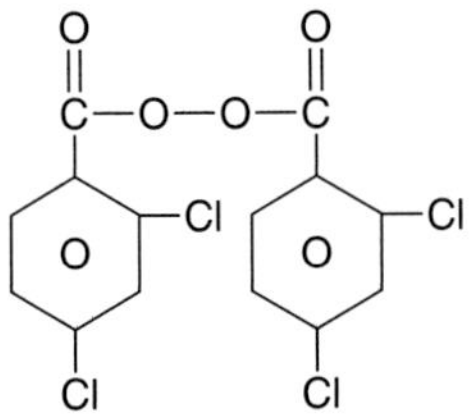

2,4-Dichlorobenzoyl peroxide

ROOM TEMPERATURE–VULCANIZED SILICONES

Because of their good physical properties and favorable processing characteristics, room temperature–vulcanized (RTV) silicones have become popular as maxillofacial materials, and are now used more often than any other material. They have good physical and mechanical properties, are easy to color and process, and allow the use of stone molds. There has been a steady improvement in the physical and mechanical properties of these materials. They are affected by accelerated aging, but not to a degree that compromises their usefulness as maxillofacial materials. These RTV silicones are similar to addition silicone impression materials in that they consist of vinyl- and hydride-containing siloxanes and are polymerized with a chloroplatinic acid catalyst.

OTHER ELASTOMERS

Several elastomers have been investigated for use as maxillofacial materials: aliphatic polyurethanes, chlorinated polyethylene, silphenylene polymers, organophosphazenes, butadiene-styrene, butadiene-acrylonitrile, and silicone-PMMA (polymethyl methacrylate) block copolymers.

FABRICATION OF THE PROSTHESES

The method for fabricating a prosthesis is similar for most materials. An impression is made of the affected area with alginate. A master cast is poured, duplicating the defect on the patient. The artificial part (such as a nose) is then carved in wax or clay on the master cast and tried on the patient to see if it fulfills the esthetic requirements for form.

The pattern is then invested in a manner similar to that used for complete dentures. Denture flasks are often used for this purpose. When the prosthesis is quite complex (such as an eye and orbit), three- or four-part molds are made. With some materials, metal molds are required because of high processing temperatures. After the pattern is invested, it is removed from the mold by use of a boiling water bath.

The mold is now ready to make the prosthesis. The patient should be present so pigments may be added to the elastomer to give a realistic appearance and match the patient's skin color. Generally, dry mineral earth pigments or artist's oil-based pigments are used. Color matching is done by mixing small amounts of the pigments into the elastomer. Some clinicians use color tabs and predetermined pigment formulations to match skin color. When a color match is achieved, the elastomer is compression molded and processed according to the manufacturer's instructions.

After processing, the prosthesis is removed from the mold and the excess flash is removed.

The prosthesis is then delivered to the patient. Surface pigmentation is generally done to give the prosthesis a more lifelike appearance. Medical grade silicone adhesives are often used to carry and bond surface colorants to the prosthesis. When mechanical undercuts are not present for retention, the patient may use adhesives to keep the prosthesis in place.

PHYSICAL PROPERTIES

The static and dynamic properties of the more popular maxillofacial materials are shown in Table 21-17. Values are representative of commercial products in each category. Heat-vulcanized silicone has the highest tensile strength at 5.87 MPa, and polyurethane the lowest at 0.83 MPa. The remaining materials have tensile strengths about 30% lower than the heat-vulcanized material. Tensile strength is important, because when the patient removes the prosthesis, high tensile forces are applied, particularly in thin areas.

Three of the materials are similar in maximum percent elongation with values from 422% to 445%. Plasticized polyvinylchloride has a lower percent elongation at 215%. Knowing the percent elongation is helpful, because different parts of the face have different requirements in terms of how far the elastomer must stretch to accommodate facial movement.

Tear resistance is important for maxillofacial materials because prostheses may be torn when patients remove them. In the *pants tear test,* a thin sheet of the elastomer is made in the shape of a pair of pants. The legs of the pants are then pulled slowly apart and the energy required to propagate a tear is measured. Heat-vulcanized silicone and RTV silicone have excellent tear resistance, because the samples do not tear but stretch, as in tensile elongation. Plasticized polyvinylchloride and polyurethane have good tear resistance at 4.3×10^6 and 6.7×10^6 dynes/cm, respectively.

The evaluation of maxillofacial materials should involve not only the static but also the dynamic physical properties, because the stress-strain curves for elastomers are nonlinear. Because of the nonlinearity of the stress-strain properties of these materials, they function differently at high and low rates of loading. The dynamic modulus is the ratio of stress to strain applied for small cyclic deformations at a given frequency at a specified point on the normal stress-strain curve, or it is the slope of the stress-strain curve at a given point corresponding to a given frequency.

In practical terms, elastomers with a high dy-

TABLE 21-17 Static and Dynamic Properties of Maxillofacial Materials

Material	Ultimate Tensile Strength (MPa)	Maximum Elongation (%)	Pants Tear Energy (dynes/cm × 10^6)	Dynamic Modulus (MPa)
Plasticized polyvinylchloride	3.99	215	4.3	4.32
Polyurethane	0.83	422	6.7	3.46
Heat-vulcanized silicone	5.87	441	Does not tear but stretches, as in tensile elongation	4.66
RTV silicone	4.20	445	Does not tear but stretches, as in tensile elongation	2.12

namic modulus are rather rigid materials, whereas materials with a low dynamic modulus are more flexible. In Table 21-17, the heat-vulcanized silicone has the highest dynamic modulus at 4.66 MPa, and the RTV silicone has the lowest at 2.12 MPa.

During the last few years there have been many significant studies on the physical properties of unpigmented and pigmented maxillofacial elastomers as a function of accelerated aging. New elastomers are also being evaluated for maxillofacial applications. It is gratifying to see renewed interest in an area of biomaterials that is often overlooked.

Efforts have been made to modify the stress-strain properties of maxillofacial materials to match living facial tissues. Medical-grade silicone adhesive has been combined with an RTV silicone base in various ratios to control the elastic properties. The stress-strain profiles of human facial tissues and various ratios of the silicone elastomers are shown in Fig. 21-18. The curves demonstrate that it is possible to formulate silicones that will match the elastic properties of facial tissues.

Major advances have been made in the last few years in the area of maxillofacial materials. New materials have made it possible to make lifelike maxillofacial prostheses that last longer in service.

PLASTIC FACINGS FOR CROWN AND BRIDGE APPLICATIONS

Before the introduction of porcelain-fused-to-metal crowns, acrylic facings were the only type of crown facing available. Porcelain facings have now replaced acrylic in all but a few applications. When used for facings, acrylic materials are similar in composition and properties to the best available denture teeth.

TEMPORARY CROWN AND BRIDGE RESTORATIONS

Chemically accelerated plastics have become popular as temporary restorations. They have decreased the use of aluminum shell and polycarbonate temporary crowns, because they are easy to fabricate and are esthetic. They are similar to chemically accelerated denture base plastics and are available in several shades to approxi-

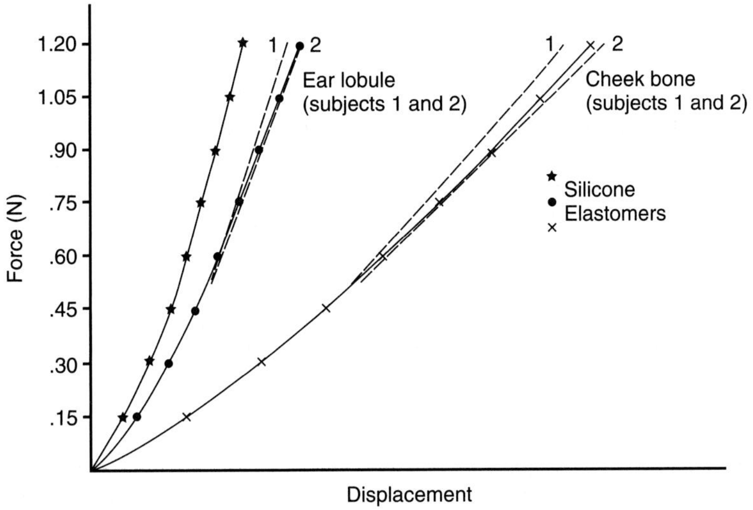

Fig. 21-18 Stress-strain properties of human facial tissues and various silicone elastomers. (Adapted from Farah JW, Robinson JC, Hood JAA, Koran A, Craig RG: *J Oral Rehabil* 15:277, 1988.)

mate the color of the patient's teeth. In one widely accepted technique, a thin polystyrene sheet is heated and then vacuum-formed over a wet gypsum model of the patient's teeth taken before tooth preparation. The thin template is then trimmed to include the teeth to be prepared and teeth on either side. In the case of a bridge, a denture tooth can be waxed to the model before vacuum forming, and this allows space in the template for the pontic of the temporary bridge. After the teeth are prepared for crowns and the final impression has been made, the thin polystyrene template is used to make the temporary restoration. The tooth preparations are lubricated, and the chemically accelerated plastic powder and liquid are mixed and placed into the template in the area of the restorations. Chemically activated temporary resins are now also available in automixing syringes and can be directly injected into the matrix. When the acrylic approaches the doughy stage, the template and acrylic are placed over the prepared teeth and seated. The patient is then asked to bring the teeth into occlusion. The temporary restoration may be removed and cooled in water several times during polymerization to control the heat and then reinserted into the mouth. When the restoration is still slightly elastic, it is removed from the mouth and allowed to continue polymerization at room temperature. The restoration is then trimmed, polished, and cemented to the prepared teeth with a temporary cement. The resulting restoration simulates the teeth as they were before preparation and has acceptable esthetics. Generally only minimal occlusal adjustment is required because the teeth are in contact during polymerization. The accuracy of various products should be considered when selecting a material. Marginal opening can be caused by polymerization shrinkage. There are reports in the dental literature of some allergic reactions to the temporary crown and bridge plastics; these reactions are believed caused by monomer or the amine accelerator. Heat generation from polymerization can also be harmful to the teeth. Using thermocouples and extracted teeth prepared for crowns, temperatures of 40° to 84° C have been recorded in the pulp chambers during polymerization. With external cooling of a restoration, the temperature rise is minimal. Silane-treated glass fibers have been used to significantly increase the flexural strength of a provisional resin. Further evaluation needs to be done to evaluate biocompatibility.

Light-activated polymers used to make temporary restorations are available in several tooth shades. The method is similar to that used for chemically activated acrylics, but has several advantages. The material can be removed from the mouth in the template, the flash can be removed before curing, and the restoration can be reinserted several times to ensure easy seating after processing. The final polymerization is done in a light chamber identical to that used for processing light-activated denture bases. The light-activated material allows fast and accurate fabrication of temporary restorations, and has the added advantage of no methyl methacrylate monomer in the formulation, thus reducing the potential for allergic reactions.

Light-activated and chemically activated composites are also gaining popularity for use as temporary restorations. A review of these materials is found in Chapter 9.

OCCLUSAL SPLINTS

The use of occlusal splints in the treatment of patients with temporomandibular joint pain or excessive bruxism has become a routine procedure. These splints are made by the same technique used for dentures. The splint is waxed on a model of the patient's teeth, usually the maxilla. The model and wax pattern are invested in a denture flask, and the wax is boiled out. After cooling, alginate separator is painted onto the mold and allowed to dry. A clear, heat-accelerated acrylic resin is packed into the mold and processed. The acrylic resin is mixed and packed when it has reached the doughy stage. Chemically accelerated acrylic resin is also used, but less often. The properties of acrylic splints are similar to those of heat-accelerated denture materials. Recently, a clear light-activated acrylic has been introduced that simplifies the construction of occlusal splints. A major advantage is that the splint can be made quickly and without flasking.

INLAY PATTERNS

Chemically accelerated acrylic is used to fabricate inlay patterns and direct posts and cores. Commercial products are brightly pigmented, have good dimensional stability, and are convenient to use. The pattern is made by painting the powder-liquid onto the die or tooth in layers and allowing it to polymerize. After polymerization, the pattern can be modified with stones and burs. If necessary, inlay wax may be added to complete the pattern. Considerably longer burnout times must be used with acrylic patterns.

IMPRESSION TRAYS AND RECORD BASES

Chemically accelerated acrylic is commonly used to produce custom impression trays. These trays provide a nearly constant distance between the tray and the tissues, allowing a more even distribution of the impression material during the impression procedure, and improved accuracy. The same material may also be used to make record bases for prosthetic applications. The principal difference in the composition of the plastics for this purpose is the addition of substantial quantities of fillers, which decrease warpage of the material during setting. Shrinkage of chemically accelerated acrylic trays can occur for up to 7 days, although the greatest shrinkage takes place during the first 24 hours. The dimensional changes of five commercially available tray materials are shown in Fig. 21-19. Significant shrinkage occurs after the initial polymerization. The products differ considerably in the length of time required to reach 90% of the total dimensional change. Although the maximum shrinkage is less than 0.4%, chemically accelerated acrylic impression trays should be allowed to stand from 2 to 9 hours, depending on the product, if dimensional changes are to be minimized. In practice, many dentists have a dental laboratory fabricate the impression trays, and the time between fabrication and use will be adequate. If trays are to be used soon after fabrication, the tray should

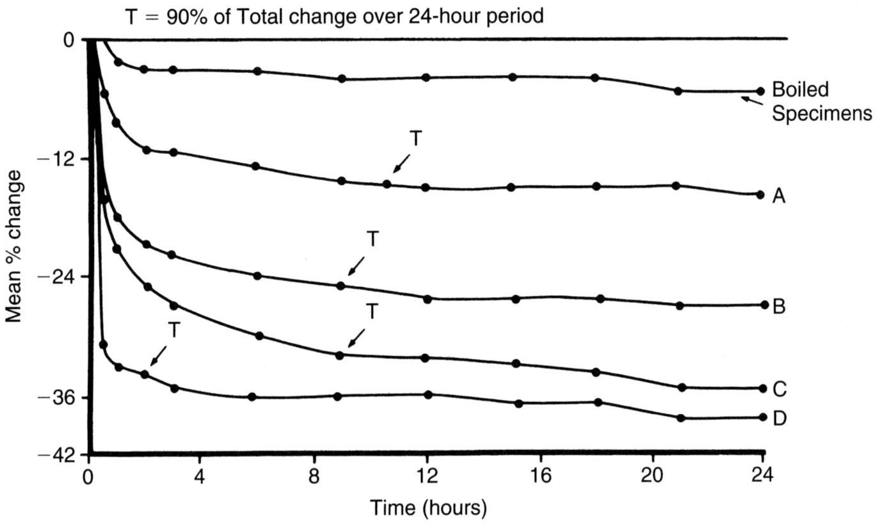

Fig. 21-19 Dimensional change of five tray materials over 24 hours.
(Adapted from Pagniano RP, Schied RC, Clowson RL, Dagefoerde RO, Zardiackas LD: *J Prosthet Dent* 47:280, 1982.)

be boiled for 5 minutes and then cooled to room temperature before use.

Vacuum-formed polystyrene is also used to make impression trays and baseplates. This material is popular with commercial laboratories because the trays and record bases can be made rapidly. These trays must be handled carefully because they are more flexible than acrylic trays and can be deformed easily by the application of heat. Prefabricated impression trays are very popular with dentists. These stock trays vary considerably between manufacturers. Stock trays are not as rigid as most custom trays and must be used with care to avoid distortion.

Light-activated tray materials have become quite popular and have many advantages over chemically accelerated acrylic. They are similar to light-activated denture base materials but are of a different color. The trays are strong, easy to make, contain no methyl methacrylate, and have negligible polymerization shrinkage in the light chamber. They can be used soon after processing because there is no clinically significant dimensional change after polymerization.

SELECTED PROBLEMS

Problem 1

A denture is to be made for a patient who has previously fractured a denture several times. How will this influence your choice of a denture base material?

Solution

A rubber-reinforced acrylic is the material of choice because this type of denture base material exhibits superior impact resistance and flexural fatigue strength. A metal base also might be used in cases where maximum strength is desired.

Problem 2

A denture is delivered from a dental laboratory with obvious porosity in the denture base. Why might this have occurred? Where is the porosity most likely to occur, and why?

Solution

Several conditions may have caused the porosity. Most commonly, the processing temperature exceeded 74° C. Other causes may be insufficient flask pressure, excessive monomer in the mix, and packing of the material before it reached the doughy consistency. Porosity almost always will occur in the thicker sections of acrylic because the polymerization reaction is exothermic and the heat cannot be dissipated as quickly from the larger mass.

Problem 3

A patient is having a maxillary denture made that opposes a natural dentition in the mandible. Should acrylic or porcelain teeth be used, and why?

Solution

Acrylic teeth should always be used when opposing natural teeth or restored teeth. Porcelain teeth are abrasive against these surfaces, and excessive wear will quickly occur.

Problem 4

A patient has a history of sensitivity to denture base materials. In making a new denture for this patient, what might decrease the potential for an allergic reaction?

Solution

Residual monomer is almost always the cause of an allergic or toxic reaction to a denture base material. To reduce the residual monomer content to a very low level, the denture should be boiled for at least 1 hour at the end of the processing cycle. Another option is to select a vinyl acrylic or a light-activated denture base material.

Problem 5

A new set of dentures is delivered to a patient, and there is no retention on the maxillary denture. At the trial-denture stage, there was good retention of the baseplate. What are the probable causes?

Solution

Assuming that a denture base material had passed the ANSI/ADA Specification test, the most probable causes are improper processing variables, such as processing too rapidly and at elevated temperatures during the early stages, deflasking before the flask has bench-cooled to near room temperature, quenching the hot flask in cold water, or overheating the denture during trimming and polishing. These processing variables can affect the accuracy of even the best denture base materials.

Problem 6

A finished denture is returned from the laboratory, and in several areas there is insufficient material in the interproximal areas. What is the probable cause?

Solution

The probable cause is packing the denture acrylic when it is not in the doughy consistency. Because of the lower viscosity, even with adequate packing pressure the material will squeeze out of the flask before it is forced into all areas of the mold cavity. Conversely, if the acrylic dough has reached the rubbery consistency, it may be too viscous to fill all areas of the mold.

Problem 7

A patient has fractured a lingual cusp and comes to the office for emergency care. You would like to prepare the tooth for a gold crown, and have your dental assistant make a custom tray for the final impression while you are preparing the tooth. In terms of the dimensional accuracy of the tray, what must be considered?

Solution

Autopolymerizing tray materials continue to change dimensionally during the first few hours after they are made. Use of a tray before this polymerization is complete can affect the accuracy of the impression. Two things can be done to eliminate this problem: (1) have the dental assistant boil the tray for a short time to force the polymerization reaction to completion, or (2) use a light-activated tray material that experiences no significant dimensional change after processing.

Problem 8

A patient has excessive wear on the anatomical areas of a denture caused by aggressive cleaning with an abrasive cleaner and a toothbrush. What instructions might you give the patient for cleaning the new denture that you will be making?

Solution

Use a soft toothbrush and soap and water (a nonabrasive hand soap) to regularly clean the denture. The patient may also soak the denture occasionally in a commercial cleanser or a solution of 1 tsp of a hypochlorite, such as Clorox, and 2 tsp of Calgon in half a glass of water. Some immersion cleansers have also been demonstrated effective as sanitizing agents.

Problem 9

A patient needs a soft denture liner for an extended period. (a) What material would you choose, and what would you tell the patient? (b) What problems are associated with these materials?

Solution a

Silicone and plasticized acrylics will both work, although silicones are generally softer with a lower Shore A hardness value. The patient should be told that any soft liner will have to be replaced occasionally because they are not as long-lasting as the denture base material.

Solution b

Growth of microorganisms, *Candida albicans* in particular; poor adhesion to the denture base; and poor tear strength are deficiencies normally associated with these materials.

Problem 10

A patient requires a maxillofacial prosthesis that includes an area of movable tissue near the mouth. How might a silicone maxillofacial material be modified to be more elastic in this instance?

Solution

Medical-grade silicone adhesive can be combined with an RTV silicone base at various ratios to control the elastic properties. By selecting the proper ratio, the stress-strain profiles of the silicone elastomer can be matched to that of human facial tissues. This is most important when the prosthesis rests on movable tissue.

BIBLIOGRAPHY

Denture Base Materials

Andreopoulos AG, Polyzois GL, Demetriou PP: Repairs with visible light-curing denture base materials, *Quint Int* 22:703, 1991.

Arab J, Newton JP, Lloyd CH: The effect of an elevated level of residual monomer on the whitening of a denture base and its physical properties, *J Dent* 17:189, 1989.

Arima T, Murata H, Hamada T: The effects of cross-linking agents on the water sorption and solubility characteristics of denture base resin, *J Oral Rehabil* 23:476, 1996.

Barclay SC, Forsyth A, Felix DH et al: Case report—hypersensitivity to denture materials, *Br Dent J* 187:350, 1999.

Benzina A, Kruft MB, van der Veen FH et al: A versatile three-iodine molecular building block leading to new radiopaque polymeric biomaterials, *J Biomed Mater Res* 32:459, 1996.

Berg E, Gjerdet NR: The effects of pressure and curing temperature on porosity of two chemically activated acrylics, *Dent Mater* 1:204, 1985.

Blanchet LJ, Bowman DC, McReynolds HD: Effects of methyl methacrylate monomer vapors on respiration and circulation in unanesthetized rats, *J Prosthet Dent* 48:344, 1982.

Chandler HH, Bowen RL, Paffenbarger GC: Physical properties of a radiopaque denture base material, *J Biomed Mater Res* 5:335, 1971.

Clark RL: Dynamic mechanical thermal analysis of dental polymers. I. Heat cured poly-(methyl methacrylate)-based materials, *Biomater* 10:494, 1989.

Craig RG: Denture materials and acrylic base materials, *Curr Opin Dent* 1:235, 1991.

Dar-Odeh NS, Harrison A, Abu-Hammad O: An evaluation of self-cured and visible light-cured denture base materials when used as a denture base repair material, *J Oral Rehabil* 24:755, 1997.

Davy KW, Anseau MR, Berry C: Iodinated methacrylate copolymers as X-ray opaque denture base acrylics, *J Dent* 25: 499, 1997.

Donovan TE, Hurst RG, Campagni WV: Physical properties of acrylic resin polymerized by four different techniques, *J Prosthet Dent* 54:522, 1985.

Ellsworth K: Fatigue failure in denture base polymers, *J Prosthet Dent* 21:257, 1969.

Firtell DN, Harman LC: Porosity in boilable acrylic resin, *J Prosthet Dent* 49:133, 1983.

Fletcher AM, Purnaveja S, Amin WM et al: The level of residual monomer in self-curing denture-base materials, *J Dent Res* 62:118, 1983.

Grant AA, Atkinson HF: Comparison between dimensional accuracy of dentures produced with pour-type resin and with heat-processed materials, *J Prosthet Dent* 26:296, 1971.

Hargreaves AS: Equilibrium water uptake and denture base resin behavior, *J Dent* 6:342, 1978.

Hargreaves AS: The effects of cyclic stress on dental polymethylmethacrylate, *J Oral Rehabil* 10:137, 1983.

Harrison WM, Stansbury BE: The effect of joint surface contours on the transverse strength of repaired acrylic resin, *J Prosthet Dent* 23:464, 1970.

Heath JR, Davenport JC, Jones PA: The abrasion of acrylic resin by cleaning pastes, *J Oral Rehabil* 10:159, 1983.

Hill RG: The crosslinking agent ethylene glycol dimethacrylate content of the currently available denture base resins, *J Dent Res* 60:725, 1981.

Hill RG, Bates JF, Lewis TT et al: Fracture toughness of acrylic denture base, *Biomater* 4:112, 1983.

Huggett R, Brooks SC, Bates JF: The effect of different curing cycles on the dimensional accuracy of acrylic resin denture base materials, *Quint Dent Technol* 8:81, 1984.

Jagger RG, Huggett R: The effect of crosslinking on sorption properties of a denture base material, *Dent Mater* 6:276, 1990.

Jagger DC, Harrison A, Jandt KD: The reinforcement of dentures, *J Oral Rehabil* 26: 185, 1999.

Kalachandra S, Turner DT: Water sorption of poly(methyl methacrylate). III. Effects of plasticizers, *Polymer* 28:1749, 1987.

Kalachandra S, Turner DT: Water sorption of plasticized denture acrylic lining materials, *Dent Mater* 5:161, 1989.

Khan Z, von-Fraunhofer JA, Razavi R: The staining characteristics, transverse strength, and microhardness of a visible light-cured denture base material, *J Prosthet Dent* 57:384, 1987.

Koda T, Tsuchiya H, Yamauchi M et al: High-performance liquid chromatographic estimation of eluates from denture base polymers, *J Dent* 17:84, 1989.

Lamb DJ, Ellis B, Priestly D: The effects of processing variables on levels of residual monomer in autopolymerizing dental acrylic resin, *J Dent* 11:80, 1983.

Latta GH Jr, Bowles WF, Conkin JE: Three-dimensional stability of new denture base resin systems, *J Prosthet Dent* 63:654, 1990.

Lorton L, Phillips RW: Heat-released stress in acrylic dentures, *J Prosthet Dent* 42:23, 1979.

Ma T, Johnson GH, Gordon GE: Effects of chemical disinfectants on the surface characteristics and color of denture resins, *J Prosthet Dent* 77:197, 1997.

May KB, Van Putten MC, Bow DA et al: 4-META polymethyl methacrylate shear bond strength to titanium, *Oper Dent* 22:37, 1997.

Messersmith PB, Obrez A, Lindberg S: New acrylic resin composite with improved thermal diffusivity, *J Prosthet Dent* 79:278, 1998.

Mutlu G, Huggett R, Harrison A et al: Rheology of acrylic denture base polymers, *Dent Mater* 6:288, 1990.

NaBadalung DP, Powers JM, Connelly ME: Comparison of bond strengths of three denture base resins to treated nickel-chromium-beryllium alloy, *J Prosthet Dent* 80:354, 1998.

Nogueira SS, Ogle RE, Davis EL: Comparison of accuracy between compression- and injection-molded complete dentures, *J Prosthet Dent* 82:291, 1999.

Ohkubo C, Watanabe I, Hosoi T et al: Shear bond strengths of polymethyl methacrylate to cast titanium and cobalt-chromium frameworks using five metal primers, *J Prosthet Dent* 83:50, 2000.

Oysaed H, Ruyter IE: Creep studies of multiphase acrylic systems, *J Biomed Mater Res* 23:719, 1989.

Phoenix RD: Introduction of a denture injection system for use with microwaveable acrylic resins, *J Prosthodont* 6:286, 1997.

Polyzois GL, Karkazis HC, Zissis AJ: Dimensional stability of dentures processed in boilable acrylic resins: a comparative study, *J Prosthet Dent* 57:639, 1987.

Powers JM, Koran A: Color of denture resins, *J Dent Res* 56:754, 1977.

Price CA, Earnshaw R: Impact testing of a polysulphone denture base polymer, *Aust Dent J* 29:398, 1984.

Rawls HR, Granier RJ, Smid J et al: Thermomechanical investigation of poly(methylmethacryate) containing an organobismuth radiopacifying additive, *J Biomed Mater Res* 31:339, 1996.

Rawls HR, Starr J, Kasten FH et al: I. Radiopaque acrylic resins containing miscible heavy-metal compounds, *Dent Mater* 6:250, 1990.

Robinson JG, McCabe JF: Impact strength of acrylic resin denture base materials with surface defects, *Dent Mater* 9:355, 1993.

Rodford RA: Further development and evaluation of high-impact-strength denture base materials, *J Dent* 18:151, 1990.

Ruyter IE, Espevik S: Compressive creep of denture base polymers, *Acta Odont Scand* 38:169, 1980.

Ruyter IE, Svendsen SA: Flexural properties of denture base polymers, *J Prosthet Dent* 43:95, 1980.

Smith LT, Powers JM: Relative fit of new denture resins polymerized by heat, light and microwave energy, *Am J Dent* 5:140, 1992.

Smith LT, Powers JM, Ladd D: Mechanical properties of new denture resins polymerized by visible light, heat and microwave energy, *Int J Prosthodont* 5:315, 1992.

Soni PM, Powers JM, Craig RG: Physical and mechanical properties of acrylic and modified acrylic denture resins, *Mich Dent Assoc J* 59:418, 1977.

Stafford GD, Huggett R, Causton BE: Fracture toughness of denture base acrylics, *J Biomed Mater Res* 14:359, 1980.

Strohaver RA: Comparison of changes in vertical dimension between compression and injection molded complete dentures, *J Prosthet Dent* 62:716, 1989.

Sykora O, Sutow EJ: Posterior palatal seal adaptation: influence of a high expansion stone, *J Oral Rehabil* 23:342, 1996.

Teraoka F, Takahashi J: Controlled polymerization system for fabricating precise dentures, *J Prosthet Dent* 83:514, 2000.

Vallittu PK: A review of fiber-reinforced denture base resins, *J Prosthodont* 5:270, 1996.

Vallittu PK: Some aspects of the tensile strength of unidirectional glass fibre-polymethyl methacrylate composite used in dentures, *J Oral Rehabil* 25:100, 1998.

Vermilyea SG, Powers JM, Koran A: The rheological properties of fluid denture base resins, *J Dent Res* 57:227, 1978.

Wang X, Powers JM, Connelly ME: Color stability of heat activated and chemically activated fluid resin acrylics, *J Prosthodont* 5:266, 1996.

Wollff EM: The effect of cross-linking agents on acrylic resins, *Aust Dent J* 7:439, 1962.

Denture Liners

Amin WM, Fletcher AM, Ritchie GM: The nature of the interface between polymethylmethacrylate denture base materials and soft lining materials, *J Dent* 9:336, 1981.

Braden M: Tissue conditioners. I. Composition and structure, *J Dent Res* 49:145, 1970.

Braden M: Tissue conditioners. II. Rheologic properties, *J Dent Res* 49:496, 1970.

Braden M, Wright PS: Water sorption and water solubility of soft lining materials for acrylic dentures, *J Dent Res* 62:764, 1983.

Dootz ER, Koran A, Craig RG: Comparison of the physical properties of eleven soft dental liners, *J Prosthet Dent* 67:707, 1992.

Duran RL, Powers JM, Craig RG: Viscoelastic and dynamic properties of soft liners and tissue conditioners, *J Dent Res* 58:1801, 1979.

El-Hadary A, Drummond JL: Comparative study of water sorption, solubility, and tensile bond strength of two soft lining materials, *J Prosthet Dent* 83:356, 2000.

Graham BS, Jones DW, Sutow EJ: An in vivo and in vitro study of the loss of plasticizer from soft polymer-gel materials, *J Dent Res* 70:870, 1991.

Graham BS, Jones DW, Sutow EJ: Clinical implications of resilient denture lining material research. II. Gelation and flow properties of tissue conditioners, *J Prosthet Dent* 65:413 1991.

Harsanyi BB, Foong WC, Howell RE et al: Hamster cheek-pouch testing of dental soft polymers, *J Dent Res* 70:991, 1991.

Hayakawa I, Hirano S, Kobayashi S et al: The creep behavior of denture-supporting tissues and soft lining materials, *Int J Prosthodont* 7:339, 1994.

Iwanaga H, Murakami S, Murata H et al: Factors influencing gelation time of tissue conditioners, *J Oral Rehabil* 22:225, 1995.

Jones DW, Sutow EJ, Hall GC et al: Dental soft polymers: plasticizer composition and leachability, *Dent Mater* 4:1, 1988.

Kawano F, Dootz ER, Koran A et al: Bond strength of soft denture liners to denture base resin, *J Prosthet Dent* 68:368, 1992.

Kawano F, Dootz ER, Koran A et al: Sorption and solubility of 12 soft denture liners, *J Prosthet Dent* 72:393, 1994.

Kawano F, Dootz ER, Koran A et al: Bond strength of six soft denture liners processed against polymerized and unpolymerized poly(methyl methacrylate), *Int J Prosthodont* 10:178, 1997.

Kawano F, Ohguri T, Koran A et al: Influence of lining design of three processed soft denture liners on cushioning effect, *J Oral Rehabil* 26:962, 1999.

McCabe JF: A polyvinylsiloxane denture soft lining material, *J Dent* 26:521, 1998.

Murata H, Shigeto N, Hamada T: Viscoelastic properties of tissue conditioners: stress relaxation test Maxwell model analogy, *J Oral Rehabil* 17:365, 1990.

Murata H, Hamada T, Taguchi N et al: Viscoelastic properties of tissue conditioners—influence of molecular weight of polymer powders and powder/liquid ratio and the clinical implications, *J Oral Rehabil* 25:621, 1998.

Murata H, Taguchi N, Hamada T et al: Dynamic viscoelastic properties and the age changes of long-term soft denture liners, *Biomater* 21:1422, 2000.

Nikawa H, Jin C, Hamada T, Murata H: Interactions between thermal cycled resilient denture lining materials, salivary and serum pellicles and Candida albicans *in vitro.* Part I. Effects on fungal growth, *J Oral Rehabil* 27:41, 2000.

Nikawa H, Yamamoto T, Hamada T: Effect of components of resilient denture-lining materials on the growth, acid production and colonization of Candida albicans, *J Oral Rehabil* 22:817, 1995.

Razavi R, Kahn Z, von Fraunhoffer JA: The bond strength of a visible light-cured reline resin to acrylic resin denture base material, *J Prosthet Dent* 63:485, 1990.

Shotwell JL, Razzoog ME, Koran A: Color stability of long-term soft denture liners, *J Prosthet Dent* 68:836, 1992.

Wright PS: Characterization of the rupture properties of denture soft lining materials, *J Dent Res* 59:614, 1980.

Wright PS: The effect of soft lining materials on the growth of *Candida albicans, J Dent* 8:144, 1980.

Wright PS: Composition and properties of soft lining materials for acrylic dentures, *J Dent* 9:210, 1981.

Denture Teeth

Cunningham JL, Benington IC: An investigation of the variables which may affect the bond between plastic teeth and denture base resin, *J Dent* 27:129, 1999.

Ekfeldt WA, Ivanhoe JR, Adrian ED: Wear mechanism of resin and porcelain denture teeth, *Acta Odont Scand* 47:391, 1989.

Huggett R, John G, Jagger RG et al: Strength of the acrylic denture base tooth bond, *Br Dent J* 153:187, 1982.

Koran A, Craig RG, Tillitson EW: Coefficient of friction of prosthetic tooth materials, *J Prosthet Dent* 27:269, 1972.

Ogle RE, Davis EL: Clinical wear study of three commercially available artificial tooth materials: Thirty month results, *J Prosthet Dent* 79:145, 1998.

Raptis CM, Powers JM, Fan PL: Frictional behavior and surface failure of acrylic denture teeth, *J Dent Res* 60:908, 1981.

Suzuki S, Sakoh M, Shiba A: Adhesive bonding of denture base to plastic denture teeth, *J Biomed Mater Res* 24:1094, 1990.

Maxillofacial Materials

Chalian VA, Drane JB, Standish SM: *Maxillofacial prosthetics,* Baltimore, 1971, Williams & Wilkins.

Craig RG, Koran A, Yu R: Color stability of elastomers for maxillofacial appliances, *J Dent Res* 57:866, 1978.

Craig RG, Koran A, Yu R: Elastomers for maxillofacial applications, *Biomater* 1:112, 1980.

Dootz ER, Koran A, Craig RG: Physical properties of three maxillofacial materials as a function of accelerated aging, *J Prosthet Dent* 71:379, 1994.

Haug SP, Moore BK, Andres CJ: Color stability and colorant effect on maxillofacial elastomers. Part II: weathering effect on physical properties, *J Prosthet Dent* 81:423, 1999.

Hulterstrom AK, Ruyter IE: Changes in appearance of silicone elastomers for maxillofacial prostheses as a result of aging, *Int J Prosthodont* 12:498, 1999.

Koran A, Craig RG: Dynamic properties of maxillofacial prostheses, *J Dent Res* 54:1216, 1975.

Kouyoumdjian J, Chalian VA, Moore BK: A comparison of the physical properties of a room temperature vulcanizing silicone modified and unmodified, *J Prosthet Dent* 53:388, 1985.

Lai JH, Hodges JS: Effects of processing parameters on physical properties of the silicone maxillofacial prosthetic materials, *Dent Mater* 15:450, 1999.

Parker S, Braden M: Soft prosthesis materials based on powdered elastomers, *Biomater* 11:482, 1990.

Polyzois GL: Color stability of facial silicone prosthetic polymers after outdoor weathering, *J Prosthet Dent* 82:447, 1999.

Polyzois GL: Mechanical properties of 2 new addition-vulcanizing silicone prosthetic elastomers, *Int J Prosthodont* 12:359, 1999.

Turner GE, Fisher TE, Castleberry DJ et al: Intrinsic color of isophorone polyurethane for maxillofacial prosthetics, *J Prosthet Dent* 51:673, 1984.

Temporary Fixed Partial Denture Materials

Chung K, Lin T, Wang F: Flexural strength of a provisional resin material with fibre addition, *J Oral Rehabil* 25:214, 1998.

Grajower R, Shaharbani S, Kaufman E: Temperature rise in pulp chamber during fabrication of temporary self-curing resin crowns, *J Prosthet Dent* 41:535, 1979.

Ireland, MF, Dixon DL, Breeding LC et al: In vitro mechanical property comparison of four resins used for fabrication of provisional fixed restorations, *J Prosthet Dent* 80:158, 1998.

Lepe X, Bales DJ, Johnson GH: Retention of provisional crowns fabricated from two materials with the use of four temporary cements, *J Prosthet Dent* 81:469, 1999.

Lui JL: Hypersensitivity to a temporary crown and bridge material, *J Dent* 7:22, 1979.

Robinson FB, Hovijitra S: Marginal fit of direct temporary crowns, *J Prosthet Dent* 47:390, 1982.

Tray Materials

Carrotte PV, Johnson A, Winstanley RB: The influence of the impression tray on the accuracy of impressions for crown and bridge work—an investigation and review, *Br Dent J* 185:580, 1998.

Goldfogel M, Harvey WL, Winter D: Dimensional change of acrylic resin tray materials, *J Prosthet Dent* 54:284, 1985.

Martinez LJ, von Fraunhofer JA: The effects of custom try material on the accuracy of master casts, *J Prosthodont* 7:106, 1998.

Millstein P, Maya A, Segura C. Determining the accuracy of stock and custom tray impression/casts, *J Oral Rehabil* 25:645, 1998.

Pagniano RP, Scheid RC, Clowson RL et al: Linear dimensional change of acrylic resins used in the fabrication of custom trays, *J Prosthet Dent* 47:279, 1982.

APPENDIX

Table of Weights and Measures

LENGTHS

1 millimeter (mm)	= 0.001 meter	= 0.03937 inch
1 centimeter (cm)	= 0.01 meter	= 0.3937 inch
1 meter (m)		= 39.37 inches
1 yard (yd)	= 0.9144 meter	= 36 inches
1 inch (in)	= 2.54 centimeters	= 25.4 millimeters
1 micrometer (μm)	= 0.001 millimeter	= 0.00003937 inch
1 micrometer (μm)	= 10,000 Angstrom units	
1 Angstrom unit (Å)	= 0.1 nanometer	= 3.937×10^{-9} inch
1 nanometer (nm)	= 0.001 micrometer	= 10 Angstrom units

WEIGHTS

1 milligram (mg)	= 0.001 gram	= 0.015 grain	
1 gram (g)	= 0.0022 pound	= 15.432 grains	
1 gram (g)	= 0.035 ounce		
1 kilogram (kg)	= 1000 grams	= 2.2046 pounds	
1 ounce (oz)	= 28.35 grams		
1 pound (lb)	= 453.59 grams	= 16 ounces	
1 pennyweight (dwt) (troy)	= 1.555 grams	= 24 grains	
1 grain (gr)	= 0.0648 gram		
1 Newton (N)	= 0.2248 pound	= 0.102 kilogram	= 100,000 dynes
1 dyne (d)	= 0.00102 gram		

CAPACITY (LIQUID)

1 milliliter (ml)	= 1 cubic centimeter	= 0.0021 pint
1 liter (l)	= 1000 cubic centimeters	= 1.057 quarts
1 quart (qt)	= 0.946 liter	= 32 ounces
1 ounce (oz)	= 29.6 milliliters	
1 cubic foot (cu ft)	= 28.32 liters	

AREA

sq in (in²)	*sq ft (ft²)*	*sq mm (mm²)*	*sq cm (cm²)*
1	0.00694	645.16	6.4516
144	1	92,903	929.03
0.00155	0.000011	1	0.01
0.155	0.0011	100	1

VOLUME

cu in (in³)	*cu mm (mm³)*	*cc (cm³)*
1	16,387	16.387
0.0000610	1	0.001
0.0610	1000	1

Note: 1 ml (or cc) of distilled water at 4° C weighs 1 g

Conversion Tables

CONVERSION FACTORS (LINEAR)

	mm	*cm*	*in*
1 Angstrom unit (Å)	0.0000001	0.00000001	0.000000003937
1 nanometer (nm)	0.000001	0.0000001	0.00000003937
1 micrometer (μm)	0.001	0.0001	0.00003937

CONVERSION FACTORS (FORCE PER AREA)

To change kilograms per square centimeter (kg/cm^2) to pounds per square inch (lb/in^2), multiply by 14.223 ($1\ kg/cm^2 = 14.223\ lb/in^2$).

To change kilograms per square centimeter (kg/cm^2) to megapascals (MPa), multiply by 0.0981 ($1\ kg/cm^2 = 0.0981$ MPa). Note $1\ MN/m^2 = 1$ MPa.

To change kilograms per square millimeters (kg/mm^2) to gigapascals (GPa) multiply by 0.00981.

To change pounds per square inch (lb/in^2) to megapascals (MPa) multiply by 0.00689.

To change meganewtons per square meter (MN/m^2) to pounds per square inch (lb/in^2), multiply by 145 ($1\ MN/m^2 = 145\ lb/m^2$).

To change meganewtons per square meter (MN/m^2) to gigapascals (GPa), divide by 1000.

CONVERSION OF THERMOMETER SCALES

Temperature Fahrenheit (° F) = 9/5 Temperature Celsius + 32°

Temperature Celsius (° C) = 5/9 Temperature Fahrenheit − 32°

or

$(°\ C \times 1.8) + 32 = °\ F$

$$\frac{°\ F - 32°}{1.8} = °\ C$$

CONVERSION FACTORS (MISCELLANEOUS)

1 foot-pound (ft-lb) = 13,826 gram-centimeters = 1.356 Newton-meters

1 radian = 57.3 degrees

1 watt = 14.3 calories/minute

CONVERSION OF EXPONENTIALS TO DECIMALS

Exponential no.	*Decimal no.*	*Exponential no.*	*Decimal no.*
1×10^{-5} (or 10^{-5})	0.00001	1×10^{1}	10
1×10^{-3}	0.001	1×10^{4}	10,000
1×10^{-1}	0.1	1×10^{7} (or 10^{7})	10,000,000
1×10^{0} (or 10^{0})	1		

Comparative Table of Troy, Avoirdupois, and Metric Weights

Grain	Troy dwt	Troy oz	Avoirdupois oz	Avoirdupois lb	G
1	1.042	0.002	0.00228	0.00014	0.065
24	1	0.05	0.0548	0.0034	1.555
480	20	1	1.097	0.0686	31.10
437.5	18.23	0.91	1	0.063	28.35
7000	291.67	14.58	16	1	453.59
15.43	0.64	0.032	0.035	0.0022	1

INDEX

A

Page numbers followed by f indicate figures; t, tables.

D

E

F

G

H

I

J

K

L

M

N

O

P

Q

R

S

T

U

V

W

X

Y

Z